OTOLARYNGOLOGY—HEAD & NECK SURGERY

VOLUME ONE
Part One: General Considerations in Head and Neck
Charles W. Cummings, Editor
K. Thomas Robbins, Associate Editor
Part Two: Face
David E. Schuller, Editor
J. Regan Thomas, Associate Editor

VOLUME TWO
Part Three: Nose
David E. Schuller, Editor
J. Regan Thomas, Associate Editor
Part Four: Paranasal Sinuses
David E. Schuller, Editor
J. Regan Thomas, Associate Editor
Part Five: Salivary Glands
Bruce H. Haughey, Editor
Part Six: Oral Cavity/ Pharynx/Esophagus
Bruce H. Haughey, Editor

VOLUME THREE
Part Seven: Larynx/Trachea/Bronchus
Paul W. Flint, Editor
Part Eight: Neck
K. Thomas Robbins, Editor
Part Nine: Thyroid/Parathyroid
K. Thomas Robbins, Editor
Part Ten: General
Lee A. Harker, Editor
Part Eleven: Infectious Processes
Lee A. Harker, Editor
Part Twelve: Vestibular System
Lee A. Harker, Editor
Part Thirteen: Facial Nerve
Lee A. Harker, Editor

VOLUME FOUR
Part Fourteen: Auditory System
Lee A. Harker, Editor
Part Fifteen: Cochlear Implants
Lee A. Harker, Editor
Part Sixteen: Skull Base
Lee A. Harker, Editor
Part Seventeen: Pediatric Otolaryngology
Mark A. Richardson, Editor

OTOLARYNGOLOGY
HEAD & NECK SURGERY

VOLUME ONE

OTOLARYNGOLOGY
HEAD & NECK SURGERY

FOURTH EDITION

Charles W. Cummings, M.D.
Distingushed Service Professor
Department of Otolaryngology—Head and Neck Surgery
Johns Hopkins University School of Medicine
Baltimore, Maryland

Paul W. Flint, M.D.
Professor
Department of Otolaryngology—Head and Neck Surgery
Director, Center for Airway, Laryngeal, and Voice Disorders
Co-Director Minimally Invasive Surgical Training Center
Johns Hopkins University School of Medicine
Baltimore, Maryland

Bruce H. Haughey, MBChB, FACS, FRACS
Professor and Director
Head and Neck Surgical Oncology
Department of Otolaryngology—Head and Neck Surgery
Washington University School of Medicine
St. Louis, Missouri

K. Thomas Robbins, M.D.
Professor and Chair
Division of Otolaryngology, Department of Surgery
Southern Illinois University School of Medicine
Springfield, Illinois

J. Regan Thomas, M.D.
Francis L.Lederer Professor and Chairman
Department of Otolaryngology—Head and Neck Surgery
University of Illinois
Chicago, Illinois

Lee A. Harker, M.D.
Deputy Director
Boys Town National Research Hospital
Vice Chairman
Department of Otolaryngology and Human
Communication
Creighton University School of Medicine
Omaha, Nebraska

Mark A. Richardson, M.D.
Professor and Chairman
Department of Otolaryngology—Head and Neck Surgery
Oregon Health and Science University
Portland, Oregon

David E. Schuller, M.D.
Professor and Chairman
Department of Otolaryngology—Head
and Neck Surgery
Director, Arthur G. James Cancer Hospital
and Richard J. Solove Research Institute
Deputy Director, Comprehensive Cancer Center
The Ohio State University
Columbus, Ohio

Illustrator:
Tim Phelps, M.S., F.A.M.I.
Medical Illustrator and Associate Professor
Johns Hopkins University School of Medicine
Baltimore, Maryland

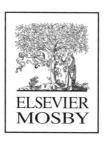

ELSEVIER
MOSBY

The Curtis Center
170 S Independence Mall W 300E
Philadelphia, Pennsylvania 19106

Cummings Otolaryngology—Head & Neck Surgery
Copyright © 2005, Mosby, Inc. All rights reserved.

NOTICE

Otolaryngology is an ever-changing field. Standard safety precautions must be followed, but as new research and clinical experience broaden our knowledge, changes in treatment and drug therapy may become necessary or appropriate. Readers are advised to check the most current product information provided by the manufacturer of each drug to be administered to verify the recommended dose, the method and duration of administration, and contraindications. It is the responsibility of the licensed prescriber, relying on experience and knowledge of the patient, to determine dosages and the best treatment for each individual patient. Neither the publisher nor the author assumes any liability for any injury and/or damage to persons or property arising from this publication.

Previous editions copyrighted 1998, 1993, 1986.

Library of Congress Cataloging-in-Publication Data
Cummings otolaryngology—head & neck surgery / [edited by] Charles W. Cummings . . . [et al.].—4th ed.
   p. ; cm
  Rev. ed. of: Otolaryngology—head & neck surgery. 3rd ed. c1998.
  Includes bibliographical references and index.
  ISBN 0-323-01985-4
   1. Otolaryngology, Operative. I. Title: Cummings otolaryngology—head and neck surgery.
  II. Title: Otolaryngology—head & neck surgery. III. Cummings, Charles W. (Charles William).
  [DNLM: 1. Otorhinolaryngologic Surgical Procedures. WV 168 C971 2005]
RF51.O86 2005
617.5'1059—dc22   2004055160

Acquisitions Editor: Rebecca Schmidt Gaertner
Developmental Editor: Mary Beth Murphy
Editorial Assistant: Suzanne Flint

Printed in the United States of America

Last digit is the print number: 9 8 7 6 5 4 3 2

Contributors

George L. Adams, M.D.
Professor and Head
Department of Otolaryngology—Head and Neck Surgery
University of Minnesota
Chair
Head and Neck Surgery
Lions 5M International Hearing Center
Minneapolis, Minnesota

Peter A. Adamson, M.D., F.R.C.S.C., F.A.C.S.
Professor
Department of Otolaryngology
University of Toronto
Adamson Associates Cosmetic Facial Surgery Clinic
Toronto, Ontario, Canada

Antoine Adenis, M.D., Ph.D.
Professor and Chairman
Department of Digestive Tract Cancer
Lille, France

Seth Akst, M.D.
Chief Resident
Department of Anesthesiology and Critical Care
The Johns Hopkins University
Baltimore, Maryland

David M. Albert, F.R.C.S.
Consultant
Paediatric Otolaryngology—Head and Neck Surgery
Great Ormond Street Hospital for Children
    NHS Trust
London, United Kingdom

William B. Armstrong, M.D.
Associate Professor
Department of Otolaryngology—Head and Neck Surgery
University of California, Irvine
Orange, California

Moisés A. Arriaga, M.D., F.A.C.S.
Director
Hearing and Balance Center
Allegheny General Hospital
Pittsburgh, Pennsylvania

Agustin J. Arrieta, M.D.
Resident
Department of Otolaryngology—Head and Neck Surgery
University of South Florida
Tampa, Florida

H. Alexander Arts, M.D., F.A.C.S.
Clinical Associate Professor
Department of Neurosurgery
Clinical Associate Professor
Department of Otorhinolaryngology
University of Michigan Medical Center
Ann Arbor, Michigan

Yasmine A. Ashram, M.D., D.A.B.N.M.
Surgical Neurophysiologist, Lecturer
Neurophysiology Division
Department of Physiology
Alexandria School of Medicine
University of Alexandria
Alexandria, Egypt

Nafi Aygun, M.D.
Assistant Professor
Department of Radiology
The Russell H. Morgan Department of Radiology and
    Radiological Sciences
The Johns Hopkins Medical Institution
Baltimore, Maryland

Douglas D. Backous, M.D.
Medical Director
The Listen for Life Center
Department of Otolaryngology—Head and Neck Surgery
Virginia Mason Medical Center
Seattle, Washington

Shan R. Baker, M.D.
Professor
Department of Otolaryngology
Professor
Center for Facial Plastic and Reconstructive Surgery
University of Michigan School of Medicine
Center for Facial Plastic Surgery
Livonia, Michigan

Thomas J. Balkany, M.D.
Chief
Division of Otology
Hotchkiss Professor
Chairman
Department of Otolaryngology—Head and
    Neck Surgery
University of Miami School of Medicine
Miami, Florida

Fuad M. Baroody, M.D.
Associate Professor
Division of Otolaryngology—Head and Neck Surgery
The University of Chicago Pritzker School of Medicine
Chicago, Illinois

Roberto L. Barretto, M.D.
Pediatric Otolaryngology—Head and Neck Surgery
St. Joseph Hospital Nasal and Sinus Center
Orange, California

Jonathan Z. Baskin, M.D.
Craniofacial Fellow
Department of Otolaryngology and Communication
    Sciences
Upstate Medical University, S.U.N.Y.
Syracuse, New York

Robert W. Bastian, M.D.
Bastian Voice Institute
Downers Grove, Illinois

Carol A. Bauer, M.D.
Associate Professor
Division of Otolaryngology—Head and Neck Surgery
Department of Surgery
Southern Illinois School of Medicine
Springfield, Illinois

Aaron Benson, M.D.
Resident
Department of Otolaryngology—Head and
    Neck Surgery
University of Illinois at Chicago
Chicago, Illinois

Nasir I. Bhatti, M.D.
Assistant Professor
Department of Otolaryngology—Head and
    Neck Surgery
The Johns Hopkins School of Medicine
Baltimore, Maryland

Carol M. Bier-Laning, M.D.
Clinical Assistant Professor
Department of Otolaryngology—Head and
    Neck Surgery
Loyola University Medical Center
Barrington, Illinois

James E. Blaugrund, M.D.
Department of Otolaryngology
Allegheny General Hospital
Allegheny Professional Building
Pittsburgh, Pennsylvania

Nikolas H. Blevins, M.D.
Assistant Professor
Department of Otolaryngology—Head and Neck
    Surgery
Tufts University New England Medical Center
Boston, Massachusetts

Andrew Blitzer, M.D., D.D.S., F.A.C.S.
Professor
Department of Clinical Otolaryngology
Columbia University
Medical Director
New York Center for Clinical Research
New York Center for Voice and Swallowing Disorders
New York, New York

Derald E. Brackmann, M.D.
House Ear Clinic
Los Angeles, California

Carol Bradford, M.D., F.A.C.S.
Director
Head and Surgery Division,
Director
Head and Neck Oncology Program
Associate Professor and Associate Chair
Department of Otolaryngology—Head and Neck Surgery
University of Michigan Health System
Ann Arbor, Michigan

Barton F. Branstetter IV, M.D.
Director
ENT Radiology
Associate Director
Radiology Informatics
Assistant Professor
Department of Radiology
University of Pittsburgh Medical Center
Pittsburgh, Pennsylvania

Hilary A. Brodie, M.D., Ph.D.
Professor and Chair
Department of Otolaryngology—Head and Neck Surgery
University of California
Davis School of Medicine
Otolaryngology Research Laboratories
Davis, California

Carolyn J. Brown, Ph.D.
Associate Professor
Department of Speech Pathology and Audiology
University of Iowa Hospitals and Clinics
Wendell Johnson Speech and Hearing Center
Iowa City, Iowa

Karla Brown, M.D.
Clinical Professor and Chief
Section of Pediatric Otolaryngology
Department of Pediatrics
Tulane Hospital for Children
Assistant Professor
Department of Otolaryngology—Head and Neck Surgery
Tulane University School of Medicine
New Orleans, Louisiana

Orval E. Brown, M.D.
Beth and Marvin C. (Cub) Culbertson Professorship in
    Pediatric Otolaryngology
Resident Selection Committee
Professor and Chairman
Department of Otolaryngology—Head and Neck Surgery
University of Texas Southwestern Medical Center
    at Dallas
Dallas, Texas

J. Dale Browne, M.D., F.A.C.S.
Professor
Department of Otolaryngology—Head and Neck Surgery
Wake Forest University School of Medicine
Winston-Salem, North Carolina

John Buatti, M.D.
Professor and Head
Department of Radiation Oncology
University of Iowa Hospitals and Clinics
Iowa City, Iowa

Daniel Buchbinder, D.M.D., M.D.
Associate Professor
Department of Otolaryngology—Head and Neck Surgery
Professor and Chair
Department of Dentistry
Professor and Chief
Division of Oral and Maxillofacial Surgery
Director of Residency Training
Division of Oral and Maxillofacial Surgery
Mount Sinai School of Medicine
New York, New York

Patrick J. Byrne, M.D.
Assistant Professor and Director
Division of Facial Plastic and Reconstructive Surgery
Department of Otolaryngology—Head and Neck Surgery
The Johns Hopkins University
Baltimore, Maryland

Joseph A. Califano III, M.D.
Associate Professor
Head and Neck Research Division
Department of Otolaryngology—Head and Neck Surgery
Associate Professor
Department of Otolaryngology
The Johns Hopkins University School of Medicine
Baltimore, Maryland

John P. Carey, M.D.
Assistant Professor
Department of Otolaryngology—Head and Neck Surgery
The Johns Hopkins University School of Medicine
Baltimore, Maryland

Eric Carlson, D.M.D., M.D.
Chief
Oral and Maxillofacial Surgery
University of Tennessee Memorial Hospital
University of Tennessee Cancer Institute
Director
Oral and Maxillofacial Surgery Residency Program
Professor and Chairman
Department of Oral and Maxillofacial Surgery
University of Tennessee Graduate School of Medicine
Knoxville, Tennessee

Ricardo L. Carrau, M.D.
Associate Professor
Department of Otolaryngology—Head and Neck Surgery
University of Pittsburgh School of Medicine
Eye and Ear Institute
Pittsburgh, Pennsylvania

Roy R. Casiano, M.D.
Director
Center for Sinus and Voice Disorders
Professor
Department of Otolaryngology—Head and Neck Surgery
University of Miami School of Medicine
Center for Sinus and Voice Disorders
Miami, Florida

Jon B. Chadwell, M.D.
Resident
Department of Otolaryngology—Head and Neck Surgery
University of Cincinnati Medical Center
Cincinnati, Ohio

Christopher Y. Chang, M.D.
Resident
Division of Otolaryngology—Head and Neck Surgery
Department of Surgery
Duke University Medical Center
Durham, North Carolina

Kristi E. Chang, M.D.
Assistant Professor
Department of Otolaryngology—Head and Neck Surgery
University of Iowa Hospitals and Clinics
Iowa City, Iowa

Burke E. Chegar, M.D.
Resident
Department of Otolaryngology and Communication
    Sciences
Upstate Medical University, S.U.N.Y.
Syracuse, New York

Sukgi S. Choi, M.D.
Associate Professor
Departments of Otolaryngology and Pediatrics
The George Washington University Medical Center
Associate Professor
Department of Otolaryngology—Head and Neck Surgery
Children's National Medical Center
Washington DC

Richard A. Chole, M.D., Ph.D.
Richard A. Lindburg Professor of Otolaryngology
Chairman
Department of Otolaryngology—Head and Neck Surgery
Washington University School of Medicine
St. Louis, Missouri

Martin J. Citardi, M.D.
Staff
Department of Otolaryngology and Communicative
    Disorders
The Cleveland Clinic Foundation
Cleveland, Ohio

Savita Collins, M.D.
Assistant Professor
Department of Otolaryngology—Head and Neck Surgery
University of Florida College of Medicine
Gainesville, Florida

Philippe Contencin, M.D.
Saint-Vincent De Paul-Hospital
Paris, France

Raymond D. Cook, M.D.
Assistant Professor
Department of Otolaryngology—Head and Neck Surgery
Wake Medical Center
Department of Otolaryngology—Head and Neck Surgery
University of North Carolina School of Medicine
Chapel Hill, North Carolina

Ted A. Cook, M.D., F.A.C.S.
Professor and Chief
Facial Plastic and Reconstructive Surgery
Department of Otolaryngology—Head and Neck Surgery
Oregon Health and Sciences University
Portland, Oregon

Robin T. Cotton, M.D.
Professor
Department of Otolaryngology—Head and Neck Surgery
University of Cincinnati Medical Center
Director
Department of Pediatric Otolaryngology—Head and Neck
    Surgery
Cincinnati Children's Hospital Medical Center
Cincinnati, Ohio

Marion Everett Couch, M.D., Ph.D.
Assistant Professor
Department of Otolaryngology—Head and
    Neck Surgery
University of North Carolina School of Medicine
Chapel Hill, North Carolina

Mark S. Courey, M.D.
Assistant Professor
Department of Otolaryngology—Head and
    Neck Surgery
Bill Wilkerson Center for Otolaryngology and
    Communication Sciences
Vanderbilt University
Nashville, Tennessee

Roger L. Crumley, M.D.
Professor and Chairman
Department of Otolaryngology—Head and Neck Surgery
University of California, Irvine Medical Center
Orange, California

Oswaldo Laércio M. Cruz, M.D.
Professor
Department of Otolaryngology
Federal University of Sao Paulo
Escola Paulista de Medicina
Sao Paulo, Brazil

**Bernard J. Cummings, M.B., Ch.B., F.R.A.N.Z.C.R.,
    F.R.C.R., F.R.C.P.C.**
Professor
Department of Otolaryngology
Professor
Department of Radiation Oncology
University of Toronto
Department of Radiation Oncology
Princess Margaret Hospital
Toronto, Ontario, Canada

Charles W. Cummings, M.D.
Distinguished Service Professor
Department of Otolaryngology—Head and Neck Surgery
Johns Hopkins University School of Medicine
Baltimore, Maryland

Calhoun D. Cunningham, III, M.D.
Costal Carolina OTO Associates
Charleston, South Carolina

Larry E. Davis, M.D.
Research Professor
Neuroscience, Microbiology, and Immunology,
Professor and Vice Chair
Department of Neurology
University of New Mexico Health Science Center
Albuquerque, New Mexico

Terry A. Day, M.D.
Associate Professor and Clinical Vice Chairman
Department of Otolaryngology—Head and Neck Surgery
Director
Division of Head and Neck Oncology Surgery
Hollings Cancer Center
Medical University of South Carolina
Charleston, South Carolina

Antonio De la Cruz, M.D.
Clinical Professor
Department of Otolaryngology—Head and Neck Surgery
University of Southern California Keck School of Medicine
Director of Education
House Ear Clinic
Los Angeles, California

Charles C. Della Santina, M.D., Ph.D.
Assistant Professor
Department of Otolaryngology—Head and Neck Surgery
Assistant Professor
Department of Biomedical Engineering
Division of Otology, Neurotology, and Skull Base Surgery
Johns Hopkins University School of Medicine
Baltimore, Maryland

Craig S. Derkay, M.D.
Professor
Departments of Otolaryngology and Pediatrics
Director
Pediatric Otolaryngology
Vice Chairman
Department of Otolaryngology—Head and Neck Surgery
Eastern Virginia Medical School
Norfolk, Virginia

Robert A. Dobie, M.D., F.A.C.S.
Clinical Professor
Department of Otolaryngology—Head and Neck Surgery
University of California, Davis
Sacramento, California

Newton O. Duncan, III, M.D.
Co-Director
Texas Pediatric Otolaryngology Center
Houston, Texas

Scott D. Z. Eggers, M.D.
Instructor of Neurology
Mayo Clinic College of Medicine
Senior Associate Consultant
Department of Neurology
Mayo Clinic
Rochester, Minnesota

David W. Eisele, M.D.
Professor and Chairman
Department of Otolaryngology—Head and Neck Surgery
University of California, San Francisco
San Francisco, California

Hussam K. El-Kashlan, M.D.
Medical Director
Vestibular Training Center
Associate Professor
Division of Otology and Neurotology
Department of Otolaryngology
University of Michigan Health System
Ann Arbor, Michigan

Ravindhra G. Elluru, M.D., Ph.D.
Assistant Professor
Department of Pediatric Otolaryngology
Cincinnati Children's Hospital Medical Center
Cincinnati, Ohio

Ramon M. Esclamado, M.D.
Vice Chairman
Department of Otolaryngology and Communicative
  Disorders
Cleveland Clinic Foundation
Cleveland, Ohio

Chun Y. Fan, M.D., Ph.D.
Assistant Professor
Department of Pathology and Otolaryngology
Department of Pathology
University of Arkansas for Medical Sciences and Central
  Arkansas Veterans Healthcare System
Little Rock, Arkansas

Edward H. Farrior, M.D., F.A.C.S.
Farrior Facial Plastic and Cosmetic Surgery
Tampa, Florida

Richard T. Farrior, M.D.
Boca Grande, Florida

Russell A. Faust, Ph.D., M.D.
Chief
Department of Otolaryngology—Head and Neck
  Surgery
Children's Hospital of Michigan
Detroit, Michigan

Willard E. Fee, Jr., M.D.
Edward C. and Amy H. Sewall Professor of
  Otolaryngology
Department of Otolaryngology—Head and Neck
  Surgery
Stanford University School of Medicine
Stanford, California

Berrylin J. Ferguson, M.D.
Associate Professor
Department of Otolaryngology—Head and Neck
  Surgery
University of Pittsburgh Medical Center
Eye and Ear Institute
Pittsburgh, Pennsylvania

Jill B. Firszt, Ph.D.
Director
Koss Cochlear Implant Program,
Director Department of Audiology
Assistant Professor
Department of Otolaryngology and Communication Sciences
Medical College of Wisconsin
Milwaukee, Wisconsin

Paul W. Flint, M.D.
Professor
Department of Otolaryngology—Head and Neck Surgery
Department of Anesthesiology and Critical Care Medicine
Director
Center for Airway, Laryngeal, and Voice Disorders
Co-Director
Minimally Invasive Surgical Training Center
Johns Hopkins University School of Medicine
Baltimore, Maryland

Robert L. Folmer, Ph.D.
Assistant Professor
Department of Otolaryngology—Head and Neck Surgery
Oregon Health and Science University Tinnitus Clinic
Portland, Oregon

Arlene A. Forastiere, M.D.
Professor
Departments of Oncology and Otolaryngology
The Johns Hopkins University School of Medicine
Baltimore, Maryland

L. Arick Forrest, M.D.
Associate Professor
Department of Otolaryngology—Head and Neck Surgery
The Ohio State University Medical Center
Columbus, Ohio

Oren Friedman, M.D.
Assistant Professor
Facial Plastic and Reconstructive Surgery
Department of Otolaryngology—Head and Neck Surgery
Mayo Clinic and Medical School
Rochester, Minnesota

John L. Frodel, Jr., M.D., F.A.C.S.
Director
Facial Plastic Surgery
Geisinger Medical Center
Danville, Pennsylvania

Gerry F. Funk, M.D.
Associate Professor
Department of Radiation Oncology
Associate Professor
Department of Otolaryngology—Head and Neck Surgery
University of Iowa Hospitals and Clinics
Iowa City, Iowa

Thomas J. Gal, M.D., M.P.H., Major, USAF-MC
Director
Head and Neck Oncology
Department of Otolaryngology—Head and Neck Surgery
Wilford Hall Medical Center
Lackland, Texas

Suzanne K. Doud Galli, M.D., Ph.D.
Adamson Associates Cosmetic Facial Surgery Clinic
Toronto, Ontario, Canada

Bruce J. Gantz, M.D.
Professor and Department Head
Department of Otolaryngology—Head and Neck Surgery
University of Iowa Hospitals and Clinics
Iowa City, Iowa

C. Gaelyn Garrett, M.D.
Associate Professor
Department of Otolaryngology
Vanderbilt Bill Wilkerson Center for Otolaryngology and Communication Sciences
Vanderbilt University Medical Center
Nashville, Tennessee

Holger G. Gassner, M.D.
Department of Otorhinolaryngology—Head and Neck Surgery
Mayo Clinic
Rochester, Minnesota

George A. Gates, M.D.
Adjunct Professor
Department of Epidemiology
Director
Virginia Merrill Bloedel Hearing Research Center
Chief Otology and Neurotology Service
Professor
Department of Otolaryngology—Head and Neck Surgery
University of Washington School of Medicine
Seattle, Washington

William Donald Gay, D.D.S., F.A.C.D.
Director
Division of Maxillofacial Prosthetics
Associate Professor
Department of Otolaryngology—Head and Neck Surgery
Washington University School of Medicine
St. Louis, Missouri

Norman Ge, M.D.
Surgery Fellow
Department of Otolaryngology—Head and Neck Surgery
University of California, Irvine Medical Center
Irvine, California

Eric M. Genden, M.D.
Associate Professor
Center for Immunobiology
Associate Professor
Department of Otolaryngology—Head and Neck
 Surgery
Mount Sinai School of Medicine
New York, New York

Elisa M. Ghezzi, D.D.S.
Adjunct Clinical Assistant Professor
Department of Dentistry
University of Michigan School of Dentistry
Ann Arbor, Michigan

Timothy G. Gillum, M.D.
Gillum Facial Plastic Surgery
Marion, Indiana

Marian Girardi, Ph.D.
Director
Clinical Research and Education
Vestibular Technologies, Inc.
Alexandria, Virginia

Douglas A. Girod, M.D.
Chairman and Professor
Department of Otolaryngology
Director
Division of Head and Neck Surgery
University of Kansas Medical Center
Kansas City, Kansas

George S. Goding, Jr., M.D.
Associate Professor
Department of Otolaryngology—Head and Neck
 Surgery
University of Minnesota, Twin Cities
Attending Staff
Department of Otolaryngology
VA Medical Center
Minneapolis, Minnesota

Andrew N. Goldberg, M.D., F.A.C.S.
Associate Professor
Department of Otolaryngology—Head and Neck
 Surgery
University of California, San Francisco
San Francisco, California

David Goldenberg, M.D.
Fellow
Department of Otolaryngology—Head and Neck
 Surgery
Johns Hopkins University School of Medicine
Baltimore, Maryland

W. Jarrard Goodwin, Jr., M.D.
Director
Sylvester Comprehensive Cancer Center
Professor
Department of Otolaryngology
University of Miami Hospital and Clinics
Sylvester Comprehensive Cancer Center
Miami, Florida

Daniel O. Graney, Ph.D.
Professor
Department of Biological Structure
University of Washington School of Medicine
Seattle, Washington

Patrick K. Ha, M.D.
Fellow
Department of Otolaryngology—Head and Neck
 Surgery
Johns Hopkins University School of
 Medicine
Baltimore, Maryland

Jeffrey R. Haller, M.D.
Rocky Mountain Ear, Nose, and Throat Center
Missoula, Montana

Jongwook Ham, M.D.
Associates in ENT Head & Neck Surgery
Elgin, Illinois

Ehab Y. Hanna, M.D., F.A.C.S.
Professor
Head and Neck Surgery
Director
Center for Skull Base Surgery
Chief
Section of Skull Base Surgery
Department of Head and Neck Surgery
MD Anderson Cancer Center
Houston, Texas

Marlan R. Hansen, M.D.
Assistant Professor
Department of Otolaryngology—Head and Neck Surgery
University of Iowa Hospital and Clinics
Iowa City, Iowa

Lee A. Harker, M.D.
Deputy Director
Boys Town National Research Hospital
Vice Chairman
Department of Otolaryngology and Human
 Communication
Creighton University School of Medicine
Omaha, Nebraska

Robert V. Harrison, Ph.D., D.Sc.
Professor
Department of Otolaryngology—Head and Neck Surgery
Professor
Department of Physiology
The Institute of Biomaterials and Biomedical Engineering
The Institute of Medical Science
The University of Toronto
Senior Scientist
Division of Brain and Behavior
Department of Otolaryngology
The Hospital for Sick Children
Toronto, Ontario, Canada

Bruce H. Haughey, MBChB, FACS, FRACS
Professor and Director
Division of Head and Neck Surgical Oncology
Department of Otolaryngology—Head and Neck Surgery
Washington University School of Medicine
St. Louis, Missouri

Gerald B. Healy, M.D., F.A.C.S.
Professor
Division of Otology and Laryngology
Department of Otolaryngology—Head and Neck Surgery
Harvard Medical School
Otolaryngologist-in-Chief
Department of Otolaryngology and Communication
    Disorders
Children's Hospital
Boston, Massachusetts

Michael L. Hinni, M.D.
Consultant
Department of Otorhinolaryngology
Head and Neck Surgeon
Mayo Clinic Scottsdale
Scottsdale, Arizona

Henry T. Hoffman, M.D.
Professor
Department of Otolaryngology—Head and Neck Surgery
Department of Radiation Oncology
Iowa City, Iowa

Eric H. Holbrook, M.D.
Instructor
Division of Otology and Laryngology
Department of Otolaryngology—Head and Neck
    Surgery
Massachusetts Eye and Ear Infirmary
Boston, Massachusetts

Lauren D. Holinger, M.D.
Professor
Department of Otolaryngology—Head and Neck Surgery
Northwestern University Feinberg School of Medicine
Professor and Chief
Division of Pediatric Otolaryngology
Children's Memorial Hospital
Chicago, Illinois

David B. Hom, M.D.
Associate Professor
Department of Otolaryngology—Head and Neck Surgery
University of Minnesota, Twin Cities
Associate Professor
Head and Neck Surgery Lions 5M International Hearing
    Center
Department of Otolaryngology
Minneapolis, Minnesota

John W. House, M.D.
Clinical Professor
Department of Otolaryngology—Head and Neck Surgery
University of Southern California Keck School of Medicine
President
House Ear Institute
House Ear Clinic
Los Angeles, California

J. W. Hudson, D.D.S.
Professor Department of Oral and Maxillofacial Surgery
University of Tennessee Graduate School of Medicine
Knoxville, Tennessee

Matthew C. Hull, M.D.
Radiation Oncologist
Mountain Radiation Oncology
Asheville, North Carolina

Timothy E. Hullar, M.D.
Assistant Professor
Department of Otolaryngology—Head and Neck Surgery
Washington University School of Medicine
St. Louis, Missouri

Kevin J. Hulett, M.D.
Clinical Assistant Professor
Department of Otolaryngology—Head and Neck Surgery
Loyola University Medical Center
Chicago, Illinois

Murad Husein, M.D., M.Sc., F.R.C.S.(C)
Assistant Professor
Department of Otolaryngology
University of Western Ontario
London, Ontario, Canada

Steven W. Ing, M.D.
Staff Attending
Department of Endocrinology
Geisinger Medical Group
Wilkes-Barre, Pennsylvania

Andrew F. Inglis, Jr., M.D.
Attending Surgeon
Division of Pediatric Otolaryngology
Children's Hospital and Medical Center
Associate Professor
Department of Otolaryngology—Head and Neck Surgery
University of Washington School of Medicine
Seattle, Washington

Robert K. Jackler, M.D.
Professor
Departments of Neurosurgery and Surgery
Edward C. and Amy H. Sewall Professor and Chair in
    Otolaryngology
Department of Otolaryngology—Head and Neck
    Surgery
Stanford University School of Medicine
Stanford, California

Herman A. Jenkins, M.D.
Professor and Chairman
Department of Otolaryngology—Head and Neck
    Surgery
University of Colorado Health Science Center
Denver, Colorado

John K. Joe, M.D.
Assistant Professor
Division of Otolaryngology—Head and Neck Surgery
Department of Surgery
Yale University School of Medicine
New Haven, Connecticut

Stephanie Joe, M.D.
Director
General Otolaryngology
Assistant Professor
Rhinology and Sinus Surgery
Department of Otolaryngology—Head and Neck
    Surgery
University of Illinois at Chicago
Chicago, Illinois

Jonas T. Johnson, M.D.
Professor
Department of Otolaryngology
University of Pittsburgh Medical Center
Eye and Ear Institute
Pittsburgh, Pennsylvania

Timothy Johnson, M.D.
William B. Taylor Professor of Dermatology
Departments of Otolaryngology, Dermatology, and Surgery
Director
Cutaneous Surgery and Oncology Unit Director
Multidisciplinary Melanoma Clinic
University of Michigan Health System
Department of Dermatology
Ann Arbor, Michigan

Kim Richard Jones, M.D., Ph.D.
Carolina ENT
Chapel Hill, North Carolina

Sheldon S. Kabaker, M.D.
Associate Clinical Professor
Division of Facial Plastic Surgery
Department of Otolaryngology—Head and Neck Surgery
San Francisco, California
Oakland, California

Lucy H. Karnell, M.D.
Associate Research Scientist
Department of Otolaryngology—Head and Neck Surgery
University of Iowa Hospitals and Clinics
Iowa City, Iowa

Matthew L. Kashima, M.D.
Assistant Professor
Department of Otolaryngology—Head and Neck
    Surgery
The Johns Hopkins University School of Medicine
Baltimore, Maryland

Robert M. Kellman, M.D.
Professor and Chairman
Department of Otolaryngology and Communication
    Sciences
Upstate Medical University, S.U.N.Y.
Syracuse, New York

Paul E. Kelly, M.D., F.A.C.S.
Private Practice
Riverhead, New York

David W. Kennedy, M.D.
Professor
Department of Otorhinolaryngology: Head and Neck
    Surgery
Vice Dean for Professional Services
Senior Vice President, University of Pennsylvania Health
    System
University of Pennsylvania School of Medicine
Philadelphia, Pennsylvania

Merrill S. Kies, M.D.
Professor of Medicine
Department of Thoracic/Head and Neck Medical Oncology
MD Anderson Cancer Center
Houston, Texas

Paul R. Kileny, Ph.D., F.A.S.H.A.
Director
Audiology and Electrophysiology
Director
Hearing Rehabilitation Program
Geriatric Center Member
Professor
Department of Pediatrics and Communicable Diseases
Professor
Department of Otolaryngology—Head and Neck Surgery
University of Michigan Medical Center
A. Alfred Taubman Health Care Center
Ann Arbor, Michigan

David W. Kim, M.D.
Assistant Professor
Department of Otolaryngology—Head and Neck Surgery
Director
Division of Facial Plastic and Reconstructive Surgery
University of California, San Francisco
San Francisco, California

John Kim, M.D., FRCPC
Assistant Professor
Department of Radiation Oncology
University of Toronto
Department of Radiation Oncology
Princess Margaret Hospital
Toronto, Ontario, Canada

William J. Kimberling, Ph.D.
Professor
Biomedical Sciences
Director
Center for the Study and Treatment of Usher Syndrome
Boys Town National Research Hospital
Omaha, Nebraska

Jeffrey L. Koh, M.D.
Director
Pediatric Pain Management Center
Associate Professor
Department of Anesthesiology and Pediatrics
Oregon Health and Sciences University
Portland, Oregon

Peter J. Koltai, M.D., F.A.C.S., F.A.A.P.
Chief of Otolaryngology
Lucile Packard Children's Hospital
Stanford University
Stanford, California

Horst R. Konrad, M.D.
Professor
Division of Otolaryngology—Head and Neck Surgery
Southern Illinois University School of Medicine
Springfield, Illinois

Frederick K. Kozak, M.D.
Clinical Instructor
Division of Otolaryngology—Head and Neck Surgery
Director
Continuing Medical Education
University of British Columbia
Staff
Division of Pediatric Otolaryngology
British Columbia's Children's Hospital
Vancouver, British Columbia, Canada

Paul R. Krakovitz, M.D.
Associate Staff
Section of Pediatric Otolaryngology
The Children's Hospital
Cleveland Clinic Foundation
Cleveland, Ohio

Russell W. H. Kridel, M.D., F.A.C.S.
Clinical Associate Professor and Fellowship Director
Division of Facial Plastics and Reconstructive
    Surgery
Department of Otolaryngology—Head and Neck Surgery
University of Texas Health Center at Houston
Facial Plastic Surgery Associates
Houston, Texas

Manoj Kumar, M.S., F.R.C.S.
Specialist
Registrar in Otolaryngology
Singleton Hospital
Swansea, Wales, United Kingdom

Parvesh Kumar, M.D.
Professor and Chair
Department of Radiation Oncology
University of Southern California Keck School of Medicine
Los Angeles, California

Dario Kunar, M.D.
Greater Baltimore Medical Center
Ear, Nose, and Throat Associates
Towson, Maryland

Ollivier Laccourreye, M.D.
Professor
Department of Otorhinolaryngology—Head and Neck Surgery
Hôpital Européen Georges Pompidou
University of Paris
Paris, France

Stephen Y. Lai, M.D., Ph.D.
Fellow
Head and Neck Surgical Oncology
Department of Otolaryngology—Head and Neck Surgery
University of Pittsburgh Medical Center
The Eye and Ear Institute
Pittsburgh, Pennsylvania

Anil K. Lalwani, M.D.
Mendik Foundation Professor of Otolaryngology
Chairman and Professor of Physiology and Neuroscience
Department of Otolaryngology—Head and Neck Surgery
New York University School of Medicine
New York, New York

Paul R. Lambert, M.D.
Professor and Chairman
Department of Otolaryngology—Head and Neck Surgery
Medical University of South Carolina
Charleston, South Carolina

George E. Laramore, M.D., Ph.D.
Chairman and Director
University Cancer Center
Professor and Chairman
Department of Radiation Oncology
University of Washington Medical Center Cancer Center
Seattle, Washington

Peter E. Larsen, D.D.S.
Professor and Chair
Department of Oral and Maxillofacial Surgery
The Ohio State University College of Dentistry
Powell, Ohio

Daniel M. Laskin, D.D.S., M.S., D.Sc.
Professor and Chairman Emeritus
Division of Oral and Maxillofacial Surgery
Professor of Psychology (Affiliate Appointment)
Virginia Commonwealth University
Richmond, Virginia

Richard E. Latchaw, M.D.
Chief
Section of Neuroradiology
Professor
Department of Radiology
University of California, Davis School of Medicine
Sacramento, California

Christine L. Lau, M.D.
Fellow
Division of Cardiothoracic Surgery
Washington University School of Medicine
St. Louis, Missouri

Ken K. Lee, M.D.
Assistant Professor
Department of Dermatology
Oregon Health and Science University
Portland, Oregon

Nancy Y. Lee, M.D.
Assistant Attending
Department of Radiation Oncology
Memorial Sloan-Kettering Cancer Center
New York, New York

Stephen Lee, M.D.
Resident
Department of Otolaryngology—Head and Neck Surgery
University of Arkansas for Medical Sciences
Fayetteville, Arkansas

Jean-Louis Lefebvre, M.D.
Professor and Chairman
Department of Head and Neck Cancer
Lille, France

Susanna Leighton, F.R.C.S.
Consultant
Paediatric Otolaryngology
Great Ormond Street Hospital for Children NHS Trust
London, United Kingdom

Donald A. Leopold, M.D.
Professor and Chair
Department of Otolaryngology—Head and Neck Surgery
University of Nebraska Medical Center
Omaha, Nebraska

Daqing Li, M.D.
Director of Gene and Molecular Therapy
Division of Otolaryngology—Head and Neck Surgery
University of Maryland School of Medicine
Baltimore, Maryland

Timothy S. Lian, M.D.
Assistant Professor
Residency Program Director
Division of Facial and Reconstructive Surgery
Department of Otolaryngology—Head and Neck Surgery
Louisiana State University Medical Center
Shreveport, Louisiana

Greg R. Licameli, M.D.
Assistant Professor
Division of Otology and Laryngology
Department of Otolaryngology—Head and Neck Surgery
Harvard Medical School
Children's Hospital
Boston, Massachusetts

Charles J. Limb, M.D.
Assistant Professor
Department of Otolaryngology—Head and Neck Surgery
Johns Hopkins University School of Medicine
Baltimore, Maryland

Jerilyn A. Logemann, Ph.D.
Director
Voice, Speech, Language, and Swallowing Center
Northwestern Memorial Hospital
Professor
Department of Otolaryngology—Head and Neck Surgery
Department of Neurology
Ralph and Jean Sundin Professor
Department of Communication Sciences and Disorders
Northwestern University Feinberg School of Medicine
Evanston, Illinois

Brenda L. Lonsbury-Martin, Ph.D.
Professor and Vice Chair of Research
Department of Otolaryngology—Head and Neck Surgery
University of Colorado Health Sciences Center
Denver, Colorado

Benjamin M. Loos, M.D.
Clinical Instructor and Fellow
Division of Facial Plastic Surgery
Department of Otolaryngology—Head and Neck Surgery
University of California, San Francisco
San Francisco, California

Manuel A. Lopez, M.D.
Fellow
Department of Otolaryngology—Head and Neck Surgery
University of Illinois at Chicago Medical Center
Chicago, Illinois

Rodney P. Lusk, M.D., F.A.C.S., F.A.A.P.
Alpine Ear, Nose, and Throat
Fort Collins, Colorado

Lawrence R. Lustig, M.D.
Associate Professor
Otology, Neurotology, Skull Base Surgery
Department of Otolaryngology—Head and Neck Surgery
Johns Hopkins University School of Medicine
Baltimore, Maryland

Anna Lysakowski, Ph.D.
Associate Professor
Department of Anatomy and Cell Biology
University of Illinois at Chicago College of Medicine
Chicago, Illinois

Richard L. Mabry, M.D.
Clinical Professor
Department of Otolaryngology—Head and Neck
   Surgery
University of Texas Southwestern Medical Center
Dallas, Texas
University of Texas Medical Branch
Galveston, Texas
University of Texas Health Science Center
San Antonio, Texas

Carol J. MacArthur, M.D.
Assistant Professor
Department of Otolaryngology—Head and Neck
   Surgery
Oregon Health and Sciences University
Portland, Oregon

Allison R. MacGregor, M.D.
Fellow
Facial Plastic and Reconstructive Surgery
Edgewood, Kentucky

Robert H. Maisel, M.D., F.A.C.S.
Professor
Department of Otolaryngology—Head and Neck
   Surgery
University of Minnesota, Twin Cities
Hennepin County Medical Center
Minneapolis, Minnesota

Patrizia Mancini, M.D.
Ear, Nose, and Throat Department
Università Degli Studi di Roma La Sapienza
Rome, Italy

Susan J. Mandel, M.D., M.P.H.
Associate Professor of Medicine and Radiology
Associate Chief for Clinical Affairs
Director Endocrinology Fellowship Training Program
University of Pennsylvania Medical Center
Division of Endocrinology, Diabetes, and Metabolism
Philadelphia, Pennsylvania

Scott C. Manning, M.D.
Associate Professor
Department of Otolaryngology—Head and Neck Surgery
University of Washington Medical Center
Chief Division of Pediatric Otolaryngology
Children's Hospital and Medical Center
Seattle, Washington

Lynette J. Mark, M.D.
Associate Professor
Department of Anesthesia and Critical Care Medicine
Associate Professor
Department of Otolaryngology—Head and Neck Surgery
Johns Hopkins University School of Medicine
Department of Anesthesiology and Critical Care Medicine
Johns Hopkins Hospital
Baltimore, Maryland

Jeffery C. Markt, D.D.S.
Assistant Professor
Department of Hospital Dentistry
University of Iowa Hospitals and Clinics
Iowa City, Iowa

Bradley F. Marple, M.D.
Associate Professor and Vice Chairman
Department of Otolaryngology—Head and Neck Surgery
University of Texas Southwestern Medical Center
Dallas, Texas

Michael A. Marsh, M.D.
Arkansas Center for Ear Nose Throat and Allergy
Sparks Medical Plaza
Fort Smith, Arkansas

Glen K. Martin, Ph.D.
Professor and Director of Research
Department of Otolaryngology—Head and Neck Surgery
University of Colorado Health Sciences Center
Denver, Colorado

Douglas D. Massick, M.D.
Assistant Professor
Department of Otolaryngology
The Ohio State University
Columbus, Ohio

Douglas E. Mattox, M.D.
Professor and Chair
Department of Otolaryngology—Head and Neck Surgery
Emory University School of Medicine
Atlanta, Georgia

Thomas V. McCaffrey, M.D., Ph.D.
Professor and Chair
Department of Otolaryngology
Program Leader
Head and Neck Cancer
University of South Florida
H. Lee Moffitt Cancer Center and Research Institute
Tampa, Florida

Timothy M. McCulloch, M.D.
Professor
Department of Otolaryngology—Head and Neck Surgery
University of Washington Medical Center
Chief
Department of Otolaryngology—Head and Neck Surgery
Harborview Medical Center
Seattle, Washington

Thomas J. McDonald, M.D.
Professor and Chairman
Department of Otolaryngology—Head and Neck Surgery
Mayo Clinic
Rochester, Minnesota

JoAnn McGee, Ph.D.
Staff Scientist
Developmental Auditory Physiology Laboratory
Boys Town National Research Hospital
Omaha, Nebraska

Trevor J. McGill, M.D., F.A.C.S.
Professor
Department of Otology and Laryngology
Harvard Medical School
Senior Associate
Department of Otolaryngology and Communication
   Disorders
Children's Hospital
Boston, Massachusetts

John F. McGuire, M.D., M.B.A.
Resident Physician
Department of Otolaryngology—Head and Neck Surgery
University of California, Irvine
Irvine, California

W. Frederick McGuirt, Sr., M.D., F.A.C.S.
James A. Harrill Professor and Chairman
Department of Otolaryngology—Head and Neck
   Surgery
Wake Forest University Baptist Medical Center
Winston-Salem, North Carolina

Sean O. McMenomey, M.D., F.A.C.S.
Associate Professor
Cochlear Implant/Implantable Hearing Aid Program
Chief
Division of Otology, Neurotology, Skull Base Surgery
Associate Professor
Department of Otolaryngology—Head and Neck
   Surgery
Oregon Health and Science University
Portland, Oregon

J. Scott McMurray, M.D., F.A.A.P., F.A.C.S.
Assistant Professor
Division of Otolaryngology—Head and Neck Surgery
Departments of Surgery and Pediatrics
University of Wisconsin School of Medicine
Madison, Wisconsin

Khosrow (Mark) Mehrany, M.D.
Fellow
Department of Dermatology
Oregon Health and Science University
Portland, Oregon

Nancy Price Mendenhall, M.D.
Rodney R. Million, M.D., Professorship for the Chairman of
   Radiation Oncology
Department of Radiation Oncology
University of Florida Health Science Center
Gainesville, Florida

Saumil N. Merchant, M.D.
Associate Professor
Department of Otology and Laryngology
Harvard Medical School
Department of Otolaryngology—Head and Neck
   Surgery
Massachusetts Eye and Ear Infirmary
Boston, Massachusetts

Jennifer L. Mertes, Au.D.
Assistant
Department of Otolaryngology—Head and Neck
   Surgery; and The Listening Center
Johns Hopkins University School of Medicine
Baltimore, Maryland

Anna H. Messner, M.D.
Service Chief and Assistant Professor
Department of Otolaryngology—Head and Neck
   Surgery
Department of Pediatrics
Lucile Packard Children's Hospital at Stanford
Pediatric Otolaryngology
Palo Alto, California

Ted A. Meyer, M.D., Ph.D.
Fellow
Department of Otolaryngology—Head and Neck
   Surgery
University of Iowa Hospitals and Clinics
Iowa City, Iowa

James Michelson, M.D.
Professor
Department of Orthopaedic Surgery
Director of Clinical Informatics
The George Washington University School of Medicine and
   Health Sciences
Washington DC

Henry A. Milczuk, M.D.
Assistant Professor
Division of Pediatric Otolaryngology
Department of Otolaryngology—Head and Neck Surgery
Oregon Health and Sciences University
Portland, Oregon

Lloyd B. Minor, M.D.
Andelot Professor and Director
Department of Otolaryngology—Head and Neck
    Surgery
Johns Hopkins University School of Medicine
Baltimore, Maryland

Steven Ross Mobley, M.D.
Assistant Professor
Facial Plastic and Reconstructive Surgery
Department of Otolaryngology
University of Utah School of Medicine
Salt Lake City, Utah

Jeffrey Morray, M.D.
Medical Director
Surgery Pain Management
PACU and Pre-Procedure Unit
Department of Anesthesiology
Phoenix Children's Hospital
Phoenix, Arizona

John B. Mulliken, M.D.
Professor
Department of Surgery
Harvard Medical School
Director of Craniofacial Center Division of
    Plastic Surgery
Children's Hospital
Boston, Massachusetts

Harlan R. Muntz, M.D., F.A.A.P., F.A.C.S.
Professor
Department of Otolaryngology—Head and Neck
    Surgery
University of Utah School of Medicine
Salt Lake City, Utah

Craig S. Murakami, M.D., F.A.C.S.
Department of Otolaryngology—Head and Neck
    Surgery
Virginia Mason Medical Center
Seattle, Washington

Charles M. Myer, III, M.D.
Professor
Department of Otolaryngology—Head and
    Neck Surgery
University of Cincinnati Medical Center
Director
Hearing Impaired Clinic
Children's Hospital Medical Center of Cincinnati
Cincinnati, Ohio

Robert M. Naclerio, M.D.
Professor and Chief
Section of Otolaryngology
The University of Chicago Pritzker School
    of Medicine
Chicago, Illinois

Joseph B. Nadol, Jr., M.D.
Walter Augustus Lecompte Professor and Chairman
Department of Otology and Laryngology
Harvard Medical School
Director Otology Service
Chief Department of Otolaryngology
Massachusetts Eye and Ear Infirmary
Boston, Massachusetts

Philippe Narcy, M.D.
Professor
Department of Otorhinolaryngology
Paris University
Hôpital Robert Debré
Paris, France

Paul S. Nassif, M.D., F.A.C.S.
Assistant Clinical Professor
Department of Otolaryngology
University of Southern California School of Medicine
Los Angeles, California
Assistant Clinical Professor
Department of Otolaryngology
University of California, Los Angeles
Attending Clinical Assistant Professor
Department of Otolaryngology
West Los Angeles VA Medical Center West
Los Angeles, California
Attending
Department of Otolaryngology
Century City Hospital
Century City, California
Spaulding Drive Cosmetic Surgery and Dermatology
Beverly Hills, California

Julian M. Nedzelski, M.D., F.R.C.S..C.
Professor and Chair
Department of Otolaryngology—Head and Neck
    Surgery
University of Toronto
Otolaryngologist-in-Chief
Sunnybrook Health Science Centre
Toronto, Ontario, Canada

John K. Niparko, M.D.
Division Director
Otology, Audiology, Neurotology, and Skull Base
    Surgery
Director
The Listening Center
Professor
Department of Otology
Johns Hopkins School of Medicine
Baltimore, Maryland

George T. Nager, M.D.
Professor
Department of Otolaryngology—Head and Neck Surgery
The Johns Hopkins University School of Medicine
Baltimore, Maryland

Susan J. Norton, Ph.D., CCC-A
Professor
Department of Otolaryngology—Head and Neck
 Surgery
University of Washington School of Medicine
Director
Research and Clinical Audiology
Division of Otolaryngology
Children's Hospital and Regional Medical Center
Seattle, Washington

Daniel W. Nuss, M.D., F.A.C.S.
Professor and Chairman
Department of Otolaryngology—Head and Neck Surgery
Louisiana State University Health Sciences Center
New Orleans, Louisiana

Brian Nussenbaum, M.D.
Assistant Professor
Department of Otolaryngology—Head and Neck Surgery
Washington University School of Medicine
St. Louis, Missouri

Bert W. O'Malley, Jr., M.D.
Chair
Department of Otorhinolaryngology—Head and Neck
 Surgery
University of Pennsylvania Medical Center
Philadelphia, Pennsylvania

Patrick J. Oliverio, M.D.
Neuroradiologist
Fairfax Radiological Consultants, P.C.
Fairfax, Virginia

Kerry D. Olsen, M.D.
Professor
Department of Otorhinolaryngology—Head and Neck
 Surgery
Mayo Medical School
Mayo Clinic
Rochester, Minnesota

Juan Camilo Ospina, M.D.
Pediatric Otolaryngology Fellow
Division of Pediatric Otolaryngology
British Columbia's Children's Hospital
Vancouver, British Columbia, Canada

Robert H. Ossoff, D.M.D., M.D.
Associate Vice Chancellor for Health Affairs
Director
Vanderbilt Bill Wilkerson Center for Otolaryngology and
 Communication Sciences
Guy M. Maness Professor and Chairman
Department of Otolaryngology—Head and Neck
 Surgery
Vanderbilt University School of Medicine
Nashville, Tennessee

Brian O'Sullivan, M.B., F.R.C.P.C.
Associate Professor
Department of Radiation Oncology
University of Toronto
Associate Director
Radiation Medicine Program
Princess Margaret Hospital
Department of Radiation Oncology
Princess Margaret Hospital
Toronto, Ontario, Canada

John F. Pallanch, M.D.
Ear, Nose, and Throat Consultant
Department of Surgery St. Lukes Medical Center
Merly Medical Center
Sioux City, Iowa

James N. Palmer, M.D.
Assistant Professor
Department of Otorhinolaryngology—Head and Neck Surgery
Hospital of the University of Pennsylvania
Philadelphia, Pennsylvania

Stephen S. Park, M.D., F.A.C.S.
Director
Division of Facial Plastic and Reconstructive Surgery
Associate Professor and Vice Chair
Department of Otolaryngology—Head and Neck Surgery
University of Virginia Health System
Charlottesville, Virginia

Nilesh Patel
Associate Adjunct Surgeon
Department of Otolaryngology—Head and Neck Surgery
New York University School of Medicine
New York, New York

G. Alexander Patterson, M.D.
Joseph C. Bancroft Professor of Surgery
Chief Section of General Thoracic Surgery Division of
 Cardiothoracic Surgery
Washington University School of Medicine
St. Louis, Missouri

Bruce W. Pearson, M.D., F.R.C.S., F.A.C.S.
Serene M. and Francis C. Durling Professor of
 Otolaryngology
Department of Otorhinolaryngology—Head and Neck Surgery
Mayo Clinic
Jacksonville, Florida

Phillip K. Pellitteri, D.O., F.A.C.S.
Associate Professor of Clinical Surgery
Penn State College of Medicine
Staff Attending
Section of Head and Neck Surgery
Department of Otolaryngology—Head and Neck Surgery
Geisinger Health System
Danville, Pennsylvania

Jonathan A. Perkins, D.O.
Assistant Professor
Department of Otolaryngology—Head and Neck Surgery
University of Washington School of Medicine
Attending Otolaryngologist
Department of Otolaryngology
Children's Hospital and Regional Medical Center
Seattle, Washington

Stephen W. Perkins, M.D., F.A.C.S.
Private Practice
Meridian Plastic Surgery Center
Department of Otolaryngology—Head and Neck Surgery
Indiana University School of Medicine
Indianapolis, Indiana
Perkins Van Natta Center for Cosmetic Surgery and
    Medical Skincare
Indianapolis, Indiana

Shirley Pignatari, M.D., Ph.D.
Associate Professor and Head
Division of Pediatric Otolaryngology
Department of Otolaryngology—Head and Neck Surgery
Federal University of São Paulo
Sao Paul, Brazil

Randall L. Plant, M.D., M.S., F.A.C.S.
Department of Otolaryngology—Head and Neck
    Surgery
Alaska Native Medical Center
Anchorage, Alaska

Steven D. Pletcher, M.D.
Resident
Department of Otolaryngology—Head and Neck
    Surgery
University of California, San Francisco
San Francisco, California

Gregory N. Postma, M.D.
Associate Professor
Department of Otolaryngology—Head and Neck
    Surgery
Wake Forest University School of Medicine
Winston-Salem, North Carolina

William P. Potsic, M.D., MM
E. Mortimer Newlin Professor
Department of Otorhinolaryngology—Head and
    Neck Surgery
University of Pennsylvania Medical Center
Medical Director
Pediatric Cochlear Implant Program
Medical Director
The Center for Pediatric Childhood
    Communication
Director
Department of Otolaryngology
The Children's Hospital of Philadelphia
Philadelphia, Pennsylvania

Vito C. Quatela, M.D.
The Lindsay House Center for Cosmetic and
    Reconstructive Surgery
Rochester, New York

C. Rose Rabinov, M.D.
Bakersfield, California

Reza Rahbar, M.D., D.M.D.
Associate in Otolaryngology
Department of Otolaryngology and Communication
    Disorders
Children's Hospital
Assistant Professor
Department of Otology and Laryngology
Harvard Medical School
Boston, Massachusetts

Gregory W. Randolph, M.D., F.A.C.S.
Assistant Professor
Department of Otolaryngology—Head and Neck
    Surgery
Harvard Medical School
Director
Endocrine Surgery
Director
General Otolaryngology
Director
General and Thyroid Services
Department of Otolaryngology—Head and Neck
    Surgery
Massachusetts Eye and Ear Infirmary
Boston, Massachusetts

Christopher H. Rassekh, M.D.
Director
Head and Neck Oncology and Reconstructive Surgery
Co-Director
Center for Cranial Base Surgery
Associate Professor
Department of Otolaryngology—Head and Neck
    Surgery
West Virginia University
Morgantown, West Virginia

Steven D. Rauch, M.D.
Associate Professor
Department of Otology and Laryngology
Harvard Medical School
Coordinator
Medical Student Education
Department of Otolaryngology—Head and Neck Surgery
Massachusetts Eye and Ear Infirmary
Boston, Massachusetts

Lou Reinisch, Ph.D.
Associate Professor
Department of Physics and Astronomy
University of Canterbury
Christchurch, New Zealand

Dale H. Rice, M.D.
Professor and Chair
Department of Otolaryngology—Head and Neck
    Surgery
University of Southern California Keck School of Medicine
Los Angeles, California

Mark A. Richardson, M.D.
Professor and Chairman
Department of Otolaryngology—Head and Neck
    Surgery
Oregon Health and Sciences University
Portland, Oregon

K. Thomas Robbins, M.D.
Professor and Chair
Division of Otolaryngology
Department of Surgery
Southern Illinois University School of Medicine
Springfield, Illinois

Kimsey Rodriguez
Resident
Department of Otolaryngology
Tulane University
New Orleans, Louisiana

Richard M. Rosenfeld, M.D., M.P.H.
Director
Department of Pediatric Otolaryngology
Long Island College Hospital
Professor
Department of Otolaryngology—Head and Neck
    Surgery
Downstate Medical Center, S.U.N.Y.
Brooklyn, New York

Jason K. Rockhill, M.D., Ph.D.
Assistant Professor
Department of Radiation Oncology
University of Washington School of Medicine
Seattle, Washington

Jay T. Rubinstein, M.D., Ph.D.
Associate Professor
Department of Otolaryngology
Associate Professor
Department of Physiology and Biophysics
Associate Professor
Department of Otolaryngology—Head and Neck
    Surgery
Iowa City, Iowa

**Michael J. Ruckenstein, M.D., M.Sc., F.A.C.S.,
    F.R.C.S.C**
Associate Professor
Department of Otorhinolaryngology—Head and Neck
    Surgery
University of Pennsylvania Medical Center
Philadelphia, Pennsylvania

Christina L. Runge-Samuelson, Ph.D.
Assistant Professor
Department of Otolaryngology and Communication
    Sciences
Koss Cochlear Implant Program
Medical College of Wisconsin
Milwaukee, Wisconsin

Cynda Hylton Rushton, D.N.Sc., R.N.
Assistant Professor
Undergraduate Instruction
Johns Hopkins School of Nursing
Baltimore, Maryland

Leonard P. Rybak, M.D., Ph.D.
Professor
Division of Otolaryngology—Head and Neck
    Surgery
Department of Surgery
Southern Illinois School of Medicine
Springfield, Illinois

Alain N. Sabri, M.D.
Assistant Professor and Consultant
Department of Otorhinolaryngology—Head and Neck
    Surgery
Mayo Clinic and Mayo Graduate School of Medicine
Rochester, Minnesota

John R. Salassa, M.D.
Assistant Professor
Department of Otorhinolaryngology—Head and Neck
    Surgery
Mayo Clinic
Jacksonville, Florida

Thomas J. Salinas, D.D.S., M.S.
Assistant Professor
Section of Maxillofacial Prosthodontics
Department of Otolaryngology—Head and Neck Surgery
University of Nebraska Medical Center
Omaha, Nebraska

Sandeep Samant, M.D., F.R.C.S.
Assistant Professor
Department of Otolaryngology—Head and Neck Surgery
University of Tennessee Health Science Center
Memphis, Tennessee

Robin A. Samlan, M.S., CCC-SLP
Department of Otolaryngology—Head and Neck Surgery
Center for Laryngeal and Voice Disorders
The Johns Hopkins University
Baltimore, Maryland

Ravi N. Samy, M.D.
Assistant Professor
Department of Otolaryngology—Head and Neck Surgery
University of Texas Southwestern Medical Center at Dallas
Dallas, Texas

Peter A. Santi, Ph.D.
Director
Cochlear Anatomy Laboratory
Professor
Department of Otolaryngology
University of Minnesota, Twin Cities
Minneapolis, Minnesota

Steven D. Schaefer, M.D.
Professor and Chairman
Department of Otolaryngology—Head and Neck Surgery
New York Eye and Ear Infirmary
New York, New York

Richard L. Scher, M.D.
Assistant Clinical
Professor Division of Otolaryngology—Head and Neck
    Surgery
Department of Surgery
Duke University Medical Center
Durham, North Carolina

David A. Schessel, Ph.D., M.D.
Associate Professor
Departments of Otolaryngology and Neurosurgery
George Washington University School of Medicine
    and Health Sciences
Washington DC

Joshua S. Schindler, M.D.
Clinical Instructor
Department of Otolaryngology
Vanderbilt University Medical Center
Nashville, Tennessee

Cecelia E. Schmalbach, M.D.
Chief Resident and House Officer
Core Otolaryngology
Department of Otolaryngology—Head and Neck
    Surgery
University of Michigan Health System
Ann Arbor, Michigan

Ilona M. Schmalfuss, M.D.
Assistant Professor
Department of Radiology
University of Florida
Gainesville, Florida

David E. Schuller, M.D.
Professor and Chairman
Department of Otolaryngology
Director
Arthur G. James Cancer Hospital and Richard J. Solove
    Research Institute
Deputy Director
Comprehensive Cancer Center
The Ohio State University
Columbus, Ohio

James J. Sciubba, D.M.D., Ph.D.
Professor
Department of Otolaryngology—Head and Neck
    Surgery
Dental and Oral Medicine
The Johns Hopkins School of Medicine
Baltimore, Maryland

Jon K. Shallop, Ph.D.
Consultant and Associate Professor
Department of Otorhinolaryngology
Mayo Clinic and College of Medicine
Rochester, Minnesota

Clough Shelton, M.D., F.A.C.S.
Medical Director
Otolaryngology Clinic
Neurotology Fellowship Program
Director
Residency Program
Professor and Assistant Chief
Division of Otolaryngology—Head and Neck
    Surgery
University of Utah Medical School
Salt Lake City, Utah

Neil T. Shepard, Ph.D.
Director
The Balance Center
University of Pennsylvania Medical Center
Professor
Department of Otorhinolaryngology—Head and Neck
    Surgery
University of Pennsylvania School of Medicine
Philadelphia, Pennsylvania

Samuel G. Shiley, M.D.
Resident
Department of Otolaryngology—Head and Neck Surgery
Oregon Health and Science University
Portland, Oregon

Edward J. Shin, M.D.
Assistant Professor
Department of Otolaryngology—Head and Neck Surgery
Mt. Sinai Medical Center
Regional Director
Department of Otolaryngology—Head and Neck
    Surgery
Elmhurst Medical Center
Elmhurst, New York

Jonathan A. Ship, D.M.D.
Professor
Departments of Oral Medicine and Medicine
Director
New York University Bluestone Center for Clinical Research
New York University College of Dentistry
New York, New York

Kevin A. Shumrick, M.D.
Professor
Department of Otolaryngology—Head and Neck Surgery
University of Cincinnati Medical Center
Cincinnati, Ohio

Kathleen C.Y. Sie, M.D.
Assistant Professor
Department of Otolarygnology—Head and Neck Surgery
University of Washington Medical Center
Assistant Professor
Division of Pediatric Otolaryngology—Head and Neck
  Surgery
Children's Hospital and Medical Center
Seattle, Washington

Patricia Silva, M.D.
Sacramento Radiology Medical Group, Inc.
Sacramento, California

Alfred Simental, M.D.
Chief
Department of Otolaryngology—Head and Neck
  Surgery
Loma Linda University School of Medicine
Loma Linda, California

Ranjiv Sivanandan, M.D.
Clinical Instructor
Department of Otolaryngology—Head and Neck
  Surgery
Stanford University School of Medicine
Stanford, California

Marshall E. Smith, M.D., F.A.A.P., F.A.C.S.
Associate Professor
Department of Otolaryngology—Head and Neck Surgery
University of Utah School of Medicine
Salt Lake City, Utah

Richard J.H. Smith, M.D.
Professor
Interdepartmental Genetics Ph.D. Program
Professor and Vice Chairman
Department of Otolaryngology—Head and Neck
  Surgery
University of Iowa Hospitals and Clinics
Iowa City, Iowa

Russell Smith, M.D.
Assistant Professor
Department of Otolaryngology—Head and Neck Surgery
University of Iowa Hospitals and Clinics
Iowa City, Iowa

Robert A. Sofferman, M.D.
Professor and Chief
Division of Otolaryngology—Head and Neck Surgery
University of Vermont School of Medicine
Burlington, Vermont

Peter S. Staats, M.D.
Associate Professor
Department of Oncology
Associate Professor
Department of Anesthesia and Critical Care Medicine
Johns Hopkins University School of Medicine
Anesthesiology and Critical Care Medicine
Division of Pain Medicine
Baltimore, Maryland

Hinrich Staecker, M.D.
Assistant Professor
Division of Otolaryngology—Head and Neck Surgery
University of Maryland Hospital-North
Baltimore, Maryland

Aldo Cassol Stamm, M.D., Ph.D.
Professor
Department of Otolaryngology—Head and Neck
  Surgery
Federal University Sao Paulo
Director ENT Sao Paulo Center
Professor
Edmundo Vasconcelos Hospital
Sao Paulo, Brazil

James A. Stankiewicz, M.D.
Professor, Vice Chairman, and Residency Program
  Director
Department of Otolaryngology—Head and Neck Surgery
Loyola University Medical Center
Maywood, Illinois

Laura M. Sterni, M.D.
Assistant Professor
Division of Pediatric Pulmonary Medicine
Department of Pediatrics
The Johns Hopkins Children's Center
Baltimore, Maryland

Holger Sudhoff, M.D.
Associate Professor and Vice Chairman
Department of Otolaryngology—Head and Neck
  Surgery
University of Bochum
St. Elisabeth Hospital
Bochum, Germany

James Y. Suen, M.D., F.A.C.S.
Professor and Chairman
Department of Otolaryngology—Head and Neck
  Surgery
University of Arkansas for Medical Sciences
Little Rock, Irkansas

John B. Sunwoo, M.D.
Assistant Professor
Department of Otolaryngology—Head and Neck Surgery
Washington University School of Medicine
St. Louis, Missouri

Neil A. Swanson, M.D.
Professor and Chairman
Department of Dermatology
Oregon Health and Science University
Portland, Oregon

Veronica C. Swanson, M.D.
Director
Pediatric Cardiac Anesthesiology
Assistant Professor
Department of Anesthesiology and Peri-Operative Medicine
Oregon Health and Science University
Portland, Oregon

Jonathan M. Sykes, M.D., F.A.C.S.
Professor
Facial Plastic and Reconstructive Surgery
Department of Otolaryngology—Head and Neck Surgery
University of California, Davis Medical Center
Sacramento, California

M. Eugene Tardy, Jr., M.D., F.A.C.S.
Professor of Clinical Otolaryngology
Division of Facial Plastic and Reconstructive Surgery
Department of Otolaryngology—Head and Neck Surgery
University of Illinois at Chicago
Chicago, Illinois

Sherard A. Tatum III, M.D.
Director
Division of Facial Plastic Surgery
Director
Center for Cleft and Craniofacial Disorders
Associate Professor
Department of Otolaryngology and Communication
   Sciences
Upstate Medical University, S.U.N.Y.
Syracuse, New York

Helene M. Taylor, M.S., CCC-SLP
Speech and Language Therapy
Primary Children's Medical Center
Salt Lake City, Utah

S. Mark Taylor, M.D., F.R.C.S.C.
Assistant Professor
Division of Otolaryngology
Department of Surgery
Dalhousie University
Halifax, Nova Scotia, Canada

Steven A. Telian, M.D.
John L. Kemink Professor of Otorhinolaryngology
Director
Division of Otology, Neurotology, and Skull Base Surgery
Medical Director
Cochlear Implant Program
Department of Otolaryngology—Head and Neck Surgery
University of Michigan Medical Center
Alfred Taubman Health Care Center
Ann Arbor, Michigan

David J. Terris, M.D., F.A.C.S.
Porubsky Distinguished Professor and Chairman
Department of Otolaryngology—Head and Neck
   Surgery
Medical College of Georgia
Augusta, Georgia

J. Regan Thomas, M.D., F.A.C.S.
Francis L. Lederer Professor and Chairman
Department of Otolaryngology—Head and Neck
   Surgery
University of Illinois at Chicago
Chicago, Illinois

James N. Thompson, M.D., F.A.C.S.
President and CEO
Federation of State Medical Boards of the United
   States
Clinical Professor
Department of Otolaryngology
University of Texas Southwestern Medical Center at
   Dallas
Dallas, Texas

Robert J. Tibesar, M.D.
Resident
Department of Otorhinolaryngology
Mayo Clinic
Rochester, Minnesota

Evan J. Tobin, M.D.
Clinical Assistant Professor
Department of Otolaryngology
The Ohio State University School of Medicine
Columbus, Ohio

Travis T. Tollefson, M.D.
Fellow
Facial Plastic and Reconstructive Surgery
Department of Otolaryngology—Head and Neck
   Surgery
University of California, Davis Medical Center
Sacramento, California

Dean M. Toriumi, M.D.
Department of Otolaryngology—Head and Neck
   Surgery
University of Illinois at Chicago Medical Center
Chicago, Illinois

Joseph B. Travers, Ph.D.
Associate Professor
Department of Psychology
College of Social and Behavioral Sciences
Professor
Section of Oral Biology
Department of Dentistry
The Ohio State University
Columbus, Ohio

Susan P. Travers, Ph.D.
Associate Professor
Department of Psychology
College of Social and Behavioral Sciences
Professor
Section of Oral Biology
Department of Dentistry
The Ohio State University
Columbus, Ohio

Robert J. Troell, M.D., F.A.C.S.
Director
The Center for Facial Plastic and Reconstructive
  Surgery
Las Vegas, Nevada

Terrance T. Tsue, M.D., F.A.C.S.
Associate Professor, Co-Vice Chairman, and Residency
  Program Director
Department of Otolaryngology—Head and Neck
  Surgery
University of Kansas Medical Center
Kansas City, Kansas

Ralph P. Tufano, M.D.
Assistant Professor
Department of Otolaryngology—Head and Neck Surgery
Johns Hopkins University School of Medicine
Baltimore, Maryland

David E. Tunkel, M.D., F.A.A.P., F.A.C.S.
Associate Professor
Department of Otolaryngology—Head and Neck Surgery
Department of Pediatrics
Director
Division of Pediatric Otolaryngology
Department of Otolaryngology—Head and Neck Surgery
Johns Hopkins University School of Medicine
Baltimore, Maryland

Ravindra Uppaluri, M.D., Ph.D.
Assistant Professor
Department of Otolaryngology—Head and Neck Surgery
Washington University School of Medicine
St. Louis, Missouri

Mark L. Urken, M.D.
Professor
Derald H. Ruttenberg Cancer Center
Professor and Chair
Department of Otolaryngology—Head and Neck Surgery
Mount Sinai School of Medicine
New York, New York

Michael F. Vaezi, M.D., Ph.D.
Staff
Center for Swallowing and Esophageal Disorders
Department of Gastroenterology and Hepatology
Cleveland Clinic Foundation
Cleveland, Ohio

Thierry Van Den Abbeele, M.D.
Chief
Department of Otolaryngology—Head and Neck Surgery
Hôpital Robert Debré
Paris, France

Jason F. Vollweiler, M.D., Ph.D.
Chief Fellow
Department of Gastroenterology and Hepatology
Cleveland Clinic Foundation
Cleveland, Ohio

Phillip A. Wackym, M.D., F.A.C.S.
Chief
Division of Otology and Neurotologic Skull Base Surgery
Medical Director Koss Hearing and Balance Center
Residency Program Director
John C. Koss Professor and Chairman
Department of Otolaryngology and Communication
  Sciences
Medical College of Wisconsin
Milwaukee, Wisconsin

David L. Walner, M.D., M.S.
Assistant Professor
Department of Otolaryngology and Bronchoesophagology
Rush Presbyterian St. Luke's Medical Center
Chicago, Illinois

Edward J. Walsh, Ph.D.
Staff Scientist
Developmental Auditory Physiology Laboratory
Boys Town National Research Hospital
Omaha, Nebraska

Tom D. Wang, M.D., F.A.C.S.
Professor
Division of Facial Plastic and Reconstructive Surgery
Department of Otolaryngology—Head and Neck Surgery
Oregon Health and Sciences University
Portland, Oregon

Randal S. Weber, M.D.
Professor and Chair
Department of Head and Neck Surgery
MD Anderson Cancer Center
Houston, Texas

Harrison G. Weed, M.S., M.D., F.A.C.P.
Associate Professor
Division of General Internal Medicine
Department of Internal Medicine
The Ohio State University Medical Center
Columbus, Ohio

Richard O. Wein, M.D.
Assistant Professor
Department of Otolaryngology and Communicative Sciences
University of Mississippi Medical Center
Jackson, Mississippi

Gregory S. Weinstein, M.D., F.A.C.S.
Associate Director
Center for Head and Neck Cancer
Associate Professor
Department of Otorhinolaryngology
University of Pennsylvania Medical Center
Philadelphia, Pennsylvania

Ralph F. Wetmore, M.D.
Professor
Department of Otorhinolaryngology—Head and Neck Surgery
University of Pennsylvania Medical Center
Director
Pediatric Otolaryngology Fellowship Program,
Attending Surgeon
Department of Otolaryngology
The Children's Hospital of Pennsylvania
Philadelphia, Pennsylvania

Ernest A. Weymuller, Jr., M.D.
Professor and Chairman
Department of Otolaryngology—Head and Neck Surgery
University of Washington Medical Center
Seattle, Washington

Brian J. Wiatrak, M.D.
Clinical Associate Professor
Department of Surgery and Pediatrics
Chief
Department of Pediatric Otolaryngology
Pediatric ENT Associates
Children's Hospital of Alabama
Birmingham, Alabama

J. Paul Willging, M.D.
Associate Professor
Department of Pediatric Otolaryngology
Cincinnati Children's Hospital Medical Center
Cincinnati, Ohio

Michael A. Williams, M.D.
Co-Chair
Ethics Committee and Consultation Service
The Johns Hopkins Hospital
Faculty Associate
The Johns Hopkins University School of Nursing
Assistant Professor
Departments of Neurology and Neurosurgery
The Johns Hopkins University School of Medicine
Baltimore, Maryland

Franz J. Wippold II, M.D., F.A.C.S.
Chief
Neuroradiology Section
Professor of Radiology
Division of Diagnostic Radiology
Department of Radiology
Mallinckrodt Institute of Radiology
Washington University School of Medicine
St. Louis, Missouri

Matthew Wolpoe, M.D.
Fellow
Department of Otolaryngology—Head and Neck Surgery
Johns Hopkins University School of Medicine
Baltimore, Maryland

Gayle Ellen Woodson, M.D.
Professor and Residency Program Director
Division of Otolaryngology
Southern Illinois University School of Medicine
Springfield, Illinois

Audie L. Woolley, M.D., F.A.C.S.
Associate Professor
Department of Surgery
Associate Professor
Department of Pediatric Otolaryngology
Medical Director
Cochlear Implant Program
Children's Hospital of Alabama
Birmingham, Alabama

Charles D. Yingling, Ph.D., D.A.B.N.M.
Department of Otolaryngology—Head and Neck Surgery
Stanford University School of Medicine
Yingling Neurophysiology Associates
Sausalito, California

Bevan Yueh, M.D., M.P.H.
Associate Professor
Department of Otolaryngology—Head and Neck Surgery
Department of Health Services
University of Washington
VA Puget Sound Health Care System
Seattle, Washington

Rex Yung, M.D., F.C.C.P.
Assistant Professor
Medicine and Oncology
Director
Bronchology and Pulmonary Oncology
Division of Pulmonary and Critical Care Medicine
Johns Hopkins University School of Medicine
Baltimore, Maryland

George H. Zalzal, M.D.
Professor
Departments of Otolaryngology and Pediatrics
The George Washington University Medical Center
Chairman
Department of Otolaryngology—Head and Neck Surgery
Children's National Medical Center
Washington DC

David S. Zee, M.D.
Director
Vestibular/Eye Movement Testing Laboratory
Professor
Department of Neurology, Otolaryngology, Ophthalmology,
    and Neuroscience
Johns Hopkins School of Medicine
The Johns Hopkins Hospital
Baltimore, Maryland

Jacob W. Zeiders, M.D.
Resident
Department of Otolaryngology—Head and Neck Surgery
University of South Florida
Tampa, Florida

Marc S. Zimbler, M.D.
Attending
Department of Otolaryngology—Head and Neck Surgery
Director
Facial Plastic and Reconstructive Surgery
Beth Israel Deaconess Medical Center
Associate Adjunct Professor
New York Eye and Ear Infirmary
New York, New York

S. James Zinreich, M.D.
Professor
Department of Otolaryngology—Head and Neck Surgery
Professor
Department of Radiology and Radiological Science
Division of Neuroradiology
The Johns Hopkins Hospital
Baltimore, Maryland

Teresa A. Zwolan, Ph.D.
Associate Professor
Department of Otolaryngology—Head and Neck Surgery
University of Michigan Medical Center
Director
Cochlear Implant Program
Hearing Rehabilitation Center
Ann Arbor, Michigan

Preface

Otolaryngology—Head & Neck Surgery was created to fill the need for a contemporary, definitive textbook on the specialty of otolaryngology—head and neck surgery. The scope of the fourth edition is a testimonial to the tremendous expansion of knowledge in this specialty. Our desire is to record this expansion in a retrievable fashion so that these volumes become indispensable reference works. The fourth edition builds on the success of the past three editions. The reader will note the continued use of algorithms and boxed lists, which serve to enhance learning.

The field of otolaryngology—head and neck surgery is represented in all of its diversity; the extensive interrelationship of its various components provided the skeleton for the table of contents. These volumes are intended as a detailed reference text and not as a surgical atlas; a definitive work, not an introductory overview. It is designed for residents and practitioners alike. We hope that our quest to document significant and up-to-date information in the specialty has been successful.

Another of our goals throughout the pages of this textbook is to acknowledge all those who have contributed to the specialty. Since significant medical expertise has no geographic boundaries, there are contributors from countries all over the world.

To ensure continuity at the editorship level, Drs. Paul Flint, Bruce Haughey, K. Thomas Robbins, and J. Regan Thomas have assumed editorship roles in this expanded effort. It is hoped that the ecumenicism which combines the effort of all the contributors will further the excellence of those now associated with otolaryngology—head and neck surgery and provide the foundation for continued progress by the generations to follow. This fourth edition builds on the success of the first three. It is more comprehensive, is of broader scope, and continues the tradition established 18 years ago.

Acknowledgment

I would like to acknowledge my father for enabling me to survive comfortably during my seemingly endless years of education. As well, my wife, Jane, and my family who have recognized the importance of and supported the mission that resulted in this resource for *Otolaryngology—Head & Neck Surgery*. I would also like to acknowledge the students and residents who are constant sources of motivation and the patients who served as the fuel that energized this project. Through their coping with illness, we are constantly aware that our search for resolution of illness must continue.

Charles W. Cummings

For those individuals privileged to serve and train under Dr. Charles Cummings, we recognize him as mentor, colleague and friend, physician and healer; we are grateful for his leadership and everlasting imprint on our mission in academic medicine.
Charlie, thank you. From your student, colleague, and friend,

Paul W. Flint

Scientific knowledge is only contemporary; a portion of what we know today is true, but much will soon be disproven or rendered obsolete. Galen was as right in his day as we are in ours. The authors have done a superb job of presenting today's knowledge. My contribution is dedicated to my wife Jill and our children Elizabeth, Robert, and Alexa.

Lee Harker

It has been a distinct honor and pleasure to be part of the editorial and publishing team assembled for this edition of *Otolaryngology—Head & Neck Surgery*. The authors have been tireless in their efforts and have worked strongly to produce chapters that are truly comprehensive in scope and depth. My sincere thanks go to each one of them and their families, who inevitably have put up with liberal amounts of "burning the midnight oil." My loyal assistant of 14 years, Debbie Turner, has kept us up to our deadlines and liaised with both authors and publishers in a highly organized way, while my office nurses Shannon Daut, Fernanda Polesel, Teresa Bieg, and Joan Martin have provided generous amounts of patient care to cover for my time away from the front lines during this textbook's creation. The residents and fellows at Washington University in St. Louis have similarly "held the fort" when necessary in the interests of this publication.

The ability to purvey knowledge starts, and continues, with one's education, for which thanks go to my parents, the late Thomas, and Marjorie Haughey, my teachers, medical professors, Otolaryngology residency mentors in Auckland, New Zealand and the University of Iowa, and colleagues in the specialty, from whom I have and will continue to learn.

My family has unswervingly endorsed the time required for this project, so heartfelt love and thanks go to my wife, Helen, as well as Rachel, Jack, Chris, Will, and Gretchen.

Finally, as we enjoy the teaching of this book and its ensuing online updates, readers are encouraged to keep in mind the source of all knowledge and truth: in the words of Proverbs 2 v.6 " . . . the Lord gives wisdom and from his mouth come knowledge and understanding." My sincere hope is that the readers everywhere will benefit from this textbook, better accomplishing our specialty's common goal of top quality patient care.

Bruce H. Haughey

The process of learning is truly lifelong. Participating in the creation of this text allows another way for me to continue to become invigorated and inspired by my specialty field. To my invaluable support mechanism, my wife, children, and family. Thank you.

Mark Richardson

It is a great honor to serve as an editor of this important textbook. I am deeply appreciative for this opportunity and the support of my co-editors. While there are many individuals who have influenced my career, I want to acknowledge the mentoring of John Fredricksen, Douglas Bryce, the late Sir Donald Harrison, Robert Byers, Oscar Guillamondegui, Helmuth Goepfert, Robert Jahrsdoerfer, Charles Cummings, and Edwin Cocke. Also, I would like to remember and honor my parents, the late Elizabeth and Wycliffe Robbins, for the values they instilled in me. Finally, and most of all, I cherish the love and support of my wife Gayle Woodson and the children, Phil, Nick, Greg, and Sarah, who together provide the caring background for making it all meaningful.

K. Thomas Robbins

I have had the privilege of being involved with this textbook since its inception. The quality of this fourth edition reflects the talent and hard work of the numerous authors and the editorial staff of Elsevier. However, special gratitude is expressed to Charlie Cummings and the other editors for their strong leadership and ability to recruit this spectacular group of authors. These projects involve a huge effort and, once again, my great family has continued to be supportive of the effort necessary to turn this project into reality. Carole, Rebecca, and Mike, you are my primary motivators. You understand the need to be supportive of this multiprong attack using patient care, research, and education to expand our ability to help our patients. Our love for one another makes this effort worthwhile.

David E. Schuller

I am pleased to thank and acknowledge the great help and assistance provided by the administrative staff in the Department of *Otolaryngology—Head & Neck Surgery* at the University of Illinois at Chicago in editing this section. I would also like to thank my co-editor, David Schuller, M.D., with whom it was a genuine pleasure to work.

J. Regan Thomas

Table of Contents

PART ONE

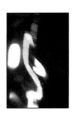

GENERAL CONSIDERATIONS IN HEAD AND NECK

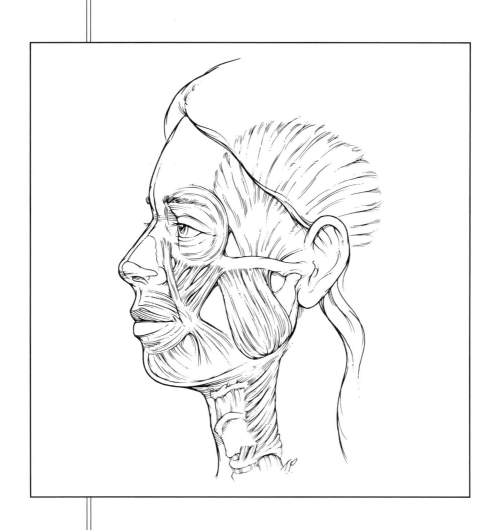

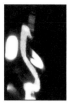

CHAPTER ONE

HISTORY, PHYSICAL EXAMINATION, AND THE PREOPERATIVE EVALUATION

Marion Everett Couch
James Blaugrund
Dario Kunar

INTRODUCTION

A physician is privileged when requested to evaluate a person and render an opinion and diagnosis. The importance of obtaining an accurate, detailed patient history cannot be overemphasized because it is the framework on which the otolaryngologist places all available information. Without this, the evaluation may be incomplete and the diagnosis flawed. Unnecessary testing may ensue, and, at the minimum, a delay in symptom management may result. In the worst scenario, a misdiagnosis may occur. Therefore, the energy expended in obtaining a complete history is always worthwhile.

Preoperative evaluation of surgical patients is, in its broadest sense, an extension of the diagnostic process. The surgeon should: strive to determine the extent of disease; prove the necessity of surgery or clearly demonstrate its benefit to the patient; optimize the choice of surgical procedure; and minimize the risk to the patient by defining concomitant health problems and instituting appropriate therapy or precautionary measures. Integral to each of these goals is an appreciation of the ideal set forth in the Hippocratic Oath—above all else, do no harm. It is the surgeon's responsibility to ensure that an appropriate patient assessment has been completed before entering the surgical suite. Surgical complications can often be avoided by recognizing the physiologic limitations of the patient preoperatively. Documentation of findings, decision making, and discussion between surgeon and patient regarding surgical risks and benefits have become medicolegal imperatives.

GATHERING A PATIENT HISTORY

The otolaryngologist should always try to request that previous medical records pertaining to the patient's current problem be sent to the office before the visit. If previous operations have been performed, operative reports can be important sources of information. In addition, pertinent radiographic imaging is helpful to obtain for review. Reports of computed tomography (CT) or magnetic resonance imaging (MRI) scans are valuable but cannot substitute for actual review of the imaging by the otolaryngologist. For head and neck cancer patients, any pathologic slide specimens from past biopsies should be sent to the pathology department for review so that a second opinion may be rendered. This is especially helpful when patients are referred with an unusual pathologic diagnosis. Finally, laboratory values can provide much information and should be carefully reviewed.

The physician should address the patient's chief complaint by determining its duration, intensity, location, frequency, factors that make the problem worse or better, any past therapy, and related symptoms. Whether the complaint is vertigo, pain, sinusitis, hearing loss, allergies, or a neck mass, the approach should entail asking many of the same basic questions followed by more specific ones designed to elucidate the full scope of the problem.

A discussion of the patient's medical history not only leads the otolaryngologist to a better understanding of the patient, but it often reveals pertinent information. For instance, a patient with an otitis externa who also is diabetic requires a high level of concern for malignant otitis externa, and this may be reflected in the management plan. If the patient requires surgery, complete knowledge of the patient's medical problems is necessary before the operative procedure.

The surgical history is equally valuable. All the past operations of the head and neck area are important to note, including surgery for past facial trauma, cosmetic facial plastic surgery, otologic surgery, and neoplasm. However, full disclosure of all past operations may be critical. The otolaryngologist needs to know if a patient scheduled for surgery has had adverse reactions to anesthetic agents or a difficult intubation.

Obviously, any known drug allergies and side effects are crucial to note prominently in the medical chart. True allergies should be distinguished from side effects of a medication. In addition, all medications and current dosages should be accurately recorded. Often, it is valuable to inquire whether the patient has been compliant with the prescribed medication regimen because the physician needs to know the doses that the patient actually is taking.

After this, it often is advantageous to assess for risk factors associated with certain disease states. Tobacco use is important to note. It is helpful to specifically ask about cigarette, cigar, and chewing tobacco consumption—either current or past use. Alcohol consumption also is occasionally difficult to quantitate unless the interviewer asks direct questions regarding frequency, choice of beverage, and duration of use. Recreational drug use should be addressed, as should risk factors for communicable diseases such as the human immunodeficiency virus (HIV) and hepatitis virus. For patients being assessed for hearing loss, major risk factors such as exposure to machinery, loud music, or gunfire should be discussed. Finally, past irradiation (implants, external beam, or by mouth) and dosage (either high or low dose) should be ascertained. A history of accidental radiation exposure also is important to document.

The patient's social history should not be overlooked because it may often reveal more occult risk factors for many diseases. For instance, a retired steel worker may have an extensive history of inhaling environmental toxins, whereas a World War II veteran may have noise-induced hearing loss from his or her military service. Family history often is equally revealing, and asking patients questions about their familial history of such conditions as hearing loss, congenital defects, atopy, or cancer may uncover useful information that they had not previously been considered.

Finally, a review of systems is part of every comprehensive history. This review includes changes in the patient's respiratory, neurologic, cardiac, endocrine, psychiatric, gastrointestinal, urogenital, cutaneous skin, or musculoskeletal systems. The otolaryngologist often may derive more insight into the patient's problem by inquiring about constitutional changes such as weight loss or gain, fatigue, heat or cold intolerance, rashes, and the like (Box 1-1).

PHYSICAL EXAMINATION

The otolaryngologist must develop an approach to the head and neck examination that allows the patient to feel comfortable while the physician performs a complete and comprehensive evaluation. Many of the techniques used by the otolaryngologist, such as fiberoptic nasopharyngolaryngoscopy, may leave a

---

BOX 1-1
HISTORY

Introduce yourself
Review:
   Questionnaire
   Medical records
   Radiographic imaging
   Laboratory values
   Pathology specimens
Inquire about chief complaints:
   Location
   Duration
   Characteristics
   Medical history
   Surgical history
   Allergies
   Medications
Risk factors:
   Tobacco, alcohol
   Social history
   Family history
Review of systems:
   Respiratory
   Neurologic
   Cardiac
   Endocrine
   Psychiatric
   Gastrointestinal
   Urogenital
   Skin
   Musculoskeletal

---

patient feeling alienated if not done correctly. Thus, it is essential to establish a rapport with a patient before proceeding with the examination. At the same time, the physician should be comfortable with a standard routine examination that allows systematic examination of every patient so that nothing is forgotten or overlooked.

A word of caution is necessary. The head and neck examination should only be done with the examiner wearing gloves and, in some instances, protective eye covering. Universal precautions are mandatory in today's practice of medicine. This has the added benefit of showing the patient that the examiner is concerned about not transmitting any diseases, which builds trust between the patient and physician.

General Appearance

Much information can be obtained by first assessing the general behavior and appearance of the patient. For instance, the patient's affect may suggest possible depression, anxiety, or even alcoholic intoxication. Psychotic behavior in the office may be a result of many factors but may indicate profound hypothyroidism in head and neck cancer patients. Astute observation of the patient's appearance is equally important. Tar-stained fingernails, teeth, or moustache are harbingers for heavy tobacco consumption. Even the gait of patients as they enter or leave the office may reveal information. Neurologic impairments, especially involving the cerebellum, may affect the patient's ability to navigate the room.

Facies

After assessing the patient's overall appearance, the face should be analyzed for facial asymmetry by positioning the head squarely in front of the examiner. For instance, in patients considering facial plastic surgery, a hemifacial microsomia may affect the final outcome, which should be discussed before the operation. In addition, a paretic facial nerve always is a serious finding that can be detected by observing the tone of the underlying facial musculature and overlying facial skin. Facial wrinkles are more prominent when the facial nerve is functioning. For patients recovering from facial nerve paralysis, the American Academy of Otolaryngology—Head and Neck Surgery (AAO—HNS) Facial Nerve Grading System is a respected standard for reporting gradations of nerve function (Table 1-1).

Facial Skeleton

The facial skeleton then should be carefully palpated for bony deformities. This is especially true in patients with recent facial trauma. The periorbital rims may be irregular as a result of fractures involving the zygomatic arches or orbital floor. The dorsum of the nose may be displaced as a result of a comminuted nasal fracture. After evaluation of the facial skeleton, the regions overlying the paranasal sinuses may be firmly palpated or tapped for tenderness, which may be present during an episode of sinusitis.

Evaluation of the temporomandibular joint (TMJ) is convenient to perform at this point in the examination. By having the examiner place three fingers over the TMJ region, which is anterior to the external auditory canal, anteromedial dislocation (caused by the action of the lateral pterygoid muscle) or clicking of the joint can be ascertained. The patient should open and close the jaw to assist in evaluating this synovial joint.

Parotid

Masses in the parotid may be benign or malignant neoplasms of the parotid, cysts, inflammatory masses, or lymph node metastasis from other areas. The tail of the parotid extends to the region lateral and inferior to the angle of the mandible. This is a common site for parotid masses to reside. The parotid-preauricular and retroauricular lymph nodes also should be systematically assessed in every patient. By facing the patient and placing both hands behind the ears before palpating the preauricular nodes, the often-neglected retroauricular nodes will not be missed.

Skin

Skin covering the face and neck should be examined, and suspicious lesions should be noted. The external auricles often receive sun exposure and are at risk for developing the skin malignancies such as basal cell and squamous cell carcinomas. The scalp should be examined for hidden skin lesions, such as melanoma, basal cell carcinoma, or squamous cell carcinoma. All moles should be inspected for irregular borders, heterogeneous color, ulcerations, and satellite lesions.

Neck

The neck, an integral part of the complete otolaryngology examination, is best approached by palpating it while visualizing the underlying structures (Figure 1-1). The midline structures such as the trachea and larynx can be easily located and then palpated for deviation or crepitus. If there is a thyroid cartilage fracture, tenderness and crepitus may be present. In thick, short necks, the "signet ring" cricoid cartilage is a good landmark to use for orientation. The hyoid bone can be inspected and palpated by gently rocking it back and forth.

TABLE 1-1

AAO-HNS FACIAL NERVE GRADING SYSTEM

Grade	Facial Movement
I. Normal	Normal facial function at all times
II. Mild dysfunction	Forehead: moderate-to-good function
	Eye: complete closure
	Mouth: slight asymmetry
III. Moderate dysfunction	Forehead: slight-to-moderate movement
	Eye: complete closure with effort
	Mouth: slightly weak with maximum effort
IV. Moderately severe dysfunction	Forehead: none
	Eye: incomplete closure
	Mouth: asymmetric with maximum effort
V. Severe dysfunction	Forehead: none
	Eye: incomplete closure
	Mouth: slight movement
VI. Total paralysis	No movement

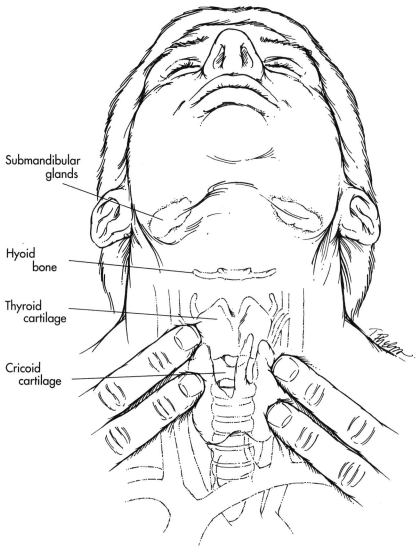

Submandibular
glands

Hyoid
bone

Thyroid
cartilage

Cricoid
cartilage

Figure 1-1. Basic anatomy of the anterior neck. Visualize structures while performing neck examination.

Thyroid Gland

Traveling more inferior in the neck, the thyroid gland, which resides below the cricoid cartilage, should be examined by standing behind the patient and placing both hands on the paratracheal area near the cricoid cartilage. Having the patient swallow or drink a sip of water often helps better delineate the thyroid lobes by having the trachea rise and fall. Pressing firmly in one tracheal groove allows the contents of the other side to be more easily distinguished by gentle palpation. Nodules or cystic structures should be carefully noted and evaluated, often by fine-needle aspiration. Adjacent adenopathy also should be carefully assessed.

Adenopathy

After assessing the thyroid gland, palpation of the supraclavicular area—from the paratracheal grooves posteriorly to the sternocleidomastoid muscle to the trapezius muscle—will help detect masses or enlarged lymph nodes, which are worrisome for metastasis from sources such as the abdomen, breast, or lung. Proceeding more superiorly, the area inferior to the angle of the mandible houses the carotid arteries and often has many lymph nodes, either "shoddy" and indistinct or firm. Palpable nodes always should be noted and may need evaluation with either fine-needle aspiration or radiologic imaging when observation is not appropriate. The carotid artery, often mistaken for a prominent node, can be assessed for the presence of bruits. The entire jugulodigastric chain of lymph nodes merits careful inspection by outlining the sternocleidomastoid muscle and palpating the soft tissue anterior and posterior to it. The submandibular and submental regions are palpated by determining the outline of the glands and any masses present. It often is difficult to distinguish masses from the normal architecture of the submandibular gland. Therefore, bimanual palpation of this area using a gloved finger in the floor of the mouth is helpful.

Triangles of The Neck

Most physicians find it helpful to define the neck in terms of triangles when communicating the location of physical findings (Figure 1-2). The sternocleidomastoid muscle divides the neck into a posterior triangle—whose boundaries are the trapezius, clavicle, and sternocleidomastoid muscles—and an anterior triangle—bordered by the sternohyoid, digastric, and sternocleidomastoid muscles. These triangles are further divided into smaller triangles. The posterior triangle houses the supraclavicular and the occipital triangles. The anterior triangle then may be divided into the submandibular, carotid, and muscular triangles.

Lymph Node Regions

Another classification system for neck masses, endorsed by the American Head and Neck Society and the AAO-HNS, uses radiographic landmarks to define six levels to depict the location of adenopathy (Figure 1-3). Level I is defined by the body of the mandile anterior belly of the contralateral digastric muscle, and the stylohyoid muscle. Level IA contains the submental nodes, and level IB consists of the submandibular nodes. They are separated by the anterior belly of the digastric muscle.

The upper third of the jugulodigastric chain is level II, whereas the middle and lower third represent levels III and IV, respectively. More specifically, the jugulodigastric lymph nodes from the skull base to the inferior border of the hyoid bone are located in level II. Sublevel IIA nodes are located medial to the plane defined by the spinal accessory nerve and sublevel IIB nodes are lateral to the nerve.

Level III extends from the inferior border of the hyoid bone to the inferior border of the cricoid cartilage, and level IV includes the lymph nodes located from the inferior border of the cricoid to the superior border of the clavicle. For levels III and IV, the anterior boundary is the lateral border of the sternohyoid muscle and the posterior limit is

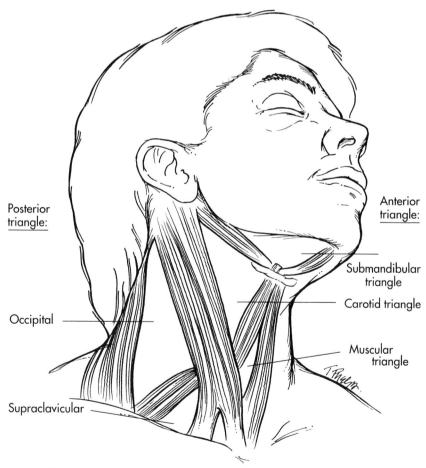

Posterior triangle:

Occipital

Supraclavicular

Anterior triangle:

Submandibular triangle

Carotid triangle

Muscular triangle

Figure 1-2. Triangles of the neck. The anterior triangle is divided from the posterior triangle by the sternocleidomastoid muscle.

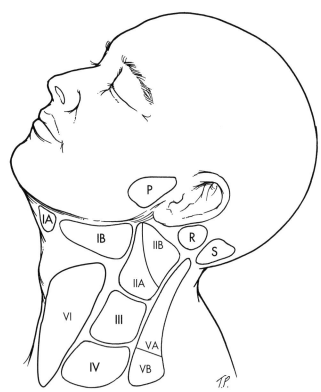

Figure 1-3. Lymph node regions of the neck.

the lateral border of the sternocleidomastoid muscle (SCM).

Level V is the posterior triangle, which includes the spinal accessory and supraclavicular nodes, and encompasses the nodes from the lateral border of the SCM to the anterior border of the trapezium muscle. Sublevel VA (spinal accessory nodes) is separated from sublevel VB (transverse cervical and supraclavicular nodes) by a plane extending from the inferior border of the cricoid cartilage. Of note, the Virchow node is not in the VB region but is located in level IV.

The pretracheal, paratracheal, precricoid (Delphian), and perithyroidal nodes are contained in level VI, which extends from the hyoid bone to the suprasternal region. The lateral borders are the common carotid arteries.

Although not part of this classification system, the parotid-preauricular, retroauricular, and suboccipital regions are commonly designated as the P, R, and S regions.

Ears
Auricles

The postauricular region, which is frequently overlooked, often has many hidden physical findings. For instance, well-healed surgical incisions signify previous otologic procedures have been performed. In children, the postauricular mastoid area may harbor important clues that mastoiditis with a subperiosteal

abscess has developed. Finally, in patients with head trauma, postauricular ecchymosis (or Battle's sign) suggests that a temporal bone fracture may have occurred.

The area anterior to the pinna, at the root of the helix, may have preauricular pits or sinuses, which may become infected. The external auricles also may show abnormalities or congenital malformations, including canal atresia, accessory auricles, microtia, and prominent protruding "bat ears." The outer ears may have edema with weeping, crusting otorrhea, which may signify an infection. Psoriasis of the auricle or external auditory canal with its attendant flaking, dry skin, and edema is another common finding.

Careful examination of the auricles may reveal conditions that require prompt management. For instance, an auricular hematoma—with a hematoma separating the perichondrium from the underlying anterior auricular cartilage—will present as a swollen auricle with distortion of the normal external anatomy. If not surgically drained, a deformed "cauliflower ear" may result. Another important diagnosis is that of carcinoma of the auricle. Because early diagnosis is important, all suspicious lesions or masses should be judiciously biopsied or cultured. A maculopapular rash on the auricle and the external auditory canal in patients with facial nerve paralysis most likely is a result of herpes zoster oticus or Ramsey-Hunt syndrome. Finally, an erythematous painful pinna may represent many diseases, such as perichondritis, relapsing polychondritis, Wegener's granulomatosis, or chronic discoid lupus erythematosus. Metabolic disorders also may have manifestations that affect the auricles. Patients with gout may have tophus on the pinna that will exude a chalky white substance if squeezed. Ochronosis is an inherited disorder of homogentisic acid that will cause the cartilage of the auricles to blacken. These examples of various diseases and syndromes illustrate the importance of routinely examining the auricles.

External Auditory Canal

The outer third (approximately 11 mm) of the auditory canal is cartilaginous. The adnexa of the skin contain many sebaceous and apocrine glands that produce cerumen. Hair follicles also are present. The inner two-thirds (approximately 24 mm) of the canal is osseous and has only a thin layer of skin overlying the bone. Cerumen is commonly found accumulating in the canal, often obstructing it. When removing cerumen, remember two points. The canal is well supplied with sensory fibers: First, CN V3, the auricular branch of CN X, C3, and CN VII. Second, the canal curves in an S-shape toward the nose. To visualize the ear canal, gently grasp the pinna and elevate it upward and backward. This will open the external auditory canal and allow atraumatic insertion of the otoscopic speculum. Cerumen impaction may be removed with many techniques, such as careful curetting, gentle suctioning, or irrigation with warm water.

An otitis externa, or "swimmer's ear," is a painful condition with an edematous, often weeping external canal. If severe, the entire canal may be so edematous and inflamed that it closes, making inspection of the tympanic membrane difficult. Gently tugging on the auricle is painful for many patients. The periauricular lymph nodes may be tender and enlarged. If the patient is immunocompromised or diabetic, the canal should be carefully inspected for the presence of granulation tissue at the junction of the cartilaginous and bony junction. This may signify that a malignant otitis externa is present, which, as an osteomyelitis of the temporal bone, requires aggressive management, including prompt intravenous antibiotics.

In older patients, atrophy of the external auditory canal skin is frequently seen and may be associated with psoriasis or eczema of the canal. If patients attempt to soothe an itch with foreign objects such as keys, hair pins, or cotton-tipped swabs, scabs or areas of ecchymosis may be present in the posterior canal wall.

Children are the most likely patients to insert foreign materials into the ear canal. Although most objects will lodge lateral to the narrowest part of the canal, the isthmus, some will be found in the anterior recess by the tympanic membrane. This makes it especially difficult for the physician to visualize with an otoscope, so have patients turn their head to view this area. In adults, cotton plugs are commonly lodged and often are impacted against the tympanic membrane. In patients of all ages, insects may find their way into the canal. An operating microscope allows excellent visualization and enables the physician to use both hands to manipulate the instruments needed to remove the object.

Otorrhea is commonly seen in the external auditory canal. The characteristics of the aural discharge may reveal the etiology of the otorrhea. For instance, mucoid drainage is associated with a middle ear chronic suppurative otitis media because only the middle ear has mucus glands. In these patients, a tympanic membrane perforation should be present to allow the mucoid otorrhea to escape. Foul-smelling otorrhea may be caused by chronic suppurative otitis media with a cholesteatoma. Bloody, mucopurulent otorrhea frequently is seen in patients with acute otitis media, trauma, or carcinoma of the ear. Otorrhea with a watery component may signify a cerebrospinal fluid leak or eczema of the canal. Black spores in the otorrhea may be present in a fungal otitis externa caused by *Aspergillus* species. Gentle

suctioning is used to clean the canal and to inspect it thoroughly.

In patients with head trauma, a temporal bone fracture is important to recognize. Bloody otorrhea in conjunction with an external canal laceration or hemotympanum are very serious findings. Longitudinal fractures often involve the external canal. Because longitudinal fractures may be bilateral, careful inspection of both canals is essential.

Tympanic Membrane

To view the tympanic membrane, the correct otoscope speculum size is used to allow a seal of the ear canal. With pressure from the pneumatic bulb, the tympanic membrane will move back and forth if the middle ear space is well aerated. Perforations and middle ear effusions are common causes for nonmobile tympanic membranes.

The tympanic membrane is oval, not round, and has a depressed central part called the *umbo*, wherein the handle of the malleus attaches to the membrane. The lateral process of the malleus is located in the superior anterior region and is seen as a prominent bony point in atelectatic membranes. Superior to this process is the pars flaccida, wherein the tympanic membrane lacks the radial and circular fibers present in the pars tensa, which is the remainder of the ear drum. This superior flaccid area is critical to examine carefully because retraction pockets may develop here, which may develop into cholesteatomas. In congenital cholesteatomas, often diagnosed in young children, the tympanic membrane is intact, and a white mass is seen in the anterior superior quadrant. Acquired cholesteatomas in adults are different in that they often are in the posterior superior quadrant and are associated with retraction pockets, chronic otitis media with purulent otorrhea, and tympanic membrane perforations.

To assess the middle ear for effusions, use the tympanic membrane as a window that allows a view of the middle ear structures (Figure 1-4). Effusions may be clear (serous), cloudy with infection present, or bloody. When the patient performs a Valsalva maneuver, actual bubbles may form in the effusion.

Hearing Assessment

Tuning fork tests, usually done with a 512-Hz fork, allow the otolaryngologist to distinguish between sensorineural and conductive hearing loss (Table 1-2). They also may be used to confirm the audiogram, which may give spurious results because of poorfitting earphones or variations in equipment or personnel. Be sure to conduct all tests in a quiet room without background noise. Also, be certain that the external auditory canal is not blocked with cerumen.

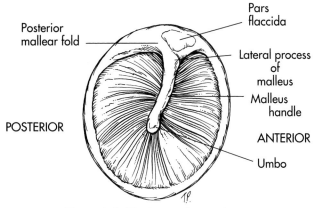

Figure 1-4. The tympanic membrane.

The Weber test is performed by placing the vibrating tuning fork in the center of the patient's forehead or at the bridge of the nose. If the patient has difficulty with these locations, the mandible or front teeth may be used, however, the patient then should tightly clench his or her teeth. The patient then is asked if the sound is louder in one ear or is heard midline. The sound waves should be transmitted equally well to both ears through the skull bone. A unilateral sensorineural hearing loss will cause the sound to lateralize to the ear with the better cochlear function. However, a unilateral conductive hearing loss will cause the Weber test to lateralize to the side with the conductive loss because the cochlea are intact bilaterally and because bone conduction causes the sound to be better heard in the ear with the conductive loss (because there is less background noise detected through air conduction). Interestingly, a midline Weber result is referred to as "negative." "Weber right" and "Weber left" refer to the direction to which the sound lateralized.

To compare air conduction with bone conduction, perform the Rinne test. The 512-Hz tuning fork is placed by the ear canal and then on the mastoid process. The patient determines whether the sound is louder when the tuning fork is by the canal (air conduction) or on the mastoid bone (bone conduction). A "positive test" result is air conduction louder than bone conduction. A conductive hearing loss will make bone conduction louder than air conduction, and this is called "Rinne negative." When the air and bone conduction are equal, it is called "Rinne equal."

The Schwabach test compares the patient's hearing with the examiner's hearing and uses multiple tuning forks such as the 256-, 512-, 1024-, and 2048-Hz forks. The stem of the vibrating tuning fork is placed on the mastoid process of the patient and then on the mastoid of the physician. This is done, alternating between the two participants, until one can no longer hear the tuning fork. Of course, this test assumes that the examiner has normal hearing. If the patient hears

TABLE 1-2

TUNING FORK TESTING

Begin with 512-Hz fork, then include 256- and 1024-Hz forks

Weber	Place tuning fork in center of patient's forehead. Ask patient if sound is louder on one side or is heard midline.		
	Weber "Negative"	**Weber Right**	**Weber Left**
Patient response	"Sound is midline"	"Sound is louder on right"	"Sound is louder on left"
Interpretation	Bone-conducted sound equal in both ears	Unilateral right conductive hearing loss; unilateral left sensorineural hearing loss	Unilateral left conductive hearing loss; unilateral right sensorineural hearing loss
Rinne	Place tuning fork lateral to ear canal, then place it firmly on mastoid process. Ask patient if sound is louder by canal or on mastoid bone.		
	Rinne "Positive"	**Rinne "Negative"**	**Rinne "Equal"**
Patient response	"Sound louder when fork by canal"	"Sound louder when fork on mastoid process"	"Sound equal"
Interpretation	Air conduction louder than bone conduction; normal	Bone conduction louder than air conduction; conductive hearing loss	Air and bone conduction equal

the sound as long as the physician, the result is "Schwabach normal." If the patient hears the sound longer than the physician, it is called "Schwabach prolonged." This may indicate a conductive hearing loss for the patient. If the patient hears the sound for less time than the physician, it is called "Schwabach shortened." This is consistent with sensorineural hearing loss for the patient.

Oral Cavity

The boundaries of the oral cavity extend from the skin-vermillion junction of the lips, hard palate, anterior two-thirds of the tongue, buccal membranes, upper-and lower-alveolar ridge, and retromolar trigone to the floor of the mouth. This region may be best seen by having the otolaryngologist use a well-directed headlight and a tongue depressor in each gloved hand. The lips should be carefully inspected. Remember that lip squamous cell carcinoma is more common on the lower lip. The commissures may have fissuring, which is seen in angular stomatitis or cheilosis. When the fissures and cracking are present on the mid-portion of the lips, this may be cheilitis.

The occlusion of the teeth and the general condition of the alveolar ridges, including the gums and teeth, should be noted. The tongue, especially the lateral surfaces where carcinomas are most common, should be inspected for induration or ulcerative lesions. Gently grabbing the anterior tongue with a gauze sponge allows the examiner to move the anterior tongue from side to side. By having the patient lift the tongue toward the hard palate, the floor of mouth and Wharton's ducts (associated with submandibular glands) can be viewed. Pooling of carcinogens in the saliva on the floor of the mouth has been postulated to cause this area to have a high incidence of carcinoma. Be sure to palpate the floor of the mouth using a bimanual approach with one gloved hand in the mouth.

The buccal membranes should be inspected for white plaques that may represent oral thrush, which easily scrapes off with a tongue blade, or leukoplakia, which cannot be removed. More worrisome for a precancerous condition is erythroplakia; therefore, all red lesions and most white lesions should be judiciously biopsied for cancer or carcinoma in situ. While examining the buccal membranes, note the location of the parotid duct, or Stenson's duct, as it opens near the second upper molar. Small yellow spots in the buccal mucosa are sebaceous glands, commonly referred to as *Fordyce spots*, and are not abnormal. Aphthous ulcers, or the common canker sore, are painful white ulcers that can be on any part of the mucosa but are commonly present on the buccal membrane.

The hard palate may have a bony outgrowth known as a *torus palatinus*. These midline bony deformities are benign and should not be biopsied, although growths that are not in the midline should be more carefully evaluated as possible cancerous lesions.

Oropharynx

The oropharynx includes the posterior third of the tongue, anterior and posterior tonsillar pillars, the soft palate, the lateral and posterior pharyngeal wall, the soft palate, and the vallecula (Figure 1-5). It is best visualized using a headlight and two tongue depressors. A dental mirror is beneficial in viewing the vallecula and the posterior pharyngeal wall, which often are obscured. Using a gloved finger to examine the base of tongue or tonsil may reveal indurated areas that may be appropriate for biopsy for neoplasm. The patient should be aware of the possibility that gagging may ensue when this is done. In patients with especially strong gag reflexes, a fiberoptic examination may be necessary to fully assess the base of tongue, posterior pharyngeal wall, and vallecula. By carefully passing the flexible fiberoptic endoscope through the anesthetized nose, the interaction of the soft palate and tongue base during swallowing also may be

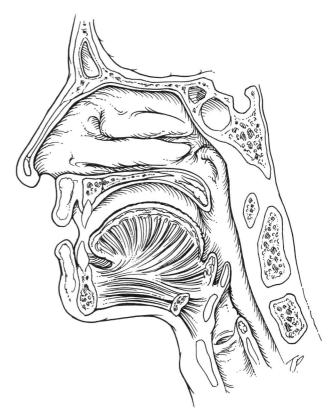

Figure 1-5. The oropharynx, which includes the posterior third of the tongue, soft palate, tonsillar pillars (anterior and posterior), lateral and posterior pharyngeal wall, and vallecula.

viewed. The uvula should be inspected because a bifid structure may signify a submucosal cleft palate. In addition, an inflamed large uvula may mean the uvula is traumatized during the night if the patient snores heavily. Small carcinomas or papilloma lesions also may be present, so careful palpation may be indicated.

The size of the tonsils usually is denoted as 1+, 2+, 3+, or 4+ (for "kissing tonsils" that meet in the midline). The tonsils and the base of tongue may contribute to upper-airway obstruction, especially if the soft palate and uvula extend posteriorly. Therefore, the oropharyngeal aperture should be carefully assessed in each patient. Tonsillitis, caused by either bacterial or viral sources such as group A streptococcus or mononucleosis, often presents with an exudate covering the cryptic tonsils. Tonsilliths are a common cause for a foreign body sensation in the back of the throat. These yellow or white concretions in the tonsillar crypts are not caused by food trapping or infection, but they often cause the patient to have halitosis and may be removed with a cotton-tipped swab.

Larynx and Hypopharynx

The larynx often is subdivided into the supraglottis, glottis, and subglottis. The supraglottic area includes the epiglottis, the aryepiglottic folds, the false vocal cords, and the ventricles. The glottis comprises the inferior floor of the ventricle, the true vocal folds, and the arytenoids. The subglottis region generally is considered to begin 5–10 mm below the free edge of the true vocal fold and to extend to the inferior margin of the cricoid cartilage, although this is somewhat controversial (Figure 1-6).

The hypopharynx can be challenging to understand. It extends from the superior edge of the hyoid bone to the inferior aspect of the cricoid cartilage by the cricopharyngeus muscle. It connects the oropharynx with the esophagus. This region comprises three areas: the pyriform sinuses, posterior hypopharyngeal wall, and the postcricoid area. This area, rich in lymphatics, may harbor tumors that often are detected only in an advanced stage. Thus, early detection of these relatively "silent" carcinomas is important and should not be missed.

The examiner should not only detect anatomic abnormalities but should observe how the larynx and hypopharynx are functioning to allow the patient to have adequate airway, vocalization, and swallow function. To survey the larynx for lesions and assess the true vocal fold function is not enough. For example, the patient with a normal-appearing larynx may have decreased laryngeal sensation with resultant aspiration and may need further diagnostic and therapeutic evaluation. Therefore, important information can

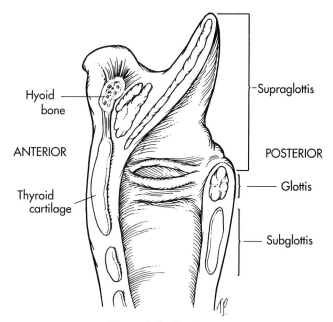

Figure 1-6. The larynx.

be obtained when the physician carefully assesses the anatomic and functional aspects of this complex area.

Correct positioning of patients increases their comfort while maximizing the examiner's view of the larynx. The legs should be uncrossed and placed firmly on the footrest. The back should be straight with the hips planted firmly against the chair. Patients, while leaning slightly forward from the waist, should place their chin upward so that the examiner's light source is sufficiently illuminating the oropharynx. After discussing the examination procedure with the patient, the patient's tongue is pulled forward by the examiner, who uses a gauze sponge between the thumb and index finger. This allows the physician's long middle finger to retract the patient's upper lip superiorly. A warm dental mirror (to prevent fogging) is placed in the oropharynx and elevates the uvula and soft palate to view the larynx (Figure 1-7). The patient with a strong gag reflex may benefit from a small spray of local anesthetic to help suppress the reflex.

Some maneuvers allow better visualization of the larynx and its related structures. Panting, quiet breathing, and phonating with a high-pitched E aid in assessing true vocal fold function.

The epiglottis should be crisp and whitish. An erythematous, edematous epiglottis may signify epiglottitis, a serious infection or inflammation that mandates consideration of airway control. The petiole of the epiglottis is a peaked structure on the laryngeal surface of the epiglottis above the anterior commissure of the true vocal folds. It may be confused for a cyst or mass but is a normal prominence. Irregular mucosal

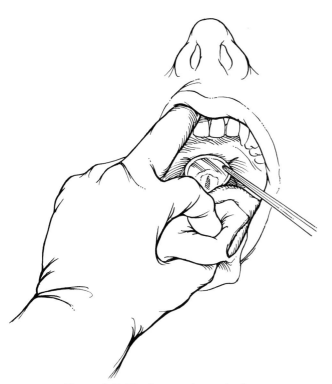

Figure 1-7. The laryngeal examination.

lesions may be carcinomas and require further evaluation.

In the posterior glottis, movement of the arytenoids allows determination of true vocal fold mobility. The interarytenoid mucosa may be edematous or erythematous, sometimes representing gastroesophageal reflux laryngitis. The mucosa over the arytenoids may be erythematous as a result of rheumatoid arthritis or as a result of recent intubation trauma. Posterior glottic webs or scars also may be present.

The true vocal folds should have translucent white, crisp borders that meet each other. Edema of the folds that extends for the entire fold length often is caused by Reinke's edema, seen in tobacco users. Actual polypoid degeneration of the vocal cord with obstructing polyps may occasionally be seen in patients and may be a result of tobacco use or hypothyroidism. Ulcerative or exophytic lesions deserve further investigation, usually requiring operative direct laryngoscopy. True vocal fold paralysis and subtle gaps present between the folds during cord adduction should be noted.

During abduction of the cords, the subglottic area may be viewed. A prominent cricoid cartilage, seen inferiorly to the anterior commissure, may be mistaken for a subglottic stenosis. It is difficult to fully inspect the subglottic area in the office setting. Any concerns about subglottic inflammatory swelling,

masses, or stenosis should be addressed in an operative setting or through radiographic imaging.

Flexible Endoscopy

Perhaps the best technique to evaluate the function of the larynx uses the flexible fiberoptic nasopharyngolaryngoscope. In conjunction with a strong light source, this allows a more complete evaluation of the structures of the larynx than a mirror examination.

A topical decongestant and anesthetic spray usually is applied to the nares. The patient is asked to gently sniff these nose sprays. Commonly used as topical anesthetics are 1% Pontocaine and 2% lidocaine. Another way to administer anesthesia is to carefully apply a viscous 2% lidocaine solution to the nares with a cotton-tipped applicator. It is important to allow time for these topical agents to anesthetize the nasal mucosa. While the physician is waiting, the scope can be prepared. The focus ring is used to get the brightest possible image. Often a small amount of residue is at the end of the fiberoptic scope. This can be carefully removed using either a pencil eraser or an alcohol swab. If the image is unclear before the scope is put in the nose, the image will be inadequate when the fiberoptic scope has been passed through the nares. Once the best possible focus has been obtained, before passing the scope through the nares, a small amount of water-soluble lubricant should be applied approximately 1 cm from the tip of the scope. This is to prevent breakage of the fiberoptic component of the scope while it is passed through the nose.

The laryngoscope then is gently passed along the floor of the nose and, with the instrument tip held above the epiglottis, the larynx may be viewed. Pooling of secretions in the pyriform sinuses is abnormal and is common in patients with decreased laryngeal sensation, neurologic impairment, or tumors. Saliva freely flowing in and out of the true cords is another indication of decreased laryngeal function. In some patients, having patients inhale and hold their breath often aids in viewing the pyriform sinuses. Asking the patient to cough and swallow and then viewing the residual saliva or phlegm also is helpful. The flexible fiberoptic examination enables the patient to freely phonate, unlike with the mirror examination. The true vocal folds may be assessed by moving the instrument tip into the laryngeal vestibule for closer inspection.

Rigid telescopic examination with 70°, 90°, and 110° telescopes is performed in a similar fashion to the mirror examination. It permits photographic documentation of the laryngeal examination. In patients with trismus, this is better tolerated than the mirror examination, and a minimal amount of local anesthetic usually is necessary.

Nose

Anterior rhinoscopy, using a headlight and nasal speculum, allows assessment of the nasal septum and inferior turbinates. The speculum should be directed laterally to avoid touching the sensitive septum with the metal edges. The point wherein numerous small branches of the external and internal carotid arteries meet, or Kiesselbach's plexus, is the most common site for epistaxis; prominent vessels in this area should be noted. Anterior septal deviations and bony spurs often are evident. The characteristics of the mucosa of the inferior turbinate may range from the boggy, edematous, pale mucosa seen in those with allergic rhinitis to the erythematous, edematous mucosa seen in those with sinusitis.

Nasal endoscopy using rigid endoscopes allows thorough examination of even the most posterior portions of the nasal cavity. After applying a local anesthetic to the nares (either lidocaine or Pontocaine spray or topical 4% cocaine), the rigid 0 degree endoscope may be passed into the nose along the floor of the nasal vault. The septum, inferior turbinate, and eustachian tube orifices in the nasopharynx may be seen this way. Often, at this time, it is necessary to spray a decongestant to shrink the nasal mucosa. It is helpful to attempt to view the nasal anatomy in both the native state and after the decongestant so that the effect of the decongestant may be seen. After inspecting both sides, the endoscope is placed above the inferior turbinate to view the middle turbinate. Accessory ostia from the maxillary sinus often are present, especially in patients with chronic sinusitis. These openings into the lateral nasal wall often are mistaken for the true maxillary ostium.

Nasopharynx

The nasopharynx extends from the skull base to the soft palate. This is a challenging area to examine, but with the available technology, there are many ways to approach this region. The technique used often will depend on the anatomy of the patient. In the patient with a high posterior soft palate and small tongue base, an otolaryngologist may use a small dental mirror and a headlight to visualize the nasopharynx. By having the patient sit upright in the chair, the physician may firmly pull the tongue forward while opening the mouth to place the mirror just posterior to the soft palate. In a manner analogous to that used to view the larynx with a mirror, the structures in the nasopharynx will be seen when the mirror is oriented upward.

Another method uses a fiberoptic nasopharyngoscope, which allows excellent visualization of this area. After anesthetizing the nares with either topical cocaine (on pledgets) or applying lidocaine spray, many otolaryngologists will spray the nares with a decongestant.

The flexible fiberoptic scope then is gently passed along the floor of the nostril beneath the inferior turbinate. The eustachian tube orifice, torus tubarius, and fossa of Rosenmüller should be inspected on each side. This may be accomplished by using the hand control to turn the tip of the scope from side to side. The midline also should be inspected for any masses, ulcerations, or bleeding areas. Rigid endoscopes offer good visualization also, although the ability to view both sides of the nasopharynx often means passing the endoscope through each nostril. The endoscopes have various angles, such as 70 degree , 90 degree , and 110 degree .

Arguably, the best view of all may be obtained using a 90° rigid scope in the oropharynx. By advancing the rigid scope through the mouth and by placing the beveled edge posterior to the soft palate, the nasopharynx may be seen in its entirety. Both sides of the nasopharynx may be compared for symmetry using this technique.

Whereas children have adenoid tissue present, adults should not have much adenoid tissue remaining in this area. Thus, adenoid tissue should not be a cause of nasal or eustachian tube obstruction in adults. One possible exception is patients with HIV infections, who may manifest adenoid hypertrophy as part of their disease. Nonetheless, adults with an otitis media, especially unilateral in nature, should have their nasopharynx inspected for possible nasopharyngeal masses. If present, it is important to diagnose nasopharyngeal carcinomas, which are most common lateral to the eustachian tube orifice in the fossa of Rosenmueller. In young male patients, nasopharyngeal angiofibromas are locally aggressive, but histologically benign masses that are most commonly present in the posterior choana or nasopharynx. These masses should not be missed. Another malignancy to consider is non-Hodgkin's lymphoma. Cysts in the superior portion of the nasopharynx may represent a benign Tornwaldt cyst or a malignant craniopharyngioma.

NEUROLOGIC EXAMINATION

Table 1-3 outlines the basics of a neurologic examination appropriate for most head and neck patients. Certainly, patients presenting with vertigo or disequilibrium require a highly specialized neurologic examination, but that is beyond the scope of this chapter. Much valuable clinical information can be obtained with an evaluation of the cranial nerves.

PREOPERATIVE EVALUATION

The patient presenting with an otolaryngologic disease process that requires surgical management must be evaluated by both general and specialty-specific criteria. Additional testing, prophylactic measures, and behavioral modification before surgery can then

TABLE 1-3

NEUROLOGIC EXAMINATION

Cranial nerves	Tests
I	Sense of smell to several substances
	Do not use ammonia (common chemical sense caused by CN V stimulation)
II	Visual acuity
	Visual fields
	Inspect optic fundi
III	Extraocular movements in six fields of gaze
IV	Pupillary reaction to light
V	Palpate temporal and masseter muscles
	Patient should clench teeth
	Test forehead, cheeks, jaw for pain, temperature, and light (cotton) touch
	Corneal reflex (blinking in response to cotton touching the cornea)
VI	Near reaction to light
	Ptosis of upper eyelids
VII	Symmetry of face in repose
	Raise eyebrows, frown, close eyes tightly, smile, puff out cheeks
VIII	Auditory—Tuning fork tests for hearing
	Vestibular—Nystagmus on lateral gaze; Hallpike-Dix test; headshaking; Caloric testing; Frenzel lenses
IX, X	Hoarseness
	True vocal cord mobility
	Gag reflex (CN IX or X)
	Movement of soft palate and pharynx
XI	Shrug shoulders against examiner's hand (trapezius muscle)
	Turn head against examiner's hand (sternocleidomastoid muscle)
XII	Stick tongue out
	Tongue deviates toward side of lesion
	Tongue atrophy, fasciculations

be implemented to maximize the surgical outcome. In addition, the patient's prior anesthetic record provides invaluable insight into issues such as airway management and overall tolerance of general, regional, local, or neuroleptic anesthesia. A social history can often be extremely beneficial as well, providing a means of anticipating postoperative needs and circumventing some prolonged admissions. Any significant issues should be raised with the departmental or hospital social worker, preferably before surgery. Last, it is important to elicit a detailed list of current medications and allergies.

In uncomplicated cases, the history and physical examination are followed by routine screening tests. Blood is drawn for a complete blood count (CBC), serum electrolytes, blood urea nitrogen (BUN), creatinine, glucose, and a clotting profile to rule out a wide range of possible occult abnormalities. In patients over 40 years of age or in those with pertinent past medical histories, chest radiography and electrocardiography (ECG) are performed. Additionally, women of childbearing age should undergo pregnancy testing.

When the need arises, consultation with appropriate specialties should be sought quickly. The consultant should be clearly informed about the nature of the proposed procedure and should be asked to comment specifically on the relative safety of performing the procedure with respect to concomitant disease processes. In cases complicated by many medical problems or those in which the establishment of a safe airway is an issue, the authors advise close consultation with the anesthesia team to avoid undue delay, cancellation of the procedure, or an undesirable outcome.

It is imperative to have copies of all laboratory results, radiographs, and pertinent tests available for review before surgery. Additional studies should be ordered by the surgeon as deemed necessary.

Consent

Although a detailed discussion of the legal ramifications of informed consent is beyond the scope of this chapter, the ethical ideal deserves consideration. An integral part of the preoperative process is the physician's thorough and candid explanation to the patient of the procedure, its risks, and the probable outcomes. The relationship that develops between the surgeon and patient at this time often does more to prevent litigation if an unfortunate circumstance occurs than any legal document detailing the risks and benefits.

Allergy

The surgeon must guard against anaphylactic reactions in all patients. The crux of this process is to have the patient identify any untoward reactions to medications, foods, or other materials. In most instances, many of the drug "reactions" described by patients do not represent true allergic phenomena. Instead, they are simply drug side effects. Nonetheless, these reactions require thorough documentation and avoidance of the allergens in the perioperative period.

Anaphylaxis results in the release of potent inflammatory agents, vasoactive substances, and proteases, all of which bring about the shock reaction. The patient may develop urticaria, profound hypotension, tachycardia, bronchoconstriction, and airway-compromising edema of the mucosal surfaces of the upper aerodigestive tract. Even in intubated patients, rapid oxygen desaturation is often a prominent feature. As the reaction progresses, cardiac arrest can ensue despite maximal resuscitative efforts. Given the potential morbidity and mortality of anaphylactic reactions, the otolaryngologist must identify all of a patient's allergens in the preoperative phase.

The incidence of serious adverse reactions to penicillin is about 1%. It is widely believed that there is a 10% to 15% chance that patients who manifest these reactions also react adversely to cephalosporins. Based on empiric observations at the authors' institution, it is believed that unless these patients have had a history of significant atopy or penicillin-induced urticaria, mucosal edema, or anaphylaxis, they can be given cephalosporins with relative impunity. Anaphylactic reactions to cephalosporins in true penicillin-allergic patients are probably less than 2%. Moreover, cephalosporins cause their own independent hypersensitivity reactions. The notion of cross-reactivity with penicillin on skin testing seems to stem from data obtained in the 1970s, in which contamination of cephalosporins with penicillin was subsequently proven. Finally, if a serious penicillin allergy is evident, alternative antibiotics such as clindamycin may be substituted for the cephalosporins.

Mucosal absorption of latex protein allergens from the surgeon's gloves can rapidly incite anaphylactic shock in patients who are highly sensitive to latex. It should be noted that about 7% to 10% of healthcare workers regularly exposed to latex and 28% to 67% of children with spina bifida demonstrate positive skin tests to latex proteins. Preoperatively, if a patient gives a history suspicious for latex allergy, it should be investigated before surgery. If the allergy is documented, perioperative precautions to avoid latex exposure must be instituted at all costs.

Similarly, patients with allergic or adverse reactions to soybean or eggs may react to propofol, a ubiquitous induction agent. Protamine and intravenous contrast agents can potentially provoke hypersensitivity responses in patients with known shellfish or other fish allergies. Although rare, some patients may have allergic reactions to ester types of local anesthetics such as cocaine, procaine, and tetracaine.

Finally, if the suspicion of allergy or adverse reaction exists, the best course of action is to avoid use of the potential offending agent altogether during surgery. If this is not feasible for some reason, then the surgeon and anesthesiologist should plan on premedicating the patient with systemic steroids, histamine antagonists, and even bronchodilators. The physicians should then be prepared to deal with the potential worst-case scenario of anaphylactic shock.

Systems
Cardiovascular

Cardiovascular complications are the most common cause of perioperative mortality. Specifically, an almost 50% mortality rate is associated with perioperative myocardial infarction. Meticulous review of the cardiovascular system is of utmost importance in determining a patient's surgical candidacy, especially those who will require a general anesthetic. Risk factors for a perioperative cardiovascular complication include jugular venous distention, third heart sounds, recent myocardial infarction (MI) (within 6 months), nonsinus heart rhythm, frequent premature ventricular contractions (>5 per minute), over 70 years of age, valvular aortic stenosis, previous vascular or thoracic surgery, and poor overall medical status. Emergency surgery poses an additional risk for cardiovascular complications. In the head and neck oncology patient population, the high incidence of tobacco and alcohol abuse leads to a relatively high incidence of coronary artery disease, cardiomyopathy, and peripheral vascular disease.

The otolaryngologist should obtain a history of previous MIs, angina, angioplasty or bypass surgery, congestive heart failure (CHF) or dyspnea on exertion, hypertension, general exercise tolerance, paroxysmal nocturnal dyspnea, claudication, stroke or transient ischemic attack, syncope, palpitations or other arrhythmias, as well as known anatomic or auscultative cardiac anomalies. The presence or suspicion of coronary artery disease, heart failure, untreated hypertension, or significant peripheral vascular disease should prompt a specific anesthesiology or cardiology consultation before surgery. This evaluation would include an assessment of the electrocardiogram, as well as possible exercise or chemical stress testing, echocardiography, and cardiac catheterization as indicated. The result of this consultation should determine the surgical and anesthetic risk and should optimize the patient's preoperative cardiovascular status. Furthermore, specific intraoperative and postoperative physiologic (e.g., invasive monitors) and pharmacologic precautionary measures should be delineated, as should the level of postoperative observation.

In general, patients are maintained on their antihypertensive, antianginal, and antiarrhythmic regimens up to the time of surgery. Certain medications such as diuretics and digoxin may be withheld at the discretion of the anesthesiologist or cardiologist. Preoperatively, serum electrolytes and antiarrhythmic levels should be checked and adjusted as necessary. Coagulation studies (prothrombin time [PT]/partial thromboplastin time [PTT]) and platelet quantification are routinely obtained in patients with cardiovascular risk factors because significant bleeding can lead to major perioperative cardiovascular complications. A relatively current chest radiograph is considered essential in this high-risk group.

Preoperatively, the otolaryngologist must be aware of the types of procedures that may have specific cardiovascular ramifications. Patients with prosthetic valves and those with a history of rheumatic fever, endocarditis, congenital heart defects, mitral valve prolapse with regurgitation, or hypertrophic cardiomyopathy should receive prophylactic antibiotics at the time of surgery. Such prophylaxis is especially important during procedures performed on the oral cavity and upper aerodigestive tract. This is also important when dealing with surgical drainage of head and neck infections, in which the risk of hematogenous bacterial seeding is high. For low-risk procedures, intravenous ampicillin—2 g given 30 minutes before surgery, followed by 1 g given 6 hours later—is sufficient prophylaxis. In high-risk procedures, intravenous gentamicin (1.5 mg/kg) and intravenous ampicillin (2 g) are administered 30 minutes before surgery, followed by the same doses of each 8 hours later. Patients with pacemakers or implanted defibrillators and those with mitral valve prolapse without regurgitation do not require endocarditis prophylaxis.

Airway, carotid, and vagus nerve manipulation can induce bradycardia and hypotension. Agents such as lidocaine, epinephrine, and cocaine, which are frequently used in sinonasal surgery, can trigger undesirable cardiovascular events. Injury to the cervical sympathetic chain may precipitate postural hypotension postoperatively. Finally, the surgeon must also be cognizant that a unipolar electrocautery device can reprogram a pacemaker during surgery.

Respiratory

Postoperative pulmonary complications are considered the second most common cause of perioperative mortality. This is not surprising considering the effects of general anesthesia and surgery on pulmonary performance. Atelectasis and ventilation/perfusion mismatch occur secondary to a number of factors, including the use of anesthetic agents and positive pressure ventilation, as well as supine positioning. Anesthetic agents, barbiturates, and opioids tend to diminish the ventilatory response to hypercarbia and hypoxia. Endotracheal intubation bypasses the warming and humidifying effects of the upper airway, leading to impaired ciliary function, thickened secretions, and subsequent decreased resistance to infection. Furthermore, postoperative pain substantially affects a patient's ability to cough, especially following thoracic or abdominal procedures (e.g., chest myocutaneous flap, gastric pull up, percutaneous endoscopic gastrostomy, rectus free-flap, iliac crest bone graft). Because of their attenuated respiratory reserve, patients with chronic pulmonary disease are much more likely to suffer postoperative pulmonary complications than are healthy patients. For instance, heavy smokers have a threefold increase in the risk of postoperative pulmonary complications when compared with nonsmokers. Hence it is imperative to identify these patients during the preoperative evaluation.

Specifically, a positive history of asthma, chronic obstructive pulmonary disease, emphysema, tobacco abuse, pneumonia, pulmonary edema, pulmonary fibrosis, or adult respiratory distress syndrome requires heightened attention before surgery. The prior treatment of these lung problems, including the number of hospitalizations and emergency room visits; the use of medications like steroids, antibiotics, and bronchodilators; and the need for intubation or chronic oxygen therapy should be addressed. The otolaryngologist should obtain an estimate of the patient's dyspnea, exercise limitation, cough, hemoptysis, and sputum production. Factors that exacerbate chronic lung disease must be identified. Once again, it is of paramount importance to investigate the tolerance of previous anesthetics in this high-risk group. Coexisting cardiac and renal disease such as CHF and chronic renal failure also impact heavily on pulmonary function. Pulmonary hypertension and cor pulmonale secondary to obstructive sleep apnea, cystic fibrosis, muscular dystrophy, emphysema, or kyphoscoliosis further complicate anesthetic management. Congenital diseases affecting the lungs such as cystic fibrosis and Kartagener's syndrome (rare) present the challenge of perioperative clearance of secretions.

On physical examination, the clinician should be attuned to the patient's body habitus and general appearance. Obesity, kyphoscoliosis, and pregnancy can all predispose to poor ventilation, atelectasis, and hypoxemia. Cachectic patients are more likely to develop postoperative pneumonia. It should be noted that clubbing and cyanosis, although suggestive, are not reliable indicators of chronic pulmonary disease. The patient's respiratory rate is determined, and the presence of accessory muscle use, nasal flaring, diaphoresis, or stridor should be documented. Auscultation that reveals wheezing, rhonchi, diminished breath sounds, crackles, rales, and altered inspiratory:expiratory time ratios should raise the suspicion of pulmonary compromise.

In patients with pulmonary disease, preoperative posteroanterior and lateral chest radiography is mandatory, because findings will often direct modification of the anesthetic technique used during surgery. Arterial blood gas (ABG) testing on room air is also indicated. Patients with an arterial oxygen tension less than 60 mm Hg or an arterial carbon dioxide tension greater than 50 mm Hg are more likely to have postoperative pulmonary complications. Serial ABG determinations can also be used to assess the overall efficacy of preoperative medical and respiratory therapy. As with chest radiography, preoperative ABG levels also provide a baseline for postoperative comparison.

Preoperative pulmonary function tests such as spirometry and flow–volume loops are quite helpful. A quantitative measure of ventilatory function can also be used to assess the efficacy of both preoperative and surgical interventions. Spirometry can be used to differentiate restrictive from obstructive lung disease, as well as to predict perioperative morbidity from pulmonary complications. Generally, a forced expiratory volume in 1 second: forced vital capacity ratio of less than 75% is considered abnormal, whereas a ratio of less than 50% carries a significant risk of perioperative pulmonary complications. Preoperative flow-volume loops can distinguish among fixed (e.g., goiter), variable extrathoracic (e.g., unilateral vocal cord paralysis), and variable intrathoracic (e.g., tracheal mass) airway obstructions.

The preoperative management of otolaryngology patients with significant pulmonary disease is vital and should follow the recommendations of a pulmonologist. Smokers are advised to cease smoking for at least a week before surgery. Chest physiotherapy aimed at increasing lung volumes and clearing secretions is instituted. This includes coughing and deep breathing exercises, incentive spirometry, and chest percussion with postural drainage. It is not advisable to operate on a patient with an acute exacerbation of pulmonary disease or with an acute pulmonary infection. Acute infections should be cleared with antibiotics and chest physiotherapy before elective surgery. Prophylactic antibiotics in noninfected patients are not recommended for fear of selecting out resistant organisms. Finally, the medical regimen, including the use of inhaled b-adrenergic agonists, cromolyn, and steroids (inhaled or systemic), must be optimized. Serum levels of theophylline, if used, should be therapeutic.

Renal

The preoperative identification and evaluation of renal problems is also imperative. Any significant electrolyte abnormalities uncovered during the routine screening of healthy patients should be corrected preoperatively, and surgery should be delayed if additional medical evaluation is warranted. Preexisting renal disease is a major risk factor for the development of acute tubular necrosis both during and after surgery. Renal failure, whether acute or chronic, influences the types, dosages, and intervals of perioperative drugs and anesthetics. An oliguric or anuric condition requires judicious fluid management, especially in patients with cardiorespiratory compromise. Furthermore, chronic renal failure (CRF) is often associated with anemia, platelet dysfunction, and coagulopathy. Electrolyte abnormalities, particularly hyperkalemia, can lead to arrhythmias, especially in the setting of the chronic metabolic acidosis that often accompanies CRF. Hypertension and accelerated atherosclerosis resulting from CRF are risk factors for developing myocardial ischemia intraoperatively. Blunted sympathetic responses may predispose to hypotensive episodes during administration of anesthesia. The otolaryngologist must also be wary of the potential for injury to demineralized bones during patient positioning. An impaired immune system can contribute to poor wound healing and postoperative infection. Finally, because patients with CRF have often received blood transfusions, they are at increased risk of carrying blood-borne pathogens such as hepatitis B and C.

The possible causes of renal disease, including hypertension, diabetes, nephrolithiasis, glomerulonephritis, polycystic disease, lupus, polyarteritis nodosa, Goodpasture's or Wegener's syndromes, trauma, or previous surgical or anesthetic insults, should be elicited. The symptoms of polyuria, polydipsia, fatigue, dyspnea, dysuria, hematuria, oliguria or anuria, and peripheral edema are recorded, as is a complete listing of all medications taken by the patient.

In dialyzed patients, it is important to document the dialysis schedule. A nephrologist should assist with the preoperative evaluation and should optimize the patient's fluid status and electrolytes before surgery. A nephrologist should also be available to help manage these issues postoperatively, especially when major head and neck, skull-base, or neurotologic surgery—which may require large volumes of fluids or blood transfusions intraoperatively—is planned.

Preoperative testing on patients with significant renal disease routinely includes ECG, chest radiography, electrolytes and chemistry panel, CBC, PT/PTT, platelet counts, and bleeding times. In addition to a nephrologic consultation, patients with significant renal disease should also receive a preoperative anesthesiology consultation, and, if indicated, further evaluation by a cardiologist.

A history of benign prostatic hypertrophy or prostate cancer, with or without surgery, may predict a difficult urinary tract catheterization intraoperatively. Finally, elective surgery should not be performed on patients with acute genitourinary tract infections because the potential for urosepsis can be increased by the transient immunosuppression associated with general anesthesia.

Hepatic Disorders

Preoperative evaluation of patients with suspected or clinically evident liver failure should begin with a history detailing hepatotoxic drug therapy, jaundice, blood transfusion, upper gastrointestinal bleeding, and previous surgery and anesthesia. The physical should include examination for hepatomegaly, splenomegaly, ascites, jaundice, asterixis, and encephalopathy. The list of blood tests is fairly extensive and includes hematocrit, platelet count, bilirubin, electrolytes, creatinine, BUN, serum protein, PT/PTT, serum aminotransferases, alkaline phosphatase, and lactate dehydrogenase. A viral hepatitis screen can be obtained as well. Of note, patients with moderate to severe chronic alcoholic hepatitis may present with relatively normal-appearing liver function tests and coagulation parameters; these patients are at risk for perioperative liver failure.

Cirrhosis and portal hypertension have wide-ranging systemic manifestations. Arterial vasodilation and collateralization leads to decreased peripheral vascular resistance and an increased cardiac output. This hyperdynamic state can occur even in the face of alcoholic cardiomyopathy. The responsiveness of the cardiovascular system to sympathetic discharge and administration of catechols is also reduced, likely secondary to increased serum glucagon levels. Cardiac output can be reduced by the use of propranolol, which has been advocated by some as a treatment for esophageal varices. By decreasing cardiac output, flow through the portal system and the esophageal variceal collaterals is diminished. Additionally, there is likely a selective splanchnic vasoconstriction. Once initiated, b-blockade cannot be stopped easily because of a significant rebound effect.

Renal sequelae vary with the severity of liver disease from mild sodium retention to acute failure associated with the hepatorenal syndrome. Diuretics given to decrease ascites can often lead to intravascular hypovolemia, azotemia, hyponatremia, and encephalopathy. Fluid management in the perioperative period should be followed closely and dialysis instituted as needed for acute renal failure.

From a hematologic standpoint, patients with cirrhosis often have an increased 2,3-diphosphoglycerate level in their erythrocytes causing a shift to the right of the oxyhemoglobin dissociation curve. Clinically, this results in a lower oxygen saturation. This situation is further compounded by the frequent finding of anemia. Additionally, significant thrombocytopenia and coagulopathy may be encountered. The preoperative use of appropriate blood products can lead to short-term correction of hematologic abnormalities, but the prognosis in these patients remains poor.

Encephalopathy stems from insufficient hepatic elimination of nitrogenous compounds. Although measurements of BUN and serum ammonia levels are useful, they do not always correlate with the degree of encephalopathy. Treatment includes hemostasis, antibiotics, meticulous fluid management, low-protein diet, and lactulose.

Endocrine Disorders
Thyroid

Symptoms of hyperthyroidism include: weight loss; diarrhea; skeletal muscle weakness; warm, moist skin; heat intolerance; and nervousness. Laboratory test results may demonstrate hypercalcemia, thrombocytopenia, and mild anemia. Elderly patients also can present with heart failure, atrial fibrillation, or other dysrhythmias. The term *thyroid storm* refers to a life-threatening exacerbation of hyperthyroidism that results in severe tachycardia and hypertension.

Treatment of hyperthyroidism attempts to establish a euthyroid state and to ameliorate systemic symptoms. Propylthiouracil inhibits both thyroid hormone synthesis and the peripheral conversion of T4 to T3. Complete clinical response may take up to 8 weeks, during which the dosage may need to be tailored to prevent hypothyroidism. Potassium iodide (Lugol's solution), which works by inhibiting iodide organification, can be added to the medical regimen. In patients with sympathetic hyperactivity, b-blockers have been used effectively. Propranolol has the added benefit of decreasing T4-to-T3 conversion. It should not be used in patients with CHF secondary to poor left ventricular function or bronchospasm because it will exacerbate both of these conditions. Ideally, medical therapy should prepare a mildly thyrotoxic patient for surgery within 7 to 14 days. If the need for emergency surgery arises, intravenous propranolol or esmolol can be administered and titrated to keep the heart rate below 90 bpm. Other medications that can be used include reserpine and guanethidine, which deplete catechol stores, and glucocorticoids, which decrease both thyroid hormone secretion and T4-to-T3 conversion. Radioactive iodine also can be used effectively to obliterate thyroid function but should not be given to women of childbearing years.

The symptoms of hypothyroidism result from inadequate circulating levels of T4 and T3 and include lethargy, cognitive impairment, and cold intolerance. Clinical findings may include bradycardia, hypotension, hypothermia, hypoventilation, and hyponatremia. There is no evidence to suggest that patients with mild to moderate hypothyroidism are at increased risk for anesthetic complications, but all elective surgery patients should be treated with thyroid hormone replacement before surgery. Severe hypothyroidism resulting in myxedema coma is a medical emergency and is associated with a high mortality rate. Intravenous infusion of T3 or T4 and glucocorticoids should be combined with ventilatory support and temperature control as needed.

Parathyroid

The prevalence of primary hyperparathyroidism increases with age. Of patients with primary hyperparathyroidism, 60% to 70% present initially with nephrolithiasis secondary to hypercalcemia, and 90% are found to have benign parathyroid adenomas. Hyperparathyroidism secondary to hyperplasia occurs in association with medullary thyroid cancer and pheochromocytoma in multiple endocrine neoplasia type IIA and, more rarely, with malignancy. In humoral hypercalcemia of malignancy, nonendocrine tumors have been demonstrated to secrete a parathyroid hormone-like protein. Secondary hyperparathyroidism usually results from chronic renal disease. The hypocalcemia and hyperphosphatemia associated with this condition lead to increased parathyroid hormone production and, over time, to parathyroid hyperplasia. Tertiary hyperparathyroidism occurs when the CRF is rapidly corrected as in renal transplantation.

In addition to nephrolithiasis, signs and symptoms of hypercalcemia include polyuria, polydipsia, skeletal muscle weakness, epigastric discomfort, peptic ulceration, and constipation. Radiographs may show significant bone resorption in 10–15% of patients. Depression, confusion, and psychosis also may be associated with marked elevations in serum calcium levels.

Immediate treatment of hypercalcemia usually combines sodium diuresis with a loop diuretic and rehydration with normal saline as needed. This becomes urgent once the serum calcium levels rise above 15 g/dl. Several medications can be used to decrease serum calcium levels. Etidronate inhibits abnormal bone resorption. The cytotoxic agent mithramycin inhibits parathyroid hormone-induced osteoclastic activity but is associated with significant side effects, and calcitonin works transiently again by direct inhibition of osteoclast activity. Hemodialysis can also be used in the appropriate patient population.

The most common cause of hypoparathyroidism is iatrogenic. Thyroid and parathyroid surgery occasionally results in the inadvertent removal of all parathyroid tissue. Ablation of parathyroid tissue can also occur after major head and neck surgery and postoperative radiation therapy. Symptoms include tetany, perioral and digital paresthesias, muscle spasm, and seizures. Chvostek's sign (facial nerve hyperactivity elicited by tapping over the common trunk of the nerve as it passes through the parotid gland) and Trousseau's sign (finger and wrist spasm after inflation of a blood pressure cuff for several minutes) are clinically important indicators of latent hypercalcemia. Treatment is with calcium supplementation and vitamin D analogs.

Adrenal

Adrenal gland hyperactivity can result from a pituitary adenoma, a corticotropin hormone (ACTH)-producing nonendocrine tumor, or a primary adrenal neoplasm. Symptoms include truncal obesity, proximal muscle wasting, "moon" facies, and changes in behavior that vary from emotional lability to frank psychosis. Diagnosis is made through the dexamethasone suppression test, and treatment is adrenalectomy or hypophysectomy. It is important to regulate blood pressure and serum glucose levels and to normalize intravascular volume and electrolytes. Primary aldosteronism (Conn's syndrome) results in increased renal tubular exchange of sodium for potassium and hydrogen ions. This leads to hypokalemia, skeletal muscle weakness, fatigue, and acidosis. The aldosterone antagonist spironolactone should be used if the patient requires diuresis.

Idiopathic primary adrenal insufficiency (Addison's disease) results in both glucocorticoid and mineralocorticoid deficiencies. Symptoms include asthenia, weight loss, anorexia, abdominal pain, nausea, vomiting, diarrhea, constipation, hypotension, and hyperpigmentation. Hyperpigmentation is caused by overproduction of ACTH and b-lipotropin, which leads to melanocyte proliferation. Measurement of plasma cortisol levels 30 and 60 minutes after intravenous administration of ACTH (250 mg) aids in diagnosis. Patients with primary adrenal insufficiency demonstrate no response. Glucocorticoid replacement is required on a twice-daily basis and should be increased with stress. Mineralocorticoid therapy can be given once daily. Of note, patients treated for more than 3 weeks with exogenous glucocorticoids for any medical condition should be assumed to have suppression of their adrenal-pituitary axis and should be treated with stress-dose steroids perioperatively.

Pheochromocytoma is a tumor of the adrenal medulla that secretes both epinephrine and norepinephrine. Of these tumors, 5% are inherited in an autosomal dominant fashion as part of a multiple endocrine neoplasia syndrome. Symptoms include hypertension (which is often episodic), headache, palpitations, tremor, and profuse sweating. Preoperative treatment begins with phenoxybenzamine (a long-acting a-blocker) or prazosin at least 10 days before surgery. A β-blocker is added only after the establishment of a-blockade to avoid unopposed β-mediated vasoconstriction. Acute hypertensive crises can be managed with nitroprusside or phentolamine.

Diabetes Mellitus

Diabetes is a disorder of carbohydrate metabolism that results in a wide range of systemic manifestations. It is the most common endocrine abnormality found in surgical patients and can be characterized as either insulin-dependent (type I or juvenile onset) or non-insulin-dependent (type II). Hyperglycemia may result from a variety of etiologies that affect insulin production and function. Management techniques seek to avoid hypoglycemia and maintain high-normal serum glucose levels throughout the perioperative period. These goals are often difficult to maintain, however, because infection, stress, exogenous steroids, and variations in carbohydrate intake can all cause wide fluctuations in serum glucose levels. Close monitoring is mandatory with correction of hyperglycemia, using a sliding scale for insulin dosage or continuous intravenous infusion in more severe cases. Fluid management should focus on maintaining hydration and electrolyte balance.

Hematologic Disorders

A history of easy bruising or excessive bleeding with prior surgery should raise suspicion of a possible hematologic diathesis. A significant number of patients will also present on anticoagulative therapy for coexisting medical conditions. After a careful history, the physician should obtain laboratory studies. PT, PTT, and platelet count are included in the routine preoperative screen. PT evaluates both the extrinsic and the final common pathways. Included in the extrinsic pathway are the vitamin K-dependent factors II, VII, IX, and X, which are inhibited by warfarin. Conversely, heparin inhibits thrombin and factors IXa, Xa, and XIa, elements of the intrinsic clotting pathway. PTT measures the effectiveness of the intrinsic and final common pathways. Relative to the normal population, some patients may demonstrate significant variation in the quantitative levels of certain factors in the absence of clinically relevant clotting abnormalities. Thrombocytopenia or platelet dysfunction can also lead to derangements in coagulation. A standard CBC includes a platelet count, which should be greater than 50,000 to 70,000 before surgery. The ivy bleeding time, a clinical test of platelet function, should be between 3 and 8 minutes. Fibrin split products may also be measured to help determine the diagnosis of disseminated intravascular coagulation.

Congenital

Congenital deficiencies of hemostasis affect up to 1% of the population. Fortunately, the majority of these deficiencies are clinically mild. Two of the more serious deficiencies involve factor VIII, which is a complex of two subunits, factor VIII:C and factor VIII:von Willebrand's factor. Gender-linked recessive transmission of defects in the quantity and quality of factor VIII:C leads to hemophilia A. Because of its short half-life, perioperative management of factor VIII:C requires infusion of cryoprecipitate every 8 hours. The disease that has a milder presentation than hemophilia A is von Willebrand's disease, in which bleeding tends to be mucosal rather than visceral.

This disease is categorized into three subtypes. Types I and II represent quantitative and qualitative deficiencies, respectively. These deficiencies are passed by autosomal dominant transmission. Type I von Willebrand's also is characterized by low levels of factor VIII:C. Type III von Willebrand's disease is much rarer and presents with symptoms similar to those of hemophilia A. Because of the longer half-life of factor VIII:von Willebrand's factor, patients with type II von Willebrand's disease can be transfused with cryoprecipitate up to 24 hours before surgery, with repeat infusions every 24 to 48 hours. Patients with type I von Willebrand's disease require additional transfusion just before surgery to boost factor VIII:C levels and normalize bleeding time.

Patients with hemophilia, von Willebrand's disease, and other less common congenital hemostatic anomalies should be followed perioperatively by a hematologist. Correction of factor deficiencies should be instituted in a timely fashion, and patients should be monitored closely for any evidence of bleeding.

Anticoagulants

Warfarin, heparin, and aspirin have become commonly used medications in the medical arsenal. Conditions such as atrial fibrillation, deep vein thrombosis, pulmonary embolism, and heart-valve replacement are routinely treated initially with heparin, followed by warfarin on an outpatient basis. This therapy markedly decreases the incidence of thromboembolic events and, when appropriately monitored, only slightly increases the risk of hemorrhagic complications. Aspirin is widely used both as an analgesic and as prophylaxis for coronary artery disease. Patients taking any of these medications need careful evaluation to assess the severity of the condition necessitating anticoagulation. The benefit of surgery relative to the risk of normalizing coagulation should be clearly established with both the patient and the physician prescribing the anticoagulant.

Warfarin should be stopped at least 3 days before surgery, depending on liver function. Patients who have been determined to be at high risk for thromboembolism should be admitted for heparinization before surgery. The infusion rate can then be adjusted to maintain the PTT in a therapeutic range. Discontinuation of heparin approximately 6 hours before surgery should provide adequate time for reversal of anticoagulation. In emergency situations, warfarin can be reversed with vitamin K in approximately 6 hours and more quickly with the infusion of fresh frozen plasma (FFP). Heparin can be reversed with protamine or FFP. Of note, a heparin rebound phenomenon in which anticoagulative effects are reestablished can occur up to 24 hours after the use of protamine. Anticoagulative therapy can be reinstituted soon after surgery if necessary. Most surgeons, however, prefer to wait several days unless contraindicated. The surgeon may often find it helpful to discuss the timing of postoperative therapy with the hematologist before surgery.

Aspirin, an irreversible inhibitor of platelet function, leads to prolonged bleeding time. No strong evidence links aspirin therapy with excessive intraoperative bleeding. However, the theoretical risk that aspirin and other nonsteroidal antiinflammatory medications present leads most surgeons to request that their patients stop taking these medications up to 2 weeks before surgery to allow the platelet population to turn over.

Liver Failure

Patients with liver failure can present with several hematologic abnormalities. Bleeding from esophageal varices secondary to portal hypertension can lead to anemia. Hypersplenism and alcoholic bone marrow suppression can result in serious thrombocytopenia. An elevated PT may indicate a deficiency in the vitamin K-dependent factors of the extrinsic clotting pathway, as well as factors I, V, and XI, which are also produced in the liver. Last, as liver failure progresses, excessive fibrinolysis may occur. All of these hematologic sequelae of hepatic failure increase the risk of operative morbidity and mortality. Preoperative management should attempt to correct anemia and thrombocytopenia as indicated and replenish deficient clotting factors with FFP. Fluid management may prove to be a difficult issue.

Another less common cause of PT elevation is the intestinal sterilization syndrome in which intestinal flora, a major source of vitamin K, are eradicated by prolonged doses of antibiotics in patients unable to obtain vitamin K from other sources. Reversal occurs rapidly with vitamin K therapy.

Thrombocytopenia

A decrease in platelet count can occur as a result of a variety of medical conditions, including massive transfusion, liver failure, disseminated intravascular coagulation, aplastic anemia, hematologic malignancy, and idiopathic thrombocytopenic purpura. With the increasing use of chemotherapeutics for a variety of malignancies, the prevalence of iatrogenic thrombocytopenia has risen. Preoperatively, the platelet count should be greater than 50,000; at levels below 20,000, spontaneous bleeding may occur. Additionally, any indication of platelet dysfunction should be evaluated with a bleeding time. Severe azotemia secondary to renal failure may lead to platelet dysfunction (uremic platelet syndrome). Dialysis should be performed as necessary.

Correction of thrombocytopenia with platelet transfusion should preferably come from human leukocyte antigen-matched donors, particularly in patients who have received prior platelet transfusions and may be sensitized. One unit of platelets contains approximately 5.5×10^{11} platelets. One unit per 10 kg of body weight is a good initial dose. The platelets should be infused rapidly just prior to surgery.

Hemoglobinopathies

Of the more than 300 hemoglobinopathies, sickle cell disease and thalassemia are by far the most common. Approximately 10% of blacks in the United States carry the gene for sickle cell anemia. The heterozygous state imparts no real anesthetic risk. There are significant clinical manifestations to the 1 in 400 blacks who are homozygous for hemoglobin S. The genetic mutation results in the substitution of valine for glutamic acid in the sixth position of the b-chain of the hemoglobin molecule, leading to alterations in the shape of erythrocytes when the hemoglobin deoxygenates. The propensity for sickling directly relates to the quantity of hemoglobin S. Clinical findings include anemia and chronic hemolysis. Infarction of multiple organ systems can occur secondary to vessel occlusion. Treatment consists of preventive measures. Oxygenation and hydration help maintain tissue perfusion. Transfusion before surgical procedures decreases the concentration of erythrocytes carrying hemoglobin S, thereby lowering the chance of sickling.

Multiple types of thalassemia exist, each caused by genetic mutations in one of the subunits of the hemoglobin molecule. Symptoms vary on the severity of the mutation. Patients with the most severe form, *b*-thalassemia major, are transfusion dependent, which often leads to iron toxicity. Other thalassemias cause only mild hemolytic anemia. If transfusion dependency exists, the patient should be screened carefully for hepatic and cardiac sequelae of iron toxicity.

Neurologic

For medicolegal reasons, it is critical to document all neurologic abnormalities. The surgeon should distinguish peripheral from central lesions, and CT or MRI is often helpful in this regard. Frequently, neurologic consultation is sought in the setting of subtle findings or confusing or paradoxic findings and for evaluation of possible nonotolaryngologic etiologies of certain complaints, such as headache and dysequilibrium. During preoperative patient counseling, the surgeon must be aware of the potential for nerve injury or sacrifice and must communicate the possible sequelae of these actions to the patient.

If the patient has a history of seizures, the surgeon needs to find out the type, pattern, and frequency of the epilepsy, as well as the current anticonvulsant medications in use and their side effects. Phenytoin therapy can lead to poor dentition and anemia, whereas treatment with carbamazepine can cause hepatic dysfunction, hyponatremia, thrombocytopenia, and leukopenia, all of which represent concerns for the surgeon and anesthesiologist. Preoperative CBC, liver function tests, and coagulation studies are thus advised. Anesthetic agents such as enflurane, propofol, and lidocaine have the potential to precipitate convulsant activity, depending on their doses. In general, antiseizure medications must be at therapeutic serum levels and should be continued up to and including the day of surgery.

Symptomatic autonomic dysfunction can contribute to intraoperative hypotension. It may be necessary to augment intravascular volume preoperatively through increasing dietary salt intake, maximizing hydration, and administering fludrocortisone.

Additional considerations must be taken into account in patients with upper motor neuron diseases, such as amyotrophic lateral sclerosis, or lower motor neuron processes affecting cranial nerve nuclei in the brainstem. In either case, the otolaryngologist may be confronted with bulbar symptoms such as dysphagia, dysphonia, and inefficient mastication. As bulbar impairment progresses, the risk of aspiration increases significantly. When respiratory muscles are affected, the patient is likely to have dyspnea, intolerance to lying flat, and an ineffective cough. Coupled with aspiration, these factors put the patient at considerable surgical risk for pulmonary complications. Hence, if surgery is necessary for these patients, preoperative evaluation should include a pulmonary workup (including chest radiography, pulmonary function tests, ABG analysis) and consultation. A video study of swallowing function may also be indicated. Finally, the patient's neurologist should be closely involved in the decision making (i.e., whether to proceed with surgery).

Parkinsonism presents the challenges of excessive salivation and bronchial secretions, gastroesophageal reflux, obstructive and central sleep apnea, and autonomic insufficiency, all of which predispose to difficult airway and blood pressure management in the perioperative period. Dopaminergic medications should be administered up to the time of surgery to avoid the potentially fatal neuroleptic malignant syndrome. Medications such as phenothiazines, metoclopramide, and other antidopaminergics should be avoided. Preoperatively, the patient's pulmonary function and autonomic stability should be investigated.

If clinically indicated, patients with multiple sclerosis should also undergo full pulmonary evaluation preoperatively, because these patients can present with poor respiratory and bulbar function. The presence of contractures can limit patient positioning on the operating table. In addition, before surgery, the patient must be free of infection because pyrexia can exacerbate the conduction block in demyelinated neurons.

The Geriatric Patient

Of all surgeries currently performed, 25% to 33% are performed on people over 65 years of age. This percentage is likely to increase as the population ages. A greater likelihood of comorbid conditions exists with increasing age. In addition, physiologic reserve is often compromised. Preoperative assessment in this population should take these considerations into account and weigh the benefit of the procedure against the often increased risks in this population. Consultation with the anesthesia service facilitates planning for high-risk elderly patients.

Approximately 50% of all postoperative deaths in the elderly occur secondary to cardiovascular events. Severe cardiac disease should be treated before any elective procedure and should be weighed against the benefit of any more urgent procedure. If surgery is required, cardiac precautions should be instituted. Patients with physical evidence or a history of peripheral vascular disease should be evaluated for carotid artery stenosis. If a critical stenosis is identified, carotid endarterectomy should be performed before any elective procedure that requires a general anesthetic. The risk of a cerebrovascular accident should be considered when evaluating patients for more urgent procedures. From a respiratory standpoint, increasing age leads to loss of lung compliance, stiffening of the chest wall, and atrophy of respiratory muscles. In many otolaryngology procedures, the surgeon should consider the risk of intraoperative or postoperative aspiration and postobstructive pulmonary edema. Patients with borderline pulmonary function may not tolerate even mild respiratory complications. The function of all the organ systems diminishes with age, necessitating a thorough preoperative evaluation to maximize elderly patient safety.

CONCLUSION

This chapter has provided a brief overview of the importance for the surgeon to gather a patient's history and complete a physical exam and preoperative evaluation. Disturbances in one organ system often have repercussions for other systems, and so an interdisciplinary approach involving the otolaryngologist, anesthesiologist, internist, and specialized consultants is often warranted. The authors have chosen to emphasize the physiologic aspects of the evaluation. This is not intended to overshadow the importance of gaining insight into a patient's psychosocial preparedness, which often requires the help of family members, social workers, psychiatrists, and support groups, as well as a keen sense of intuition on the part of the surgeon. Furthermore, the surgeon's preoperative discussions with the patient provide a means to reinforce the patient's postoperative expectations and coping mechanisms. Finally, it must be reiterated that the responsibility of ensuring an appropriate preoperative evaluation lies with the surgeon and that the expediency of this process should be in keeping with the best interest of the patient.

REFERENCES

Adkins Jr RB: *Preoperative assessment of the elderly patient.* In Cameron JL, editor: *Current surgical therapy,* St Louis, Mosby, 1992.

Buckley FP: *Anesthesia and obesity and gastrointestinal disorders.* In Barash PG, Cullen BF, Stoelting RK, editors: *Clinical anesthesia,* Philadelphia, JB Lippincott, 1989.

Curzen N: *Patients with permanent pacemakers in situ.* In Goldstone JC, Pollard BJ, editors: *Handbook of clinical anesthesia,* New York, Churchill Livingstone, 1996.

Davies W: *Coronary artery disease.* In Goldstone JC, Pollard BJ, editors: *Handbook of clinical anesthesia,* New York, Churchill Livingstone, 1996.

Ellison N: *Hemostasis and hemotherapy.* In Barash PG, Cullen BF, Stoelting RK, editors: *Clinical anesthesia,* Philadelphia, JB Lippincott, 1989.

Gelman S: *Anesthesia and the liver.* In Barash PG, Cullen BF, Stoelting RK, editors: *Clinical anesthesia,* Philadelphia, JB Lippincott, 1989.

Goldstone JC: *COPD and anesthesia.* In Goldstone JC, Pollard BJ, editors: *Handbook of clinical anesthesia,* New York, Churchill Livingstone, 1996.

Graf G, Rosenbaum S: *Anesthesia and the endocrine system.* In Barash PG, Cullen BF, Stoelting RK, editors: *Clinical anesthesia,* Philadelphia, JB Lippincott, 1989.

Hirsch NP, Smith M: *Central nervous system.* In Goldstone JC, Pollard BJ, editors: *Handbook of clinical anesthesia,* New York, Churchill Livingstone, 1996.

Hurford WE: *Specific considerations with pulmonary disease.* In Firestone LL, Lebowitz PW, Cook CE, editors: *Clinical anesthesia procedures of the Massachusetts General Hospital,* ed 3, Boston/Toronto, Little, Brown, 1988.

Kovatsis PG: *Specific considerations with renal disease.* In Davidson JK, Eckhardt III WF, Perese DA, editors: *Clinical anesthesia procedures of the Massachusetts General Hospital,* ed 4, Boston/Toronto/London, Little, Brown, 1993.

Long TJ: *General preanesthetic evaluation.* In Davidson JK, Eckhardt III WF, Perese DA, editors: *Clinical anesthesia procedures of the Massachusetts General Hospital,* ed 4, Boston/Toronto/London, Little, Brown, 1993.

Morgan C: *Cardiovascular disease, general considerations.* In Goldstone JC, Pollard BJ, editors: *Handbook of clinical anesthesia,* New York, Churchill Livingstone, 1996.

Robbins KT and others: Neck dissection classification update. Revisions proposed by the American Head and Neck Society and the American Academy of Otolaryngology–Head and Neck Surgery, *Arch Otolaryngol Head Neck Surg* 128:751, 2002.

Rotter S: *Specific considerations with cardiac disease.* In Davidson JK, Eckhardt III WF, Perese DA, editors: *Clinical anesthesia procedures of the Massachusetts General Hospital,* ed 4, Boston/Toronto/London, Little, Brown, 1993.

Strang T, Tupper-Carey D: *Allergic reaction.* In Goldstone JC, Pollard BJ, editors: *Handbook of clinical anesthesia,* New York, Churchill Livingstone, 1996.

Sussman GL, Beezhold DH: Allergy to latex rubber, *Ann Intern Med* 122:43, 1995.

Vandam LD, Desai SP: *Evaluation of the patient and preoperative preparation.* In Barash PG, Cullen BF, Stoelting RK, editors: *Clinical anesthesia,* Philadelphia, JB Lippincott, 1989.

CHAPTER TWO

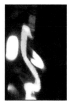

OVERVIEW OF DIAGNOSTIC IMAGING OF THE HEAD AND NECK

Nafi Aygun
Patrick J. Oliverio
S. James Zinreich

INTRODUCTION

Diagnostic medical imaging has changed medical and surgical diagnosis in ways never imagined. Every area of clinical medicine has been affected in a profound way. Medical imaging specialists are able, through their consultations, to assist the otolaryngologist in a variety of ways, including providing primary diagnosis, confirming a clinical impression, evaluating regional anatomy, assessing response to treatment, and assisting in definitive treatment of patients.

Neuroradiologists are subspecialty trained diagnostic radiologists who specialize in the imaging of the head and neck, skull base, temporal bone, brain, and spine. They are the primary imaging consultants for otolaryngologists.

This chapter provides an introduction and overview of head and neck imaging for the otolaryngologist. The various available imaging modalities are discussed. Imaging strategies for various regions and clinical questions are reviewed. The basic approach to the radiologist's image acquisition and interpretation are described so that the referring physician will gain a measure of understanding of this field. This is intended to maximize the usefulness of diagnostic imaging in the care of patients.

The scope of head and neck imaging is too broad a topic to be covered in one chapter. The authors provide the clinician with an outline and brief synopsis of the field. Definitive textbooks for each area of head and neck imaging are available.[13,47,49,53]

AVAILABLE IMAGING MODALITIES
Conventional Radiography

Since the discovery of the x-ray, it has been used in imaging the head and neck region. The traditional projections obtained with conventional radiography that are applicable to head and neck imaging are described below.

Views of the Facial Bones and Sinuses: Lateral, Caldwell, Waters, and submentovertex (SMV or base) views are attainable. The lateral view shows the frontal, maxillary, and sphenoid sinus. It is best obtained 5 degrees off the true lateral position to avoid superimposition of the posterior walls of the maxillary sinuses. The Caldwell view displays the frontal sinuses and posterior ethmoid air cells. It is obtained in the posteroanterior (PA) projection with 15 degrees of caudal angulation of the x-ray beam. The Waters view can show the maxillary sinuses, anterior ethmoid air cells, and orbital floors. It is obtained in the PA projection with the neck in 33 degrees of extension. The SMV view can show the sphenoid sinuses and the anterior and posterior walls of the frontal sinuses. It is obtained in the anteroposterior (AP) projection with the head in 90 degrees of extension.

Views of the Neck: AP and lateral views of the neck exposed for soft-tissue detail are useful for the evaluation of the overall contour of the soft tissues of the neck. These views are essentially the same projections used in the evaluation of cervical trauma, but they are not exposed for bone detail.

Cervical Spine Imaging: The complete plain film assessment of the cervical spine requires AP, lateral, right anterior oblique (RAO) and left anterior oblique (LAO) views, and an open-mouth AP view of the upper cervical spine to visualize the odontoid process of the second cervical vertebra. Specialized views such as the "swimmer's" (Twining) or "pillar" views can be used as needed. A "swimmer's" view is used to identify the lower cervical vertebral bodies when they cannot be seen from a routine lateral view. The "pillar" view is used to visualize the cervical articular masses *en face*.

Temporal Bone Imaging: Several projections are acceptable for visualizing portions of the temporal bone, including the Schüller projection, a lateral view of the mastoid obtained with 30 degrees of cephalocaudad angulation. The Stenvers projection is an oblique projection of the petrous bone obtained with the patient's head slightly flexed and rotated 45 degrees toward the side opposite the one under study. The beam is angulated 14 degrees. The transorbital projection is a frontal projection of the mastoids and petrous bones. Conventional imaging of the temporal bone has largely been replaced by computed tomography (CT) scanning.

Computed Tomography

CT was developed for clinical use in the mid-1970s by Hounsfield. CT uses a tightly collimated x-ray beam that is differentially absorbed by the various body tissues to generate highly detailed cross-sectional images. The degree of attenuation of the x-ray photons is assigned a numeric readout. These units of attenuation are known as *Hounsfield units* (*HU*) and generally range from −1000 HU to +1000 HU. Water is assigned a value of 0 HU.

To create images, CT uses complex mathematical reconstruction algorithms. Bone disease and bone trauma are best visualized with a bone detail algorithm (Figure 2-1). The raw data generated from the scan can be used in any number of ways. Images from a given reconstruction algorithm can be displayed in various ways to highlight differences in attenuation of different structures. In CT scanning, *window width* refers to the range of attenuation values in HU that make up the gray scale for a given image. The *window level* refers to the center HU value for that given window width. The various types of CT scans have standard window width and level settings.

Computed Tomography Image Display

Multiple options for displaying the image (adjusting the window level and width parameters on the imaging console) and recording it permanently on radiographic film are available. Each pixel (picture

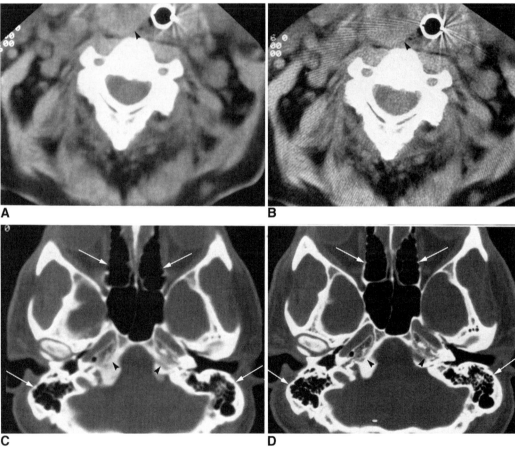

Figure 2-1. Comparison of various computed tomography algorithms and windows. **A,** Soft-tissue algorithm and, **B,** bone algorithm images of a laryngeal hematoma *(arrowheads)* using soft-tissue windows (350 HU width). The bone algorithm image has a grainier appearance, whereas the standard algorithm gives a smoothed image. **C,** Soft-tissue algorithm and, **D,** bone algorithm images of the skull base using bone windows (4000 HU width). Note the improved sharpness of the petrous apex trabeculae *(arrowheads)* and bony walls of the mastoid and ethmoid sinus air cells *(arrows)*.

element) of the CT image is given a density value. Water has been assigned a value of 0 on this scale developed by Hounsfield, and fat is approximately –80 to –100 HU. Calcium and bone are in the 100 to 400 HU range, and most fluids are in the 0 to 30 HU range. The window level is simply the midpoint of the densities chosen for display. The range of densities chosen above and below the window level defines the window width. A narrow window width of 80 HU and a level of +40 HU is frequently used for brain imaging because it centers the density at the common density of brain tissue, and displays only those densities 40 HU greater than and 40 HU less than the window level. Thus any density greater than +80 HU will be displayed as white, and any density less than 0 will be displayed as black on the gray scale. Any intermediate density will be spread out evenly along the gray scale. For imaging of the soft tissues of the head and neck, a window level of approximately 40 to 70 HU is usually chosen, at a midpoint approximately equal to the density of muscle. The window width frequently is in the 250 to 400 HU range, thus displaying a wider range of densities including calcification, intravenous contrast, muscle, and fat to best advantage. For imaging bony structures such as paranasal sinuses and temporal bone, window levels from 0 to +400 HU and a wide window width of 2000 to 4000 HU may be chosen. The reason for a wide bone window width is that a wide range of densities ranging from cortical bone (approximately +1000 HU) down to gas (–1000 HU) need to be displayed on the same image. However, structures of intermediate density between bone and gas occupy a narrow range on the gray scale at this window width and are poorly discriminated (appear washed-out) on

these settings. The terminology commonly used to describe the previously mentioned windows includes *soft-tissue windows* (window width of 250–400 HU) and *bone windows* (2000–4000 HU).

It is important to understand that these display windows are completely independent of the mathematical imaging algorithm chosen for creation of the image. In other words, an image created by a soft-tissue algorithm can be displayed with soft tissue and bone window widths (Figures 2-1, *A*, *C*). Conversely, the image may be computer reconstructed using a bone algorithm and displayed with either soft-tissue or bone window width (Figure 2-1, *B*, *D*). To optimize the imaging of the soft tissue lesion and the adjacent bone, a soft-tissue and a bone algorithm may be used, generating images with the appropriate soft-tissue and bone windows (see also Figures 2-12, *A*, *C*).

Patient Cooperation

Patient cooperation is necessary to obtain optimal image quality. The patient is instructed not to swallow and to stop breathing or to maintain quiet breathing during each slice acquisition to minimize motion artifact from the adjacent airway and pharyngeal structures. Occasionally, provocative maneuvers such as blowing through a small straw or using a cheek-puffing (modified Valsalva) maneuver to distend the hypopharynx, or phonating to assess vocal cord movement, may be necessary (Figures 2-2 and 2-3).

CT scanners have evolved over time such that the most advanced scanners now scan in a "helical" fashion, in which the scanner uses a slip-ring technique. This allows the table to move as the scan is performed, resulting in complete volumes of tissue being

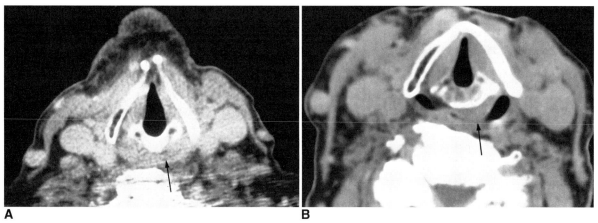

A　　　　　　　　　　　　　　　　　　**B**

Figure 2-2. Larynx without and with modified Valsalva maneuver. **A,** Axial contrast-enhanced computed tomography (CECT) performed during quiet breathing does not allow discrimination of the retrocricoid carcinoma *(arrow)* because the posterior pharyngeal wall is collapsed against the mass. **B,** Axial CECT in the same patient (a few minutes later) obtained with a modified Valsalva maneuver causes distension of the now air-filled hypopharynx, permitting tumor detection *(arrow)*.

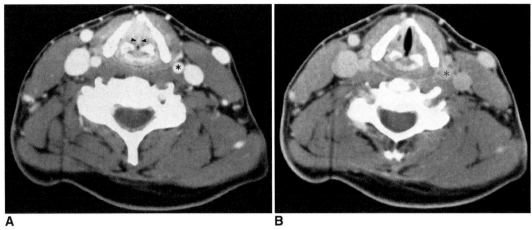

Figure 2-3. Axial contrast-enhancing computed tomography during breath holding and while phonating. **A,** This axial computed tomography, obtained during breath holding, shows the true vocal cords adducting and approximating each other *(arrowheads)*. Note the superb high-contrast density in common carotid artery *(asterisk)* and jugular veins. **B,** Phonating "eeee" causes the vocal cords to partially adduct into the paramedian position. Note that the contrast density has significantly decreased in the common carotid artery *(asterisk)* and the jugular veins in this delayed image, obtained well after contrast infusion had finished.

imaged without skipping tissue between slices. Multirow-multislice CT allows a greater amount of data to be gathered in a shorter time. At present, CT scanners can obtain slices 0.5 to 1-mm thick. A neck examination from skull base to the mediastinum can be performed in less than a minute. More importantly, enhanced computer technology permits real time manipulation of these data, allowing multiplanar and various forms of 3D reconstructions. CT is no longer an imaging modality confined to the axial (transverse) plane.

Contrast enhancement often is used to opacify blood vessels and to identify regions of abnormal tissue as identified by abnormal enhancement patterns (Figure 2-4). As it relates to head and neck imaging, contrast is particularly useful in CT scans of the neck and orbits. Contrast often is not needed in evaluation of the temporal bones, although it can be necessary on occasion. CT of the facial bones and paranasal sinuses usually does not require intravenous contrast.

As a brief review, the radiation exposure (dose) that a patient receives is known as the *radiation absorbed dose*. This radiation absorbed dose is a measure of the total radiation energy absorbed by the tissues, and it is expressed in an international system (SI) unit known as the Gray (Gy). One Gy is the amount of radiation needed to deposit the energy of 1 Joule (J) in 1 kg of tissue (1 Gy = 1 J/kg). Formerly, the unit used to express radiation absorbed dose was the rad (1 rad = amount of radiation needed to deposit the energy of 100 ergs in 1 g of tissue). The conversion of rads to Gy is: 1 Gy = 100 rad.

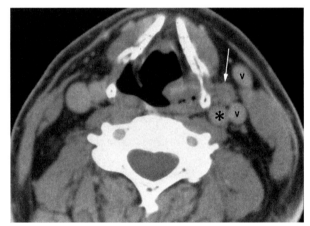

Figure 2-4. Contrast-enhancing computed tomography (CECT) with suboptimal contrast infusion. This axial CECT of a patient with a left piriform sinus tumor was obtained with insufficient contrast infusion, resulting in poor discrimination of the common carotid artery *(asterisk)* and jugular vein *(v)* from the isodense adjacent metastatic lymph node *(arrow)*. Inadequate contrast infusion also reduces the likelihood of identifying the focal defect in nodal metastasis.

Radiation dose equivalent is a more useful term as it considers the "quality factor" (Q) of the radiation involved (radiation dose equivalent = radiation absorbed dose × Q). The quality factor considers the varying biologic activity of various types of ionizing radiation. For x-rays, Q = 1. Thus, when discussing diagnostic x-rays, the radiation dose equivalent equals the radiation absorbed dose. The SI unit for the radiation dose equivalent is the Sievert (Sv). The former unit was the Roentgen equivalent for man (rem). In summary, 1 Gy = 1 Sv, and 1 Sv = 100 rem.

Radiation dose equivalent depends on the kVp and mAs of the exposure. For a given kVp, radiation dose equivalent varies linearly with the mAs. At 125 kVp, the radiation dose equivalent for a CT slice is approximately 1.1 to 1.2 cSv/100 mAs (1.1–1.2 rem/100 mAs). The actual dose will vary from machine to machine. Table 2-1 illustrates that the dose can be reduced by the use of low mAs technique when possible.

In contiguous CT imaging, the dose to the region scanned is approximately equal to the per-slice dose. The dose will be slightly lower if a gap is maintained between slices and it will be slightly higher if overlap occurs between slices.

The effective dose equivalent was developed as a means of representing the fraction of the total stochastic risk of fatal cancers and chromosomal abnormalities resulting from the irradiation of a particular organ or tissue when the body is uniformly irradiated. A system of weighting is used to consider the individual sensitivity of the body's major tissues and organs. A full discussion of this is beyond the scope of this chapter. Suffice to say that, for a given examination, the effective dose to the patient is less than the dose (radiation dose equivalent) received by the area under examination. A list of common radiographic procedures and their effective dose equivalents is in Table 2-2.

Magnetic Resonance Imaging

Magnetic resonance imaging (MRI) is an imaging modality that uses the response of biologic tissues to an applied and changing magnetic field to generate images. It is not possible to completely describe the principles of MRI in an introductory chapter of all head and neck imaging. A brief summary of MRI follows.

Two types of magnets are used to perform clinical MRIs: permanent and superconducting. Permanent

---

TABLE 2-1

RELATIVE RADIATION DOSE FOR SINUS CT (USING 125 KVP)

mAs	Radiation Dose Equivalent
450	4.95–5.40 cSv (4.95–5.40 rem)
240	2.64–2.88 cSv (2.64–2.88 rem)
160	1.76–1.92 cSv (1.76–1.92 rem)
80	0.88–0.96 cSv (0.88–0.96 rem)

From Zinreich S: Imaging of inflammatory sinus disease, *Otolaryngol Clin North Am* 26:535, 1993.

TABLE 2-2

ESTIMATED EFFECTIVE DOSE EQUIVALENT OF COMMON EXAMINATIONS

Examination	Effective Dose Equivalent
Sinus series, four views	7.0 mrem
Chest, PA and lateral	7.2 mrem
Kidneys and upper bladder	8.7 mrem
Lumbar spine, five views	125.1 mrem
CT, brain*	112.0 mrem
CT, sinus (160 mAs)[†]	51.2 mrem
CT, sinus (80 mAs)[‡]	25.6 mrem

From Zinreich S: Imaging of inflammatory sinus disease, *Otolaryngol Clin North Am* 26:535, 1993; and Zinreich S, Abidin M, Kennedy D: Cross-sectional imaging of the nasal cavity and paranasal sinuses, *Operative Techniques Otolaryngol Head Neck Surg* 1:93, 1990.
*120 kVp, 240 mAs, 10-mm slice thickness, contiguous.
[†]125 kVp, 160 mAs, 3-mm slice thickness, contiguous.
[‡]125 kVp, 80 mAs, 3-mm slice thickness, contiguous.

---

magnets do not require continual input of energy to maintain the magnetic field. They are composed of large magnetic metallic elements set up to generate a uniform magnetic field between components. Superconducting magnets are electromagnets usually composed of niobium-titanium wire. They require input of energy to start them, but once they are up to strength, they are maintained in a super conductive state by means of an encasing system of liquid nitrogen and liquid helium shells.

The earth has a magnetic field strength of 0.5 Gauss (G). The tesla (T) is another unit of magnetic strength that is related to G by the equation 1 T = 10,000 G. Clinical MRI units usually operate at magnetic field strengths of between 0.3 and 1.5 T. Small bore research scanners of strengths of 4.0 T are in use.

Many MR pulse sequences are available to generate images. The most common pulse sequence in MRI is the spin-echo technique.

MRI is one of the most active areas of development and research within diagnostic radiology. MRI derives its signal from hydrogen protons, most abundant in tissue fat and water, by placing them in a high magnetic field. This tends to align the spinning protons in the direction of the magnetic field. Radio frequency pulses are transmitted into the subject to excite the spinning protons, changing their orientation with respect to the magnetic field. As the protons realign with the magnetic field, they lose energy and give off a signal, which the MR scanner measures and reconstructs into an image. The quality of MRI depends on a high signal-to-noise ratio, which improves image contrast and spatial resolution.[14] In general, the higher the field strength of the magnet, the higher the signal-to-noise ratio. Thus MRI scanners with field strengths of 0.5 to 2.0 T are commonly used for imaging.

Surface coils significantly improve the quality of head and neck imaging by increasing the signal-to-noise ratio. A surface coil is a receiving antenna for the radio frequency signal that is emitted from the imaging subject after the initial radio frequency stimulation. The standard head coil is usually adequate for studying head and neck disease above the angle of the mandible. A head coil allows imaging of the adjacent brain and orbits, an advantage when head and neck lesions extend intracranially. Neck coils cover a larger area from the skull base to the clavicles and come in various configurations, for example, volume neck coil, anterior neck coil, 5-in flat coil placed over the anterior neck, and bilateral temporomandibular joint (TMJ) coil. Slice thickness on MRI is most commonly 5 mm, with 3-mm sections used for smaller regions of interest. However, a thinner slice has a smaller signal-to-noise ratio. Occasionally, 1- to 2-mm sections may be needed for small structures (e.g., facial nerve), requiring a volume acquisition technique. The number of slices is limited in MRI (as opposed to CT) by the specific sequence used, ranging from 6 to 8 slices with STIR (inversion recovery technique) up to 14 to 18 slices with a T2-weighted sequence. Volume acquisition techniques will allow 60 or more thin slices.

Magnetic Resonance Imaging Artifacts

Motion artifact, chemical shift artifact, dental work (e.g., amalgam, implants, braces, etc.), and eyelid mascara degrade MRI (Figure 2-5). Motion artifact becomes more prominent with increased field strength, increased length of individual pulse sequences, and the total length of the imaging study. A typical imaging sequence may last from 2 to 8 minutes. To limit motion artifact, sequences fewer than 4 minutes are preferred, and the patient should be instructed not to swallow and to breath shallowly and quietly.

Chemical shift artifact arises from the differences in resonance frequencies of water and fat protons. The result is an exaggerated interface (spatial misregistration) in areas where fat abuts structures containing predominantly water protons such as the posterior globe or a mass. Chemical shift artifact may produce the appearance of a pseudocapsule around a lesion or cause obscuration of a small-diameter structure such as the optic nerve. Chemical shift artifact may be identified as a bright band on one side of the structure and a black band on the opposite side. This is usually most noticeable on T1-weighted images (T1WIs).

Metallic artifact from dental work varies in severity depending on amount and composition of the metal in the mouth, as well as the pulse sequence and field strength of the MRI scanner. Most dental amalgam causes mild distortion to the local magnetic field, resulting in a mild dropout of signal around the involved teeth. Extensive dental work, metallic implants, and braces may cause more severe distortion of the image,

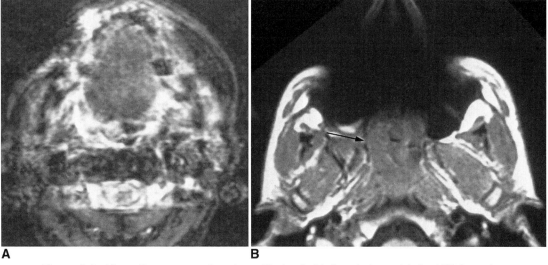

A   **B**

Figure 2-5. Magnetic resonance imaging artifacts. **A,** Motion during axial short T1 inversion recovery sequence caused significant degradation of the image with anatomic distortion and mismapping of the signal intensity. **B,** Metallic dental braces cause artifacts distorting anterior facial structures in this T1-weighted image of a boy with juvenile angiofibroma filling the nasal cavity *(arrow)* and nasopharynx. Anterior maxilla and portion of the nose have been distorted.

precluding visualization of the maxilla, mandible, and floor of the mouth. Mascara containing metallic compounds can also cause localized signal loss in the anterior orbit and globe.

Magnetic Resonance Imaging Pulse Sequences

Numerous pulse sequences are available on clinical MRI units. The details of the physics of MRI may be found in most radiology-MRI textbooks.[6] Commonly used imaging protocols include T1-weighted, spin (proton) density, T2-weighted, gadolinium-enhanced T1-weighted, fat-suppressed, and gradient echo imaging. Magnetic resonance angiography is infrequently obtained (Figures 2-6 and 2-7). The abbreviations used to identify sequence parameters on hard copy film or in journal articles are repetition time (TR), echo time (TE), and inversion time (TI) and are measured in milliseconds. The following description of pulse sequences is presented to assist the clinician in identifying and understanding the commonly performed sequences and in determining their respective use in the head and neck.

T1-weighted images. T1-weighted (short TR) sequences (see Figures 2-6, A and 2-7, A) use a short TR (500–700 ms) and a short TE (15–40 ms). T1-weighted imaging is the fundamental head and neck sequence because it provides excellent soft-tissue contrast with a superior display of anatomy, a high signal-to-noise ratio, and a relatively short imaging time (2–5 min), minimizing motion artifacts. Fat is high signal intensity (bright or white) on T1WIs and provides natural contrast in the head and neck. Air, rapid blood flow, bone, and fluid-filled structures

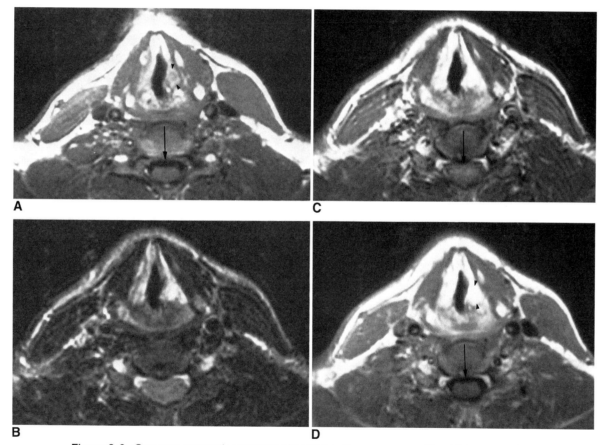

Figure 2-6. Common magnetic resonance imaging pulse sequences without fat suppression. **A,** Axial T1-weighted image (T1WI) of the left glottic tumor *(arrowheads)*, which is intermediate in signal intensity and thickens the true cord. Note that the cerebrospinal fluid (CSF) surrounding the spinal cord *(arrow)* is black, indicating that this is a T1WI. **B,** Spin density–weighted image also reveals high signal intensity (caused by increased water content) of the vocal cord tumor. CSF is now isointense to the spinal cord *(arrow)*, indicating this is a spin density sequence. **C,** T2-weighted image demonstrates a high signal intensity mass clearly demarcated against the dark background of fat and muscle. **D,** Postgadolinium T1WI shows enhancement of the cord tumor *(arrowheads)*. CSF remains black *(arrow)*.

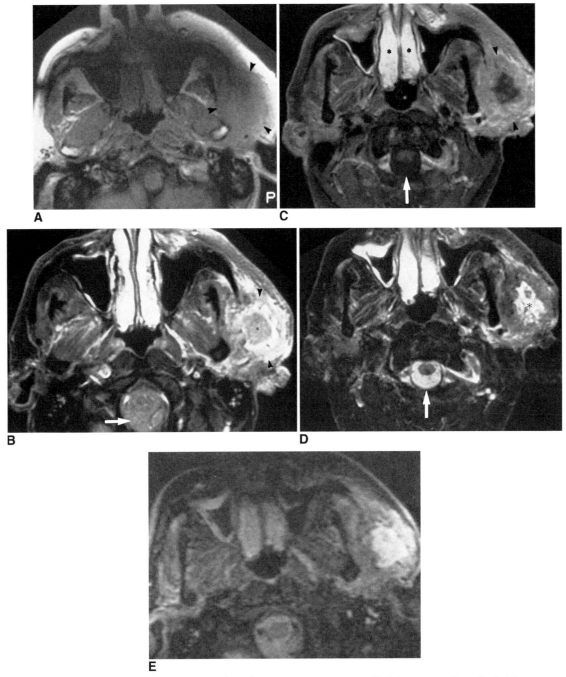

Figure 2-7. Magnetic resonance imaging pulse sequences with fat suppression. **A,** Axial T1-weighted image (T1WI) without contrast in a patient with squamous cell cancer shows a poorly defined mass in the left parotid gland *(arrowheads)*. Suboptimal signal in the image is the result of a signal drop-off at the edge of the anterior neck surface coil. **B,** Axial postgadolinium T1WI with fat saturation has adequate suppression of subcutaneous fat (compared with **A**) and enhancement of the tumor *(arrowheads)*. Center of the mass enhances less and likely is necrotic. Cerebrospinal fluid (CSF) is black *(arrow)*, indicating a T1WI. Note the marked enhancement of the inferior turbinates *(asterisks)* compared with the precontrast T1WI. **C,** Axial postgadolinium spin density image with fat saturation shows a high signal in the mass *(arrowheads)* with a lower-intensity necrotic center *(asterisk)*. Fat signal is suppressed and the image is similar to **B**. CSF is isointense with the spinal cord indicating the use of a spin density sequence. Turbinates are very bright. **D,** Axial T2-weighted image with fat saturation demonstrates nearly ideal fat suppression, almost as good as a short T1 inversion recovery (STIR) sequence. Necrotic or cystic center of the mass *(asterisk)* and CSF *(arrow)* have become very bright. **E,** On this axial STIR image with excellent fat suppression, the margin and center of the mass are bright.

[e.g., vitreous and cerebrospinal fluid (CSF)] are low signal intensity (dark or black) on T1WIs. Muscle is low to intermediate in signal intensity on T1WIs. The inherent high contrast of fat relative to adjacent structures allows excellent delineation of the muscles, globe, blood vessels, and mass lesions that border on fat. Surrounding bone is black, except for the enclosed bone marrow (e.g., sphenoid wing, mandible, and thyroid cartilage), which is bright from fat within the marrow. The aerated paranasal sinuses are black, whereas retained mucous or mass lesions are of low to intermediate signal intensity. Most head and neck mass lesions will show a low to intermediate signal intensity on T1WIs. Fewer slices are available with a short TR compared with a long TR sequence. (To quickly identify a T1WI: fat is white, CSF and vitreous are black, and nasal mucosa is low signal.)

Spin (proton) density-weighted images. Spin density-weighted sequences (also known as proton density, balanced, or mixed sequences) use a long TR (2000–4000 ms) and a short TE (20–40 ms). Spin density images (see Figure 2-6, *B*) show air and bone as low signal intensity and fluid-containing structures and muscles as intermediate signal intensity, with fat remaining moderately high in signal intensity but somewhat decreased in signal from T1WI. A solid mass or fluid-filled lesion with a high protein content will demonstrate moderate to high signal intensity, which may improve its visibility relative to muscle but may obscure it relative to the adjacent fat. Paranasal sinus inflammation typically appears very bright on spin density images. (To quickly identify a spin density image: CSF and vitreous are intermediate in signal.)

T2-weighted images. T2-weighted images (see Figure 2-6, *C*) use a long TR (2000–4000 ms) and a long TE (50–90 ms) and are sometimes referred to as long TR/long TE images. Note that spin density and T2WI are acquired simultaneously from a single sequence that produces two sets of images with the same TR but different TEs. For example, spin density = 2000/30 and T2WI = 2000/80. T2WIs are most useful for highlighting pathologic lesions. T2WIs show the vitreous and CSF as high signal intensity (bright) relative to the low to intermediate signal intensity of head and neck fat and muscle. Fat loses signal intensity with increased T2 weighting. Most head and neck masses are higher signal intensity on a T2WI compared with their low-to-intermediate signal intensity on T1WI. The combination of the T1WI and T2WI is often useful for characterizing fluid-containing structures, solid components, and hemorrhage. Bone, rapid vascular flow, calcium, hemosiderin, and air-containing sinuses are black. Inflammatory sinus disease and normal airway mucosa appear very bright. (To quickly identify a T2WI: CSF, vitreous, and nasal mucosa are white. Fat is low to intermediate in signal.)

Gadolinium enhancement. Paramagnetic gadolinium compounds are commonly used in central nervous system (CNS) imaging for lesion enhancement. Gadolinium is used in conjunction with T1WI sequences (gadolinium shortens the T1) and, with the dose used, it has little effect on T2WI. The advantages of gadolinium enhancement are increased lesion conspicuity and improved delineation of the margins of a mass relative to the lower signal of muscle, bone, vessel, or globe.[8] However, gadolinium enhancement (without concomitant fat suppression) has had limited usefulness within the head and neck, as well as in the orbit, because of the large amount of fat present within these regions (see Figure 2-6, *D*). After gadolinium injection, the signal increases within a lesion, often obscuring the lesion within the adjacent high signal intensity fat.[39] Therefore, for head and neck imaging, gadolinium is optimally used with specific fat suppression techniques that turn fat dark or black. Gadolinium enhances normal structures including nasal and pharyngeal mucosa, lymphoid tissue in Waldeyer's ring, extraocular muscles, and slow-flowing blood in veins, all of which may appear surprisingly bright, especially if combined with fat suppression techniques. (To quickly identify a gadolinium-enhanced T1WI: nasal mucosa is white, fat is white, and CSF and vitreous are black. Also look for Gd-DTPA printed directly on the image or on adhesive study labels.)

Fat suppression methods. Several sequences have been developed that suppress fat signal intensity. T2WIs, short TI inversion recovery (STIR), spectral presaturation inversion recovery (SPIR), and chemical shift selective presaturation (fat saturation) are some of the more common clinically available methods of fat suppression. One advantage of fat suppression is reduction or elimination of chemical shift artifacts by removing fat signal from the image while preserving water signal. Additionally, some fat suppression techniques take advantage of gadolinium enhancement by eliminating the surrounding high intensity signal from fat while retaining the high intensity enhancement produced by gadolinium. Most pathologic lesions have increased water content, and gadolinium exerts its paramagnetic effects while in blood vessels and in the increased extracellular fluid of the lesion, but gadolinium does not enhance fat. The fat signal can be manipulated in the following manners:

1. T2WIs provide a moderate degree of fat suppression and discrimination of fat from water

protons, yet enough fat signal persists to obscure some head and neck inflammatory and neoplastic lesions, especially lymph nodes. This sequence may be used before or after gadolinium and, because of the long TR used, yields the highest number of slices.

2. STIR (see Figure 2-7, *E*) is superior to T2WI for suppressing fat signal.[2] The inversion time (e.g., TI = 140 ms) is individually "tuned" for each patient to place fat at the null point of signal intensity and thus eliminates fat signal by turning it completely black. STIR images show the mucosa, vitreous, and CSF as very high signal intensity. Most mass lesions in the head and neck will have similar high signal intensity on STIR and T2WI. The disadvantage of STIR is image degradation secondary to a decreased signal-to-noise ratio, an increased susceptibility to motion artifacts, and increased scan time. It is inadvisable to perform STIR after gadolinium administration because the gadolinium can result in a "paradoxical" signal loss (rather than enhancement) by shortening the T1. The longer the T1 of a structure, the brighter it becomes on STIR. STIR is often limited to six to eight slices, making full neck evaluation difficult, unless a concatenated technique is used, which increases slices acquired but requires a doubling of scan time. (To quickly identify a STIR image: fat is almost completely black; CSF, vitreous, and mucosa are white. A TI is listed with the TR and TE times on the image.)

3. Chemical shift selective presaturation sequences (see Figure 2-7, *B*) used with a spin echo technique (Chem-Sat, General Electric) or with an inversion recovery technique (SPIR, Phillips) selectively suppress either water or fat signal, but fat saturation (suppression) is the most clinically useful technique. (Note that for the remainder of this chapter, the terms *fat suppression* and *fat saturation* are used interchangeably and refer to chemical shift selective presaturation techniques.) T1-weighted fat saturation sequences take full advantage of gadolinium enhancement. A gadolinium-enhancing lesion within the head and neck retains its high signal intensity and is not obscured, because fat is suppressed to become low to intermediate signal intensity. Enhancing masses within the head and neck and orbit are particularly well imaged with this technique.[26]

The disadvantages of fat saturation sequences are that non-gadolinium–enhancing lesions may be less well discriminated, that these sequences are more susceptible to artifacts, and that nonuniform fat sup-

pression occurs. Also, two or three fewer slices are acquired than with T1WI, unless the TR time is lengthened. (To quickly identify a gadolinium-enhanced T1WI with fat saturation: mucosa and small veins are white, fat is low to intermediate intensity, and CSF and vitreous are black.)

Fat saturation can optimize long TR (spin density and T2WI) sequences (see Figures 2-7, *C*, *D*). The advantage occurs when the spin density image is performed after gadolinium, since moderate T1-shortening effects by gadolinium occur with this sequence. Most lesions and vascular structures will show a mild degree of enhancement, with an image almost equivalent to a post-gadolinium fat saturation T1WI. Fat-saturated T2WIs provide excellent fat suppression almost equivalent to STIR, optimizing the high signal from normal structures and lesions that are high in water content contrasted against a black background of fat.

Gradient-echo techniques. Numerous gradient echo sequences are available that have a variety of applications. Gradient echo scans have a very short TR (30–70 ms), a very short TE (5–15 ms), and a flip angle of less than 90 degrees. They have a variety of proprietary acronyms including GRASS, MPGR, and SPGR (General Electric) and FLASH and FISP (Siemens). Gradient echo sequences take advantage of the phenomenon of flow-related enhancement. That is, any rapidly flowing blood will appear extremely bright. These sequences are useful for localizing normal vessels, detecting obstruction of flow in compressed or thrombosed vessels, or showing vascular lesions that have tubular, linear, or tortuous bright signal representing regions of rapid blood flow (Figure 2-8). Gradient echo sequences may be obtained faster than conventional spin-echo techniques, although their increased susceptibility to motion artifact decreases the benefits of a short scan time. Gradient echo techniques also permit volume, that is, 3D vs 2D acquisition of images, allowing increased spatial resolution and computer workstation reconstruction of any imaging plane at various slice thicknesses. The disadvantage of gradient echo sequences is the increased magnetic susceptibility artifact from bone or air, thus limiting their role near the skull base or paranasal sinuses. (To quickly identify a gradient echo image: arteries and often veins are white; fat, CSF, vitreous, and mucosa may have variable signal intensities depending on the technique used.)

Magnetic Resonance Angiography

Magnetic resonance angiography (MRA) is a technique that takes advantage of phase or time-of-flight differences in flowing blood relative to motionless structures and selectively produces images of structures

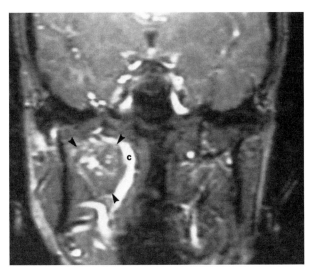

Figure 2-8. Gradient echo sequence in patient with right vagal paraganglioma. Coronal multiplanar gradient echo image demonstrates a mass *(arrowheads)* displacing the internal carotid artery *(c)* medially. Arterial blood flow is very high in signal intensity in the medially displaced internal carotid artery, as well as within the feeding vessels deep inside mass.

with rapid blood flow. MRA can generate 2D and 3D images of normal vessels and vascular lesions. At present, MRA does not equal the spatial resolution of conventional angiography, but the technology is in rapid evolution. Experience in the head and neck indicates that MRA is useful for evaluating vascular compression and vessel encasement and patency, but full characterization of tumor vascularity and vascular malformations is suboptimal.[35]

Magnetic Resonance Imaging Disadvantages

Several disadvantages of MRI of the head and neck bear consideration. MRI frequently requires 45 to 90 minutes of scanning time, during which time the patient must remain motionless, a process difficult for a sick patient to accomplish. Motion artifacts are more frequently encountered than with CT, although dental artifacts may be less problematic. Although no harmful effects are known to occur during pregnancy, MRI is used sparingly during a pregnant patient's first trimester. (MRI uses no ionizing radiation, and no harmful effects have been shown with its use at current field strengths.) Absolute contraindications to MRI include patients with cardiac pacemakers, cochlear implants, and ferromagnetic intracranial aneurysm clips. Those patients at risk for metallic orbital foreign bodies should be screened with plain films or CT before MRI. Generally, ocular prostheses and ossicular implants are safe. Unfortunately, MRI is one of the more expensive imaging modalities.

Ultrasound

High-resolution diagnostic ultrasound uses the properties of reflected high-frequency sound waves to produce cross-sectional images, obtainable in almost any plane. The transducer, a high-frequency 5- or 10-MHz probe, scans over the skin surface of the region of interest. Fat has a moderate degree of internal echoes (echogenicity). Skeletal muscle is less echogenic than fat. A solid mass has well-defined margins and variable echogenicity but is usually less echogenic than fat. A cyst has few, if any, internal echoes, a strongly echogenic back wall, and strong through-transmission of sound behind the cyst. Both calcium and bone are strongly echogenic, thus obscuring adjacent structures by an acoustic shadow. Ultrasound has no known harmful effects and no contraindications. High-resolution ultrasound is quick and accurate. Furthermore, it is relatively inexpensive compared with CT or MRI.

Nuclear Medicine
Positron Emission Tomography

As opposed to the imaging modalities already discussed in this chapter, which allow detailed anatomic information, positron emission tomography (PET) imaging provides physiologic and biochemical data. A positron emitting radiopharmaceutical is intravenously injected and its distribution in the body is measured. Positron emitting radiopharmaceuticals can be developed from naturally occurring substances such as ^{15}O water, ^{11}C carbon monoxide, or ^{13}N ammonia, or radioactive analogues of other biologic substances such as ^{18}F fluoro-2-deoxy-2-glucose (FDG). After being emitted from the atom, the positron travels in the tissue for a short distance until it encounters an electron and forms a *positronium*, which immediately annihilates (converts its mass to energy) forming two 511 keV photons. These annihilation photons travel away from each other at 180 degrees and are picked up by the detectors placed around the patient. Simultaneous detection of these photons relates them to the same annihilation event and allows spatial localization. Annihilation coincidence detection can be accomplished by very expensive dedicated PET scanners, yielding superior spatial resolution and sensitivity. Less costly gamma camera–based hybrid systems allow utilization of PET imaging outside the academic centers.

Attenuation of the photons in tissues they travel through decreases the apparent activity picked up by the detectors. Attenuation correction methods provide improved anatomic detail and better lesion localization but they result in noisier images. The effect of attenuation correction on visual image quality is controversial and, in many centers, the images are generated both with and without attenuation correction. For semi-quantitative and quantitative evaluation, however, attenuation correction is necessary.

Depending on the radiopharmaceutical chosen, PET imaging can provide information regarding blood flow, ischemia, deoxyribonucleic acid metabolism, glucose metabolism, protein synthesis, amino acid metabolism, and receptor status. Radiopharmaceutical development requires sophisticated knowledge and equipment which, combined with the very short half-life of most of these substances, limit clinical utility. The relatively long half-life of FDG (110 minutes) accounts for its widespread use. FDG can be delivered to PET imaging facilities through commercial vendors obviating the need for an on-site cyclotron.

Glucose metabolism in growing neoplastic cells is enhanced and accounts for the increased uptake on FDG-PET studies. Molecular studies have revealed that several genetic alterations responsible for tumor development also have direct effects on glycolysis. It has also been shown that increased tumoral FDG uptake is strongly related to the number of viable tumor cells, but not clearly associated with their proliferative rate. The glucose analogue 2-deoxy-D-glucose is transported into the cell and metabolized in the glycolytic cycle. After phosphorylation with hexokinase to DG-6-phosphate, the compound is metabolically trapped in the cell. Because of this trapping mechanism, FDG concentration steadily increases in metabolically active cells, yielding a high contrast between tumor and normal tissue. Bear in mind that increased glucose metabolism is not unique to malignant cells and can be seen in benign tumors, inflammatory or infectious lesions, and even normal tissues. Also, some malignant cells may not have increased glucose metabolism for a variety of reasons.

A typical PET scan is started 30 to 60 minutes after the intravenous administration of 10 mCi of ^{18}F-FDG. A 6- to 12-hour period of fasting is required before injection. Patients are encouraged to drink water before the FDG injection to minimize collection in the urinary system. The patients are told not to speak or chew before PET scanning. Since normal FDG uptake in muscle may mimic tumor, muscle relaxants such as benzodiazepines are used in some centers. Scanning is performed in the supine position at multiple table positions to cover the entire body. Scan time is 30 to 60 minutes.

Qualitative evaluation of FDG-PET images is sufficient for most clinical purposes, but quantitative measurement of FDG concentration is possible. Several approaches of different complexity can be applied for this purpose. Some of these require complex computation, data acquisition, and arterial blood sampling during scanning. The most commonly used method, standardized uptake values (SUV), is simple and confined to the measurement of radioactivity concentrations at a single time point. The activity concentration is normalized to the body weight or body surface area. SUV may allow differentiation of malignant tissue from benign causes of increased uptake and can be used to measure the response to treatment. A downside of SUV calculation in therapy monitoring is that it only allows comparison of two measurements obtained at the same time point after tracer injection.

A major disadvantage of PET is lack of anatomic information, resulting in poor lesion localization. A number of software applications are used to "fuse" PET images with CT or MR images, which are obtained at different time points. Fusion of anatomic and functional images significantly improves lesion localization, but it is still subject to many technical difficulties and errors. Combined PET/CT units permit acquisition of both CT and PET images using a single piece of equipment in the same session. Experience with these combined units is very promising. Errors in lesion localization are minimized, although they do occur in certain body regions where physiologic or involuntary motion is unavoidable.

Another major limitation of PET is poor spatial resolution. Currently, the maximum spatial resolution of dedicated PET scanners is about 5 to 6 mm. It is substantially inferior for more commonly used hybrid scanners. PET is an evolving technology and improvements in spatial resolution will surely be accomplished. Because of fundamental limitations inherent to the method, however, the maximum achievable spatial resolution is 1 to 2 mm. Therefore, PET is incapable of showing microscopic disease.

Radionuclide Imaging

Scintigraphy has several applications in the head and neck. In salivary gland imaging, technetium-99m (^{99m}Tc)-pertechnetate imaging may be useful for assessing salivary gland function in autoimmune and inflammatory disease of the salivary glands. If the salivary glands are obstructed, the degree of obstruction, as well as the follow-up of obstruction after treatment, can be assessed. In evaluating neoplasms of the salivary glands, the findings of the ^{99m}Tc-pertechnetate scan are almost pathognomonic of Warthin's tumor and oncocytoma. Spatial resolution is approximately limited to 1.5 cm, so accurate localization of the mass within the gland is difficult. Single photon emission computed tomography (SPECT) may be useful in some cases.

Techniques of thyroid imaging and thyroid therapy are described in several textbooks.[31,52] Many centers use I-123 to obtain a thyroid update determination, and ^{99m}Tc-pertechnetate is used to obtain whole gland images. It is these images that determine whether thyroid nodules are "hot" or "cold." I-131 is used for therapy of hyperthyroidism and in follow-up to detect and treat residual, recurrent, and metastatic thyroid cancers.

Medullary carcinoma of the thyroid is difficult to visualize, but ^{99m}Tc-DmSA has been used. In-111 pentetreotide has been used with some success.

Identification of parathyroid adenomas has been done for several years with a subtraction technique using ^{99m}Tc-pertechnetate and Tl-201 (Figure 2-9). The basis of this test is that thallium is taken up by thyroid tissue and parathyroid tissue. Thyroid tissue is the only tissue that uptakes ^{99m}Tc-pertechnetate. Therefore, the subtraction of the ^{99m}Tc-pertechnetateimage from the thallium-201 image should leave only parathyroid tissue. The sensitivity of this technique is believed to be excellent for lesions larger than 1 g. Sensitivity decreases for smaller lesions, and the subtraction technique can be hampered by patient motion. To identify parathyroid adenomas, ^{99m}Tc-sestamibi has also been used.[20] A single radiopharmaceutical double-phase protocol is the most recent improvement in identification of parathyroid adenomas.

CSF leaks can be detected with ^{111}In DTPA placed into the subarachnoid space. This technique is described and illustrated in Chapter 62.

Reconstruction Techniques—3D

Image data from either CT or MRI can be processed to create 3D reconstructions, but a separate computer workstation with appropriate imaging software is necessary.

CT data are loaded as a stack of contiguous 2D slices that define the scanned volume. Reconstructions are created either by choosing a specific range of densities for display or by manually tracing the outline of the desired structure. Improvements offered by multislice–multirow CT scanners and enhanced computational capacity of imaging workstations have led to a paradigm shift in radiology; volume imaging has replaced axial imaging. CT data from a large body part can be gathered in a very short time as a whole and the obtained "volumetric" data set can be displayed in various planes and 3D reconstructions.

Magnetic resonance data for image analysis are best acquired using a "volume acquisition" method, in which data are acquired as a complete 3D block rather than as individual slices. Because volume acquisition takes longer, gradient echo techniques are usually required to reduce the imaging time. Once acquired, the data are displayed in any desired plane and, by

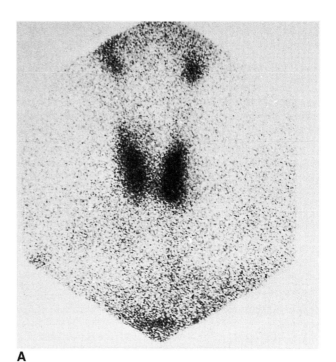

A

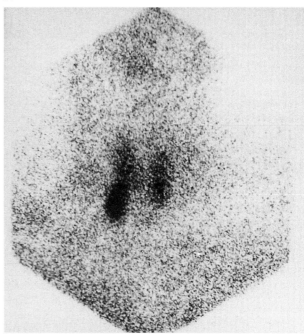

B

Figure 2-9. A, Technetinum-99m (^{99m}Tc)-pertechnetate scintigraphy in a patient with suspected parathyroid adenoma is essentially normal. **B,** Corresponding Tl-201 scintigraphy reveals an apparent area of increased uptake adjacent to the lower pole of the right lobe.

selecting a range of signal intensities or by tracing specific structures with a cursor, 3D surface models are created.

The utility of 3D reconstruction is best appreciated with craniofacial reconstructions.[16,30] Directly

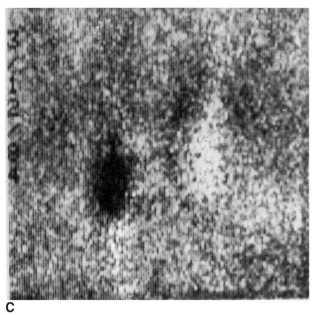

C

Figure 2-9, cont'd **C,** Subtraction of the ^{99m}Tc-pertechnetate study from the T1-201 study confirms the presence of a parathyroid adenoma.

visualizing the 3D relationships of the facial structures aids surgical planning. Instructors find 3D models of the face and orbital structures useful for teaching medical students, residents, and anatomy students. Virtual endoscopy is a computer-generated simulation of endoscopic perspective. The virtual endoscopic images of the trachea, larynx, pharynx, nasal cavity, and paranasal sinuses and ear have demonstrated clinical utility (Figure 2-10).

At present, the spatial resolution of CT is superior to MRI in the head and neck for displaying bony relationships. However, MRI provides a superior display of transcranial soft-tissue structures, such as the entire visual pathway, and has better tissue contrast resolution than CT. Thus CT and MRI will likely have complementary roles in 3D image display.

APPLICATIONS OF CT, MRI, AND ULTRASOUND IN THE HEAD AND NECK

Each anatomic region requires a different imaging approach to optimize the detection and characterization of the structure or lesion of interest. The following is a description of the indications for using CT, MRI, or ultrasound in specific head and neck regions, plus a general imaging approach relevant to each anatomic region in terms of imaging planes, slice thickness, contrast agents, and pulse sequences. Whenever possible, CT and MRI are performed before biopsy or resection of lesions because the resulting edema may obscure the true margins of a mass.

Application of Computed Tomography in Head and Neck Region
Suprahyoid Neck

Suprahyoid neck CT is often performed for simultaneous evaluation of the deep extent of mucosal-based tumors and to evaluate associated metastatic disease to the cervical lymph node chains. To cover the region from the skull base down to the root of the neck, contiguous axial 3- to 5-mm sections from the bottom of the sella down to the hyoid bone, followed by 3- to 5-mm sections at 5-mm intervals from the hyoid bone

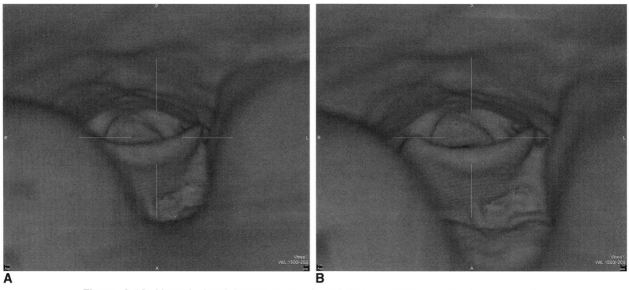

A   **B**

Figure 2-10. Normal virtual laryngoscopy. A real-time navigation in the larynx can be performed with ease using a workstation and special software.

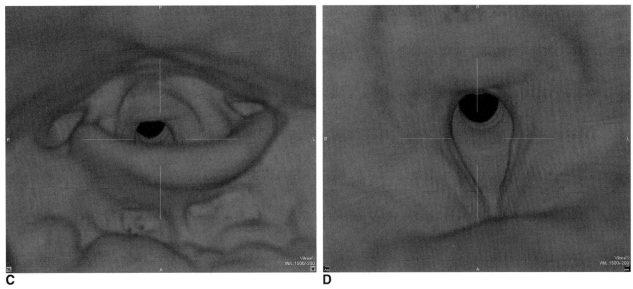

Figure 2-10, cont'd.

down to the sternal notch (thoracic inlet), are required. Because streak artifacts from dental fillings frequently obscure the oropharynx and nasopharynx, it is usually necessary to obtain additional angled sections to assess the pharynx directly posterior to the dental work (Figure 2-11). Direct coronal 3- to 5-mm images are very useful in defining craniocaudal relationships in lesions of the oral cavity and facial bones. The use of intravenous contrast is critical for adequate performance and interpretation of this study, especially the axial sections. Optimally, contrast is continuously infused during the entire scanning sequence so that a high concentration of intravascular (both arterial and venous) contrast allows differentiation of vessels (see Figures 2-3 and 2-4) from other higher density structures such as lymph nodes and muscle. Otherwise, determination of vascular invasion, compression, and discrimination of vessels from nodes and small muscle bundles can be extremely difficult. Contrast is best administered with a mechanical pump infusion (although a drip-infusion technique may also be effective), giving a single dose (40 g iodine) up to a double dose (80 g iodine) of contrast. Frequently, only a soft-tissue algorithm is necessary for each slice photographed with both soft-tissue and bone windows. However, sections of the skull base and mandible may need reconstruction using a bone algorithm if a suspicion of bone erosion or destruction by tumor or inflammation exists. Coronal images are advantageous when assessing lesions of the tongue, floor of mouth, retromolar trigone, mandible, or skull base.

Cervical Lymphadenopathy

Lymph node CT evaluation is concomitantly performed during CT investigation of most suprahyoid and infrahyoid tumors or inflammation. Axial 3- to 5-mm slices must extend from the skull base to the clavicles to encompass the many node chains that extend the length of the neck. As mentioned earlier in this chapter, the quality of lymph node assessment depends very much on the success of achieving a high concentration of contrast in the arterial and venous structures of the neck. Otherwise, nodes and vessels may appear remarkably similar.

Postoperative Neck

Imaging the postoperative neck uses the same techniques as the suprahyoid-infrahyoid neck. Thinner sections or supplemental coronal images in the region of suspected recurrence may be required.

Salivary Glands

Salivary gland CT is most frequently performed with the axial plane parallel to the infraorbitomeatal line and can be used for assessment of both the parotid and the submandibular gland. However, dental amalgam can cause significant streak artifacts that obscure the parotid or submandibular gland parenchyma. If the dental work is identified on the lateral scout view (scanogram), dental artifacts can usually be avoided if an oblique semi-axial projection is chosen with the scanner gantry angled in a negative direction (between a coronal and an axial plane), thus avoiding the teeth. This plane has the advantage of visualizing both parotid

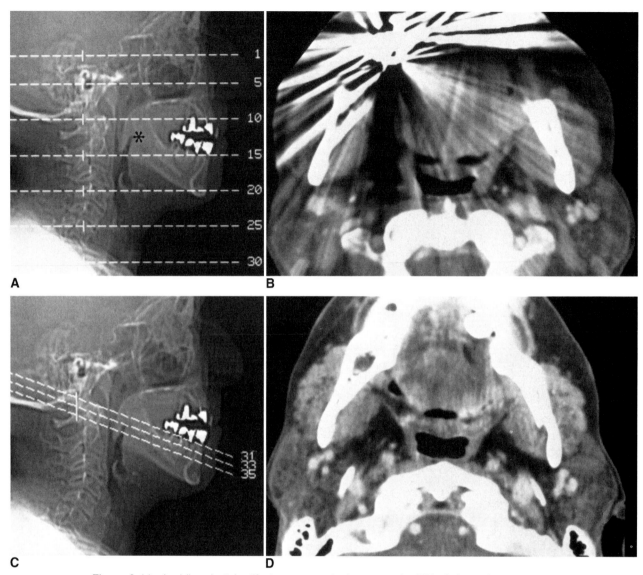

Figure 2-11. Avoiding dental artifacts on computed tomography (CT). **A,** Lateral scout image without angulation of the CT gantry (dotted lines represent selected axial images) in a patient with numerous metallic densities in teeth from dental work. Posterior tongue *(asterisk)* and soft palate lie directly posterior to metal. **B,** Axial contrast-enhanced computed tomography (CECT) at the level of the dental work is not interpretable because of the numerous streak artifacts caused by metallic fillings and crowns. **C,** Scout view depicting additional slices with the CT gantry angled to avoid dental work. **D,** Angled axial CECT at the same level as **B** shows a significant improvement in image quality of the posterior tongue and oropharynx.

and submandibular glands in the same slice and is parallel to the posterior belly of the digastric muscle.[54] The direct coronal projection may yield additional anatomic information for evaluating both the parotid and the submandibular glands and avoids creating dental artifacts through the parotid gland, but the dental artifacts may still compromise visualization of the submandibular duct and gland. A slice thickness of 3 to 5 mm is generally adequate for evaluating the gland parenchyma. Occasionally, supplemental 1- to 2-mm slices are required for evaluating smaller lesions.

With the current generation of high-resolution scanners, noncontrast computed tomography (NCCT) may suffice for the salivary glands. However, contrast-enhanced computed tomography (CECT) is preferable to NCCT in most cases because CECT maximizes the tissue contrast resolution between a salivary lesion and the adjacent normal gland, fat, and muscle.[10,48] CECT is also essential for assessment of salivary tumor metastases to the lymph node chains of the neck. A normal parotid gland is a relatively fatty structure with a density intermediate between the low density facial fat and the higher density adjacent masseter muscle. However, the parotid gland has a wide variation in normal density and may have increased density, approaching that of muscle in children and adults or in patients with chronic inflammation. The submandibular gland normally has density just slightly less than skeletal muscle and lymph nodes. In those occasional cases in which the gland parenchyma is similar to muscle in density, MRI, CECT, or even CT sialography (CTS) may be necessary to discriminate the margins of a suspected mass from the surrounding glandular tissue.

Sialography and Computed Tomography Sialography

Conventional sialography remains the best radiographic method for evaluating ductal anatomy in obstructive, inflammatory, and autoimmune salivary gland diseases. Supplemental CTS may be performed when routine sialography shows an unexpected mass lesion or in the infrequent situation when NCCT (or CECT) shows a dense, enlarged gland in which a mass is suspected but not clearly demarcated. CTS is unnecessary in most salivary tumor cases because of the much improved capabilities and thin sections of the high resolution third- and fourth-generation CT scanners compared with early generation scanners. However, MRI may be the preferred alternative method of studying dense salivary glands. CTS may be obtained at the time of intraductal injection of fat-soluble or water-soluble contrast or after a routine sialogram (the gland may be reinjected during the CT with the catheter left in place). The plane of study is the same as that used for NCCT and should be similarly angled to avoid dental filling artifacts. The use of concentrated sialographic contrast material may cause significant streak artifacts if too much contrast collects in dilated ducts, acini, or large pools, all of which can obscure smaller masses in the gland. For optimal CTS, the injection is extended into the acinar phase to maximize parenchymal opacification and thereby silhouette mass lesions within the parenchyma.[15]

Larynx and Infrahyoid Neck

Laryngeal and infrahyoid neck CT is most commonly requested to evaluate squamous cell carcinoma of the larynx or hypopharynx, associated cervical lymph node metastasis, trauma, and inflammation. Thus axial imaging from the angle of the mandible down to the sternal notch is required to survey the lymphatic chains and infrahyoid neck, using 3- to 5-mm contiguous sections and intravenous contrast infusion.

However, the fine detail of the larynx and vocal cords requires thinner contiguous sections of 2 to 3 mm. When assessing the true vocal cords and the arytenoid cartilages, 1- to 1.5-mm contiguous sections may occasionally be necessary to get adequate spatial resolution. Sections through the vocal cords are optimally obtained parallel to the plane of the cords by angling the scanner gantry parallel to the plane of the hyoid bone or the closest adjacent cervical disk space. Because assessment of vocal cord mobility is important in staging glottic carcinoma, various provocative techniques may facilitate laryngeal imaging in those cases where the vocal cords are obscured on physical examination. Quiet breathing places the cords in a partially abducted position. By having the patient blow through a straw or do a modified Valsalva maneuver (puffing out the cheeks) the hypopharynx and supraglottic larynx can be distended, allowing better separation of the aryepiglottic folds from the hypopharynx, while simultaneously abducting the cords (see Figure 2-3). The vocal cords can be assessed during phonation ("eeee"), which causes the cords to adduct and move to a paramedian position (see Figure 2-3). Breath holding will also adduct the vocal cords, close the glottis, and significantly reduce motion artifacts. By scanning the larynx twice, once to adduct and a second time (sections limited to the glottis) to abduct the vocal cords, the radiologist can assess vocal cord motion and identify fixation. Intravascular contrast should be given to differentiate vascular structures from adjacent nodes and muscles and to assess tumor margins. Evaluation of laryngeal trauma may not require intravenous contrast. Bone windows are helpful for assessing cartilage fractures or tumor erosion. Coronal images to assess the configuration of the true and false vocal cords, yielding similar information to that obtained by conventional AP tomography of the larynx, can easily be obtained.

Thyroid and Parathyroid Glands

Thyroid gland CT is performed in the same manner as the scanning of the larynx. The indication for performing CT arises when physical examination, ultrasound, or a nuclear medicine study suggests an unusually large or fixed mass. CT can help determine the extent of invasion and compression of adjacent structures in the larynx, hypopharynx, and mediastinum. The 3- to 5-mm sections are obtained from the hyoid bone to the top of the aortic arch to cover potential sites of ectopic thyroid and parathyroid tissue. Although the normal thyroid is hyperdense because of its natural iodine content on NCCT, a CECT is preferred for this study. The normal thyroid enhances intensely on CECT, with most mass lesions of the thyroid appearing less enhanced. The parathyroids are rarely imaged primarily by CT because nuclear medicine and ultrasound techniques are excellent procedures for localizing these small glands.

Paranasal Sinuses

Paranasal sinus CT can be approached in several ways depending on the anticipated disease process. Plain films may be used as the initial screening device for evaluating sinusitis or facial trauma. Once a mass or inflammatory lesion is detected within the sinuses, CT is the method of choice for further evaluation. A better substitute for the plain film sinus series is a screening axial sinus NCCT (Figure 2-12, *A*), which gives superior information on specific sinus involvement by inflammatory processes as well as better delineation of bony sclerosis or destruction. One method is to use 5-mm thick sections obtained at 10-mm intervals (5-mm gap), which can cover the entire paranasal sinuses with six to eight slices. Using a bone algorithm and photographing using bone windows, an accurate assessment of the presence or absence of sinus disease can be made. Another advantage of using the axial plane rather than the coronal plane for screening the sinuses is the inclusion of the mastoid air cells and middle ear, which can be another source of infection in a patient with a fever of unknown origin.

When endoscopic sinus surgery is anticipated, direct coronal NCCT imaging of the sinuses is mandatory for pre-operative evaluation of the extent of sinus disease, to detect anatomic variants, and for planning the surgical approach (Figure 2-12, *B*). This study is done with thin sections ranging from 2 to 3 mm of thickness. Frequently suboptimal is the 5-mm slice thickness, causing volume averaging of small structures and obscuring the fine details of ostiomeatal anatomy. Coronal imaging may be performed with the neck extended in either the prone or the supine position. An advantage of the prone position is that free fluid in the maxillary sinus layers dependently in the inferior portion of the sinus. In the supine position, fluid and mucus layer superiorly at the maxillary sinus ostium and may cause confusion with inflammatory mucosal thickening. Frequently, only the bone algorithm with its edge enhancement properties is needed for evaluating the detailed anatomy of the ostiomeatal complex. Contrast-enhanced sinus CT is usually not necessary for routine sinusitis, although when severe nasal polyposis is suspected, contrast may be useful to demonstrate the characteristic "cascading" appearance of the enhancing polyps or to characterize an associated mucocele. A soft-tissue algorithm with soft-tissue windows may be useful when using CECT for intracranial complications from

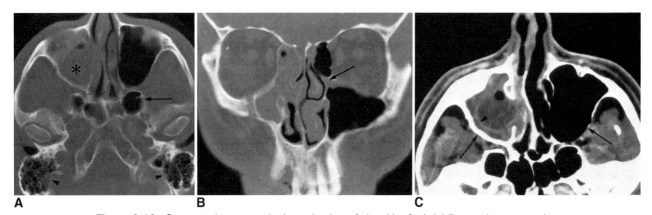

A   B   C

Figure 2-12. Computed tomography in evaluation of sinusitis. **A,** Axial 5-mm sinus screening noncontrast computed tomography (NCCT) using bone algorithm and bone windows in a patient with chronic right maxillary sinusitis. Excellent bony detail is obtained of both maxillary sinuses (posterior wall thickening and sclerosis are present on right) and mastoids. Clear discrimination of soft-tissue opacification of the right maxillary sinus *(asterisk)* is achieved compared with the normal air-filled left maxillary sinus. Pneumatized pterygoid process *(arrow)* is an extension of sphenoid sinus pneumatization. **B,** Coronal 3-mm NCCT with bone algorithm and bone windows in the same patient clearly demonstrates mucosal thickening and opacification of the right maxillary and ethmoid sinuses, and left maxillary infundibulum *(arrow)*. Sharp anatomic detail of the bony architecture and the use of coronal plane are essential for preoperative planning before endoscopic sinus surgery. **C,** Axial 3-mm contrast-enhanced computed tomography with soft-tissue algorithm and soft-tissue windows exaggerates the right maxillary sinus posterior wall thickness *(arrows)*. Thickened mucosa has a thin rim of enhancement along its luminal margin *(arrowhead)*. Combination of bony sclerosis and mucosal thickening is often seen in chronic sinusitis.

sinus inflammatory processes. A nasal decongestant may be used to help decrease normal but asymmetric nasal mucosa congestion (normal nasal mucosal cycle) from a mucosal-based mass.

The assessment of sinus tumors requires the most detailed imaging. Both axial CECT and coronal CECT with 3-mm sections are used to precisely determine the extent of sinus tumor spread into adjacent compartments, including the anterior and middle cranial fossa, orbit, and parapharyngeal space. For an optimal study, both soft-tissue and bone algorithms are used. This differentiates the soft-tissue component, as well as evaluating subtle bony destruction (Figure 2-12, A, C). The coronal plane is best for evaluating the cribriform plate. CECT is used to maximize the enhancement characteristics of the tumor and differentiate it from adjacent soft-tissue structures. In some cases, it may be necessary to extend the axial sections beyond the sinuses to include the cervical lymph node chains of the neck. If this is the case, a constant infusion technique is performed, scanning from the sternal notch up to the top of the paranasal sinuses, followed by the coronal images through the paranasal sinuses. This permits the optimal concentration of intravascular contrast to be obtained in the lower neck, to distinguish vessels from lymph nodes.

Facial Trauma

Facial trauma CT characterizes fractures and facial soft tissue injury very well. Both axial NCCT and coronal NCCT are obtained to optimally determine the 3D relationships of fracture fragments. Scanning may be performed with either 3-mm sections in both planes, or alternatively, contiguous 1.5-mm sections with coronal reformatted images when the patient cannot tolerate the coronal position because of other trauma or cervical spine instability. However, reformatted images are frequently degraded by motion artifact, and spatial resolution is usually unsatisfactory unless thin sections are used. Bone algorithm is preferred. Images are photographed with bone and soft-tissue windows. Soft-tissue algorithm for assessing orbital and facial soft-tissue injury is optional and requires additional image reconstruction time. The surgeon may find 3D reconstruction helpful when planning facial restoration.

Temporal Bone and Skull Base

In the past, evaluation of the skull base and temporal bones was principally performed using plain films and conventional tomography performed in the AP and lateral projections to assess bone destruction and mastoid or middle ear opacification. Tomograms are now rarely done or needed. The development of CT has completely eliminated the need for tomography in this region since the spatial and contrast resolution is superior. Also, overlapping structures do not degrade the CT image. CT of the temporal bones requires imaging, preferably in two planes using thin sections. Contiguous 1- to 1.5-mm sections are frequently obtained in the axial and the direct coronal planes. In some cases, if the need for reformatted images is anticipated, scanning in the axial plane with a 0.5-mm overlap may optimize reformatted coronal and sagittal images. Rotationally reformatted images are most helpful in displaying an entire semicircular canal in a single plane to aid in the diagnosis of dehiscent superior semicircular canal. In general, intravenous contrast is not necessary for temporal bone imaging, although vascular tumors or squamous cell carcinoma invading the temporal bone may require the use of intravenous contrast plus supplemental soft-tissue algorithms to best image the extracranial and intracranial soft-tissue component of the lesion. However, bone algorithm with bone windows is used in all temporal bone imaging. CECT of other lesions of the skull base proper may require both axial and coronal 3-mm sections. Bone and soft-tissue algorithms are necessary for assessing skull base tumor spread.

Application of Magnetic Resonance Imaging in Head and Neck Region
Suprahyoid Neck

MRI is ideally suited for imaging the suprahyoid neck (including nasopharynx, oropharynx, oral cavity, and tongue). Surface coils that improve signal detection may be used for imaging this area. The standard head coil will permit visualization of the suprahyoid neck structures caudally down to approximately the level of the inferior margin of the mandible and floor of mouth. For imaging the oral cavity, floor of mouth, submandibular space, and cervical lymph node chains, a head coil will not suffice. Either an anterior or volume neck coil is needed to visualize the entire neck from the skull base to the thoracic inlet (from dura to pleura). Several pulse sequences and imaging planes using 5-mm thick sections are required to adequately assess the deep and superficial structures of the neck. (Implicit in this discussion of MRI technique for all areas of the head and neck is the fact that a sagittal T1WI is obtained as the initial sequence in all of the authors' studies and is used primarily as a scout view for the proper positioning in other imaging planes, as well as for anatomic information.) A precontrast axial T1WI, and often a coronal T1WI, are required to optimally assess fat planes in the neck. Fat provides an excellent white background from which muscle and fascial planes, bone, sinus, and vascular structures can easily be discriminated. The coronal plane is particularly useful for visualizing the relationships of the suprahyoid neck structures to the skull base and also for delineating the anatomy of the tongue and floor of mouth. A T2WI, usually obtained in the axial plane, is required to detect structures with a long T2 (e.g., water, tumors, edema, proteinaceous cysts) that appear brighter than the background muscle and fat (fat loses signal intensity with increased T2 weighting). Postgadolinium T1WIs with fat saturation (suppression) in the axial and coronal plane are frequently helpful to discriminate the enhancing margins of a lesion or to detect perineural spread of tumor. The T2WI may also be combined with fat suppression and gadolinium usage to optimize the information obtained by this more time-consuming long TR sequence.

Lymphadenopathy

Before the widespread use of gadolinium and fat suppression techniques, MRI was often less sensitive and less specific than CT in detecting cervical lymph node metastases. However, improved MRI scanner technology, gadolinium enhancement, and fat suppression sequences have allowed considerable progress toward that goal. Also, the MRI detection of carotid artery invasion by extracapsular spread of tumor from nodes is often superior to CECT. Controversy still exists in defining the role of MRI in cervical lymph node imaging. Prospective studies of MRI in head and neck tumor and node staging are planned.

An anterior or volume neck coil using 5-mm thick sections with a small 1- to 2-mm interslice gap is necessary to encompass the entire lymph node chains throughout the neck from the skull base to the clavicles within the imaging field of view. The axial plane is frequently used, but the full craniocaudal extent of nodal disease is often better appreciated on coronal and sagittal views. Because the primary tumor is being scanned concomitantly, a choice between pulse sequences for characterizing both the lymph nodes and primary lesion must be made, yet with a minimum number of sequences (shortening the total scan time). Although most of the following sequences are quite sensitive for detecting adenopathy, few of them are specific in discriminating malignant metastatic nodes from reactive (inflammatory) adenopathy. The detection of cervical lymphadenopathy with MRI may be accomplished with (in decreasing order of sensitivity) a STIR sequence, a fat saturation T2WI, a fat saturation postgadolinium T1WI, a conventional T2WI, or a precontrast T1WI. Although STIR is the most sensitive sequence, it also yields the fewest slices, making full nodal evaluation problematic. However, a fat saturation T1WI can be obtained in a much shorter time than either a STIR or T2WI, and the fat saturation T1WI promises improved MRI specificity in

metastatic node differentiation from inflammatory disease. The significance of a ring-enhancing node on MRI should be analogous to ring enhancement of a metastatic node seen with the current gold standard, CECT.

Salivary Glands

MRI of the parotid gland can be accomplished with a standard head coil using 3- to 5-mm slices, but at the risk of excluding a portion of the submandibular gland that lies at the edge of the usable field of view. A volume neck coil is the better coil for imaging both parotid and submandibular glands within the same field of view, especially if a malignancy is suspected and cervical lymph node metastases are sought lower in the neck. A smaller TMJ coil may be necessary for evaluation of perineural tumor spread along with facial nerve into the mastoid segment of the facial nerve canal. As discussed earlier in this chapter, in assessing the suprahyoid neck (in which the salivary glands also reside) the MRI sequences that are most suited to salivary imaging include axial or coronal precontrast T1WI or both, axial and coronal fat saturation postgadolinium T1WI, axial T2WI (precontrast or postgadolinium with fat saturation), and often an axial or coronal STIR (for lymph node detection). T1WIs allow for detection of a low-intensity mass within the high-intensity background of a fatty parotid gland or for assessment of the adjacent fat planes.[10] The fat saturation postgadolinium T1WI is used for detecting the margins of a mass within a less fatty parotid or submandibular gland, for detecting extension beyond the margins of the gland, and especially for detecting perineural tumor spread along the fifth and seventh cranial nerves (best appreciated in the coronal plane). T2WIs are useful for localizing a tumor with a high water content or one with cystic or necrotic areas.[46] More recently, magnets with superior gradient performance allowed MR sialography images. This technique eliminates the need for intraductal injection of a contrast agent and uses the naturally present fluid within the ductal system as the basis of image generation. The intraparotid ductal system can be visualized up to the second-order branches. Despite its limitation in spatial resolution compared with conventional sialography, MR sialography is a viable alternative for the diagnosis of ductal disease in many clinical scenarios.

Larynx and Infrahyoid Neck

The larynx and infrahyoid neck require either an anterior or a volume neck coil, preferably using no thicker than 3-mm sections for the larynx. The field of view should include the area from the inferior margin of the mandible to the clavicles. Although the larynx can be examined well by both axial CECT and MRI, laryngeal MRI has a higher proportion of suboptimal studies. Laryngeal MRI is more susceptible to motion artifacts than MRI of other regions of the neck because of a combination of swallowing, breathing, and vascular pulsation from the adjacent common carotid arteries. A brief training session instructing the patient how to minimize swallowing and breathing artifacts may significantly improve results if it is done immediately before scanning. Additionally, shorter pulse sequences (i.e., T1WI) are more likely to be free of swallowing artifacts. Precontrast axial and coronal T1WIs are essential to assess the paralaryngeal (paraglottic) fat planes. The coronal plane, angled parallel to the airway, is especially useful for determining transglottic tumor spread.[51] Fat saturation postgadolinium T1WIs in the axial and coronal planes are best for detecting lesion margins, invasion of adjacent cartilage, and associated malignant nodes. T2WI in the axial plane may help detect moderately increased tumor signal and improve detection of high signal cystic or necrotic neck lesions. The longer T2WI and STIR sequences are more prone to motion artifacts and are occasionally suboptimal in quality.

Thyroid and Parathyroid Glands

The same techniques and slice thickness as those of the larynx are used for the thyroid and parathyroid glands. The field of view may need lower centering to include the upper mediastinum and ensure complete evaluation of the inferior extent of a thyroid tumor or an ectopic parathyroid gland. Coronal and sagittal views aid understanding of the craniocaudal extent of the lesion relative to the aortic arch, great vessels, and mediastinum. This information is especially useful to the surgeon. Although MRI may detect an unsuspected thyroid or parathyroid lesion during routine neck or cervical spine imaging, MRI is less frequently used for primary evaluation of these lesions because of the cost of the study and susceptibility to motion artifacts. The normal thyroid gland will enhance mildly on both gadolinium-enhanced MRI and CECT. A solid mass in the thyroid or parathyroid is usually low intensity on T1WI and high signal on T2WI, and it may enhance with gadolinium. Cystic lesions are bright on T2WI.

Paranasal Sinuses

Sinus MRI is primarily indicated for evaluating sinus tumors (and occasionally inflammatory disease such as a mucocele) and may be accomplished with a standard head coil, using 3- to 5-mm slices. The principal value of MRI over CT for sinus tumors is the ability of MRI to distinguish between tumor and obstructed sinus secretions and to predict the true extent of the tumor. A precontrast sagittal, axial, or coronal T1WI will provide a good demonstration of the sinuses, nasal cavity, cribriform plate, masticator and parapharyngeal spaces, and orbits. T1WI may differentiate hydrated from viscous sinus secretions. Secretions are low signal when hydrated or fluid-like and are intermediate to high signal when viscous and desiccated. Coronal T2WIs or axial T2WIs (either pre gadolinium, or postgadolinium with fat saturation) are useful for detecting inflammatory sinus secretions, which are high signal when hydrated or fluid and are low signal when viscous and desiccated. However, tumors tend to be intermediate in signal on T2WI. Because fat is not present to any significant degree in the paranasal sinuses, a STIR sequence frequently adds little over a T2WI and is unnecessary. Sagittal, coronal, or axial fat saturation T1WI is recommended to better define the sinus tumor margins when the tumor extends directly or by perineural spread beyond the sinus into the anterior cranial fossa, orbit, parapharyngeal space, or pterygopalatine fossa. The sagittal and coronal planes are very helpful for evaluating cribriform plate extension. The coronal and axial planes are best for orbital, cavernous sinus, pterygopalatine fossa, and parapharyngeal space spread.

Temporal Bone

MRI has significantly improved the detection of internal auditory canal (IAC), facial nerve canal, and jugular foramen lesions. Gadolinium-enhanced MRI has eliminated the need for air-contrast CT cisternography to detect a small intracanalicular acoustic schwannoma. MRI is useful, in combination with CT, for assessing expansile or destructive lesions of the temporal bone and external auditory canal. A standard head coil is adequate for most temporal bone lesions, but a smaller 5- to 10-cm TMJ coil may be needed for evaluating the mastoid and parotid segments of the facial nerve. The small size of the temporal bone structures and their respective lesions requires high spatial resolution images, which may be accomplished by using thinner slices of 0.5 to 3.0 mm (preferably without an interslice gap), smaller surface coils (higher signal-to-noise ratio), volume acquisition, or T1WI (higher signal-to-noise ratio). Precontrast T1WI in the sagittal and axial planes is useful for defining anatomy and for detection of high-signal lesions such as fat, methemoglobin, and viscous or proteinaceous cysts. Postgadolinium T1WIs (without or with fat saturation) in the axial and coronal planes are essential for detecting small enhancing lesions and determining the extent of larger lesions. In fact, for routine evaluation of a suspected acoustic schwannoma, only a post-gadolinium axial and coronal T1WI study may be required. T2WIs are frequently unnecessary for IAC tumors but may be helpful when brainstem ischemic or demyelinating disease, meningioma, blood products, proteinaceous secretions, or a large destructive tumor is suspected or is being further evaluated after a preliminary temporal bone CT. A facial nerve lesion in the mastoid segment of the facial nerve canal is best evaluated for proximal and distal extension using a TMJ coil with sagittal and coronal pre gadolinium and postgadolinium T1WIs.

Skull Base

MRI may be indicated for primary lesions of the skull base or for intracranial and extracranial lesions that secondarily involve the skull base. A standard head coil using 3- to 5-mm slices images this region well. Pregadolinium sagittal, axial, or coronal T1WI allows for assessment of the fat planes of the suprahyoid neck and detection of high signal intensity blood breakdown products, proteinaceous fluids, or fat within the lesion. Postgadolinium axial and coronal (occasionally sagittal) fat saturation T1WIs are excellent for determining the extent of an enhancing lesion above, below, and within the skull base. T2WI in the axial or coronal plane may be helpful for detecting a high signal lesion. STIR images usually give similar information to T2WIs in the skull base and may not be necessary.

Ultrasound Applications in the Head and Neck

High-resolution ultrasound evaluation of the suprahyoid neck, salivary glands, and infrahyoid neck is limited to the more superficial neck structures because of the impediment to sound transmission caused by the highly reflective facial bones, mandible, mastoid tip, and air within the oral cavity and pharynx. The ultrasound technique, using a high-frequency 5- to 10-MHz probe and multiple imaging planes, is similar for all these regions. A small superficial lesion is best seen with a high-frequency probe, whereas a larger and deeper lesion may require a lower frequency probe. Color flow Doppler technique may help differentiate vascular structures from a cystic or solid lesion. Head and neck ultrasound is performed less frequently in North America than in Europe, perhaps because of the common availability of CT in North America and the perception of the greater accuracy of CT. Head and neck ultrasound has no role as a staging modality for skull base and sinus neoplasms.

Suprahyoid Neck

Ultrasound may be used for the assessment of tumors of the floor of the mouth, anterior two-thirds of the tongue, malignant adenopathy, and invasion of the carotid artery and jugular vein. The deep structures centered in the parapharyngeal space are inade-

quately assessed by this technique and are better investigated by CT and MRI. Ultrasound can assess tumor extent in the floor of the mouth and tongue but has limitations: The mandible obscures the pterygoid muscles, and pharyngeal air hides the posterior pharyngeal wall and epiglottis.[17] Ultrasound excels in differentiating cystic from solid masses. A cyst has few internal echoes, a strongly echogenic back wall, and strong through-transmission of sound, whereas a solid mass has many internal echoes and no additional through-transmission.

Metastatic Lymphadenopathy

Ultrasound is very sensitive in detecting metastatic involvement of the lower two-thirds of the internal jugular, spinal accessory, submental, and submandibular nodes. Its accuracy may exceed CT for detecting enlarged lymph nodes, but ultrasound does not reliably differentiate large reactive nodes from metastatic nodes.[22] The upper one-third of the internal jugular, retropharyngeal, and tracheoesophageal groove nodes are poorly evaluated because of obscuration by bone or airway structures. Ultrasound may be the best method (possibly better than MRI or CT) for determining the presence of tumor invasion of the common or internal carotid artery and internal jugular vein by adjacent primary tumor or extracapsular spread from metastatic nodes. Invasion of the carotid artery is characterized by loss of the echogenic fascial plane between the vessel wall and the tumor.

Salivary Glands

Ultrasound has indications for both inflammatory and neoplastic disease. It may detect salivary duct stones as small as 2 mm. An obstructed dilated duct may appear as a tubular cystic structure. An abscess may be detected and drained under ultrasound guidance during the acute stage of sialadenitis, a time during which sialography is contraindicated. A mass in the superficial parotid gland is easily assessed by ultrasound, but the deep lobe of the parotid gland is obscured by the mandible, styloid process, and mastoid tip. Ultrasound is also very sensitive for a mass in the submandibular gland. Although ultrasound can determine the sharpness of margins of the lesion, an aggressive neoplasm or inflammatory process extending beyond the margins of the gland is better evaluated by MRI or CECT because the deep landmarks are more easily demonstrated with these methods. Well-defined margins usually indicate a benign mass, and infiltrative margins suggest malignancy.

Infrahyoid Neck

Ultrasound using a high-frequency transducer is usually the first imaging modality for evaluating superficially located thyroid gland and parathyroid gland masses because it is relatively inexpensive and easily performed. In the infrahyoid neck, ultrasound is not used for the larynx, retropharyngeal space, or thoracic inlet because overlying cartilage, airway structures, sternum, and clavicles cause acoustic shadows that may obscure lesions. The right, left, and pyramidal lobes may be evaluated by scanning in the axial, sagittal, and oblique planes. A thyroid mass and highly echogenic calcification are easily assessed. A parathyroid adenoma is readily evaluated if its location is cranial to the sternum. Ultrasound-guided fine needle biopsy of a thyroid or parathyroid mass is possible at the time of scanning. Large cystic and solid masses of the infrahyoid neck may be differentiated by ultrasound. Lymphoma of the neck may appear weakly echogenic, sometimes simulating a cyst.

FDG-PET APPLICATIONS IN HEAD AND NECK CANCER

PET is evolving and its exact role in imaging head and neck carcinoma is yet to be determined. Most of the available data are from retrospective studies, which involve limited numbers of patients. Nonetheless, PET has demonstrated great potential in this field.

Staging
T-staging

The detection rate of a primary tumor in the setting of squamous cell carcinoma of the head and neck (SCCHN) with FDG-PET is slightly superior to MRI and CT and comparable to panendoscopy. For the superficial mucosal lesions, however, the limitations of all imaging modalities including PET are well recognized and panendoscopy remains the best way to evaluate such lesions. PET, because of limited spatial resolution and lack of anatomic detail, appears inappropriate for the assessment of submucosal extent of disease and involvement of adjacent structures. MRI and CT remain the modality of choice for this purpose. FDG-PET may identify a primary tumor that is not detected by other diagnostic modalities in the setting of cervical nodal metastasis with unknown primary, although false positive results are also frequent in this setting. In a study by Regelink and others, 50 patients with nodal metastasis with no apparent primary were evaluated using FDG-PET, MRI or CT, and panendoscopy with directed biopsy.[38] They found 16 primary tumors. Of these, 4 were demonstrated by FDG-PET imaging only.

N-staging

The sensitivity of FDG-PET in detection of metastatic lymph nodes in the neck is slightly higher than in other modalities. The impact of this increased sensi-

tivity on patient management remains to be seen. A modality that would reliably differentiate N0 necks from N1 disease is very much needed, but it is unrealistic to expect PET to diagnose microscopic metastasis—even in the future—because of inherent technical limitations of spatial resolution. Currently available data do not justify the routine use of FDG-PET for nodal staging.

M-staging

FDG-PET imaging is suitable for detection of distant disease because of its great sensitivity and ability to examine virtually the entire body in a single study. Synchronous lesions in the upper aerodigestive tract and lungs are also detected with FDG-PET more accurately than other modalities, although false positive results remain problematic.

Therapy Monitoring

Tracer uptake can be quantified and changes in tumor metabolism can be monitored by PET imaging during treatment. Whether these changes can predict response to treatment is an active area of research. Early data suggest that, very early FDG-PET study performed days after initiation of treatment may separate responders from non-responders even before any structural changes have occurred. If this is proved to be true, it may permit modification of treatment very early in the process.

Detection of Recurrent Disease

Evaluation of the neck after surgery and radiotherapy is limited both clinically and radiologically. PET is definitely superior to anatomic imaging modalities and clinical exam in distinguishing recurrent disease from fibrosis or scar tissue (Figure 2-13). It is, however, well recognized that false positive results are common in the first months after therapy. It is generally recommended to defer FDG-PET studies at least 4 months after treatment.

PRINCIPLES OF IMAGE INTERPRETATION
Strategy for Image Interpretation and Differential Diagnosis

This section is included to aid the beginning surgeon or oncologist in developing a basic strategy for image interpretation. Normally, the radiologist chooses and supervises the appropriate imaging study, evaluates and interprets the images, and communicates its significance to the referring physician. However, frequent dialogue between the referring physician and the radiologist will significantly improve interpretation of the imaging study. Accurately interpreting an imaging study of the head and neck requires a systematic method of observation, knowledge of the complex anatomy, spaces, and pathophysiology, and an

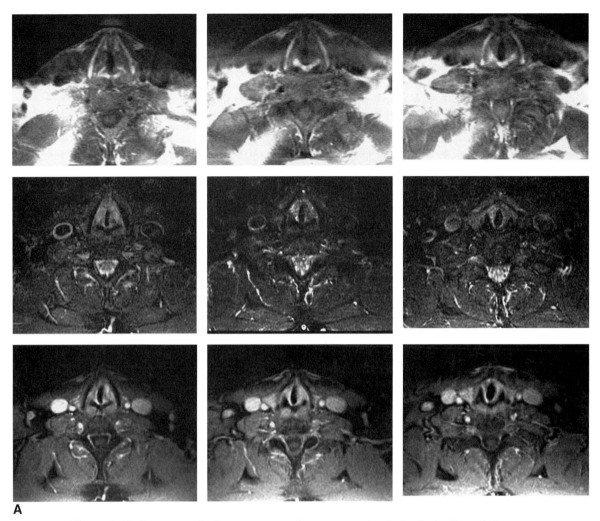

A

Figure 2-13. Recurrent glottic squamous-cell cancer previously treated with radiotherapy. **A**, T1-weighted, T2-weighted (STIR) and contrast enhanced, fat-saturated T1-weighted MRIs show mild fullness in the left true vocal cord without a discrete mass. It is impossible to differentiate post-therapy changes from the recurrent tumor.

understanding of imaging principles. The differential diagnosis of lesions of the head and neck requires a systematic approach as well. One such diagnostic imaging process is summarized below:

1. Obtain clinical data: age, sex, history, physical findings.
2. Survey the films for all abnormalities and summarize these findings.
3. Compartmentalize the lesion.
4. Interpret the chronicity and aggressiveness of the observations: acute or chronic, nonaggressive or aggressive, benign or malignant.
5. Develop a differential diagnosis. Use pathologic categories: congenital, inflammatory, tumor, trauma, vascular. Use clinical and radiographic

information to narrow the choices and arrive at the most appropriate diagnosis.

By using such a strategy, it is unlikely that important findings will be missed because all the images have been evaluated. This may be done by looking at all the anatomic spaces on each slice and proceeding sequentially through all the slices. Alternatively, each anatomic space can be evaluated on serial slices, followed by the next anatomic space, and so on. Characterizing a lesion requires specific observations: location, anatomic space of the epicenter, size, definition of margins, extent of spread in each direction, invasion of adjacent compartments, involvement of neurovascular structures, enhancement pattern, cysts, calcification, density, signal intensity, echogenicity, hemorrhage, and lymphadenopathy. Next, summariz-

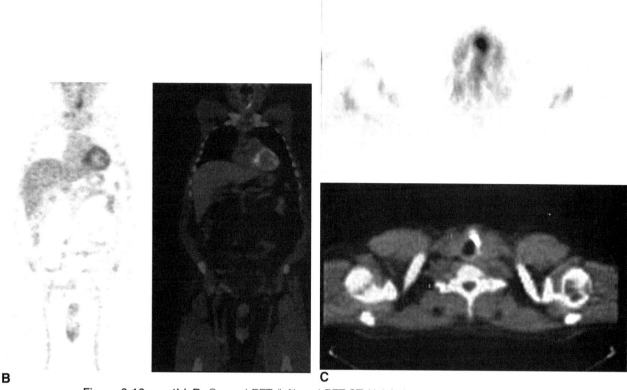

Figure 2-13, cont'd B, Coronal PET (left) and PET-CT (right) demonstrate increased metabolic activity in the left glottic and subglottic region. **C**, Axial PET (above) and PET-CT (below) show uptake anterior to the cricoid, compatible with extra-laryngeal involvement not visualized on the MRI (surgery-pathology proven).

ing the findings helps to tie them together into a logical pattern. Compartmentalizing a lesion is the last step in the observational process and requires placing the epicenter or site of origin of the lesion in a specific anatomic space, although some lesions may be multicompartmental. The origin of a lesion is limited by the types of tissue that reside in each specific space. An example of such a summary would be, "A 35-year-old male has a cystic, nonenhancing mass in the sublingual space." A frequent cause of misdiagnosis is the failure to make all the observations first. Interpretation and differential diagnosis of the lesion are the final steps.

The interpretation of the significance of a lesion uses both its radiologic and clinical features. For example, the interpretation might use the following descriptions: inflammatory (edema, abscess cavity, fever), nonaggressive (remodeling of bone, slow progression of symptoms), aggressive (destruction of bone, rapid progression), benign neoplastic (well-defined margins, displacement of adjacent structures, nonpainful), malignant (poorly defined margins, invasion and destruction of adjacent structures, pain and neuropathies), or cystic (low-density center with a thin rim of enhancement, fluctuant). The differential

diagnosis is narrowed by further refining the interpretation, "A 35-year-old male has an asymptomatic cystic, nonenhancing mass in the sublingual space that appears chronic and nonaggressive." With knowledge of the relevant clinical findings, the proper differential diagnosis, which is specific for each anatomic space, can then be constructed and limited to one (or at least a few) possible pathologic causes. In this example, a ranula would be the most likely consideration.

IMAGING ANATOMY, SITE-SPECIFIC LESIONS, AND PSEUDOTUMORS OF HEAD AND NECK
Spaces of Suprahyoid Neck

The traditional approach to radiographic interpretation of the head and neck region has been to follow a surgical compartmental approach: nasopharynx, oropharynx, oral cavity, pharynx, and larynx. The nasopharynx extends vertically from the skull base to the soft palate. The oropharynx encompasses the area from the soft palate-hard palate to the hyoid bone. The oral cavity is located anterior to the oropharynx. Below the hyoid bone reside the larynx anteriorly and the hypopharynx more posteriorly. With the advent of cross-sectional imaging in radiology, first with CT and later with MRI, the radiologic interpretive approach changed from a pattern based on surgical compartmental anatomy to one dependent on fascial spaces. However, a combination of the two interpretive approaches, for example, parapharyngeal space at the nasopharyngeal level (with the compartmental designation serving as a modifier) may be more helpful in precisely defining a lesion location.

The head and neck region, the anatomic territory that extends from the skull base to the thoracic inlet, is best and most conveniently divided into the suprahyoid and infrahyoid neck with the hyoid bone serving as the divisional point.[24] Figures 2-14 through 2-16 demonstrate normal cross-sectional CT and MRI anatomy of the suprahyoid neck. The suprahyoid neck may be divided into a series of fascial spaces based on the division and layers of the superficial and deep cervical fascia. The superficial cervical fascia surrounds the face and neck, providing a fatty layer on which the skin is able to slide. The underlying deep cervical fascia is separated into three distinct layers: superficial (investing) layer, middle (visceral) layer, and deep (prevertebral) layer. (Space limitations and the complexity of the fascial spaces do not allow for a detailed description or explanation of the deep cervical fascia.) Although not usually visualized on CT or MRI, these fascial layers divide the suprahyoid neck into distinct anatomic and surgically defined spaces:

1. Parapharyngeal space (PPS)
2. Pharyngeal mucosal space (PMS)
3. Parotid space (PS)
4. Carotid space (CS)
5. Masticator space (MS)
6. Retropharyngeal space (RPS)
7. Prevertebral space (PVS)
8. Oral cavity (OC)
9. Sublingual space (SLS)
10. Submandibular space (SMS)

Inflammatory and neoplastic disease, the major pathophysiologic processes of the head and neck territory, tend to grow and spread in the boundaries and confines of these fascial spaces.[5] Nevertheless, this approach based on the use of fascial anatomy allows delineation of specific anatomic spaces, with identification of disease-specific lesions for each of these spaces. As a consequence, a more accurate differential diagnosis and resulting final diagnosis are attained.

Parapharyngeal Space

The crucial anatomic center point to understanding suprahyoid anatomy is the parapharyngeal space (PPS). This fibrofatty fascial space extends from the skull base to the level of the hyoid bone and serves as a marker space around which the remaining fascial

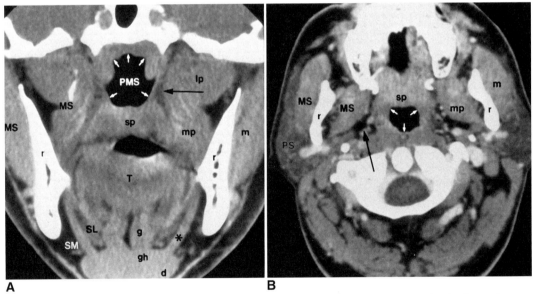

A   **B**

Figure 2-14. The normal computed tomography anatomy of suprahyoid neck. **A,** Coronal contrast-enhanced computed tomography (CECT) and, **B,** axial CECT demonstrate low-fat density of the parapharyngeal space *(arrow)*. Note its central position as a marker space. The following structures can be identified: anterior belly of digastric muscle *(d)*, genioglossus muscle *(g)*, geniohyoid muscle *(gh)*, lateral pterygoid muscle *(lp)*, masseter muscle *(m)*, medial pterygoid muscle *(mp)*, masticator space *(MS)*, mylohyoid muscle *(asterisk)*, nasopharyngeal mucosal space *(PMS, small arrows)*, parotid space *(PS)*, ramus of mandible *(r)*, sublingual space *(SL)*, submandibular space *(SM)*, soft palate *(sp)*, and intrinsic tongue musculature *(T)*.

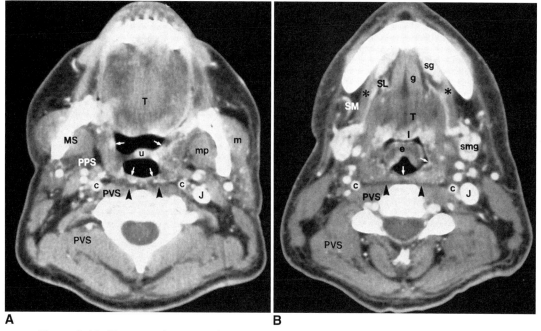

Figure 2-15. The normal computed tomography anatomy of sublingual space, submandibular space, and oral cavity. **A,** Axial contrast-enhanced computed tomography at superior and, **B,** inferior tongue levels, respectively. Note the following structures: internal carotid *(c)*, epiglottis *(e)*, genioglossus muscle *(g)*, jugular vein *(J)*, lingual tonsil *(l)*, masseter muscle *(m)*, medial pterygoid muscle *(mp)*, masticator space *(MS)*, mylohyoid muscle *(asterisk)*, pharyngeal mucosal space of oropharynx *(small arrows)*, prevertebral space *(PVS)*, retropharyngeal space *(arrowheads)*, sublingual space *(SL)*, submandibular space *(SM)*, submandibular gland *(smg)*, intrinsic musculature of tongue *(T)*, and uvula of soft palate *(u)*.

spaces are arranged. It contains fat, portions of the third division of cranial nerve V, the internal maxillary artery, the ascending pharyngeal artery, and the pterygoid venous plexus. In the axial plane, this space has a triangular configuration and demonstrates bilateral symmetry. In the coronal plane, the PPS has an hourglass shape, thicker at the skull base and hyoid level and thinner in the mid suprahyoid neck.

The PPS is clearly defined and located on both the axial and coronal planes with both CT and MRI.[42] With the former technique, the predominant fat content serves as a low-density marker between the medial muscles of deglutition found in the pharyngeal mucosal space and the muscles of mastication, located more laterally. With MRI, the PPS has a bright signal intensity on T1WI (the scanning sequence that best highlights fat and muscle tissue differences). With longer TR times and more T2 weighting, this fatty space becomes less intense in signal.

Because this space is the epicenter around which the other fascial spaces are arranged, it serves as a potential marker or pivotal space. By noting the position and direction of displacement of the PPS, one can determine the epicenter and fascial space origin of a suprahyoid lesion. Because the PPS contains few

structures from which lesions arise, most lesions found in this space have spread here secondarily from an adjacent fascial space.[43]

The fascial spaces that are centered about the parapharyngeal space include the pharyngeal mucosal space (PMS), the carotid space (CS), the parotid space (PS), the masticator space (MS), the retropharyngeal space (RPS), and the prevertebral space (PVS). Each space has well-defined anatomic boundaries, contains major structures of importance, and gives rise to pathologic processes that are site selective for that space. For consideration of pathologic processes in each fascial space, it is convenient to use the following outline: congenital, inflammatory, neoplastic (benign and malignant), pseudo lesions, and miscellaneous. This approach, using these few disease categories, elicits most of the major lesions to be found in the head and neck and is used in the following discussion of suprahyoid and infrahyoid lesions.

Pharyngeal Mucosal Space

The PMS lies medial to the PPS and anterior to the PVS. It encompasses the mucosal surfaces of the inner boundaries of the nasopharynx and oropharynx and includes lymphoid (adenoidal) tissue, minor salivary

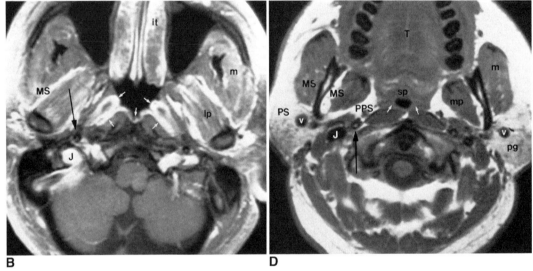

Figure 2-16. The normal magnetic resonance imaging anatomy of suprahyoid neck. **A,** Sagittal mid-line noncontrast T1-weighted image (T1WI). **B,** Axial noncontrast T1WI at the level of jugular foramen. **C,** Axial postgadolinium T1WI at the same level of **B** demonstrates enhancement of the nasopharyngeal mucosa and jugular veins. **D,** Axial noncontrast T1WI at the level of C2 vertebral body and mid tongue demonstrates high signal intensity of parapharyngeal space fat. The following structures are labeled: cerebellum *(cb)*, clivus *(cl)*, hard palate *(hp)*, internal carotid artery *(arrow)*, inferior turbinates *(it)*, jugular vein *(J)*, lateral pterygoid muscle *(lp)*, masseter muscle *(m)*, medulla *(md)*, masticator space *(MS)*, nasopharyngeal mucosal space *(small arrows)*, pons *(p)*, parotid gland *(pg)*, parapharyngeal space *(PPS)*, parotid space *(PS)*, retropharyngeal space *(arrowheads)*, sphenoid sinus *(s)*, soft palate *(sp)*, intrinsic musculature of tongue *(T)*, temporalis muscle *(tp)*, and retromandibular vein *(v)*.

glands, portions of the constrictor muscles, and muscles of deglutition. The medial portion of the eustachian tube passes through it. These structures lie medial to or on the airway side of the buccopharyngeal fascia. This fascial structure may be seen on MRI as a band of low signal intensity. On CECT or gadolinium-enhanced MRI studies, the overlying pharyngeal mucosa enhances.

The PMS extends from the skull base to the lower margin of the cricoid cartilage, extending into the upper portion of the infrahyoid neck. It encompasses the nasopharynx, oropharynx, and portions of the hypopharynx. Lesions in this space displace the PPS laterally.

In general, caution is used when interpreting the mucosal surfaces of the pharynx, oral cavity, and larynx. The normal mucosa is high signal on T2WI and STIR and enhances on postgadolinium T1WI (and with CECT). It may be confused with a superficial mucosal-based malignancy. Likewise, a small superficial mucosal-based tumor may be indistinguishable from the adjacent normal mucosa. The direct clinical examination of the mucosal surfaces is still superior to cross-sectional CT or MR imaging in detecting superficial tumor; however, both CT and MRI excel in detecting submucosal tumor and deep invasion. Mucosal irregularity and slight asymmetry are common, especially near the fossa of Rosenmüller (the lateral pharyngeal recesses of the nasopharynx), and care is taken in ascribing abnormality. Repeat studies with a modified Valsalva maneuver to distend the airway may be helpful. Involvement of the submucosal muscles and adjacent deep structures, such as the PPS, will confirm the presence of a suspected neoplastic mucosal lesion. Lymphoid (adenoidal) tissue is often hypertrophic and prominent, especially in children and young adolescents, and may encroach on the airway. On CT, lymphoid tissue is isodense to muscle. With MRI, it has a similar intensity to muscle on T1WI but has a bright signal on T2WI. It lies superficial to the buccopharyngeal fascia and is relatively homogeneous.

Inflammatory lesions of the PPS include pharyngitis, abscess (especially tonsillar abscess), and postinflammatory retention cysts (Figure 2-17). Benign mixed salivary tumor is the most common benign neoplasm.

A Thornwaldt cyst is a common congenital lesion of the midline posterior nasopharyngeal mucosa and only rarely becomes secondarily infected. It is very bright on long TR sequences on MRI.

Squamous cell carcinoma (SCC), the most common tumor of the upper aerodigestive tract, originates from the PMS. The majority of lesions arise from squamous epithelium in the region of the lateral pharyngeal recess (Figures 2-18 and 2-19). Small submucosal lesions may be missed on the clinical examination but may be detected with cross-sectional imaging. Involvement of the adjacent musculofascial spaces confirms the presence of a mucosal lesion. It may become large and lead to extensive invasion and destruction of the neighboring fascial spaces or extend medially to involve the PPS. With CT, SCC demonstrates inhomogeneous lesion enhancement, commonly with extension into adjacent spaces. With MRI, it is of intermediate intensity on T1WI and high intensity on T2WI and enhances after gadolinium infusion.[37] It may cause serous otitis media and mastoid cell opacification because of dysfunction of the eustachian tube from invasion or mass effect. Extension superior to the skull base is common. The foramen lacerum, foramen ovale, carotid canal, jugu-

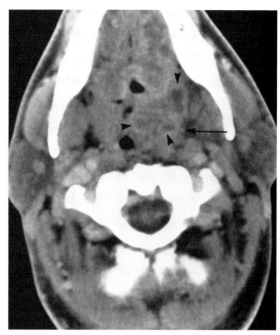

Figure 2-17. Tonsillar abscess. Axial contrast-enhanced computed tomography demonstrates a low-density left tonsillar lesion *(arrowheads)* with thin peripheral rim enhancement. The left tonsil is increased in size. Partially effaced left parapharyngeal space *(arrow)* is lateral in position.

lar foramen, and clivus may be affected. Perineural tumor spread along cranial motor nerve V is common and its presence should be diligently sought, especially if there is unilateral atrophy of the muscles of mastication innervated by the mandibular division of the fifth cranial nerve. Inferiorly, nasopharyngeal SCC may extend to involve the soft palate, tonsillar pillars, and nasal cavity. Asymptomatic cervical adenopathy with involvement of the superior internal jugular and spinal accessory lymph node chains is the presenting mode in more than 50% of patients. Lymph nodes are usually considered positive when larger than 1.5 cm in diameter. An enhancing lymph node rim with necrotic low-density center on CECT indicates neoplastic involvement. On MRI, lymph nodes have bright signal intensity on T2WI. On T1WI, after gadolinium administration, lymph node enhancement may be seen.

The extensive lymphoid tissue in this space is a source for development of non-Hodgkin's lymphoma (Figure 2-20). Both SCC and lymphoma may have extensive lymph node involvement. The nodes associated with SCC commonly have necrotic centers, whereas those of lymphoma are usually non-cavitary and homogeneous. Malignant minor salivary gland tumors also occur in this space. These three malignant lesions are difficult to separate radiologically.

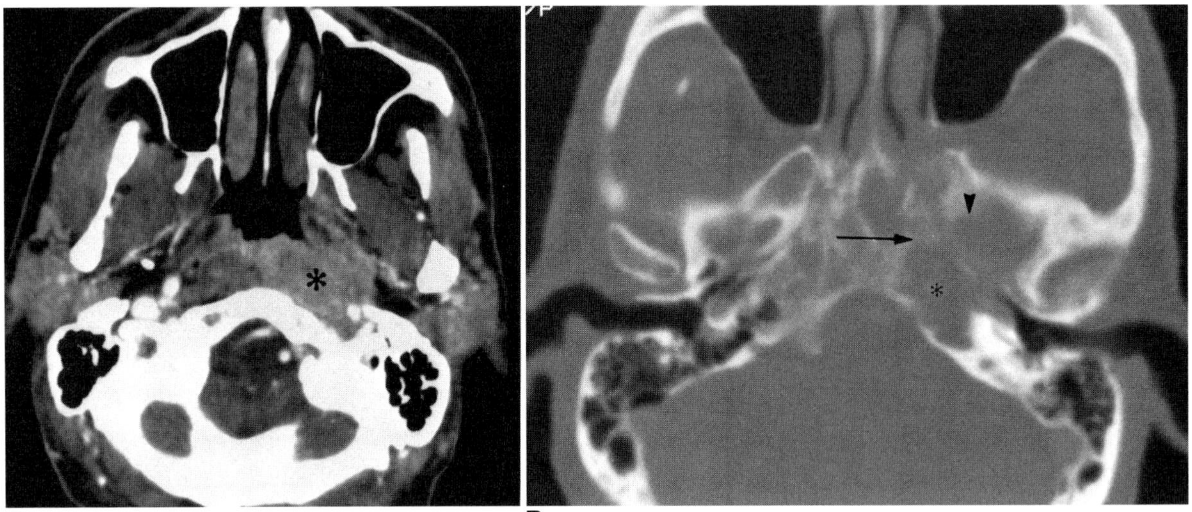

Figure 2-18. Nasopharyngeal carcinoma. **A,** Axial contrast-enhanced computed tomography (CECT) demonstrates enhancing lesion *(asterisk)* involving the pharyngeal mucosa space, retropharyngeal spaces, and prevertebral space. A tumor abuts the skull base. **B,** Axial CECT image with bone settings at the level of the skull base demonstrates a lytic destructive lesion involving the anteromedial left petrous bone *(asterisk)*, medial portion of greater sphenoid wing *(arrowhead)*, and adjacent clivus *(arrow)*.

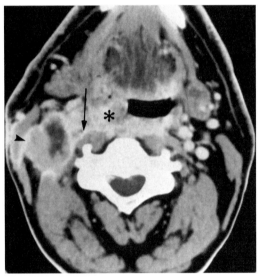

Figure 2-19. Squamous cell carcinoma of oropharynx. Axial contrast-enhanced computed tomography demonstrates a mixed-density enhancing lesion *(asterisk)* in the right oropharynx. The tumor has extended posterolaterally to surround the carotid vessels *(arrow)*. Enhancing lymph node *(arrowhead)* with low-density necrotic center is noted posterior to the carotid space, lying just beneath the sternocleidomastoid muscle. Enhancement of the adjacent sternocleidomastoid muscle indicates muscle invasion.

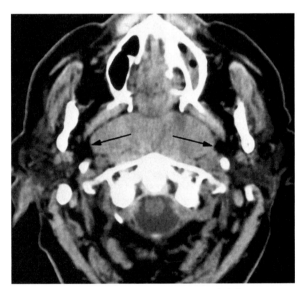

Figure 2-20. Nasopharyngeal lymphoma. Axial non-contrast computed tomography demonstrates a large homogeneous pharyngeal mucosal space with a nasopharyngeal mass lesion, displacing prevertebral and retropharyngeal spaces posteriorly. The lesion bulges into parapharyngeal space bilaterally *(arrows)*.

Parotid Space

The PS, the home of the parotid gland and the extracranial portion of the facial nerve, lies lateral to both the PPS and the CS and posterior to the masti-cator space. It extends superiorly from the level of the mid squamous temporal bone to the angle of the mandible inferiorly. It contains the parotid gland, multiple lymph nodes (within and outside the parotid gland parenchyma), the facial nerve, the retromandibular vein, and branches of the external carotid artery. The parotid gland overlies the posterior portion of the masseter muscle. Its deep retromandibular portion lies posterior to the mandible and lateral to the PPS and the CS. The posterior belly of the digastric muscle separates the PS from the CS.

Because of its high fat content, especially in the adult, the parotid gland parenchyma is frequently low density on CT but may vary and approach muscle density. It is high intensity on T1WI (slightly less than subcutaneous fat) and has decreased intensity on T2WI but often retains its bright T2 signal intensity relative to muscle. The retromandibular vein lies just posterior to the lateral margin of the mandibular ramus. The diagonal course of the facial nerve, paralleling a line drawn from the stylomastoid foramen to a point just lateral to the retromandibular vein, divides the parotid gland into superficial and deep portions. Although this is not a true anatomic division, it is useful for surgical planning. The facial nerve may be seen on some MRI studies. Its course must be considered and determined when removal of deep parotid lobe lesions is planned.

Lesions in the parotid space are usually surrounded by parotid gland tissue and are better defined with MRI than CT.[48] With NCCT, lesions are usually isodense to the normal gland or increased density. With MRI, lesions are muscle intensity on T1WI and usually hyperintense to normal parotid gland on T2WI.[42] When small, parotid lesions tend to be homogeneous. With increase in lesion size, areas of hemorrhage, necrosis, and calcification may develop. If the lesion extends or originates from the deep portion of the gland, it displaces the PPS medially and occasionally anteriorly. Large lesions in the parotid gland proper will cause widening of the stylomandibular notch, the space between the posterior border of the mandible and the styloid process. Comparison with the contralateral side will make subtle widening of this space evident.[23] Deep lobe lesions, if large, may displace the carotid artery posteriorly. Benign lesions as a general rule are well defined. Malignant lesions have indistinct margins and may invade adjacent structures. Lesions in the PPS or CS may extend laterally into the parotid space, mimicking a parotid lesion clinically.

Congenital lesions of the PS include hemangioma, lymphangioma, and first and second branchial cleft cyst, the latter presenting as a cystic-appearing lesion with smooth walls.[25] Enhancing margins of the cyst indicate it is secondarily infected. Inflammatory disease may present as diffuse swelling or as a localized abscess. Infection of the adjacent skull base is best demonstrated with CT. Infection may occur secondary to calculus disease.

Calculi are also best demonstrated by sialography as intraluminal filling defects or by CT because of its tenfold higher sensitivity over plain films for detecting calcified calculi. Sialadenitis, autoimmune disease, and strictures are still best evaluated by conventional sialography, which best demonstrates ductal anatomy. Chronic sialadenitis will cause the affected parotid gland CT density to approach that of muscle. This appears as lower parotid gland signal on T1WI and brighter signal on T2WI than that of the contralateral parotid gland. Autoimmune diseases, such as Sjögren's syndrome, demonstrate bilateral parotid enlargement. Bilateral gland enlargement by benign lymphoepithelial cysts is seen in acquired immunodeficiency syndrome.

Benign pleomorphic adenoma (benign mixed tumor), the most common benign neoplasm of the parotid gland, is well defined and demonstrates variable degrees of contrast enhancement (Figure 2-21). It is usually ovoid in configuration and may involve either the superficial or deep lobe of the parotid gland or, less commonly, both. Rarely, benign mixed tumors may arise from salivary rest tissue medial to the deep lobe and have a fat border on both their medial and lateral margins. Calcification is occasionally seen within the tumor. The tumor is hypointense on T1WI and hyperintense on T2WI. Both the superficial and deep lobes of the parotid gland may be involved, leading to a dumbbell configuration of the mass and associated widening of the stylomandibular notch.

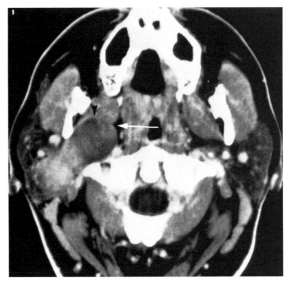

Figure 2-21. Benign pleomorphic adenoma of the right parotid gland. Axial contrast-enhanced computed tomography demonstrates a dumbbell-shaped tumor with enhancement of its superficial portion. Its deep portion is predominantly low density. Parapharyngeal space is displaced medially *(arrow)*. The lateral pterygoid muscle is indented and lies anteriorly *(arrowhead)*. The lesion has displaced the ramus of mandible anteriorly.

Malignant lesions include mucoepidermoid carcinoma, adenoid cystic carcinoma, acinic cell carcinoma, and malignant mixed tumor (Figure 2-22). High-grade malignant lesions have infiltrative borders. MRI is superior to CT for showing lesion margins and extent. Because of the abundant lymph node tissue within the parotid gland, lymph node involvement may be seen with non-Hodgkin's lymphoma, and metastatic involvement may be seen with SCC and malignant melanoma. Basal cell carcinoma of the adjacent ear and cheek may metastasize to the parotid lymph nodes.

Carotid Space

The CS—the space of vessels, nerves, and lymph nodes—lies posterior to the PPS, lateral to the retropharyngeal space, anterolateral to the prevertebral spaces, and medial to the PS and styloid process. The posterior belly of the digastric muscle separates the CS from the parotid space. The CS is formed from portions of all three layers of the deep cervical fascia. The CS extends from the temporal bone and base of the skull superiorly to the mediastinum inferiorly.[18] It contains the common carotid artery, its major divisions, the internal and external carotid artery, the jugular vein, cranial nerves IX to XII, sympathetic plexus, and lymph nodes. The jugular vein lies lateral

and posterior to the carotid artery. The vagus nerve lies in the posterior groove between the two vessels. Cranial nerves IX, XI, and XII migrate to the anteromedial portion of the CS lower in the neck. Lesions of the CS displace the PPS anteriorly and, if large, may remodel the styloid process, displacing it anterolaterally.

Infection of the CS occurs most commonly secondary to spread of infection from adjacent fascial spaces. Reactive inflammatory lymph nodes, which are characteristically homogeneous and less than 1 cm in size, may be seen in any portion along the carotid space and be seen with such varied infectious processes as sinusitis, infectious mononucleosis, and tuberculosis. Suppurative lymph nodes may have low-density centers and may not be distinguished from malignant lymph nodes. Clusters or groups of lymph nodes lumped into large masses are not uncommon. Cellulitis causes a loss of normal soft-tissue planes. Abscesses are characterized by focal fluid collections with enhancing margins.

On CECT, normal blood vessels demonstrate contrast enhancement. With dynamic CECT, a wash-in phase (early visualization of contrast) may be demonstrated within normal vessels and within the feeding or draining vessels of a mass, which further indicates the vascular etiology of a lesion. On MRI, blood vessels

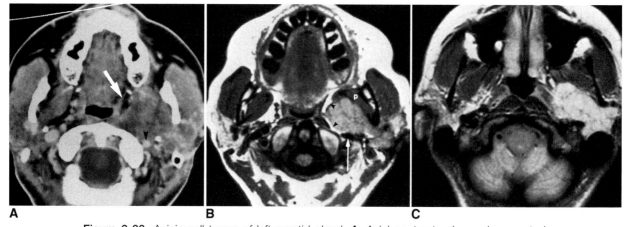

Figure 2-22. Acinic cell tumor of left parotid gland. **A,** Axial contrast-enhanced computed tomography at level of C1 and C2 demonstrates an inhomogeneous irregular mass lesion involving both the superficial and deep portions of the left parotid gland. Lesion displaces the parapharyngeal space anteriorly and medially *(arrow)*. Stylomandibular distance is increased. Areas of patchy enhancement are noted around the periphery and throughout the lesion. Lesion has displaced the carotid artery posteriorly *(arrowhead)*. **B,** Axial T1-weighted image demonstrates superior contrast resolution of magnetic resonance imaging. Both superficial and deep portions of the lesion are well outlined. The margin of the lesion can be separated from the lateral pterygoid muscle *(p)*, which is displaced anteriorly and laterally. PPS *(arrowheads)*, indicated by its high-intensity fat, is displaced medially. The flow void marks the site of the left carotid artery *(arrow)*. **C,** Axial spin density magnetic resonance imaging image at the level of the skull base demonstrates a well-defined lesion of increased signal intensity. Involvement of both superficial and deep lobes is well delineated.

appear as circular or linear areas of flow void, because of flow of fast-moving blood. Turbulent or slow flow may lead to areas of mixed signal intensity. Vessel ectasia, dissection, aneurysm, pseudoaneurysm, and thrombosis may be diagnosed readily with either cross-sectional imaging technique. Assessment of adjacent sectional images will demonstrate a tubular configuration to the lesion. An ectatic carotid artery or an asymmetrically enlarged jugular vein may present clinically as a lateral neck mass, but is readily discernible radiologically. The right jugular vein is usually larger than the left and at times may be several times larger than the left, reflecting its greater venous drainage from the brain. Thrombosis, either arterial or venous in nature, appears as a linear or tubular intraluminal filling defect with or without associated mass effect on CECT because the vasa vasorum of the vessel wall enhances in a ring-like fashion.[1] Subacute thrombosis or vessel wall hemorrhage secondary to dissection or trauma will yield a bright signal on T1WI because of the T1 shortening effects of paramagnetic methemoglobin, a blood breakdown product.

Most mass lesions originating in the CS are of neoplastic origin. Most neurogenic tumors are schwannomas (Figure 2-23). A schwannoma arises from Schwann cells that form the covering of nerves and most commonly originate from the vagus nerve (less

commonly from the sympathetic plexus). A neurofibroma contains mixed neural and Schwann-cell elements and arises from the peripheral nerves. Neurofibromas are rare; when present, they usually are multiple and part of neurofibromatosis, type two. Both tumors are well defined with CT, with either tumor having a low-density component because of fat infiltration. On CECT, neurofibromas demonstrate variable degrees of enhancement. On MRI, they have a similar appearance. On both CT and MRI, most neural tumors have similar density and intensity characteristics to salivary gland tumors and often may not be differentiated. Neural tumors may have dense enhancement and simulate paragangliomas. On angiography, neuromas characteristically are hypovascular in contrast to paragangliomas, which are hypervascular. Neurogenic lesions arise posterior to the internal carotid artery and thus cause anterior displacement of the latter.

Paragangliomas—lesions developing from neural crest cell derivatives—may arise in the jugular foramen (glomus jugulare), along the course of the vagus nerve (glomus vagale), or at the carotid bifurcation (carotid body tumor) (Figures 2-24 and 2-25). Paragangliomas are multiple in up to 5% of patients. The lesion is ovoid with smooth margins. Because of its marked hypervascularity, it is densely enhancing on CT. Angiography reveals a very vascular tumor with dense capillary staining. At the skull base, it erodes the jugular spine and causes permeative bone erosion of the jugular foramen in contradistinction to a schwannoma, which causes a smooth expansion with intact cortical margins. A jugular foramen paraganglioma may extend into the temporal bone or infiltrate through the skull base, presenting as a posterior fossa mass. In the mid neck, a paraganglioma causes characteristic displacement of the carotid artery anteriorly and the jugular vein posterolaterally. At the carotid bifurcation, a lesion causes splaying of the internal and external carotid arteries. On MRI, it is recognized by its hypervascularity, characterized by multiple areas of signal void and flow-related enhancement from enlarged feeding and draining vessels.[33]

Lymph node involvement in the CS may be seen most commonly with metastases from SCC or as part of a general involvement by non-Hodgkin's lymphoma. Lymph node involvement may be the initial manifestation of squamous cell carcinoma. Extracapsular spread of disease may occur. Complete encasement of the carotid artery (carotid fixation) may indicate inoperability. However, the carotid artery may be sacrificed at operation if the patient successfully tolerates a carotid balloon occlusion test. Metastatic lymph nodes are characteristically inhomogeneous, especially after contrast enhancement.

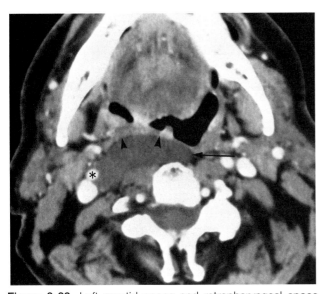

Figure 2-23. Left carotid space and retropharyngeal space ganglioneuroma. Axial contrast-enhanced computed tomography at the level of mid tongue demonstrates a C- or sausage-shaped, well-defined, low-density lesion in the anteromedial portion of the left carotid space. The lesion partially encases the left carotid artery *(asterisk)* and displaces it posterolaterally. It extends medially into the left retropharyngeal space *(arrow)*. Parapharyngeal space has been displaced laterally. Pharyngeal mucosal space *(arrowheads)* lies anterior to the lesion.

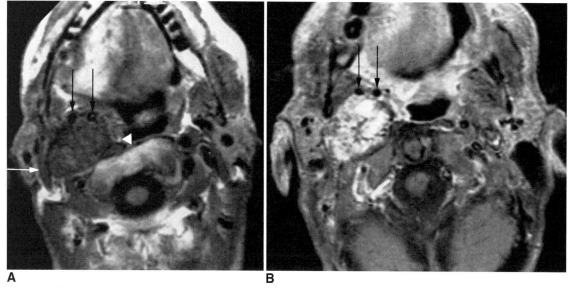

Figure 2-24. Glomus vagale (paraganglioma) of right carotid space. **A,** Axial T1-weighted image (T1WI) at the level of C2 demonstrates a mixed-density, predominantly low-density lesion involving the posterior aspect of the left carotid space. The lesion displaces the posterior belly of the digastric muscle laterally *(white arrow)* and the internal and external carotid arteries anteriorly *(black arrows)*. Parapharyngeal fat is displaced medially *(arrowhead)*. The lesion bulges into the medial aspect of the airway. The small areas of punctate low intensity noted along the margin and in the anterior portion of the lesion represent the tumor vessel flow voids. **B,** Axial T1WI at the same level postgadolinium injection demonstrates dense patchy enhancement of the lesion. Again noted are multiple punctate vascular flow voids within the lesion and around the periphery. Carotid vessels *(arrows)* are noted overlying the anterior lesion margin.

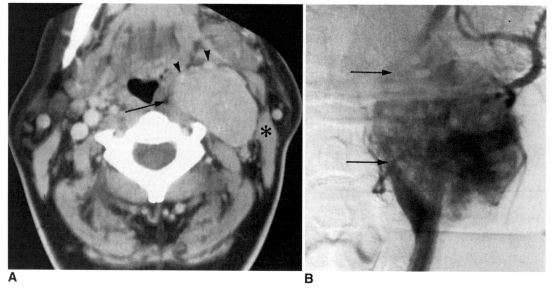

Figure 2-25. Glomus vagale of left carotid space. **A,** Axial contrast-enhanced computed tomography at the level of mid tongue demonstrates a relatively homogeneous, well-defined enhancing lesion in the left carotid space. Carotid vessels lie on the anteromedial margin of the lesion *(arrowhead)*. Parapharyngeal space is displaced medially *(arrow)*. The lesion lies deep to the sternocleidomastoid muscle *(asterisk)*. **B,** Anteroposterior digital subtraction angiogram demonstrates a densely vascular staining tumor displacing the internal carotid artery medially *(arrows)*. Vascularity and dense tumor stain indicate the lesion is paraganglioma.

Masticator Space

The MS, the space of the muscles of mastication and the posterior portion of the mandibular ramus, lies anterior to the PS and is separated from the muscles of deglutition in the pharyngeal mucosal space by the PPS.[10] It contains the masseter, temporalis, and medial and lateral pterygoid muscles, motor branch of the third division of cranial nerve V, inferior alveolar nerve (sensory second division of cranial nerve V), internal maxillary artery and its branches, pterygoid venous plexus, and the ramus and posterior body of the mandible. It includes the temporal fossa (supra zygomatic MS) superiorly, encompasses the zygomatic arch, and extends inferiorly to include the infratemporal fossa and structures on both sides of the mandible. A mass in the MS displaces the PPS posteriorly and medially.

Infection (cellulitis, abscess, osteomyelitis) may involve the mandible or the muscles of mastication. Extension through the skull base or involvement of the supra zygomatic masticator space may occur and should be ruled out (Figure 2-26). Abscesses commonly arise from an odontogenic focus or from poor dentition. The bone changes of osteomyelitis are best demonstrated with CT.

Benign lesions include hemangioma and lymphangioma (Figure 2-27). Nasopharyngeal angiofibroma, a

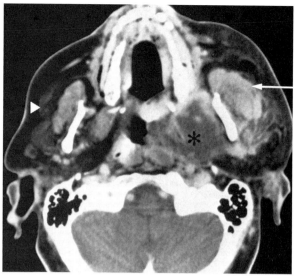

Figure 2-26. Left masticator space abscess. Axial contrast-enhanced computed tomography at the level of the superior alveolar ridge demonstrates a low-density lesion *(asterisk)* in the medial aspect of the left masticator space, involving the left lateral pterygoid muscle. The abscess is surrounded by a rim of irregular enhancement. Edema has infiltrated and obscured the parapharyngeal space. Left masseter muscle *(arrow)* is thickened and edema is present in the soft-tissue planes, lateral to the masseter muscle and in the buccal space anteriorly. Note the accessory parotid gland overlying the right masseter muscle *(arrowhead)*.

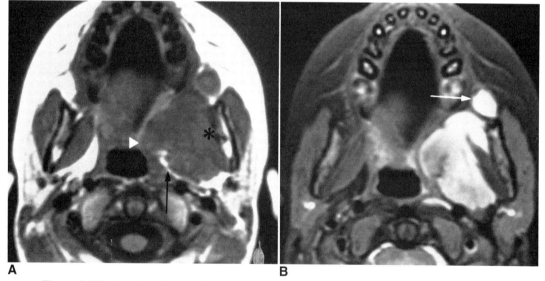

A   **B**

Figure 2-27. Lymphangioma of left masticator space. **A,** Axial T1-weighted image at the level of the base of the tongue and tonsillar region of the oropharynx demonstrates an inhomogeneous low-density soft-tissue mass involving the left lateral pterygoid muscle *(asterisk)*. It displaces parapharyngeal space medially and anteriorly *(arrow)*. The mass extends to the anterior medial wall of the left oropharynx *(arrowhead)*. **B,** Axial spin density image with fat suppression demonstrates a lesion with bright signal intensity. The lesion margins are now better defined. The lesion can now be separated from the lateral pterygoid muscle. The lesion abuts the anteromedial wall of oropharynx. Anteriorly, the lesion extends into the buccal space *(arrow)*, anterior to the cortical margin of mandible.

tumor of young adolescent males, arises in the pterygopalatine fossa and commonly extends into the masticator space (Figure 2-28). Primary bone neoplasms may arise from the mandible. Chondrosarcoma and osteosarcoma present with chondroid calcification and new bone formation, respectively. The bone lesion is characteristically muscle intense on T1WI and hyperintense with T2WI. Postgadolinium T1WI demonstrates extensive enhancement. An infiltrating mass with mandibular destruction may be indistinguishable from metastatic disease. Non-Hodgkin's lymphoma

may present with bone involvement, with a soft-tissue mass, or as a lymph node mass. SCC presents as an infiltrating mass and occurs secondary to extension from a neighboring fascial space (Figure 2-29). Perineural spread of tumor is common in the MS. The fifth nerve should be assessed for thickening and enhancement along its course as it passes from the brainstem to the cavernous sinus, through the foramen ovale, and eventually below the skull base as it passes inferiorly to innervate the individual muscles of mastication (Figure 2-30). The foramen ovale may

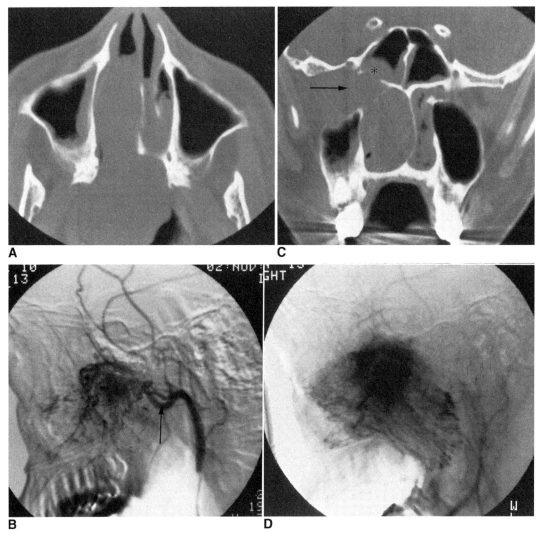

Figure 2-28. Nasopharyngeal angiofibroma. **A,** Axial noncontrast computed tomography (NCCT) demonstrates a homogeneous soft-tissue mass enlarging the right nasal aperture. A large component of the tumor projects posteriorly into the nasopharynx and oropharynx. **B,** Coronal NCCT also demonstrates the complete opacification and expansion of the right nasal aperture by a soft-tissue mass. The tumor extends into and widens the right infraorbital fissure *(arrow)*. The tumor *(asterisk)*, having destroyed right floor, is present in the sphenoid sinus. **C** and **D,** Lateral subtraction angiograms (early arterial and capillary phase) demonstrate a vascular mass in the nasopharynx and nasal aperture. Internal maxillary artery *(arrow)* gives rise to leash of tumor vessels. Dense tumor stain is noted in the capillary phase.

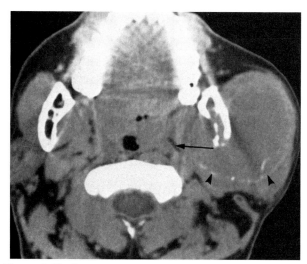

Figure 2-29. Squamous cell carcinoma (SCC) of mandibular ramus. Axial contrast-enhanced computed tomography at the level of C2 demonstrates a large soft-tissue tumor destroying the central portion and medial margin of the left mandibular ramus with an extension of the soft-tissue tumor into the masseter and lateral pterygoid muscles. Parapharyngeal space has been displaced medially *(arrow)*. Thin rim of circular enhancement is noted posteriorly and laterally *(arrowheads)*.

be increased in size, and a tumor may be found within the cavernous sinus. Tumor involvement of the inferior alveolar nerve may cause erosion, irregular enlargement, or destruction of the inferior alveolar canal of the mandible.[3]

Pseudotumors may mislead the unwary. An accessory parotid gland overlying the anterior border of the masseter muscle or asymmetric enlargement of the parotid gland may simulate tumor. In both situations the parotid gland variant retains MRI signal characteristics identical to the normal parotid gland. Hypertrophy of the masseter muscle may occur secondary to teeth grinding, mimic a mass lesion, or be bilateral. If the fifth cranial nerve is injured or invaded by a tumor resulting in denervation of the muscles, ipsilateral atrophy of the muscles of mastication and fat infiltration ensue. The normal contralateral muscle group may be incorrectly considered enlarged and misinterpreted as tumor involvement.

Retropharyngeal Space

The RPS, a potential space between the middle and deep layers of the deep cervical fascia, lies posterior to the pharyngeal mucosal space, anterior to the PVS, and medial to the carotid space. It extends from the skull base superiorly to the T3 level of the upper mediastinum inferiorly.[12] The importance of the RPS derives from its potential to serve as a passageway for infection to spread among the head, neck, and

mediastinum. Its contents are fat and lymph nodes, the principal nodes being the nodes of Rouviere (the classic lateral retropharyngeal nodes) and the medial retropharyngeal nodes. This nodal group is commonly involved in children, and up to 1 cm in size is considered normal. But a node larger than 5 mm is viewed with suspicion in an adult. A mass lesion in the RPS will displace the PPS anterolaterally. Infection, either pharyngitis or tonsillitis, may give RPS lymph node involvement. Diffuse cellulitis or abscess may occur, the latter usually secondary to infection of the pharyngeal mucosal space or prevertebral space. Infection or mass in the lateral alar portion of the infrahyoid RPS may have a "bow-tie" appearance on axial imaging (Figure 2-31). SCC may invade the RPS directly or may present solely with lymph node involvement. The pattern is one of inhomogeneous enhancement, commonly with necrotic low-density centers. With non-Hodgkin's lymphoma, lymph nodes are homogeneous and multiple, commonly involving more than one of the fascial spaces.

Prevertebral Space

The PVS, also defined by the deep layers of the deep cervical fascia, is divided into anterior and posterior compartments. The former encompasses the anterior cervical vertebral bodies, extending from one transverse process to another. The posterior compartment surrounds the posterior spinal elements. The PVS contains the prevertebral, scalene, and paraspinal muscles, the brachial plexus, the phrenic nerve, the vertebral body, and the vertebral artery and vein. Similar to the anatomy of the RPS, the PVS extends from the skull base superiorly to the mediastinum inferiorly.

The PVS lies directly posterior to the RPS and posteromedial to the carotid space. An anterior compartment PVS mass causes thickening of the prevertebral muscles and displaces the prevertebral muscles and the PPS anteriorly. A mass in the posterior compartment of the PVS displaces the paraspinous musculature and the posterior cervical space fat laterally, away from the posterior elements of the spine. Infection and malignant disease, the common disease processes of the PVS, usually involve the vertebral body.

Infection, including tuberculosis and bacterial pathogens, characteristically involves the vertebral body, as well as the adjacent intervertebral disk space. Benign processes, although much less common, include chordoma, osteochondroma, aneurysmal bone cyst, giant cell tumor, and plexiform neurofibroma. Malignant disease processes include metastatic disease, leukemia, lymphoma, and direct invasion by SCC. Vertebral body destruction with associated

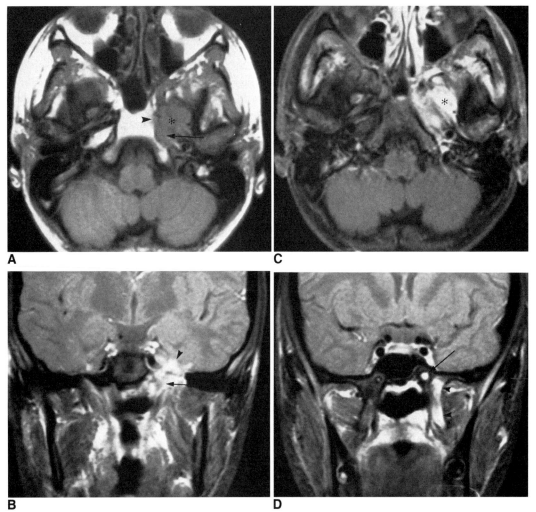

Figure 2-30. Adenoid cystic carcinoma of masticator space invading left skull base. **A,** T1-weighted (T1WI) magnetic resonance image demonstrates a low-density, well-defined lesion *(asterisk)* abutting the lateral border of the clivus and destroying the medial apex of the left petrous temporal bone *(arrow)*. Lateral cortical margin of the clivus has been eroded *(arrowhead)*. **B,** Axial postgadolinium fat-suppressed T1WI demonstrates diffuse patchy enhancement of the left middle fossa lesion *(asterisk)*. On this sequence, the normal high signal intensity of fat has been suppressed. **C,** Coronal postgadolinium fat-suppressed spin density image demonstrates an enhancing tumor *(arrowhead)* below the skull base with the extension through the foramen ovale into the left middle fossa *(arrow)*. **D,** Coronal spin density with fat suppression postgadolinium infusion demonstrates an enhancing tumor in the expanded vidian canal *(arrow)* and pterygoid fossa *(arrowheads)*.

soft-tissue mass may be seen. The spinal canal and dural sac may be compromised.

Oral Cavity

The oral cavity, the space of the anterior two-thirds of the tongue and the floor of the mouth, lies below the hard palate, medial to the superior and inferior alveolar ridge and teeth, anterior to the oropharynx, and superior to the mylohyoid muscle, the muscle stretch-ing between the inferomedial margins of the mandible. The oral cavity is separated from the oropharynx posteriorly by the circumvallate papillae, tonsillar pillars, and soft palate. The oral cavity includes the oral tongue (the anterior two-thirds of the tongue), whereas the oropharynx contains the base of the tongue (the posterior one-third of the tongue), the soft palate, the tonsils, and the posterior pharyngeal wall.

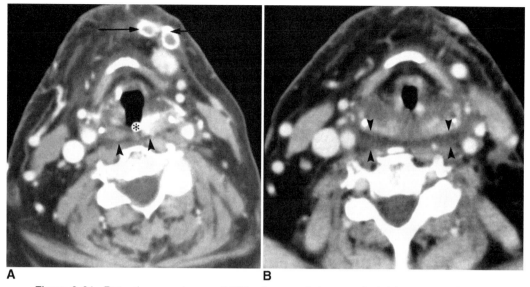

A   **B**

Figure 2-31. Retropharyngeal space (RPS) edema and abscess. **A,** Axial contrast-enhanced computed tomography (CECT) at the level of the superior margin of the hyoid bone demonstrates a nasogastric tube *(asterisk)* in the posterior wall of the oropharyngeal airway and mild thickening of the lateral wall of the larynx. RPS is normal *(arrowhead)*. Two lymph nodes *(arrows)* with rim enhancement lie anterior to the left submandibular gland. **B,** Repeat axial CECT at the same level 6 months later demonstrates a well-defined "bow-tie" appearance of edema in the RPS *(arrowheads)*.

The oral cavity can be divided into two major spaces, the sublingual space (SLS) and the submandibular space (SMS). The mylohyoid muscle, which constitutes the floor of the mouth, is the boundary marker between these two spaces. Other areas of the oral cavity include the floor of the mouth, oral tongue, hard palate, buccal mucosa, upper alveolar ridge, lower alveolar ridge, retromolar trigone, and lip. Assessment of these regions is also needed.

Most masses in the oral cavity and oropharynx are amenable to direct clinical assessment. Mucosal lesions are readily visualized. The purpose of sectional imaging is to evaluate the degree of submucosal involvement. The majority of neoplasms of the oral cavity are readily detected on clinical examination. SCC accounts for approximately 90% of oral cavity and oropharyngeal neoplasms (Figures 2-32 through 2-34). Cross-sectional imaging has an important role to play in estimation of tumor size, identification of tumor invasion, and assessment of nodal metastasis.

Congenital lesions include lingual thyroid and cystic lesions (epidermoid, dermoid, and teratoid cysts). Most infections of the oral cavity are dental in origin. Dental infections anterior to the second molar tend to involve the sublingual space and lie superior to the mylohyoid muscle. Infections of the posterior molars usually involve the SMS and lie inferior to the mylohyoid muscle. Knowledge of which space is involved is crucial to plan adequate surgical drainage.

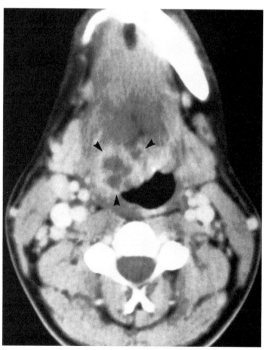

Figure 2-32. Right base of tongue and tonsillar abscess. Axial contrast-enhanced computed tomography of the suprahyoid neck demonstrates an inhomogeneous mixed low-density enhancing mass *(arrowheads)* in the base of the tongue and in the right tonsillar region. Low-density area of the lesion indicates pus within the abscess.

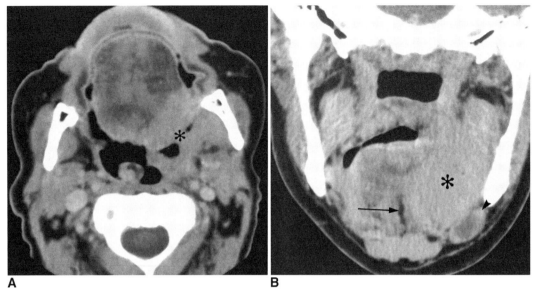

A   B

Figure 2-33. Squamous cell carcinoma of the base of tongue and the floor of the mouth. **A,** Axial contrast-enhanced computed tomography (CECT) at the level of the mid tongue demonstrates a homogeneous lesion *(asterisk)*, isodense relative to the muscles of mastication, involving lateral and posterior margins of the left side of tongue, left lateral pterygoid muscle, and tonsillar region of oropharynx. **B,** Coronal CECT demonstrates a homogeneous mass involving the lateral portion of the tongue, extending from the floor of mouth inferiorly to the tonsillar region superiorly *(asterisk)*. Midline septum *(arrow)* of the tongue is displaced laterally. Necrotic lymph node *(arrowhead)* lies inferior to the tongue.

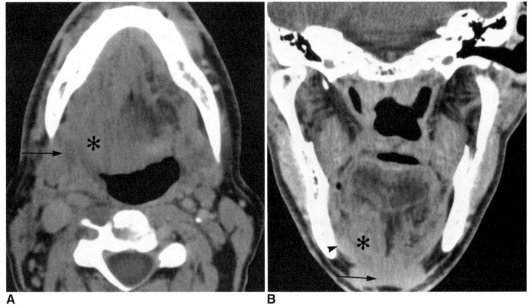

A   B

Figure 2-34. Non-Hodgkin's lymphoma of the base of tongue and the floor of the mouth. **A,** Axial contrast-enhanced computed tomography (CECT) at the midlevel of the tongue demonstrates an enlargement of the right side of the tongue by a homogeneous mass lesion *(asterisk)*, isodense to the normal tongue musculature. Submandibular space *(arrow)*, located more laterally, is also involved. **B,** Coronal CECT demonstrates homogeneous involvement of the right inferior lateral base of the tongue *(asterisk)*, mylohyoid muscle *(arrowhead)*, and floor of the mouth. Lesion lies above the anterior belly of digastric muscle *(arrow)*. Homogeneous nature of the lesion favors lymphoma.

Sublingual Space

The SLS is located in the anterior tongue, lateral to the intrinsic muscles of the tongue (genioglossus and geniohyoid) and superior and medial to the mylohyoid muscle. Anteriorly, it extends to the genu of the mandible and, posteriorly, it connects freely with the SMS at the posterior margin of the mylohyoid muscle. It contains the anterior portion of the hyoglossus muscle, the lingual nerve (sensory division of cranial nerve V), the chorda tympani branch of cranial nerve VII, the lingual artery and vein, the deep portion of the submandibular glands and ducts, and the sublingual glands and ducts.

Congenital lesions of the sublingual space include epidermoid, dermoid, lymphangioma, and hemangioma. Lingual thyroid tissue will result if there is failure of normal descent of developing thyroid tissue from the base of the tongue into the lower neck. On CT, the lingual thyroid is midline in the posterior portion of the tongue and demonstrates dense contrast enhancement. Nuclear medicine thyroid scans demonstrate functioning thyroid tissue.

Cellulitis and abscess may occur secondary to dental or mandibular infections or arise as a consequence of calculus disease of either the submandibular or sublingual glands. Abscess is characterized by central areas of low density with or without boundary enhancement (Figure 2-35). As with parotid gland calculi, CT readily identifies calcified stones and demonstrates bone destruction and sequestra of mandibular osteomyelitis. Ranula, a postinflammatory retention cyst of the sublingual gland, presents as a cystic low-density lesion. As it enlarges, it extends posteriorly and inferiorly into the submandibular space, where it is referred to as a "diving ranula" (Figure 2-36).

SCC, the most common malignancy of the SLS, may spread from the oropharynx, oral cavity, alveolar ridge, or anterior portion of the tongue. A mass with irregular areas of enhancement, ulceration, central necrosis, and lymph node involvement is characteristic. Normal fat planes may be obscured. Tumor spread across the midline of the tongue, along the lingual or mandibular nerve, or invasion of the cortex or medulla of the mandible is an important finding that alters treatment planning.

Submandibular Space

The SMS lies inferior and lateral to the SLS. It is located inferior to the mylohyoid bone and superior to the hyoid bone. It contains the anterior belly of the digastric muscle, fat, submandibular and submental lymph nodes, the superficial portion of the submandibular gland, the inferior portion of the hypoglossal nerve, and the facial artery and vein.

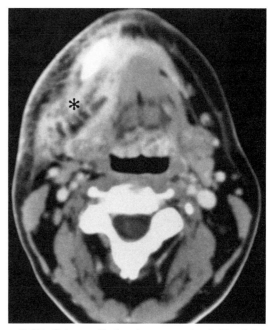

Figure 2-35. Submandibular abscess and cellulitis. Axial contrast-enhanced computed tomography demonstrates a mixed low-density and enhancing lesion *(asterisk)* involving the right submandibular space (SMS). Abscess displaces the midline structures of the tongue to the left. Edema extends laterally from the SMS into overlying soft tissues. Fat is of increased density because of infiltration by edema.

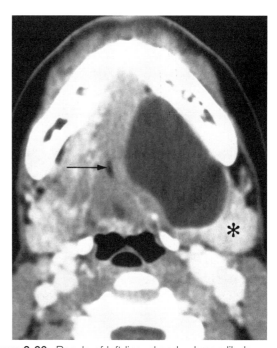

Figure 2-36. Ranula of left lingual and submandibular space. Axial contrast-enhanced computed tomography at the level of the body of the mandible demonstrates a large, low-density lesion with well-defined margins involving both sublingual and submandibular space. Lesion displaces the midline tongue structures *(arrow)* to the right. Submandibular gland is displaced posteriorly and laterally *(asterisk)*.

Congenital lesions are not uncommon and include second branchial cleft cyst, thyroglossal duct cyst, and cystic hygroma (lymphangioma). Branchial cleft cyst occurs most commonly at the angle of the mandible, posterior to the submandibular gland, anterior to the sternocleidomastoid muscle, and anterolateral to the carotid space (Figure 2-37). It may have an associated fistula or sinus tract. Thyroglossal duct cysts are midline in location and are found anywhere from the tongue base to the midportion of the thyroid gland. Cystic hygroma, a malformation of lymphatic channels, is a multilocular fluid density lesion that may involve both the SLS and SMS in the adult.

Ranula, a retention cyst of the sublingual gland, commonly extends into and may predominantly involve the SMS. It is unilocular in configuration. Its tail of origin should be carefully searched for in the SLS because this will aid in establishing its origin and diagnosis.

Benign tumors include benign mixed cell tumor, lipoma, dermoid, and epidermoid. Most malignant disease represents secondary submandibular and submental nodal involvement, commonly from SCC of the oral cavity and face. Multiple enlarged lymph node involvement may be seen with non-Hodgkin's lymphoma.

Spaces of Infrahyoid Neck

The infrahyoid neck extends superiorly to the hyoid bone and inferiorly to the clavicles and contains the following spaces:

1. Infrahyoid RPS
2. Infrahyoid PVS
3. Anterior and posterior (lateral) cervical spaces
4. Hypopharyngeal mucosal space (PMS)
5. Visceral space and larynx
6. CS

Normal cross-sectional anatomy of the infrahyoid neck is presented in Figures 2-38 through 2-40. The PPS ends at the hyoid bone and does not continue into the infrahyoid neck. The mucosal, carotid, retropharyngeal, prevertebral, and posterior cervical spaces are all continuous superiorly with the suprahyoid neck and extend inferiorly to the thoracic inlet.[46] These spaces are discussed in more detail in the suprahyoid neck section of this chapter. The posterior cervical space is described in the next section. Lesions may secondarily invade the structures of the infrahyoid neck from the cranial margin (submandibular, parapharyngeal, carotid, retropharyngeal, and oropharyngeal mucosal spaces), posterior margin (prevertebral space and vertebrae), and inferior margin (mediastinum and chest wall).

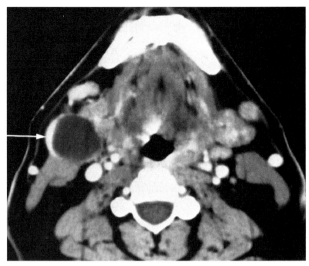

Figure 2-37. Infected branchial cleft cyst. Axial contrast-enhanced computed tomography at the midlevel of the tongue and base of the mandible demonstrates a well-defined, low-density lesion in the lateral portion of the submandibular space lying anterior to the right sternocleidomastoid. A thin rim of peripheral enhancement is noted anteriorly and medially. The lateral wall demonstrates thick enhancement *(arrow)*. Location favors the second branchial cleft cyst. Enhancement of the cyst wall indicates that it is infected.

Infrahyoid Retropharyngeal Space

The infrahyoid RPS, a potential space containing a thin layer of fat and no lymph nodes, is bounded by the middle layer of deep cervical fascia anteriorly, the alar fascia of the carotid sheath laterally, and the deep layer of deep cervical fascia posteriorly.[11] Unlike the suprahyoid RPS, which contains both fat and lymph nodes, the infrahyoid RPS only contains fat. On CT and MRI, the normal infrahyoid RPS is an inconsistently demonstrated fat stripe overlying the anterior margin of the longus colli muscles, nestled between the two carotid sheaths.

The infrahyoid RPS may be involved by processes arising from tissues within this space, but more commonly it is affected by external invasion from the adjacent spaces. Lesions within this space have a characteristic "bow-tie" configuration and lie anterior to the longus colli muscles (Figure 2-41). Lipomas and lymphangiomas are two low-density congenital lesions arising primarily in, or secondarily extending into, the infrahyoid RPS. Inflammation of this space may arise from pharyngeal mucosal laceration, discitis, or osteomyelitis from the PVS, or from infections tracking in through the posterior cervical space. Gas in this space suggests laceration of the pharynx, larynx, or trachea, pneumomediastinum, or the presence of gas-forming organisms (Figure 2-42). Edema from inflammation in an adjacent space may track

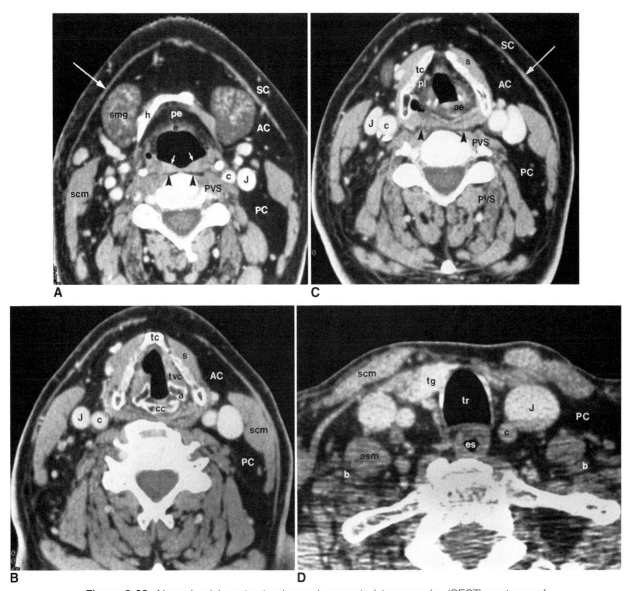

Figure 2-38. Normal axial contrast-enhanced computed tomography (CECT) anatomy of infrahyoid neck. CECT obtained at: **A,** hyoid bone; **B,** false vocal cord; **C,** true vocal cord; and **D,** thyroid gland levels. (Streaky densities in the superficial fat of the right neck area in **A** and **B** are from earlier radiation of the right parotid mass.) Note the following structures: arytenoid cartilage (a), anterior cervical space (AC), aryepiglottic fold (ae), anterior scalene muscle (asm), brachial plexus (b), carotid artery (c), cricoid cartilage (cc), epiglottis (e), esophagus (es), hyoid bone (h), jugular vein (J), posterior cervical space (PC), preepiglottic fat (pe), paralaryngeal fat (pl), prevertebral space (PVS), pharyngeal mucosal space (small arrows), platysma muscle (large arrow), retropharyngeal space (arrowheads), strap muscle (s), superficial cervical space (SC), sternocleidomastoid muscle (scm), submandibular gland (smg), thyroid cartilage (tc), thyroid gland (tg), trachea (tr), and true vocal cord (tvc).

into the RPS and occasionally mimic a true fluid collection or abscess. Neoplasms arising in the hypopharyngeal MS, CS, posterior thyroid gland, and larynx may involve the RPS. Extracapsular spread of internal jugular and spinal accessory metastatic nodes, as well as recurrent visceral space neoplasms, occasionally may invade the RPS. One common pseudomass that

indents into this space is a tortuous common or internal carotid artery, usually seen in the middle-aged and elderly populations.

Infrahyoid Prevertebral Space

The infrahyoid PVS continues superiorly into the suprahyoid PVS and inferiorly to the mediastinum.

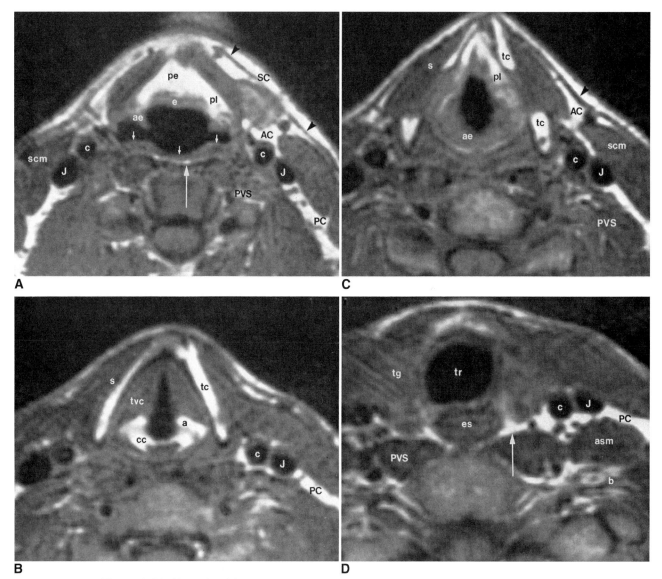

Figure 2-39. Normal axial magnetic resonance anatomy of infrahyoid neck. Noncontrast T1-weighted images obtained at: **A,** hyoid bone; **B,** false vocal cord; **C,** true vocal cord; and **D,** thyroid gland levels. The following structures are labeled: arytenoid cartilage *(a)*, anterior cervical space *(AC)*, aryepiglottic fold *(ae)*, anterior scalene muscle *(asm)*, branchial plexus *(b)*, carotid artery *(c)*, cricoid cartilage *(cc)*, epiglottis *(e)*, esophagus *(es)*, jugular vein *(J)*, posterior cervical space *(PC)*, preepiglottic fat *(pe)*, paralaryngeal fat *(pl)*, prevertebral space *(PVS)*, pharyngeal mucosal space *(small arrows)*, platysma muscle *(arrowheads)*, retropharyngeal space *(large arrow)*, strap muscle *(s)*, superficial cervical space *(SC)*, sternocleidomastoid muscle *(scm)*, thyroid cartilage *(tc)*, thyroid gland *(tg)*, trachea *(tr)*, and true vocal cord *(tvc)*.

This space is susceptible to the same pathologic processes as the suprahyoid component, which include inflammatory and infectious processes (arthritis, discitis, osteomyelitis), as well as neoplasms arising in the spinal canal, brachial plexus, paraspinous musculature, or vertebral bodies (Figure 2-43).

Anterior and Posterior Cervical (Lateral Cervical) Spaces

The posterior cervical (lateral cervical) space corresponds to the posterior triangle and is a fibrofatty layer containing the internal jugular, spinal accessory, and transverse cervical lymph node chains, as well as

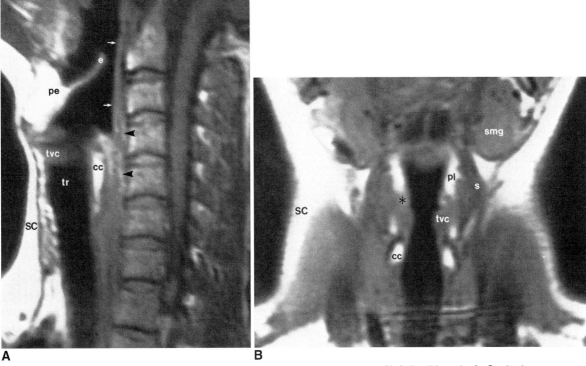

Figure 2-40. Normal sagittal and coronal magnetic resonance of infrahyoid neck. **A,** Sagittal T1-weighted image (T1WI) and, **B,** coronal T1WI obtained through the larynx. Note the following structures: cricoid cartilage *(cc)*, epiglottis *(e)*, false vocal cord *(asterisk)*, pharyngeal mucosal space *(small arrows)*, preepiglottic fat *(pe)*, paralaryngeal fat *(pl)*, retropharyngeal space *(arrowheads)*, strap muscle *(s)*, superficial cervical space *(SC)*, submandibular gland *(smg)*, trachea *(tr)*, and true vocal cord *(tvc)*.

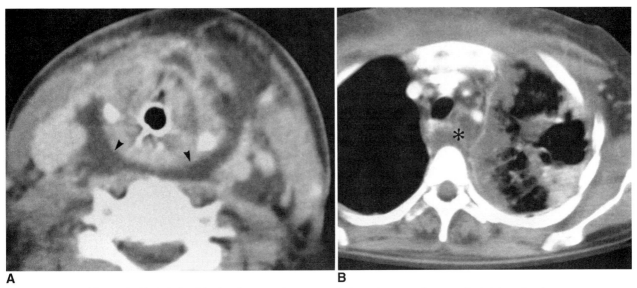

Figure 2-41. Infrahyoid retropharyngeal space and visceral space abscess. **A,** Axial contrast-enhanced computed tomography at the level of the false vocal cords demonstrates a low-density abscess in the retropharyngeal space *(arrowheads)* creating a "bow-tie" configuration. The abscess extends laterally to the left posterior cervical space and anteriorly into the visceral and anterior cervical spaces. **B,** Communication between the retropharyngeal space and mediastinum is well demonstrated by cephalad extension of this mediastinal abscess *(asterisk)* posterior to the trachea.

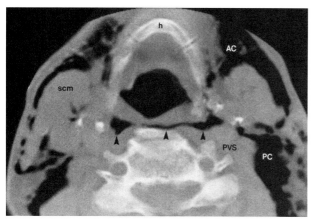

Figure 2-42. Axial non-contrast computed tomography of subcutaneous emphysema highlighting cervical spaces. Gas from a pneu-mono mediastinum has dissected into the anterior cervical space *(AC)*, posterior cervical space *(PC)*, and retropharyngeal space *(arrowheads)*. Note the "bow-tie" pattern of the retropharyngeal space. Other labeled structures include the hyoid bone *(h)*, sternocleidomastoid muscle *(scm)*, and prevertebral space *(PVS)*.

the spinal accessory and phrenic nerves. The posterior cervical space is limited by the sternocleidomastoid muscle and investing layer of deep cervical fascia anterolaterally, the carotid sheath anteriorly, and the prevertebral fascia posteromedially. It extends superiorly from the mastoid process and skull base down to the first rib and clavicles inferiorly.[34] Thus, a small

portion of the posterior cervical space extends into the suprahyoid neck, with the majority occupying the infrahyoid neck.

A trans spatial lesion (lymphangioma, plexiform neurofibroma, lipoma, hemangioma) may invade two or more anatomic compartments, without respect for fascial boundaries.[55] Congenital lesions of the posterior cervical space include a second branchial cleft cyst, which tends to lie along the anterior margin of the sternocleidomastoid muscle, and a lymphangioma or cystic hygroma (Figure 2-44). Both lesions are CSF density on CT, low intensity on T1WI, high intensity on T2WI, and may ring-enhance if secondarily infected. Inflammation may enter this space from cutaneous lesions or from abscessed lymph nodes. Benign neoplasms include neurogenic tumors (plexiform neurofibroma, schwannoma), a lipoma, or a hemangioma. Malignant neoplasms in the posterior cervical space are most commonly metastatic to the spinal accessory or internal jugular lymph nodes, with SCC representing the largest group of both primary and secondary tumors involving this space. Less commonly, sarcomas such as liposarcoma, leiomyosarcoma, or malignant fibrous histiocytoma arise here. Normal structures such as the scalene muscles, poorly opacified vessels on CT, and high-signal, flow-related enhancement in vessels on MRI may be misinterpreted as a pseudomass. Denervation atrophy of the sternocleidomastoid muscle or other neck muscles may occasionally cause an incorrect interpretation of

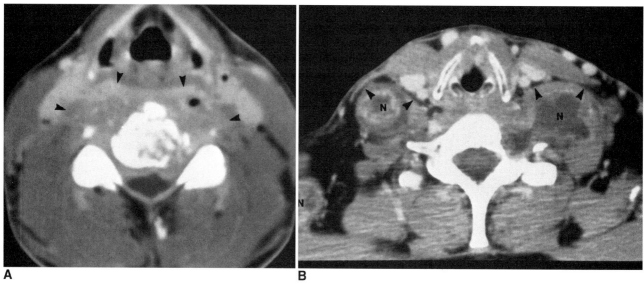

A   B

Figure 2-43. Prevertebral space (PVS) lesions. **A,** Axial contrast-enhanced computed tomography (CECT) of the prevertebral abscess extends anteriorly from C5-6 discitis. Anterolateral margins of the abscess *(arrowheads)* displace pharyngeal mucosa and posterior cervical spaces anteriorly. A small amount of gas is present in the abscess on the left. **B,** Axial CECT of bilateral plexiform neurofibromas *(N)* arising from the brachial plexus in the PVS shows anterior displacement of fat in the posterior cervical spaces *(arrowheads)*.

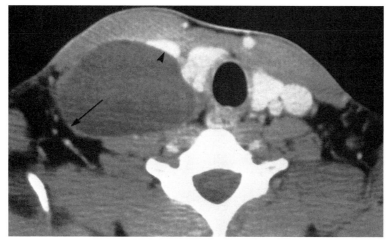

Figure 2-44. Posterior cervical space lymphangioma. Contrast-enhanced computed tomography reveals a homogeneous, bright, low-density mass with sharp margins displacing the posterior cervical space fat *(arrow)* posterolaterally and internal jugular vein *(arrowhead)* anteriorly.

the contralateral (normal-sized) muscles as representing masses.

Hypopharyngeal Mucosal Space

The hypopharyngeal mucosal space forms the walls of the hypopharynx and includes the continuation of the pharyngeal mucosal space below the hyoid bone posteriorly, the piriform sinuses laterally, the aryepiglottic folds and epiglottis anteriorly, and the cricopharyngeus muscle inferiorly. The hypopharyngeal mucosal space, piriform sinuses, and aryepiglottic folds are frequently challenging to evaluate on CECT and MRI because they are relatively thin membranous spaces that are normally collapsed together when the pharynx is relaxed. A modified Valsalva maneuver is usually required to distend the hypopharynx enough to obtain adequate imaging (see Figure 2-2).

As with the suprahyoid pharyngeal mucosal space, caution must be exercised in assigning abnormality to this space, since redundancy of the mucosa and incomplete distension may mimic a tumor. Foreign bodies, inflammation, and SCC are the most common lesions in this space. Inflammation may cause ulceration or swelling of the mucosa, with gas or a ring-enhancing fluid collection suggesting the diagnosis. Reactive lymph nodes are common. The best indicator of hypopharyngeal malignancy is a bulky mass with invasion and destruction of submucosal and deep structures including the retropharyngeal space, aryepiglottic folds, cricoid cartilage and larynx, as well as associated necrotic lymph nodes (Figure 2-45).

Visceral Space and Larynx

The visceral space, corresponding to the muscular triangle, is confined by the middle layer of deep cervical

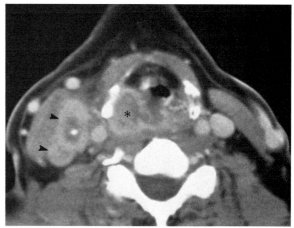

Figure 2-45. Piriform sinus squamous cell carcinomas. Axial contrast-enhanced computed tomography shows a mildly enhancing mass in the right piriform sinus *(asterisk)* displacing the aryepiglottic fold anteromedially. Focal defects in the internal jugular and spinal accessory nodes *(arrowheads)* indicate metastatic tumor spread. Calcification is noted in the internal jugular node.

fascia with the anterior fascial layer splitting around the thyroid gland. The visceral space contains the larynx, trachea, hypopharynx, esophagus, parathyroid glands, thyroid gland, recurrent laryngeal nerve, and tracheoesophageal lymph nodes.[4] The superior margin is the hyoid bone, and the inferior border is the mediastinum. The skeleton of the larynx includes the thyroid, cricoid, arytenoid, cuneiform, and corniculate cartilages. These cartilages may reveal a variable degree of calcification or ossification. These findings progress with the patient's age. Ligaments from the stylohyoid and stylohyoid muscles frequently calcify. Knowledge of the normal patterns of calcification is helpful for distinguishing opaque foreign bodies, such as chicken bones, from normal structures on plain films or CT.

Larynx

The hyoid bone supports the laryngeal skeleton and is occasionally fractured in blunt trauma or destroyed by neoplasms. Fractures of the laryngeal skeleton appear on CT as linear lucencies, often with displacement or distortion of the cartilage. A fracture is best appreciated (on bone windows) in well-ossified cartilage, but its identification is more challenging in noncalcified cartilage requiring, the use of a narrower window width and careful scrutiny of cartilage configuration. Laryngeal trauma may result in hematomas of the aryepiglottic folds, false cords, true cords, or subglottis, and may potentially compromise the airway (Figure 2-46). Adjacent subcutaneous emphysema may result from trauma to the laryngopharyngeal mucosa, from a penetrating injury to the neck, or from upward dissection from the chest wall or mediastinum.

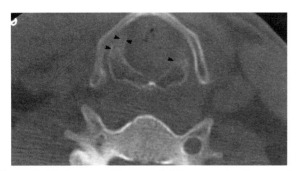

Figure 2-46. Laryngeal trauma. Axial non-contrast computed tomography at the level of cricothyroid articulation shows a laterally displaced cricoid ring *(arrowheads)* fracture and subglottic hematoma obstructing the airway.

Laryngoceles are formed by increased intraglottic pressure (e.g., in horn players and glass blowers) or from obstruction of the laryngeal ventricle and its distal appendix by inflammatory or neoplastic lesions (Figure 2-47). An internal laryngocele tracks superiorly within the paralaryngeal (paraglottic) fat, is air- or fluid-filled (obstructed laryngocele), and causes variable compromise of the supraglottic larynx. A mixed (external) laryngocele extends further superolaterally, piercing the thyrohyoid membrane, and may present as a neck mass. A mucocele (mucous retention cyst) of the supraglottic laryngeal mucosa may be indistinguishable from an obstructed internal laryngocele. Inflammation of the supraglottic larynx may lead to epiglottitis, thickening the epiglottis and aryepiglottic folds, and compromising the airway (Figure 2-48).

Apart from routine evaluation of adenopathy from suprahyoid neck and sinus tumors, laryngeal and hypopharyngeal SCC is the most common indication for imaging the infrahyoid neck. Because both CECT and MRI are relatively insensitive to superficial mucosal-based lesions, knowledge of the physical examination findings and specific locations of concern is mandatory to facilitate lesion localization and characterization. Findings that help identify SCC of the superficial mucosa of the larynx or pharynx are a mass, mucosal irregularity or asymmetry, and ulceration. Fat planes in the laryngopharynx are critical for determining the extent of deep invasion or inflammation. The fat in the preepiglottic space, epiglottis, and aryepiglottic folds and paralaryngeal fat of the supraglottic larynx are major landmarks that are easily identified on axial CT and MRI. Coronal T1WIs are particularly useful for evaluating the configuration of the airway and for determining the craniocaudal margins of a supraglottic, glottic, infraglottic, or transglottic lesion because the vertically oriented paralaryngeal fat plane terminates inferiorly at the true vocal cords

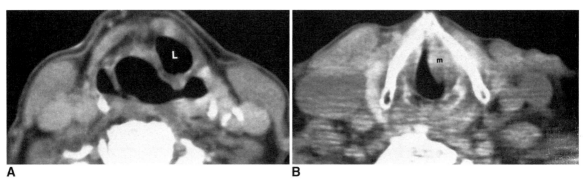

A   **B**

Figure 2-47. Laryngocele. **A,** Axial contrast-enhanced computed tomography (CECT) at the level of the thyrohyoid membrane demonstrates an air-filled internal laryngocele *(L)* displacing the preepiglottic fat and aryepiglottic fold. Note that the thyrohyoid membrane is separated from the piriform sinus by the aryepiglottic fold. **B,** Axial CECT at the true cord level reveals the cause of the laryngocele—an obstructing transglottic carcinoma *(m)*.

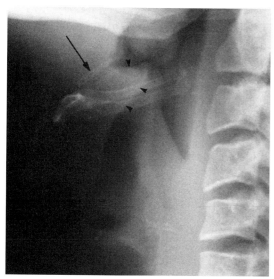

Figure 2-48. Epiglottitis. Lateral plain film of the neck demonstrates the swollen epiglottis *(arrowheads)* and aryepiglottic folds. The lower portion of the stylohyoid ligament *(arrow)* has ossified bilaterally.

(thyroarytenoid muscle). A lesion becomes transglottic when the fat interface between the thyroarytenoid muscle (true vocal cord) and the paralaryngeal fat (false vocal cord) is eliminated, indicating the tumor has crossed the laryngeal ventricle (Figure 2-49, *A*). The anterior commissure should be less than 1-mm

thick. Greater thickness in this area represents tumor spread from the anterior margin of one cord to another. A diagnosis of vocal cord fixation may be made when the involved cord remains paramedian during quiet breathing or with a modified Valsalva maneuver (Figure 2-49, *B*).

Cartilage invasion or destruction by aggressive infections or tumors is an important part of staging, and is often difficult to predict on CECT or MRI when the cartilage is incompletely calcified. If the cartilage has ossified, CECT and MRI are relatively sensitive for detecting cartilage erosion. MRI, using a combination of T1WI, T2WI, and postgadolinium fat saturation T1WI, may be more sensitive than CECT to invasion of the central layer of the thyroid cartilage, especially if the cartilage has ossified and the central fatty marrow has been locally replaced by an invading tumor. The best indicator of cartilage invasion is the presence of a tumor on the external margin of the cartilage in the strap muscles (Figure 2-50).

Thyroid Gland

The thyroid gland lies within the anterior leaves of the middle layer of deep cervical fascia (within the visceral space), anterior and lateral to the thyroid, cricoid, and upper tracheal cartilages. It consists of the lateral thyroid lobes, isthmus, and pyramidal lobe. Normal iodine content of the thyroid gland makes it higher density than muscle on NCCT. The gland is

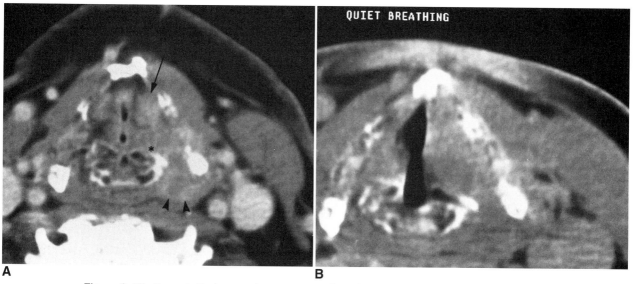

A   **B**

Figure 2-49. Transglottic laryngeal squamous cell carcinoma with vocal cord fixation. **A,** True vocal cords are adducted on an axial contrast-enhanced computed tomography (CECT) obtained during breath holding, with the tumor extending anteriorly and superiorly from the left true cord into adjacent paralaryngeal fat *(arrow)* and posteriorly into the cricoarytenoid joint *(arrowheads)*. Anterior corner of the calcified left arytenoid cartilage *(asterisk)* has been eroded by the tumor. **B,** Repeat axial CECT, performed during quiet breathing, reveals fixation of the left true cord in midline. Right cord is partially abducted.

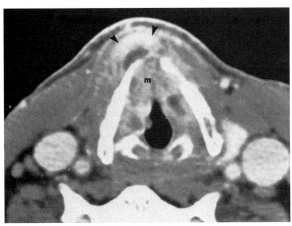

Figure 2-50. Transglottic squamous cell carcinoma with cartilage invasion. Axial CECT at the true vocal cord level shows an enhancing mass *(m)* originating in the left vocal cord, crossing the anterior commissure, and invading the anterior third of the right cord. The tumor has invaded through the anterior thyroid cartilage and displaces the thyroid strap muscles anteriorly *(arrowheads)*.

normally homogeneous with enhancement on both CECT and MRI, but internal inhomogeneity from calcification, goiter, colloid cyst, or a solid mass is occasionally encountered on routine neck imaging. When physical examination, ultrasound, or thyroid scintigraphy raises the suspicion of a thyroid carcinoma or thyroid lymphoma, CECT or MRI may be used for further characterization, especially if it is a low thoracic inlet thyroid or parathyroid mass.

Absence of the thyroid gland at the level of the thyroid cartilage should redirect attention to the tongue for an ectopic lingual thyroid gland (Figure 2-51). A thyroglossal duct cyst is a remnant of the embryonic thyroglossal duct and may occur anywhere along its migratory path from the foramen cecum in the tongue to the pyramidal lobe, although most occur just inferior to the hyoid bone (Figure 2-52). Inflammatory thyroiditis may enlarge the thyroid gland. Benign enlargement may also result from colloid cysts and goiters. Thyroid calcification is nonspecific and occurs in goiters, as well as in benign thyroid adenomas.

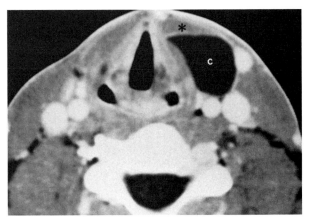

Figure 2-52. Thyroglossal duct cyst. Low-density thyroglossal duct cyst *(c)* elevates the thyroid strap muscles *(asterisk)* and laterally displaces the sternocleidomastoid muscle in this axial contrast-enhanced computed tomography.

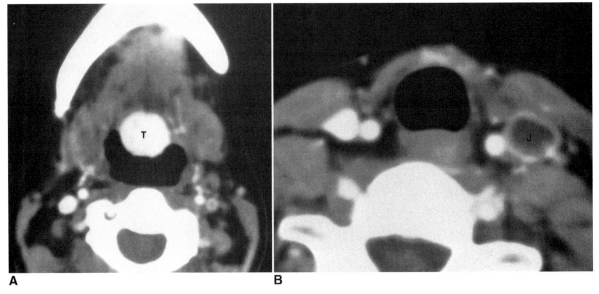

A **B**

Figure 2-51. Lingual thyroid gland. **A,** Densely enhancing mass of ectopic thyroid tissue *(T)* bulges posteriorly from the tongue at the level of the foramen cecum on the axial contrast-enhanced computed tomography. **B,** CECT at the upper tracheal level reveals that the thyroid gland is absent from its normal location. Note the pseudotumor of the thrombosed internal jugular vein *(J)* mimicking ring-enhancing node metastasis.

Primary malignancies of the thyroid include papillary, follicular, mixed, and anaplastic carcinomas, as well as non-Hodgkin's lymphoma, all of which may have a similar imaging appearance (Figure 2-53). Indistinct margins of a thyroid mass, infiltration of adjacent tissues, and necrotic lymph nodes are all indications of thyroid malignancy. Metastasis to the thyroid gland more commonly arises from extracapsular spread of SCC in adjacent nodes than from hematogenous deposits.

Parathyroid Glands

The parathyroid glands are usually four to six in number and underlie the posterior surface of the thyroid gland. Because they are quite small, normal parathyroid glands are frequently not visualized on routine neck imaging. An ectopic parathyroid gland may occur in the mediastinum (Figure 2-54). A parathyroid adenoma is usually a discrete mass lying deep to the thyroid lobes. Occasionally, an adenoma may be detected on routine CT or MRI as a nodular, enhancing mass that may be differentiated from lymph nodes by its location posterior to the thyroid gland.

Lymphadenopathy
Lymph Node Anatomy and Classification

The nodes of the superficial triangles of the neck are organized by major lymphatic chains. The traditional classification of lymph nodes of the head and neck includes 10 groups: lateral cervical, anterior cervical, submandibular, submental, sublingual, parotid, facial, mastoid, and occipital. The lateral cervical chains are further subdivided into the deep and superficial

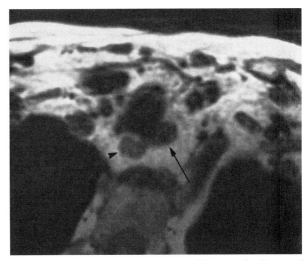

Figure 2-54. Parathyroid adenoma. Retrotracheal ectopic parathyroid adenoma *(arrowhead)* looks similar to the adjacent normal esophagus *(arrow)* on an axial T1-weighted image.

chains. The deep lateral cervical chain includes the internal jugular, spinal accessory, and transverse cervical (supraclavicular) nodes. The superficial lateral cervical chain consists of the external jugular nodes. The anterior cervical (juxtavisceral) group contains the prelaryngeal (Delphian), pretracheal, prethyroid, and lateral tracheal (tracheoesophageal or paratracheal) nodes.[45] The cervical lymph node chains are found throughout several of the spaces of the neck:

1. Posterior cervical space: spinal accessory, transverse cervical, and internal jugular (posterior to the internal jugular vein) nodes
2. Carotid space: internal jugular nodes (anterior to the internal jugular vein posterior margin)
3. Submandibular space: submandibular and submental nodes
4. Parotid space: parotid nodes
5. Suprahyoid retropharyngeal space: medial and lateral retropharyngeal nodes
6. Visceral space: prelaryngeal, prethyroid, pretracheal, and tracheoesophageal nodes
7. Subcutaneous tissues of the scalp and face: occipital, mastoid, and facial nodes

A condensation of this nomenclature into seven groups with Roman numerals (levels I to VII) has been proposed and is a useful shorthand for node documentation and statistical analysis. Because this latter classification is not standard at all institutions, to prevent confusion its use should be agreed to by the head and neck surgeons, radiation therapists, oncologists, and radiologists. Som and others[48] have proposed an imaging based nodal classification to find a common

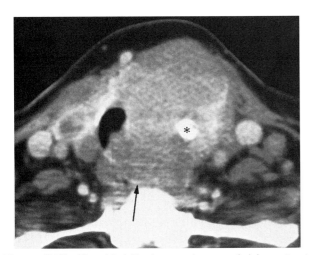

Figure 2-53. Thyroid follicular carcinoma. Axial contrast-enhanced computed tomography just below the cricoid shows a large mass with nodular calcification *(asterisk)* displacing the trachea to the right and distorting the airway. Posteriorly it has invaded the retropharyngeal space *(arrow)*.

ground between anatomical imaging criteria and the two most commonly used clinical nodal classifications: The American Joint Committee on Cancer and the American Academy of Otolaryngology–Head and Neck Surgery.

In this classification, Level I combines the submandibular and submental lymph nodes. Levels II to IV divide the internal jugular chain roughly into thirds, using landmarks that are easily recognizable on cross-sectional imaging. Level II is the jugulodigastric nodes (upper internal jugular), including the nodes from the skull base down to the bottom of the body of the hyoid bone. Level III is the supraomohyoid internal jugular chain (middle internal jugular), from the bottom of the body of the hyoid bone to the level of the bottom of the cricoid cartilage. Level IV includes the infra omohyoid (low internal jugular), nodes from the level of the bottom of the cricoid to the level of the clavicles. Level V includes the spinal accessory and transverse cervical nodes from the skull base to the clavicles, which lie posterior to the sternocleidomastoid muscle. Level VI includes the upper visceral nodes, which lie between the carotid arteries from the level of the bottom of the hyoid bone to the level of the top of the manubrium. Level VII nodes are located in the superior mediastinum between the carotid arteries, below the level of the manubrium and above the level of the innominate vein.

Subdivisions of the levels I, II, and V are also defined. Level Ia nodes are the submental nodes; they lie medial to the lateral margin of the anterior belly of the digastric muscle. Level Ib nodes lie lateral to the digastric muscle about the submandibular gland. Level IIa nodes are located at the level of, or anterior to, the internal jugular vein. Level II nodes that are posterior to and separate from the internal jugular vein are in Level IIb. Level Va nodes lie above the level of the bottom of the cricoid arch. Level Vb nodes are below the level of the cricoid and above the level of the clavicle. The levels Ib and IIa are divided by an arbitrarily selected imaginary coronal plane that follows the posterior border of the submandibular gland. The posterior margin of the sternocleidomastoid muscle separates the levels II, III, and IV from the level V.

It must be noted that the retropharyngeal, supraclavicular and parotid nodes are not included in the level classification. The retropharyngeal nodes lie medial to the internal carotid arteries within 2 cm form the skull base. Supraclavicular nodes lie at the level of, or caudal to, the clavicle and lateral to the carotid arteries. Separation of the supraclavicular nodes from low Level IV and Level V nodes may be difficult on the transverse images because of the oblique course of the clavicle.

Lymph Nodes: Normal and Pathologic

CECT remains the gold standard for detecting and classifying cervical lymphadenopathy as benign or malignant. The important considerations in radiographic lymph node detection and characterization are location, size, number, clustering, enhancement pattern, calcification, sharpness of margins, and invasion or displacement of adjacent structures. First, the nodes must be detected and localized to a specific nodal chain or level using one of the conventions for labeling node regions discussed previously. Node involvement is described as unilateral or bilateral and in terms of the specific level(s) or chain(s) affected.

Inflammatory (reactive) lymph nodes on CECT tend to be less than 10 mm (rarely larger than 20 mm), have central hilar or mild homogeneous enhancement, and have well-defined margins (Figure 2-55). Node margins should remain sharp in reactive adenopathy, except in cases with large abscessed nodes that elicit an inflammatory reaction in the adjacent fat, obscuring the node margins (Figure 2-56). Calcification is a common finding in previously infected or healed nodes and frequently occurs in tuberculosis or bacterial infections. Multiple nodes may be present, but they tend not to cluster. On MRI, these reactive nodes are enlarged and have well-defined margins on all sequences. They are muscle intensity on T1WI, enhance moderately and homogeneously on postgadolinium fat-suppressed T1WI, and are bright on T2WI and STIR.

The correlation of lymph node size with sensitivity and specificity in predicting malignant metastasis has been performed for different neck regions in patients with head and neck carcinoma, allowing more appropriate size criteria for distinguishing normal from abnormal lymph nodes.[45] Although CT can readily detect lymph node enlargement, it has also proven capable of accurately diagnosing metastases in "normal size" nodes from head and neck primary SCC. The upper range of normal for cervical lymph node size is between 5 and 10 mm, with the jugular digastric node ranging up to 15 mm. The exceptions are the submandibular and submental nodes, which are usually abnormal if larger than 5 mm, and the retropharyngeal nodes when larger than 10 mm in children or larger than 5 mm in adults. Generally, cervical nodes larger than 10 to 15 mm are potentially malignant and nodes smaller than this are considered reactive or inflammatory. Nodes larger than 20 mm are frequently malignant because the average size of a clinically positive metastatic node is 21 mm by physical examination and 20 mm by CT. Clinically occult neck disease occurs in 15 to 40% of patients with head and neck SCC. Clinically occult nodes average 12 mm (Figure 2-57). Studies comparing clinical and CT staging

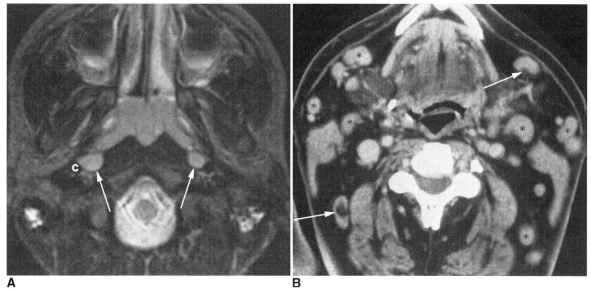

Figure 2-55. Normal lymph node anatomy. **A,** In this 8-year-old child, normal lateral retropharyngeal nodes *(arrows)* lie medial to the internal carotid arteries *(c)* and demonstrate a moderately high signal on the T2-weighted images. High-signal adenoidal tissue is commonly prominent at this age. **B,** Multiple mildly enlarged nodes *(asterisks)* are present in the submandibular, anterior jugular, internal jugular, and spinal accessory lymphatic chains on this contrast-enhanced computed tomography. Note the eccentric fatty hilum *(arrows)* in two nodes, a potential pitfall in the diagnosis of focal defect in the metastatic node.

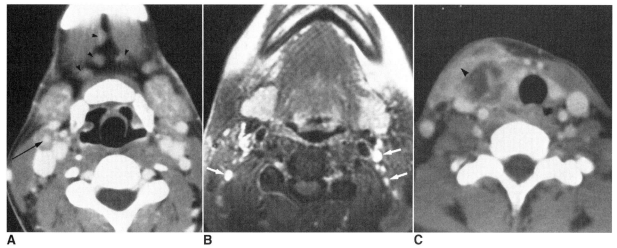

Figure 2-56. Reactive and inflammatory lymph nodes on contrast-enhanced computed tomography (CECT) and magnetic resonance imaging. **A,** Axial CECT of the hyperplastic nodes in a patient with acquired immunodeficiency syndrome-related complex displays multiple submental nodes *(arrowheads)* and an enlarged internal jugular node with central hilar enhancement *(arrow)*. **B,** Small, normal, or reactive lymph nodes *(arrows)* enhance on this fat saturation postgadolinium T1-weighted image. **C,** Axial CECT of a tuberculous nodal mass (scrofula) with peripheral enhancement and invasion of the sternocleidomastoid muscle *(arrowhead)* is difficult to distinguish from the cluster of metastatic nodes.

of nodal metastases have shown that physical examination of the neck has an accuracy of 70 to 82% compared with 87 to 93% for CT. In patients with no nodal disease on examination, CT is likely to upstage an N0 neck to N1 in 20 to 46% of cases and upstage clinical staging of the neck between 5 and 67% of cases overall. CT may downstage the clinical neck examination in 3 to 36% of cases.[7,29]

The enhancement pattern on CT is very helpful, but not infallible, in distinguishing inflammatory nodes

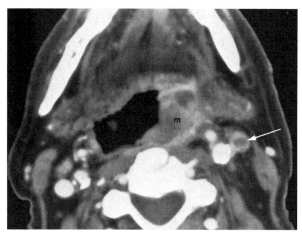

Figure 2-57. Metastatic node on contrast-enhanced computed tomography (CECT). Axial CECT in a patient with a left piriform sinus squamous cell carcinoma *(m)* and a "normal-sized" 9-mm node *(arrow)* with a focal defect (ring enhancement with "necrotic" center) is diagnostic of metastasis.

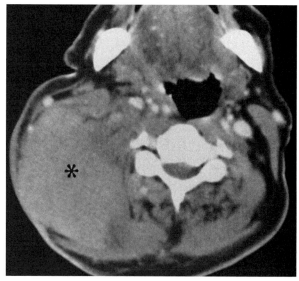

Figure 2-58. Node involvement by non-Hodgkin's lymphoma. Axial contrast-enhanced computed tomography shows a very large, homogeneous spinal accessory node *(asterisk)* invading both the skin and prevertebral space paraspinous musculature. The absence of central necrosis or focal defects in a mass this large is suggestive but not diagnostic of lymphoma.

from metastatic nodes. Node detection is improved by performing CECT with a constant infusion technique. The presence of a focal defect (central low density) or peripheral enhancement is characteristic of malignancy even in normal-sized nodes less than 15 mm. A focal defect in an enlarged node is a strong indication of a necrotic node metastasis, although tuberculosis or an abscessed node may mimic this appearance. Central dense or linear enhancement of the hilum of an enlarged node without ring enhancement is usually a distinguishing sign of a reactive node. Nodes larger than 20 to 40 mm without central necrosis often indicate lymphoma or sarcoidosis (Figure 2-58). Treated lymphomatous nodes may have dystrophic calcification and, rarely, calcium matrix-forming tumors (osteosarcoma, chondrosarcoma) may have radiodense metastases. When margins of an enlarged node with central necrosis are indistinct, extracapsular penetration of the tumor through the node capsule has likely occurred (Figure 2-59). This sign may decrease the 5-year survival by 50%. The number of nodes involved is important. Multiple nodes suggest a more widespread inflammatory or neoplastic process. Clustering of multiple nodes—sometimes into a seemingly single, complex mass—suggests malignancy and may be palpable as a single large mass. Round, rather than bean-shaped nodes, clusters of nodes, and indistinct margins suggest malignancy but are less specific than having a size larger than 15 mm, ring enhancement, or focal defect.

MRI of malignant adenopathy has both advantages and limitations compared with CECT. Malignant nodes appear as muscle intensity on T1WI, may show ring enhancement on postgadolinium fat-suppressed

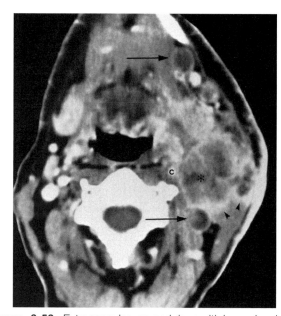

Figure 2-59. Extracapsular spread in multiple nodes in a patient with tonsillar squamous cell carcinoma (SCC). Left submandibular and spinal accessory node metastases *(arrows)* have typical ring enhancement and central low density on this axial contrast-enhanced computed tomography. The large cluster of metastatic nodes *(asterisk)* in the left internal jugular chain shows central low-density focal defects. Note the poorly defined infiltrative margins of this mass of nodes characteristic of extracapsular tumor spread. Tumor is invading the sternocleidomastoid muscle *(arrowheads)* posterolaterally and prevertebral space medially. About 40% of the left internal carotid artery *(c)* circumference is surrounded by tumor, which may still allow surgical preservation of the carotid artery.

T1WI, are very bright on STIR, and are usually bright on T2WI (although necrosis may give both a high and low signal on long TR sequences) (Figure 2-60). Fat-suppressed long TR sequences will diminish background fat signal, further improving detection. The STIR image is superior to CECT in sensitivity for any enlarged lymph node, but is nonspecific for metastases. MRI and CECT rely on the same criteria of size, clustering, margin sharpness, and shape for characterization of abnormal nodes. The specificity of ring enhancement on CECT is the main advantage of CT for diagnosis of metastases. The same finding of ring enhancement on postgadolinium fat-suppressed T1WI likely represents a focal tumor or central necrosis as well. Otherwise, the other MRI sequences described are nonspecific. MRI may better demonstrate invasion of adjacent structures, especially muscles, than does CECT.

Adjacent fat, bone, cartilage, and muscle are commonly compressed or invaded with extracapsular spread. Secondary invasion of adjacent structures and anatomic spaces by aggressive lymph node lesions may develop in the carotid sheath structures, skull base, PVS and vertebrae, and mandible. The superficial nodes may invade adjacent muscle and skin. Internal jugular and spinal accessory nodes may invade the carotid, parapharyngeal fat, prevertebral, and infrahyoid visceral spaces. Parotid nodes may violate the surrounding parotid parenchyma, skin, masticator space,

and parapharyngeal space. Suprahyoid retropharyngeal nodes may extend laterally into the CS, posteriorly into the PVS, anteriorly into the mucosal space, and superiorly into the skull base. The tracheoesophageal nodes may involve the common carotid artery and the internal jugular vein in the CS, the recurrent laryngeal nerve, the visceral space structures of the larynx and thyroid, and the mediastinum.

Invasion of the carotid artery carries a poor prognosis, with local recurrence rate of 46% and a distant metastatic rate of 56 to 68%. For patients with a tumor involving the carotid artery, the 5-year survival rate decreases to 7%, and the mean survival decreases to less than 1 year. Prolonged survival is possible if the involved carotid artery is resected. Detection of carotid artery invasion by MRI may be more accurate than ultrasound. The best imaging modality among CECT, MRI, or ultrasound for evaluating carotid fixation remains controversial.[28] Surprisingly, criteria for carotid invasion are not well established in the literature. CT and MRI criteria, based on the work of Picus and others on aortic invasion by esophageal carcinoma, include effacement of the fascial plane surrounding greater than 25% of the vessel circumference.[36] Additional criteria suggest that a very high likelihood of fixation exists if the tumor involves 75% or more of the circumference of the carotid and if nodal extracapsular penetration has occurred (see Figure 3-59). Ultrasonography is a potentially valuable adjunctive

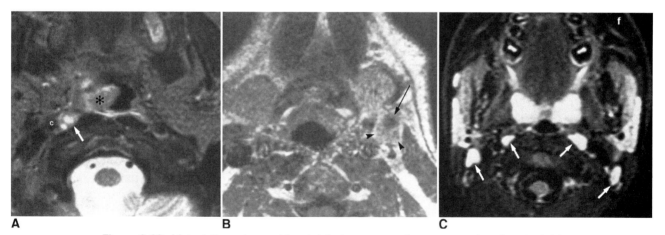

A   **B**   **C**

Figure 2-60. Metastatic nodes and focal defects on magnetic resonance imaging. **A,** Axial T2-weighted image at the soft-palate level depicts high-signal intensity at the right tonsillar squamous cell carcinoma (SCC) *(asterisk)*. A 10-mm metastatic lateral retropharyngeal node of Rouviere with a high-signal intensity central defect *(arrow)* lies medial to the internal carotid artery *(c)*. **B,** Left jugular digastric node *(arrowheads)* with low-signal intensity focal defect *(arrow)* on gadolinium-enhanced T1-weighted image is analogous to focal defect seen with metastases on a contrast-enhanced computed tomography. **C,** Axial short T1 inversion recovery (STIR) image achieves excellent fat suppression of subcutaneous fat *(f)*. Metastatic neuroblastoma is demonstrated in the bright internal jugular and spinal accessory nodes *(arrows)*. Note the bright appearance of the normal tonsillar and parotid gland tissues on STIR.

technique capable of demonstrating invasion of the common and internal carotid artery, as well as the internal jugular vein.

SINUSES AND SKULL BASE
Nose and Paranasal Sinuses

The sinonasal region can be divided into three major regions: the sinuses, the ostiomeatal complex, and the nasal cavity. The paranasal sinuses are mucosal-lined, air-filled cavities that are named after the bones of the face in which they develop. This mucosa is prone to both inflammatory and neoplastic disease. The frontal, maxillary, ethmoid, and sphenoid sinuses all drain through ostia into the nasal cavity. The frontal, maxillary, anterior ethmoid, and middle ethmoid sinuses drain into the semilunar hiatus under the middle turbinate. This area represents the ostiomeatal complex or unit. A small lesion here can cause obstruction to multiple sinus ostia. The posterior ethmoids and sphenoid sinus drain under the superior turbinate or sphenoethmoidal recess. The nasal cavity extends from the nares anteriorly to the choana posteriorly, and from the hard palate inferiorly to the cribriform plate superiorly. The midline nasal septum, lateral turbinates, and maxillary and ethmoid sinuses form the walls.

The compartments adjacent to the sinuses that are at risk for invasion by aggressive inflammatory or neoplastic processes include the anterior cranial fossa, orbits, cavernous sinus (from the sphenoid sinus), MS, pterygopalatine (pterygomaxillary) fossa, oral cavity, and anterior soft tissues of the face. These compartments are carefully viewed for dural or brain invasion, optic nerve and extraocular muscle compromise, perineural spread into the skull base, or direct extension into the deep compartments of the suprahyoid neck and oral structures. Involvement of any one of these secondary compartments can significantly alter treatment planning and surgical approach.

Paranasal Sinuses

Congenital and developmental anomalies of the sinonasal cavities are sought on all CT examinations. Common anatomic variants include pneumatization or paradoxical curvature of the turbinates, deviated septum, sinus hypoplasia, and Haller air cells (Figure 2-61). Sinus underdevelopment may range from aplasia to hypoplasia. Pneumatization implies sinus development has occurred. Aeration indicates that the pneumatized portion of the sinus is air-filled. Mucosal thickening or opacification signifies the pneumatized section is filled with soft-tissue inflammation or fluid. Either hypoplasia or the reactive new bone formation (chronic inflammation) may cause thickening and sclerosis of the sinus walls.

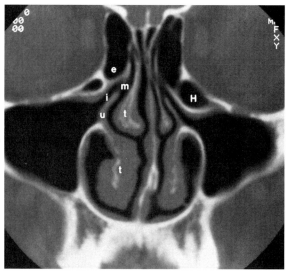

Figure 2-61. Normal ostiomeatal complex. Coronal noncontrast computed tomography demonstrates the ostiomeatal complex to the best advantage. Normal mucociliary drainage is from the maxillary sinus up through the infundibulum *(i)* and maxillary sinus ostium into the middle meatus *(m)*. Ethmoid bulla *(e)* and uncinate process *(u)* form the lateral and medial walls of the infundibulum, respectively. Normal anatomic variant of a Haller air cell *(H)* underlying the orbit causes a mild narrowing of the left infundibulum. Smaller Haller cell is present on the right. Note the mildly asymmetric mucosa of the turbinates *(t)*, which is part of the normal nasal cycle.

In general, evaluation of the paranasal sinuses involves assessment of two components: (1) the sinus contents (including the mucosa) and (2) the bony walls. Normal sinus mucosa is very thin and not seen on CT or MRI, and the bone is normally thin and delicate in the posterior maxillary, ethmoid, and sphenoid sinuses. CT or MRI readily reveals the presence of a normally aerated sinus, mucosal thickening (chronic sinusitis, retention cysts, or polyps), an air-fluid level (acute sinusitis, intubation, and trauma), or complete opacification (mucocele, trauma, and acute or chronic sinusitis) (Figure 2-62). The normally delicate posterolateral maxillary sinus wall is a much better indicator of bony sclerosis than the anterior wall. The normally thick anterior wall of the maxillary (and frontal) sinus may range from 1 to 3 mm (see Figure 2-12, A, C). Beginning observers frequently forget to assess the bone for important clues such as thickening and sclerosis (chronic sinusitis or hypoplasia), fractures, remodeling (slowly expanding mucocele or neoplasm), or destruction (malignancy or aggressive infection such as mucormycosis).

Deciding which portion of the opacified sinus, sinuses, or nasal cavity contains tumor and which contain obstructed mucous secretions is clinically important with a sinus or nasal tumor. The question is

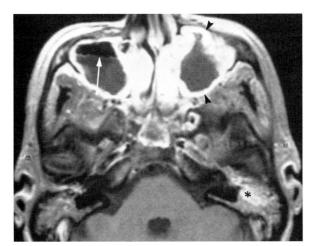

Figure 2-62. Acute and chronic sinusitis. Postgadolinium fat saturation T1-weighted image demonstrates an air-fluid level *(arrow)* in the right maxillary sinus and is diagnostic of acute sinusitis (superimposed on chronic sinusitis). Left maxillary sinus is filled with low-intensity secretions and has a peripheral ring of enhancing inflamed mucosa *(arrowheads)* typical of chronic sinusitis. Mastoid air cells and the left middle ear cavity *(asterisk)*, which normally appear black, are filled with enhancing inflammatory tissue.

ate signal intensity on T1WI and intermediate signal intensity on T2WI, although minor salivary tumors and adenoid cystic carcinoma may be of high signal intensity.[41] The highly cellular aggressive neoplasms tend to have a lower water content and are less bright on T2WI. Tumors enhance moderately and, more or less, uniformly with gadolinium. Sinus secretions are complex in their patterns. Hydrated, nonviscous mucus is low intensity on T1WI and high intensity on T2WI. Desiccated, viscous mucus tends to be high intensity on T1WI and low-to-intermediate intensity on T2WI. Extremely desiccated mucus may lack signal intensity on T1WI or T2WI, simulating bone or air. Both an obstructed sinus and an expansile mucocele frequently have two or more layers of mucus in a concentric ring pattern with the most desiccated, viscous secretions located centrally. The peripheral mucosa of an obstructed sinus enhances in chronic sinusitis or with a pyomucocele, but does not enhance with a simple mucopyocele. The presence of tumor vs obstructed secretion is best solved by comparing the respective change in signal intensity of each component on the T1WI, T2WI, and postgadolinium T1WI, and is rarely answered by a single sequence. A minimum of a T1WI and a T2WI is required.

Ostiomeatal Complex

The ostiomeatal complex has become an area of active radiologic and pathophysiologic investigation with the development of endoscopic sinus surgery for inflammatory sinus disease. Coronal thin section NCCT is the best means of demonstrating the

more problematic with NCCT or CECT because tumor and sinus secretions are frequently similar in density, and both the tumor and the mucosa may enhance; however, MRI is usually much more informative (Figure 2-63). Evaluation of this problem requires a knowledge of signal intensity patterns of tumor vs mucus. Sinonasal tumors tend to be low-to-intermedi-

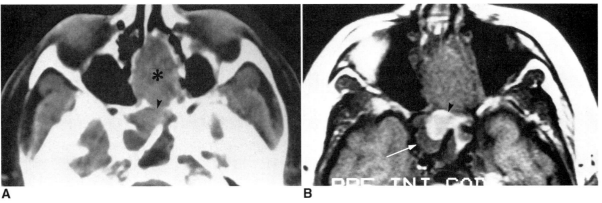

A B

Figure 2-63. Comparison of computed tomography and magnetic resonance imaging for separating sinonasal small cell tumor from sphenoid pyomucocele. **A,** Axial contrast-enhanced computed tomography shows a mildly enhancing mass *(asterisk)* in the left posterior nasal cavity and ethmoids, which appears to extend into the sphenoid sinus. Sphenoid sinus contents actually represent two different viscosities of mucus, with higher density mucus anteriorly *(arrowhead)* correlating with most desiccated or viscous mucus. **B,** Axial noncontrast T1-weighted image demonstrates an intermediate-signal nasal tumor. Anterior, high-signal, viscous mucus *(arrowhead)* in the sphenoid sinus is clearly discriminated from the nasal tumor anteriorly and from the low-signal hydrated mucus *(arrow)* posteriorly.

Continued

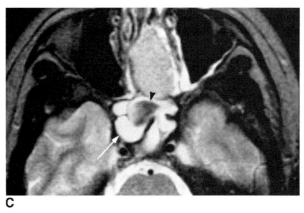

C

Figure 2-63, cont'd C, On axial noncontrast T2-weighted image, the nasal tumor signal is intermediate, similar to the brain. Anterior viscous mucus *(arrowhead)* in the sphenoid sinus has reversed signal to become low intensity, whereas hydrated mucus *(arrow)* posteriorly has now become very bright.

anatomy of this area (see Figure 2-61). Pertinent observations include: (1) the individual's sinonasal anatomy and the presence of any anatomic variants (hypoplastic maxillary sinus, concha bullosa, agger nasi air cells, Haller air cells, deviated septum, deviated uncinate process, prominent ethmoid bulla, paradoxical curvature of the middle turbinate); (2) the location of obstructed air cells; (3) the extent of the chronic or acute sinus disease and whether this pattern is consistent with the obstruction of the ostiomeatal complex; and (4) the presence of any earlier surgical alterations (Caldwell-Luc, internal or external ethmoidectomy, uncinatectomy, etc.). Ostiomeatal complex obstruction may result from

anatomic compression, mucosal inflammation, polyps, benign neoplasms, and SCCA. Mucoceles, indicated by sinus expansion and low-density mucus on CECT, or by concentric rings of variably desiccated mucus in an expanded sinus on MRI, are a complication of chronic sinus obstruction (Figure 2-64). A mucopyocele only shows peripheral enhancement when it is infected, and is then called a pyomucocele.

Nasal Cavity

The nasal cavity is occasionally the site of symptomatic disease. Anatomic variants include choanal atresia, concha bullosa, paradoxical curvature of the middle turbinate, wide nasal cavity from a hypoplastic maxillary sinus, and septal deviation. The nasal mucosa of the turbinates may be asymmetric in thickness because of the normal nasal cycle or the presence of polyps or inflammation. Obstruction of the ostiomeatal complex and other sinuses may occur with benign (antrochoanal polyp, neural tumors, inverting papilloma) or malignant (SCC, adenocarcinoma, adenoid cystic carcinoma) tumors (Figure 2-65). If a nasal mass is present, the extent of the mass within the nasal cavity, adjacent sinuses, or orbits, or involvement of the cribriform plate, may be determined by coronal CECT or sagittal and coronal MRI because this may affect the surgical approach and postoperative therapy.

Facial Trauma

Facial trauma is briefly included here because of the intimate relationship of the facial bones and sinuses. Thin-section axial and direct coronal NCCT is the ideal method for determining the full extent of facial

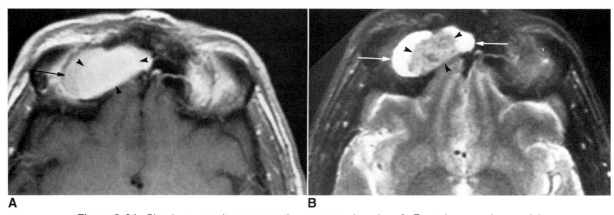

A   **B**

Figure 2-64. Simple mucocele on magnetic resonance imaging. **A,** Frontal mucocele on axial T1-weighted image expands the right frontal sinus and has a very high-signal central viscous or desiccated component *(arrowheads)* and a lower-intensity peripheral concentric ring of less viscous mucus *(arrow)*. **B,** Axial T2-weighted image reversal of signal intensities in concentric rings, with peripheral hydrated mucus *(arrow)* becomes bright and the central viscous mucus *(arrowheads)* loses signal.

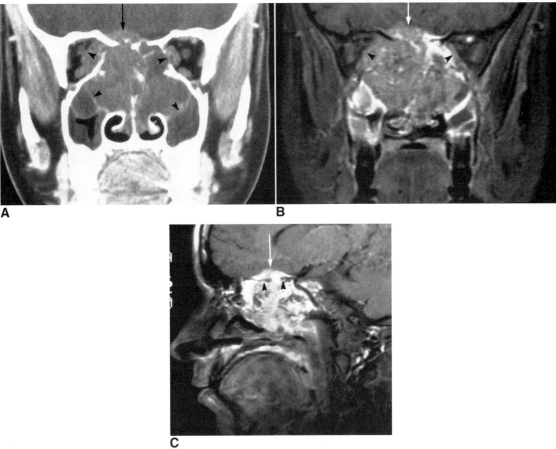

Figure 2-65. Invasive small cell carcinoma of cribriform plate and orbits. **A,** Coronal contrast-enhanced computed tomography shows (more clearly than magnetic resonance imaging) a mass centered in the posterior ethmoid sinuses with bone destruction of the cribriform plate *(arrow)* and medial orbits. The tumor has invaded both orbits and maxillary sinuses *(arrowheads).* **B,** Anterior cranial fossa extension *(arrow)* through the cribriform plate and orbital invasion *(arrowheads)* are well seen on this coronal fat saturation postgadolinium T1-weighted image. **C,** Sagittal fat saturation postgadolinium T1WI depicts the anterior-posterior dimension of the tumor and extension of enhancing tumor *(arrow)* through the low-intensity cribriform plate and planum sphenoidale *(arrowheads).*

trauma. One strategy for evaluating the extent of sinus trauma is to visually trace each bony outline on consecutive slices in both imaging planes, looking for fractures, normal fissures and canals, and displacements. However, the quickest way to locate sinus fractures is to search for indirect signs of fracture (Figure 2-66): an air-fluid level, complete opacification of a sinus with blood, and the presence of gas outside the sinus (pneumocephalus, subcutaneous emphysema, infratemporal fossa, or orbital gas). Identification of the fractures allows determination of fracture classification: nasal, orbital blowout, trimalar or tripod, Le Fort (I, II, III, and complex), or nasoethmoidal complex fracture (Figure 2-67). Assessment is made of the extent of soft-tissue trauma, particularly the orbital soft tissues of the lens, globe, extraocular muscles,

and optic nerve. Displaced orbital floor fractures may entrap fat or the extraocular muscles and result in enophthalmos or dysfunction of ocular motility.

Skull Base

Anatomically, the skull base can be divided into the anterior, middle, and posterior fossae. The lesser and greater wings of the sphenoid bone divide the anterior fossa from the middle fossa, while the petrous pyramid and mastoid portions of the temporal bone divide the middle and posterior fossae. The parietal and occipital lobes of the brain do not directly contact the skull base.

The skull base is formed from five bones: frontal, ethmoid, temporal, sphenoid, and occipital. The frontal and temporal bones are paired. Each of these bones can be subdivided into component bones. For

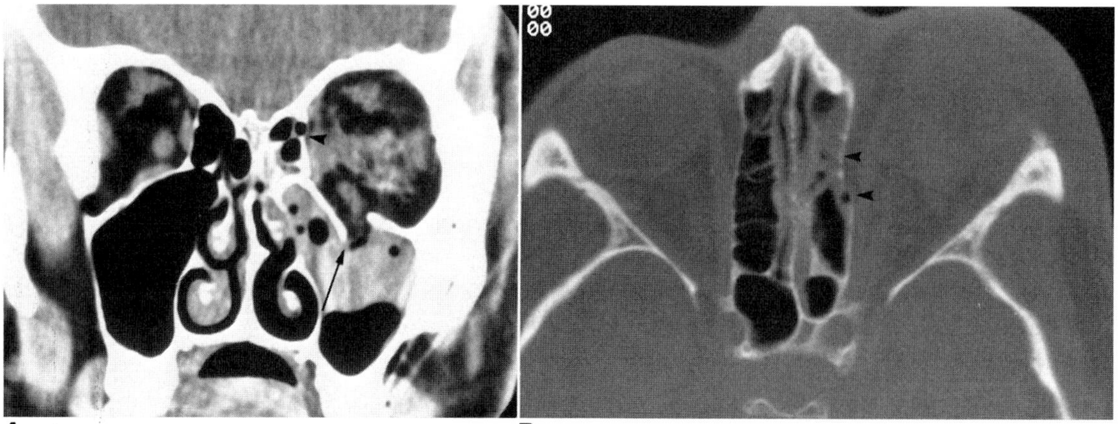

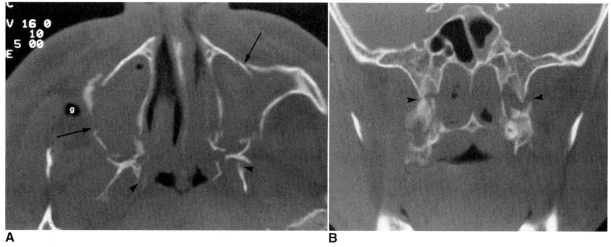

Figure 2-66. Medial and lateral orbital blowout fractures. **A,** Coronal noncontrast computed tomography (NCCT) with soft-tissue windows shows an orbital blowout fracture with displacement of the floor *(arrow)*, distortion of the inferior rectus, and herniation of orbital fat through the orbital floor defect. Both intraconal hemorrhage and high-density maxillary sinus hemorrhagic air-fluid level are well demonstrated on these windows. Medial orbital blowout fracture *(arrowhead)* is suspected as well. **B,** Axial NCCT using bone windows shows opacified left anterior ethmoid air cells that help direct the observer to the displaced medial orbital fracture *(arrowheads)*.

Figure 2-67. Facial fractures. **A,** Bilateral Le Fort type II fractures of the maxillary sinus anterior and posterior walls *(arrows)* and the pterygoid plates *(arrowheads)* appear as discontinuities or lucencies of the bone on this 3-mm axial noncontrast computed tomography (NCCT). Indirect signs of facial fracture are opacified maxillary sinuses, gas *(g)* in the right buccal fat pad, and pre malar facial swelling. **B,** Coronal NCCT clearly demonstrates bilateral pterygoid plate fractures *(arrowheads)*.

example, the occipital bone has basioccipital, condylar, and squamosal portions. The skull base has its longest diameter in the AP plane, extending from the region of the crista galli to the posterior margin of the foramen magnum posteriorly. It is the thinnest in its superior-inferior direction, ranging between 3 and 5 mm in most areas, with the exception of the much thicker petrous temporal bone.

With CT, the skull base may be imaged using the axial or the coronal plane (only a modified coronal plane is possible because of limited gantry tilt). The coronal plane is excellent for delineating the superior inferior extent of a lesion. CT gives excellent visualization of bone detail, especially when bone algorithm techniques are used. In addition to the axial plane, MRI allows imaging both in a true coronal plane and in the sagittal plane, the latter especially useful for the study of midline lesions (e.g., chordoma). MRI also yields improved lesion contrast and conspicuity and more accurate delineation of lesion extent.

Using an anatomic approach, clinicians may classify skull base lesions as anterior, middle, or posterior fossa. They may then develop a unique differential for the medial and lateral portions of each fossa. Lesions may also be categorized as primary, those arising within the skull base itself, and secondary, those extending down from the cranial cavity above (endocranial lesions) or growing up from below (exocranial lesions). Endocranial masses are extracerebral and intracerebral lesions, whereas the exocranial lesions are secondary to extension superiorly from a disease process of the orbit, suprahyoid head and neck, cervical spine, and prevertebral muscles.

The skull base contains multiple foramina that allow the exit of cranial nerves and inflow and outflow of arteries and veins. These foramina also provide an access route for disease processes to spread from the cranial cavity to the infra calvarial structures and vice versa.[5] MRI performed after gadolinium infusion and with the use of fat suppression techniques allows sensitive detection of perineural spread, most readily seen with involvement of the fifth and seventh cranial nerves.[27]

Skull base fractures are readily detected with CT using thin slice sections and reformation techniques.

Sinus air-fluid levels, sinus opacification, and clouding of the temporal bones may herald the presence of a fracture. Similarly, sinus opacification and fracture location may indicate the site of a CSF leak.

Inflammatory skull base lesions are now less common. Osteitis is seen as sclerosis of bone margins. Osteomyelitis usually involves all three skull tables and is characterized by irregular serpiginous lytic areas, occasionally with areas of bone sequestration present.

The osseous changes of neoplastic disease may be erosive, infiltrative, expansive, lytic, sclerotic, or of mixed density. Primary skull neoplastic lesions are uncommon. Benign conditions include osteoma, chondroma, giant cell tumor, cholesterol granuloma, and aneurysmal bone cyst (Figure 2-68). Osteosarcoma, chondrosarcoma, fibrosarcoma, and rarely Ewing's sarcoma and lymphoma, are examples of malignant lesions. Metastatic lesions are more common than primary skull base lesions and frequently have an associated soft-tissue component (Figure 2-69). Osteoblastic metastases are most commonly caused by carcinoma of the prostate or breast; sclerotic changes may be seen occasionally in lymphoma (Figure 2-70). Lytic lesions are more common than osteoblastic findings and are usually secondary to carcinoma of the lung, breast, kidney, or colon.

Intracerebral neoplastic processes may have associated osseous changes. Cerebral gliomas rarely cause

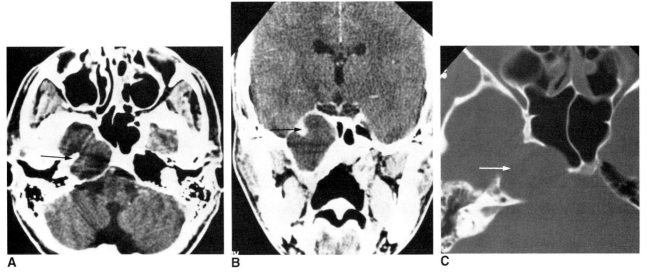

A   B   C

Figure 2-68. Cholesterol granuloma. **A** and **B,** Axial and coronal contrast-enhanced computed tomography (CECT) images demonstrate expansile lesion of the right petrous apex and greater wing of sphenoid. Lesion is homogeneously low density in nature. Displaced right internal carotid artery *(arrows)* lies in the lateral aspect of the lesion. **C,** Axial CECT bone algorithm image using bone windows demonstrates truncation of the anteromedial portion of the right petrous temporal bone *(arrow)* and adjacent posterolateral portion of the sphenoid bone. The lesion bulges into the right sphenoid sinus.

Continued

Figure 2-68, cont'd D, Coronal T1-weighted image and **E,** T2-weighted image demonstrate a lesion that is high intensity on both sequences, consistent with methemoglobin. Right internal carotid artery is noted in the midlateral portion of the lesion *(arrow)*. The lesion extends above and below the skull base and invaginates into the sphenoid sinus.

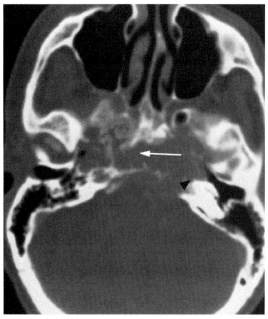

Figure 2-69. Skull base metastasis from adenocarcinoma of the breast. Axial noncontrast computed tomography demonstrates a metastatic tumor infiltrating and destroying a majority of the middle fossa. Clivus *(arrow)* and anteromedial left temporal bone *(arrowhead)* are especially affected.

local bone erosion or expansion; however, optic gliomas may cause expansion of the optic canal. Neuromas (nerve sheath tumors) may cause smooth expansion of skull base foramina: internal auditory canal (cranial nerve VIII), jugular foramen (cranial nerves IX, X, and XI), hypoglossal canal (cranial nerve XII), and lateral wall clivus and foramen rotundum (cranial nerve V). Paragangliomas cause irregular erosive changes in the

skull base foramina (Figure 2-71). A meningioma is often heralded by hyperostosis (bone sclerosis), especially common with a lesion of the middle fossa involving either the greater or lesser sphenoid wing. Chordoma, a tumor of notochordal remnants, typically causes destruction of the clivus (basisphenoid and basiocciput) with associated soft-tissue mass and calcification.[32,50] Erosion of the sella floor and sella expansion are characteristic of pituitary adenomas.

Temporal Bone

Determination of temporal bone abnormality requires assessment of the external ear, middle ear, mastoid air cells, petrous apex, inner ear, IAC, facial nerve canal, and vascular compartment (jugular foramen and carotid canal). The adjacent compartments into which an aggressive temporal bone lesion can spread, or from which a lesion can invade the temporal bone, include cerebellopontine angle (meningioma, acoustic schwannoma), middle cranial fossa (geniculate schwannoma, cholesteatoma), jugular foramen (schwannoma, paraganglioma, glomus tumor), skull base and clivus (chordoma), carotid space (aneurysm, schwannoma), parotid space (adenoid cystic carcinoma), and soft tissues of the external ear and scalp (SCC).

For the external ear and external auditory canal (EAC), the search for abnormality may be accomplished with either high-resolution CT or MRI. Abnormal development (external ear hypoplasia, fibrous or bony EAC atresia), soft-tissue opacification (cerumen, EAC cholesteatoma, SCC), bone erosion (EAC cholesteatoma, mucormycosis, squamous cell carcinoma), bone formation (exostoses), or scutum

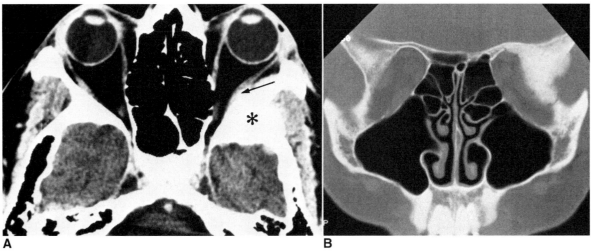

Figure 2-70. Metastatic prostate carcinoma to left orbit. **A,** Axial contrast-enhanced computed tomography (CECT) demonstrates sclerotic metastasis of the posterolateral margin of the left orbit *(asterisk)*. Small soft-tissue component *(arrow)* lies deep to the hyperostosis, displacing the lateral rectus muscle medially. **B,** Coronal CECT with bone settings demonstrates a marked sclerotic reaction of the superior lateral portion of the left orbit. Intraorbital volume is decreased.

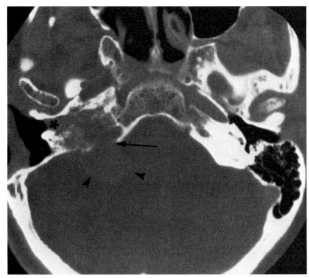

Figure 2-71. Glomus tumor (paraganglioma) of the right petrous temporal bone. Axial contrast-enhanced computed tomography with bone windows demonstrates an infiltrative destructive lesion of the middle and superior portions of the right petrous temporal bone *(arrow)*. Poorly defined margin of the lesion is characteristic of a glomus tumor. Soft-tissue mass *(arrowheads)* is noted in the right cerebellopontine angle cistern and in the inferior portion of the right middle ear cavity *(asterisk)*. Previous right mastoidectomy has been performed.

erosion (par flaccida cholesteatoma) can easily be detected and their extent defined by CT. MRI may add additional information on soft-tissue involvement below the skull base or on infiltration of the auricle and scalp.

The middle ear is best evaluated with high-resolution CT. Ossicular chain anomalies (fusion, dislocation, prosthesis, stapedial foot-plate sclerosis), air-fluid level (trauma, acute otitis media), soft-tissue opacification (acute or chronic otitis media, cholesteatoma, trauma, chronic endotracheal or nasogastric intubation), and tympanic membrane thickening (otitis media) may all be characterized (Figure 2-72). The radiographic approach to the mastoid air cells and petrous apex is similar to that of the paranasal sinuses, consisting of the evaluation of the mastoid and petrous apex soft-tissue contents and the bony walls. Assessment is made of development or pneumatization of these regions (pneumatization or opacification by soft tissue), the bony septae and walls (hypoplasia or sclerosis from chronic otomastoiditis), the margins of the mastoid or petrous apex [expanded by a primary or secondary cholesteatoma (Figure 2-73) or a cholesterol granuloma], bone destruction (SCC, malignant fibrous histiocytoma, glomus tumor). MRI may complement CT for assessment of larger petrous apex or mastoid masses. A normal unpneumatized, fatty (marrow-filled) petrous apex is high signal on T1WI and low signal on T2WI, but a cholesterol granuloma is high signal on T1WI and T2WI from the methemoglobin (see Figure 2-68). Mucus in an air cell is low intensity on T1WI, is very high intensity on T2WI, and enhances mildly with gadolinium. A primary cholesteatoma is similar to CSF in intensity, appearing low intensity on T1WI and moderately high signal on T2WI, and does not enhance with gadolinium. Postoperative findings encountered on CT and MRI include metallic ossicular

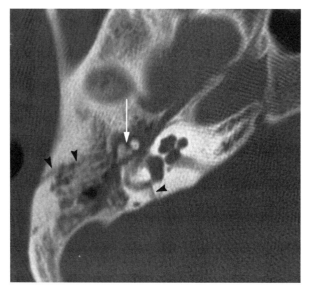

Figure 2-72. Transverse petrous fracture with ossicular dislocation. High-resolution 1.5-mm noncontrast computed tomography using a bone algorithm and bone windows shows a transverse petrous fracture *(arrowheads)* extending through the mastoid bone and semicircular canals. Ossicular dislocation of the head of malleus from its articulation with the fractured body of incus *(arrow)* is seen. Middle ear opacification also confirms presence of temporal bone trauma.

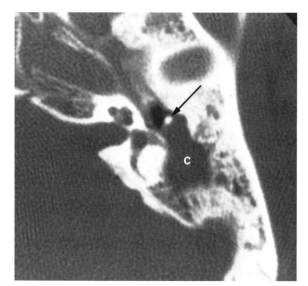

Figure 2-73. Pars flaccida cholesteatoma. Middle ear cholesteatoma *(c)* expands the mastoid antrum and epitympanic recess on this axial noncontrast computed tomography. The absence of incus and soft tissue abutting the head of malleus *(arrow)* confirm ossicular erosion.

prostheses, cochlear implants, and various types of mastoidectomies.

The inner ear structures are best assessed by high-resolution CT with attention to anatomic variants and bone density. A saccular vestibule is one of the more common congenital anomalies. A cochlea with less than 2 ½ to 2 ¾ turns represents a Mondini malformation (Figure 2-74). The basal turn of the cochlea and round window may be identified on both axial and coronal CT images. The horizontal (lateral) semicircular canal cortex may be eroded by a cholesteatoma. The oval window and foot plate of the stapes are thickened in stapedial otosclerosis, and the ring of the otic capsule is demineralized in labyrinthine otosclerosis (otospongiosis). The entire petrous bone may be abnormally low density with dysplasias such as osteogenesis imperfecta or sclerotic in osteopetrosis and Paget's disease. Inflammatory or neoplastic lesions may involve the cochlea and vestibule without obvious bony changes on CT; however, MRI with gadolinium-enhanced T1WI may show an enhancing lesion.

The IAC and facial nerve canals are best evaluated by high-resolution CT for bony detail and by gadolinium-enhanced MRI for the soft-tissue abnormality. On CT, the findings might include widening (acoustic schwannoma, surgery) or narrowing (bone dysplasia, hyperostosis from a meningioma) of the IAC. The facial nerve canal may be traced along its entire course in both axial and coronal planes for areas of erosion (facial neuroma, paraganglioma, hemangioma) or abnormal position (anterior location of mastoid segment with EAC atresia). Gadolinium-enhanced MRI is the modality of choice for evaluating the seventh and eighth cranial nerves within the IAC and temporal bone (schwannomas of the facial nerve, of the vestibular nerve, or within the cochlea) or for demonstrating seventh cranial nerve inflammation (Bell's palsy) (Figures 2-75 and 2-76). Note that the facial nerves

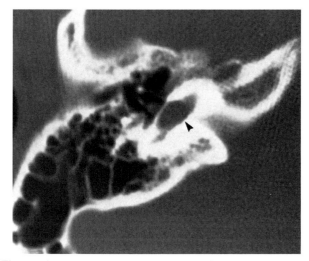

Figure 2-74. Mondini malformation. Saccular combined vestibule and cochlea *(arrowhead)* reveal a severe form of Mondini malformation on this axial noncontrast computed tomography.

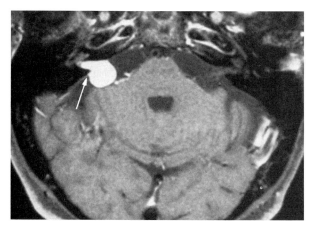

Figure 2-75. Acoustic schwannoma. Axial fat saturation post-gadolinium T1-weighted image demonstrates a brightly enhancing right cerebellopontine angle mass with intracanalicular (characteristic of acoustic schwannoma) and extracanalicular components. Note the acute angle that the mass makes with the petrous ridge *(arrow)*.

may normally enhance mildly and usually symmetrically within the facial nerve canal. Asymmetric enhancement is more likely to be abnormal.

POSTOPERATIVE NECK AND FACE

A preoperative CECT or MRI is extremely helpful for interpreting the postoperative neck, skull base, or face

for sites of concern and potential tumor recurrence. Likewise, a baseline CECT or MRI 3 to 6 months after surgery and radiation further improves the ability of imaging to detect posttreatment tumor recurrence. The posterior cervical space is the most frequently altered neck space, and part or all of its contents may be resected for staging and treatment of head and neck carcinoma. Note is made of missing structures.[19] A radical neck dissection (Figure 2-77, *A*) removes the sternocleidomastoid muscle, internal jugular vein, regional lymph nodes, and most of the fibrofatty tissue that comprises this space. Modified radical, functional, and supraomohyoid neck dissections remove less.

The oral cavity and face also are affected by surgery. Facial trauma is frequently treated by internal fixation with metallic screws and plates. Internal fixation also is performed as part of composite reactions where the mandible is split, or when the mandible is partially resected for invasion by tumor. Metal wires, screws, and plates may cause artifacts obscuring sites of posttraumatic CSF leak or potential tumor recurrence. Sinus and palate tumors may require resection of the maxilla, palate, orbital walls and soft tissue, and cribriform plate. The fat, muscle, or bone contained in free flaps, myocutaneous flaps, and osteocutaneous flaps placed in the surgical cavity further complicates image interpretation (Figure 2-77, *B*). Laryngeal

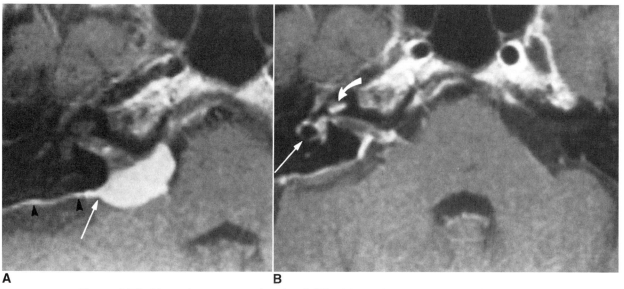

A   **B**

Figure 2-76. Magnetic resonance imaging (MRI) of internal auditory canal (IAC) and facial nerve. **A,** Axial postgadolinium T1-weighted image shows a broad-based brightly enhancing meningioma overlying the IAC. Note its obtuse angle *(arrow)* with the petrous ridge and dural "tail" extending posteriorly *(arrowhead)*, which are characteristic of a meningioma. **B,** In the same patient, postoperative labyrinthitis has developed on this follow-up axial postgadolinium T1-weighted images. Abnormal enhancement of the vestibule, semicircular canals *(straight arrow)*, and cochlea *(curved arrow)* are new findings (which can only be observed by gadolinium-enhanced MRI).

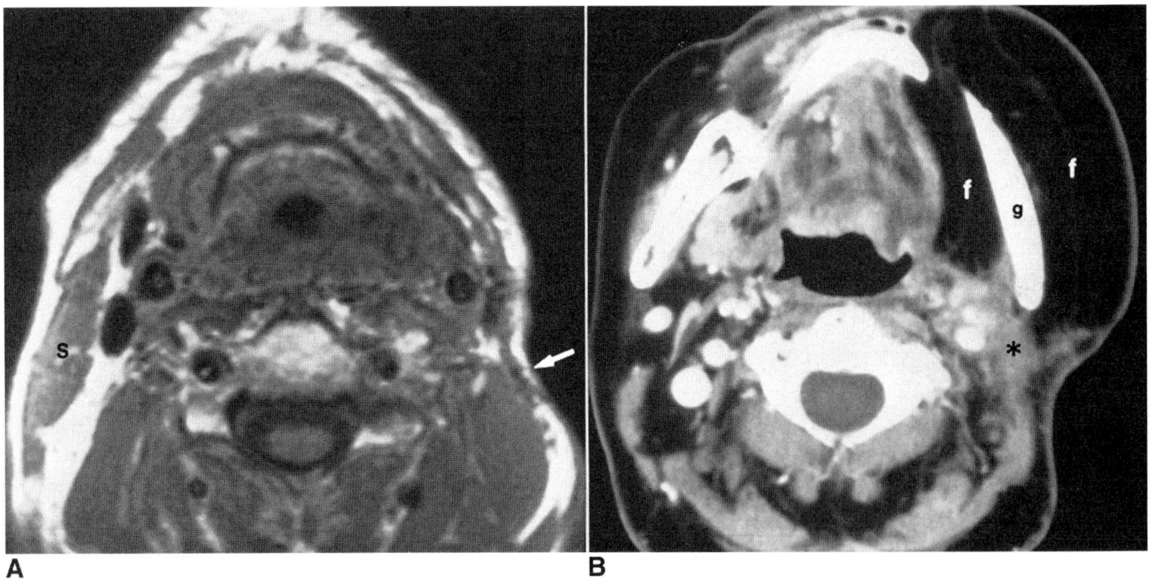

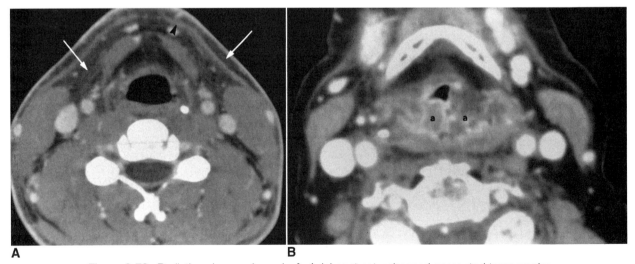

Figure 2-77. Postoperative appearance of neck. **A,** Axial T1-weighted image demonstrates an earlier left neck dissection *(arrow)* with removal of the sternocleidomastoid muscle *(s)* and posterior cervical space fat. **B,** Patient with an osteocutaneous flap, with thick fat *(f)* on deep and external margins of the mandibular graft *(g)*, has developed a deep recurrent tumor *(asterisk)* around the carotid sheath.

surgery may remove part or all of the laryngeal skeleton, often with placement of a tracheostomy. The remaining soft tissues of the collapsed visceral space are difficult to accurately evaluate.

Radiotherapy frequently causes an edematous pattern, characterized on CT by a streaky increase in the density of the subcutaneous, parapharyngeal, and posterior cervical space fat planes (Figure 2-78, *A*). On MRI it may have an increased signal on T2WI. The mucosal space of the pharynx and larynx may also develop swelling and edema, appearing as diffuse mucosal thickening and enhancement on CECT, while

Figure 2-78. Radiation changes in neck. **A,** Axial contrast-enhanced computed tomography (CECT) demonstrates streaky densities in fat throughout the superficial cervical and anterior cervical spaces *(arrows)* and a thickening of the platysma muscle *(arrowhead)*. **B,** Different patient who had radiation therapy for glottic carcinoma has developed a thickening of the epiglottis and aryepiglottic folds *(a)* on this axial CECT. This finding may persist for many months after therapy.

MRI may show high signal on long TR sequences and on gadolinium-enhanced T1WI (Figure 2-78, *B*). Postradiation edema, particularly of the larynx and pharynx, may mimic recurrent neoplasm for as long as 6 months to 7 years after radiotherapy.[20] Finally, treated lymph nodes may decrease in size or totally disappear, leaving a "dirty fat" appearance.

Recurrent tumor spread often produces strands or nodules of soft-tissue density within or replacing the normal fat planes. However, CECT has difficulty detecting small (less than 1 cm) or mucosal-based tumors, and reliably differentiating between recurrent carcinoma and fibrosis or edema. A new bulky, ring-enhancing mass, local tissue invasion, or further bone destruction is a strong sign of recurrent tumor. MRI is reportedly capable of distinguishing tumor from radiation-induced fibrosis in some cases. Posttreatment fibrosis or scarring is similar to or lower in signal than muscle on all sequences (particularly on T2WI), is usually linear, is not mass-like, and may enhance mildly in a linear fashion. MRI is superior to CT (particularly NCCT) in discrimination of recurrent tumor from muscle and vascular structures. In the posttreatment neck, gadolinium-enhanced MRI may have the potential to identify tumor recurrence and allow separation of tumor from fibrosis because recurrent tumor may ring-enhance, a pattern not seen with scar. Finally, PET/CT is better able to differentiate the metabolically active tumor tissue from postoperative changes.

REFERENCES

1. Albertyn LE, Alcock MK: Diagnosis of internal jugular vein thrombosis, *Radiology* 162:505, 1987.
2. Atlas SW and others: STIR MR imaging of the orbit, *Am J Neuroradiol* 9:969, 1988.
3. Ator GA and others: Evaluation of mandibular tumor invasion with magnetic resonance imaging, *Arch Otolaryngol Head Neck Surg* 116:454, 1990.
4. Babbel RW, Smoker WRK, Harnsberger HR: The visceral space: the unique infrahyoid space, *Semin Ultra CT MR* 12:204–223, 1991.
5. Batsakis JG: *Tumors of the head and neck: clinical and pathological considerations*. Baltimore, Williams & Wilkins, 1979.
6. Brant-Zawadzki M: *Magnetic resonance imaging principles: the bare necessities*. In Brant-Zawadzki M, Norman D, editors: *Magnetic resonance imaging of the central nervous system*, New York, Raven Press, 1987.
7. Close LG and others: Computed tomographic evaluation of regional lymph node involvement in cancer of the oral cavity and oropharynx, *Head Neck* 11:309, 1989.
8. Crawford SC and others: The role of gadolinium-DTPA in the evaluation of extracranial head and neck mass lesions, *Radiol Clin North Am* 27:219, 1989.
9. Curtin HD: Assessment of salivary gland pathology, *Otolaryngol Clin North Am* 21:547, 1988.
10. Curtin HD: Separation of the masticator space from the parapharyngeal space, *Radiology* 163:195, 1987.
11. Davis WL, Smoker WRK, Harnsberger HR: The normal and diseased infrahyoid retropharyngeal, danger, and prevertebral spaces, *Semin Ultra CT MR* 12:241, 1991.
12. Davis WL and others: Retropharyngeal space: evaluation of normal anatomy and diseases with CT and MR imaging, *Radiology* 174:59, 1990.
13. Delblasio AM, editor: *Maxillofacial imaging*, Philadelphia, WB Saunders, 1990.
14. Elliot DO: Magnetic resonance imaging fundamentals and system performance, *Radiol Clin North Am* 25:409, 1987.
15. Evers K and others: CT sialography: utilising acinar filling, *Br J Radiol* 58:839, 1985.
16. Fishman EK and others: Three-dimensional reconstruction of the human body, *Am J Roentgenol* 150:1419, 1988.
17. Fruehwald FX: Clinical examination, CT and US in tongue cancer staging, *Eur J Radiol* 8:236, 1988.
18. Fruin ME, Smoker WRK, Harnsberger HR: The carotid space of the infrahyoid neck, *Semin Ultra CT MR* 12:224, 1991.
19. Glazer HS and others: Neck neoplasms: MR imaging. II. Posttreatment evaluation, *Radiology* 160:349, 1986.
20. Glazer HS and others: Radiation fibrosis: differentiation from recurrent tumor by MR imaging, *Radiology* 156:721, 1985.
21. Gordon BM and others: Parathyroid imaging with Tc-99m sestamibi, *Am J Roentgenol* 167:1563, 1996.
22. Hajek PC and others: Lymph nodes of the neck: evaluation with US, *Radiology* 158:739, 1986.
23. Harnsberger HR: CT and MRI of masses of the deep face, *Curr Probl Diagn Radiol* 16:141, 1987.
24. Harnsberger HR: *Head and neck imaging: handbooks in radiology*, Chicago, Mosby, 1990.
25. Harnsberger HR and others: Branchial cleft anomalies and their mimics: CT evaluation, *Radiology* 152:739, 1984.
26. Hendrix LE and others: MR imaging of optic nerve lesions: value of gadopentetate dimeglumine and fat-suppression technique, *Am J Neuroradiol* 11:749, 1990.
27. Laine FJ and others: Perineural tumor extension through the foramen ovale: evaluation with MR imaging, *Radiology* 174:65, 1990.
28. Langman AW and others: Radiologic assessment of tumor and the carotid artery: correlation of magnetic resonance imaging, ultrasound, and computed tomography with surgical findings, *Head Neck* 11:443, 1989.
29. Mancuso AA, Dillon WP: The neck, *Radiol Clin North Am* 27:407, 1989.
30. Marentette LJ, Maisel RH: Three-dimensional CT reconstruction in midfacial surgery, *Otolaryngol Head Neck Surg* 98:48, 1988.
31. Mettler FA, Gulberteau MJ: *Essentials of nuclear medicine imaging*, ed 3. Philadelphia, WB Saunders, 1991.
32. Moore T, Ganti SR, Lindfors KK: CT appearance of clival chordomas, *J Comput Assist Tomogr* 10:34, 1986.
33. Olsen WL and others: MR imaging of paragangliomas, *Am J Roentgenol* 148:201, 1987.
34. Parker GD, Harnsberger HR, Smoker WRK: The anterior and posterior cervical spaces, *Semin Ultra CT MR* 12:257, 1991.
35. Pernicone JR and others: Three-dimensional phase-contrast MR angiography in the head and neck: preliminary report, *Am J Neuroradiol* 11:457, 1990.
36. Picus D and others: Computed tomography in the staging of esophageal carcinoma, *Radiology* 146:433, 1983.
37. Rafto SE, Gefter WB: MRI of the upper aerodigestive tract and neck, *Radiol Clin North Am* 26:547, 1988.
38. Regelink and others: Detection of unknown primary tumours and distant metastases in patients with cervical metastases: value of FDG-PET versus conventional modalities, *Eur J Nuc Med* 29:1024, 2002.

39. Robinson JD and others: Extracranial lesions of the head and neck: preliminary experience with Gd-DTPA-enhanced MR imaging, *Radiology* 172:165, 1989.

40. Schwartz JD and others: MR imaging of parotid mass lesions: attempts at histopathological differentiation, *J Comput Assist Tomogr* 13:789, 1989.

41. Shapiro MD, Som PM: MRI of the paranasal sinuses and nasal cavity, *Radiol Clin North Am* 27:447, 1989.

42. Silver AJ and others: CT of the nasopharynx and related spaces. I. Anatomy, *Radiology* 147:725, 1983.

43. Silver AJ and others: CT of the nasopharynx and related spaces. II. Pathology, *Radiology* 147:733, 1983.

44. Smoker WRK: Normal anatomy of the infrahyoid neck: an overview, *Semin Ultra CT MR* 12:192, 1991.

45. Som PM: Lymph nodes of the neck, *Radiology* 165:593, 1987.

46. Som PM: *Salivary glands.* In Som PM, Bergeron RT, editors: *Head and neck imaging,* St Louis, Mosby, 1990.

47. Som PM, Curtin HD, editors: *Head and neck imaging,* ed 3. St Louis, Mosby, 1996.

48. Som PM and others: Benign and malignant parotid pleomorphic adenomas: CT and MR studies, *J Comput Assist Tomogr* 12:65, 1988.

49. Swartz JD, Harnsberger HR: *Imaging of the temporal bone,* ed 2. New York, Thieme Medical Publishers, 1992.

50. Sze G and others: Chordoma: MR imaging, *Radiology* 166:187, 1988.

51. Teresi LM, Lufkin RB, Hanafee WN: Magnetic resonance imaging of the larynx, *Radiol Clin North Am* 27:393, 1989.

52. Thrall JH, Ziessman HA: *Nuclear medicine, the requisites,* St Louis, Mosby, 1995.

53. Valvassori GE, Mafee MF, Carter BL: *Imaging of the head and neck.* New York, Thieme Medical Publishers, 1995.

54. van den Akker HP: Diagnostic imaging in salivary gland disease, *Oral Surg Oral Med Oral Pathol* 66:625, 1988.

55. Vogelzang P, Harnsberger HR, Smoker WRK: Multispatial and transpatial diseases of the extracranial head and neck, *Semin Ultra CT MR* 12:274, 1991.

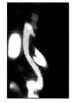

CHAPTER THREE

BIOPHYSIOLOGY AND CLINICAL CONSIDERATIONS IN RADIOTHERAPY

Jason K. Rockhill
George E. Laramore

INTRODUCTION

The use of ionizing radiation in medicine dates back almost to the very date of its discovery. In 1895, Wilhelm Roentgen discovered x-rays, and 3 years later, Pierre and Marie Curie announced that they had isolated radium from pitchblende. The first documented radiation biology experiment was performed inadvertently at about this time when Antoine Becquerel developed a "burn" on his chest from carrying a vial of radium salt in his vest pocket. It soon became apparent that this newly discovered entity—"radiation"—had the ability to affect profound biological changes. The public embraced this new agent, and it was touted as a cure for almost every ailment known. The results of these early clinical trials are not well documented, but it is probably safe to assume that most were not very successful. However, the first "cure" of a malignant neoplasm achieved with ionizing radiation was reported in the 1899 in Stockholm.[1] Thor Stenbeck treated a 49-year-old woman's basal-cell carcinoma of the skin on her nose. He delivered 100 treatments in the course of 9 months and she was alive and well 30 years after the treatment. In 1901, Dr. Frand Williams in Boston reported on the successful treatment of a lip cancer.[1]

During the early 1900s, most clinical radiotherapy was done by surgeons who used it as another form of cautery. Radiation was used in large doses to produce a "tissue slough" and the adverse side effects associated with its early use still color the attitudes many physicians have toward radiotherapy. Used properly, ionizing radiation produces selective modifications of cells through subtle changes introduced into deoxyribonucleic acid (DNA) and other cellular elements. Special training is required to understand these effects and how to best use them in clinical settings. From this need, radiation oncology has emerged as a separate medical specialty.

The capabilities of the radiation oncologist have increased in keeping with advancing technology.

Initially, only low-energy x-rays were available, and these were capable of treating only superficial tumors, without causing severe side effects to the intervening healthy tissues. High-energy linear accelerators were then developed for research purposes and soon were used to produce "megavoltage" x-rays for medical use in a few large centers, although the "megavoltage" era in radiotherapy really began with the use of γ-ray beams from ^{60}Co sources. Now compact linear accelerators are used routinely in radiotherapy departments. Similarly, research into nuclear physics made it possible to produce many artificial radioisotopes that have had application in medicine; the field is no longer restricted to ^{226}Ra as it was in the past. Also, specialized, high-dose rate brachytherapy devices have been developed, which reduce the duration of the implant and simplify the radiation protection problem. Improved treatment modalities such as particle beam radiotherapy, intensity-modulated radiation therapy (IMRT), and chemotherapy–radiotherapy combination treatments have recently emerged into routine clinical use and have the potential for changing the field of radiotherapy as much in the future as it has been changed in the past.

The purpose of this chapter is to provide the clinician with an overview of the basic principles of physics and biophysiology that underlie modern radiotherapy. Limitations of space necessitate the presentation of the overall picture only, rather than a detailed chronological account of the development of the field. Topics are covered in a manner that assumes no previous experience on the part of the reader. The references cited are representative and illustrative in nature rather than comprehensive.

BASIC OVERVIEW OF PHYSICS
Conventional Types of Radiation

Radiotherapy is performed most commonly using high-energy photons (or quanta) of electromagnetic radiation. The electromagnetic spectrum is a continuum with radiowaves 10^3–10^5 cm in length lying at one end and energetic cosmic rays 10^{-12} cm in length lying at the other end. The γ-rays produced from a ^{60}Co source are about 1.3 million electron volts (MeV) in energy, which corresponds to a wavelength of 10^{-10} cm. Energies of 3 to 5 electron volts (eV) are needed to break chemical bonds, and this typically requires wavelengths shorter than 10^{-4} cm. Microwaves (12 cm, 1.03×10^{-5} eV) used for heating purposes are much less energetic than γ-rays produced from a ^{60}Co source and act by rotating water molecules in an electromagnetic field.

High-energy photons used in radiotherapy initially interact in matter (i.e., tissue) to produce high-energy electrons by one of three principal processes: photoelectric effect, Compton scattering, or pair production. In the photoelectric effect, a photon excites a tightly bound, inner-shell electron and is completely annihilated. This process scales like Z^3/E^3 per gram of material, where Z is the "effective" nuclear charge of the material, and E is the photon energy. This process is most important for photon energies in the range of 10 to 50 kiloelectron volts (keV), which is the range typically used in diagnostic radiology. A higher effective Z of bone relative to soft tissue causes it to show up well on diagnostic films.

The Compton Effect is most important in the 500-keV to 10-MeV range of photon energies used in therapy. It scales like Z^0 per gram of material and decreases in a complex way with increasing energy. Physically, a photon can be thought of as transferring a part of its energy to a loosely bound outer electron and emerging at a lower energy and longer wavelength. Within this energy range, all tissues absorb photons at about the same rate on a gram-for-gram basis. This is important for therapeutic purposes, such as when managing soft-tissue tumors adjacent to bone. On films exposed with megavoltage x-rays, much of the distinction between bone and soft tissue is lost.

Pair production refers to a high-energy photon being annihilated in the strong electromagnetic field of an atomic nucleus and producing an electron–positron pair. The threshold energy for this process is 1.02 MeV. It scales like Z per gram of material and increases with increasing photon energy. For a 10-MeV photon, this accounts for about 28% of the total absorption cross-section in tissue. Other processes also can take place at higher photon energies.

Once one of these primary processes has occurred, a high-energy electron is produced, which creates secondary ionization events as it travels through tissue. Typically, about 34 eV of energy is lost for each ion pair that is produced. The resulting ionization clusters

are relatively isolated on a scale of typical cellular distances. Most of the events involve water molecules in the cell cytoplasm, and their reaction products initiate complex sequences of chemical reactions that generally involve free radicals. The biologic properties of different megavoltage photon beams are essentially equivalent per unit of energy deposited.

Radiation doses are specified in terms of the energy deposited in a unit quantity of material. In the past, the conventional dose unit was the *rad*, which was equivalent to 100 ergs being deposited per gram of material. More recently, an international commission[62] has agreed that radiation doses should be specified in terms of *gray* (Gy), which corresponds to 1 joule being deposited per kilogram of material. The older literature specifies radiation doses in terms of rad, whereas the newer literature specifies doses in terms of Gy. Doses in this chapter are specified in terms of Gy. Numerically, doses in rad can be converted to equivalent doses in Gy by dividing by 100 (i.e., 100 rad = 1 Gy).

Typical depth-dose curves for photon beams used in the therapy of head and neck cancers are shown in the upper panel of Figure 3-1. The plots are for the dose along the central axis for a 10 cm x 10 cm field size. The energy of the beam is specified by the energy to which the incident electron beam is accelerated before impacting the target and actually producing the x-rays. The x-ray beam is a continuum with the maximum energy equal to that of the electron beam. To express that a range of x-ray energies is produced, the term *MV* is used rather than *MeV*. Appropriate filtering elements also are used to "harden" and "shape" the beam, but for most practical purposes, at a given source-axis distance (SAD), the beams from given energy linear accelerators are essentially equivalent. The three curves have the same general shape but vary somewhat in specific details. Note that the curves do not start out at their maximum value, but rather build-up, which occurs because the initial, high-energy electrons produced by the photon beam are directed primarily in the forward direction. The number of these electrons increases with depth until a distance equal to the average electronic path length is reached. The deposited dose is low at the surface and then increases to a maximum, after which it decreases with depth because of attenuation of the radiation field. The distance of the dose maximum from the surface is referred to as D_{max}. It varies from 1.2 cm for the 4-MV (80-cm SAD) beam, to 1.3 cm for the 6-MV (100-cm SAD) beam, and to 3 cm for the 15-MV (100-cm SAD) beam. The skin and subcutaneous tissues are spared within this build-up region, enabling the delivery of a higher dose of radiation to a deeper tumor. Higher energy photon beams can be used with even

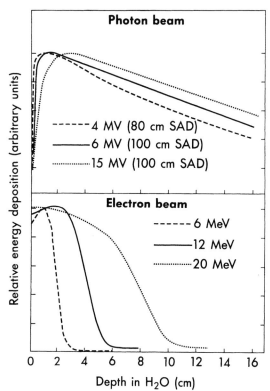

Figure 3-1. Typical depth-dose curves for megavoltage photon and electron beams commonly used in the therapy of head and neck cancers. The upper panel shows curves for 10 cm × 10 cm fields for a 4-MV (80-cm SAD) linear accelerator *(dashed line)*, a 6-MV (100-cm SAD) linear accelerator *(solid line)*, and a 15-MV (100-cm SAD) linear accelerator *(dotted line)*. The lower panel shows depth-dose curves for 10 cm × 10 cm fields for 6-MeV *(dashed line)*, 12-MeV *(solid line)*, and 20-MeV *(dotted line)* electron energies.

greater values of D_{max}, but these mainly have increased usefulness for the more deeply seated tumors of the thorax, abdomen, or pelvis.

Alternatively, the high-energy electron beam produced by the linear accelerator can be used directly in patient treatments. Typical depth-dose curves for various electron energies are shown in the lower panel of Figure 3-1. Note that these beams typically penetrate a given distance and then fall off rapidly. There is a slight amount of skin sparing for the 6-MeV beam, but not for the others. These beams are useful for treating skin cancers, tumors of the buccal mucosa, or even superficial tumors of the oral cavity, provided that appropriate applicator cones are used.[58] Optimal treatment of a given lesion may require some combination of electron and photon beams,[53] and this in turn requires the services of a comprehensive radiation treatment facility. Megavoltage electron beams have the same biologic properties as megavoltage photon beams for an equivalent dose of absorbed radiation.

Particle Radiation

In the strictest sense, the electron beams used in conventional radiotherapy facilities are a type of particle radiation, but this section will be devoted to the heavier charged particles (e.g., protons, α-particles, heavy ions, π-mesons, and fast neutrons) used experimentally at a small number of radiotherapy centers throughout the world. These particles are of special interest because of their different radiobiologic properties or their better depth-dose characteristics, which allow for higher tumor doses without causing a commensurate increase in the dose to the surrounding healthy tissues.

One particle for which there has been a great amount of clinical work is the fast neutron. A depth-dose curve for a beam from the cyclotron facility at the University of Washington is shown in the upper panel of Figure 3-2. Note that this is similar in general appearance to the photon beam curves in Figure 3-1. Fast neutrons are of clinical interest because of their radiobiologic properties, which occur because of the

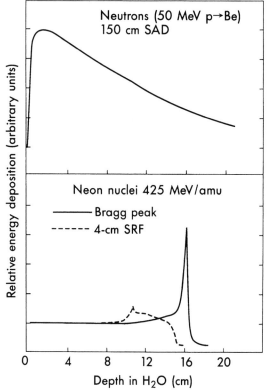

Figure 3-2. The upper panel shows a typical depth-dose curve for a neutron beam used in therapy. It is for a 10 cm × 10 cm field size and was generated from a 50-MeV p → Be reaction at 150 cm SAD. The lower panel shows the pure Bragg curve *(solid line)* for a neon ion beam of energy 425 MeV/amu and the resulting curve *(dotted line)* when a 4-cm spiral ridge filter (SRF) is used to broaden the beam for therapy. The data in the lower panel are from the BEVALAC facility at the Donner Laboratories.

much greater amount of energy they deposit when they go through tissue. Neutrons are neutral particles and interact with the atomic nuclei, producing "heavy" charged particles such as protons, α-particles, or nuclear fragments that in turn create a dense chain of ionization events as they go through tissue. The distribution of these secondary particles depends on the energy spectrum of the neutron beam, and hence the biologic properties of the beam strongly depend on its energy spectrum. Neutrons used in therapy generally are produced by accelerating charged particles, such as protons or deuterons, and impacting them on a beryllium target. To a first approximation, the beam can be specified by indicating the charged particle that is accelerated, the energy of the particle when it impacts the target, the amount of energy absorbed by the target, and the distance between the target and the treatment axis (SAD). The curve in Figure 3-2, for example, is for a 10 cm × 10 cm field for a beam produced by accelerating a stream of protons to 50 MeV and impacting them on a beryllium target of a thickness that absorbs about 50% of the beam energy. The resulting neutron beam has approximately the same penetration characteristics as the photon beam from a 6-MV linear accelerator. Most often, cyclotrons are used to accelerate the charged particle beams, but special linear accelerators can be used as well.

Neutrons can also be produced using deuterium-tritium (DT) generating tubes that yield a quasi mono-energetic beam of 14- or 15-MeV neutrons. Although the cost of systems using the DT reaction is lower than cyclotron-based systems, their lower neutron output makes them less suitable for therapy. Although once popular, such DT systems now are rarely used clinically. Neutrons in the energy range most commonly used in therapy deposit most of their energy via a "knock-on" reaction, whereby a hydrogen nucleus is impacted, producing a recoil proton. This process is more efficient in tissues that contain a greater quantity of hydrogen, such as adipose or nerve tissue, and is less efficient in bone. Compared with muscle, the absorption can vary by ~10%.[13] Typically, the recoil fragments produced by therapy neutron beams deposit 50 to 100 times more energy than the electrons created by megavoltage photon beams. The energy deposited by a radiation beam is characterized by its linear energy transfer (LET) spectrum. The primary high-energy electrons produced by megavoltage photons have LETs in the range of 0.2 to 2 keV per micron traversed, whereas the recoil protons produced by fast neutrons have LETs in the range of 20 to 100 keV per micron. It is this difference in LETs that results in the special radiobiologic properties discussed in the next section.

Considerable interest is being shown in using charged particle beams directly for therapeutic purposes, which generally requires beams of much higher energy than those used to produce neutrons. The lighter particles, such as protons and α-particles, are of interest because of their extremely favorable depth-dose characteristics. The radiobiologic properties of these beams are similar to those of conventional photon or electron beams. In the United States, proton beam radiotherapy is carried out at Northeast Proton Therapy Center (Harvard), LLUMC Proton Treatment Center (Loma Linda), Midwest Proton Radiotherapy Institute (Indiana University), and Crocker Nuclear Laboratory (UC Davis). Heavy charged particles combine the favorable depth-dose properties of the proton and α-particle beams with the favorable biologic properties of the neutron beams. Energies are on the order of several hundred MeV per nucleon rather than the few MeV per nucleon for the recoil fragments produced by neutrons. These highly energetic particles do not deposit much energy in tissue until they reach the end of their path, where they are moving slowly. Hence, they do not produce much radiation damage in the intervening tissues.

The lower panel of Figure 3-2 shows a "pure" Bragg peak for a neon beam (solid line) and for its spread form (dotted line). These data are from the BEVALAC facility at the Donner Laboratories in Berkeley, CA. Note the high ratio of the energy deposited at the peak compared with that deposited at shallower depths for the directed beam. The Bragg peak itself is narrow. It must therefore either be "scanned" across a tumor while its penetration depth is being varied, or it must be spread out by passing it through appropriate filters. The dotted curve shows the result after the beam is passed through a 4-cm spiral ridge filter (SRF). Note that this lowers the peak-to-plateau ratio of energy deposition and, at the same time, broadens the trailing edge of the peak. Clearly, both effects are undesirable for therapeutic purposes; however, the dose of radiation deposited along the initial portion of the path is still lower than that deposited across the spread peak, which represents an advantage over the other types of radiation discussed thus far in this chapter. The broadening of the trailing edge of the peak occurs because of fragmentation of the neon nuclei in the filter, and this does not occur with protons or α-particles. Thus, the spread peaks for the latter two particles have somewhat better localization than the curve shown here. A more sophisticated approach is to use true three-dimensional scanning, which changes the particle energy as the beam is swept across the target. Currently, heavy ion radiotherapy is available only at the Heavy Ion Medical Accelerator (HIMAC) facility in Chiba, Japan, and at the GIS in Darmstadt, Germany.

Another type of charged particle that has been used in radiotherapy is the π-meson. The biologic properties of a π-meson beam are complex because of the large number of processes involved, but in a crude sense, they can be thought of as behaving like a mixture of low-LET and high-LET radiation. These beams have been studied in the past but are no longer used clinically.

FUNDAMENTALS OF RADIOBIOLOGY
Cell Killing by Radiation

Within the cell, there are certain key "targets" that must be affected by the radiation before the cell is killed. The nuclear DNA is probably the most critical target, but other elements, such as the nuclear membrane and mitochondria, also may be important. When any form of radiation interacts with the cell material, there is some probability that one or more of the key target areas will be directly affected. This is the "direct" mechanism of action. Conversely, the radiation interaction may be with some other element such as a molecule in the cell's cytoplasm, and the loss of this molecule may not be critical to the cell's continued function. However, the reaction products may be capable of damaging the critical targets, provided that they can diffuse to them and interact before being converted to nontoxic elements by other chemical interactions. (For the OH radical produced by the interaction of radiation with H_2O in the cell, the diffusion distance is about 2 nm.) This is the "indirect" mechanism of action. All forms of radiation interact by both mechanisms, but because of the smaller amount of energy deposited by low-LET radiation, it primarily interacts through the indirect mechanism. High-LET radiation kills a significant number of cells via the direct mechanism. Comparing the biologic effects of low- and high-LET radiation provides a way of studying the results of these two processes.

Perhaps the simplest biologic experiment is to irradiate a colony of cells with different amounts of a given type of radiation and see how many are alive and able to reproduce afterward. This is done by plating the cells out on a new growth medium and counting the resulting colonies. This assays for a reproductive viability that is the quantity of paramount importance in tumor control. The radiation is given in a single dose, and the cells are plated out immediately.

A plot of the surviving fraction of cells as a function of the radiation dose is shown in Figure 3-3. By convention, the surviving cell fraction is plotted on a logarithmic scale, and the radiation dose is plotted on a linear scale. This curve is representative of most mammalian cells. Consider the solid curve, which represents the survival data. Note that there are two distinct regions to the curve. There is an initial region for low

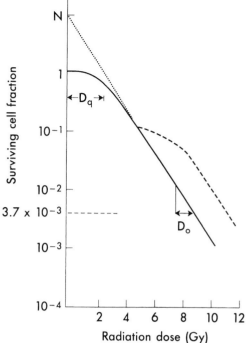

Figure 3-3. A representative cell survival curve *(solid line)* for mammalian cells exposed to single doses of radiation. The surviving cell fraction is plotted on a logarithmic scale, and the radiation dose is plotted on a linear scale. D_q characterizes the width of the shoulder region, which in target theory also may be characterized by the extrapolation number, N. D_o characterizes the slope of the "straight line" portion of the curve. The *dotted line* shows the extrapolation of the linear portion of the curve back to the abscissa. The *dashed line* shows the regeneration of the cell survival curve if, after giving a certain amount of radiation, 6 to 8 hours are allowed to pass before additional radiation is given. (Redrawn from Hall EJ: *Radiobiology for the radiologist,* Philadelphia, 1994, JB Lippincott.)

radiation doses, where the slope of the curve is shallow. In this region, small incremental changes in the amount of radiation are not very effective at increasing the number of cells that are killed. This is called the *shoulder* region, and its width is characterized by the parameter D_q. It is the distance along the dose axis at a surviving fraction of unity between the abscissa and the point where the extrapolated linear portion of the curve is intersected. It is a measure of the ability of the cells to repair small amounts of radiation damage.

At higher doses of radiation, the curve becomes a straight line on a semilog plot. Its slope is characterized by D_o, which is the incremental dose change required to reduce the surviving cell fraction to $1/e$ of its value. The steeper the slope in this region, the smaller is the value of D_o and the more radiosensitive is the cell line. When extrapolated back to a zero radiation dose, it intersects the abscissa at a value N. A curve of this type can be modeled using the equation

$$S = 1 - [1 - \exp(-D/D_0)]^N$$

where S is the surviving fraction, D is the radiation dose, and N and D_0 are as indicated in the figure. In target theory, N can be thought of as the number of distinct targets in the cell that should receive one radiation "hit" before the cell is inactivated. Other parameters also can be introduced into the analysis by requiring more than one radiation hit to inactivate a given target, but such refinements are beyond the scope of this overview. Radiobiologic data also can be analyzed using a linear-quadratic model of the form

$$S = \exp(-\alpha D - \beta D^2)$$

where α and β are simply parameters used to fit the curve over some restricted dose range.[40] Large $\beta{:}\alpha$ ratios correspond to curves with large shoulder regions. There is one final point to note from Figure 3-3. If 5 Gy are given, resulting in a 10% cell survival, and then 6 to 8 hours pass before giving additional radiation, the shoulder region of the survival curve is regenerated as shown by the dashed curve. During the waiting period, the cells have regained most of their original ability to recover from small doses of radiation. This is called *sublethal damage repair.*

The basic features of the cell survival curves can be qualitatively understood in terms of the DNA repair processes as outlined in Figure 3-4. The complementary strands of the helix are represented by the parallel straight lines, and the base pairings between the strands are represented by the open circles and dots that link the lines. In the upper panel, a photon schematically interacts with one strand of the DNA, which could either be via the direct or the indirect mechanism, with the particular nature of the damage event being irrelevant to the present discussion. What is important is that only one strand of the DNA is affected. Most cells contain repair enzymes that can excise the damaged portion and then, using the information on the complementary strand, can reproduce the damaged portion. This is what is taking place in the shoulder region of the cell survival curve. If small amounts of radiation are given, there is a likelihood that many cells will experience only one damage event that can be repaired in this manner. However, when larger amounts of radiation are given, a situation as shown in the lower panel occurs. Now many of the cells experience multiple damage events, and there is increased probability that some cells will have damage to both DNA strands. When the cell attempts to repair the radiation damage, a portion of both strands is excised, and a portion of the genetic information is lost. If this information loss occurs in a "silent" region of the DNA, the cell continues to live. If the information loss occurs in a key area of the genome, then the cell ultimately dies. This is the situation that occurs in the straight portion of the cell survival curve.

Relative Biologic Effectiveness and Oxygen Enhancement Ratio

High-LET radiation deposits so much energy as it goes through the cell that radiation damage events are

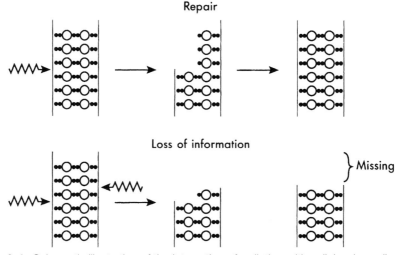

Figure 3-4. Schematic illustration of the interaction of radiation with cellular deoxyribonucleic acid (DNA). In the upper portion, the radiation interacts with one strand of the DNA, and using the appropriate repair enzymes, the cell can excise the damaged portion and reproduce the affected region using the genetic information on the complementary strand. In the lower portion, the radiation interacts with both strands of the DNA. When the cell attempts to repair the radiation damage, genetic information is lost.

clustered closely in space and time, which means that if one strand of the DNA is damaged, there is a high probability that the other strand also will be damaged. Thus, the situation as shown in the lower panel of Figure 3-4 occurs, with an increasing portion of the radiation damage being irreparable. As the LET of the radiation is increased, we expect to see the shoulder of the cell survival curve decrease (i.e., $D_q \rightarrow 0$) and the slope of the straight portion of the curve become steeper (i.e., $D_o \rightarrow 0$). This effect is shown in Figure 3-5, which shows survival curves for human kidney cells exposed to 250 kVp x-rays, 15 MeV neutrons from a DT generator, and 4 MeV α-particles. The LET of the radiation increases as indicated, and the curves change as expected.

Because the shapes of the cell survival curves shown in Figure 3-5 differ according to the type of radiation used, it is difficult to define biologically equivalent doses for therapeutic purposes. Consider the neutron and the x-ray curves, for example. If one chooses as an endpoint the amount of radiation required to kill 99% of the cells, this requires about 9.3 Gy of x-rays but only about 4.2 Gy of neutrons. Hence on a physical dose basis, the neutrons are more effective, and a relative biologic effectiveness (RBE) of 9.3/4.2 = 2.2 can be defined. If one chooses as an endpoint the amount of radiation required to kill 50% of the cells, then the respective doses are 2.8 Gy of

x-rays and 1.1 Gy of neutrons for an RBE of 2.5. This situation illustrates a general phenomenon: because of the increased shoulder on the cell survival curves for low-LET radiation, the RBE for neutrons and other high-LET radiation increases with lower dose increments. The change is greatest for cell lines that have the largest shoulders on the low-LET curves (e.g., gut, nerve tissue) and is smallest for cell lines having small shoulders (e.g., bone marrow, germ cells).[38] In the early days of neutron radiotherapy, physicians did not appreciate the dependence of the RBE on dose size and tissue type, which led to a high incidence of treatment-related complications. These effects now are being considered, and the incidence of complications is much lower.

Previously in this chapter, it was noted that low-LET radiation primarily killed cells through the indirect mechanism, which involved the radiation interacting with molecules in the cell cytoplasm. The sequence of chemical reactions that can take place is complex, but at some point, a free radical generally is involved. A free radical is a chemical species that contains an unpaired electron and is highly reactive. Oxygen acts to stabilize the free radicals, thus allowing them to diffuse to the DNA or other target regions where they react chemically to produce damage. An obvious question is how great an oxygen concentration is required. Experiments have been performed on many species of bacteria, yeasts, and mammalian cells. The overall conclusions are summarized in Figure 3-6, which shows the relative radiosensitivity as a function of the oxygen concentration in torr (1 torr = 1 mm Hg). Note that the radiosensitivity does not change much until the oxygen concentration decreases below about 20 torr, and then it decreases

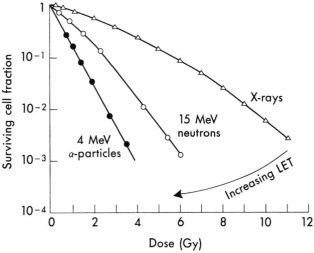

Figure 3-5. Survival curves for cultured human cells exposed to radiation having different linear energy transfers (LETs). The *triangles* indicate data for 250 kVp x-rays, the *open circles* indicate data for 15 MeV neutrons from a DT reaction, and the *closed circles* indicate data for 4 MeV α-particles. Note that with increasing LET, the shoulder on the curve decreases, and the slope of the straight portion increases. (Redrawn from Hall EJ: *Radiobiology for the radiologist,* Philadelphia, 1994, JB Lippincott; original data from Broerse JJ, Bardensen GW, van Kersen GR: *Int J Radiat Biol* 13:559, 1967.)

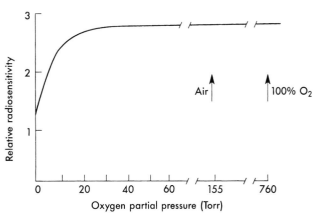

Figure 3-6. Plot of relative radiosensitivity of cells as a function of the oxygen concentration in Torr. Well-oxygenated cells are 2.5 to 3.0 times more sensitive than their hypoxic counterparts. Oxygen concentrations for room air and 100% O_2 at 1 atmosphere of pressure are indicated by the arrows. This curve is schematic and is not meant to represent any particular cell line.

fairly rapidly. At essentially 0 torr, the cells are 2.5 to 3.0 times less radiosensitive than they are on the flat portion of the curve. Healthy tissues of the body are at oxygen concentrations between that of arterial and venous blood—40 to 100 torr—and so are on the radiosensitive portion of the curve. However, large tumors tend to outgrow their blood supply and develop regions of necrosis surrounded by cells in a very hypoxic state. These tumor cells lie on the radioresistant portion of the curve, and this is thought to be one reason why large tumors are not as well controlled by radiotherapy as small ones.

One way of avoiding this problem is to use a mode of radiotherapy that is not as dependent on the presence of oxygen for cell killing. One possibility is to use high-LET radiation, for which the direct mechanism of cell killing is more important. Figure 3-7 shows cell survival curves for human kidney cells irradiated in well-oxygenated conditions (open circles) and

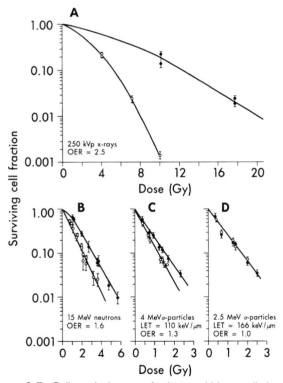

Figure 3-7. Cell survival curves for human kidney cells irradiated during hypoxic and well-oxygenated conditions for radiation beams having different LET values. The *open circles* represent the well-oxygenated cells, and the *closed circles* represent the hypoxic cells. **A,** 250 kVp x-rays; **B,** 15 MeV neutrons from a DT generator; **C,** 4 MeV a-particles; and **D,** 2.5 MeV a-particles. Values of the oxygen enhancement ratio (OER) are indicated in the respective panels. The OER decreases as the LET increases. (Redrawn from Hall EJ: *Radiobiology for the radiologist,* Philadelphia, 1994, JB Lippincott; original data from Broerse JJ, Bardensen GW, van Kersen GR: *Int J Radiat Biol* 13:559, 1967.)

hypoxic conditions (closed circles). If a 90% cell kill is chosen as the endpoint, then for 250 kVp x-rays, it takes 2.5 times as much radiation to kill hypoxic cells as it does well-oxygenated cells. The oxygen enhancement ratio (OER) is 2.5. As the LET of the radiation increases—going to 15 MeV neutrons from a DT reaction, then to 4 MeV α-particles, and finally to 2.5 MeV α-particles—the OER decreases to 1. This shows the effect of the increasing importance of the direct mechanism as the LET of the radiation increases. In general, the OER decreases with increasing LET until a value of 1 is reached, for a LET of about 150 keV/micron.

Cell Cycle Effects

Cycling mammalian cells proliferate by undergoing mitotic divisions. To define terms, take mitosis or M phase as a starting point. After this comes a "resting" phase, G_1, before the cell starts undergoing DNA synthesis. After DNA synthesis (S), there is another resting phase, G_2, before the cell again enters mitosis. Actively proliferating cells will enter G_1 again after mitosis. Some cells can enter a quiescent or G_0 phase after mitosis, where they are actively producing proteins but not preparing for proliferation.

Although it is well recognized that many chemotherapeutic agents act at specific points along the cell cycle, it is not commonly appreciated that cells also vary in their degree of radiosensitivity according to their position in the cell cycle. Synchronously dividing cell populations are needed in experiments that measure this effect. One way of producing such a cell population is to exploit the fact that, at the time of mitosis, many cells growing in monolayers attached to the surface of culture containers will take on a spherical shape and become loosely attached to the vessel wall. If the container is subjected to a gentle shaking motion, these cells will become detached and float to the surface of the growth medium where they can be collected. These cells can then be inoculated into a fresh growth medium, wherein they will grow in synchrony through several cell cycles. Radiobiologic experiments can be performed on these cells at different times after "shake-off," and they can be caught at different points along the cycle.

The result of radiosensitivity measurements for typical mammalian cells is shown in Figure 3-8. Relative radioresistance is shown along the abscissa as a function of position along the cell cycle. The position of the cells along the cycle is shown at the top of the figure. The cells are radiosensitive early in the M phase but become more resistant toward the end of this phase. They are resistant in the early G_1 phase but then become more sensitive in the late G_1 and early S phases. They then become more resistant

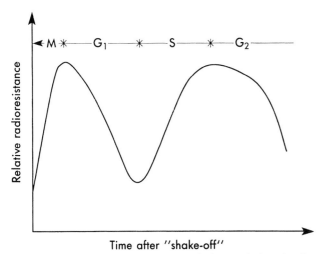

Figure 3-8. Schematic illustration of the variation in the radiosensitivity of mammalian cells with their position along the cell cycle. The abscissa shows relative radioresistance as a function of time after "shake-off." The relative position along the cell cycle is indicated along the top of the curve. The curve is schematic and not meant to represent any particular cell line.

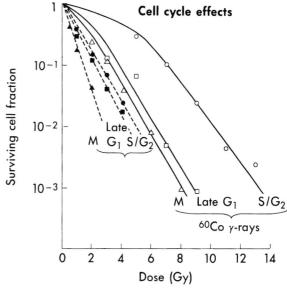

Figure 3-9. Cell survival curves for synchronously dividing Chinese hamster ovary cells at different points along the cell cycle. The *open symbols* indicate cells irradiated with ^{60}Co γ-rays, and the *closed symbols* indicate cells irradiated with a 50 MeV D→Be neutron beam from the TAMVEC facility. The *circles* represent cells in late S and early G_2; the *squares* represent cells in late G_1; and the *triangles* represent cells in mitosis. (Redrawn from Gragg RL and others: *Radiat Res* 76:283, 1978; and Meyn RE: personal communication, 1984.)

again in the late S and early G_2 phases. Cell lines vary in the time they require to go through the cycle, but this is mostly caused by different lengths of the G_1 phase. The exact mechanisms underlying this change in radiosensitivity are not clear, but it is interesting to note that at the beginning of mitosis, the DNA in the chromosomes aggregates into a discrete state; in the late S phase, the DNA content of the cell has doubled. These points in the cycle correspond, respectively, to the points of maximum and minimum radiosensitivity.

Other variations in radiosensitivity may correlate with different amounts of sulfhydryl compounds in the cell. Sulfhydryl compounds act as free radical scavengers and so act to protect the cell from the indirect effects of radiation. These levels can be modified by radioprotectors that generally contain a thiol group.

Figure 3-9 shows specific cell survival curves for Chinese hamster ovary cells at different points along the cell cycle.[30,31,46] The open symbols are for cells exposed to γ-rays from a ^{60}Co source, and the closed symbols are for cells exposed to a fast neutron beam. Note that for each form of radiation there is the same type of variation along the cell cycle, but the degree of variation is about a factor of 4 less for the neutron beam. OERs are about the same for different points along the cycle, so this represents an effect apart from this.

Many tumor systems contain an appreciable number of cells in a "noncycling" or G_o phase. Radiation damage to cells in this phase cannot be monitored

until the cells are recruited back into the cycle and until it can be seen whether they produce viable progeny. Noncycling cells can be produced in the laboratory by allowing them to grow in a medium until some key nutrient is exhausted. Cell proliferation then stops, and, if the cells are kept in this suboptimal medium, the number of cells remains constant. Such cells are said to be in the plateau phase of growth[37] and are mostly in the G_o phase. These cells can be irradiated and then can either be immediately inoculated into fresh growth medium or can be incubated for a period in the suboptimal medium before the inoculation takes place. Once they are placed in the fresh growth medium, they return to their normal cycling mode, although the cell survival curve varies depending on whether they have been incubated for a time before being placed in the fresh medium.

This effect is shown in Figure 3-10. The circular data points indicate cells treated with ^{60}Co radiation, and, for a given dose of radiation, there are more surviving cells after an 8-hour delay than if the cells immediately started cycling. This effect is called *potentially lethal damage repair* because the effect of the radiation damage depends on what happens to the cell after the irradiation. The dose is only potentially—but not necessarily—lethal to the cell because

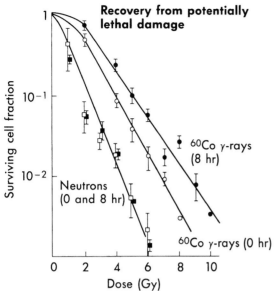

Figure 3-10. Potentially lethal damage repair for Chinese hamster ovary cells irradiated in the plateau phase. The circular data points correspond to cells irradiated with ^{60}Co photons, and the square data points correspond to cells irradiated with a 50 MeV D→Be neutron beam from the TAMVEC facility. The *open symbols* indicate cells plated out immediately, and the *closed symbols* represent cells plated out after an 8-hour delay. Surviving cell fraction is plotted along the abscissa as a function of the radiation dose. (Redrawn from Gragg RL, Humphrey RM, Meyn RE: *Radiat Res* 71:461, 1977.)

the cell can repair itself before reentering the mitotic cycle where the damage is expressed. The square data points are for cells irradiated with 50 MeV D → Be neutrons. For high-LET radiation, potentially lethal damage cannot be repaired (or can be repaired only to a limited extent), a fact that may be important in certain clinical settings.

THERAPEUTIC WINDOW CONCEPT

Dose-response curves for tumor control and normal tissue damage are sigmoidal in shape. Whether radiation can safely control a given tumor depends on the relative positions of these two curves. Dose-response curves for a "radiosensitive" tumor are shown in Figure 3-11. Here, giving a therapeutic dose of radiation results in a 95% probability of tumor control and only a 5% probability of normal tissue complication. A large gap exists between the two curves (i.e., a wide "therapeutic window"). This should be contrasted with the situation shown in Figure 3-12 for a "radioresistant" tumor. In this situation, a dose of radiation that would result in a 95% probability of tumor control would result in an unacceptably high probability of normal tissue damage. Giving doses that are within the limits of normal tissue tolerance would yield only a low likelihood of tumor control, and the separation

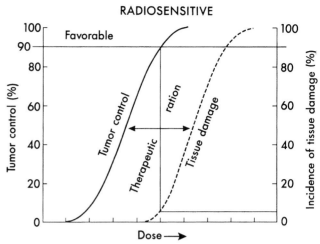

Figure 3-11. Dose-response curves for tumor control *(solid line)* and for healthy tissue damage *(dashed line)* for a "radiosensitive" tumor. This corresponds to a wide "therapeutic window," in that doses that yield a high probability of tumor control have a low probability of causing healthy tissue damage.

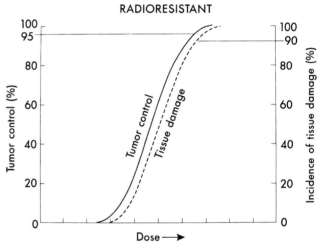

Figure 3-12. Dose-response curves for tumor control *(solid line)* and for healthy tissue damage *(dashed line)* for a "radioresistant" tumor. This corresponds to a narrow "therapeutic window," in that doses that yield a high probability of tumor control have a high probability of causing healthy tissue damage.

between the two curves is narrow. Clearly, the concept of a therapeutic window depends on the radiobiological properties of the tumor and the healthy tissue in the irradiated volume.

In general, local control of tumors can be improved by better dose localization. This means moving higher on the tumor-response curve without moving higher on the normal tissue-complication curve, or by exploiting some intrinsic difference in the properties of the tumor and normal tissues, which effectively widens the gap between the two curves. Three-dimensional treatment planning and delivery, brachytherapy, intraoperative radiotherapy, and the use of charged particle radiation are examples of better dose localization; the use of high-LET radiation, altered fractionation schedules, radiosensitization agents, and radioprotective agents are examples of exploiting some intrinsic difference in the properties of the tumor and normal tissues. Treatment paradigms are rapidly developing in the use of radiotherapy to treat head and neck cancers as the physics of the delivery combine with the biology of the tumors and normal tissues.

CLINICAL CORRELATION
Fractionated Radiotherapy

The intent of clinical radiotherapy is to sterilize tumors and at the same time to avoid untoward damage to the healthy tissues in the treatment volume. To accomplish this goal, different ways of parceling out the daily dose of radiation or fractionation have evolved over time. The spectrum of response to different dose fractionation between normal tissues and tumors can be summarized by what are known as the four R's of radiotherapy: (1) Repair (of sublethal damage); (2) Redistribution (across the cell cycle); (3) Repopulation; and (4) Reoxygenation. Fractionated radiotherapy has evolved to exploit the differences in these effects between tumors and healthy tissues. With few exceptions, radiotherapy works not because tumors are intrinsically more radiosensitive than normal tissue (i.e., a smaller value of D_o) but because normal tissues are better at repair and repopulation. These four R's also account for different response rates between tumors.

The tumor and the healthy tissue consist of heterogeneous populations in regard to the timing of the cells in the cycle. In addition, the tumor may have an appreciable number of its cells in a hypoxic state. Figure 3-13 shows what happens when such a mixture of cells is irradiated with equal-dose fractions of magnitude D. The first dose increment preferentially kills the cells that are well oxygenated and are in radiosensitive portions of the cell cycle. If several hours pass before delivering the next dose increment, during this period, there is repair of sublethal damage. With the killing of a substantial number of cells, there is less competition for the available oxygen, hence some of the formerly hypoxic cells can reoxygenate. Also, some of the cells can proceed along the cell cycle and thus be in a more radiosensitive phase when the next dose of radiation is delivered. Assuming that both effects occur, the result is the solid curve shown in Figure 3-13. If there is no reoxygenation or redistribution throughout the cell cycle, then the result is the dotted curve, which shows less cell kill because the remaining cells are in a radioresistant state.

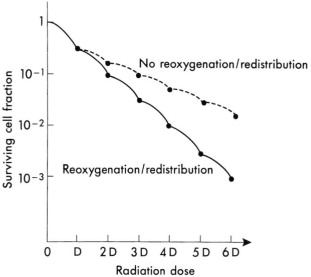

Figure 3-13. Illustration of the effects of fractionated radiotherapy on a heterogeneous cell population. Surviving cell fraction is plotted along the abscissa as a function of the radiation dose. The dose is given in increments, D, with the time interval between successive doses being long enough to allow for sublethal damage repair. The initial dose increment kills a greater fraction of well-oxygenated cells than it does their hypoxic counterparts. It also preferentially kills those cells in the radiosensitive phases of the cell cycle. The *solid curve* indicates when the remaining cells reoxygenate and redistribute along the cell cycle before the next radiation dose is given. The *dashed curve* indicates when there is no reoxygenation or redistribution, and successive radiation doses are delivered to a more radioresistant cell population. The figure is schematic and is not meant to represent any particular cell line.

These are not the only effects; there is continued cell division and regrowth during the time interval between radiation fractions. These tumor repopulation kinetics have not been considered in Figure 3-13. To maximize the cell kill, it is important that the size of the dose fractions be greater than D_q—the width of the shoulder region of the single fraction cell survival curve.

Time-dose considerations are important in estimating the effect of a given total radiation dose. If the dose were given in a single fraction, then the healthy tissues would experience more cell killing than if it were given in a fractionated manner. This difference occurs because single fractions allow no opportunity for sublethal damage repair. In general, smaller total radiation doses given over shorter total treatment times produce the same normal tissue effects as larger total radiation doses given over longer time intervals. The classic measurements that illustrate this point are the isoeffect measurements on skin that were made by Strandquist.[52] He showed that the isoeffect lines for various degrees of skin damage and for curing skin cancer were straight when plotted on a log-log scale of total dose versus time. Moreover, the lines appeared to have the same slope (i.e., were parallel). The required dose to produce a given effect was proportional to time to the 0.33 power. Ellis[23] extended this concept to clinical radiotherapy by allocating a portion of the exponent 0.33 to the overall treatment time, T, and a portion to the number of fractions, N. He defined the nominal standard dose (NSD) by

$$NSD = D_t/T^{0.11}N^{0.24}$$

where D_t is the total radiation dose. The exponents in this expression are for skin and no doubt vary for other tissues.

The linear-quadratic model discussed earlier in this chapter provides another way of comparing the biologic effectiveness of different radiation schedules. Assuming that there are n separated doses of radiation of magnitude, D, and neglecting the effect of cellular proliferation, the cumulative biologic effect of the treatments can be given by

$$E = nD(\alpha + \beta D) = \alpha D_t(1 + D\beta/\alpha)$$

where D_t is the total dose of radiation. Dividing through by α the following is obtained

$$E/\alpha = D_t(1 + D\beta/\alpha)$$

where E/α is the biologically effective dose. For purposes of comparing radiation schedules, $\alpha/\beta = 3$ can be used for late-responding tissues, and $\alpha/\beta = 10$ can be used for early-responding tissues (i.e., acute effects). It is also possible to modify this expression to crudely account for tumor proliferation (repopulation) during the radiation course.[38]

Altered Fractionation Schedules

The highly fractionated radiotherapy schemes used today are the result of many years of clinical experience, but radiobiologic considerations may provide guidance for their improvement. For example, acute radiation side effects, such as mucositis and pharyngeal edema, are caused by changes in tissues that are composed of rapidly proliferating cells. Late effects, such as subcutaneous fibrosis, vascular damage, radiation necrosis, and spinal cord injury, are caused by changes in tissues composed of more slowly proliferating cells. Radiobiologic measurements indicate that for low-LET radiation, the tissues experiencing late effects are characterized by cell survival curves having large shoulders.[61] The late effects limit the total dose that can be delivered in the treatment of head and neck cancer. Hence, a logical approach would be to give smaller radiation treatment fractions so as not to exceed the shoulder on the late effects tissue curves and then give a higher total dose, which modeling pre-

dicts would yield greater tumor control. This would effectively widen the therapeutic window. Note that the assumption is implicitly made that the tumor will behave like the rapidly proliferating healthy tissues and thus will not have a large shoulder on its cell survival curve. To avoid too great a prolongation of the overall treatment time and hence allowing tumor repopulation kinetics to dominate, multiple daily fractions must be given. A sufficient time interval (generally ~6 hours) should elapse between the multiple daily treatments to allow for adequate repair of sublethal and potentially lethal damage in the healthy tissues. Several possible fractionation schemes are outlined in Figure 3-14. Discussion of these schemes follows.

Hyperfractionation is the administration of multiple daily doses of radiation of such a size that the overall treatment time is about the same as for a conventionally fractionated course of once-a-day radiotherapy. Several randomized phase III clinical trials recently have been completed using the hyperfractionation approach.* None of these trials has shown a significant improvement in overall survival, but local and regional control is better by 10% to 15% compared with standard fraction radiotherapy. More important, several radiobiological principles have been verified, including the ability of normal tissue to repair much of the radiation damage in time intervals of approximately 4 to 6 hours. The acute side effects of hyperfractionation are generally slightly greater than with standard fractionation, but the long-term effects appear to be very similar.

Accelerated fractionation is the administration of multiple daily radiation doses of larger size to reduce the overall treatment time. Where there are innumerable schemes that can be used, we will discuss three basic types utilizing the nomenclature of Ang.[5]

Type A

One of the more extreme accelerated schedules is the continuous hyperfractionated accelerated radiotherapy treatment (CHART) regimen.[17] This regimen consists of giving three daily radiation treatments of 1.5 Gy each for a total dose of 54 Gy without giving any weekend breaks. This was compared in a randomized study with standard fractionation (66 Gy in 33 fractions) for head and neck cancers. As might be expected, acute radiation reactions in the CHART arm have been severe, but resolve more rapidly. There was a trend toward improved primary tumor control in the CHART arm but no significant difference in overall survival. This study does demonstrate that tumor repopulation can be addressed by hyperfrac-

---

*References 4, 15, 17, 28, 54, 59, 60.

FRACTIONATION SCHEMES

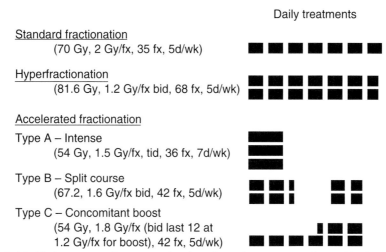

Daily treatments

Standard fractionation
(70 Gy, 2 Gy/fx, 35 fx, 5d/wk)

Hyperfractionation
(81.6 Gy, 1.2 Gy/fx bid, 68 fx, 5d/wk)

Accelerated fractionation

Type A – Intense
(54 Gy, 1.5 Gy/fx, tid, 36 fx, 7d/wk)

Type B – Split course
(67.2, 1.6 Gy/fx bid, 42 fx, 5d/wk)

Type C – Concomitant boost
(54 Gy, 1.8 Gy/fx (bid last 12 at
1.2 Gy/fx for boost), 42 fx, 5d/wk)

Figure 3-14. Various types of treatment fractionation schemes currently used in the treatment of head and neck cancer.

tionation since the local control with CHART is slightly better than standard course radiotherapy, even at a lower dose. Further studies with CHART revealed that dose escalation was possible and became the bases for a phase III study to be discussed later.[15]

Type B

To reduce the acute effects of treatment, some fractionation schemes build a "planned break" into the regime to allow for recovery of the mucosa. Wang has used such a schema in the treatment of advanced head and neck tumors.[59,60] He used 1.6 Gy fractions twice daily, which resulted in an acute mucosal reaction that required a planned two-week break in the middle of therapy. Unfortunately, one would also expect the tumor to repopulate during this time.

Type C

Another version of accelerated radiation that attempts to limit the healthy tissue acute reactions is the concomitant boost regimen proposed by Ang and others, which delivers the accelerated portion of the radiation only during the last phase of treatment.[4] In this approach, the volume of tissue receiving the twice-daily treatments is limited to the primary target volume, and no breaks in treatment are given. A further theoretical advantage is that the accelerated portion of the radiation is given at a time when the proliferation rate has been increased for the tumor and the healthy tissues.

In 1991, the Radiation Therapy Oncology Group (RTOG) undertook a national, multi-centered randomized study comparing conventional fractionation

(70 Gy in 2 Gy fractions a day, 5 days a week for 7 weeks) vs hyperfractionation (81.6 Gy in 1.2 Gy fractions twice a day, 5 days a week for 7 weeks) vs accelerated fractionation with break (67.2 Gy in 1.6 Gy fractions twice a day, 5 days a week for 6 weeks with a 2-week break after 38.4 Gy) vs concomitant boost (72 Gy in 1.8 Gy fractions, 5 days a week for 6 weeks with a concomitant boost of 1.5 Gy delivered as a second daily fraction for the last 12 treatments).[28] A total of 1073 analyzable patients with locally advanced head and neck cancers were evaluated. The overall survival was not significantly different in each arm. The hyperfractionation and concomitant boost arms had significantly better local-regional control than those treated with standard fractionation and accelerated fractionation with break. As expected, patients in the non-standard fractionation arms had increased acute toxicity, but the late toxicity was similar across all treatment arms.

Intensity Modulated Radiation Therapy

The goal in the delivery of radiation therapy is to determine what is tumor or has a significant risk for harboring tumor (i.e., lymph nodes) and what is normal healthy tissue. The ultimate delivery of radiotherapy would be to deliver the entire dose to the tumor and none to normal tissue. In some situations, this is possible by placing radioactive sources directly into the tumor, but this is impossible if the area of concern involves too large of a region. When radiation therapy is given externally, the goal is to maximize the dose to the targeted area and minimize the dose to normal tissue. Our technical ability to accomplish this has significantly improved with the use of Intensity Modulated Radiation Therapy (IMRT).

IMRT is the logical progression in developing improved conformal therapy. Figure 3-15 illustrates this. During the early years of radiotherapy, fields were limited in shape and in direction they could be aimed (i.e., AP/PA and right and left laterals). Our subsequent ability to shape the beam with either customized Cerrobend blocks or multileaf collimators allowed the field to be shaped to cover the target of interest. When multiple beams are used in three-dimensional (3D) conformal therapy, the resulting isodose curves can conform closely to the shape of the tumor (Figure 3-15, *B*). However, there are still times when 3D conformal therapy is not able to deliver a better therapeutic dose because the tumor is in close proximity to normal tissues that should be spared.

IMRT allows the dose across a treatment field to be delivered as a gradient. This can be accomplished in several ways. Dynamic IMRT delivers the treatment much like a tomotherapy unit that circles around the patient in thin slices. As the gantry goes around the patient, the blocking leaves in the treatment machine move to change shape with the tumor as the beam moves. Each slice is treated before moving on to the next slice. "Step and shoot" IMRT is similar to more traditional 3D conformal therapy in that multiple beam arrangements are used during the treatment. Each beam arrangement then has multiple field shapes. The field shape can be changed in a stepwise manner or dynamically. In a stepwise delivery system, each beam arrangement will start with a large field and a portion of the daily dose will be delivered. The field shape will then be modified and another portion of the dose delivered. Usually critical or normal structures are blocked when the field is modified. The result is a much steeper dose gradient between target areas and normal–critical areas. The other type of delivery system is step and shoot IMRT that is a hybrid of the stepwise system and true dynamic IMRT. Multiple beam arrangements are used but the leaves that control the field shape are changed in real time. Thus, when a specific beam is to be used for treatment, the shape of the field is changed so that normal/critical tissue can be spared. The result with any one of these three techniques is a sharper gradient between target tissue and normal–critical tissue. True dynamic IMRT is much quicker in its ability to deliver treatment, but technically more difficult to do quality assurance. Although the step and shoot techniques can be a little slower, verifying quality is easier since a single point can be used to reference the isocenter of the treatment.

The University of California at San Francisco has developed an extensive IMRT program for treating nasopharyngeal carcinoma.[44] Lee and others have reported on 67 patients that were treated with some variation of IMRT as discussed earlier. The patient population had some heterogeneity in treatment in that some patients also received chemotherapy (50 patients) and some had brachytherapy or gamma knife boost (27 patients). The four-year estimated overall survival was 88%, which appears to be better than previously reported results of around 60 to 80%. More important, they were able to deliver between 65 to 70 Gy to the primary targeted volume with less acute and long-term toxicity. The nasopharynx is a challenging area anatomically to target with increased doses because of its close proximity to critical structures (e.g., optic apparatus) and normal tissues (e.g.,

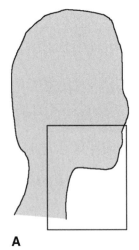
A

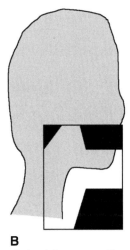
B

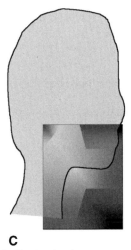
C

Figure 3-15. A, Initially there was little ability to modify radiotherapy fields. **B,** Customized blocking allowed the fields to be shaped to conform to the area of interest. **C,** IMRT allows the intensity of the dose to be varied across the field.

parotid glands) being in the path of externally delivered radiotherapy.

The use of IMRT is still developing. There is now a paradigm shift in how head and neck cancers are to be treated with IMRT. With 3D conformal therapy, a large initial field was treated to a specific dose that was intended to be homogeneous across the field. That field may have included lymphatics at risk, as well as normal tissue such as salivary glands. The primary tumor could then be boosted, but the total dose would be limited by nearby critical structures. Researchers hope that IMRT will afford the flexibility of better sparing of normal tissues, increased dose delivery to targeted tissue, and steeper gradients between targeted tissue and critical structures. It will also be important to better define the areas at risk that need to be treated.

Intraoperative Radiotherapy

During the late 20th and early 21st centuries, researchers in Japan and the United States have been increasingly interested in radiotherapy directly administered to the exposed tumor bed at the time of surgery. Intraoperative radiotherapy (IORT) is given as a single, large fraction using either orthovoltage x-rays or megavoltage electrons. In this approach, it is often possible to move critical structures outside the radiation fields, and the surgeon can aid in identifying the areas at highest risk for residual tumor. A few institutions have dedicated equipment in operating rooms, but the majority of facilities offering IORT transport patients from the operating room to a sterilized unit in the radiation oncology center where the radiation actually is delivered.

Because the biologic effectiveness of a single large dose of radiation is much greater than if the same amount of radiation was given in multiple increments, the total dose given intraoperatively should be reduced compared with that given in a course of fractionated radiotherapy. Most of the IORT experience is for tumors of the abdomen and pelvis, but some general guidelines can be given regarding the tolerance of certain classes of normal structures of importance in the head and neck region. Major blood vessels tolerate single doses in the range of 20 to 25 Gy, whereas damage to peripheral nerves has been noted at doses higher than 20 Gy.[41,48]

IORT has shown benefit in case-specific situations. A Japanese group reported on 25 patients with advanced or recurrent head and neck cancer treated with IORT at the time of surgery.[55] Their two-year cumulative local control was 0% for gross residual disease, 54.5% for microscopic residual disease, and 81.8% in patients with a close margin after their resections. Of the 22 patients, 5 experienced late complications that included osteoradionecrosis and carotid artery rupture. The incidence of complications increased in those patients that received over 20 Gy in a single dose. There may also be some benefit in the use of IORT in patients who undergo surgical resection with palliative intention in that the time-to-tumor progression may be delay with IORT.[50] Clinicians from Mayo have suggested that a dose of 12.5 Gy is safe and improves tumor control and survival in patients with microscopic residual disease in areas that are difficult to resect (i.e., the skull base).[48]

Brachytherapy

Many radioactive isotopes are used in modern radiotherapy practice. Although ^{226}Ra and ^{137}Cs needles may still be used for implants in certain cases, the trend now is toward afterloading techniques using ^{192}Ir sources. These sources produce a lower-energy γ-ray, thus simplifying the radiation protection requirements associated with routine patient care. These sources are left in place for a specified time and then are removed. Alternatively, permanent implants using ^{198}Au and ^{125}I can be used. These implants deliver their total radiation dose over the effective lifetime of the radioactive material.

One obvious advantage to using implants for a portion of the planned radiotherapy is better dose localization, which results in less radiation damage to the healthy tissue surrounding the tumor. Another advantage is the relatively prolonged time over which the radiation is delivered. External-beam radiation is given at the rate of 1.5 to 2.0 Gy per minute. A typical ^{192}Ir implant delivers its dose at the rate of 0.4 to 0.8 Gy per hour. This can be thought of as continuous fractionation, and it allows for healthy tissue repair and reoxygenation of the tumor throughout the time course of the implant. A typical ^{125}I implant delivers its dose at an even slower rate. Often high total doses in the range of 100 to 200 Gy are given, but one half of the total dose is given during the first 60-day half-life, one-fourth of the total dose is given during the next 60-day half-life, and so on. The actual radiobiology of such extremely low-dose rates is somewhat uncertain.

More recently, high-dose-rate remote afterloading devices have been developed. These devices push a single, high-activity ^{192}Ir source through a set of interstitial catheters, and a computer program controls the source dwell time at various points throughout the implant. Typically, about 3.0 to 3.5 Gy is given to a distance of about 1 cm from the periphery of the catheters each treatment, and two daily treatments are given about 6 hours apart. Each treatment takes about 15 to 30 minutes, depending on the strength of the radioactive source and the complexity of the implant. There are approximate guidelines to determine how a radiation dose delivered in this manner corresponds to the more familiar doses delivered via low-dose-rate implants, but long-term late effects data are still being accrued.[10,57] Because these treatments are given in a shielded area in the radiation oncology department, no radioactive material is left in the catheters when patients return to their rooms, and the radiation protection problem is greatly reduced.

High-Linear Energy Transfer Radiation

Most clinical data on the use of high-LET radiation in the management of head and neck tumors are for fast neutrons. This will be the topic of this section.

Squamous Cell Carcinomas

The usefulness of fast neutron radiotherapy in the treatment of squamous cell carcinomas of the head and neck has been a controversial subject. The first reported work dates back to the 1940s when Stone and others conducted a series of clinical studies using an early cyclotron at Berkeley.[51] A total of 249 patients were treated, and about half of these patients had head and neck tumors. Although many dramatic tumor responses were reported, the late complication rate was unacceptably high. Interest in fast neutron radiotherapy waned until the late 1950s when a better understanding of fast neutron radiobiology indicated that most of Stone's patients had inadvertently received extremely high doses of radiation. Investigation of fast neutron radiotherapy then began at Hammersmith Hospital, and an early report again noted dramatic tumor response, but this time with a more acceptable complication rate.[12] Unfortunately, other trials in Europe and the United States failed to confirm this benefit.[21,22,33,34] They showed no improvement with neutron radiation in either local control at the primary site or in survival rates. However, they seemed to show improved local control for clinically positive neck nodes (45% vs 26%, $P = .004$).[32,34] This now can be qualitatively understood in terms of the basic radiation biology of these tumors. Using fast neutrons and conventional photon irradiation, Battermann and others measured the response rates of pulmonary metastases from various tumor histologies.[7] They found that the RBE for squamous cell tumors was about the same as for the normal tissue side effects (e.g., RBE of 3.0–3.8), so a therapeutic gain would not necessarily be expected if some other factor such as tumor hypoxia was not a problem or if OER effects would come into play. Guichard and others[36] have demonstrated in animal models that metastatic lymph nodes often have a greater fraction of hypoxic cells than primary tumors of equal size. Measurements of oxygen partial pressure in humans show that hypoxic regions within cervical lymph node metastases constitute

approximately 20% of their volume.[29] Hence, it may be that tumor hypoxia in enlarged cervical lymph nodes, and not at the primary tumor site, accounted for the clinical observations that were reported. In an attempt to resolve this matter, the RTOG undertook yet another randomized trial to study squamous cell tumors of the head and neck. These studies utilized modern neutron radiotherapy facilities and sophisticated treatment techniques, but again no overall benefit was noted for fast neutron radiotherapy for those with squamous cell tumors.[45]

Tumors that recur after initial radiotherapeutic or after surgical treatment represent another situation wherein high-LET radiotherapy may offer some benefits over conventional radiotherapy. Such recurrences may derive from clones of cells exhibiting a resistance to conventional photon irradiation. Furthermore, the initial treatment may have compromised the vascularity, and the recurrent tumors may have a greater degree of hypoxia than tumors treated *de novo*. Two nonrandomized clinical trials support this hypothesis. Fermi Laboratories reported an 85% initial response rate, a 45% complete response rate, and an ultimate local control rate of 35% in 20 patients irradiated with neutrons for squamous cell carcinoma recurrent in regions that had received previous photon irradiation.[49] A report from Hammersmith on nine similar patients showed an 89% complete remission rate and a 56% local control rate at 1 year.[24] The rate of major treatment complications was about 25%.

Salivary Gland Malignancies

Based on the radiobiologic data of Battermann and others, salivary gland tumors exhibit high RBEs for neutron irradiation.[7] They found an RBE of 8 for fractionated neutron radiation of adenoid cystic carcinoma metastatic to lung, which would indicate a large therapeutic gain factor in using neutrons to treat this tumor system. Phase II clinical trials and a randomized phase III study support this conclusion.

The randomized trial and the historical series are summarized in Table 3-1.[35,43] The data in this table are for patients treated for gross disease, either *de novo* or for tumor recurrent after surgery. Patients with microscopic residual disease after a surgical resection are not included. Although the number of patients in the randomized trial is small, the difference in the local control rates at 2 years is statistically significant ($P = .005$). The rates of complete tumor clearance in the cervical lymph nodes were six of seven (86%) for the neutron group and one of four (25%) for the photon group. There was an association between improved local control and survival rate at 2 years: 62% for the neutron group vs 25% for the photon group ($P = .1$). Given the dramatic differences

post-operative radiotherapy vs induction chemotherapy with cisplatin and fluorouracil followed by radiotherapy. Those patients on the sequential chemotherapy followed by radiotherapy were re-evaluated after the modality and were taken to surgery if there was not significant disease regression. A functioning larynx was maintained in 62% of the surviving patients in the chemotherapy followed by radiotherapy. Survival was not significantly different in the two treatment arms.

Intergroup trial R91-11 built on the results of the VA Laryngeal Study.[27] The three arms of this trial were induction chemotherapy vs radiotherapy alone vs radiotherapy with concurrent cisplatin. At two years, 88% of the concurrent chemoradiotherapy group had preserved their larynx, 74% for the induction chemotherapy followed by radiotherapy group, and 69% for the radiotherapy only group.

Currently, clinicians have shown more interest in using chemotherapy concomitantly with radiotherapy, which has greater potential for giving a synergistic rather than an additive effect. However, this regimen is also associated with increased acute toxicity. Large-scale, randomized clinical trials using this approach are only now being done. An early success of this approach is Intergroup Study 0099 for locally advanced nasopharyngeal cancer, which stopped early because an interim analysis showed a statistically significant advantage to the experimental arm.[3] In the experimental arm, patients were given concomitant chemotherapy consisting of cisplatinum at 100 mg/m^2 every 3 weeks along with radiotherapy followed by 4 cycles of consolidation chemotherapy with cisplatinum and 5-fluorouracil. In the control arm, patients were treated with standard fractionated radiotherapy. A significant improvement in overall survival was seen at 3 years with 78% survival in the chemoradiotherapy arms vs 47% in the radiotherapy only arm. Nasopharynx appears to behave differently from other head and neck cancers.

The second-generation chemoradiotherapy trials from the Intergroup looked at three different treatment arms in unresectable head and neck cancers (hypopharynx, larynx, oral cavity, base of tongue, and tonsil.)[2] The first arm was radiotherapy alone. The second arm was standard radiotherapy and concurrent cisplatin at 100 mg/m^2 on days 1, 22, and 43. The third arm was split course radiotherapy with concurrent cisplatin and fluorouracil. After two cycles of chemotherapy and 30 Gy, those patients with a complete response or who were still unresectable received another cycle of chemotherapy and another 30 to 40 Gy. Those who had a partial response went on to be resected. The projected 3-year overall survival was 23% for the radiotherapy alone group, 37% for the combined chemoradiotherapy group, and 27% for the split course chemoradiotherapy. Toxicity was much more significant for the combined modality groups. The role of combining chemotherapy and radiotherapy is still evolving. Work is continuing on ways to combine altered fractionation schemes and chemotherapy.

REFERENCES

1. http://www.xray.hmc.psu.edu/rci/ss9/ss9_2.html, http://www.xray.hmc.psu.edu/rci/ss9/ss9_1.html (Interesting review of the history of radiation therapy.)
2. Adelstein DJ and others: Phase III comparison of standard radiation therapy and two schedules of concurrent chemoradiotherapy on patients with unresectable squamous cell head and neck cancer, J Clin Oncol 21:92, 2003.
3. Al-Sarraf M and others: Chemoradiotherapy versus radiotherapy in patients with advanced nasopharyngeal cancer: phase III randomized intergroup study 0099, J Clin Oncol 16:1310, 1998.
4. Ang KK and others: Concomitant boost radiotherapy schedules in the treatment of carcinoma of the oropharynx and nasopharynx, Int J Radiat Oncol Biol Phys 19:1339, 1990.
5. Ang KK: Altered fractionation trials in head and neck cancer, Semin Radiat Oncol 8:230, 1998.
6. Austin-Seymour and others: Fractionated proton radiation therapy of chordoma and low grade chondrosarcoma of the base of skull, J Neurosurg 70:13, 1989.
7. Battermann JJ and others: Observations on pulmonary metastases in patients after single doses and multiple fractions of fast neutrons and cobalt-60 gamma rays, Eur J Cancer 17:539, 1981.
8. Berson AM and others: Charged particle irradiation of chordoma and chondrosarcoma of the base of skull and cervical spine: the Lawrence Berkeley Laboratory experience, Int J Radiat Oncol Biol Phys 15:559, 1988.
9. Bhattacharyya N and others: Successful treatment of esthesionneuroblastoma and neuroendodrine carcinoma with combined chemotherapy and proton radiation. results in 9 cases Arch Otolaryngol Head Neck Surg 123:34, 1997.
10. Brenner DJ, Hall EJ: Conditions for the equivalence of continuous to pulsed low dose rate brachytherapy, Int J Radiat Oncol Biol Phys 20:181, 1991.
11. Brizel DM and others: Phase III randomized trial of amifostine as a radioprotector in head and neck cancer J Clin Oncol. 18:3339, 2000.
12. Catterall M, Bewley DK, Sutherland I: Second report on a randomized clinical trial of fast neutrons compared with X- or gamma ray in treatment of advanced cancers of the head and neck, BMJ 1:1942, 1977.
13. Catterall M, Bewley DK: Fast neutrons in the treatment of cancer. London, Academic Press, 1979.
14. Constine LS and others: Protection by WR 2721 of human bone marrow function following irradiation, Int J Radiat Oncol Biol Phys 12:1505, 1986.
15. Cox JD and others: Dose-response for local control with hyperfractionated radiation therapy in advanced carcinomas of the upper aerodigestive tracts: preliminary report of Radiation Therapy Oncology Group protocol 83-13, Int J Radiat Oncol Biol Phys 18:515, 1990.
16. Department of Veterans Affairs Laryngeal Cancer Study Group: Induction chemotherapy plus radiation compared with surgery plus radiation in patients with advanced laryngeal cancer, N Engl J Med 324:1685, 1991.

17. Dische S and others: A randomized multicentre trial of CHART versus conventional radiotherapy in head and neck cancer, *Int J Radiat Oncol Biol Phys* 44:123, 1997.

18. Dische S: Chemical sensitizers for hypoxic cells: a decade of experience in clinical radiotherapy, *Radiother Oncol* 3:97, 1985.

19. Douglas JG and others: Neutron radiotherapy for the treatment of locally advanced major salivary gland tumors, *Head Neck* 21:255, 1999.

20. Douglas JG and others: Treatment of locally advanced adenoid cystic carcinoma of the head and neck with neutron radiotherapy, *Int J Radiat Oncol Biol Phys* 46:551, 2000.

21. Duncan W and others: Fast neutron therapy for squamous cell carcinoma in the head and neck region: results of a randomized trial, *Int J Radiat Oncol Biol Phys* 13:171, 1987.

22. Duncan W and others: Fast neutrons in the treatment of head and neck cancers: the results of a multi-centre randomly controlled trial, *Radiother Oncol* 2:293, 1984.

23. Ellis F: *Fractionation in radiotherapy*. In Delly T, Wood C, editors: *Modern trends in radiotherapy*, vol 1. London, Butterworth, 1967.

24. Errington RD, Catterall M: Re-irradiation of advanced tumors of the head and neck with fast neutrons, *Int J Radiat Oncol Biol Phys* 12:191, 1986.

25. Fazekas JT and others: Failure of misonidazole-sensitized radiotherapy to impact upon outcome among stage III-IV squamous cancers of the head and neck, *Int J Radiat Oncol Biol Phys* 13:1155, 1987.

26. Fazekas JT and others: The role of hemoglobin concentration in the outcome of misonidazole-sensitized radiotherapy of head and neck cancers: based on RTOG trial 79-15, *Int J Radiat Oncol Biol Phys* 17:1177, 1989.

27. Forastiere AA and others: Phase III trial to preserve the larynx: induction chemotherapy and radiotherapy versus concomitant chemoradiotherapy versus radiotherapy alone, intergroup trial R91-11, *Prog Proc Am Soc Clin Oncol* [abstract] 20:2a, 2001.

28. Fu KK and others: A radiation therapy oncology group (RTOG) phase III randomized study to compare hyperfractionation and two variants of accelerated fractionation to standard fractionation radiotherapy in head and neck squamous cell carcinomas: first report of RTOG 9003, *Int J Radiat Oncol Biol Phys* 48:7, 2000.

29. Gatenby RA and others: Oxygen distribution in squamous cell carcinomas and its relationship to outcome of radiation therapy, *Int J Radiat Oncol Biol Phys* 14:831, 1988.

30. Gragg RL and others: The response of Chinese hamster ovary cells to fast neutron radiotherapy beams III: variation in relative biological effectiveness with position in the cell cycle, *Radiat Res* 76:283, 1978.

31. Gragg RL, Humphrey RM, Meyn RE: The response of Chinese hamster ovary cells to fast-neutron radiotherapy beams II: sublethal and potentially lethal damage recovery capabilities, *Radiat Res* 71:461, 1977.

32. Griffin TW and others: Fast neutron irradiation of metastatic cervical adenopathy: the results of a randomized RTOG study, *Int J Radiat Oncol Biol Phys* 9:1267, 1983.

33. Griffin TW and others: Fast neutron radiation therapy for unresectable squamous cell carcinomas of the head and neck: the results of a randomized RTOG study, *Int J Radiat Oncol Biol Phys* 10:2217, 1984.

34. Griffin TW and others: Mixed neutron/photon irradiation of unresectable squamous cell carcinomas of the head and neck: the final report of a randomized trial, *Int J Radiat Oncol Biol Phys* 17:959, 1989.

35. Griffin TW and others: Neutron vs photon irradiation of inoperable salivary gland tumors: results of an RTOG-MRC cooperative randomized study, *Int J Radiat Oncol Biol Phys* 15:1085, 1988.

36. Guichard M and others: Radiosensitivity of lymph node metastases versus initial subcutaneous tumors in nude mice, *Radiat Res* 78:278, 1979.

37. Hahn GM, Little JB: Plateau phase cultures of mammalian cells, *Curr Top Radiat Res Q* 8:39, 1972.

38. Hall EJ: *Radiobiology for the radiologist*. Philadelphia, JB Lippincott, 1994.

39. Hug EB and others: Locally challenging osteo- and chondrogenic tumors of the axial skeleton: results of combined proton and photon radiation therapy using three-dimensional treatment planning, *Int J Radiat Oncol Biol Phys* 31:467, 1995.

40. Kellerer AM, Rossi HH: RBE and the primary mechanism of radiation action, *Radiat Res* 47:15, 1971.

41. Kinsella TJ and others: Tolerance of peripheral nerve to intraoperative radiotherapy (IORT): clinical and experimental studies, *Int J Radiat Oncol Biol Phys* 11:1579, 1985.

42. Laramore GE and others: Neutron versus photon irradiation for unresectable salivary gland tumors: final report of an RTOG-MRC randomized clinical trial, *Int J Radiat Oncol Biol Phys* 27:235, 1993.

43. Laramore GE: Fast neutron radiotherapy for inoperable salivary gland tumors: is it the treatment of choice? *Int J Radiat Oncol Biol Phys* 13:1421, 1987.

44. Lee NL and others: Intensity-modulated radiotherapy in the treatment of nasopharyngeal carcinoma: an update of the UCSF experience, *Int J Radiat Oncol Biol Phys* 53:12, 2002.

45. Maor MH and others: Fast neutron therapy in advanced head and neck cancer: a collaborative international randomized trial, *Int J Radiat Oncol Biol Phys* 32:599, 1995.

46. Meyn RE: Personal communication, 1984.

47. Overgaard J and others: Misonidazole combined with split course radiotherapy in the treatment of invasive carcinoma of the larynx and pharynx: report from the DAHANCA study, *Int J Radiat Oncol Biol Phys* 15:1065, 1989.

48. Pinheiro AD and others: Intraoperative radiotherapy for head and neck and skull base cancer, *Head and Neck* 25:217, 2003.

49. Saroja KR and others: Re-irradiation of locally recurrent tumors with fast neutrons, *Int J Radiat Oncol Biol Phys* 15:115, 1988.

50. Schleicher UM and others: Intraoperative radiation therapy for pre-irradiated head and neck cancer, *Radiother Oncol* 50:77, 2001.

51. Stone RS: Neutron therapy and specific ionization, *Am J Roentgenol* 59:771, 1948.

52. Strandquist M: Studien uber die Kumulative urkung der roentgenstrahlen bei fractionerung, *Acta Radiol Suppl* 55:1, 1944.

53. Tapley ND: Electron beam. In Fletcher GH, editor: Textbook of radiotherapy, ed 3, Philadelphia, 1980, Lea & Febiger.

54. Thames HD and others: Accelerated fractionation vs. hyperfractionation: rationales for several treatments per day, *Int J Radiat Oncol Biol Phys* 9:127, 1983.

55. Toita T and others: Intraoperative radiation therapy (IORT) for head and neck cancer, *Int J Radiat Oncol Biol Phys* 30:1219, 1994.

56. van der Bogaert V and others: Early results of the EORTC randomized clinical trial on multiple fractions per day (MFD) and misonidazole in advanced head and neck cancer, *Int J Radiat Oncol Biol Phys* 12:587, 1986.

57. Visser AG, van den Aardweg GJMJ, Levendag PC: Pulsed dose rate and fractionated high dose rate brachytherapy: choice of brachytherapy schedules to replace low dose rate treatments, *Int J Radiat Oncol Biol Phys* 34:497, 1996.
58. Wang CC, Doppkes KP, Biggs PJ: Intra-oral cone radiation therapy for selected carcinomas of the oral cavity, *Int J Radiat Oncol Biol Phys* 9:1185, 1983.
59. Wang CC, Suite HD, Blitzer PH: Twice-a-day radiation therapy for supraglottic carcinoma, *Int J Radiat Oncol Biol Phys* 12:3, 1986.
60. Wang CC: Local control of oropharyngeal carcinoma after two accelerated hyperfraction radiation therapy schemes, *Int J Radiat Oncol Biol Phys* 14:1143, 1988.
61. Withers HR, Thames HD, Peters LJ: Biological basis for high RBE values for late effects of neutron irradiation, *Int J Radiat Oncol Biol Phys* 8:2071, 1982.
62. Wyckoff HO, Allisy A, Liden K: The new special names of SI units in the field of ionizing radiations, *Phys Med Biol* 20:1029, 1975.

SUGGESTED READINGS

Forastiere A and others: Head and neck cancer, *N Engl J Med* 345:1890, 2001.
Hall EJ: *Radiobiology for the radiologist*. Philadelphia, Lippincott Williams & Wilkins, 2000.
Laramore GE: *Radiation therapy of head and neck cancer*. Berlin, Springer-Verlag, 1989.
Nias AHW: *Clinical radiobiology*. NewYork, Churchill Livingstone, 1988.
Steel GG, Adams GE, and Peckham MJ: *The biological basis of radiotherapy*. New York, Elsevier, 1983.

CHAPTER FOUR

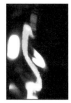

CHEMOTHERAPY FOR HEAD AND NECK CANCER

Arlene A. Forastiere
Merrill S. Kies

INTRODUCTION

The otolaryngologist frequently cares for patients with head and neck cancer who will receive chemotherapy as a component of their treatment (Table 4-1). Most often, these patients have locally advanced squamous cancer or metastatic disease not amenable to curative therapy with surgery or radiation. Many patients have recurrent disease after earlier surgery and radiotherapy. Chemotherapy may also be indicated for patients with advanced carcinomas of the oropharynx or larynx as an aspect of primary management. Of course, chemotherapy is also administered in experimental protocols as an induction regimen, or it can be given concomitantly with radiotherapy for patients with a high risk of tumor relapse. The focus of this chapter will be on chemotherapy for squamous cell carcinomas of the head and neck, although salivary gland cancers, melanomas, and sarcomas are other processes that may be treated with systemic therapy.

Surgeons should be familiar with: (1) the principles of administering chemotherapy in a clinical trial; (2) the appropriate dose and expected side effects of specific chemotherapeutic agents; (3) the basic principles of combination chemotherapy in combined modality programs; and (4) the standard use and experimental approaches of chemotherapy for squamous cell carcinomas and salivary gland tumors.

PRINCIPLES OF CLINICAL TRIALS

The efficacy of chemotherapy or combined modality programs is investigated through clinical trials.[201] To evaluate the use of a particular treatment, clinicians establish at the onset the parameters to be evaluated: objective response rate, survival, disease-free survival or duration of response, and toxicity are commonly identified. The parameters of interest for a specific trial design are defined before the initiation of the study and analyzed at the completion of the study.

The primary end points depend on the nature of the clinical trial or phase of testing.

The evaluation of chemotherapeutic agents occurs in three steps or phases. The goals of phase I trials are to determine the toxic effects associated with a new drug and to establish the highest dose of the drug that can be safely administered. Patients with different tumor types refractory to conventional chemotherapy are enrolled. The purpose of phase II trials is to determine whether a drug or drug combination tested in patients with the same tumor type has enough activity to warrant further testing in a comparative trial. The primary end point is response rate. Phase III trials are randomized comparisons of two or more treatment options, often comparing a standard treatment to a new or more complex therapy. Response rate, progression-free survival, or response duration and survival are primary end points. The determination of sample size and patient entry criteria and the follow-up evaluation and monitoring of patients are critical for a valid interpretation of a phase III trial.[168]

Standard definitions exist for the various end points in clinical trials that allow objective reporting of results. Definitions of response are complete, partial, minor, stable, and progressive disease (Box 4-1). The most meaningful response in terms of prolongation of survival is the attainment of a complete response in which no tumor is detectable after a clinical and radiographic examination. By convention, a partial response indicates that the disease has regressed by at least 50% as determined by serial bidimensional measurements and that no new lesions have appeared elsewhere for at least 4 weeks. The response rate represents the percentage of complete and partial responders. Minor responses and stabilization of disease have historically been of little value but may become significant as newer "targeted" treatments are tested.

TABLE 4-1		
CHEMOTHERAPEUTIC AGENTS WITH ACTIVITY IN HEAD AND NECK CANCERS		
Agent	**Mechanism**	**Toxicity**
Alkylators		
Cyclophosphamide	DNA cross-linker	Neutropenia, nausea, cystitis
Ifosfamide	DNA cross-linker	Myelosuppression, cystitis, confusion, alopecia
Antimetabolities		
Methotrexate	Binds dihydrofolate reductase	Mucositis, myelosuppression
5-Fluorouracil	Inhibits thymidylate synthetase	Mucositis, myelosuppression, diarrhea
Antibodies		
Bleomycin	Scission of DNA	Pulmonary fibrosis, rash, mucositis
Adriamycin	DNA intercalator	Cardiotoxicity, mucositis, myelosuppression, alopecia
Vinca alkaloids		
Vincristine	Mitotic arrest	Neurotoxicity, myelosuppression, alopecia
Vinblastine	Mitotic arrest	Neurotoxicity, myelosuppression, alopecia
Miscellaneous		
Cisplatin	DNA intercalator	Nephrotoxicity, vomiting, ototoxicity, neuropathy
Carboplatin	DNA intercalator	Myelosuppression
Taxanes		
Paclitaxel	Microtubule stabilizer	Myelosuppression, neuropathy
Docetaxel	Microtubule stabilizer	Edema, neutropenia, neuropathy

BOX 4-1	
CRITERIA FOR RESPONSE	
Complete response	Complete disappearance of all evidence of tumor for at least 4 weeks.
Partial response	Disease regression by at least 50% of the sum of the product of the perpendicular diameters of all measurable tumor for at least 4 weeks. No simultaneous increase in the size of any lesion or appearance of new lesions may occur.
Minor response	Regression by less than 50% of the sum of the products of the perpendicular diameters of all measurable lesions.
Stable disease	No appreciable change in dimensions of all evaluable lesions.
Progressive disease	Increase in the size of any detectable lesions by at least 25% or the appearance of new lesions.

When a study is completed, there are several ways to compute the response rate. In calculating the fraction of responders, the numerator should always be the number of patients who qualify in a particular response category, but the denominator often varies from study to study. Some investigators compute response rate using all patients entered into a study, whereas others evaluate response rates after eliminating early death or patients failing to receive a specific number of cycles of treatment. The latter method of computing a response rate results in a much larger value than the former.

Survival is usually calculated from date of study entry until date of death. Progression-free survival is calculated from study entry until disease progression and disease-free survival from achievement of complete response until disease progression. Duration of response is calculated from response date until date of disease progression. Toxicity should be strictly defined for every study before initiation. The National Cancer Institute (NCI) has developed a comprehensive set of standardized drug-induced toxicity criteria. Using a 0 to 4 grading scale, toxicity to each organ system can be objectively assessed. All toxic reactions should be reported in detail in the final results.

In planning a clinical trial, particularly a phase III trial, having comparable patients in each group is critical. This requirement often is accomplished by randomization with stratification for important prognostic variables. Prognostic variables are those factors known to influence response, regardless of treatment. One of the more well-known, important prognostic variables is the Karnofsky Performance Status. In 1948, a 0-to-100 performance scale was devised by David Karnofsky to describe a patient's functional ability. This scale is used today interchangeably with a 0-to-5 point scale (Box 4-2) adapted by several cooperative groups. Performance status is an established prognostic variable that directly correlates with response to chemotherapy. Those patients with a performance status greater than 2 or less than 50% are poor candidates for phase II and III clinical trials and are poor candidates for chemotherapy with palliative intent. These patients usually have a large tumor burden, are malnourished, and have a very short survival time regardless of treatment. By definition, they are nonambulatory for more than 50% of their waking hours and require special care and assistance. If a trial is randomized but not stratified for performance status, a large number of patients with poor Karnofsky Performance Status could be randomly assigned to one of the treatment groups and make it appear less efficacious than a second, when it

actually may be equal or better. Important prognostic variables should be defined at the onset of a study and should be analyzed in the results.

It is important in designing and drawing conclusions from trials to note whether the trial is prospectively randomized with concurrent controls or is a clinical trial with historical controls. Proponents of randomized trials believe that one is more certain of equality between the two groups by a concurrent randomization process.[201] This will reduce the bias of selecting control subjects from a historical pool and will also reduce the influence of improvements in management or changes in treating physicians with time.

SQUAMOUS CELL CARCINOMA
Overview of Current Concepts

Before 1970, chemotherapy had a limited role in the management of squamous cell cancer of the head and neck in community practice and at academic centers. In part, this was because of the paucity of available drugs with documented antitumor activity for this disease. The only drug with clearly established activity, used worldwide, was the folic acid analog methotrexate. Many other drugs had been tested, although the assessment criteria used to define response were not uniform. Hence, the reported response rates were unreliable, representing an accumulation of observations of any degree of tumor regression. In contrast,

---

BOX 4-2
PERFORMANCE STATUS

ECOG, SWOG, Zubrid Scales

0 Fully active, able to carry on all predisease performance without restriction

1 Restricted in physical strenuous activity but ambulatory and able to do work of a light or sedentary nature, (e.g., light housework, office work)

2 Ambulatory and capable of all self-care but unable to do any work activities; up and about more than 50% of waking hours

3 Capable of only limited self-care, confined to bed or chair more than 50% of waking hours

4 Completely disabled; cannot do any self-care; totally confined to bed or chair

5 Dead

Karnofsky Scale

100 Normal; no complaints; no evidence of disease

90 Able to carry on normal activity; minor signs or symptoms

80 Normal activity with effort; some signs or symptoms of disease

70 Cares for self; unable to do normal activity or active work

60 Requires occasional assistance, but is able to care for most needs

50 Requires considerable assistance and frequent medical care

40 Disabled; requires special care and assistance

30 Severely disabled; hospitalization indicated; death not imminent

20 Very sick; hospitalization and active support treatment necessary

10 Moribund; fatal process; progressing rapidly

0 Dead

ECOG, Eastern Cooperative Oncology Group; SWOG, Southwestern Oncology Group.

during the past two decades, a rigid system has been applied to the testing of potentially useful drugs. There are now clearly defined parameters for the objective evaluation of response and survival time and statistical guidelines for the design of clinical research trials to establish efficacy or to show improvement compared with standard therapies.

The serendipitous identification of the metal compound cisdiamine-dichloroplatinum (II) (cisplatin) as a potential anticancer agent by Rosenberg[183] in 1968 spurred clinical research efforts to test new agents and combination chemotherapy regimens for the palliation of patients with locally recurrent and metastatic cancers. Several highly effective chemotherapy regimens were identified and then incorporated into a combined modality approach to treating the newly diagnosed patient. The ultimate goal was to improve survival time with squamous cancers of the head and neck. It became clear that chemotherapy administered before definitive surgery or radiotherapy could result in rapid regression of tumor in the majority of patients without substantially increasing the morbidity of subsequent surgery or radiation. Further, a proportion of the responding patients would have no histologic evidence of tumor in the resected specimen. This increased the possibility of altering the standard surgical approach at some sites to preserve organ function. In addition to investigative trials using chemotherapy before definitive local therapy, traditional adjuvant chemotherapy administered after surgical resection and chemotherapy used as a radiosensitizer concomitant with radiotherapy have been under active investigation.

Prognostic Factors

Many chemotherapy trials have been analyzed to determine factors that would predict response to chemotherapy and prolonged survival time. Because squamous cell cancer of the head and neck is a heterogeneous disease, each factor should be evaluated in the context of multiple primary sites. Most single-institution trials have only modest numbers of patients and therefore lack the statistical confidence to draw firm conclusions. For patients with recurrent disease, poor prognostic factors are a low performance status, poor nutrition, a large tumor burden, and extensive previous radiotherapy and surgery.[12] Tumor progression during or shortly after surgery or radiotherapy is also an ominous sign. In these circumstances, any response to chemotherapy is likely to be marginal and brief, without impact on overall survival time. However, it seems clear that survival time may be prolonged in patients who achieve a complete response to chemotherapy. These patients, in general, have a good performance status; they are not malnourished and have not received previous chemotherapy for recurrent disease.

For newly diagnosed patients treated with induction chemotherapy, the most consistent prognostic factor for overall response and complete response is T and N stage. There is a significant correlation between tumor size and response, with lower response rates observed in T4 and N3 stage disease, in particular.[39,73,106] The importance of primary site as a prognostic factor for response to chemotherapy is unclear. One investigator, in an analysis of 208 patients, reported that cancers within the oral cavity and nasopharynx were significantly associated with high response rates.[108] Nasopharynx cancer was found to be significant in two other trials.[6,73] The pattern of failure for patients with nasopharyngeal carcinoma is also different than that of cases at other sites, with metastatic sites assuming a larger proportion. Besides nasopharyngeal carcinoma, most trials have failed to demonstrate differences by site, which may relate to inadequate patient numbers and only modestly effective chemotherapy regimens.

Because of the importance of performance status as a predictor of outcome for patients with recurrent disease, induction chemotherapy trials have excluded patients with poor performance status (<50% on the Karnofsky scale). Within the range of 50% to 100%, no clear differences have been observed. Tumor differentiation does not appear to be a predictive factor in studies that have used cisplatin-based combination chemotherapy regimens. It is well established that overall survival time correlates with performance status, T and N stage, primary site,[5,73,106] and nodal extracapsular extension of tumor.[124,203] The survival time of patients with cancers of the nasopharynx and larynx is longer than that of those with oral cavity and hypopharyngeal primary cancers after researchers correct for other factors in multivariate analyses of patients receiving induction chemotherapy.

The application of biologic factors (e.g., DNA content,[71] immunologic status, and circulating immune complexes[195]) to predict response and survival outcome is under investigation. Evidence exists that DNA ploidy and DNA content can predict survival and disease-free survival times.[222,249] Molecular markers (such as *p53* and *p16*) that act as predictors for response and survival time are also under investigation.[21,22]

CHEMOTHERAPY FOR PALLIATION

Systemic management of recurrent head and neck cancer is a major concern because 30% to 50% of patients diagnosed this year will die with recurrent local and regional disease within 5 years. Distant metastases will be clinically present in 20% to 40% of patients, but occult disease determined at autopsy may be present in up to 60%.[135] The primary goal of conventional chemotherapy used for palliation should be to prolong survival time. Patients with locally advanced or disseminated recurrent squamous cell carcinomas of the head and neck have a median survival time of 6 to 8 months, and 20% survive 1 year. Chemotherapy has not yet altered these statistics, although it has been useful in palliation. One often hears that pain relief can be achieved with chemotherapy, but this should not constitute the sole reason for treatment. Tumor regression may be associated with a transient diminution of pain, although the aggressive use of a variety of available oral analgesics (tablet and elixir preparations) is a much more rational approach to pain management.

Single Agents

The response rate (complete and partial) of recurrent or metastatic squamous cell cancer to commonly used agents is provided in Table 4-2. In general, about one third of patients respond. The majority are partial responses, with less than 5% of patients achieving a complete response. Response duration tends to be brief, on the order of 2 to 4 months, and median survival time is 6 to 9 months.

Methotrexate

Methotrexate is a folic acid analog that is S-phase specific. Its mechanism of action involves binding to the enzyme dihydrofolate reductase, which blocks the reduction of dihydrofolate to tetrahydrofolic acid. Tetrahydrofolic acid is necessary for the synthesis of thymidylic acid and purine. This then interrupts the synthesis of DNA, RNA, and protein. The cytostatic

effects of methotrexate can be circumvented by the administration of reduced folates, such as leucovorin, which can be converted to the tetrahydrofolate coenzyme required for purine biosynthesis. The therapeutic index of methotrexate can be increased if leucovorin is administered at intervals after methotrexate is given. This results from a selective rescue of nonmalignant cells and forms the basis for the use of high doses of methotrexate followed by leucovorin to ameliorate methotrexate toxicity to healthy cells. Cancer cells may lack transport sites for leucovorin and are subject to the lethal effects of methotrexate. Mechanisms for resistance to methotrexate include the selection of cells with decreased transport of methotrexate into cells and increased dihydrofolate reductase activity.

Methotrexate can be administered by intramuscular injection or subcutaneous, intravenous, or oral routes. Weekly or biweekly administration is the preferred schedule. A conventional dose of intravenous methotrexate is 40 to 60 mg/m^2 weekly. When higher doses of methotrexate are used, they may be in the moderate-dose range (250–500 mg/m^2, intravenous) or the high-dose range (5–10 g/m^2). These are both followed by leucovorin rescue, usually beginning at 24 hours and continuing until the plasma methotrexate level is less than 10^{-8} mol/L. At this dose range, the toxicity for patients with normal renal function usually is limited to mild stomatitis and myelosuppression. More severe, life-threatening reactions consisting of confluent mucositis, pancytopenia, liver function abnormalities, and an exfoliative maculopapular rash occur rarely and require intensive medical support. Renal dysfunction may occur with high-dose methotrexate administration because of precipitation of the drug, especially in the case of acidic urine. Hydration and alkalinization of the urine before and after methotrexate administration can reduce the risk.

Methotrexate was previously widely used for management of squamous cancers of the head and neck. Therapy with this drug is relatively nontoxic, inexpensive, and convenient. Response rates to conventional doses vary between 8% and 50%, averaging 30%.[16] Weekly treatment, if tolerable, is superior to twice monthly or monthly treatments. Levitt and others[141] have shown in vitro that when moderate-to-high doses of methotrexate are used with leucovorin rescue, an enhanced therapeutic index results from the high intracellular levels of drug associated with selective rescue of healthy tissue. The initial results of pilot trials of moderate- or high-dose methotrexate suggested improvement in response rates for those with head and neck cancers. However, there is no clear benefit to the higher dose (e.g., as much as 5000 mg) from prospective randomized trials comparing conventional

TABLE 4-2

ACTIVITY OF SINGLE AGENT CHEMOTHERAPY

Agent	Dosing Schedule	Response Rate (%)
Methotrexate	40–50 mg/m^2 weekly	30
Cisplatin	80–120 mg/m^2 every 3-4 weeks	33
Carboplatin	400 mg/m^2 every 4 weeks	24
Paclitaxel	135–200 mg/m^2 every 3-4 weeks	38
Docetaxel	75 mg/m^2 every 3 weeks	38
Ifosfamide	1.5–2.5 g/m^2 every 4 weeks	26
Bleomycin	15 mg/m^2 twice weekly	18
5-Fluorouracil	500 mg/m^2 weekly	15

with moderate- or high-dose methotrexate, with or without leucovorin rescue.[233,248]

Cisplatin

Cisplatin is an inorganic metal coordination complex with major antitumor activity in a number of diseases. The drug behaves as a bifunctional alkylating agent binding to DNA to cause interstrand and intrastrand cross-linking. Cisplatin also binds to nuclear and cytoplasmic proteins. Resistance is believed to develop through increased metabolic inactivation. Cisplatin is administered by the intravenous route and requires aggressive hydration and diuresis to prevent renal tubular damage. A dose range of 80 to 120 mg/m^2 every 3 or 4 weeks[105] or by 24-hour infusion[117] have been administered. More often, the 80 to 100-mg/m^2 dose is used. The drug is not schedule dependent, although it has been shown that 5-day continuous infusion increases exposure to the active platinum species when compared with bolus dosing.[84]

The major toxic reaction is renal dysfunction, manifested by an increase in serum creatinine levels or a decrease in creatinine clearance. The peak serum creatinine level occurs at 1 or 2 weeks and returns to baseline by 3 or 4 weeks. An increase in serum creatinine level to 2 mg/dL has been noted in up to 20% of patients in several series. This drug should not be used in patients with a creatinine clearance below 40 mL/min. Nausea and vomiting are almost universal. Ototoxicity can occur, usually in the 4000- to 8000-Hz range. It tends to be dose-related and cumulative and may be permanent. Hematologic toxicity, including neutropenia and thrombocytopenia, is mild, with a nadir at 2 weeks. Anemia is common and appears to be a result of bone marrow suppression; rarely, patients manifest an acute hemolytic anemia. Hypomagnesemia can occur in part because of renal wasting. A peripheral neuropathy with predominantly sensory deficits occurs and is related to cumulative cisplatin dosage. Ototoxicity and peripheral neuropathy are very common toxicities when the cumulative cisplatin dose approaches or exceeds 600 mg/m^2. These toxicities preclude long-term management with cisplatin in chemotherapy responders and dose intensification. This led to a search for analogs with similar efficacy but a different spectrum of toxicity.

Cisplatin has the same response rate as methotrexate, approximately 30%, with some reported complete responses and a duration of response of approximately 4 months.[117,247] Two controlled trials comparing methotrexate with cisplatin found no difference in response rate or survival time between the two but noted quite different toxicities.[98,110] Advantages of cisplatin over methotrexate are its relatively rapid response rate and the fact that it needs to be given only once every 3 or 4 weeks. Cisplatin has been studied at different doses to determine whether a dose/response effect exists. In a comparison of 60 mg/m^2 and 120 mg/m^2, Veronesi and others[228] found no difference in response rates. Forastiere and others[81] conducted a pilot trial evaluating 200 mg/m^2 and observed a 73% response rate or double that expected with conventional dosing. Although this suggested benefit from the higher dose, ototoxicity and neurotoxicity occurred frequently and limited treatment duration.

Carboplatin

More than one dozen derivatives of cisplatin have been evaluated for clinical development. Of these, carboplatin (cis-diamine-cyclobutane dicarboxylato-platinum II) was the first to become widely available. Carboplatin appears to have a mechanism of action similar to the parent compound, but it has a different toxicity profile. The dose-limiting toxicity is myelosuppression, primarily leukopenia and thrombocytopenia, which should be considered when carboplatin is combined with other myelosuppressing agents. Renal toxicity, ototoxicity, and neurotoxicity are rare, and the emetogenic potential of carboplatin is less. The drug can be administered in the outpatient setting without the need for hydration. Based on pharmacokinetic parameters, an intravenous dose of 400 mg/m^2 is considered the equivalent in potency to 100 mg/m^2 of cisplatin and can be safely administered to patients with creatinine clearance of 60 mg/mL or more. Most clinicians calculate carboplatin dose using the Calvert[31] formula, which accounts for delayed renal excretion leading to increased drug exposure.

Carboplatin has a 24% response rate in phase II trials in patients with recurrent squamous cell cancer of the head and neck. It may not be as active as cisplatin; one comparative trial in patients with untreated disease has documented an inferior outcome for carboplatin.[10] Thus, carboplatin is often reserved for patients who are not candidates for cisplatin therapy because of excessive nausea, renal impairment, or preexisting peripheral neuropathy. Carboplatin can be administered in the outpatient setting and requires no prehydration. The major toxicity caused by carboplatin is myelosuppression, which limits the total dose that can be given and the frequency of drug administration. The availability of colony-stimulating factors that can lessen the degree and duration of myelosuppression may provide a means to compensate for marrow toxicity.

Taxanes

The taxanes are a new class of compounds that include paclitaxel (Taxol) and docetaxel (Taxotere). These drugs act by stabilizing microtubules after binding to the *b* subunit of tubulin, thereby inhibiting microtubule depolymerization, which results in a cell cycle arrest at G_2. Preclinical studies showed that the taxanes were active against a variety of solid tumors and that prolonged infusions were more effective.[90,99,176,230] Trials involving patients with head and neck cancer have shown response rates of approximately 30% to 40%.[34,66,80,83,219]

Paclitaxel has been administered at doses of 135 to 250 mg/m² given over 3 or 24 hours, and docetaxel has been given at 60 to 100 mg/m² by bolus injection every 3 weeks. The major toxicity is neutropenia, particularly with high doses, and infection is a chief concern. Growth factors such as granulocyte-macrophage colony-stimulating factor (GM-CSF) and granulocyte colony-stimulating factor (G-CSF) may be used to shorten the neutropenic nadir duration and hopefully lessen the risk of infection.[184] Given this risk, patients with good performance status are better candidates for treatment at 175 to 200 mg/m². Paclitaxel has been given over several schedules, and the optimal dosing schedule is being investigated. Docetaxel is a semisynthetic agent and may be more effective than paclitaxel. In two small phase II studies, response rates of 32% and 50% were observed.[34,63]

Ifosfamide

Ifosfamide is structurally related to cyclophosphamide (to be discussed) and has a similar mechanism of action, leading to DNA interstrand and intrastand cross-linking that disrupts DNA replication. It is activated by hepatic p-450 mixed-function oxidase, and its metabolites are excreted in the urine. Ifosfamide in total doses of 7 to 10 g/m² is usually administered as a 5-day continuous infusion or over 3 to 5 days in equally divided doses. The drug is repeated at 3- or 4-week intervals. Sodium mercaptoethane sulfonate (MESNA) is a thiol compound that should be administered concomitantly with ifosfamide to limit urothelial toxicity. The total daily dose of MESNA should equal the daily dose of ifosfamide. It may be administered as a continuous infusion or in divided doses. Patients need to be well hydrated before drug administration. The major dose-limiting toxicity is hemorrhagic cystitis, although with the use of MESNA, myelosuppression, nausea, vomiting, and hyponatremia are more frequent toxicities. Central nervous system toxicities, which include cerebellar dysfunction, seizures, confusion, and lethargy, occur in up to 30% of patients treated with doses of 8 to 10 g/m² over 5 days. Early phase II results with this drug are promising, with reported response rates ranging from 6% to 43% with a median of 26%.*

---

*References 53, 56, 95, 127, 136, 138, 167, 172, 200.

Bleomycin

Bleomycin (Blenoxane) is an antineoplastic antibiotic that binds to DNA and produces DNA strand breaks by generating oxygen free radicals. The conventional dose of bleomycin is 10 to 20 U/m² once or twice weekly given intramuscularly or intravenously. It also may be given by a continuous 24-hour infusion over 5 or 7 days at a dose of 10 Us/m² each 24 hours. The major metabolism of bleomycin is via the kidneys. It is important that the dose of bleomycin be reduced if the level of serum creatinine is abnormal. A 50% dose reduction is recommended for a creatinine clearance of 15 to 30 mL/min, and a 75% reduction is recommended if the creatinine clearance is below 15 mL/min. Approximately half of the patients receiving this drug will develop fever or chills during the first 24 hours, which can be reduced with the use of antipyretics. A rare complication is an anaphylactic reaction. It has been recommended that a dose of 1 U be given several hours before the first dose of bleomycin. Alopecia can occur, particularly with the higher dosage of drug. Skin toxicity, including erythema, thickening, and hyperpigmentation, is common. Patients may develop stomatitis, which necessitates discontinuing a prolonged infusion.

Pulmonary toxicity is potentially one of the most serious complications of bleomycin administration. Patients may develop pneumonitis, a dry cough, and rales. Pulmonary function tests most commonly show a decreased carbon monoxide diffusion capacity. Pulmonary fibrosis with associated hypoxia and restrictive lung disease can result. Bleomycin pulmonary toxicity is more common in elderly patients, in patients who have had previous lung irradiation, and in patients who have had a total dose higher than 200 U. Patients should be closely monitored with serial tests of diffusion capacity when the cumulative dose exceeds 150 U. Giving the drug by continuous infusion may lessen pulmonary toxicity.[240]

Bleomycin has undergone testing using an intermittent bolus dosing schedule with response rates of 18%. A pharmacokinetic advantage may be achieved by continuous infusion because both agents have a short plasma half-life. Bleomycin is most frequently used in combination with other agents, and is not currently in common usage.

5-Fluorouracil

5-Fluorouracil (5-FU) is a fluorinated pyrimidine similar to uracil. 5-FU competes for the enzyme thymidylate synthetase by displacing uracil, which in turn inhibits the formation of thymidine, an essential factor in DNA synthesis. The conventional intravenous dose of 5-FU is 10 to 15 mg/kg weekly. An alternate method of delivery is a loading dose of 400 to 500 mg/m^2 daily for 5 days, followed by a weekly intravenous dose of 400 to 500 mg/m^2. It is recommended that no more than 800 mg be given as a single bolus. The therapeutic index of 5-FU may be enhanced by giving it by continuous infusion, which allows delivery of up to 1 g/m^2 per day for 5 days, repeated every 3 or 4 weeks, without marked enhanced toxicity. Continuous infusion of 5-FU has been studied primarily in patients with adenocarcinomas of the gastrointestinal tract. However, the results of one randomized trial studying patients with head and neck cancer and comparing bolus with continuous infusion of 5-FU showed improved response rates with continuous infusion.[131] 5-FU toxic reactions include myelosuppression with neutropenia and thrombocytopenia occurring at 1 or 2 weeks. Nausea, vomiting, and diarrhea may occur, and stomatitis is common with higher doses. Patients may develop alopecia, hyperpigmentation, or a maculopapular rash. In patients with head and neck carcinomas, treatment with 5-FU can produce response rates of 15%, thus it has most often been used in combination with other agents, particularly cisplatin.[8,169]

Other Single Agents with Activity in the Treatment of Head and Neck Cancer

Several other chemotherapeutic agents were reported to have response rates in excess of 15% for patients with recurrent disease. They include Adriamycin, cyclophosphamide, hydroxyurea, and vinblastine.[9] Several of these are only marginally effective as single agents for recurrent disease, although when used in combinations or in patients with no previous treatment, they may be more efficacious. These agents will be discussed.

Cyclophosphamide

Cyclophosphamide is activated in the liver by microsomal enzymes. Its major mechanism of action is cross-linking DNA strands, preventing further division. Cyclophosphamide can be given orally or intravenously. When given intravenously, it usually is given as a single dose of 500 to 1000 mg/m^2 repeated every 3 or 4 weeks. It is important to hydrate patients well before and after giving cyclophosphamide. Drugs that stimulate liver enzymes, such as barbiturates, should be avoided, or the cyclophosphamide dose should be modified. After an intravenous dose, bone marrow suppression, predominantly neutropenia, can occur within 1 or 2 weeks, with a recovery at 2 or 3 weeks. Many patients have some degree of nausea and vomiting. Alopecia and ridging of the nails can occur. Azoospermia and cessation of menses, often with permanent infertility, can occur with most alkylating agents.

Acute hemorrhagic cystitis occurs most commonly in patients who are poorly hydrated. It is recommended that patients drink at least 2 quarts of fluid per day while taking cyclophosphamide. Toxicity may occur as microscopic hematuria or gross bleeding. This can eventually result in a fibrotic bladder, and a few cases of bladder carcinoma have been described in patients who have received cyclophosphamide.

Adriamycin

Adriamycin (doxorubicin) is an anthracycline derivative that intercalates between nucleotide pairs in DNA to interfere with nuclei acid synthesis. This drug is given intravenously, usually at doses of 60 to 75 mg/m^2 every 3 weeks. Alternate schedules that are associated with a much lower risk of cardiac toxicity include doses of 20 to 30 mg/m^2 daily for 3 days repeated every 3 weeks, low doses given weekly, or prolonged infusions.[15] The patient's urine may be red for 1 or 2 days after Adriamycin treatment.

If Adriamycin infiltrates subcutaneous tissue, it can cause severe necrosis of skin and subcutaneous tissue. The drug causes alopecia, which can be decreased by using scalp hypothermia. Stomatitis, nausea, vomiting, and diarrhea are common. Adriamycin, like actinomycin D, can cause radiation recall in patients who have had previous radiotherapy. The drug can also cause neutropenia and thrombocytopenia with a nadir at 1 or 2 weeks and a return to normal values by 3 weeks.[17]

The most dose-limiting toxic effect of Adriamycin is cardiac toxicity, which manifests as a cardiomyopathy,[238] leading to congestive heart failure in approximately 10% of patients who receive a cumulative dose greater than 550 mg/m^2. Other predisposing factors include age, previous cardiac irradiation, other cardiotoxic chemotherapeutic agents, and a previous history of heart disease. Many methods of observing patients have been used, including endomyocardial biopsy. Radionuclide ejection fraction is a relatively easy and accurate way to determine the amount of damage to the heart from Adriamycin.

Vinca Alkaloids

Vinblastine and vincristine are vinca alkaloids. These agents act by disrupting microtubular spindle formation, causing mitotic arrest. Vinblastine (Velban) can be given weekly at 5 mg/m^2, or it may be given by continuous infusion over several days. The major toxic reactions are myelosuppression, alopecia, and myalgia. Vincristine (Oncovin) is usually given at 1.0 to 1.5 mg/m^2 once or twice monthly. It is recommended for adults that a single dose not exceed 2 mg. The drug is neurotoxic, which is most commonly manifested as a sensory motor peripheral neuropathy or hoarseness that will progress if the drug is not discontinued. Most patients will experience constipation, and they should take stool softeners with the drug. Vincristine causes alopecia, but it has almost no myelosuppressive effects.

Hydroxyurea

Hydroxyurea (Hydrea) inhibits ribonucleotide reductase, interfering with the conversion of ribonucleotide to deoxyribonucleotide and causing inhibition of DNA synthesis. The drug is given orally. The major toxic responses are neutropenia and thrombocytopenia, so the dose should be reduced or delayed if the leukocyte count decreases to less than $2500/mm^3$ or the platelet count decreases to less than $100,000/mm^3$. The nadir occurs approximately 10 days after starting the drug. Nausea and diarrhea are common. Stomatitis can occur, particularly if there is concurrent irradiation. Patients also may develop a maculopapular rash. This drug is most commonly used as a radiation sensitizer.

New Single Agents

Many new drugs are being investigated for their activity in patients with head and neck cancer in phase I and II studies. Topoisomerase I inhibitors are under study.[180]

Gemcitabine is a pyrimidine antimetabolite that may have antitumor activity in patients with head and neck carcinomas. This agent is converted to an active triphosphate metabolite, which is then incorporated into DNA and terminates transcription. Early phase II results have demonstrated only modest activity with response rates of 18%.[35]

Vinorelbine is a semisynthetic vinca alkaloid with dramatically less neurotoxicity than other agents of its class. Early studies have demonstrated response rates of 22%.[94,218] Finally, analogs of methotrexate have been evaluated for response in small series. Trimetrexate, edatrexate, and piritrexim are active in squamous cell carcinomas of the head and neck but offer no special advantage over methotrexate.[55,179,188,223,236]

COMBINATION CHEMOTHERAPY FOR RECURRENT DISEASE

In an effort to improve response rates and, hopefully survival time, combination chemotherapy was developed. Many combination chemotherapy regimens have been evaluated in phase II trials involving a few patients with recurrent head and neck cancer. Often, the results indicate a high response rate that suggests improvement over that expected from single agent methotrexate or cisplatin. However, the median duration of response ranges from 2 to 6 months, and no one has yet documented improved survival time over single-agent chemotherapy. Many of the regimens are complex, often with additional toxic effects.

Only through large comparative trials with patients randomized and stratified for prognostic variables can it be determined whether therapeutic benefit exists with combination chemotherapy. The results of 12 trials comparing combination chemotherapy to single-agent cisplatin or methotrexate are shown in Table 4-3. Some of the studies had small numbers of patients and lacked balance between treatment groups for prognostic factors such as performance status and extent of previous treatment. However, four large multiinstitutional trials that were well designed with respect to prognostic factors showed a significant difference in response rates between the combination treatment and the single-agent control arm.[41,79,86,119,232]

The Eastern Consortium Oncology Group (ECOG) compared an outpatient regimen of cisplatin, bleomycin, and methotrexate to weekly methotrexate.[232] The response to single-agent therapy with methotrexate was 35%, and to the combination 48%—a significant improvement ($P = .04$). However, toxicity was greater for the combination, with no difference in survival time.

The Southwestern Oncology Group (SWOG) reported a comparison of cisplatin and 5-FU vs carboplatin and 5-FU to weekly methotrexate.[79,86] The response rates for the three arms were 32%, 21%, and 10%, respectively. There was a significant difference comparing the cisplatin combination with methotrexate ($P < .001$); the difference between the response to the carboplatin combination and the response to methotrexate approached statistical significance ($P = .05$). The cisplatin and 5-FU arm was associated with significantly more toxicity than methotrexate; carboplatin and 5-FU were intermediate in toxicity. Despite these findings, the median survival times were not different, varying between 4.7 and 6.6 months.

The third study to show a difference in response rates compared the combination of cisplatin and 5-FU with each drug used alone.[119] The response rate to the combination was 40% compared with 18% for cisplatin and 15% for continuous infusion 5-FU ($P < .01$). Although the median survival times were not different, an analysis of patients surviving longer than 9 months showed a 40% survival rate for the combination treatment group compared with 27% and 24% for the single-drug treatments ($P < .05$).

The latter two trials are also of interest because of the similar response rates observed for cisplatin and 5-FU, which were administered using the same dose and schedule in both studies. Cisplatin with 5-FU is a commonly used drug regimen for the treatment of patients with head and neck cancer for palliation and in combined modality programs. Response rates to this combination reported from small phase II trials in patients with recurrent disease range from 11% to 79%.[224] The results of these two large multiinstitutional

TABLE 4-3

RANDOMIZED TRIALS OF CHEMOTHERAPY FOR RECURRENT HEAD AND NECK CANCER

Author	Regimens	CR + PR (%)	Survival (months)
Davis and Kessler, 1979[52]	PMB	11	
	P	13	
Jacobs, 1983[118]	PM	33	6.3
	P	18	6.9
Drelichman, 1983[63]	P		
	Vb	41	5.6
	M	33	4.0
Vogl, 1985[232]	PMB	48	5.6
	M	35	5.6
Morton, 1985[162]	PB	24	4.0
	P	13	4.2
	B	14	2.8
	No chemotherapy		2.1
Williams, 1986[246]	PVbB	23	6.8
	M	16	7.2
Campbell, 1987[32]	PF	19	2.7
	PM	40	8.7
	P	31	5.3
	M	33	6.7
Eisenberger, 1989[68]	CM	25	6l
	M	25	6l
Liverpool Study, 1990[146]	P	14	6l
	PF	12	6l
	M	6	2l
	PM	11	6l
Forastiere, 1992[86]	PF	32	6.6
	CF	21	5.0
	M	10	5.6
Jacobs, 1992[119]	PF	32	5.5
	P	17	5.0
	F	13	6.1
Clavel, 1994[41]	PMBVb	34	7.0
	PF	31	7.0
	P	15	7.0

(Reprinted with permission from *Tumors of the nasal cavity and paranasal sinuses, nasopharynx, oral cavity, and oropharynx.* In Schantz SP, Harrison LB, Forastive AA: *Cancer-principles and practice of oncology*, ed 5. Philadelphia, Lippincott-Raven, 1997.)
CR, Complete response; PR, partial response; P, cisplatin; M, methotrexate; B, bleomycin; Vb, vinblastine; C, carboplatin; F, fluorouracil.

trials have served to establish a response rate of 32% that can be expected from the cisplatin and 5-FU combination in patients with recurrent head and neck cancer.

Clavel and others[41] also observed significant differences between combination chemotherapy and single agents. They found significant differences in response rates for two cisplatin-containing combinations compared with single agent methotrexate—34%, 31%, and 15%, respectively. These data corroborate the work of Vogl, Jacobs, and Forastiere.

Two comparative trials listed in Table 4-3 showed significant differences in median survival time.[32,162] Morton and others[162] compared the combination of cisplatin and bleomycin to each single agent and to a control arm featuring no treatment. The response rate to each of the three chemotherapy arms was low, although the two cisplatin arms had median survival times of 4.0 and 4.2 months, which was improved over a 2.1-month survival time for the no-treatment arm. In the four-arm trial reported by Campbell and others,[32] survival time was significantly longer for single-agent cisplatin compared with methotrexate, and there was no advantage for the combination treatments. Both of these trials had small numbers of patients and were unevenly balanced for prognostic factors, which serves to decrease the reliability of the statistical interpretation. Thus, from these randomized trials, it appears that higher response rates can be achieved with some combination chemotherapy regimens. Toxicity is more severe, and overall survival time as measured by median survival time is not improved. However, one study did find that a significantly greater proportion of patients treated with cisplatin and 5-FU lived longer than 9 months when compared with those receiving single-agent therapy. The patients who are more likely to be in the subset showing improvement have a better performance status.

As for other sites, the most effective combinations for treating those with nasopharyngeal carcinoma are cisplatin-based regimens. Higher complete and partial response rates than those from other sites have been reported in several phase II trials.* A few long-term disease-free survivors have been seen as a result of cisplatin-based combinations.[20,40,76] French investigators have formed a collaborative group to study nasopharyngeal cancer. They have reported a series of studies evaluating cisplatin combination chemotherapy. Their regimen of cisplatin, bleomycin, and 5-FU resulted in a 20% complete response rate and an 86% overall response rate. Four patients with metastatic disease were long-term, disease-free survivors for 52 to 58 months.[20,50,150] In their series, 131 patients with metastatic nasopharyngeal carcinoma were treated between 1985 and 1991. Ten percent of the members of this group were long-term, disease-free survivors. Thus, this disease entity shows a unique chemosensitivity even in patients with either bone or visual metastasis.[76] Browman and Cronin[25] summarized all of the available data regarding combination therapy by use of a metaanalysis. They analyzed all randomized trials published between 1990 and 1992 and concluded that cisplatin was the most effective single agent. Further, they found that the combination cisplatin and 5-FU was more efficacious than any single agent or other reported combinations. The combination of cisplatin and 5-FU is the gold standard to which all new combinations should be compared. Response rates achieved with this combination are approximately 32%, and the complete response rate ranges from 5% to 15%. Given these low response rates, one of the goals of clinical trials is to find new single agents and new combinations that may be more effective. Patients with locally advanced or metastatic disease should be considered for trials in an effort to improve on these statistics. Patients who have undergone previous surgery and radiation with good performance status and no previous chemotherapy are the best candidates to test new treatment protocols.

COMBINED MODALITY THERAPY

Although surgery and radiotherapy cure a high percentage of patients with early-stage squamous cell carcinoma of the head and neck, conventional treatment will not cure the majority of those with advanced disease. Because treatment for recurrent disease with chemotherapy is far from satisfactory, much effort has been directed toward improvements in the primary treatment program by using combined modality therapy. To this end, three general approaches have been undertaken: (1) induction, also known as neoadjuvant therapy, in which chemotherapy is given before surgery or radiation; (2) chemoradiation, in which chemotherapy is given simultaneous with radiation to enhance its effect; and (3) adjuvant therapy, in which chemotherapy is given after surgery or radiation in an effort to decrease metastatic disease burden.

Induction Chemotherapy

Theoretically, treatment with chemotherapy before surgery or radiation—known as induction chemotherapy—has several advantages. This neoadjuvant chemotherapy allows for the delivery of drugs to the best possible host in terms of medical condition, which leads to increased compliance and better tolerance of therapy. Chemotherapy, when given first, can reduce tumor burden and downstage patients, resulting in the preservation of organ function by obviating the need for surgery. Further, induction therapy can reduce metastatic seeds and eliminate problems with poor vascularity that often occur after surgery or radiation, thus reducing a potential pharmacologic sanctuary.

One of the first uses of induction chemotherapy involved methotrexate with leucovorin rescue given twice before surgery.[215] It was reported that 77% of patients had some tumor shrinkage, although by strict criteria of tumor response (>50% in all sites), the response rate was only 20%. Although it could not be concluded that the result was better than with surgery alone, no increased incidence of postoperative complications occurred. Many other studies followed using single-agent methotrexate and bleomycin. The complete response rate was approximately 5% in these studies.

With the introduction of cisplatin into clinical trials in the mid-1970s, combination therapy consisted of cisplatin followed by a 5- to 7-day continuous infusion of bleomycin. Early series[111,173] reported overall response rates of 71% to 76%, with a 20% complete response rate. Other investigators added vinblastine, vincristine, or methotrexate to the two-drug combination with similar results.[9] An alternate and probably more effective regimen tested in the 1980s at Wayne State University was cisplatin (100 mg/m^2) followed by a 5-day infusion of 5-FU (1 g/m^2 per day by continuous infusion).[182] In phase II trials, this regimen was associated with an overall response rate as high as 93% and a 54% complete response rate when three cycles were administered. Although the toxicity from cisplatin is the same, 5-FU appears to be better tolerated than bleomycin, without the associated allergic phenomena or lung toxicity.

Ensley and others[69,70] from Wayne State University have reported a high complete response rate using five or six courses of cisplatin and 5-FU alternating with methotrexate, leucovorin, and 5-FU. In one study, the complete response rate was 65% in 31 patients completing the protocol, although toxicity was formidable, and approximately one third of patients withdrew from the study early. Despite the potential for improvement in response rate, the feasibility of this approach has yet to be demonstrated.

Investigators at the Dana Farber Cancer Center[64] and at the University of Chicago[235] have used leucovorin to biochemically modulate the cytotoxic effects of 5-FU. Leucovorin results in an increase in intracellular-reduced folate levels and inhibition of thymidylate synthase.[159] Dreyfuss and others[64] administered cisplatin, 5-FU, and high-dose leucovorin (500 mg/m^2), all by continuous infusion, over 6 days to 35 patients with local regionally advanced head and neck cancer. The overall response rate was 80%, and 66% had a complete response by clinical assessment. A pathologic complete response was documented in 14 of 19 patients (74%). Moderate-to-severe mucositis occurred in the majority of patients, although with dosage adjustment, the regimen was tolerable and acceptable to patients. Vokes and others[235] treated 31 patients with similar disease with a less intensive regimen of cisplatin, 5-FU, and leucovorin. Leucovorin was administered orally in a dose of 100 mg every 4 hours during the 5-day infusion of 5-FU. After two courses, the overall response rate in 29 evaluable patients was 90%, and the complete response rate was 30%.

Since the early 1980s, the many uncontrolled trials of induction chemotherapy before surgery or radiotherapy have shown that this approach is feasible for those with locally advanced disease and does not add to the morbidity of subsequent definitive local treatment.[137,207] With the cisplatin plus 5-FU regimen, a response can be expected in 80% to 90% of patients with, on average, a 40% complete response rate. Approximately two-thirds of complete responses by clinical examination will be confirmed pathologically. Response to induction chemotherapy correlates with response to subsequent radiotherapy.[72,96,113]

Thus, patients who are resistant to cisplatin-based induction chemotherapy have a high likelihood of not responding to radiotherapy. Large randomized trials that consider all the important prognostic variables and have long-term follow-up periods are necessary to draw conclusions regarding disease-free survival and overall survival benefit.[85] The results of 17 randomized controlled trials of induction chemotherapy before surgery, radiotherapy, or both have been published.

Three of the most important trials are listed in Table 4-4; The Head and Neck Contracts program,[106] the SWOG trial,[190] and the Veterans Affairs Laryngeal Cancer Study Group trial[231] were large multiinstitutional randomized studies. The patients had advanced resectable head and neck cancer, and the treatment arms were well balanced to TN stage and primary site. The Head and Neck Contracts program randomly assigned patients to receive one of three treatments: (1) surgery followed by radiation, (2) induction chemotherapy with one cycle of cisplatin plus bleomycin followed by surgery and radiation, or (3) induction chemotherapy, surgery, radiation, and maintenance chemotherapy with cisplatin for 6 months. The 5-year survival rates for the three regimens were 35%, 37%, and 45%, respectively; the differences were not significant. However, the time to development of distant metastases and the frequency of distant metastases as a site of first recurrence were significantly less in patients in the maintenance chemotherapy arm compared with the other two groups. On subgroup analysis, there was a significant difference in disease-free survival time for patients receiving maintenance chemotherapy for oral cavity primary tumors and for N1 or N2 disease.[120] In retrospect, it is not surprising that this trial did not show any improvement in overall survival time because only one cycle of cisplatin and bleomycin was administered before surgery, resulting in a low response rate of 37%.

In the SWOG[190] trial, patients were randomly assigned to receive either three cycles of cisplatin, bleomycin, methotrexate, and vincristine before surgery and radiotherapy or standard treatment with surgery and radiotherapy. The median survival time was 30 months for patients in the standard treatment arm compared with 18 months for the induction chemotherapy arm. The distant metastatic rate was 49% with standard treatment and 28% with induction chemotherapy. Although differences in survival time and pattern of recurrence are striking, statistical significance was not reached. This trial fell short of its accrual goals and had a high rate of noncompliance, with only 56% of patients assigned to induction chemotherapy completing the treatment per protocol.

TABLE 4-4

RANDOMIZED TRIALS OF NEOADJUVANT CHEMOTHERAPY BEFORE SURGERY OR RADIOTHERAPY

Author	Regimen	Sites	Number of Patients	Operability	Survival Benefit	Other Outcomes
HN Contracts, (1987, 1990)[106]	PB	OC,L,HP	443	O	For N$_2$ disease in subset analysis	Disease in distant metastases
Carugati (1988)[33]	PB ± M	OC,OP,L	120	O	None	
Toohill (1987)[220]	PF	OC,OP,HP,NP	60	O + I	None	
Jaulerry (1992)[121]	PFV		108	NS	None	
	PBVM	OC,OP,HP,L	100	NS	None	
Szpirglas (1987)[212]	DVcBP	OC,OP	114	I	None	
Mazeron (1992)[155]	PFBM	OC,OP	107	O + I	None	
Martin (1990, 1995)[153,154]	PF	OC,OP,HP,L	75	O + I	None	Decrease in distant metastases
Schuller (1988)[190]	PBMF	OC,OP,HP,L	158	O	None	Larynx preserved in 64% at 2 years
VA Study (1991)[231]	PF	L	332	O	None	Decrease in distant metastases
Paccagnella (1994)[164]	PF	OC,OP,HP	237	O + I	For inoperable patients in subset analysis only	Decrease in distant metastases; improved L-R control for inoperable patients
Depondt (1993)[57]	CF	OC,OP,HP,L	324	O	None	
DiBlasio (1994)[59]	PF	NS	69	O	Significantly worse with chemotherapy	Larynx preserved in 42% at 3 years
Hasegawa (1994)[103]	PF	OC,OP,HP,L	50	O	None	
Chan (1995)[37]	PF	HP	82	NA	None	
Eschwege (1995)[75]	BEP	NP	339	NA	Significant improvement Survival at 7 years	
Dalley (1995)[51]	PF	HP	91	O		
Lefebvre (1996)[140]	PF	HP	202	O	Statistically equivalent survival	Decrease in distant metastases
Domenge (2000)[61]	PF		318	O+I	Yes	

(Reprinted with permission from *Tumors of the nasal cavity and paranasal sinuses, nasopharynx, oral cavity, and oropharynx*. In Schantz SP, Harrison LB, Forastive AA: *Cancer-principles and practice of oncology*, ed 5. Philadelphia, Lippincott-Raven, 1997.)

P, Cisplatin; B, bleomycin; OC, oral cavity; L, larynx; HP, hypopharynx; O, operable; M, methotrexate; OP, oropharynx; F-5, fluorouracil; NP, nasopharynx; I, inoperable; V, vinblastine; Vc, vincristine; L-R, locoregional; C, carboplatin; NS, not specified; NA, not applicable; E, epirubicin.
Shigematsu (1971)[198] Chemotherapy 000 (tongue) Response Yes-DFS.

Domenge and others[61] have recently reported a phase III trial in which 318 patients with locally advanced oropharyngeal squamous cancers were randomly assigned to receive induction chemotherapy with cisplatin and 5-FU followed by locoregional treatment or locoregional therapy alone. Overall survival was better in the chemotherapy group (median, 5.1 vs 3.3 years; $P = .03$).

Encouraging data emerge from induction chemotherapy trials in the area of organ preservation (see Organ Preservation section to follow). The Veterans Affairs Laryngeal Cancer Study Group[231] completed a randomized trial in patients with resectable stage III and IV squamous cell cancer of the larynx. Patients were randomly assigned to receive standard therapy with total laryngectomy and postoperative radiotherapy or to receive a maximum of three cycles of cisplatin and 5-FU chemotherapy followed by radiotherapy. Surgery was reserved for salvage patients with persistent or recurrent disease. If patients did not have at least a partial response at the primary site after two cycles of chemotherapy, they underwent immediate surgery. The complete and partial response rate after two cycles of chemotherapy was 85%, and after three cycles it was 98%. The pathologically confirmed complete response rate at the primary site was 64%. At a median follow-up period of 33 months, there was no significant difference in survival time. However, the patterns of relapse differed: recurrence at the primary site was 2% with surgery vs 12% with chemotherapy ($P = .0005$); regional node recurrence rates were similar ($P = .305$); distant metastases were 17% with surgery vs 11% with chemotherapy ($P = .016$); and the rate of second primary malignancies was 6% with surgery vs 2% with chemotherapy ($P = .029$). After 3 years of follow-up, 66% of surviving patients in the induction chemotherapy treatment group had a preserved, functional larynx. Similar results were reported by the EORTC comparing cisplatin and 5-FU induction chemotherapy followed by radiotherapy to laryngopharyngectomy and radiation in patients with locally advanced cancer of the hypopharynx. No survival time differences were observed, and 28% of patients were alive with a functional larynx. The larynx preservation rate was 42% at 3 years, considering only deaths from local disease as failure.[140]

In follow-up to the VA study, the Head and Neck Intergroup has conducted a prospective three-arm study comparing induction chemotherapy with cisplatin and 5-FU followed by radiotherapy; radiotherapy alone; and radiotherapy with concomitant cisplatin.[87] For entry, patients had stage III/IV disease, but T1 and advanced T4 lesions conferred ineligibility. Infiltrating tumors greater than 1 cm into the tongue base or the demonstration of thyroid cartilage

destruction were not allowed. Five hundred ten patients were entered, 65% of whom had stage III disease. Two thirds of patients had supraglottic primary sites. No unexpected toxicity was observed. With no difference in overall survival, the concomitant treatment arm resulted in superior larynx preservation, 88% compared with 74% resulting from sequential chemotherapy and radiation and 69% with radiotherapy alone. Notably, patients with destructive T4 primary tumors were excluded from this study. Long-term outcomes including quality of life and functional data are awaited.

The Domenge trial[61] in Table 4-4 demonstrated a survival benefit from induction chemotherapy. Two trials showed an improvement in survival time for chemotherapy-treated patients after subset analysis. In a large Italian study, Paccagnella and others[163,164] observed an improvement in local control, metastatic rate, and survival time for inoperable patients. In a follow-up study to the Head and Neck Contracts Program, Jacobs and others[119] reported an improvement in survival time for the subgroup with oral cavity primaries and limited nodal disease. In terms of patterns of failure, five trials showed a decrease in the rate of distant metastasis.[119,140,164,190]

These trials have helped to clarify many issues. First, the overall response rates range from 60% to 90% with complete response rates of 20% to 50%. Survival time is improved in patients with a complete response compared with nonresponders, and pathologic complete response can be seen in 30% to 70%. Second, response to chemotherapy predicts for response to radiotherapy. Patients who fail to respond to chemotherapy do not respond well to radiation. Third, neoadjuvant chemotherapy increases neither surgical nor radiotherapy complication rates. Fourth, the most critical prognostic factors for response are TN stage and type of chemotherapy. Biologic behavior appears to differ per site. Fifth, although no benefit in overall survival time has yet been shown, a significant reduction in the rate of distant metastases has been observed. Finally, organ preservation and improved quality of life can result with induction chemotherapy. For patients with advanced laryngeal cancer who would require a total laryngectomy, the available data indicate that laryngeal function can be preserved in two thirds without jeopardizing survival time.

Neoadjuvant chemotherapy has been used to manage advanced nasopharyngeal carcinoma similarly to other sites. To date, two randomized prospective trials have been conducted. The International Nasopharyngeal Study Group[116] randomly assigned 339 patients, who were at high risk for relapse (i.e., N_2, N_3 disease), to receive three cycles of bleomycin, epirubicin, and cisplatin chemotherapy followed by radiotherapy or radiotherapy alone. At a median follow-up period of 49 months, there was a significant difference in disease-free survival time, 42% vs 29% at 4 years (P = .006) in favor of the chemotherapy arm. No difference in overall survival time was observed, 50% vs 42%, although median survival time was superior for the chemotherapy and radiation arm compared with radiation alone, 50 and 37 months, respectively.

In the second study, Chan and others[37] randomly assigned 82 patients to receive either radiotherapy alone or two cycles of cisplatin and 5-FU followed by radiotherapy. These patients had tumors 4 cm or large or N_3 nodal disease. The overall response rate to chemotherapy was 81%, and this increased to 100% after radiation vs 95% for radiation alone. However, at a median follow-up period of 28.5 months, 2-year survival and disease-free survival time were not significantly altered by the addition of chemotherapy. This lack of difference may be accounted for partly by the less intensive nature of the chemotherapy with the 5-FU being given at 1000 cy/m² per day over 3 days.

Concurrent Radiotherapy and Chemotherapy

Concurrent radiotherapy and chemotherapy have been used primarily in patients with unresectable disease to improve local and regional control. The major drugs with efficacy for this tumor type and in vitro evidence of radiation enhancement capability have been tested as single agents since the 1960s. The theoretic rationale and mechanism for the interaction between cytotoxic drugs and radiation that results in additive or synergistic enhancement have been reviewed in detail.[91,205,213] This biologic phenomenon rests on several mechanisms. These include (1) inhibition of DNA repair, (2) redistribution of cells in sensitive phases of the cell cycle, and (3) promoting oxygenation of anoxic tissues. The net effect is to improve cellular cytotoxicity.[235] Most of the single agents used to treat patients with head and neck cancer have been combined with radiation.

Nearly all reported trials of concomitant chemotherapy and radiotherapy have noted enhanced acute radiation-induced toxicity, primarily mucosal, which often has resulted in dose reductions and lengthy interruptions in radiation without evidence of survival benefit. Thus, in combining these two treatment modalities, it is essential that toxicity not preclude the use of chemotherapy and radiation in the optimal dose and schedule.

Single Agents and Radiotherapy

For an outline of randomized trials of simultaneous single-agent chemotherapy with radiotherapy vs radiotherapy, see Table 4-5.

TABLE 4-5

RANDOMIZED TRIALS OF SIMULTANEOUS SINGLE AGENT CHEMOTHERAPY WITH RADIOTHERAPY VS RADIOTHERAPY

Investigations	Chemotherapy	Number of Patients	Response Rate	Survival Benefit
Richards (1969)[175]	HU	40	Yes	NR
Stefani (1971)[206]	HU	150	No	No
Hussey (1975)[115]	HU	42	No	No
Condit (1968)[44]	MTX	40	Yes	NR
Gupta (1987)[100]	MTX	313	Yes	Yes
Kapstad (1978)[126]	Bleomycin	29	Yes	NR
Shanta (1980)[193]	Bleomycin	157	No	Yes
Morita (1980)[160]	Bleomycin	45 (tongue)	No	No
Scandolaro (1982)[187]	Bleomycin	30	No	No
Parvinen (1985)[166]	Bleomycin	46	NR	No
Shetty (1985)[196]	Bleomycin	38	No	No
Vermund (1985)[227]	Bleomycin	222	Yes	No
Fu (1987)[92]	Bleomycin	104	No	Yes-DFS
Eschwege (1988)[74]	Bleomycin	199	NR	No
Shigematsu (1971)[198]	5-FU	63	Yes	Yes-DFS
Lo (1976)[147]	5-FU	163	Yes	Yes
Browman (1993)[26]	5-FU	175	Yes	No
Weissberg (1989)[241]	Mitomycin-C	117	Yes	Yes
Haselow (1990)[104]	CDDP	319	Yes	NR

(Reprinted with permission from *Tumors of the nasal cavity and paranasal sinuses, nasopharynx, oral cavity, and oropharynx*. In Schantz SP, Harrison LB, Forastive AA: *Cancer-principles and practice of oncology*, ed 5. Philadelphia, Lippincott-Raven, 1997.)
HU, hydroxyurea; MTX, methotrexate; 5-FU, 5-fluorouracil; DFS, disease-free survival; CDDP, cisplatin.
Adelstein (1990b)[2] Sequential VBM ± F → RT Number of Significant increase Significant improvement in DFS.

Chapter 4 Chemotherapy for Head and Neck Cancer **129**

Methotrexate plus radiotherapy. Methotrexate can produce an S-phase block of the cell cycle, resulting in accumulation of cells in the G1 phase and causing increased radiosensitivity.[13] In one early study, 96 patients with inoperable disease were randomly assigned to receive radiotherapy alone or radiation preceded by intravenous methotrexate.[133] The complete response rate was the same in both groups, as was the 3-year survival rate. However, the incidence of mucositis increased in those patients who received chemotherapy. A second large study of patients with stage III and IV squamous cell carcinoma, similar to the previous study, again showed no difference in the 3-year survival rate, although the rate of distant metastases was only 19% in patients who received chemotherapy plus radiation compared with 33% of patients who received radiotherapy alone.[149] The Radiation Therapy Oncology Group (RTOG) randomly assigned 712 patients to receive radiotherapy alone or radiation plus pretreatment methotrexate.[77] No difference occurred in survival time between the treatment groups, and more patients failed to complete irradiation in the combined therapy group. In a randomized study published by Condit,[44] there was no improvement in survival time in the combined group. In another study, Gupta and others[100] observed an improvement in survival time and better control of the primary tumor. This was especially true for those with oropharyngeal tumors. Thus, three randomized series with adequate patient numbers showed negative results, and a fourth study showed improved survival time.

Hydroxyurea plus radiotherapy. Hydroxyurea kills cells in the S-phase and synchronizes cells into the more radiosensitive G_1 phase. Despite good theoretic activity, three randomized trials have shown no advantage of hydroxyurea in addition to radiotherapy. In one series, 12 patients with advanced cancer were randomly assigned to receive radiation alone or with hydroxyurea (80 mg/kg biweekly).[206] The complete response rate at the primary site was 40% in both groups, but survival time was inferior in the combination group. In addition, distant metastases developed in 23% of patients receiving combined treatment as compared with 8% receiving irradiation alone. Another study of 40 patients comparing radiotherapy alone or with hydroxyurea (80 mg/kg three times per week) showed no difference in complete response rate or survival times, but it did show a 40% incidence of mucositis in the combined group.[175]

Bleomycin plus radiotherapy. Bleomycin and irradiation have been studied in vitro, and the enhanced effects are believed to be caused by interference with cellular repair after irradiation. Nine randomized trials have compared radiotherapy alone with radiation plus bleomycin. The first series included 227 patients with advanced oropharyngeal carcinomas.[29] Bleomycin was given at 15 mg twice weekly for 5 weeks. No difference in response rate or survival time was noted, and bleomycin was not well tolerated, causing a significant amount of mucositis. The results were unchanged in a recent update of this trial.[74] Similar results were reported by Vermund and others.[227] In contrast, a third large series from India[194] included patients with advanced buccal mucosa cancers and compared radiotherapy given alone with radiation plus bleomycin (10 to 15 mg three times per week for 6 weeks). The complete response rate in the radiotherapy group was 21% compared with 77% in the combined therapy group.

An improvement in disease-free survival time, local and regional control, and complete response rate, but not overall survival time, was reported by Fu and others.[92] In this Northern California Oncology Group trial, patients received either radiotherapy alone or radiation with bleomycin (5 mg twice weekly) followed by 16 weeks of maintenance bleomycin and methotrexate. The complete response rates were 45% with radiotherapy alone and 67% for the combined treatment (P = .056). The 2-year local and regional control rate was significantly improved with the addition of bleomycin, 26% vs 64% (P = .001). The incidence of distant metastases as a site of failure was similar in both treatment groups, indicating that the bleomycin and methotrexate maintenance regimen was ineffective in controlling micrometastatic disease. In this trial, in contrast to the others reported, the dose of bleomycin used with radiotherapy was well tolerated. A significant reduction in radiation dose or treatment delays did not occur as a result of enhancement of acute radiation toxicity.

Nine randomized trials of bleomycin and radiation have been completed. Only three of these showed a response benefit.[92,126,193]

5-Fluorouracil plus radiotherapy. Several early trials indicated that 5-FU was an active radiosensitizer for patients with head and neck cancer. Three randomized trials have been published. Lo and others[147] randomly assigned 134 patients with advanced head and neck cancer to receive radiotherapy with or without 5-FU (10 mg/kg per day for 3 days, 5 mg/kg per day for 4 days, 5 mg/m² three times per week). The 5-year survival rate for radiation alone was 14%, and for combined treatment it was 32%. This improvement in survival time occurred for patients with primary lesions in the tongue or tonsil only. In another study, Shigematsu and colleagues[198] used intraarterial 5-FU with radiotherapy to treat patients with maxillary sinus carcinoma and observed an improvement in disease-free survival time. Browman and others[26] randomly assigned patients to receive infusional 5-FU and radiation or radiation alone and observed a higher complete response rate but no change in survival time.

Mitomycin and radiotherapy. Mitomycin is an antibiotic that during hypoxic conditions is enzymatically reduced to form an active alkylating species.[185] It is selectively toxic to hypoxic cells. Therefore, because hypoxic cells within tumors have reduced sensitivity to the effects of radiation, it has been hypothesized that combined treatment could improve the therapeutic ratio.[181] This concept was tested by Weissberg and others[241] in a randomized trial by treating 120 patients with advanced head and neck cancer with radiotherapy alone or with radiation with mitomycin (15 mg/m²). Disease-free survival time at 5 years was 49% for the radiotherapy-alone patients and 75% for those treated with mitomycin (P < .07). Local and regional control rates were significantly improved with administration of mitomycin, 55% vs 75% (P < .01). There was no difference in the incidence of distant metastases or overall survival time between treatment groups.

Cisplatin and radiotherapy. The exact mechanism of interaction between cisplatin and radiation is not known. Hypoxic and aerobic cell sensitization and the inhibition of cellular repair processes for sublethally damaged cells contribute to the effects observed in in vitro systems.[58] In a phase II trial, the RTOG administered cisplatin (100 mg/m²) every 3 weeks to 124 patients with locally advanced, unresectable head and neck cancer.[6] Sixty percent of patients completed the combined treatment per protocol, and 69% of all patients achieved a complete response. Separate analysis of the disease-free and overall survival times for those with nasopharynx and non-nasopharynx primary sites with more than 5 years of follow-up have been published.[7,151] A comparison to RTOG patients treated with radiotherapy alone suggested improvement in survival time for the combined treatment.

Wheeler and others[244] piloted a study involving the administration of high-dose cisplatin (200 mg/m²) every 4 weeks with concurrent radiotherapy in 18 patients with unresectable disease and observed complete responses in 94%. The median survival time was 23 months with 56% and 41% alive and disease-free at 1 and 2 years, respectively. A high rate of distant relapse was observed. Only one randomized trial has been conducted to evaluate concomitant cisplatin and radiotherapy.[104] Through the Head and

Neck Intergroup mechanism, 371 patients with unresectable local regional squamous cell head and neck cancer were randomly assigned to receive radiotherapy alone or radiation plus weekly low-dose cisplatin, 20 mg/m².

There was a significant difference in overall response rate (complete and partial), 59% for those receiving radiation alone and 73% for those receiving the combined treatment (P = .007). However, there was no significant difference in complete response or survival time. The lack of survival benefit may be because of the low total dose of cisplatin received—only 120 to 140 mg/m² over the 6 to 8 weeks of radiation treatment.

Concomitant chemotherapy and radiotherapy have been useful for the treatment of patients with nasopharyngeal carcinoma. A head and neck intergroup trial closed in November 1995 demonstrating favorable results for the combined approach in this disease.[7] In this study, patients received either radiotherapy alone or cisplatin (100 mg/m² days 1, 22, and 43) during radiotherapy followed by adjuvant chemotherapy with cisplatin and 5-FU (three cycles). An analysis of 147 randomized patients revealed significant differences in 3-year survival time (78% vs 47%) and progression-free survival time (69% vs 24%) favoring the chemotherapy group. This exciting result has now changed the standard of care for those with nasopharyngeal carcinoma in the United States. Patients with stage III or IV disease should be treated with concomitant chemoradiotherapy followed by adjuvant chemotherapy.

Randomized trials of single agents and radiotherapy have shown improved survival time with methotrexate, bleomycin, and 5-FU.[147,194] Improved disease-free survival, but not overall survival time, has been shown in two other trials with use of bleomycin and mitomycin.[92,241] Because mucosal toxicity is enhanced with these regimens and because overall survival time, although improved, remains poor, none of these regimens has become a standard therapy. The exciting results of the intergroup trial using concurrent cisplatin in patients with locally advanced nasopharyngeal cancer cannot be generalized to other sites, but they will form a basis for further investigation.

The favorable results from concurrent cisplatin treatment and radiotherapy followed by adjuvant chemotherapy establish this as a standard management approach for locally advanced nasopharyngeal cancer in the United States.

Multiple Agents and Radiotherapy

Combining several drugs with radiation will enhance acute toxicity, which may be severe. Therefore, investigators have piloted trials designed with split-course radiation to allow for healthy tissue recovery. Most of these studies are limited to patients with stage III and IV locally advanced unresectable squamous cell cancer and have improved survival time as the primary goal. These regimens alternate chemotherapy and radiotherapy or use split-course radiotherapy to maximize tumor cell kill and to minimize tissue toxicity. For those with head and neck cancer, protracted radiation results in decreased local control rates because of accelerated repopulation of cancer cells that survive the initial insult.[11,165] Thus, alternating two non–cross-resistant agents may potentially eliminate not only tumor cell repopulation but primary drug resistance.

Early phase I and II studies have used infusional 5-FU as originally reported by Byfield and others,[28] adding cisplatin[1,216] or hydroxyurea[234] with concurrent split-course single daily fraction radiation. Alternatively, cisplatin and fluorouracil with leucovorin modulation have been combined with split-course accelerated radiotherapy.[242] Several studies with long follow-up periods reported promising survival and response data but also severe toxicity.[3,102,216,237,242]

Mature data were reported by Taylor and others[216] using cisplatin plus continuous-infusion 5-FU and radiotherapy and alternating 1 week of treatment with 1 week of rest. The median survival time for 53 patients with a median follow-up period in excess of 4 years was 37 months. The complete response rate was 55%. The total dose received of radiation and 5-FU but not cisplatin correlated with outcome. Local control was poorest in stage IV patients with N3 disease.

Although these pilot trials all report encouraging data for improved survival time, randomized trials that use radiotherapy alone as the control are needed before these approaches can be recommended outside the research setting. Data from selected randomized trials are shown in Table 4-6. The South-East Cooperative Oncology Group (SECOG)[204] compared alternating with sequential chemotherapy and radiotherapy. The chemotherapy selected was vincristine, bleomycin, and methotrexate with a further randomization to inclusion of 5-FU or not. Survival rates were lower than observed in a previous pilot trial, and a significant improvement in disease-free survival time was observed on subset analysis for larynx primaries managed with the alternating schedule. The alternating regimen was associated with a higher frequency of severe mucosal reactions.

Merlano and others[156] published the final report of a randomized comparison of alternating and sequential chemotherapy (vinblastine, bleomycin, methotrexate) and radiotherapy followed by surgical salvage if feasible. Four courses of chemotherapy were alternated with three courses of radiotherapy (20 Gy each). All patients had unresectable stage III or IV squamous cell cancer. The complete response rate before and after surgical intervention and the overall survival time at 4 years were significantly superior for patients receiving concomitant treatment. Severe mucosal toxicity was observed in 30.5% of patients in the alternating regimen compared with only 6% of those receiving chemotherapy before radiotherapy. The results of a follow-up trial reported by Merlano and others[156,157] showed a significant difference in relapse-free and overall survival time for patients treated with alternating cisplatin plus 5-FU and radiotherapy compared with radiotherapy alone. All patients had unresectable locally advanced squamous cell cancer of the head and neck.

In a small randomized trial, Adelstein and others[2] compared simultaneous cisplatin plus 5-FU and radiotherapy to sequential treatment. Patients with stage II, III, or IV, either resectable or unresectable disease, were eligible. In the simultaneous treatment, patients were evaluated for surgery after chemotherapy and 30 Gy. Complete responders and those with unresectable disease continued treatment with chemotherapy and radiotherapy. In the sequential treatment, surgical evaluation occurred after three cycles of chemotherapy and before radiotherapy. The results with follow-up period ranging from 9 to 41 months showed a significant difference in disease-free survival time but not overall survival time. At this point in follow-up, 18 of 48 patients were complete responders and had not required surgery. Taylor,[217] similarly to Adelstein and others,[3] compared cisplatin plus 5-FU and concomitant radiotherapy with sequential treatment. They found a significant improvement in local and regional control in patients receiving concomitant treatment.

The use of concurrent combination chemotherapy and radiation has continued to be under intense study in recent years.[130] There has been clear demonstration of enhancement of tumor control and improvement of survival over radiation treatment alone (see Table 4-6). There has also been a substantial increase in acute toxicities, especially dermatitis and mucositis, and longer follow-up evidence for increased late toxicity has begun to emerge.

As a generalization, patients admitted to these studies have had variable head and neck primary T sites, although oropharynx primaries tend to predominate. Brizel and others[24] have compared a hyperfractionated radiotherapy arm to a total dose of 75 Gy with the same radiation schedule, to 70 Gy, and concurrent cisplatin and 5-fluorouracil. The concurrent treatment was followed by two cycles of adjuvant chemotherapy. There was a statistically significant

TABLE 4-6

RANDOMIZED TRIALS OF CONCOMITANT OR ALTERNATING COMBINATION CHEMOTHERAPY AND RADIATION

Author (Ref)	Treatment	Number of Patients	Survival other Outcomes
Keane (1993)[128]	Concurrent MMC + F/RT	104	NS
	RT	105	
Merlano (1992)[158]	Alternating PF/RT	80	Significant increase
	RT	77	Significant improvement in CR + L-R control with PFS/RT
Taylor (1994)[217]	Concurrent PF/RT	108	NS
	Sequential PF → RT	107	Significant improvement L-R control for $T_{3-4}N_2$ subset with PFS/RT
Adelstein (1990)[2]	Concurrent PF/RT	24	NS
	Sequential PF → RT	24	Significant improvement in DFS with concurrent PFS/RT
Merlano (1991)[156]	Alternating VBM/RT	61	Significant increase
	Sequential VBM → RT	55	Significant increase in CR and PFS with concurrent VBM/RT
SECOG (1986)[204]	Concurrent VBM ± F/RT	136	
	Sequential VBM ± F → RT	NS	DFS improved for larynx with concurrent VBM ± F/RT
Brizel (1998)[24]	Concurrent PF/RT	56	L-R Control improved ($P = .1$)
	HFRT	60	
Wendt (1998)[243]	Concurrent PFL/RT	130	Improved survival ($P = .0003$)
	HFRT	140	
Calais (1999)[30]	Concurrent Pc/RT	109	Improved survival ($P = .02$)
	RT	113	
Jeremic (2000)[123]	Concurrent C/RT	65	Improved survival ($P = .008$)
	HFRT	65	

(Reprinted with permission from *Tumors of the nasal cavity and paranasal sinuses, nasopharynx, oral cavity, and oropharynx.* In Schantz SP, Harrison LB, Forastive AA: *Cancer-principles and practice of oncology*, ed 5. Philadelphia, Lippincott-Raven, 1997.) MMC, Mitomycin C; F-5, fluorouracil; L, leucovorin; Pc, carboplatin; RT, radiotherapy; NS, not significant; PFS, progress-free survival; CR, complete response; DFS, disease-free survival; SECOG, Southeast Cooperative Oncology Group; P, cisplatin; V, vinblastine; B, bleomycin; M, methotrexate; L-R, locoregional.

improvement in local disease control and a strong trend toward improved overall survival. In this trial, neck dissection was recommended in patients with N2/3 disease. Clayman and others[42] reviewed the M.D. Anderson experience examining the indication for neck dissection in this patient population. This report suggests that neck dissections are required only when there is radiographic evidence of residual disease 6 to 8 weeks after the completion of definitive chemoradiation. Wendt and others[243] reported a statistically significant 3-year survival advantage after the concurrent use of cisplatin, 5-FU and leucovorin given as a single therapeutic modality. Calais and others[30] compared a more standard once-daily fractionation radiation schedule with the same radiotherapy and concurrent carboplatin and 5-FU, demonstrating a statistically significant advantage in local regional tumor control and overall survival at 3 years. This report is particularly germane because the study group consisted of oropharyngeal patients only. Finally, Jeremic and colleagues[123] investigated the value of adding cisplatin given daily to a hyperfractionated radiation therapy program vs the same radiation schedule given alone in patients with locally advanced squamous cell cancers of the head and neck. In this recent report, locoregional and distant disease control, as well as overall survival were improved at the 5 years. The clearest benefit in all four studies was an improvement in locoregional control that translated into a survival advantage. Acute toxicity was increased, especially mucositis and hematologic effects, but there was no obvious escalation of long-term sequelae. However, this potential problem area has not been fully studied. In aggregate, overall 3-year survival exceeded 50% in these experimental programs, underscoring the potential therapeutic efficacy of concomitant chemotherapy and radiation in advanced head and neck cancers.

Concurrent chemotherapy, particularly with multiple drugs, leads to a marked increase in acute toxicity. "In-field" mucositis and dermatitis can be severe, are associated with much discomfort, and may lead to increased risk of infection, poor nutritional intake, and interruption of radiotherapy or chemotherapy dose reductions. This may compromise tumor control and ultimate survival. There also is the potential for an increase in serious long-term toxicities as survival increases after these intensive treatment programs. For optimal results, concurrent treatments should be administered in centers with sufficient training and expertise and with experienced supportive care teams available.

The results of these trials indicate that improved disease-free and overall survival times were obtained for patients with locally advanced squamous cell head and neck cancer using alternating or concomitant chemotherapy and radiotherapy. Well-designed clinical trials are needed to determine optimal chemotherapy and radiotherapy schedules. Randomized trials are currently in progress to help clarify these issues.

Adjuvant Chemotherapy

Adjuvant chemotherapy after primary surgery has been shown to be effective in patients with breast cancer and osteogenic sarcoma. To date, three randomized trials have been designed to address this question in those with head and neck cancer. Adjuvant chemotherapy has several potential advantages over neoadjuvant treatment. With adjuvant treatment, surgery is not delayed, and a patient with resectable disease can undergo surgery sooner. Secondly, induction therapy can blur the margins of disease, making the degree of surgical resection less obvious. Finally, induction chemotherapy, if successful, can lead to symptom abatement, resulting in patient refusal of surgery afterward.

Through the Head and Neck Intergroup mechanism, a large multiinstitutional trial was conducted to test whether the addition of chemotherapy to surgery and radiotherapy prolonged survival time or altered the pattern of recurrence.[139] Patients with stage III or IV squamous cell carcinoma of the oral cavity, oropharynx, or larynx and those with stage II, III, or IV of the hypopharynx who had negative pathologic margins of resection were eligible.

Randomization was to immediate postoperative radiotherapy or to three cycles of cisplatin plus 5-FU chemotherapy followed by radiotherapy. A preliminary analysis of the 503 patients in the study has shown no significant difference in disease-free survival time, overall survival time, and local and regional control. However, there was a significantly lower rate of distant metastases as a site of failure ($P = .016$) at any time for patients treated with adjuvant chemotherapy. Perhaps more important was the finding that a high-risk subset of patients (those with extracapsular extension, carcinoma in situ, or close

surgical margins) appears to benefit from adjuvant chemotherapy with increased survival time and local control that approached statistical confidence when compared with those receiving radiation alone.

Two trials testing induction chemotherapy added maintenance chemotherapy to one treatment group and observed differences in outcome. The Head and Neck Contracts Program[106] trial of one course of cisplatin and bleomycin induction chemotherapy before surgery and radiation included 6 months of maintenance chemotherapy in one of the three treatment arms. There was a significant decrease in the distant metastatic rate observed for those patients. Ervin and others[73] randomly assigned patients showing a response to cisplatin, bleomycin, and methotrexate induction chemotherapy to receive three additional cycles or observation after definitive surgery and radiotherapy. The 3-year disease-free survival time for patients receiving maintenance chemotherapy was 88% compared with 57% for the control subjects ($P = .03$). In a phase II pilot, Johnson and others[124] treated 42 patients with extracapsular spread of tumor in cervical lymph node metastases with 6 months of methotrexate and 5-FU after resection and radiotherapy. The 2-year disease-free survival rate was 66%, which was improved from an expected control rate of 38% based on historical experience.

Shin and others[199] have recently reported the potential benefit of adjuvant cis retinoic acid interferon-α and vitamin E in advanced-stage patients treated for 1 year after completion of primary therapy. In a phase II experience with eligible patients considered disease-free at the start of the adjuvant program, they reported 90% failure-free survival at median 2-year follow-up. This adjuvant regimen is currently being tested in a prospective phase III trial.

Considered together, the results of these trials indicate that adjuvant chemotherapy can affect micrometastatic disease and decrease the rate of distant recurrence. The data also suggest that disease-free survival time may be improved. The major impediment to successfully conducting adjuvant or maintenance chemotherapy trials in patients with head and neck cancer is patient noncompliance and physician fatigue. The morbidity of the primary treatment, combined with the medical and social situations of this group of patients, makes classical adjuvant chemotherapy difficult or not feasible for many patients. In addition, there appears to be no role for adjuvant chemotherapy in low-risk patients, although high-risk patients may benefit.

ORGAN PRESERVATION

Many squamous cell cancers of the head and neck are diagnosed at a late stage. Stage III and IV tumors often necessitate extensive or radical surgery that can alter function. Problems with radical surgery include loss of speech, loss of swallowing function, or disfigurement without a concomitant improvement in survival time. Therefore, preservation of function became one of the major challenges of the 1990s. A role for combined modality treatment in preserving organ function has already been noted for laryngeal preservation as in the VA larynx study.[231] In this study, neoadjuvant chemotherapy followed by radiotherapy was more successful in preserving voice function compared with surgery without a loss in survival time.

Neoadjuvant chemotherapy has been used to preserve organ function for patients with hypopharyngeal, laryngeal, and oropharyngeal cancers. Several nonrandomized studies have been completed using cisplatin-based chemotherapy. In these studies, patients were required to have achieved either partial or complete response to go on to conventional radiotherapy. Nonresponders then went on to undergo radical surgery. In these pilot studies, there were no survival differences between the surgical groups and the groups that avoided surgery, suggesting that quality of life may be improved without worsening survival.

In addition to the VA larynx study,[231] another large randomized study has been completed. This study[140] was done in Europe by the European Organization for Research and Treatment of Cancer (EORTC) beginning in 1990 and compared a larynx-preserving therapy (induction chemotherapy plus radiation) with conventional surgery plus postoperative radiation. The design of the EORTC study was similar to the VA larynx study; the patients were randomly assigned to either treatment, and patients receiving induction chemotherapy received cisplatin plus 5-FU. After two cycles of chemotherapy, only responders (i.e., partial or complete responders) received a third cycle. Patients achieving a complete response then received definitive radiotherapy. Nonresponding patients or those with partial response underwent conventional surgery followed by postoperative radiation. As in the VA study, the overall survival data were not different between the two arms, and the median duration of survival time was longer for the chemotherapy arm. Local failures occurred more commonly in the chemotherapy arm, but the distant metastatic rate was lower. In both studies, a large number of patients were enrolled, and of the surviving patients, a significant percentage were able to retain their larynx.

The intergroup study, previously discussed, further supports the concept that for selected patients definitive treatment with chemotherapy and radiation may allow for organ preservation with no compromise in terms of survival. In the R91-11 trial, there was comparison between induction chemotherapy, radiotherapy alone, and radiotherapy with concurrent cisplatin. The results indicated a significant advantage for concomitant cisplatin treatment with preservation of the larynx in 88% of patients treated in the concomitant arm. It can be concluded that the option of organ preservation therapy with chemotherapy and radiation therapy is becoming a reality for many patients with squamous cancers of the head and neck. Certainly, enrollment of patients with advanced cancers of the oropharynx and hypopharynx to clinical trials of multimodel therapy.

INTRAARTERIAL CHEMOTHERAPY

Poor response to chemotherapy after surgery or radiotherapy may be caused by impaired drug delivery into the region. Intraarterial chemotherapy has been used in attempts to overcome this for almost three decades. The rationale for intraarterial therapy is based on the steep dose-response curve exhibited by most cytotoxic drugs.[88] Maximum cell kill occurs when the tumor exposure to a high concentration of drug is optimized. Drug toxicity also follows a steep curve. Therefore, regional drug delivery has the potential to increase tumor drug exposure and reduce systemic exposure that affects critical healthy tissues.[38,43] The principal determinant of a drug's therapeutic advantage is the ratio of total body clearance to the regional exchange rate.

Several factors should be considered when choosing a drug for intraarterial delivery: (1) drug concentration, not time of exposure, is the major factor in cell killing; (2) the drug should be deactivated in the systemic circulation; (3) there should be a high tissue extraction; and (4) a drug should not require activation in the liver.

Intraarterial cisplatin has been shown to be effective and relatively nontoxic in patients with several solid tumors. Pharmacokinetic studies have shown a regional increase in plasma and tissue platinum concentrations in the infused area. Several studies indicate significant palliation in patients with head and neck squamous cancers in whom irradiation and surgery failed to eradicate the tumor. A response rate of 87% using intraarterial 5-FU, methotrexate, and bleomycin was reported by Donegan and Harris.[62] Tumor regression lasted up to 13 months. Intraarterial methotrexate and bleomycin have been used before irradiation for patients with advanced head and neck cancer, with a 28% partial response rate.[250] Intraarterial cisplatin given before surgery or radiation has produced responses in the 70% to 80% range.[161]

One of the major drawbacks of intraarterial therapy is catheter-related complications: air and plaque emboli, sepsis, and patient immobility during chemotherapy administration. These problems have been overcome by the introduction of an implantable infusion pump.[14] This system has been used successfully to treat patients with recurrent head and neck cancer with continuous infusion of dichloromethotrexate and fluorodoxyuridine.[82,245]

One primary site for which intraarterial chemotherapy has been more extensively studied is paranasal sinus cancer. Japanese investigators have favored cannulation of the superficial temporal artery and infusion of 5-FU integrated with surgery and radiotherapy.[186,197] More recently, investigators in the United States have evaluated superselective arterial catheterization and short-term intraarterial chemotherapy to debulk locally advanced resectable and unresectable paranasal sinus carcinoma. This approach minimizes potential toxic effects to adjacent healthy tissues.

Dimery and colleagues[60] reported evaluating intraarterial cisplatin and bleomycin by this technique combined with intravenous 5-FU. A complete response rate of 23% was achieved in those receiving the chemotherapy alone. After surgery or radiotherapy, 63% of patients were disease free, and 61% were spared orbital exenteration. Papadimitrakopoulou and others[97] further evaluated intraarterial cisplatin with systemic paclitaxel and ifosfamide induction therapy for maxillary cancers in an attempt to determine the efficacy of the regimen in patients who otherwise would require orbital exenteration or a major cranial facial resection. The organ preservation rate was 74% with 17 of 24 patients disease free at 1.6 years' medial follow-up.

More recently, Robbins and colleagues[177,178] have reported an extensive experience in 213 patients with stage III/IV squamous cell carcinomas treated with weekly intraarterial infusion of cisplatin, simultaneous intravenous thiosulfate, and external beam radiotherapy. Complete tumor response in the primary and regional sites was observed in 80% and 61% of patients, respectively. Cancer-specific 5-year survival was 54%, and six treatment-related deaths occurred.

Although intraarterial therapy has several theoretic advantages over systemic chemotherapy, it has not been established as a superior approach. Most series contain small numbers of selected patients. This therapy should not be viewed as a standard of care by the community, and further investigation appears to be warranted.

SALIVARY GLAND CANCERS

Cancers of the salivary gland represent approximately 3% of all neoplasms in the head and neck region. The majority originate in the parotid gland. Despite optimal treatment with surgery and postoperative radiotherapy, patients with advanced salivary gland cancers have a poor prognosis, with survival times ranging from 0% to 32% at 10 years. Survival time varies with histology, with 10-year survival rates of 96% reported for low-grade mucoepidermoid carcinoma and 29% reported for adenoid cystic carcinoma.[89] The probability of recurrence also varies with site. Local or distal recurrence occurs in up to 66% of patients with cancers of the major salivary glands and in up to 92% of patients with cancers of the minor salivary glands.[45] The reasons for recurrence include failure of local control and spread of disease to distant sites, particularly the lung.

Chemotherapy in the management of salivary gland cancers has been used mainly for the treatment of patients with recurrent disease. Because of the relatively small number of patients, trials often contain few patients with a variety of histologic findings. Many reports document single cases, leaving uncertainty as to the number of patients who may have been treated. Suen and Johns[211] reported that response to chemotherapy varies with histologic findings. They also found that response varies with the site of recurrence, with local and regional disease having a higher response rate than distant disease. In addition, patients without previous radiotherapy had a better response to chemotherapy. Drawing conclusions from most series is difficult because they usually include a group of patients treated for many years with a variety of combinations and single agents. In addition, some cancers with distal spread, such as adenoid cystic carcinoma, can grow at such a slow rate that responses and impact on survival time are difficult to interpret.

Suen and Johns[211] reported large series of patients treated at their institutions and at others in an attempt to define the best single agents or combinations of drugs for salivary gland cancers of specific histologic categories. For those with adenoid cystic carcinoma, the best single agents are cisplatin, 5-FU, and doxorubicin. Cisplatin has been reported to have a complete response rate of 29% and an overall response rate of 64% in 14 treated patients.[189,211] Complete responses lasted from 7 to 18 months. 5-FU has been reported to have a partial response rate of 46% in 13 patients.[125,214] Adriamycin was noted to have a response rate of 13% in seven patients.[174,226] Methotrexate, vincristine, and cyclophosphamide appear to have little activity for adenoid cystic carcinoma. The combination of Adriamycin and cyclophosphamide has been used in five patients with a 40% partial response rate.[171] Because of poor prognosis of patients with advanced disease and the activity of cisplatin, Sessions and others[191] treated four patients with intraarterial cisplatin before further therapy. All patients had some tumor shrinkage, but only two had a partial response. There was minimal toxicity.

Very few studies of single-agent chemotherapy for mucoepidermoid carcinoma exist. Several of the studies were done before the widespread use of cisplatin, and data on its use as a single agent for the management of this carcinoma are not available. Methotrexate has been used in four patients, with one achieving a complete response and one having a partial response. Posner and others[171] used two different combinations for recurrent mucoepidermoid carcinoma. Two of three patients responded to a combination of cisplatin, bleomycin, and methotrexate. Three patients failed to respond to a combination of cyclophosphamide and Adriamycin. Further studies need to be done to determine the most active agents for mucoepidermoid carcinoma.

Only scattered reports of the use of chemotherapy for the other salivary gland cancers exist. The combination of Adriamycin, cisplatin, and cyclophosphamide achieved one complete response and two partial responses in three treated patients with adenocarcinoma.[4] The small numbers of patients in each series preclude firm conclusions regarding the true level of antitumor activity of these drugs. However, the data provide an indication of which drugs are reasonable to choose for single-agent or combination chemotherapy. Creagan and others[49] reported the results of cisplatin-based chemotherapy in 34 patients with locally recurrent or metastatic cancers originating from the salivary gland or contiguous structures. Most patients received cyclophosphamide or mitomycin, plus Adriamycin and cisplatin combination chemotherapy. A 38% response rate was observed, listing a median of 7 months. The median survival time was 18 months for responders to chemotherapy and 15 months for nonresponders. Thus, response to treatment did not appear to confer a survival advantage. Dreyfuss and others[65] also evaluated cyclophosphamide, Adriamycin, and cisplatin in a series of 13 patients (nine with adenoid cystic carcinoma and four with adenocarcinoma), observing responses in 46% (three complete and three partial responses). In another combination chemotherapy trial, Venook and others[225] treated 17 patients with advanced or recurrent salivary cancer with cisplatin, Adriamycin, and 5-FU. Thirty-five percent of patients responded to chemotherapy. In this small series, response rate was not influenced by the extent of previous treatment.

Whether combination chemotherapy can improve survival time in patients with recurrent disease is not clear. In some patients with recurrent disease, particularly adenoid cystic carcinoma, the pace of disease can be so slow that patients often do not need to be treated with chemotherapy for a prolonged period. This slow growth rate in some patients may be one of the factors accounting for the poor response to chemotherapy. New agents need to be evaluated in adequate numbers of patients to determine activity with statistical confidence. A recent paclitaxel trial showed evidence of activity in mucoepidermoid and adenocarcinoma of salivary origin with 7 of 29 (25%) patients achieving partial response.[122] In contrast, adenoid cystic carcinomas were not responsive to therapy. Studies of adjuvant chemotherapy in salivary cancer have not been undertaken because of the small numbers of patients and relatively ineffective chemotherapy. Clearly, collaborative efforts will be necessary before conclusions can be drawn concerning the use of chemotherapy for salivary gland cancers.

CHEMOPREVENTION OF HEAD AND NECK CANCER

Chemoprevention is defined as the administration of pharmacologic agents to inhibit the events occurring during the multistep process of carcinogenesis or the reversal of a premalignant condition. The biology of carcinogenesis leading to upper aerodigestive tract malignancies is not well understood. Tumor formation is believed to be a multistep process involving biochemical and molecular changes that result in dysregulated differentiation and proliferation.[78] Chromosomal alterations and mutations of specific oncogenes are associated with epithelial cancers. Investigators studying various genomic, proliferation, and differentiation biomarkers have found alterations in specific markers (keratin, involucrin, transglutaminase) during the process of abnormal squamous differentiation. These biomarkers can be useful as intermediate end points in future chemoprevention trials.[143] Our understanding of the biology of carcinogenesis for head and neck cancer and other aerodigestive tract tumors is expected to rapidly expand in the next decade.

Chemoprevention is particularly relevant to patients who are curatively treated for an early stage head and neck squamous cell cancer. It is recognized that second primary malignancies develop at a rate of 3% to 4% per year in these patients.[46,129,142] The explanation for this risk is based on the concept of field cancerization first formulated in the 1950s.[202,210] Repeated exposure of the entire epithelial surface to carcinogens, such as tobacco and alcohol, can lead to the development of multiple sites of premalignant and malignant change. The ability of retinoids and carotenoids to affect epithelial growth and differentiation is supported by in vitro, animal, and epidemiologic studies.[19] Although the exact mechanism by which retinoids inhibit carcinogenesis is not known, retinoids have been shown to modify genomic expression at the level of messenger RNA synthesis and to regulate transcription of specific genes.[148,239] Clinically, retinoids and carotenoids have been used to prevent malignant transformation of dysplastic leukoplakia lesions. Most recently, retinoids have been studied in the prevention of second primary cancers. Retinoids are the synthetic and natural analogs of vitamin A. β-carotene is the major source of vitamin A in the diet.

The major limitation in the use of retinoids is associated toxicity. Acute toxicity includes dryness of conjunctival and oral mucous membranes, cheilitis, skin desquamation, hypertriglyceridemia, bone tenderness, arthralgias, and myalgias. Chronic toxicities include hepatotoxicity and bone remodeling.[107] These compounds are teratogenic, causing multiple malformations. Because of these toxicities, a number of retinoids have been synthesized. Four that are used clinically are vitamin A (retinol); β-all-transretinoic acid (retinoid); 13-cis retinoic acid (isotretinoin); and an aromatic ethyl ester derivative, etretinate.[107] In contrast to the retinoids, the major toxicity of the carotenoids is yellowing of the skin. Other compounds that may have use in chemoprevention based mainly on in vitro and animal data are α-tocopherol (vitamin E), selenium, and N-acetyl cysteine. The latter compound is a precursor of intracellular glutathione that enhances its antioxidant activity as a free-radical scavenger. N-acetyl cysteine is nontoxic and currently under investigation in Europe for the prevention of second malignancies in patients with a previous head and neck or lung carcinoma.[107] EGFR, farnesyl transferase, and COX-2 inhibitors are also under study as potential chemoprevention agents.

Studies with retinoids and carotenoids in patients with leukoplakia are listed in Table 4-7. Stich and others[208,209] reported two trials conducted in India and

the Philippines in betel nut chewers. In one placebo-controlled trial, β-carotene was compared with β-carotene plus vitamin A. Complete response was observed in 3% of the patients taking placebo, in 15% of β-carotene–treated patients, and in 28% of those taking the combination. These patients demonstrated significant suppression of micronuclei expression and index of DNA damage on serial cytologic examinations. In a subsequent study, patients were randomly assigned to receive placebo or twice the dose of vitamin A (200,000 IU/wk) received in the first trial. A 57% complete response rate was observed with total suppression of the development of new leukoplakic lesions. In the placebo group, the complete response rate was 3%, and there was a 21% rate of new lesion formation.[209] In a small pilot study, Garewal and others[93] observed a 71% complete and partial response rate in 24 patients treated with β-carotene. There was no significant toxicity. Other investigators reported complete and partial response rates ranging from 60% to 100% with 13-cis retinoic acid.[134,192]

These results led Hong and others[109] to conduct a randomized placebo-controlled trial of 13-cis retinoic acid (1 or 2 mg/kg per day) in oral leukoplakia with dysplastic change. All patients were assessed with pretreatment and posttreatment biopsies. Patients were treated for 3 months and observed for 6 months. There was a highly significant difference in response rate, 67% vs 10%, comparing the treated group with those taking placebo. Histologic reversal of dysplastic change was documented in 54%. Unfortunately, after stopping treatment, the relapse rate was high within 2 or 3 months, and the regimen was associated with considerable toxicity. In a follow-up trial,[144] 56 patients received 13-cis retinoic acid (1.5 mg/kg

TABLE 4-7

RESULTS OF RANDOMIZED CHEMOPREVENTION TRIALS IN THE HEAD AND NECK

Study	Design	Number of Patients	Intervention and Dose	Results
Oral premalignancy				
Hong and others, 1986[109]	Induction	44	Isotretinoin (2 mg/kg/d)	Positive
Lippman and others, 1993[145]	Maintenance	70	Isotretinoin (0.5 mg/kg/d)	Positive
Stich and others, 1988[209]	Induction	65	Vitamin A (200,000 IU/wk)	Positive
Han and others, 1990[101]	Induction	61	Retinamide (40 mg/d)	Positive
Costa and others, 1994[48]	Maintenance	153	Fenretinide (200 mg/d)	Positive
Previous cancer				
Hong and others, 1990[112]	Adjuvant	103	Isotretinoin (50 to 100 mg/m²/d)	Positive
Bolla and others, 1994[18]	Adjuvant	316	Etretinate (50 mg/d; 25 mg/d)	
Pinto and other, 2001[170]	Adjuvant	189	Isotretinoin (7.5-10mg/d)	Negative
Khuri and others, 2003[129]	Adjuvant	1190	Isotretinoin (300mg/d)	Negative

(Reprinted with permission from Lippman and others: Strategies for chemoprevention study of premalignancy and second primary tumors in the head and neck, *Curr Opin Oncol* 7:234, 1995.)

per day) for 3 months, followed by randomization to low-dose 13-cis retinoic acid (0.5 mg/kg per day) or β-carotene maintenance therapy. cis-Retinoic acid proved superior in maintaining remissions and had an acceptable level of toxicity in this low dosage.

Hong and others[112] reported the results of using 13-cis retinoic acid to prevent second primary malignancies in patients with squamous cell cancer of the head and neck rendered disease free with surgery and radiotherapy. This placebo-controlled chemoprevention trial randomly assigned 103 patients to receive high-dose 13-cis retinoic acid (50 to 100 mg/m² per day) or placebo for 1 year. At a median follow-up period of 32 months, second primary tumors had developed in 4% of those receiving retinoic acid compared with 24% of the placebo group ($P = .005$). The results of this trial have led to the initiation of two multiinstitutional confirmatory trials in the United States; two chemoprevention trials are in progress in Europe.[23] In the United States, the North Central Cancer Treatment Group and ECOG have randomly assigned patients with stage I and II squamous cancers of the head and neck rendered disease free with surgery or radiotherapy to placebo or low-dose 13-cis retinoic acid (0.15 mg/kg per day) for 2 years.[170] Preliminary results suggest no benefit for the experimental regimen, with respect to the incidence of second primary tumors or survival. The M.D. Anderson Cancer Center and Radiation Therapy Oncology Group have conducted a placebo-controlled trial for the same patient group testing a higher dose of cis-retinoic acid, 30 mg/day, for 3 years. Dose reductions for toxicity were allowed. Khuri and others[129] have recently reported that no long-term disease-free or survival benefit was clearly demonstrated.

SUMMARY

Tumors of various histologic types occur in the head and neck. Excluding thyroid malignancies, approximately 80% are squamous cell carcinomas. Data evaluating the impact of chemotherapy on survival time, particularly for combined modality treatments, are limited to this common histologic type for which patient numbers are available for randomized comparative trials. Phase I, II, and III studies in patients with locally recurrent or metastatic disease have shown that chemotherapy can produce response rates of 30% to 40%, and combination chemotherapy is more effective than single agents. However, responses tend to be brief (2 to 4 months) and may not be associated with longer survival time. Thus, chemotherapy for these patients is palliative. An exception to this is for patients with tumors of the nasopharynx in whom higher response rates and a small proportion of long-term disease-free survivors are observed. Prognostic

factors have been identified that should be used by the physician to select patients most likely to benefit from palliative treatment.

In newly diagnosed patients with locally advanced disease, high response rates have been achieved with induction chemotherapy; and this approach remains under study. An important role for chemotherapy may be to preserve organ anatomy and function at selected sites. Three large multicenter randomized trials were successfully conducted with preservation of laryngeal function. Chemotherapy administered concurrently with radiotherapy has improved local control and survival time in selected series. The increase in toxicity associated with these regimens should be carefully considered when selecting patients for this combined treatment. Chemotherapy for those with parotid cancers has been studied only for recurrent disease. Response rates are modest, and impact on survival time has not been demonstrated.

Figure 4-1 shows an algorithm for management of late-stage (locally advanced) squamous cell carcinomas of the head and neck. Patients with earlier-stage disease (i.e., stage I or II) should receive conventional therapy with either surgery, radiotherapy, or both. Patients with stage III or IV disease can be divided into those with resectable or unresectable disease. Those with unresectable disease should often be treated with chemotherapy and radiation or entered into a combined chemoradiation treatment protocol. Those with stage III disease also benefit from combination treatment as part of a clinical trial. Patients with metastatic disease should receive chemotherapy with palliative intent if performance status is favorable. Patients with "resectable" disease can be further divided by site. Those with primary oral cavity tumors would be best served by surgery followed by radiotherapy, whereas patients with oropharynx, hypopharyngeal, or laryngeal tumors are treated with radiation, with or without chemotherapy depending on the site and stage.

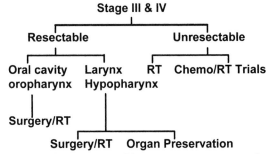

CANCER OF THE HEAD AND NECK

Figure 4-1. Management of late-stage squamous cell carcinomas of the head and neck.

Chemoprevention will continue to be an important area of research in the coming decade. One randomized trial has shown a decreased rate of second primary tumors in patients with curatively treated upper aerodigestive tract primary tumors. Confirmatory trials have been unsuccessful thus far, but multiple new strategies are to be considered for further testing.

The management of head and neck cancer is a multidisciplinary activity. The identification of effective chemotherapeutic agents and their integration into the initial curative therapy of head and neck cancer has the potential to improve survival time and preserve organ function. Through well-designed and well-executed clinical trials, coupled with basic research of the biology of upper aerodigestive tract tumors, further advances in the management and prevention of these cancers can be achieved.

REFERENCES

1. Adelstein DJ and others: Long-term results after chemoradiotherapy for locally confined squamous cell head and neck, *Am J Clin Oncol* 13:440, 1990.
2. Adelstein DJ and others: Simultaneous versus sequential combined technique for squamous cell head and neck cancer, *Cancer* 65:1685, 1990.
3. Adelstein DJ and others: Concurrent radiation therapy and chemotherapy for locally unresectable squamous cell head and neck cancer: an Eastern Cooperative Oncology Group pilot study, *J Clin Oncol* 11:2136, 1993.
4. Alberts DS and others: Adriamycin, cis-platinum, cyclosphosphamide combination chemotherapy for advanced carcinoma of the parotid gland, *Cancer* 47:645, 1981.
5. Al-Sarraf M and others: *Adjuvant chemotherapy for patients with locally advanced head and neck cancer: RTOG and Wayne State University experiences.* In Salmon SE, editor: *Adjuvant therapy of cancer*, vol 5. Philadelphia, Grune & Stratton, 1987.
6. Al-Sarraf M and others: Concurrent radiotherapy and chemotherapy with cisplatin in inoperable squamous cell carcinoma of the head and neck, *Cancer* 59:259, 1987.
7. Al-Sarraf M and others: Chemoradiotherapy versus radiotherapy in patients with advanced nasopharyngeal cancer: phase III randomized Intergroup Study 0099. *J Clin Oncol* 16:1310-1317, 1998.
8. Al-Sarraf M: Chemotherapeutic management of head and neck cancer, *Cancer Metast Rev* 6:191, 1987.
9. Al-Sarraf M: Head and neck cancer: chemotherapy concepts, *Semin Oncol* 15:70, 1988.
10. Al-Sarraf M: *Management strategies in head and neck cancer: the role of carboplatin.* In Bunns PA Jr and others, editors: *Current perspectives and future directions*, Philadelphia, WB Saunders, 1990.
11. Amdur RJ and others: Split-course versus continuous-course irradiation in the postoperative setting for squamous cell carcinoma of the head and neck, *Int J Radiat Oncol Biol* 17:279, 1989.
12. Amer MH and others: Factors that affect response to chemotherapy and survival of patients with advanced head and neck cancer, *Cancer* 43:2202, 1979.
13. Bagshaw MA, Doggett RLS: A clinical study of chemical radiosensitization, *Front Radiat Ther Oncol* 4:164, 1969.
14. Baker SR and others: Intraarterial infusion chemotherapy for head and neck cancer using a totally implantable infusion pump, *Head Neck Surg* 4:118, 1981.
15. Benjamin RS and others: *Adriamycin cardiac toxicity: an assessment of approaches to cardiac monitoring and cardioprotection.* In Hacker MP, Lazo LS, Tritton TR, editors: *Organ directed toxicities of anticancer drugs*, Boston, Martinus Nijhoff, 1988.
16. Bertino JR, Mosher MB, DeConti RC: Chemotherapy of cancer of the head and neck, *Cancer* 31:1141, 1973.
17. Blum RH: An overview of studies with adriamycin (NSC-123127) in the United States, *Cancer Chemother Rep* 6:247, 1975.
18. Bolla M and others: Prevention of second primary tumours with etretinate in squamous cell carcinoma of the oral cavity and oropharynx: results of a multicentric double-blind randomized study, *Eur J Cancer* 30A:767, 1994.
19. Boone CW, Kelloff GJ, Malone WE: Identification of candidate cancer chemopreventive agents and their evaluation in animal models and human clinical trials: a review, *Cancer Res* 50:2, 1990.
20. Boussen H and others: Chemotherapy of metastatic and/or recurrent undifferentiated nasopharyngeal carcinoma with cisplatin, bleomycin, and fluorouracil, *J Clin Oncol* 9:1675, 1991.
21. Boyle JO and others: The incidence of p53 mutations increases with progression of head and neck cancer, *Cancer Res* 53:4477, 1993.
22. Brennan JA and others: Molecular assessment of histopathologic staging in squamous cell carcinoma of the head and neck, *N Engl J Med* 332(26):1787, 1995.
23. Briggs RJS, Forastiere AA: Isotretinoin for prevention of second squamous cell carcinoma of the head and neck, *Otolaryngol Head Neck Surg* 105:752, 1991.
24. Brizel DM and others: Hyperfractionated irradiation with or without concurrent chemotherapy for locally advanced head and neck cancer, *N Engl J Med* 338: 178-1804, 1998.
25. Browman GP, Cronin L: Standard chemotherapy in squamous cell head and neck cancer: what we have learned from randomized trials, *Semin Oncol* 21:311, 1994.
26. Browman GP and others: Placebo-controlled randomized trial of iv infusional 5-fluorouracil concurrent with standard radiotherapy in stage III and IV head and neck cancer, *Proc Am Soc Clin Oncol* 12:891, 1993.
27. Buesa JM and others: Phase II trial of ifosfamide in recurrent and metastatic head and neck cancer, *Ann Oncol* 2:151, 1991.
28. Byfield JE and others: Phase I and II trial of 5-day infused 5-fluorouracil and radiation in advanced cancer of the head and neck, *J Clin Oncol* 2:406, 1984.
29. Cachin Y and others: Preliminary results of a randomized EORTC study comparing radiotherapy and concomitant bleomycin to radiotherapy alone in epidermoid carcinomas of the oropharynx, *Eur J Cancer* 13:1389, 1977.
30. Calais G and others: Randomized trial of radiation therapy versus concomitant chemotherapy and radiation therapy for advanced-stage oropharynx carcinoma, *J Natl Cancer Inst* 91:2081-2086, 1999.
31. Calvert AH: Dose optimization of carboplatin in adults, *Anticancer Res* 14(6A):2273, 1994.
32. Campbell JB and others: A randomized phase III trial of cisplatinum, methotrexate, cisplatin + methotrexate, and cisplatinum + 5-fluorouracil in end-stage head and neck cancer, *Acta Otolaryngol* 103:519, 1987.
33. Carugati A, Pradier R, de la Torre A: Combination chemotherapy pre-radical treatment for head and neck

squamous cell carcinoma, *Proc Am Soc Clin Oncol* 7:152, 1988.

34. Catimel G and others: A phase II study of gemcytabine (LY188011) in patients with advanced squamous cell carcinoma of the head and neck, *Ann Oncol* 5:543, 1994.

35. Catimel G and others: Docetaxel (Taxotere): an active drug for the treatment of patients with advanced squamous cell carcinoma of the head and neck, *Ann Oncol* 5:533, 1994.

36. Cervellino JC and others: Ifosfamide and MESNA for the treatment of advanced squamous cell head and neck cancer, *Oncology* 48:89, 1991.

37. Chan ATC and others: A prospective randomized study of chemotherapy adjunctive to definitive radiotherapy in advanced nasopharyngeal carcinoma, *Int J Radiat Oncol Biol Phys* 33:761, 1995.

38. Chen HG, Gross JF: Intraarterial infusion of anticancer drugs: theoretic aspects of drug delivery and review of responses, *Cancer Treat Rep* 64:31, 1980.

39. Choksi AJ, Dimery IW, Hong WK: Adjuvant chemotherapy of head and neck cancer: the past, the present, and the future, *Semin Oncol* 15(Suppl 3):45, 1988.

40. Choo R, Tannock I: Chemotherapy for recurrent or metastatic carcinoma of the nasopharynx: a review of the Princess Margaret Hospital experience, *Cancer* 68:2120, 1991.

41. Clavel M and others: Randomized comparison of cisplatin, methotrexate, bleomycin, and vincristine (CABO) versus cisplatin and 5-fluorouracil (CF) versus cisplatin (C) in recurrent or metastatic squamous cell carcinoma of the head and neck, *Ann Oncol* 5:521, 1994.

42. Clayman GL and others: The role of neck dissection after chemoradiotherapy for oropharyngeal cancer with advanced nodal disease, *Arch Otolaryngol Head Neck Surg* 127:135-139, 2001.

43. Collins JM: Pharmacologic rationale for regional drug delivery, *J Clin Oncol* 2:498, 1984.

44. Condit PT: Treatment of carcinoma with radiation therapy and methotrexate, *MO Med* 65:832, 1968.

45. Conley J, Dingman DL: Adenoid cystic carcinoma in the head and neck (cylindroma), *Arch Otolaryngol* 100:81, 1974.

46. Cooper JS and others: Second malignancies in patients who have head and neck cancer: incidence, effect on survival and implications based on RTOG experience, *Int J Radiat Oncol Biol Phys* 17:449, 1989.

47. Cortes EP and others: Chemotherapy for head and neck cancer relapsing after chemotherapy, *Cancer* 47:1966, 1981.

48. Costa A and others: Prospects of chemoprevention of human cancers with the synthetic retinoid fenretinide, *Cancer Res* 54:2032, 1994.

49. Creagan ET and others: Cisplatin-based chemotherapy for neoplasms arising from salivary glands and contiguous structures in the head and neck, *Cancer* 62:2313, 1988.

50. Cvitkovic E and others: 5-fluorouracil (5FU), mitomycin (M), epirubicin (E), cisplatin (P) in recurrent and/or metastatic undifferentiated nasopharyngeal carcinoma (UCNT) (abstract), *Proc Am Soc Clin Oncol* 10:200, 1991.

51. Dalley D and others: The value of chemotherapy prior to definitive local therapy in patients with locally advanced squamous cell carcinoma of the head and neck, *Proc Am Soc Clin Oncol* 14:297, 1995.

52. Davis D, Kessler W: Randomized comparison of cisdiaminedichloroplatinum versus cisdiaminedichloro-platinum, methotrexate and bleomycin in recurrent squamous cell carcinoma of the head and neck, *Cancer Chemother Pharmacol* 3:57, 1979.

53. de Andres L and others: Function preservation in stage III squamous laryngeal carcinoma: results with an induction chemotherapy protocol, *Laryngoscope* 105:822, 1995.

54. Decker DA and others: Chemotherapy for nasopharyngeal carcinoma: a ten year experience, *Cancer* 52:602, 1983.

55. Degardin M and others: Phase II piritrexim study in recurrent and/or metastatic head and neck cancer, *Proc Am Soc Clin Oncol* 11:244, 1992.

56. Demard F and others: *Induction chemotherapy for larynx preservation in laryngeal and hypopharyngeal cancers.* In Johnson JT, Didolkar MS, editors: *Head and neck cancer,* vol 3, Amsterdam, Excerpta Medica, 1993.

57. Depondt J and others: Neoadjuvant chemotherapy with carboplatin/5-fluorouracil in head and neck cancer, *Oncology* (Suppl 50):23, 1993.

58. Dewit L: Combined treatment of radiation and cisdiaminedichloroplatinum (II): a review of experimental and clinical data, *Int J Radiat Oncol Biol Phys* 13:403, 1987.

59. Di Blasio B and others: A prospective randomized trial in resectable head and neck carcinoma: loco-regional treatment with and without neoadjuvant chemotherapy (abstract), *Proc Am Soc Clin Oncol* 13:279, 1994.

60. Dimery IW and others: Neoadjuvant therapy of advanced paranasal sinus carcinoma with combined intraarterial and systemic chemotherapy (abstract 8.5). Presented at the Third International Head and Neck Oncology Research Conference, Las Vegas, Sept 26-28, 1990.

61. Domenge C and others: Randomized trial of neoadjunctive chemotherapy in oropharyngeal carcinoma. French Croupe d'Etude des Timeur: de la Tete et du Cou (GETTEC) (abstract), *Br J Cancer* 12:1594-1598, 1983.

62. Donegan WL, Harris HS: Factors influencing the success of arterial infusion chemotherapy for cancer of the head and neck, *Am J Surg* 123:549, 1972.

63. Drelichman A, Cummings G, Al-Sarraf M: A randomized trial of the combination of cis-platinum, oncovin and bleomycin (COB) versus methotrexate in patients with advanced squamous cell carcinoma of the head and neck, *Cancer* 52:399, 1983.

64. Dreyfuss AI and others: Continuous infusion high-dose leucovorin with 5-fluorouracil and cisplatin for untreated stage IV carcinoma of the head and neck, *Ann Int Med* 112:167, 1990.

65. Dreyfuss AI and others: Cyclophosphamide, doxorubicin, and cisplatin combination chemotherapy for advanced carcinomas of salivary gland origin, *Cancer* 60:2869, 1987.

66. Dreyfuss AI and others: Doxetaxel (Taxotere): an active drug for squamous cell carcinoma of the head and neck, *J Clin Oncol* 14:1672, 1996.

67. Egorin MJ and others: Prospective validation of a pharmacologically based dosing scheme for the cis-diamminedi-chloroplatinum (II) analogue diaminecyclobutanedicarboxylatoplatinum, *Cancer Res* 45:6502, 1985.

68. Eisenberger M and others: A comparison of carboplatin plus methotrexate versus methotrexate alone in patients with recurrent and metastatic head and neck cancer, *J Clin Oncol* 7:1341, 1989.

69. Ensley JF and others: An intensive five course, alternating combination chemotherapy induction regimen used in patients with advanced, unresectable head and neck cancer, *J Clin Oncol* 6:1147, 1988.

70. Ensley JF and others: An intensive six course alternating induction regimen for patients with advanced squamous cell cancers of the head and neck: a Wayne State University and

Southwest Oncology Group pilot study, *Proc Am Soc Clin Oncol* 10:205(A-682), 1991.

71. Ensley JF and others: Cellular DNA content parameters in untreated and recurrent squamous cell cancers of the head and neck, *Cytometry* 10:334, 1989.

72. Ensley JF and others: Correlation between response to cisplatinum-combination chemotherapy and subsequent radiotherapy in previously untreated patients with advanced squamous cell cancers of the head and neck, *Cancer* 54:811, 1984.

73. Ervin TJ and others: An analysis of induction and adjuvant chemotherapy in the multidisciplinary treatment of squamous cell carcinoma of the head and neck, *J Clin Oncol* 5:10, 1987.

74. Eschwege F and others: Ten-year results of randomized trial comparing radiotherapy and concomitant bleomycin to radiotherapy alone in epidermoid carcinomas of the oropharynx: experience of the European Organization for Research and Treatment of Cancer, *NCI Monogr* 6:275, 1988.

75. Eschwege F and others: Randomized multicentric international phase III trial of neoadjuvant chemotherapy with bleomycin, epirubicin, cisplatin, followed by radiotherapy versus radiotherapy alone in undifferentiated carcinoma of naso-pharyngeal type: preliminary results, *Int J Radiat Oncol Biol Phys* 82(Suppl):192, 1995.

76. Fandi A and others: Nasopharyngeal cancer: epidemiology, staging, and treatment, *Semin Oncol* 21:382, 1994.

77. Fazekas JT, Sommer C, Kramer S: Adjuvant intravenous methotrexate or definitive radiotherapy alone for advanced squamous cancers of the oral cavity, oropharynx, supraglottic larynx or hypopharynx, *Int J Radiat Oncol Biol Phys* 6:533, 1980.

78. Fearon ER, Vogelstein B: A genetic model for colorectal tumorigenesis, *Cell* 61:759, 1990.

79. Forastiere AA: *Carboplatin plus 5-fluorouracil trials in advanced head and neck cancer.* In Bunn PA and others, editors: *Carboplatin (JM-8): current perspectives and future directions,* Philadelphia, WB Saunders, 1990.

80. Forastiere AA: *Head and neck malignancies.* In McGuire WP, Rowinsky EK, editors: *Paclitaxel in cancer treatment,* New York, Marcel Dekker, 1995.

81. Forastiere AA and others: High-dose cisplatin in advanced head and neck cancer, *Cancer Chemother Pharmacol* 19:155, 1987.

82. Forastiere AA and others: Intraarterial cisplatin and FUDR in advanced malignancies confined to the head and neck, *J Clin Oncol* 5:1601, 1987.

83. Forastiere AA: Paclitaxel (taxol) for the treatment of head and neck cancer, *Semin Oncol* (Suppl 21):49, 1994.

84. Forastiere AA and others: Pharmacokinetic and toxicity evaluation of 5-day continuous infusion versus intermittent bolus cisdiamine-dichloroplatinum (II) in head and neck cancer patients, *Cancer Res* 48:3869, 1988.

85. Forastiere AA: Randomized trials of induction chemotherapy: a critical review, *Hematol/Oncol Clin North Am* 5:725, 1991.

86. Forastiere AA and others: Randomized comparison of cisplatin and 5-fluorouracil versus carboplatin + 5-FU versus methotrexate in advanced squamous cell carcinoma of the head and neck, *J Clin Oncol* 10:1245, 1992.

87. Forastiere AA and others: Phase III trial to preserve the larynx: induction chemotherapy and radiotherapy versus concomitant chemoradiotherapy versus radiotherapy alone, Intergroup Trial R91-11 (abstract). *Proc Am Soc Oncol* 20:2a, 2001.

88. Frei E III, Canellos GP: Dose: a critical factor in cancer chemotherapy, *Am J Med* 69:583, 1980.

89. Friedman M and others: Malignant tumors of the major salivary glands, *Otolaryngol Clin North Am* 19:625, 1986.

90. Fromes Y and others: Differential effects of taxol or taxotere on tau and MAP2 containing microtubules, *Proc AACR* 33:551, 1992.

91. Fu KK: Biological basis for the interaction of chemotherapeutic agents and radiation therapy, *Cancer* 55:2123, 1985.

92. Fu KK and others: Combined radiotherapy and chemotherapy with bleomycin and methotrexate for advanced inoperable head and neck cancer: update of a Northern California Oncology group randomized trial, *J Clin Oncol* 5:1410, 1987.

93. Garewal HS and others: Response of oral leukoplakia to beta-carotene, *J Clin Oncol* 8:1715, 1990.

94. Gebbia V and others: Chemotherapeutic treatment of recurrent and/or metastatic nasopharyngeal carcinoma: a retrospective analysis of 40 cases, *Br J Cancer* 68:191, 1993.

95. Giglio R and others: Organ preservation (LP) in resectable stage III and IV epidermoid carcinoma of the larynx (LC) with sequential chemotherapy (CT) + radiation therapy (RT) (abstract), *Proc Am Soc Clin Oncol* 12:282, 1993.

96. Glick JH and others: The adjuvant treatment of inoperable stage III and IV epidermoid carcinoma of the head and neck with platinum and bleomycin infusions prior to definitive radiotherapy, *Cancer* 46:1919, 1980.

97. Glover KY and others: Intraarterial cisplatin, intravenous paclitaxel, and ifosfamide as an organ preservation approach in paranasal sinus squamous cell cancer (abstract), *Proc Am Soc Clin Oncol* 22:505, 2003.

98. Grose WE and others: Comparison of methotrexate and cisplatin for patients with advanced squamous cell carcinoma of the head and neck region: a Southwest Oncology Group study, *Cancer Treat Rep* 69:577, 1985.

99. Gueritte-Voegelein F and others: Relationships between the structure of taxol analogues and their antimitotic activity, *J Med Chem* 34:992, 1991.

100. Gupta NK, Pointon RCS, Wilkinson PM: A randomized clinical trial to contract radiotherapy with radiotherapy and methotrexate given synchronously in head and neck cancer, *Clin Radiol* 38:575, 1987.

101. Han J and others: Evaluation of N-4-(hydroxycarbophenyl) retinamide as a cancer prevention agent and as a cancer chemotherapeutic agent, *In Vivo* 4:153, 1990.

102. Haraf DJ and others: Survival and analysis of failure following hydroxyurea, 5-fluorouracil, and concomitant radiation therapy in poor prognosis head and neck cancer, *Am J Clin Oncol* 14:419, 1991.

103. Hasegawa Y and others: A randomized trial in resectable head and neck carcinoma: loco-regional treatment with and without neoadjuvant chemotherapy (abstract), *Proc Am Soc Clin Oncol* 13:286, 1994.

104. Haselow RE and others: *Radiation alone versus radiation plus weekly low-dose cis-platinum in unresectable cancer of the head and neck.* In Fee WE Jr and others, editors: *Head and neck cancer,* vol 2. Philadelphia, Mosby, 1990.

105. Hayes DM and others: High-dose cis-platinum diaminedichloride: amelioration of renal toxicity by mannitol diuresis, *Cancer* 39:1372, 1977.

106. Head and Neck Contracts Program: Adjuvant chemotherapy for advanced head and neck squamous carcinoma, *Cancer* 60:301, 1987.

107. Heyne KE, Lippman SM, Hong WK: Chemoprevention in head and neck cancer, *Hematol Oncol Clin North Am* 5:783, 1991.

108. Hill BT, Price LA: *The significance of primary site in assessing chemotherapy response and survival in*

advanced squamous cell carcinomas of the head and neck treated with initial combination chemotherapy without cisplatin: analysis at nine years. In Salmon S, editor: *Adjuvant therapy of cancer*, vol 5. Philadelphia, Grune & Stratton, 1987.

109. Hong WK and others: 13-cis retinoic acid in the treatment of oral leukoplakia, *N Engl J Med* 315:1501, 1986.

110. Hong WK and others: A prospective randomized trial of methotrexate versus cisplatin in the treatment of recurrent squamous cell carcinoma of the head and neck, *Cancer* 52:206, 1983.

111. Hong WK and others: Induction chemotherapy in advanced squamous head and neck carcinoma with high-dose cis-platinum and bleomycin infusion, *Cancer* 44:19, 1979.

112. Hong WK and others: Prevention of second primary tumors with isotretinoin in squamous cell carcinoma of the head and neck, *N Engl J Med* 323:795, 1990.

113. Hong WK and others: Sequential response patterns to chemotherapy and radiotherapy in head and neck cancer: potential impact to treatment in advanced laryngeal cancer, *Prog Clin Oncol Res* 201:191, 1985.

114. Huber MH and others: A phase II study of ifosfamide in recurrent squamous cell carcinoma of the head and neck, *Am J Clin Oncol* 19:379, 1996.

115. Hussey D, Abrams J: Combined therapy in advanced head and neck cancer with hydroxyurea and radiotherapy, *Prog Clin Cancer* 6:79, 1975.

116. International Nasopharynx Cancer Study Group: VUMCA I Trial: preliminary results of a randomized trial comparing neoadjuvant chemotherapy (cisplatin, epirubicin, bleomycin) plus radiotherapy vs. radiotherapy alone in stage IV (≥ N2, M0) undifferentiated nasopharyngeal carcinoma: a positive effect on progression-free survival, *Int J Rad Oncol Biol Phys* 35:463, 1996.

117. Jacobs C and others: 24-hour infusion of cis-platinum in head and neck cancers, *Cancer* 42:2135, 1978.

118. Jacobs C and others: A randomized phase III study of cisplatin with or without methotrexate for recurrent squamous cell carcinoma of the head and neck: a Northern California Oncology Group study, *Cancer* 52:1563, 1983.

119. Jacobs C and others: A phase III randomized study comparing cisplatin and fluorouracil as single agents and in combination for advanced squamous cell carcinoma of the head and neck, *J Clin Oncol* 10:257, 1992.

120. Jacobs C, Makuch R: Efficacy of adjuvant chemotherapy for patients with resectable head and neck cancer: a subset analysis of the Head and Neck Contracts Program, *J Clin Oncol* 8:838, 1990.

121. Jaulerry C and others: Induction chemotherapy in advanced head and neck tumors: results of two randomized trials, *Int J Radiat Oncol Biol Phys* 23:483, 1992.

122. Jennings T and others: Phase II trial of paclitaxel in advanced or metastatic salivary gland malignancies: an Eastern Cooperative Oncology Group Study (abstract), *Proc Am Soc Clin Oncol* 20:236a, 2003.

123. Jeremic B and others: Hyperfractionated radiation therapy with or without concurrent low-dose daily cisplatin in locally advanced squamous cell carcinoma of the head and neck: a perspective randomized trial, *J Clin Oncol* 18:1458-1464, 2000.

124. Johnson JT and others: Adjuvant chemotherapy for high-risk squamous cell carcinoma of the head and neck, *J Clin Oncol* 5:456, 1987.

125. Johnson RO and others: Infusion of 5-fluorouracil in cylindroma treatment, *Arch Otolaryngol* 79:625, 1964.

126. Kapstad B and others: Combined preoperative treatment with cobalt and bleomycin in patients with head and neck carcinoma: a controlled clinical study, *Int J Radiat Oncol Biol Phys* 4:85, 1978.

127. Karp DD and others: Larynx preservation using induction chemotherapy plus radiation therapy as an alternative to laryngectomy in advanced head and neck cancer, *Am J Clin Oncol* 14:273, 1991.

128. Keane TJ and others: A randomized trial of radiation therapy compared to split course radiation therapy combined with mitomycin and 5-fluorouracil as initial treatment for advanced laryngeal and hypopharyngeal squamous carcinoma, *Int J Radiat Oncol Biol Phys* 25:613, 1993.

129. Khuri F and others: Isotretinoin effects on head and neck cancer recurrence and second primary tumors (abstract), *Proc Am Soc Clin Oncol* 22:90, 2003.

130. Kies MS, Bennett CL, Vokes EE: Locally advanced head and neck cancer, *Curr Treatment Options Oncol* 2:7-13, 2001.

131. Kish JA and others: A randomized trial of cisplatin (CACP)+ 5-fluorouracil (5-Fu) infusion and CACP + 5-Fu bolus for recurrent and advanced squamous cell carcinoma of the head and neck, *Cancer* 56:2740, 1985.

132. Kish JA and others: Activity of ifosfamide (NSC-109724) in recurrent head and neck cancer patients (abstract), *Proc Am Assoc Cancer Res* 31:190, 1990.

133. Knowlton AH and others: Methotrexate and radiation therapy in the treatment of advanced head and neck tumors, *Radiology* 116:709, 1975.

134. Koch H: Biochemical treatment of precancerous oral lesions: the effectiveness of various analogues of retinoic acid, *J Maxillofac Surg* 6:59, 1978.

135. Kotwall C and others: Metastatic patterns in squamous cell cancer of the head and neck, *Am J Surg* 154:439, 1987.

136. Kraus DH and others: Larynx preservation with combined chemotherapy and radiation therapy in advanced hypopharynx cancer, *Otolaryngol Head Neck Surg* 111:31, 1994.

137. Kun LE and others: A randomized study of adjuvant chemotherapy for cancer of the upper aerodigestive tract, *Int J Radiat Oncol Biol Phys* 12:173, 1986.

138. Laccourreye O and others: *Preservation of the larynx following neoadjuvant chemotherapy: a preliminary report.* In Banzet P and others, editors: *Neoadjuvant chemotherapy*, Paris, Springer-Verlag, 1991.

139. Laramore G and others: Adjuvant chemotherapy for resectable squamous cell carcinomas of the head and neck: report on Intergroup study 0034, *Int J Radiat Oncol Biol Phys* 23:705, 1992.

140. Lefebvre JL and others: Larynx preservation in hypopharynx and lateral epilarynx cancer: preliminary results of EORTC randomized phase III trial 24891, *J Natl Cancer Inst* 88:890, 1996.

141. Levitt M and others: Improved therapeutic index of methotrexate with leucovorin rescue, *Cancer Res* 33:1729, 1973.

142. Licciardello JT, Spitz MR, Hong WK: Multiple primary cancer in patients with cancer of the head and neck: second cancer of the head and neck, esophagus, and lung, *Int J Radiat Oncol Biol Phys* 17:467, 1989.

143. Lippman SM and others: Biomarkers as intermediate end points in chemoprevention trials, *J Natl Cancer Inst* 82:555, 1990.

144. Lippman SM and others: Low-dose 13-cis-retinoic acid maintains remission in oral premalignancy: more effective than b-carotene in randomized trial (abstract), *Proc Am Soc Clin Oncol* 9:59, 1990.

145. Lippman SM and others: Comparison of low-dose isotretinoin with beta-carotene to prevent oral carcinogenesis, *N Engl J Med* 328:15, 1993.
146. Liverpool Head and Neck Oncology Group: A phase III randomized trial of cisplatinum, methotrexate, cisplatinum + methotrexate and cisplatinum + 5-FU in end stage squamous cell carcinoma of the head and neck, *Br J Cancer* 61:311, 1990.
147. Lo TCM and others: Combined radiation therapy and 5-fluorouracil for advanced squamous cell carcinoma of the oral cavity and oropharynx: a randomized study, *Am J Roentgenol* 126:229, 1976.
148. Lotan R: Effects of vitamin A and its analogs (retinoids) on normal and neoplastic cells, *Biochem Biophys Acta* 605:33, 1980.
149. Lustig RA, Demare PA, Kramer S: Adjuvant methotrexate in the radio-chemotherapeutic management of advanced tumors of the head and neck, *Cancer* 37:2703, 1976.
150. Mahjoubi R and others: Metastatic undifferentiated carcinoma of nasopharyngeal type treated with bleomycin (B), epirubicin (E), and cisplatin (C): Final report (abstract), *Proc Am Soc Clin Oncol* 11:240, 1992.
151. Marcial VA and others: Concomitant cisplatin chemotherapy and radiotherapy in advanced mucosal squamous cell carcinoma of the head and neck: long-term results of the Radiation Therapy Oncology Group study 81-17, *Cancer* 66:1861, 1990.
152. Martin M and others: Ifosfamide in advanced epidermoid head and neck cancer, *Cancer Chemother Pharmacol* 31:340, 1993.
153. Martin M and others: Randomized study of 5-fluorouracil and cisplatin as neoadjuvant therapy in head and neck cancer: a preliminary report, *Int J Radiat Oncol Biol Phys* 19:973, 1990.
154. Martin M and others: A randomized prospective study of CDDP and 5-FU as neoadjuvant chemotherapy in head and neck cancer: a final report, *Proc Am Soc Clin Oncol* 14:294, 1995.
155. Mazeron JJ and others: Induction chemotherapy in head and neck cancer: results of a phase III trial, *Head Neck* 14:85, 1992.
156. Merlano M and others: Combined chemotherapy and radiation therapy in advanced inoperable squamous cell carcinoma of the head and neck, *Cancer* 67:915, 1991.
157. Merlano M and others: Five-year update of a randomized trial of alternating radiotherapy and chemotherapy compared with radiotherapy alone in treatment of unresectable squamous cell carcinoma of the head and neck, *J Natl Cancer Inst* 88:58, 1996.
158. Merlano M and others: Treatment of advanced squamous-cell carcinoma of the head and neck with alternating chemotherapy and radiotherapy, *N Engl J Med* 327:1115, 1992.
159. Moran RG: Leucovorin enhancement of the effects of fluoropyrimidines on thymidylate synthase, *Cancer* 63(suppl):1008, 1989.
160. Morita K: Clinical significance of radiation therapy combined with chemotherapy, *Strahlentherapie* 156:228, 1980.
161. Mortimer JE and others: Feasibility and efficacy of weekly intraarterial cisplatin in locally advanced (stage III and IV) head and neck cancers, *J Clin Oncol* 6:969, 1988.
162. Morton RP and others: Cisplatinum and bleomycin for advanced or recurrent squamous cell carcinoma of the head and neck: a randomized factorial phase III controlled trial, *Cancer Chemother Pharmacol* 15:283, 1985.
163. Paccagnella A and others: Chemotherapy before locoregional treatment in stage III & IV head and neck cancer: intermediate results of an ongoing randomized phase III trial. AGSTIC study, *Proc Am Soc Clin Oncol* 9:173, 1990.
164. Paccagnella A and others: A phase III trial of initial chemotherapy in stage III or IV head and neck cancer: a study by the gruppo di studio sui tumori della testa e del collo, *J Natl Cancer Inst* 86:265, 1994.
165. Pajak TF and others: Elapsed treatment days: a critical item for radiotherapy quality control review in head and neck trials: RTOG report, *Int J Radiat Oncol Biol Phys* 20(1):13, 1991.
166. Parvinen LM and others: Combined bleomycin treatment and radiation therapy in squamous cell carcinoma of the head and neck region, *Acta Radiol Oncol* 24:487, 1985.
167. Pfister DG and others: Larynx preservation with combined chemotherapy and radiation therapy in advanced but resectable head and neck cancer, *J Clin Oncol* 9:850, 1991.
168. Piantadosi S: Principles of clinical trial design, *Semin Oncol* 15:423, 1988.
169. Pinto HA, Jacobs CJ: Chemotherapy for recurrent and metastatic head and neck cancer, *Hematol Oncol Clin North Am* 5:667, 1991.
170. Pinto HA and others: Phase III trail of low-dose 13-cis-retinoic acid for prevention of second primary cancers in Stage I-II head and neck cancer: an Eastern Cooperative Oncology Group Study (abstract), *Proc Am Soc Clin Oncol* 20:222a, 2001.
171. Posner MR and others: Chemotherapy of advanced salivary gland neoplasms, *Cancer* 50:2261, 1982.
172. Price LA, Hill BR: Larynx preservation after initial chemotherapy plus radiation therapy as opposed to surgical intervention with or without radiation therapy in previously untreated advanced head and neck cancer: final analysis (abstract), *Proc Am Soc Clin Oncol* 11:244, 1992.
173. Randolph VL and others: Combination therapy of advanced head and neck cancer: induction of remissions with diaminedichloroplatinum (II) bleomycin and radiation therapy, *Cancer* 41:460, 1978.
174. Rentschler R, Burgess MA, Byers R: Chemotherapy of malignant major salivary gland neoplasms, *Cancer* 40:619, 1977.
175. Richards GJ Jr, Chambers RG: Hydroxyurea: a radiosensitizer in the treatment of neoplasms of the head and neck, *Am J Roentgenol* 105:555, 1969.
176. Ringel I, Horwitz SB: Studies with RP 56976 (taxotere): a semi-synthetic analog of taxol, *J Natl Cancer Inst* 83:288, 1991.
177. Robbins KT and others: Efficacy of targeted supradose cisplatin and concomitant radiation therapy for advanced head and neck cancer: the Memphis experience, *Int J Radiat Oncol Biol Phys* 38:263-271, 1997.
178. Robbins KT and others: Targeted chemoradiation for advanced head and neck cancer: analysis of 213 patients, *Head Neck* 22:687-693, 2000.
179. Roberts F: Trimetrexate as a single agent in patients with advanced head and neck cancer, *Semin Oncol* 15:22, 1988.
180. Roberts F and others: Phase II study of topotecan in advanced head and neck cancer: identification of an active new agent, *Proc Am Soc Clin Oncol* 13:281, 1994.
181. Rockwell S, Sartorelli AC: *Mitomycin C and radiation*. In Hill B, Bellamy A, editors: *The interactions between antitumor drugs and radiation*, Boca Raton, Fla, CRC Press, 1989.
182. Rooney M and others: Improved complete response rate and survival in advanced head and neck cancer after three-course induction therapy with 120-hour 5-FU infusion and cisplatin, *Cancer* 55:1123, 1985.

183. Rosenberg B: *Cisplatin: its history and possible mechanisms of action.* In Prestayko AW, Crooke ST, Carter SK, editors: *Cisplatin: current status and new developments,* New York, Academic Press, 1980.

184. Rowinsky EK and others: Taxol: the first of the taxanes, an important new class of antitumor agents, *Semin Oncol* 19:646, 1992.

185. Sartorelli AC: Therapeutic attack of hypoxic cells of solid tumors, *Cancer Res* 48:775, 1988.

186. Sato Y and others: Combined surgery, radiotherapy, and regional chemotherapy in carcinoma of the paranasal sinuses, *Cancer* 25:571, 1967.

187. Scandolaro L, Bertoni F: Tolleranza cutanea e mucosa e risposte cliniche a breve termine nella associazione tra radioterapia e bleomycina per tumori del distretto cervico-cefalico, *Acta Otorhinol Ital* 2:213, 1982.

188. Schornagel JH and others: Randomized Phase III trial of edatrexate versus methotrexate in patients with metastatic and/or recurrent squamous cell carcinoma of the head and neck: a European organization for research and treatment of head and neck cancer cooperative group study, *J Clin Oncol* 13:1649, 1995.

189. Schramm VL, Strodes C, Myers EN: Cisplatin therapy for adenoid cystic carcinoma, *Arch Otolaryngol* 107:739, 1981.

190. Schuller DE and others: Preoperative chemotherapy in advanced resectable head and neck cancer: final report of the Southwest Oncology Group, *Laryngoscope* 98:1205, 1988.

191. Sessions RB and others: Intra-arterial cisplatin treatment of adenoid cystic carcinoma, *Arch Otolaryngol* 108:221, 1982.

192. Shah JP and others: Effects of retinoids on oral leukoplakia, *Am J Surg* 146:466, 1983.

193. Shanta Y, Krishnamurthi S: Combined bleomycin and radiotherapy in oral cancer, *Clin Radiol* 156:228, 1980.

194. Shanta V, Krishnamurthi S: Combined therapy of oral cancer bleomycin and radiation: a clinical trial, *Clin Radiol* 28:427, 1977.

195. Shantz SP and others: Immunologic determinants of head and neck cancer: response to induction chemotherapy, *J Clin Oncol* 7:857, 1989.

196. Shetty P and others: Controlled study in squamous cell carcinoma of base of tongue using conventional radiation, radiation with single drug, and radiation with multiple drug chemotherapy (abstract), *Proc Am Soc Clin Oncol* 4:152, 1985.

197. Shibuya H and others: Reappraisal of trimodal combination therapy for maxillary sinus carcinoma, *Cancer* 50:2790, 1982.

198. Shigematsu Y, Sakai S, Fuchihata H: Recent trials in the treatment of maxillary sinus carcinoma with special reference to the chemical potentiation of radiation therapy, *Acta Otolaryngol* 71:63, 1971.

199. Shin DM and others. Phase II trail of bioadjuvant therapy with interferon-alpha2a (IFN-α2a), 13-cis-retinoic acid (13-cRA) and alpha tocopherol (α-TF) for locally advanced squamous cell carcinoma of the head and neck (SCCHN): long-term follow-up (abstract), *Proc Am Soc Clin Oncol* 22:496, 2003.

200. Shirinian MH and others: Laryngeal preservation by induction chemotherapy plus radiation therapy in locally advanced head and neck cancer: the MD Anderson Cancer Center experience, *Head Neck* 16:39, 1994.

201. Simon RM: *Design and conduct of clinical trials.* In Devita VT Jr, Hellman S, Rosenberg SA, editors: *Cancer principles and practice of oncology,* ed 3. Philadelphia, JB Lippincott, 1989.

202. Slaughter DP, Southwick HW, Smejkal W: Field cancerization in oral stratified squamous epithelium, *Cancer* 6:193, 1953.

203. Snow GB and others: Prognostic factors of neck node metastasis, *Clin Otolaryngol* 7:185, 1982.

204. South-East Cooperative Oncology Group: A randomized trial of combined multidrug chemotherapy and radiotherapy in advanced squamous cell carcinoma of the head and neck, *Eur J Surg Oncol* 12:289, 1986.

205. Steel GG, Peckham MJ: Exploitable mechanisms in combined radiotherapy-chemotherapy: the concept of additivity, *Int J Radiat Oncol Biol Phys* 5:85, 1979.

206. Stefani S, Eells RW, Abbate J: Hydroxyurea and radiotherapy in head and neck cancer, *Radiology* 101:391, 1971.

207. Stell PM and others: Sequential chemotherapy and radiotherapy in advanced head and neck cancer, *Clin Radiol* 34:463, 1983.

208. Stich HF and others: Remission of oral leukoplakia and macronuclei in tobacco/betal quid chewers treated with beta-carotene and beta-carotene plus vitamin A, *Int J Cancer* 42:195, 1988.

209. Stich HF and others: Response of oral leukoplakias to the administration of vitamin A, *Cancer Lett* 40:93, 1988.

210. Strong MS, Incze J, Vaughan CW: Field cancerization in the digestive tract: its etiology, manifestation and significance, *J Otolaryngol* 13:1, 1984.

211. Suen JY, Johns ME: Chemotherapy for salivary gland cancer, *Laryngoscope* 92:235, 1982.

212. Szpirglas H and others: Neo-adjuvant chemotherapy: a randomized trial before radiotherapy in oral and oro-pharyngeal carcinomas: end results. In *Proceedings of the 2nd International Head and Neck Oncology Research Conference.* Arlington, Va, September 10-12, 1987.

213. Tannock IF, Rotin D: Keynote address: mechanisms of interaction between radiation and drugs with potential for improvements in therapy, *NCI Monogr* 6:77, 1988.

214. Tannock IF, Sutherland DJ: Chemotherapy for adenocystic carcinoma, *Cancer* 46:452, 1980.

215. Tarpley JL and others: High-dose methotrexate as a preoperative adjuvant in the treatment of epidermoid carcinoma of the head and neck: a feasibility study and clinical trial, *Am J Surg* 130:481, 1975.

216. Taylor SG IV and others: Combined simultaneous cisplatin/fluorouracil chemotherapy and split course radiation in head and neck cancer, *J Clin Oncol* 7:846, 1989.

217. Taylor SG IV and others: Randomized comparison of neoadjuvant cisplatin and fluorouracil infusion followed by radiation versus concomitant treatment in advanced head and neck cancer, *J Clin Oncol* 12:385, 1994.

218. Testolin A and others: Vinorelbine in pretreated advanced head and neck squamous cell carcinoma: a phase II study, *Proc Am Soc Clin Oncol* 13:289, 1994.

219. Thornton D and others: A phase II trial of taxol in squamous cell carcinoma of the head and neck, *Proc Am Soc Clin Oncol* 13:288, 1994.

220. Toohill RJ and others: Cisplatin and fluorouracil as neoadjuvant therapy in head and neck cancer: a preliminary report, *Arch Otolaryngol Head Neck Surg* 113:758, 1987.

221. Troizzi PL and others: 5-Fluorouracil, cyclophosphamide, and vincristine for adenoid cystic carcinoma of the head and neck, *Cancer* 59:887, 1987.

222. Truelson JM and others: DNA content and histologic growth pattern correlate with prognosis in patients with advanced squamous cell carcinoma of the larynx. The Department of Veterans Affairs Cooperative Laryngeal Cancer Study Group, *Cancer* 70:56, 1992.

223. Uen WC and others: A phase II study of piritrexim in patients with advanced squamous head and neck cancer, *Cancer* 69:1008, 1992.

224. Urba SG, Forastiere AA: Systemic therapy of head and neck cancer: most effective agents, areas of promise, *Oncology* 3:79, 1989.

225. Venook AP and others: Cisplatin, doxorubicin, and 5-fluorouracil chemotherapy for salivary gland malignancies: a pilot study of the Northern California Oncology Group, *J Clin Oncol* 5:951, 1987.

226. Vermeer RJ, Pinedo HM: Partial remission of advanced adenoid cystic carcinoma obtained with adriamycin, *Cancer* 43:1604, 1979.

227. Vermund H and others: Bleomycin and radiation therapy in squamous cell carcinoma of the upper aero-digestive tract: a phase III clinical trial, *Int J Radiat Oncol Biol Phys* 11:1877, 1985.

228. Veronesi A and others: High-dose versus low-dose cisplatin in advanced head and neck squamous cell cancer: a randomized study, *J Clin Oncol* 3:1105, 1985.

229. Verweij J, Alexiera-Figresch J, DeBoer MF: Ifosfamide in advanced head and neck cancer: a phase II study of the Rotterdam Cooperative Head and Neck Cancer Study Group, *Eur J Cancer Clin Oncol* 24:795, 1988.

230. Verweij J, Clavel M, Chevalier B: Paclitaxel (taxol) and docetaxel (taxotere): not simply two of a kind, *Ann Oncol* 5:495, 1994.

231. Veterans Affairs Laryngeal Cancer Study Group: induction chemotherapy plus radiation in patients with advanced laryngeal cancer, *N Engl J Med* 324:1685, 1991.

232. Vogl SE and others: A randomized prospective comparison of methotrexate with a combination of methotrexate, bleomycin, and cisplatin in head and neck cancer, *Cancer* 56:432, 1985.

233. Vogler WR and others: Methotrexate therapy with or without citrovorum: factor in carcinoma of the head and neck, breast and colon, *Cancer Clin Trials* 2:227, 1979.

234. Vokes EE and others: Hydroxyurea, fluorouracil, and concomitant radiotherapy in poor prognosis head and neck cancer: a phase I-II study, *J Clin Oncol* 7:761, 1989.

235. Vokes EE and others: Induction chemotherapy with cisplatin, fluorouracil, and high-dose leucovorin for locally advanced head and neck cancer: a clinical and pharmacologic analysis, *J Clin Oncol* 8:241, 1990.

236. Vokes EE and others: A phase II study of piritrexim in combination with methotrexate in recurrent and metastatic head and neck cancer, *Cancer* 67:2253, 1991.

237. Vokes EE and others: Induction chemotherapy followed by concomitant chemoradiotherapy for advanced head and neck cancer: impact on the natural history of the disease, *J Clin Oncol* 13:876, 1995.

238. Von Hoff DD, Rozencweig M, Piccart M: The cardiotoxicity of anticancer agents, *Semin Oncol* 9:23, 1982.

239. Wang SY, LaRosa GJ, Gudas LJ: Molecular cloning of gene sequences transcriptionally regulated by retinoic acid and dibutyrl AMP in cultured mouse teratocarcinoma cells, *Dev Biol* 107:75, 1985.

240. Weiss RB, Muggia FM: Cytotoxic drug-induced pulmonary disease: update 1980, *Am J Med* 68:259, 1980.

241. Weissberg JB and others: Randomized clinical trial of mitomycin C as an adjunct to radiotherapy in head and neck cancer, *Int J Radiat Oncol Biol Phys* 17:3, 1989.

242. Wendt TG and others: Cisplatin, fluorouracil with leucovorin calcium enhancement, and synchronous accelerated radiotherapy in the management of locally advanced head and neck cancer: a phase II study, *J Clin Oncol* 7:471, 1989.

243. Wendt TG and others: Simultaneous radiochemotherapy versus radiotherapy alone in advanced head and neck cancer: a randomized multicenter study, *J Clin Oncol* 16:1318-1324, 1998.

244. Wheeler RH and others: High dose cisplatin and concomitant conventional fractionation radiation with or without prolonged infusion 5-fluorouracil in patients with unresectable stage III or IV squamous cell carcinoma of the head and neck. Presented at the Third International Head and Neck Oncology Research Conference, Las Vegas, Nev, Sept 26-28, 1990 (abstract 6.3).

245. Wheeler RH, Baker SR, Medvec BR: Single-agent and combination-drug regional chemotherapy for head and neck cancer using an implantable infusion pump, *Cancer* 54:1504, 1984.

246. Williams SD and others: Chemotherapy for head and neck cancer: comparison of cisplatin + vinblastine + bleomycin versus methotrexate, *Cancer* 57:18, 1986.

247. Wittes RE and others: cis-Dichlorodiammine platinum (II) in the treatment of epidermoid carcinoma of the head and neck, *Cancer Treat Rep* 61:359, 1977.

248. Woods RL, Fox RM, Tattersall MHN: Methotrexate treatment of squamous cell head and neck cancers: dose response evaluation, *BMJ* 282:600, 1981.

249. Zatterstrom UK and others: Prognostic factors in head and neck cancer: histologic grading, DNA ploidy, and nodal status, *Head Neck* 13:477, 1991.

250. Zielke-Temme BC and others: Combined intraarterial chemotherapy, radiation therapy and surgery for advanced squamous cell carcinoma of the head and neck, *Cancer* 45:1527, 1980.

CHAPTER FIVE

SKIN FLAP PHYSIOLOGY AND WOUND HEALING

Patrick J. Byrne
George S. Goding, Jr.

INTRODUCTION

A comprehensive discussion of the physiology of the skin as it applies to surgery is essentially one of vascular supply. Local skin flaps, like pedicled flaps and free tissue transfer, are dependent on the maintenance of adequate perfusion to meet the metabolic demands of mobilized tissue. An understanding of this physiology allows the surgeon to plan flaps intelligently to ensure a favorable outcome. In addition, an understanding of flap physiology provides a conceptual basis on which to optimize the management of the challenging defect or the tenuous flap.

The vascular supply to the skin serves two purposes: thermoregulation and nutritional support. Nutritional support is regulated largely by the capillary network, which is under the control of the precapillary sphincters. Local hypoxemia causes vasodilation of the precapillary sphincters. Thermoregulation is controlled by arteriovenous shunts, which are located more superficially in the skin. The sphincters of the arteriovenous shunts are under sympathetic control. When body temperature increases, the resulting decrease of norepinephrine leads to lesser sphincteric contraction, thus allowing greater blood flow to the skin. The opposite occurs with decreased body temperature.

The creation of a flap applies specific stresses to healthy skin. These stresses include local tissue trauma and reduced neurovascular supply to the affected tissue. The extent to which skin can survive these injuries is a reflection of the anatomy and physiology of skin and of the cutaneous response to injury. Knowledge of these principles has led to improved skin flap survival rate by means of improved flap design. Increasing cutaneous flap survival rate by minimizing the deleterious physiologic effects of flap transposition is an area of active research that has yet to produce techniques that have widespread clinical application.

An important concept in skin vascular physiology as it applies to flaps is that of the angiosome. In 1987, Taylor and Palmer[357] coined the term *angiosome* to refer to the tissue supplied by a named artery. The head and neck region has several such angiosomes, including the important thyroid, facial, buccal, ophthalmic, superficial temporal, and occipital.[65] Adjacent angiosomes are in communication with each other via choke vessels. This relationship becomes important in the design of various flaps. It has been demonstrated that axial pattern flaps (to be discussed in this chapter) are capable of supplying adequate blood flow to an adjacent angiosome. The incorporation of tissue on an additional angiosome beyond this adjacent angiosome, however, invites vascular compromise and likely flap failure. Techniques such as delay to extend this vascular supply may be necessary.

ZONES OF PERFUSION

Maintenance of cell function and viability is the objective of the circulatory system at macrocirculatory, capillary, interstitial, and cellular levels. The importance of tissue vascularity is well recognized, but the complexity and diversity of tissue perfusion mechanisms require that the process be divided into components. Each level of perfusion has unique physiologic characteristics, and optimal management is possible only if these differences are recognized. Johnson and Barker[165] described two levels of risk zones for flap failure, making a distinction between thrombosis at the arterial and capillary levels. By extension of this concept, four zones of the circulatory system can be considered for all hazards (Figure 5-1). Proper function of each zone is crucial to tissue viability.

Zone I consists of the cardiopulmonary system, the conduits for blood flow (arteries and veins), neural control of those conduits, and the lymphatic system. Zone I has historically been recognized as essential for flap survival. The delay phenomenon is primarily a zone I effect. The development of the pedicled flap[14] underscores the importance of zone I in extending flap survival time. Free microvascular tissue transfer also is a zone I manipulation.

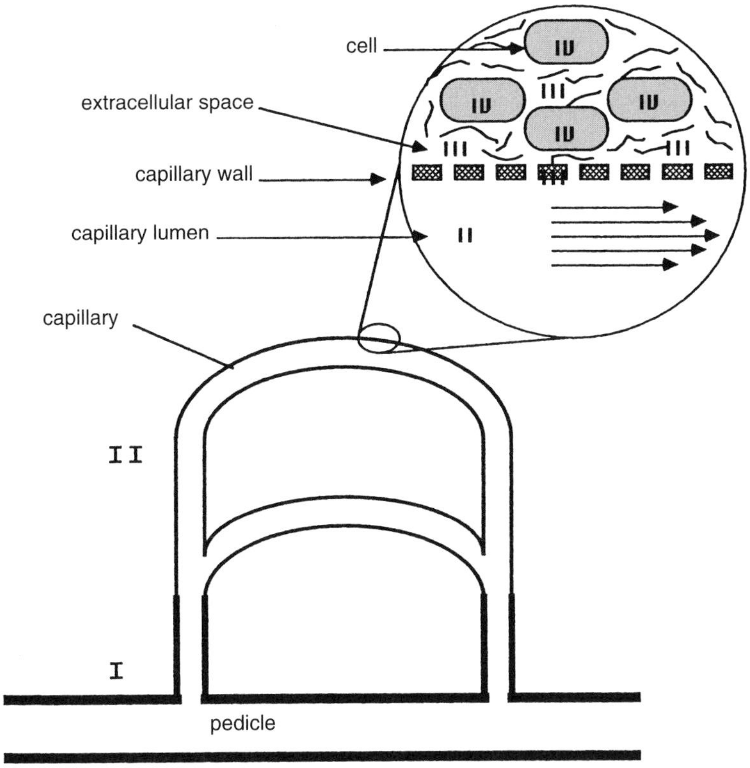

Figure 5-1. Zones of perfusion. Zone I is the macrocirculatory system consisting of cardiopulmonary, neurovascular, and lymphatic function. Zone II is the capillary circulatory systems composed of arterioles, capillaries, venules, and arteriovenous shunts. The interstitial system is zone III and entails the capillary membranes and interstitial ground substance. The cell membrane, organelles, and intracellular space comprise zone IV, the cellular system.

Zone II comprises the capillary circulation. The importance of the capillary circulation is shown by the "no-reflow phenomenon," wherein a loss of nutritive blood flow occurs in the presence of an adequate vascular supply.[5]

Zone III is the interstitial space and its mechanisms of nutrient delivery. The capillary wall is included in zone III because capillary permeability is a main determinant of interstitial space properties. Failure of metabolites to enter and traverse the interstitial space can result in loss of cell viability, even though there is adequate zone I and even zone II function. Interstitial systems are an important link in skin flap survival rate.[274]

The cell and its membranes comprise zone IV. Maintaining viable cells is the ultimate determinant of flap survival. Prolongation of cell survival by selective changes in cell permeability and uptake is a potential intervention that may improve flap survival rate.

ANATOMY AND PHYSIOLOGY OF SKIN

The skin serves as a sensory and as a protective organ. The thick epidermal layers are largely impermeable to gases and most liquids. Because of this, many agents that could result in beneficial effects to skin flaps are ineffective when applied topically to intact skin.

The epidermis of the skin is derived from ectoderm in the early embryo. The glandular appendages of the skin (i.e., sebaceous glands and hair follicles) develop from tubes and solid cords that invaginate from the covering ectoderm.[248] The epidermis is a metabolically active, but avascular, stratified squamous epithelium. The average epidermal thickness for most of the body is 0.1 mm. The majority of cells undergo keratinization and form the various epithelial layers.[163] The superficial keratinized cells of the skin are continuously replaced by cells originating from the mitotic activity in the basal layer of the epidermis. Melanocytes derived from neural crest cells also are found in the epithelium of skin and comprise a second cell type.

The dermis is derived from embryonic mesoderm and consists primarily of noncellular connective tissue. This relatively noncellular layer has metabolic requirements far less than those of the epidermis. Nerves, blood vessels, lymph vessels, and the base of the epidermal glandular appendages are found within the dermis.[163] The dermis is 15–40 times thicker than the epidermis, with a maximum width of 4 mm on the back.[167] The outer surface of the dermis has an uneven border contacting the epidermis and is known as the papillary layer. The papillary dermis is characterized by an abundant ground substance, irregularly arranged collagen bundles, and a highly developed microcirculation. The reticular dermis is composed of thick bundles of collagen and coarse elastic fibers. Fibrocytes and blood vessels are proportionally less numerous.

Deep to the reticular layer of the dermis, the anatomy of loose-skin and fixed-skin animals diverges. In fixed-skin animals (e.g., humans, swine), the subcutaneous layer consists of loose connective tissue and a varying amount of fat cells. It is a deeper continuation of the dermis and collagenous fibers continuous with those in the dermis. The density of the collagenous fibers is related to the degree of cutaneous mobility over the underlying structures. In the palms and soles, for example, these fibers are particularly numerous. The deep surface of the subcutaneous layer is attached to the superficial fascia of underlying muscle where it is present.

In loose-skin animals (e.g., rats, rabbits, dogs), the panniculus carnosus muscle is firmly attached to the reticular dermis. The panniculus carnosus is separated from the superficial fascia of underlying muscles by a loose areolar tissue layer. This layer allows for increased mobility of the superficial cutaneous–panniculus carnosus complex relative to the underlying tissue. This mobility afforded by the loose areolar tissue layer creates a greater dependence on direct cutaneous arterial supply than is seen in humans.

Zone I: Macrocirculatory System

Blood vessels travel by one of two main routes to terminate in the cutaneous circulation. Musculocutaneous arteries pass through the overlying muscle to which they provide nutrition; septocutaneous arteries[67] (also referred to as direct cutaneous arteries) travel through fascial septa that divide the muscular segments (Figure 5-2).

The cutaneous portion of a septocutaneous artery typically runs parallel to the skin surface, providing nutrition to a large area of skin. Septocutaneous arteries typically have a pair of veins accompanying them and run above the superficial muscular fascia.[373] The more common musculocutaneous arteries leave the muscle and enter the subcutaneous tissue to supply a smaller region of skin.

Septocutaneous and musculocutaneous arteries empty into a diffuse interconnecting vascular network of dermal and subdermal plexi. This network provides a redundancy in the vascular supply to the skin. A col-

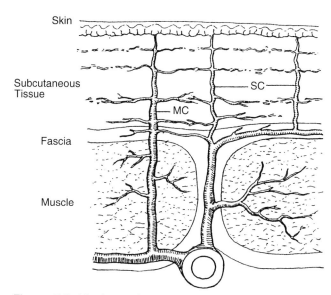

Figure 5-2. Varying pathways to skin define musculocutaneous (*MC*) and septocutaneous (*SC*) arteries.

lateral blood supply supports the vascular territory of each artery. Lymphatic vessels form a plexus running parallel and deep to the network of blood capillaries. The lymphatic capillaries end in blind sacs and conduct extracellular fluid back into the bloodstream. Lymphatic function is affected by inflammation and loss of blood vessel pulsations.[285]

The neural supply to the skin originates from sensory nerves and sympathetic nerves. The sensory nerves are distributed in segmental fashion, forming dermatomes, and participate in the skin's protective function. The postganglionic terminals of cutaneous sympathetic nerves contain the neurotransmitter norepinephrine and are found in the area of cutaneous arterioles.[5,238]

Zone II: Capillary System

The cutaneous capillary system, along with the arteriovenous shunts, serves the two important functions of nutritional support and thermoregulation. Primarily because of its thermoregulatory function, the rate of blood flow through the skin is one of the most variable in the body. During ordinary skin temperatures, the amount of blood flowing through the skin (approximately 9 ml/min/100 g of tissue) is greater than the flow required for nutritional support.[380] Blood flow can increase to 20 times this value with maximal vasodilation. When the body is exposed to extreme cold, blood flow can be reduced to levels that are marginal for cutaneous nutrition.

Before entering the capillary bed, the arterioles branch into small vessels (e.g., terminal arterioles or metarterioles) that are surrounded by a discontinuous layer of smooth muscle. A simple ring of smooth muscle forms a sphincter at the point where the capillaries originate from the metarteriole. This sphincter can completely stop blood flow within the capillary. The capillary bed can be bypassed by arteriovenous shunts that allow the arterioles to empty directly into venules. During conditions of adequate systemic vascular pressure, preshunt and precapillary sphincters regulate the distribution of cutaneous blood flow.[126]

The preshunt sphincters are involved in regulating the changes in blood flow that affect thermoregulation and systemic blood pressure.[98,334] Release of norepinephrine by the postganglionic sympathetic fibers results in contraction of the preshunt sphincters. This diverts blood away from the skin surface wherein heat loss can occur. With increased body temperature, the sympathetic vasoconstrictor impulses decrease, allowing for increased blood flow to the skin.

Local production of bradykinin may play a role in regulating skin blood flow by causing vasodilation.[130] The cutaneous circulation also is extremely sensitive to circulating norepinephrine and epinephrine. Even in areas of skin that have lost their sympathetic innervation, a mass discharge of the sympathetic system will still result in intense vasoconstriction in the skin.

The precapillary sphincter, which controls the amount of nutritive blood flow to the skin, responds to local hypoxemia and increased metabolic byproducts by dilation.[125,384] Capillary blood flow also is affected by elevated interstitial pressure, which can compress the capillary and decrease transcapillary flow. Conversely, as pressure decreases in the interstitium, the capillary expands and flow increases.[308] Acute increases in systemic blood pressure cause an immediate increase in local blood flow followed by return of flow to near normal levels in less than 1 minute. This normalization of capillary blood flow is called *autoregulation*.[130] The metabolic theory for autoregulation proposes that an excess of oxygen and nutrients results in arteriolar constriction. This process is believed to be the primary functional mechanism of autoregulation. The myogenic theory suggests that stretching of the arteriolar muscle results in reflex contraction and may be a mechanism to protect capillaries from excessively high blood pressures. Reduction of blood flow also may occur as a result of increased interstitial pressure.

Zone III: Interstitial System

The interstitial space is filled with proteoglycans and collagen.[308] In many tissues, hyaluronic acid filaments make up the interstitial ground substance. These filaments normally are woven through the interstitium, producing a medium that exhibits high resistance to fluid movement unless the tissue is well hydrated.[133]

In tissues with excess edema, the filaments do not overlap, which will produce shear planes of free fluid within the interstitium.[132]

Two processes by which substances can move across the interstitial space are diffusion and convection.[28] *Diffusion* is the process wherein a molecule passively moves to a lower concentration. Molecular movement by diffusion is affected by many factors. An important characteristic is lipid solubility. Lipid-soluble molecules tend to traverse cell membranes more easily and quickly than nonlipid-soluble agents. Large molecules diffuse more slowly than small ones. As molecules diffuse away from the capillary, the concentration of that molecule decreases by the inverse square law. As edema occurs, diffusion distances increase.[148] The concentration of a molecule within the interstitium also varies from the arteriolar side to the venular side of a capillary.[237]

Convective flow, or bulk flow, is another way for molecules to move across the interstitium. Rather than a given agent diffusing to a lower concentration, the agent is swept along with the current of plasma that flows across the interstitial space in microchannels. The agents then diffuse the short distance from the microchannels to the cells.

The relative importance of diffusion and convective flow is controversial. Some authors believe diffusion is primarily responsible for cell nutrition. Convection becomes relatively more important for certain tissues, molecules, or pathologic states.

Convective flow of nutrient-laden plasma out of the capillaries and across the interstitial space is produced by a combination of hydrostatic and osmotic pressures as described by Starling in 1896.[241] The formula is:

$$Jv/A = Lp[(P_c - P_i) - \sigma_s(\pi_c - \pi_i)]$$

In descriptive terms, flow of plasma out of the capillary per unit area (Jv/A) is related to the product of the water permeability of the membrane (Lp) multiplied by the difference between hydrostatic pressure in the capillary (P_c) and interstitial space (P_i) minus the difference between osmotic pressure in the capillary (π_c) and the osmotic pressure in the interstitial space (π_i). The osmotic pressures are adjusted by the osmotic coefficient, σ_s, a measure of the "leakiness" of a semipermeable membrane.

In functional terms, over the length of the capillary, hydrostatic pressure decreases as fluid exits the capillary and hydraulic resistance is overcome. At the same time, oncotic pressure within the capillary increases as fluid exits the capillary and plasma proteins are retained. These changes in gradients favor return of fluid at the venular end of the capillary and in the immediately postcapillary venule. Pressure gradients also are responsible for bulk flow of fluid across the interstitial space in fluid microchannels.

A net change of 2 mOsm is sufficient to increase interstitial pressure beyond transmural capillary pressure,[202] thereby compressing the capillary. Increased venous pressure limits interstitial resorption of fluid and contributes to formation of an interstitial transudate.[308] Inflammation in a flap is probably a result of nociceptor pathway stimulation by handling of the flap. Even the relatively minor trauma of inserting a fine needle causes a "very large" increase in capillary permeability within minutes after insertion, as evidenced by rapid influx of proteins into the interstitium.[34] Ischemia also will produce inflammation. Capillary hyperpermeability has been found throughout ischemic flaps.[380] The lymphatic system has two functions that affect zone III: to remove excess fluid and to remove interstitial protein. There is some controversy in the physiology literature regarding the magnitude of the latter function.[137] If the lymphatic system is malfunctioning, interstitial fluid and interstitial protein will accumulate.[210]

Zone IV: Cellular Systems

The intracellular space is the endpoint for nutrient transport and the origin of metabolic waste. The cell wall is a fluid lipid bilayer, 7.5 to 10.0 nm thick. The lipid bilayer is a major barrier to movement of solutes across the membrane. The primary function of the cell membrane is to maintain or to vary in a controlled fashion the separation of the extracellular and intracellular environments. This separation is achieved by specific membrane proteins, which act as solute pumps and solute and solvent leaks. The osmotic pressure between the two environments also should be maintained to preserve normal cell volume. The sodium–potassium pump is important in maintaining osmotic equilibrium across the cell membrane and has a requirement for energy in the form of adenosine triphosphate (ATP).[206] A loss of energy substrate (oxygen and consequently ATP) produces an intracellular movement of sodium and an increase in intracellular osmotic pressure.[222] These changes occur quickly,[95,96,209,386] within 10 minutes after arterial occlusion.[158] Within seconds of hypoxia, levels of adenosine triphosphate begin to decrease, and cells begin to swell.[209] Relatively brief periods of ischemia result in a reversible swelling of the cell and organelles. If the ischemic insult is severe and prolonged, cell lysis and flap necrosis occur.

CLASSIFICATION OF FLAPS

Flaps are commonly classified according to their principle blood supply. These include random flaps, arterial cutaneous flaps (i.e., axial flaps), fasciocutaneous, musculocutaneous, and venous (Figure 5-3). Venous flaps to this point have had no application in head and neck reconstruction. Flaps may also be described according to site of origin relative to the area to be reconstructed. Thus, flaps utilized in the head and neck include local, regional, and distant. Distant flaps may be pedicled or free flaps (microvascular free tissue transfer).

Random Cutaneous Flaps

The vascular supply to a random flap is from the subdermal plexus. The subdermal vascular plexus is supplied by unnamed musculocutaneous artery perforators near the base of the flap. The random cutaneous flap is commonly used in local flap reconstruction. The plane of dissection is through the subcutaneous fat. Examples of local random flaps include advancement, rotation, a combination of rotation-advancement, transposition, and tubed flaps. The survival of such flaps is determined by the perfusion pressure supplying the flap, and is not necessarily related to simple length to width ratios. While not without usefulness, such ratios are indirectly related to the actual vascular physiology.

Arterial Cutaneous (Axial) Flaps

Arterial cutaneous flaps (also called axial pattern flaps) are supplied by a defined septocutaneous artery that runs beneath the longitudinal axis of the flap. These flaps typically have an improved survival length relative to random cutaneous flaps. The plane of dissection must include the septocutaneous vessel within the subcutaneous fat. The axial flap may be designed to include tissue distal to that supplied directly by the artery. In such a case, the more distal portion of the flap is essentially a random flap, and caution must be exercised to avoid overextending the design beyond viability.

Use of arterial cutaneous flaps is limited by the availability of direct cutaneous arteries. Examples of arterial cutaneous flaps used in head and neck reconstruction are the deltopectoral flap, based on the anterior perforators of the internal mammary, and the paramedian forehead flap, based on the supratrochlear vessels.

Myocutaneous and Fasciocutaneous Flaps

Myocutaneous flaps represent an additional modification to improve flap survival. Myocutaneous flaps are based on distal segmental vessels leaving the local vasculature (perforators and cutaneous vessels) intact, which requires incorporation of muscle with the flap. Myocutaneous flaps are typically named for the donor muscle. Examples include the pectoralis myocutaneous flap, based on the pectoral branch of the thoracoacromial artery, and the latissimus dorsi

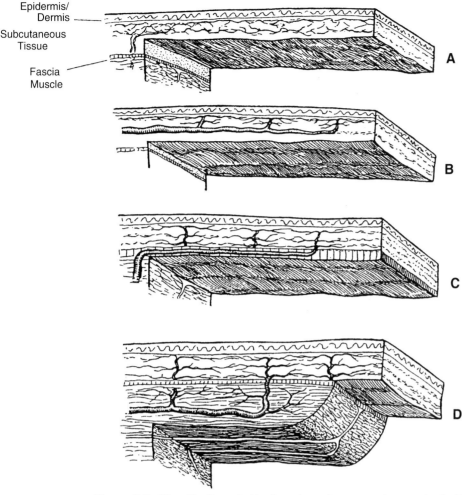

Epidermis/
Dermis
Subcutaneous
Tissue
Fascia
Muscle

Figure 5-3. Classification of skin flaps based on vascular supply. **A,** Random. **B,** Arterial cutaneous. **C,** Fasciocutaneous. **D,** Musculocutaneous.

myocutaneous flap, based on the thoracodorsal artery.

The increased blood flow and higher tissue oxygen tensions available with myocutaneous flaps[124] make this design superior in the management of contaminated or infected defects. Improved phagocytotic and bactericidal activity of leukocytes is seen in myocutaneous flaps relative to random pattern flaps in the canine model.[89] These physiologic benefits contribute to the ability of myocutaneous flaps to resist bacterial inoculation more effectively than random pattern flaps.

Like for arterial flaps, it often is desirable to extend the surface area of the flap in clinical situations. A random portion of the flap can be incorporated based on the subdermal plexus. This random extension usually is the portion of the flap most at risk of ischemic necrosis.

Fasciocutaneous flaps use direct arterial (septocutaneous) vessels with the cutaneous branches at the level of the deep fascia forming a plexus, which supplies the subdermal plexus.[71] The appropriate size of fasciocutaneous flaps is less well-defined than axial pattern flaps with their obvious arterial supply. Fasciocutaneous flaps appear to rely more on potential skin vascular territories. Four types of fasciocutaneous flaps have been described based on the pattern of blood supply incorporated into the fascial component of the flap. Examples include the parascapular flap and the radial forearm flap.

Free Microvascular Flaps

Free flaps have become the standard of care for many types of reconstruction and hold several advantages over regional flaps. Free flaps may be fasciocutaneous, musculocutaneous, myofascial, osseous, or osteocutaneous, or a combination of these. Tissue from a distant site can be harvested based on the characteristics of the donor site and the needs of the defect. Vascularity of the flap is maintained by microvascular anastomosis of the artery and vein. The flap can be harvested and customized to the defect in terms of absolute size and relative amounts of bone, muscle, skin, or nerve that is needed. Careful design of a free flap can eliminate a risk of partial necrosis caused by a random extension.

PHYSIOLOGY OF ACUTELY RAISED FLAPS

A number of changes detrimental to skin survival occur when a cutaneous flap is created. That flaps survive at all is a testimony to the minimal nutritional requirements of skin. The primary insult affecting flap survival is impaired vascular supply and the resultant ischemia. In the presence of adequate blood flow, complete flap survival occurs. Nerve section and inflammation influence flap survival primarily by affecting blood flow. Recovery from ischemia also can occur by the timely formation of new vascular channels between the transposed flap and the recipient bed.

Impairment of Vascular Supply

Partial interruption of the vascular supply (zone I) to the skin is the most obvious and critical change that occurs with elevation of a cutaneous flap. Myers[253] has emphasized that "fresh flaps are always both viable and ischemic." Flap survival depends on the degree of ischemia and the amount of time before recovery of nutrient blood flow. Flaps can tolerate an average of 13 hours of complete avascularity and survive.[180] Limitation of the vascular supply results in a local decrease in perfusion pressure to the skin. In arterial or myocutaneous flaps, the blood supply to the skin overlying the vascular pedicle usually is adequate.[123] In random flaps or random extensions of flaps, the

decrease in perfusion pressure becomes more pronounced with increasing distance from the base of the flap.[64,203] When perfusion is reduced in one area of a random flap, the adjacent vascular territories supplied by a separate perforating vessel can provide a low pressure blood supply through the subdermal plexus (Figure 5-4). Because the nutritional requirements of skin are relatively low, a number of vascular territories can be compromised before necrosis will result.

The surviving length of the random portion of the flap depends on the physical properties of the supplying vessels (intravascular resistance) and the perfusion pressure.[68] When the perfusion pressure decreases below the pressure in the interstitial space, capillary blood flow ceases. The pressure at which there is no longer enough intravascular blood pressure to maintain capillary blood flow is called the *critical closing pressure.*

In the past, random cutaneous flaps often were designed relative to a desired length-to-width ratio, with a wider base needed to successfully transfer a longer flap. The wider random flap only includes additional vessels with the same perfusion pressure. The relationship between perfusion pressure and critical closing pressure is not altered, and no change in survival length occurs (Figure 5-5).[242]

In free flaps, a secondary ischemia can occur when thrombus formation occurs at the anastomosis. Anastomosis failure is related to exposure of the vascular intima to platelets.[165,377] Platelet activation is caused by superficially exposed subendothelium or, with deeper vessel injury, exposure to collagen types I and III.[22] The geometry of the vascular arrangement often is a critical factor when experienced surgeons lose a free flap.

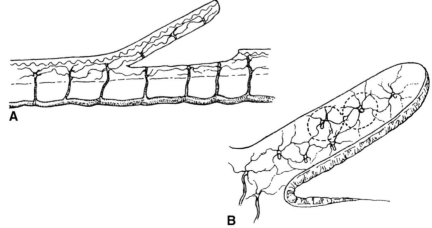

Figure 5-4. A and **B**, Vascular territories in skin flaps. Multiple perforating vessels exist and are interconnected at the periphery of their vascular territory. When some of these vessels are cut, blood supply can be replaced from nearby perforating vessels, and then tissue necrosis does not occur.

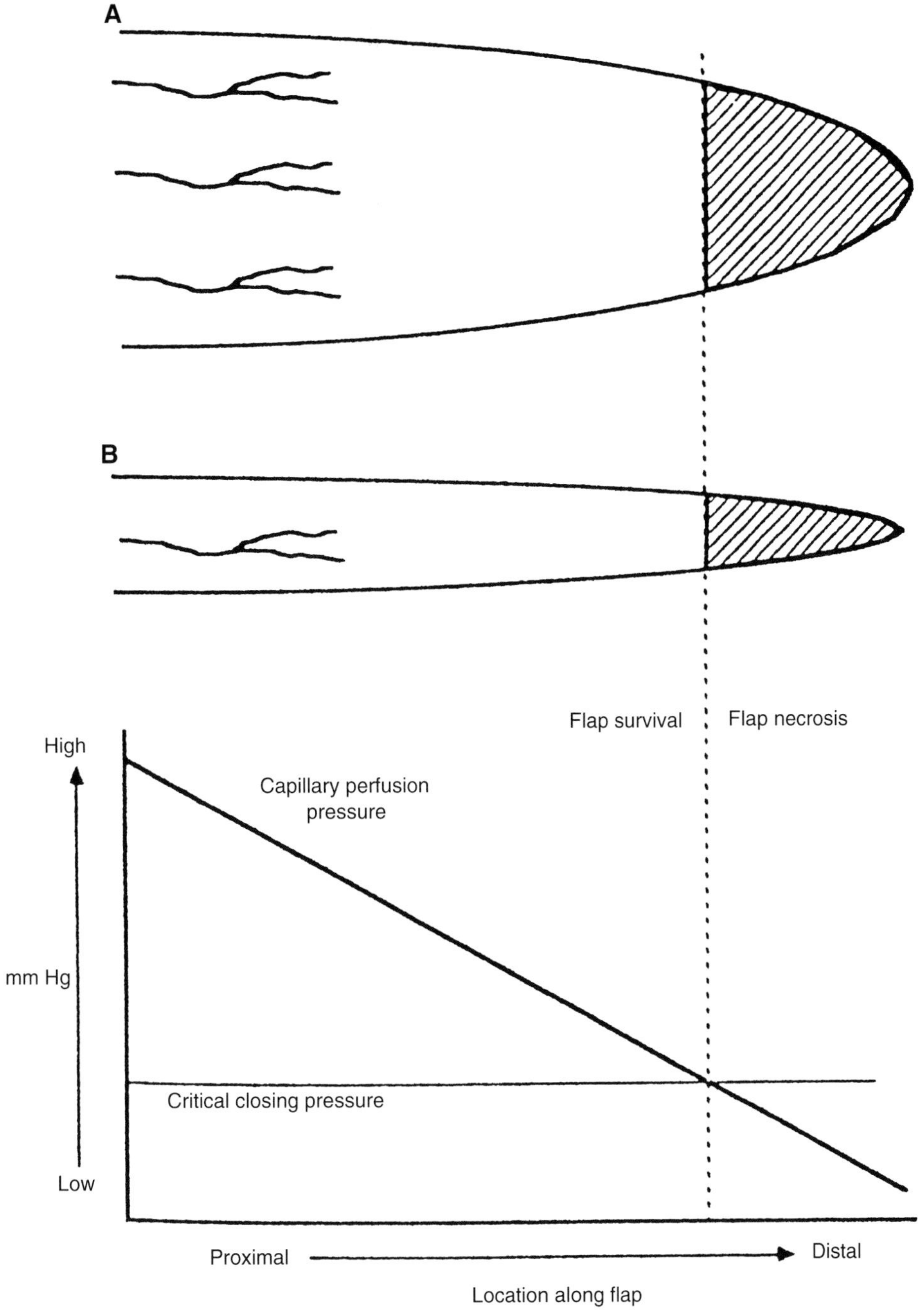

Figure 5-5. Fallacy of the length-to-width ratio. The slope of decreasing perfusion pressure versus flap length does not change with incorporation of additional vessels (flap **a** versus flap **b**) with the same perfusion pressure. Flap necrosis occurs when perfusion pressure decreases below critical closing pressure of the capillary bed.

The venous outflow from the skin also is impaired with flap elevation. Venous flow can occur through the subdermal plexus or by venous channels that accompany the feeding artery in the pedicle. Complete venous occlusion in the early postelevation period may be more damaging to flap survival than inadequate arterial supply.[349] Fortunately, the subdermal plexus alone often is adequate to provide adequate venous outflow. Care should be taken to preserve venous outflow in flaps pedicled solely on the feeding vessels.

Impairment of lymphatic drainage with flap elevation also occurs. Reduction of the cutaneous lymphatic drainage results in an increase in interstitial fluid pressure that is compounded by increased leakage of intravascular protein associated with inflammation. The resulting edema leads to increased interstitial pressure, which decreases capillary perfusion by increasing the critical closing pressure (Figure 5-6).[111,307] Alterations in the Starling's forces result in further ischemic swelling of cells and the interstitial space, setting a positive feedback cycle in motion.

Microcirculatory Changes

Necrosis in flaps is caused by prolonged loss of nutritional blood flow.[247,253,281] There are several proposed mechanisms for loss of nutritional flow, each of which may play a role. Erythrocyte sludging frequently has been noted in capillaries undergoing ischemia, often without thrombus formation.[313,348] Therefore, sludging is not necessarily caused by platelet activation unless there is a microvascular anastomosis or other vessel injury involved, such as tearing, stretching, laceration, or crushing. Microemboli are commonly generated from a microvascular anastomosis.[22]

The reason for the erythrocyte sludging is multifactorial. Erythrocytes become turgid and lose the flaccid, biconcave disk in the acidic environment of ischemia. Narrowing of the capillaries,[317] presumably a result of external compression, also contributes to stacking of erythrocytes within the lumen of ischemic tissue capillaries. Sludging is seen less often if the hematocrit is kept below 30%.[20]

Capillary blood flow is further hindered by leukocyte adherence to the capillary wall.[317] The leukocytes probably are responding to cytokines released from the cells in response to initial injury. The leuko-

cytes first roll along the capillary wall and then begin to stick. As time progresses, the leukocytes flatten onto the endothelial cell and eventually pass into the interstitium. Each step of the way has biochemical mediators. Carolina rinse solution will decrease sticking but not rolling.[300] Leukocyte depletion in patients undergoing heart transplantation prevents ultrastructural evidence of reperfusion injury.[287] Schemic cells of all tissues swell because of the loss of energy substrate needed to continue maintaining the osmotic gradient. Swelling of extravascular cells causes compression of the vascular lumen,[17] but endothelial cell swelling has a greater effect on capillary blood flow.[348] The effect of cell swelling is most dramatic in bone microcirculation, wherein a relatively small increase in cellular edema has a profound effect on vascular resistance.[249] A similar relationship between edema and increased vascular resistance has been shown in cardiac reperfusion studies.[2] Histologic evidence of edema can be used to grade the severity of free flap injury.[218] Nitric oxide synthase, an endothelial-derived vasodilator, has been studied for its effect in skin flaps.[195,198]

Neovascularization

In surviving flaps, blood flow gradually increases. If the flap is in a favorable recipient site, a fibrin layer forms within the first 2 days. Neovascularization of the flap begins 3 or 4 days after flap transposition.[112,359,366] Revascularization adequate for division of the flap pedicle has been shown as early as 7 days in animal models and humans.[59,193]

During revascularization, vascular endothelial cells play a major role in the formation of new vessels. Normally, endothelial cells are in a quiescent state, although when stimulated by angiogenic growth factors, these cells can dramatically proliferate. This normally occurs only during certain conditions, such as wound healing and ovulation.

Beginning with an angiogenic stimulus, the angiogenic process involves a number of discrete yet overlying steps (Figure 5-7). Initially, the vessels become dilated and permeable with retraction of the endothelial cells and a decrease in endothelial junctions. The basement membrane then is dissolved by proteases, and the endothelial cells migrate from the vascular wall toward the angiogenic stimulus. Behind the leading front of migrating endothelial cells, endothelial cell replication begins forming a capillary sprout that elongates toward the angiogenic source. The nearby capillary sprouts then anastomose to each other, forming capillary loops. As capillary loops and sprouts continue, the loops become patent, developing newly formed blood vessels. These blood vessels differentiate and lay down basement membrane consisting of type IV collagen, laminin, and proteoglycans.

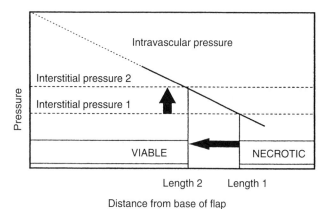

Figure 5-6. The relationship between increased interstitial pressure and decreased surviving flap length. Intravascular perfusion pressure decreases along the length of the flap. At the distal end of the flap, intravascular perfusion pressure will become less than interstitial pressure, causing the capillaries to collapse (critical closing pressure). As edema is generated by ischemia and inflammation, interstitial pressure increases, which results in a decrease in surviving length from length 1 to length 2.

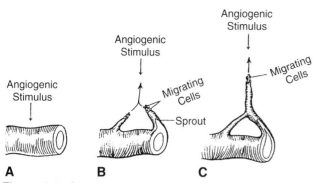

Figure 5-7. Steps in angiogenesis. **A,** Initial stimulus with retraction of endothelial cells and thinning of basement membrane. **B,** Migration of endothelial cells and formation of capillary sprout. **C,** Formation of capillary loops, which become patent to form new blood vessels.

Pericytes and fibroblasts then migrate to the capillary loop sites.[107]

With the continued presence or absence of the angiogenic stimulus, substantial remodeling, regression, and rearrangement of the new capillaries occur.[107] Some capillaries join preexisting flap vessels (inosculation), but the majority of revascularization appears to involve direct ingrowth of recipient vessels into the flap (Figure 5-8).[219] New capillaries can grow toward an angiogenic source at a mean rate of 0.2 mm/day. When the angiogenic stimulus is discontinued, the capillary vessels regress and eventually disappear over a period of weeks. Angiogenic growth factors can stimulate capillary growth over distances of 2 to 5 mm.[97] To prevent an uncontrollable cascade of neovascularization, mechanisms to inhibit angiogenesis are believed to exist. Evidence suggests that pericytes can suppress endothelial growth by direct

contact.[66] Thus, the physiologic response of angiogenesis may be analogous to the blood coagulation pathway that should be maintained at a constant steady state of control. In soft-tissue wound repair, macrophages, lymphocytes, mast cells, and platelets are involved in releasing various factors that modulate angiogenesis.[107] Tissues that are particularly high in angiogenic factors are bovine brain,[221] corpus luteum[122] retina,[90] salivary glands,[157] and lymphatic tissues.[3] Benign and malignant tumors also can be sources of angiogenic growth factors.

Nerve Section

Sensory and sympathetic nerves are severed in the process of flap elevation. Although loss of sensation may limit the usefulness of the flap after transfer, adrenergic denervation has implications for flap survival. When a sympathetic nerve is divided, catecholamines are released from the nerve terminal, and the mechanism for catecholamine reuptake is eliminated[170,276,288] A local "hyperadrenergic state" exists, which produces vasoconstriction mediated by α-adrenergic receptors in the cutaneous vasculature.[276]

The vasoconstricting effect of sympathectomy further reduces the total flap blood flow[183,281] that has already been decreased by division of supplying vessels. This negatively affects the ratio of perfusion pressure to the critical closing pressure of the arterioles in the subdermal plexus. A greater proportion of the distal flap is excluded from the blood supply, and necrosis becomes more likely. The stored transmitter is depleted within 24 to 48 hours,[170,171] and blood flow increases as the concentration of norepinephrine declines.[281] In critical areas of the flap, the time to recovery of nutrient blood flow may be delayed sufficiently to produce additional necrosis.

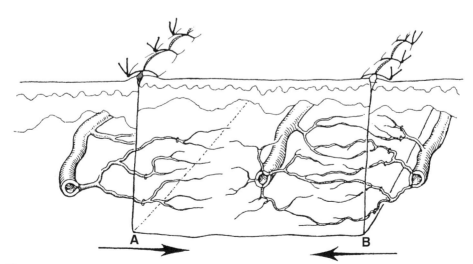

Figure 5-8. Ingrowth of angiosomes. Cross-section of the flap showing **A,** direct ingrowth vs **B,** inosculation.

Inflammation/Prostaglandins

The surgical trauma and ischemia associated with an acutely raised flap result in an inflammatory response. Histamine, serotonin, and kinins are released into the extracellular compartment after flap elevation, increasing the permeability of the microcirculation. The result is an increase in the concentration of proteins and cells within the extracellular space. The presence of nonbacterial inflammation beginning a few days before flap elevation has been shown to improve flap survival.[216,220] This is presumably the result of an increase in local blood flow.

The inflammation created during flap elevation may have deleterious effects because of the resultant edema formation. In addition to compromising capillary blood flow and altering the relationships of the Starling equation, interstitial edema increases the diffusion distances between cells. The effect is enhanced as a result of the inverse square law for diffusion. Edema also can constitute a direct barrier to diffusion.[146]

The action of the primary mediators of the inflammatory response (histamine, serotonin, and kinins) is short-lived. After kinin formation and in the presence of complement, prostaglandins are synthesized by injured cells. Prostaglandins play an important role in the later stages of the inflammatory reaction, while simultaneously initiating the early phases of injury repair.

Prostaglandins are derived from essential fatty acids that are incorporated in membrane phospholipids (Figure 5-9). Activation of phospholipases results in the production of prostaglandin H_2 (PGH_2) by cyclooxygenase. Prostaglandin E_1 (PGE_1) and prostaglandin E_2 (PGE_2) can be synthesized from prostaglandin H_2 by isomerases in the vascular endothelium. PGE_1 and PGE_2 produce vasodilation. Prostaglandin D_2 (PGD_2) also is formed by an isomerase reaction and is the principal cyclooxygenase product of the mast cell. Its effects on the cutaneous microvasculature are similar to PGE_1. Prostacyclin (PGI_2) is a vasodilating agent and inhibitor of platelet

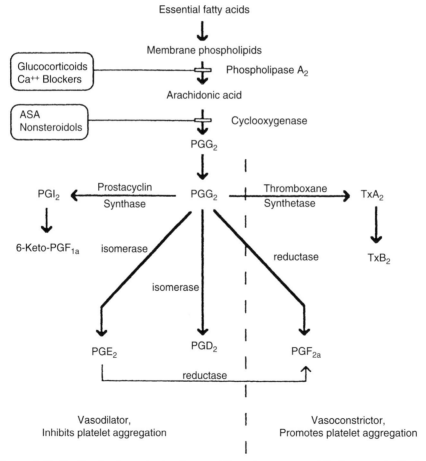

Figure 5-9. Synthesis of prostaglandins and thromboxanes and their general effects in the cutaneous circulation.

aggregation that is derived from PGH_2 through the action of prostacyclin synthase. In the skin, PGI_2 is primarily produced in the endothelial cells of blood vessels.[138,172] Prostacyclin is metabolized to 6-keto-PGF_{1a}.

Thromboxane synthetase converts PGH_2 into thromboxane A_2 (TxA_2) and is primarily located in the platelets. Its effects include vessel constriction and promotion of platelet aggregation.[176] TxA_2 is unstable and rapidly converted into thromboxane B_2 (TxB_2). Prostaglandin F_{2a} (PGF_{2a}) is derived from PGH_2 by a reductase reaction. A marked increase in resistance is seen in cutaneous arteries, arterioles, and venules in the presence of PGF_{2a}.[257] The synthesis of prostaglandins and thromboxane can be altered by pharmacologic manipulation. The action of phospholipase A_2 can be inhibited by drugs that reduce the availability of Ca^{++}. Glucocorticoids also affect phospholipase A_2 activity by inducing the synthesis of a protein that inhibits the enzyme.[41] Aspirin and other nonsteroidal antiinflammatory drugs (NSAIDs) interfere with the cyclooxygenase enzyme inhibiting the synthesis of PGH_2.

Prostaglandins clearly play a role in the inflammatory response after flap surgery. Prostacyclin levels increase after flap elevation with a peak concentration around 7 days and then decrease to postoperative day 21.[138] PGE_2, PGF_{2a}, and TxB_2 also increase after the creation of a flap. The increase of PGE_2, PGF_{2a}, and TxB_2 can be blunted by creating a bipedicled flap. Conversion to a single pedicle flap ("delay") results in decreased levels of thromboxane and an increased PGE_2, which remain at least to 7 days.[252] Whether these changes in prostaglandin levels represent a cause or a side effect of the observed phenomenon remains to be seen.

Reperfusion Injury

Controversy and often confusion surround the terms *no-reflow* and *reperfusion injury*. *No-reflow* is a term connoting the condition when zone I perfusion has been reestablished, but zone II or III failure prevails. *Reperfusion injury* describes the observation that tissues tolerate short periods of total ischemia fairly well but exhibit histologic injury after return of perfusion—thus injury apparently caused by reperfusion.[386] Both terms imply a period of ischemia, and both conditions result in microcirculatory failure.

All flaps experience some ischemia, and return of blood flow may result in microcirculatory impairment.[253,321] Free radicals form during reperfusion and result in tissue injury, but other causes, such as hyperosmosis from lactic acid accumulation,[349] have been implicated.[386]

Free Radical Formation

When oxygen becomes available with reperfusion, an additional menace to flap survival is produced—the free radical. This byproduct of reperfusion can cause damage at the cellular and subcellular levels,[184,344] contributing to postischemic tissue necrosis. The neutrophil appears to play a major role in the mediation of reperfusion injury.[211]

Free radicals are extremely reactive compounds because of an unpaired electron in their outer orbits. Oxygen free radicals are formed by the sequential univalent reduction of molecular oxygen. The superoxide anion radical (O_2^-) is formed by the addition of a single electron to molecular oxygen. Superoxide is a byproduct of ATP production in the mitochondria and other oxidation reduction reactions.[344] Polymorphonuclear cells are a second source of superoxide radicals that are released in response to bacterial inflammation.[18]

A major source of free radicals in ischemic tissue is the enzyme xanthine oxidase (Figure 5-10).[235] With ischemia, high energy phosphate compounds are converted to hypoxanthine that accumulates in the tissues. When oxygen becomes available with reperfusion, xanthine oxidase catalyzes the conversion of hypoxanthine into uric acid, producing superoxide in the process. This reaction is believed to be an important mechanism in ischemic tissue injury in skin flaps.[234] The role of xanthine oxidase has been brought into question by the ability of some investigators to find xanthine oxidase activity in ischemic skin,[159,385] but others have not.[295] Xanthine oxidase activity has been found in normal rat skin and increases its activity after venous occlusion, reperfusion,[159] and flap elevation with the highest levels being present distally.[9] Tissue damage resulting from free radical production can occur from lipid peroxidation of the cellular membrane and denaturation of the intracellular matrix.[251,348] Delayed neovascularization has been proposed as another consequence of free radical damage affecting proliferating endothelial cells.[160]

Capillary Obstruction (No-Reflow)

Arterial and random flaps can tolerate several hours of total avascularity and remain viable.[180] When the critical ischemia time for a flap is exceeded, an ischemia-related obstruction to blood flow, known as the *no-reflow phenomenon*, develops. Even though large vessels (zone I) have adequate flow, there is no perfusion in zone II or III. The no-reflow phenomenon was described in skin flaps by May and others.[232] Swelling of the endothelial and parenchymal cells, coupled with intravascular stasis and eventual thrombosis, leads to loss of nutritive flow. Interactions between polymorphonuclear cells and endothelial cells appear to play a fundamental role in the generation of

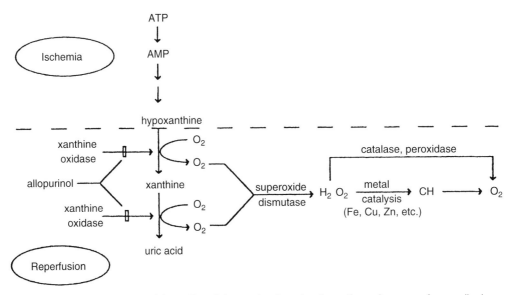

Figure 5-10. Xanthine oxidase. Possible mechanism for formation of oxygen-free radicals during reperfusion after ischemia and the subsequent reduction of the superoxide.

a reperfusion injury.[282,331] Both cell groups produce cytokine and proadhesive molecules that affect the inflammatory response.[298] Polymorphonuclear cells adhere to the vascular wall and generate proteases and oxygen free radicals that injure the endothelial cells.[378]

A unique aspect of free flap physiology is microcirculatory failure related to showers of microemboli from the anastomosis[22] These microemboli will flow through the microcirculation and sometimes will transiently occlude capillaries before finally clearing the microcirculation. Microemboli generated from the anastomosis have importance in management of microcirculatory failure and the no-reflow phenomenon as it applies to free flaps.[147]

FLAP BIOMECHANICS

Skin flap biomechanics are governed principally by collagen and elastin.[115,205] The interplay of these components has a direct influence on the results of flap wound closure. Collagen I and II comprise the principal structural framework of the extracellular matrix.[115] Elastic fibers, meanwhile, are responsible primarily for the elasticity and compliance of the skin. When skin is stretched, the fine elastin network initially allows easy deformation. This is demonstrated on the stress-strain curve (section I)[87] (Figure 5-11). As the force (stress) applied to the skin increases, randomly arranged collagen fibers begin to lengthen in the direction of the force and deformation becomes more difficult (section II). Further lengthening becomes difficult. Once the collagen fibers have all become oriented longitudinally with the force, little

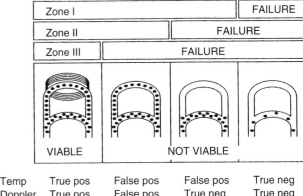

Figure 5-11. Perfusion types. Zones of circulatory impairment. The relationship of microcirculatory impairment and anomalous readings of common measurements of flap perfusion is shown. All zones should be functioning for cell viability, and zone III is the first to fail. Zone III failure is shown as a loss of interstitial flow; whereas capillary blood flow is potentially still present. Zone II failure occurs with loss of capillary blood flow. Arteriovenous shunt flow may still be present, but it is not nutritive. Finally, with zone I failure, the flap is ischemic. See text for a discussion of monitors of perfusion.

further deformation is possible with increasing stress (section III). Section III behaves similarly to elderly skin, suggestive of the maintenance of collagen biomechanics with aging. As patients age, there is a progressive decrease in elastic fibers.[115] Thus, less force is necessary to produce lengthening. Older patients can therefore be expected to have less wound tension.

Wound tension is an important factor in flap survival, as well as scar formation. Excessive tension in skin flaps is associated with increased flap necrosis.[115] This is likely secondary to a decrease in blood flow with increasing wound tension.[115]

The term *creep* refers to the increase in strain (change in length relative to original length) seen when a constant stress (force) is applied to the skin.[363] Stress relaxation, on the other hand, refers to the decrease in stress that occurs when skin is held under tension at a constant strain.[110] Thus, the physiology of skin is altered over time by the application of a constant stress. These properties are responsible for the effects with tissue expansion and serial excisions of lesions.

Flap undermining is routinely performed during flap elevation and wound closure. It is the release of the attachments of the skin to the underlying tissue that results in a decreased wound tension when undermining is performed.[205] The force required to counteract the resistance between the dermis and underlying tissue is the shearing force.[115] In an animal model, the reduction in the shearing force, and thus wound tension, was found to decrease with undermining up to 4 cm.[197] Further undermining did not produce further improvement in wound tension.

ATTEMPTS TO ALTER SKIN FLAP VIABILITY
Increased Blood Supply

Skin flap failure can occur from extrinsic and intrinsic causes.[150] Extrinsic reasons for flap necrosis are those not resulting from the design of the raised flap. Examples include systemic hypotension, infection, and pedicle compression. These factors often can be overcome in the clinical situation. The primary intrinsic factor affecting flap survival is inadequate blood flow. Numerous experimental attempts have been made to influence flap microcirculation or decrease the deleterious effects of inadequate flap blood flow (Figure 5-12). The most successful has been flap delay. Table 5-1 shows the affected zones of perfusion for various interventions to increase flap survival.

Delay

Four things are accepted about the delay phenomenon. First, it requires surgical trauma. Second, a large percentage of the neurovascular supply to the flap should be eliminated. Third, delay results in increased flap survival at the time of tissue transfer. Fourth, the beneficial effects can last up to 6 weeks in humans.[289] To explain this phenomenon, three theories regarding the mechanism of delay have been developed: (1) delay improves the blood flow; (2) delay conditions

TABLE 5-1	
ZONES OF PERFUSION AFFECTED BY VARIOUS INTERVENTIONS TO INCREASE FLAP SURVIVAL	
Intervention	**Affected Zones**
Flap design	I
Delay	I, II
Vasodilators	II
Neovascularization	II
Rheology	II
Inflammation	II, III
Antioxidants	II, III, IV
Metabolic manipulation	II, IV
Increased oxygenation	IV

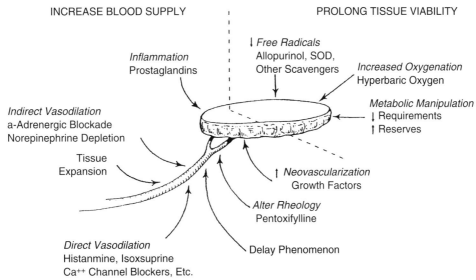

Figure 5-12. Experimental attempts to affect flap survival.

the tissue to ischemia[236]; and (3) delay closes arteriovenous shunts.[306] Most recent studies support a mechanism resulting in increased circulation to the flap. How this occurs remains to be proven.

The percentage of arteriovenous shunt flow to total blood flow is similar in delayed and acute flaps.[278] Delayed flaps simply have an increase in total blood flow. The addition of systemic norepinephrine decreases the blood flow in delayed flaps to the level seen in acute flaps. Thus, one effect of delay is a decrease in vasoconstriction in the distal portion of the flap.

Flaps delayed as few as 24 hours survive to a greater length[218] and can tolerate longer periods of ischemia.[11,374,376] Distal perfusion in the pig flank flap increases with a bipedicle flap delay up to 4 days. No further increase in perfusion occurs, extending delay up to 14 days.[281] Pang and others[281] theorized that after a delay, a reduced vasoactivity of the small arteries allows delivery of more blood to the distal portion of the flap. This modulation could occur by release of vasoconstrictive substances (i.e., norepinephrine, thromboxane, and serotonin) during elevation of the bipedicled flap. Degeneration release of norepinephrine occurs soon after flap elevation with norepinephrine stores largely depleted in the first 24–48 hours.[170,171] In bipedicle flaps, Cutting and others[60] found the catecholamine level beginning to increase 4 days after flap construction; others[170,171] have found the catecholamine levels to be depressed over a greater period. Necrosis is not seen with the first stage of delay because the bipedicled flap has an adequate blood supply. After depletion of the catecholamines, a relative state of sympathectomy develops. Because of the catecholamine depletion, conversion of the delayed flap to a single pedicle is not accompanied by the same degree of vasoconstriction.[278]

Early after elevation, the vasculature to the flap has an increased sensitivity to the effects of adrenergic drugs.[276] Intravenous norepinephrine will decrease blood flow to a myocutaneous flap, even in the presence of increased blood flow to control skin.[247] This hypersensitivity to exogenous norepinephrine can be partially blocked by management with phenoxybenzamine, an a-adrenergic blocking agent. The period of hypersensitivity to norepinephrine lasts slightly less than 1 week[247] and correlates with the period of decreased tissue norepinephrine found after flap elevation.[60] Recovery from the hyperadrenergic state also appears to play a role in the delay phenomenon.

Reorientation of the major vascular channels is another mechanism to increase blood flow to the distal portion of the single pedicle flap.[59,128] The effect of delay is greater in narrow flaps than in wide flaps.[351] The longitudinal channeling is greater in narrow flaps

because more of the transverse vessels are cut. Dilation of existing vessels is most evident in transitional areas between vascular territories of adjacent perforating arteries.[39] The effects of delay have been produced by inducing collateral blood flow by vessel occlusion in the laboratory setting[40,80,273,272] and clinically.[356] Longitudinal flow also is enhanced by vasodilating substances released by inflammation and mild ischemia.[351] Pang and others[278] believed that the depletion of vasoconstricting substances played a role in the early stage of delay, whereas locally released vasodilating substances were involved in the later stages.

Vasodilators
Indirect Vasodilators

The intense vasoconstriction associated with the release of norepinephrine after flap elevation should hinder flap survival. One of the benefits of flap delay seems to be depletion of norepinephrine before creation of the flap to be transferred. If this vasoconstriction could be blocked or reversed, the duration and severity of distal flap ischemia should be lessened. The result would be increased flap survival without the need for delay.

a-Adrenergic blocking agents are directed against the catecholamine-induced vasoconstriction seen after flap elevation. Using the rat model, phenoxybenzamine resulted in improved flap survival in some studies.[92,254,383] Phenoxybenzamine and phentolamine ointments applied topically also were found to be effective in increasing flap survival in the rat model.[121] Other investigators have been unable to reproduce beneficial effects in the rabbit or pig.[181,254] Depletion of norepinephrine stores before flap elevation with reserpine[62,168,177,181] and guanethidine[1,91,136] also has met with mixed results and systemic toxicity.

Several anesthetic agents have vasoactive properties and may influence flap survival. Because general anesthetics often are used during the creation of larger flaps, any potential effects on flap survival are important. Isoflurane (a sympatholytic vasodilator) was found to significantly improve flap survival compared with nitrous oxide, which induces vasoconstriction.[77] Verapamil and lidocaine have also been found to decrease skin flap necrosis when used locally in the vicinity of the pedicle of axial pattern flaps.[115]

Direct Vasodilators

Multiple topical anti-ischemic agents have been found to have beneficial effect on skin flaps in experimental models.[204] This has not yet translated into widespread clinical use however, as the experimental and clinical results have been mixed. Direct vasodilators such as histamine, hydralazine, nitroglycerin, pentoxifylline, and topical dimethylsulfoxide have shown a beneficial result and no effect on skin flap survival.[181] Isoxsuprine is a phenylethylamine derivative of epinephrine having *a*-adrenergic receptor antagonistic and *b*-adrenergic receptor agonistic properties, resulting in relaxation of vascular smooth muscle. In high doses, isoxsuprine can decrease viscosity and inhibit platelet aggregation. Isoxsuprine was found to increase blood flow in the area of the dominant artery in porcine myocutaneous and arterial flaps. Unfortunately, no improvement in blood flow was seen in the distal random portion of the flaps or in flap survival.[183,260,279,390] The smaller vessels in the distal random portion of a flap were theorized to have a different sensitivity than muscular or axial arteries to vasodilator drugs. Manipulation of these distal vascular channels appears to be critical in increasing flap survival.

Calcitonin gene-related peptide (CGRP) is a bioactive neuropeptide found in primary sensory neurons. It is a potent vasodilator and is thought to stimulate smooth muscle relaxation by an endothelial-dependent mechanism. CGRP administration improves blood flow and survival in ischemic skin flaps[252] and delays the onset of the no-reflow phenomenon.[253] Pretreatment with capsaicin, which depletes neuropeptides from primary sensory neurons, results in a decreased flap survival.[190] These findings suggest a potential role for primary sensory neurons in cutaneous vascular control and flap survival.

Prostaglandins have multiple effects on healing wounds and the vasculature to the skin, including vasodilation and decreased platelet aggregation. Prostaglandins E1 and E2 have been found to decrease skin necrosis in random skin flaps.[363] Prostaglandin E1 also effects leukocyte-endothelial cell adhesion, a factor in ischemia reperfusion injury. Administration of prostaglandin E1 may increase flap survival by decreasing the expression of anti-intercellular adhesion molecule-1, thus limiting the leukocyte-endothelial cell adhesion.[110] The mechanism of delivery for these substances has been via topical application with absorption through the skin, or injections subcutaneously or intravenously. Attempts to improve delivery have shown promise in the laboratory. The vasoactive drug buflomedil has been delivered bound to liposomes with a measured therapeutic effect on ischemic skin flaps.[204] Topical application of nitroglycerin was found to increase flap survival in some studies[56,301,312,361] but not in all.[7,22] Nitroglycerin acts as a vasodilator with more potent venodilator than arteriodilator effects. The action on the veins was believed to contribute to the increased flap survival. The ability to decrease platelet aggregation may be the main therapeutic benefit of nitroglycerin and other direct vasodilators that affect platelet function. Nitroglycerin and nifedipine have been found effective in improving random

pattern skin flaps in laboratory animals exposed to cigarette smoke.[70]

Neovascularization

The identification of a host of biologically active growth factors and the continued development of improved methods of delivery of these agents into target sites have generated enthusiasm for the application of these technologies to aid in flap outcomes. The stimulation of angiogenesis through gene transfer techniques offers hope to the treatment of ischemic tissues of various types, including flaps. Vascular endothelial growth factor (VEGF) is a potent angiogenic molecule, as is basic fibroblast growth factor (FGF-2). VEGF has shown promise to improve flap survival and has been demonstrated in the laboratory to improve flap survival in random flaps,[341] axial flaps,[155] and flaps treated preoperatively.[367] Nitric oxide synthase may increase VEGF levels and improve ischemic flap survival.[367] Application of fibroblast growth factors results in increased endothelial cell proliferation and vascular tube formation. The application of fibroblast growth factor has improved the survival of prefabricated myocutaneous flaps in animal studies.[71] Application of growth factor can generate functional blood vessels and nonsurgically anastomose divided vessels within 2 or 3 weeks.[36] The increased neovascularization also allows earlier ligation of the original vascular pedicle with complete tissue survival.[154,277] Growth factors have a short half-life and are more effective when delivered in a sustained release manner using a gelatin sponge.[153,347] The delay phenomenon does not work by an angiogenic mechanism, and attempts to increase survival of the random portion of a pedicled flap with fibroblast growth factors have had mixed results.[82,143,161,364] Growth factors may have their greatest clinical potential when a flap is transferred into an area of vascular compromise (e.g., irradiated soft tissue, diabetes, and steroid dependency).[154]

Rheology

In a homogeneous fluid that exhibits equal shear stress at different rates of shear, flow (Q) in a vessel can be approximated by Poiseuille's equation:

$$Q = \$PI\$gDP \cdot r^4 \cdot \$PI\$gpl \cdot 8 \cdot n$$

where $\$PI\$gDP$ equals pressure gradient; r^4 equals the fourth power of the vessel radius; l equals vessel length; and n equals viscosity.[131] Although blood is a non-Newtonian fluid, the qualitative relationships in the equation remain. In larger vessels, the radius is a dominant factor, but in the capillary microcirculation, viscosity becomes more important. By decreasing the viscosity of blood, it may be possible to increase flow to the distal random portion of the acutely raised flap and beneficially affect flap survival. Viscosity is influenced by the hematocrit, serum proteins, temperature, erythrocyte deformability, aggregation, and other factors.[315] Each of these factors can be potentially manipulated with a resultant change in viscosity.

Hemodilution has been shown to decrease viscosity and have a beneficial effect on flap survival.[84,259,302] Reducing blood viscosity by protein depletion also results in increased flap survival in rats.[316]

Pentoxifylline and low viscosity whole blood substitutes (Fluosol-DA) will also lower viscosity. Pentoxifylline is a hemorheologic agent that results in increased erythrocyte deformability[276] and decreased platelet aggregability.[315] When given 7 to 10 days before flap elevation, pentoxifylline improves flap survival.[315,391] Beneficial effects with limited preoperative dosing of pentoxifylline have not been uniform.[45,138,151,244,262] Fluosol-DA administration also has failed to consistently increase flap survival.[302,342]

Inflammation

The surgical trauma associated with an acutely raised or delayed flap results in an inflammatory response. This response results in a local increase in blood flow that could benefit flap survival. Improved flap blood flow and survival can occur with different methods of creating an inflammatory response before flap creation.[207,216] The beneficial effects of inflammation on flap survival also can be seen on a flap raised adjacent to a previously delayed flap.[166] Attempts to increase flap blood flow and survival with 5 days of low power laser burns have had mixed results.[173,342] These studies show that the inflammatory response has the potential to improve survival without sympathectomy or vascular division.

The mechanism by which inflammation produces a beneficial effect appears to involve the products of cyclooxygenase metabolism of arachidonic acid. Administration of PGI_2 results in dilation of the arterial pedicle and increased flap blood flow.[194] The result is increased flap survival.[87,309,320] Systemic administration of PGE_1 increases flap survival at low doses but can hinder flap survival at higher doses, causing hypotension.[350] Topical administration of PGE_1 also improves flap survival[323] but should be applied to the critical ischemic area to be effective.[324] Additional prostaglandin effects, such as increased erythrocyte deformity[208] and decreased platelet aggregation,[325] have been proposed as the mechanism of increased survival with prostaglandin administration.

Cyclooxygenase inhibitors, such as indomethacin and ibuprofen, have been shown to increase skin flap

viability[311,320] and prolong tolerance of ischemia.[81] Glucocorticoids, which inhibit phospholipase activity, also have increased flap survival in some studies[200,239,240] but not in others.[258] Blocking TxA_2 synthesis has had mixed results.[176,275]

Tissue Expansion

Tissue expansion has been shown to increase the size of the transferred flap in experimental animals and humans. Examination of expanded skin in the guinea pig has shown an increase in the thickness[15] and mitotic activity[102] of the epidermal layer, indicating epidermal proliferation. Blood flow in expanded tissue is greater than in skin overlying a noninflated expander 1 hour after creation of a pedicled flap.[225] The increase in blood flow to expanded skin seems to be short-lived.[118,310] Apart from the acute changes seen with expander manipulation, flap viability and blood flow in expanded skin appear to be similar to those seen in delayed flaps.[322]

Other Method

A number of drugs with multiple effects that should alter the blood flow to the flap have been tried with varying results. Ancrod, a defibrinogenating enzyme from the pit viper, has a selective affinity for fibrinogen and stimulates release of plasminogen activator with a resultant decrease in viscosity. The drug also causes increased endothelial generation of prostacyclin. When given postoperatively for 7 days, ancrod was unable to increase the viable surface area of porcine myocutaneous flaps.[246]

Chlorpromazine's effects include α-adrenergic blockade, stabilization of cell membranes, serotonin antagonism, metabolic depression, and cooling. All of these effects should be beneficial to the ischemic flap, but the results from experimental studies have been mixed.[13,29,152]

Parenteral pentoxifylline has decreased the ischemic areas of random pattern skin flaps in rats.[70]

An interesting manipulation to increase survival of thin axial pattern skin flaps was proposed by Morrison and others.[250] In their study, the femoral artery and vein were implanted into the subdermal layer of skin in the rabbit model. After 8 to 12 weeks, sufficient neovascularization occurred to allow creation of a large skin flap based on the transferred pedicle. If confirmed in other laboratories, this technique may allow greater flexibility in the design of axial pattern flaps.

PROLONGED VIABILITY
Protection Against Harmful Agents

The formation of free radicals with reperfusion and the return of molecular oxygen to ischemic tissue place an increased burden on flap survival. Research has focused on decreasing the production of free radicals and using agents that remove free radicals (free radical scavengers) from the immediate environment.

Nitric oxide is a radical with vasodilating properties that protects tissues from neutrophil-mediated ischemia-reperfusion injury.[129] L-arginine, a nitric oxide precursor, is converted into nitric oxide by the enzyme nitric oxide synthase. L-arginine has been found to have a protective effect on myocutaneous island flaps,[129] as well as random pattern skin flaps.[129] Nitric oxide inhibition decreases skin flap survival.[369]

Ischemia-reperfusion injury occurs in zones II and III, where a cascade of events may lead to flap failure upon the re-establishment of blood flow after prolonged ischemia. Platelets play a role in this cascade of events. Inhibition of platelet activation by a platelet glycoprotein IIb/IIIa inhibitor has shown promise in the enhancement of skin flap survival after a long period of ischemia.[129]

Administration of allopurinol (a xanthine oxidase inhibitor) preoperatively prevents the increased xanthine oxidase activity seen with acute flap elevation.[385] Improved survival of dorsal rat flaps has been accomplished with allopurinol when given at high doses,[7,299] with lower doses having no effect.[296] The high doses required to obtain a beneficial effect have led to concern about the use of allopurinol to increase flap survival in the clinical setting.

A number of free radical scavengers are available to protect the tissues from destruction by free radicals. Superoxide dismutase (SOD), an intracellular free radical scavenger, catalyzes the conversion of superoxide to hydrogen peroxide (H_2O_2) and molecular oxygen. When given systemically, SOD is an effective scavenger of the superoxide radical regardless of its source.[234] SOD treatment has resulted in improved flap survival[106,246,397] and increased tolerance of flaps to ischemia.[229,318] Improved flap survival also has been shown with a number of other naturally occurring compounds with free radical scavenging properties. These include deferoxamine[8], vitamin E, vitamin A, vitamin C, glutathione,[140] various amino acids,[283] and amino acid derivatives.[187]

The hydrogen peroxide formed by the dismutation of superoxide is not particularly harmful. In the presence of chelated metal complexes, hydrogen peroxide can be converted into a hydroxyl radical ($OH\cdot$).[72] The hydroxyl radical is much more reactive and may be responsible for much of the damage inflicted by oxygen free radicals.[141,344] The presence of a hematoma under a flap may decrease flap survival by increasing the available iron, which acts as a catalyst in the formation of free radicals.[10]

Hyperbaric Oxygen

Improvement in flap survival with hyperbaric oxygen treatment has been documented,[179,290,293] but this has not been a consistent finding.[39] Hyperbaric oxygen treatment increases blood oxygen-carrying capacity by 20%.[178] This relative increase is greater with a low hematocrit because the additional oxygen is dissolved in the plasma rather than carried by hemoglobin. A greater effect of hyperbaric oxygen treatment may be increasing oxygen diffusion from surrounding perfused tissue to the ischemic portion of the flap.[63] Increased flap survival also occurs with treatments using hyperbaric air, showing that increased oxygen can be delivered with an increase in ambient pressure alone.[355]

The beneficial effect of hyperbaric oxygen in pedicled flaps includes decreased leukocyte adherence,[396] reduction of edema caused by vasoconstriction,[268] and neovascularization in irradiated tissue.[228] Animal studies have confirmed that it should be given early,[261] and one study suggested often.[290] Hyperbaric oxygen may increase the length of island flaps with vascular insufficiency.[129] The benefit on pedicled island flaps may be most profound in those flaps with arterial insufficiency in particular.[368] There is little benefit from hyperbaric oxygen if the treatment is delayed by 24 hours or more after flap elevation.[169]

In a retrospective study of 65 patients with pedicled flaps that were determined by the surgeon to be in a high-risk group, hyperbaric oxygen was beneficial.[33] Although there is evidence that hyperbaric oxygen is effective for impaired flaps, it is not cost effective to treat every flap. Determining which flaps need treatment and which flaps will benefit is key. French investigators found that a hyperbaric oxygen challenge test (test dive) was predictive of successful outcome if the transcutaneous oxygen measurement rose 50 mm Hg or more. Still, the authors noted the need for further studies to determine indications for hyperbaric oxygen.[230]

Metabolic Manipulation

Additional strategies for increasing flap survival include decreasing the metabolic requirements or increasing the metabolic reserves of skin. These approaches are based on the idea that flap necrosis occurs when tissue metabolic demand is greater than what the blood supply can deliver. Decreasing temperature is an effective way to reduce metabolic activity and delay necrotic changes, but improvement in flap survival is not seen.[117,186]

Administration of adenosine triphosphate-magnesium chloride complex increased survival in the rat abdominal flap.[397] The metabolic support provided by this compound was believed to delay the onset of irreversible cell damage. Difluoromethylornithine (DFMO) was found to increase survival of abdominal flaps in rats.[292] DFMO appears to decrease metabolic demand by inhibiting the synthesis of polyamines, which are required for protein synthesis and cellular proliferation.

Increasing the individual cell's tolerance to ischemia also can be accomplished through stress conditioning. The production of heat-shock proteins can protect cells from a subsequent stress as long as an adequate recovery period (6–8 hours) from the initial stress occurs.[291] In an initial study, induction of heat-shock proteins resulted in improved flap survival.[196]

IMPAIRED FLAPS

In the majority of flaps, carefully designed and accomplished in healthy patients, flap survival is the rule, and methods improving survival or extensive monitoring or treatment of the flap are not warranted. The exceptions to the rule should be identified so extra efforts to ensure survival are reasonable and cost effective. Several factors place the patient in a higher risk category.

Smoking tobacco is associated with an increased chance of flap necrosis in facelift operations.[304] Exposure to tobacco smoke resulted in increased flap necrosis of dorsal flaps in rats[267] and hamsters.[57] The deleterious effects of nicotine appear to increase with prolonged exposure. The mechanism of tobacco or nicotine producing decreased flap survival is unknown but may involve direct endothelial damage, vasoconstriction caused by catecholamine release, or local concentrations of prostaglandins.[99] Long-term, low-dose nicotine (comparable with human smoking exposure) was used in a rat model[101] to document decreased capillary blood flow and survival; these effects could be avoided if the nicotine was withdrawn 2 weeks before raising the flap.

Radiation has been shown to be deleterious to flap survival in some studies[286,395] but not in others.[192,261,379] The reason for this discrepancy is probably because of differences in the radiation regimen administered (i.e., radiation dosage, fractionation, and surgical timing in respect to the radiation). Radiation treatment results in endarteritis obliterans and altered wound healing. Despite previous radiation, the delay phenomenon continues to improve flap survival.[94] Flap neovascularization is delayed but not eliminated after radiation. The use of angiogenic growth factors has the potential to increase the viability of irradiated skin flaps by means of accelerating revascularization.

The ischemia time occurring during the transfer of free flaps (called primary ischemia) appears to hinder the flap's ability to tolerate a second ischemic insult. The longer the period of perfusion after the microvascular anastomosis (called reperfusion period), the better a flap will tolerate secondary ischemia.[17] Porcine ventral arterial island flaps initially exposed to 2 hours of ischemia followed by 12 hours of blood flow had a 50% survival rate after a subsequent 7.2 hours of "secondary ischemia."[182] This is compared with 13 hours for the initial ischemic event needed to produce a 50% survival rate.[77]

Vascularity of the recipient bed is an important factor in free flaps. Experimentally, a pedicle can be divided at 6 days out[51] Typically in clinical situations, the pedicle is no longer monitored after 1 week, although there are cases of late flap failure.[377] If the flap is placed into a bed with poor vascularity, dependence on the pedicle may be prolonged. If there is late pedicle failure combined with a poor vascular bed in which neovascularization has not occurred, there could be an increased incidence of late complications.

Diabetes may be considered a risk factor because of the small vessel disease, although investigators did not find decreased flap survival in streptozotocin-induced diabetic rats. They did find slower endothelial growth at the anastomosis, but concluded diabetes is not a contraindication to the use of a free flap.[53] Ketamine and pentobarbital were found to decrease blood flow in the distal flap.[365] In a study on rats, older rats were found to have decreased tolerance to muscle ischemia than young rats, and this was assumed to be related to decreased mitochondrial function.[218] Fluid management also can have an impact on flap survival. Fluid overload will increase flap edema, and at the other extreme, intraoperative systemic hypotension has been shown to be detrimental.[336]

Central venous pressure monitoring was not found to be helpful.[164] Other miscellaneous injuries documented in an isolated, perfused porcine flap include phototoxicity[245] and exposure to organic solvents.[188]

FLAP SALVAGE

Once a flap is identified as being at risk for necrosis, action can be taken to improve survival. Zone I manipulations are the most effective. In pedicled flaps, efforts to enhance zone I perfusion are limited to preoperative planning, flap execution and design, and surgical delay. If effectively executed, pedicled flap loss is a result of failure of zone II and III, which will develop slowly and involve the distal or random portion of the flap. Clinical efforts to improve zone II or III failure are limited to methods such as hyperbaric oxygen or leeching. Of the hundreds of pharmacologic agents that have been tested, none have gained widespread clinical use.

In contrast, the global ischemia of free flap failure often relates to a zone I failure—thrombosis or compression of the pedicle. This failure often is acute and relatively easy to detect and repair. If the zone I failure is not quickly resolved, the injury will progress to zones II and III.

Free flaps need intensive postoperative monitoring. There are several different methods of monitoring free flaps, but none are foolproof, and frequent observation by experienced personnel is still the gold standard. Pedicle failure can be determined early, and the flap can be salvaged by exploring the anastomosis and clearing the thrombus in many cases.

Because of the accessibility of the vessels and a short period of nonperfusion (primary ischemia), the question was raised whether washing out flap vessels could potentially improve survival in the event of secondary ischemia,[313] analogous to organ transplantation. University of Wisconsin solution has been used to effectively decrease perivascular swelling in the microvasculature of organ systems.[256] The solution has been used as a washout solution to improve survival in free flaps by Babajanian and others.[16,17]

An intriguing application of perfusion washout technology is extracorporeal circulation,[224] which investigators theorize could be used if there were no suitable donor site vessels. Extracorporeal circulation was studied in a flow-through venous free flap. Only a plasma solution was able to maintain viability over 3 days of extracorporeal infusion, although 3 other test perfusates caused massive edema and total obstruction to perfusion.

Perfusion washout also has been studied for its ability to improve survival after the thrombosis is cleared from the anastomotic site. University of Wisconsin solution caused greater improvement when used during secondary ischemia than during primary ischemia, indicating that it may be better for flap salvage than prophylaxis.[15] Urokinase has been used for the antithrombotic effects at the anastomosis and, because of microemboli, at the capillaries (zone II).[147] Intravascular heparin was not useful after thrombus formation.[215] Medicinal leeches have been used clinically.[142] The leeches are thought to relieve microcirculatory congestion during active feeding and for several hours afterwards because of the antithrombotic effect of the leeches' salivary fluid. There is a risk of aeromonas infection. The "chemical leech"[377] and mechanical leeches have been described.[343] Relief of vascular congestion and edema also may be possible with microdialysis techniques, which have been used to reduce skin flap edema in a rat model.[271]

Hyperbaric oxygen has been used for free flap salvage. In a study of a rat epigastric free flap after 8 hours of global ischemia, hyperbaric oxygen increased survival and increased distal blood flow by laser Doppler.[396] In a similar model, hyperbaric oxygen inhibited the xanthine oxidase system and improved free flap survival after 18 hours of nonperfused storage.[353] Hyperbaric oxygen therapy will not be effective treatment unless the thrombosis has been cleared, but it may prolong viability and increase neovascularization.

SUMMARY

The blood flow required for nutritional support of the skin is dramatically less than what is available to carry out its thermoregulatory function, which allows skin to survive a compromise of its blood supply during creation of local flaps. The surviving length of a particular flap depends on the relationship between the proximal perfusion pressure (zone I) and the critical closing pressure of the arterioles, capillaries, and venules in the subdermal and subpapillary plexi (zone II). The interstitial space (zone III) is a critical link in this process. Cell viability (zone IV) is the ultimate determinate of flap survival. Appropriate flap design is the most critical factor in maintaining an adequate relationship between the zones of the circulatory system and avoiding tissue necrosis.

During the first 48 hours after raising a flap, the transferred tissue must survive a number of hazards. After the initial ischemia that all flaps undergo, reperfusion injury occurs by the formation of free radicals and other factors that can further damage tissue. An inflammatory response begins the process of wound healing, but also may impair perfusion in zones II and III. Beyond the first few days, neovascularization and wound healing lessen the surviving flap's dependence on the pedicle.

The several types of skin flaps may be classified on the basis of their blood supply. These include random flaps, arterial cutaneous flaps (i.e., axial flaps), fasciocutaneous flaps, and musculocutaneous flaps. In addition, one may classify them on the basis of the origin of the soft tissue relative to the defect. Thus there are local, regional, and distant flaps. Distant flaps may be pedicled or transferred via microvascular free tissue transfer. Regardless of the type of flap or site of origin, each flap involving skin is governed by certain biomechanical properties. Stress and strain are controlled by the collagen and elastin components of the skin. These biomechanical properties change with time, both with the aging process and over the shorter term. Creep and stress relaxation influence wound healing and are particularly important in tissue expansion. Attempts to improve flap survival have involved improving flap design, altering the early physiologic impairment of blood flow, and increasing tissue resistance to ischemia. The most effective efforts to improve survival have been focused on zone I—surgical delay to decrease distal ischemia in pedicled flaps and revision of a microvascular anastomosis to avoid global ischemia in free flaps. Treatment of zones II to IV includes pharmacologic manipulations designed to improve blood flow or increase tissue tolerance of ischemia. These treatments have not achieved sufficient and reproducible results required for incorporation into common clinical usage.

WOUND HEALING

The creation of a surgical flap results in a cutaneous wound that requires repair. A series of overlapping and closely coordinated events is initiated with disruption of the skin surface. The events associated with wound repair are relatively consistent regardless of the causative agent. Multiple cell types participate in wound repair (Table 5-2).

Disruption of the protective layer of skin results in exposure of the subepithelial layers and vascular endothelium along with extravasation of blood products. A blood clot is formed that provides a wound matrix for cell migration, as well as initiates the inflammatory response. This is the beginning of tissue repair. After establishment of an inflammatory phase, a phase of tissue proliferation occurs that includes the formation of granulation tissue, reepithelialization, and wound contraction. Finally, a prolonged phase of tissue remodeling completes the healing process. All three phases of wound healing overlap in time and appear to be tightly coordinated. Much of the recent work in wound repair has involved the regulation and communication between the involved cell types that result in a well-healed wound.

TABLE 5-2

CELL TYPES SHOWN TO BE INVOLVED WITH
WOUND REPAIR

Tissue	Cell Types
Vascular	Platelets, macrophages, neutrophils, endothelial cells, smooth muscle
Epidermis	Keratinocytes, malanocytes, Langerhans cells
Adnexal structures	Outer root sheah cells, hair dermal papilla cells
Dermis	Fibroblasts, myofibroblasts
Nervous system	Neurons
Subcutaneous fatty layer	Adipocytes

INFLAMMATORY PHASE

The initial injury to the skin results in disruption of blood vessels and extravasation of blood constituents. The vascular response to injury begins with a brief period of vasoconstriction that aids in hemostasis.[345] Platelets respond by aggregating at the injury site; they along with fibrinogen, fibrin, and fibronectin, form a blood clot that reestablishes hemostasis. The clot covers the wound and provides an initial matrix for cell attachment and migration.[46,78] The clot contains a variety of cytokines and growth factors. Platelets release platelet-derived growth factor (PDGF), transforming growth factor–β (TGF-β) and epidermal growth factor (EGF).[227] PDGF plays roles in chemotaxis for macrophages and fibroblasts, macrophage activation, fibroblast proliferation, matrix production, and angiogenesis.[145,314] TGF-β is involved in keratinocyte migration, chemotaxis for macrophages and fibroblasts, and fibroblast matrix synthesis and remodeling.[32,269] EGF plays a role in keratinocyte migration and replication.[114,372]

Tissue injury is associated with the onset of acute inflammation and the arrival of polymorphonuclear granulocytes (neutrophils). One day after tissue injury, neutrophils constitute nearly 50% of all cells at the wound site.[88] Neutrophils help to remove foreign material and bacteria from the wound. They are subsequently extruded with the eschar or cleared by macrophages.[338] Neutrophils[189] also release interleukin (IL)–1α and IL-1β and tissue necrosis factor-α (TNF-α). Both are early activators of growth factor expression in macrophages, keratinocytes, and fibroblasts.[156]

Neutrophils are highly abundant in the circulation, and quite a number are collected passively along with platelets at the wound site in the blood clot. Neutrophils also appear to be specifically attracted by a subset of cytokines referred to as chemokines. Along with growth factors, platelets release the chemokine-connective tissue-activating peptide-III (CTAP-III), which is converted into neutrophil-activating peptide-2 (NAP-2) by proteases released from neutrophils already attached to the thrombus.[35] NAP-2 stimulates migration and extravasation of neutrophils via the chemokine receptor 2 (CXCR2). In addition, vascular endothelial cells and pericytes secrete growth-related oncogene-α (GRO-α),[119] which supports movement of neutrophils to the wound. An additional method of attracting neutrophils involves the strong and selective expression of IL-8 under the wound surface that stimulates the CXCR2 and CXCR1 (not targeted by GRO-α) receptors. IL-8 is expressed by neutrophils and macrophages immediately below the denuded wound surface. The expression of IL-8 is induced by pro-inflammatory cytokines such as IL-1, TNF-α (expressed initially by neutrophils and later by macrophages), bacterial products (lipopolysaccharides), and hypoxia.[156]

Monocytes infiltrate the wound early after injury and become activated macrophages. On the third day following an injury, with wound closure and the decline of neutrophils, monocytes represent the most frequent blood-cell population.[88] Monocytes/macrophages are attracted to the wound by the chemokine monocyte chemoattractant protein-1 (MCP-1). MCP-1 is produced by resident and infiltrating mononuclear cells, keratinocytes at the wound edge, and endothelial cells. Macrophages[189] play a central role in the inflammatory phase of wound healing. In addition to their immunological functions as antigen-presenting cells and phagocytes, macrophages are an important source of growth factors. Macrophages release TGF-α. TGF-β, insulin-like growth factor I (IGF-I), heparin-binding epidermal growth factor (HB-EGF), fibroblast growth factor (FGF), PDGF, and vascular endothelial growth factor (VEGF).[392] TGF-α, like EGF, has a stimulatory effect on keratinocyte migration and replication.[303] IGF-I—also produced by keratinocytes, fibroblasts, and platelets—promotes reepithelialization and granulation tissue formation.[31] HB-EGF, basic FGF (bFGF), PDGF, and VEGF promote angiogenesis.[392] As its name implies, FGF also enhances fibroblast growth.

Lymphocytes are attracted to the wound site and after 14 days are the dominating leukocyte subset. Lymphocytes interact with Langerhans cells in the epidermis and nerve endings in the dermis to play an antimicrobial role. Leukocytes also produce growth factors (e.g., HB-EGF and bFGF).[116] Lymphocytes are attracted to wound sites initially by MCP-1. After day 4, lymphocytes are attracted to wound sites by interferon-γ-inducible protein-10 (IP-10) and monokine induced by interferon-γ (Mig). The presence of IP-10 and Mig after day 4 reflects a shift in the cytokine profile form TNF-α/IL-1 to interferon–γ.[116]

Nitric oxide (NO) is a short-lived free radical that exerts its effects at many levels. Nitric oxide synthase (NOS) is frequently produced in response to acute inflammatory stimuli such as wounding. NO may have a capacity for selective regulation of gene expression.[85] This would be important during the inflammatory phase of wound healing, when NO production is greatest. Production of NO is catalyzed by nitric oxide synthases (NOSs), a group of three isoenzymes: neuronal (nNOS), endothelial (eNOS), and inducible (iNOS).[3,243] NOS catalyses the oxidation of the amino acid L-arginine to release citrulline and NO.[24] NO appears to participate in the regulation of skin homeostatic functions such as circulation, UVB-mediated melanogenesis, sunburn erythema, and the mainte-nance of the protective barrier against microorganisms.[37] During the inflammatory phase, iNOS is elevated, with infiltrating macrophages being a major source of iNOS expression.[104,305]

PROLIFERATION PHASE

The successful development of an inflammatory phase results in the recruitment of keratinocytes, fibroblasts, and endothelial cells. The arrival of these cells marks the transition from a process of clearing and stabilizing the wound to one of proliferation and repair. The proliferation phase consists of re-epithelialization, formation of granulation tissue, and wound contraction. Similar to the three major phases of wound healing, these three aspects of the proliferation phase overlap in time and are closely interrelated.

Re-epithelialization

Re-epithelialization attempts to restore the protective barrier of the skin; it begins within hours of injury. It is the result of keratinocyte migration and proliferation.

Keratinocyte Migration

Changes leading to keratinocyte migration begin early after wounding. Growth factors that enhance keratinocyte migration are EGF, TGF-α, FGF7 (keratinocyte growth factor), TGF-β1, HGF, IGF-I, and insulin.[392] IL-8 is also capable of stimulating keratinocyte migration and proliferation.[134] IL-8 is highly expressed along the denuded wound surface. Keratinocytes express the receptor for IL8 and GRO-α. These findings suggest that the interaction of the keratinocyte with its ligand plays a role in re-epithelialization.

Under the influence of these growth factors and cytokines, epithelial cells at the wound margin undergo changes that set the stage for cell movement. These changes include filament reorganization, reduction of the number of intercellular attachments, and the expression of members of the integrin superfamily of cell surface receptors.[120]

Integrin receptors are transmembrane, heterodimeric glycoproteins consisting of one α chain and one β chain. Keratinocytes, at the leading edge of the wound, express integrins that allow them to interact with fibronectin ($\alpha v\beta6$, $\alpha5\beta1$), vitronectin ($\alpha v\beta5$), and collagen ($\alpha2\beta1$)[398] present at the wound margin and interwoven with the fibrin clot.[47] The keratinocytes are guided into the wound migrating between the fibrin clot and the collagenous dermis by the interaction of the integrin receptors and the extracellular matrix proteins. Keratinocytes produce plasminogen activators,[38] which activate plasmin and collagenase-1 (matrix metalloproteinase-1; MMP-1).[297] Plasmin and MMP-1 are necessary to dissolve fibrin and collagen type I, respectively, for migration to occur. In partial thickness wounds, keratinocyte migration also occurs from skin appendages, including the hair follicle.[392]

The relationship between the enzyme production of matrix metalloproteinases (MMPs), extracellular matrix proteins, integrins, and keratinocyte migration was recently summarized by Parks.[284] Plasmin and collagenase-1 break down matrix barriers that impede cell migration. Keratinocytes migrate along a path of least resistance driven and oriented by collagenase-1.[297] Collagenase-1, acting on its principal substrate in the dermis (i.e., type I collagen), provides migrating keratinocytes with a mechanism to maintain their course and directionality in the wound environment during re-epithelialization. In wounds, basal keratinocytes dislodge from the basement membrane and contact dermal collagen type I. The integrin $\alpha2\beta1$ becomes concentrated at the forward-basal tip of the migrating keratinocyte. $\alpha2\beta1$ binds dermal collagen with high affinity and this interaction induces collagenase-1 expression. Collagenase-1 cleaves type I collagen and converts it to a gelatin, allowing the cell to migrate. The high affinity of $\alpha2\beta1$ with dermal collagen, but not with gelatin, favors establishment of attachment to native, uncleaved, and exposed dermal collagen in the open wound surface. When continually repeated, this process provides the migrating cells with a mechanism to control their direction and to remain superficial to the dermis but deep to the fibrin clot during re-epithelialization.

Keratinocyte Proliferation

Migrating keratinocytes are found on the advancing epithelial margin. Proliferating keratinocytes are found within the epithelial margin and the nearby hypertrophic epithelium behind the actively migrating cells.[398] Keratinocyte proliferation begins 1 to 2 days after injury. The growth factors known to enhance keratinocyte replication are EGF, TGF-α, FGF7, IGF-I, IL-1, IL-6, HGF, nerve growth factor,[392] and IL-8.[134] Neuropeptides are also thought to have growth stimulatory effects on keratinocytes through the activation of cyclic adenosine-5-monophosphate. Examples include calcitonin gene-related peptide, vasoactive intestinal polypeptide, peptide histidine-methionine, and growth hormone releasing factor.[354] Leptin, produced in the subcutaneous layer, is reported to have growth stimulatory effects on keratinocytes as well.[105]

Keratinocytes can express all three forms of NOS.[103] NO serves as a mediator that regulates gene expression and proliferation in keratinocytes. Proliferating keratinocytes at the wound margin and, to a lesser extent, fibroblasts express iNOS.[104] Wound closure in iNOS-deficient mice[393] and inhibition of iNOS in normal mice[346] is delayed. These findings suggest an important role for iNOS in the regulation of epithelial movements and the re-epithelialization process.

With the re-establishment of an epithelial layer, basement membrane proteins re-emerge, progressing inward from the wound margin.[48] Keratinocyte behavior returns to normal with adhesion of basal keratinocytes to the basal lamina and restoration of intercellular attachments.[338]

Formation of Granulation Tissue

At approximately 3 to 4 days following injury, a new stromal framework, known as granulation tissue, begins to enter the wound and replace the fibrin clot. Granulation tissue consists of a dermal matrix that provides a framework for cell migration that is enhanced by new vessels that migrate into the wound (i.e., angiogenesis).

Dermal Matrix

The cell that is most important in the production of the dermal matrix is the fibroblast.[392] Fibroblasts enter the wound by 2 to 3 days, and within the first week become the dominant cell population in the wound. As fibroblasts invade, the fibrin clot is lysed and fibronectin and hyaluronic acid are deposited, forming early granulation tissue. These molecules serve as scaffolding on which the fibroblasts can migrate and adhere.

To facilitate migration into a wound filled with cross-linked fibrin or later with a tightly woven extracellular matrix (ECM), migratory fibroblasts secrete a range of proteolytic enzymes[338] (i.e., collagenase-1, gelatinase-A, and stromelysin-1 or MMP-1, -2, and -3, respectively). This process initially occurs in the periphery of the clot and later more centrally as the granulation tissue grows into the wound space. At any given time, the ECM of the wound margin differs from the ECM located centrally.

The fibroblast is critical in the production of the dermal matrix producing type I and III collagens, fibronectin, elastin, and proteoglycans. Fibroblasts also contribute to growth factor production, providing connective tissue growth factor (CTGF). CTGF stimulates migration and proliferation of fibroblasts. Keratinocyte growth factor stimulates epidermal cell motility and proliferation. VEGF stimulate angiogenesis.[162] MCP-1, involved in neutrophil recruitment early in the inflammatory process, also attracts mast cells. The mast cells produce high levels of IL-4, which in turn stimulates proliferation of fibroblasts[362] and decreases the expression of MCP-1 and IL-8.[42] This limits the inflammatory reaction.

NO in granulomas seems to exert an organizing influence, allowing the host to assemble macrophages, directing vascular ingrowth, and compartmentalizing the inflammatory nidus.[199,335] Peak NOS activity is noted 24 hours after wounding declines but remains subsequently elevated for at least 14 days.[213] The macrophage is the primary cell type implicated in inducible NOS activity and NO production during inflammation. Fibroblasts may also participate during the time coincidental with active collagen synthesis.[327,388] Fibroblasts are able to produce NO linked either to eNOS or, after stimulation with interferon-gamma or bacterial lipopolysaccharide (LPS), to iNOS.[103]

When NO is inhibited experimentally, granulomas tend to become larger and have a higher bacterial load.[199] NO deficient states (diabetes and protein-calorie malnutrition) are associated with decreased wound extracellular matrix deposition and impaired wound healing.[329,330] Excessive delivery of NO can also inhibit wound healing.[25] NO also affects wound collagen accumulation and the acquisition of wound mechanical strength. Inhibition of wound NO synthesis is accompanied by a lowered wound breaking strength and decreased collagen deposition.[326,327,328] NO likely mediates an antiproliferative effect on skin fibroblasts in addition to its effects on collagen synthesis.[389]

Angiogenesis

The process of angiogenesis is closely related to the formation of granulation tissue. The newly formed granulation tissue requires a vascular supply to provide for its metabolic needs. The process of angiogenesis begins at the time of injury. Cell disruption and hypoxia, hallmarks of tissue injury, are strong inducers of angiogenesis factors. Acidic fibroblast growth factor (aFGF or FGF-1) and basic fibroblast growth factor (bFGF or FGF-2) are released from disrupted cells and have potent angiogenic activity.[360] Hypoxia stimulates macrophages and keratinocytes to produce the angiogenic growth factor VEGF.[83] bFGF may set the stage for angiogenesis during the first 3 days of wound repair, while VEGF may be critical for angiogenesis during granulation tissue formation from day 4 through 7.[265] eNOS appears to contribute to granulation tissue formation by triggering endothelial migration, proliferation, and differentiation, thus participating in capillary ingrowth into the wound site during repair.[212] NO stimulates VEGF production and vascular endothelial growth factor-mediated endothelial cell migration and helps to redistribute microvascular blood flow.[266,400] This encourages vasodilation and angiogenesis. Other growth factors known to enhance angiogenesis include PDGF, HB-EGF, IGF-I, and hepatocyte growth factor (HGF).[392]

Mast cells are frequently found near capillary sprouting sites, suggesting an association between mast cells and angiogenesis. Mast cells may act at sites of new vessel formation by secreting tryptase, which also functions as an angiogenesis factor.[30] Heparin, leptin, and fibronectin also enhance angiogenesis.[392]

The process of angiogenesis was recently reviewed by Tonnesen and others.[360] Following stimulation by growth factors and other angiogenic agents, vessels adjacent to the wound transiently (3–5 days after injury) deposit fibronectin within their vascular walls. Endothelial cells release plasminogen activator and procollagenase, resulting in the digestion of the basement membrane by plasmin and collagenase. On the fourth day after injury, with disruption of the confining basement membrane, the endothelial cells are able to enter the ECM as capillary sprouts.[233] The fibrin and fibronectin surrounding the tips of capillary sprouts are released from the plasma rather than being derived from wound fibroblasts.

The fibrin- and fibronectin-rich provisional ECM induces capillary sprouts to express $\alpha v \beta 3$ integrin with the most pronounced expression at the capillary tips. Appearing to have a functional role in wound angiogenesis,[50] $\alpha v \beta 3$ allows the capillary sprouts to migrate through the basement membrane (infiltrated with fibronectin) and into the fibrin- and fibronectin-rich wound clot.

The endothelial sprouts extend, branch, and create networks, pushed by cell proliferation (stimulated by FGF and VEGF) from the rear and pulled by chemotaxis from the front. These events require an interaction between endothelial cells, angiogenesis factors, and surrounding ECM proteins. At first, the developing blood vessels are surrounded by a provisional matrix containing fibronectin and proteoglycans, but eventually a mature basement membrane is formed. Blood flow begins with the formation of capillary arcades. VEGF, FGF, and mast cell tryptase induce new sprouts to extend from these loops, further extending into the dermal matrix.[360] With maturation of wound granulation tissue and accumulation of collagen, most of the new vessels degenerate and the density of blood vessels declines.[360] The coverage of endothelial cells by periendothelial cells (smooth muscle cells) is necessary for vascular maturation.[42] This appears to be regulated by PDGF and VEGF.[27] The mature vessels no longer express $\alpha v \beta 3$.[360]

Wound Contraction

During the second week of healing, fibroblasts acquire smooth muscle cell features by presenting cytoplasmic microfilament bundles.[108] These fibroblasts are called myofibroblasts. Myofibroblasts contain α-smooth muscle (αSM) actin and provide the contractile forces produced in wound granulation tissue.[109,333] During wound healing, αSM actin is transiently expressed by fibroblasts (myofibroblasts). The staining intensity of αSM actin increases from the 6th to the 15th day of injury. It decreases thereafter and disappears at the 30th day in a mouse model.[69] TGF-β1 is thought to induce αSM actin expression in fibroblasts.[74]

Fibronectin plays a role in wound contraction by binding to fibrin in the provisional and forming a scaffold for fibroblast and keratinocyte migration and tissue support.[332] Fibronectin binds to cell surface integrin receptors to form fibrils allowing interaction between the cell and ECM. The fibroblasts, having already migrated into the wound, begin to interact with each other and the matrix, resulting in wound contraction.

REMODELING PHASE

By the third week after an uncomplicated injury, wound closure has been completed and local infections overcome. Collagen synthesis and degradation is in balance and the remodeling phase begins. Myofibroblasts and vascular cells undergo apoptosis (programmed cell death) and are removed.[75] Granulation tissue is transformed into a scar. Lymphocytes constitute the most frequent leukocyte subset in human skin wounds during this phase,[88] but it is unknown whether lymphocytes are associated intimately with tissue remodeling. Tissue collagenases (MMPs) degrade and digest the excess collagen fibers. Other enzymes (hyaluronidase, bacterial collagenase, and lysosomal proteases) also function to remodel granulation tissue. A more ordered pattern of collagen arrangement is achieved under the influence of local mechanical forces.

The wound gradually increases in strength, ultimately attaining 80% of the tensile strength of normal skin.[223] Type III collagen, synthesized early in the repair process, is replaced by type I collagen until the normal skin ratio of 4:1 (type I to III collagen) is realized.[345]

REFERENCES

1. Aarts HF: Regional intravascular sympathetic blockade for better results in flap surgery: an experimental study of free flaps, island flaps and pedicle flaps in the rabbit ear, *Plast Reconstr Surg* 66:690, 1980.
2. Acar C and others: Studies of controlled reperfusion after ischemia XIX: reperfusate composition: benefits of blood cardioplegia over Fluosol DA cardioplegia during regional reperfusion—importance of including blood components in the initial reperfusate, *J Thorac Surg* 101:248, 1991.
3. Alderton WK, Cooper CE, Knowles RG: Nitric oxide synthases: structure, function and inhibition, *Biochem J* 357: 593-615, 2001.
4. Ames A and others: Cerebral ischemia. II: the no-reflow phenomenon, *Am J Pathol* 52:437, 1968.
5. Angel M and others: Augmentation of skin flap survival with allopurinol, *Ann Plast Surg* 18:494, 1987.
6. Angel MF and others: The critical relationship between free radicals and degrees of ischemia: evidence for tissue intolerance of marginal perfusion, *Plast Reconstr Surg* 81:233, 1988.
7. Angel MF and others: The etiologic role of free radicals in hematoma-induced flap necrosis, *Plast Reconstr Surg* 77:795, 1986.
8. Angel MF and others: A biochemical study of acute ischemia in rodent skin free flaps with and without prior elevation, *Ann Plast Surg* 26:419, 1991.
9. Angel MF and others: The beneficial effect of chlorpromazine on dorsal skin flap survival, *Ann Plast Surg* 23:492, 1989.
10. Ariyan S: The pectoralis major myocutaneous flap. A versatile flap for reconstruction in the head and neck area, *Plast Reconstr Surg* 63:73, 1979.
11. Austad E and others: Histomorphic evaluation of guinea pig skin and soft tissue after controlled tissue expansion, *Plast Reconstr Surg* 70:704, 1982.
12. Babajanian M and others: Prolongation of secondary critical ischemia time of experimental skin flaps using UW solution as a normothermic perfusate, *Otolaryngol Head Neck Surg* 108:149, 1993.
13. Babajanian M and others: Temporal factors affecting the secondary critical ischemia of normothermic experimental skin flaps, *Arch Otolaryngol Head Neck Surg* 117:1360, 1991.
14. Babior B, Kipnes R, Curnutte J: Biological defense mechanisms: the production by leukocytes of superoxide, a potential bactericidal agent, *J Clin Invest* 52:741, 1973.
15. Barker JH and others: Direct monitoring of capillary perfusion following normovolemic hemodilution in an experimental skin-flap model, *Plast Reconstr Surg* 86:946, 1990.
16. Barker JH and others: Microcirculatory disturbances following the passage of emboli in an experimental free-flap model, *Plast Reconstr Surg* 90:95, 1992.
17. Bassingthwaighte JB: Discussion of Hjortdal VE, Hansen ES and others: The microcirculation of myocutaneous island flaps in pigs studied with radioactive blood volume tracers and microspheres of different sizes, *Plast Reconstr Surg* 89:116, 1992.
18. Bauer JA, Rao W, Smith DJ: Evaluation of linear polyethylenimine/nitric oxide adduct on wound repair: therapy versus toxicity, *Wound Rep Reg* 6: 569, 1998.
19. Benjamin LE, Hemo I, Keshet E: A plasticity window for blood vessel remodeling is defined by pericyte coverage of the preformed endothelial network and is regulated by PDGF-B and VEGF, *Development* 125:1591, 1998.
20. Bert JL, Pearce RH: *The interstitium and microvascular exchange.* In *Handbook of physiology,* ed. 4, Bethesda, MD, American Physiologic Society, 1984.
21. Bibi R, Ferder M, Strauch B: Prevention of flap necrosis by chlorpromazine, *Plast Reconstr Surg* 77:954, 1986.
22. Blair RJ and others: Human mast cells stimulate vascular tube formation. Tryptase is a novel, potent angiogenic factor, *J Clin Invest* 99: 2691, 1997.
23. Blakytny R and others: Lack of insulin-like growth factor 1 (IGF1) in the basal keratinocytes layer of diabetic skin and diabetic foot ulcers, *J Pathol* 190:589, 2000.
24. Border WA, Noble NA: Transforming growth factor-β in tissue fibrosis, *N Engl J Med* 331:1286, 1994
25. Bowersox J, Strauss MB, Hart GB: Clinical experience with hyperbaric oxygen therapy in the salvage of ischemic flaps and grafts, *J Hyperbar Med* 1:141, 1986.

26. Brace RA: Progress toward resolving the controversy of positive vs. negative interstitial fluid pressure, *Circ Res* 49:281, 1981.

27. Brandt E and others: The beta-thromboglobulins and platelet-derived CXC chemokines with divergent roles in early neutrophil regulation, *J Leukoc Biol*, 67:471, 2000.

28. Brown DM and others: Platelet-derived growth factor BB induces functional vascular anastomoses in vivo, *Proc Natl Acad Sci USA* 92:5920, 1995.

29. Burch-Gerharz D, Ruzicka T, Kolb-Bachofen V: Nitric oxide and its implications in skin homeostasis and disease – a review, *Arch Dermatol Res* 290:643, 1998.

30. Burge TH and others: Loss of fibrinogen rescues mice from the pleiotropic effects of plasminogen deficiency, *Cell*, 87:709, 1996.

31. Caffe H, Gallagher T: Experiments on the effects of hyperbaric oxygen on flap survival in the pig, *Plast Reconstr Surg* 81:954, 1988.

32. Callegari PR and others: An anatomic review of the delay phenomenon: I. experimental studies, *Plast Reconstr Surg* 89:397, 1992.

33. Campbell WB: *Lipid-derived autacoids: eicosanoids and platelet-activating factor*. In Gilman AG and others, editors: *Goodman and Gilman's the pharmacologic basis of therapeutics*, New York, Pergamon Press, 1990.

34. Carmeliet P: Mechanisms of angiogenesis and arteriogenesis, *Nat Med* 6:389, 2000.

35. Chu B, Deshmukh N: The lack of effect of pentoxifylline on random skin flap survival, *Plast Reconstr Surg* 83:315, 1989.

36. Clark RA and others: Fibronectin and fibrin provide a provisional matrix for epidermal cell migration during wound reepithelialization, *J Invest Dermatol* 79:64, 1982.

37. Clark RA and others: Reepithelialization of normal human excisional wounds is associated with a switch from $\alpha v \beta 5$ to $\alpha v \beta 6$ integrins, *Br J Dermatol* 135:46, 1996.

38. Clark RA and others: Fibronectin and fibrin provide a provisional matrix for epidermal cell migration during wound reepithelialization *J Invest Dermatol* 79: 264, 1982.

39. Clark RA and others: Collagen matrices attenuate the collagen synthetic response of cultured fibroblasts to TGF-β, *J Cell Sci* 108:1251, 1995.

40. Clark RA and others: Transient functional expression of $\alpha v \beta 3$ on vascular cells during wound repair, *AM J Path* 148:1407, 1996.

41. Clarke H, Chen G: Peripheral neovascularization of muscle and musculocutaneous flaps in the pig, *Plast Reconstr Surg* 89:109, 1992.

42. Cooley BC and others: The influence of diabetes on free flap transfer: I. flap survival and microvascular healing, *Ann Plast Surg* 29:58, 1992.

43. Cox K, Larrabee W: A study of skin flap advancement as a function of undermining, *Arch Otolaryngol* 108, 1982.

44. Craig S, Rees T: The effects of smoking on experimental skin flaps in hamsters, *Plast Reconstr Surg* 75:842, 1985.

45. Cummings C, Trachy R: Measurement of alternative blood flow in the porcine panniculus carnosus myocutaneous flap, *Arch Otolaryngol* 111:598, 1985.

46. Cutting C and others: Changes in quantitative norepinephrine levels in delayed pig flank flaps, *Plast Reconstr Surg* 69:652, 1982.

47. Cutting C, Robson M, Koss N: Denervation supersensitivity and the delay phenomenon, *Plast Reconstr Surg* 61:881, 1978.

48. Cutting C: *Skin flap physiology*. In Cummings CW, editor: *Otolaryngology—head and neck surgery*, St. Louis, Mosby, 1986.

49. Cutting C: Critical closing and perfusion pressures in flap survival, *Ann Plast Surg* 9:524, 1982.

50. Daley CH, Odland G. Age-related changes in the mechanical properties of the skin, *J Invest Dermatol* 73:84–87, 1979.

51. D'Amore PA: *The role of growth factors and cell-cell communication in the control of angiogenesis*. In Cederholm-Williams SA, Ryan TJ, Lydon MJ, editors: *Fibrinolysis and angiogenesis in wound healing*, Princeton, NJ, Excerpta Medica, 1987.

52. Daniel RK, Kerrigan CL: *Principles and physiology of skin flap surgery*. In McCarthy JG, editor: *Plastic surgery*, vol. 1, Philadelphia, WB Saunders, 1990.

53. Daniel RK: *The anatomy and hemodynamics of the cutaneous circulation and their influence on skin flap design*. In Grabb WC, Myers MB, editors: *Skin flaps*, Boston, Little, Brown, 1975.

54. Darby I, Skalli O, Gabbiani G: α-smooth muscle actin is transiently expressed by myofibroblasts during experimental wound healing, *Lab Invest* 63:21, 1990.

55. Davies BW and others: The impact of vasodilators on random pattern skin flap survival in the rat following mainstream smoke exposure, *Ann Plast Surg* 40(6)630–636, 1998.

56. Davis RE and others: Comparison of topical anti-ischemic agents in the salvage of failing random-pattern skin flaps in rats, *Arch Facial Plas Surg* 1(1):27, 1999.

57. Desmouliere A and others: Transforming growth factor-β1 induces α-smooth muscle actin expression in granulation tissue myofibroblasts and in quiescent and growing cultured fibroblasts, *J Cell Biol* 122:103, 1993.

58. Desmouliere A and others: Apoptosis mediates the decrease in cellularity during the transition between granulation tissue and scar, *Am J Pathol* 146:56, 1995.

59. Dohar J, Goding G, Azarshin K: The effects of inhalation anesthetic agents on survival in a pig random skin flap model, *Arch Otolaryngol* 118:37, 1992.

60. Donaldson DJ, Mahan JT: Keratinocyte migration and the extracellular matrix, *J Invest Dermatol*, 90:623, 1988.

61. Dorion D, Boyd J: Augmentation of transmidline skin perfusion and viability in transverse rectus abdominis myocutaneous (TRAM) flaps in the pig, *Plast Reconstr Surg* 88:642, 1991.

62. Douglas B and others: Beneficial effects of ibuprofen on experimental microvascular free flaps: pharmacologic alteration of the no-reflow phenomenon, *Plast Reconstr Surg* 79:366, 1987.

63. Dunn CL and others: A single postoperative application of nitroglycerin ointment does not increase survival of cutaneous flaps and grafts, *Dermatol Surg* 26(5):425, 2000.

64. Dvorak HF and others: Vascular permeability factor/vascular endothelial growth factor, microvascular hyperpermeability, and angiogenesis, *AM J Pathol* 146:1029, 1995.

65. Earle A, Fratianne R, Nunez F: The relationship of hematocrit levels to skin flap survival in the dog, *Plast Reconstr Surg* 54:341, 1974.

66. Efron DT, Most D, Barbul A: Role of nitric oxide in wound healing, *Curr Opin Clin Nutr Metab Care* 3:197, 2000.

67. Emerson D, Sykes P: The effect of prostacyclin on the experimental random skin flap in the rat, *Br J Plast Surg* 34:264, 1981.

68. Engelhardt E and others: Chemokines IL-8, Groα, MCP-1, IP-10, and Mig are sequentially and differentially expressed during phase-specific infiltration of leukocyte subsets in human wound healing, *Am J Pathol* 153:1849, 1998.

69. Eshima I, Mathes SJ, Paty P: Comparison of the intracellular bacterial killing activity of leukocytes in musculocutaneous and random-pattern flaps, *Plast Reconstr Surg* 86:541, 1990.

70. Federman JL and others: Experimental ocular angiogenesis, *Am J Ophthalmol* 89:231, 1980.

71. Finseth F, Adelberg MG: Prevention of skin flap necrosis by a course of treatment with vasodilator drugs, *Plast Reconstr Surg* 61:738, 1978.

72. Finseth F, Zimmerman J: Prevention of necrosis in island myocutaneous flaps in the pig by treatment with isoxsuprine, *Plast Reconstr Surg* 64:536, 1979.

73. Fishman RA: Brain edema, *N Engl J Med* 292:706, 1975.

74. Flores J and others: The role of cell swelling in ischemic renal damage and the protective effect of hypertonic solute, *J Clin Invest* 51:118, 1972.

75. Folkman J: How is blood vessel growth regulated in normal and neoplastic tissue? *Cancer Res* 46:467, 1986.

76. Folkow B: Role of the nervous system in the control of vascular tone, *Circulation* 21:760, 1960.

77. Forrest C, Pang C, Lindsay W: Dose and time effects of nicotine treatment on the capillary blood flow and viability of random pattern skin flaps in the rat, *Br J Plast Surg* 40:295, 1987.

78. Forrest C and others: Pathogenesis of ischemic necrosis in random-pattern skin flaps induced by long-term nicotine treatment in the rat, *Plast Reconstr Surg* 87:518, 1991.

79. Francis A, Marks R: Skin stretching and epidermopoiesis, *Br J Exp Pathol* 58:35, 1977.

80. Frank S and others: Nitric oxide drives skin repair: novel functions of an established mediator, *Kidney International* 61:882, 2002.

81. Frank S and others: Induction in inducible nitric oxide synthase and its corresponding tetrahydrobiopterin-cofactor-synthesizing enzyme GTP-cyclohydrolase I during cutaneous wound repair, *J Invest Dermatol*, 111:1058, 1998.

82. Frank S and others: Leptin enhances wound re-epithelialization and constitutes a direct function of leptin in skin repair, *J Clin Invest* 106:501, 2000.

83. Freeman TJ and others: Inhibition of endogenous superoxide dismutase with diethyldithiocarbamate in acute island skin flaps, *Otolaryngol Head Neck Surg* 103:938, 1990.

84. Furcht LT: Critical factors controlling angiogenesis: cell products, cell matrix, and growth factors, *Lab Invest* 55:505, 1986.

85. Gabbiani G and others: Granulation tissue as a contractile organ, *J Exp Med* 135:719, 1972.

86. Gabbiani G: Evolution and clinical implications of the myofibroblast concept *Cardiovasc Res* 38:545, 1998.

87. Gaboriau H, Murakami C: Skin Anatomy and flap physiology, *Otol Clin North Am* 34(3), 2001.

88. Gaskell P, Krisman AM: Critical closing pressure of vessels supplying the capillary loops of the nail fold, *Circ Res* 7:461, 1958.

89. Gatti J and others: Assessment of neovascularization and timing of flap division, *Plast Reconstr Surg* 73:396, 1984.

90. Gibbs S and others: Epidermal growth factor and keratinocyte growth factor differentially regulate epidermal migration, growth, and differentiation, *Wound Repair Regen*, 8:192, 2000.

91. Gillitzer R, Goebeler M: Chemokines in cutaneous wound healing, *J Leukoc Biol* 69:513, 2001.

92. Goding G, Cummings C, Bright D: Effects of local hypothermia on the porcine myocutaneous flap. In Stucker FJ, editor: Plastic and reconstructive surgery of the head and neck, proceedings of the fifth international symposium, Philadelphia, BC Decker, 521, 1991.

93. Goding G, Cummings C, Trachy R: Tissue expansion and cutaneous blood flow, *Laryngoscope* 98:1, 1988.

94. Goebeler M and others: The chemokine repertoire of human dermal microvascular endothelial cells and its regulation by inflammatory cytokines, *J Investig Dermatol*, 108:445, 1997.

95. Goliger JA, Paul DL: Wounding alters epidermal connexin expression and gap junction mediated intercellular communication, *Mol Biol Cell* 6:381, 1996.

96. Goshen J, Wexler M, Peled I: The use of two alpha blocking agents, phenoxybenzamine and phentolamine, in ointment and injection form to improve skin flap survival in rats, *Ann Plast Surg* 15:431, 1985.

97. Gospodarowicz D, Thakoral KK: Production of a corpus luteum angiogenic factor responsible for the proliferation of capillaries and revascularization of the corpus luteum, *Proc Natl Acad Sci U S A* 75:874, 1978.

98. Gottrup F and others: A comparative study of skin blood flow in musculocutaneous and random-pattern flaps, *J Surg Res* 37:443, 1984.

99. Gottrup F and others: The dynamic properties of tissue oxygen tension in healing flaps, *Surgery* 95:527, 1983.

100. Grange H, Goodman A, Grange N: Role of resistance and exchange vessels in local microvascular control of skeletal muscle oxygenation in the dog, *Circ Res* 38:379, 1976.

101. Guba A: Study of the delay phenomenon in axial pattern flaps in pigs, *Plast Reconstr Surg* 63:550, 1979.

102. Gurunluoglu R and others: Effect of transfection time on the survival of epigastric skin flaps pretreated with adenovirus encoding the VEGF gene, *Ann Plast Surg* 49(2):161, 2002.

103. Guyton A, Hall J: *Local control of blood flow by the tissues, and humoral regulation.* In *Human physiology and mechanisms of disease,* ed 9, Philadelphia, WB Saunders, 142, 1997.

104. Guyton A, Hall J: *Overview of the circulation: medical physics of pressure, flow, and resistance.* In *Textbook of medical physiology,* ed 9, Philadelphia, WB Saunders, 1996.

105. Guyton A, Hall J: *The body fluid compartments: extracellular and intracellular fluids: interstitial fluid and edema.* In *Textbook of medical physiology,* ed 9, Philadelphia, WB Saunders, 1996.

106. Guyton A, Schell K, Murphres D: Interstitial fluid pressure: III. its effect on resistance to tissue fluid mobility, *Circ Res* 19:412, 1966.

107. Gyulai R and others: Chemotaxis of freshly separated and cultured human keratinocytes, *Clin Exp Dermatol*, 19:309, 1994.

108. Hannington-Kiff J: Intravenous regional sympathetic block with guanethidine, *Lancet* 1(7865):1019–1020 1974.

109. Hargens AR: *Introduction and historical perspectives.* In Hargens AR, editor: *Tissue fluid pressure and composition,* Baltimore, Williams & Wilkins, 1, 1971.

110. Hauben D, Aijlstra F: Prostacyclin formation in delayed pig flank flaps, *Ann Plast Surg* 13:304, 1984.

111. Hayden R and others: The effect of glutathione and vitamins A, C, and E on acute skin flap survival, *Laryngoscope* 97:1176, 1987.

112. Hayden R and others: The effect of hydroxyl radical scavenging on acute axial-random skin flap survival, *Laryngoscope* 98:106, 1988.

113. Hayden RE, Pillips JG, McLear PW: Leeches. Objective monitoring of altered perfusion in congested flaps, *Arch Otolarynol Head Neck Surg* 114:1395, 1988.

114. Hayward PG and others: Local infiltration of an angiogenic growth factor does not stimulate the delay phenomenon, *Br J Plast Surg* 44:526, 1991.

115. Heldin CH, Westemark B: Mechanism of action and in vitro role of platelet-derived growth factor, *Physiol Rev* 79:1283, 1999.

116. Henrich DE and others: The influence of arterial insufficiency and venous congestion on composite graft survival, *Laryngoscope* 105:565, 1995.

117. Hirigoyen MB and others: Improved efficacy of urokinase further prolongs ischemic skin-flap survival, *J Reconstr Microsurg* 11:151, 1995.

118. Hjortdal VE and others: Differential release of endothelin in myocutaneous island flaps in response to gradually insetting venous stasis or arterial ischemia, *Metabolism* 43:1201, 1994.

119. Hochberg J and others: Development and evaluation of an in vivo mouse model for studying myocutaneous flap microcirculation and viability before and after suturing or stapling, *Int J Microcirc* 14:67, 1994.

120. Hodgson R, Brummett R, Cook T: Effects of pentoxifylline on experimental skin flap survival, *Arch Otolaryngol Head Neck Surg* 113:950, 1987.

121. Hoft HD and others: Can chlorpromazine prevent flap necrosis? *Br J Plast Surg* 43:587, 1990.

122. Hom D and others: Utilizing angiogenic agents to expedite the neovascularization process in skin flaps, *Laryngoscope* 98:521, 1988.

123. Hom D, Assefa G: Effects of endothelial cell growth factor on vascular compromised skin flaps, *Arch Otolaryngol Head Neck Surg* 118:624, 1992.

124. Hong JP and others: The effect of prostaglandin E1 versus ischemia-reperfusion injury of musculocutaneous flaps, *Ann Plast Surg* 47(3):316, 2001.

125. Hubner G and others: Differential regulation of pro-inflammatory cytokines during wound healing in normal and glucocorticoid-treated mice, *Cytokine* 8:548, 1996.

126. Huffman H and others: An endothelial growth stimulating factor from salivary glands, *Exp Cell Res* L02:269, 1976.

127. Iannotti Y, Crowell RM, Klato I: Brain tissue in focal cerebral ischemia, *J Neurosurg* 62:83, 1975.

128. Im MJ and others: Effect of allopurinol on the survival of hyperemic island skin flaps, *Plast Reconstr Surg* 73:276, 1984.

129. Im MJ and others: Effects of sympathetic denervation and oxygen free radicals on neovascularization in skin flaps, *Plast Reconstr Surg* 92:736, 1993.

130. Ishiguro N and others: Basic fibroblast growth factor has a beneficial effect on the viability of random skin flaps in rats, *Ann Plast Surg* 32:356, 1994.

131. Iyer VR and others: The transcriptional program in the response of human fibroblasts to serum, *Science* 283:83, 1999.

132. Jakubovic HR, Ackerman AB: *Structure and function of skin*. In Moschella SL, Hurley HJ, editors: *Dermatology*, Philadelphia, WB Saunders, 1992.

133. Jensen NF and others: The efficacy of routine central venous monitoring in major head and neck surgery: a retrospective review, *J Clin Anesth* 7:119, 1995.

134. Johnson P, Barker J: Thrombosis and antithrombotic therapy in microvascular surgery, *Clin Plast Surg* 19:799, 1992.

135. Jonsson K and others: Tissue oxygen measurements in delayed skin flaps: a reconsideration of the mechanisms of the delay phenomenon, *Plast Reconstr Surg* 82:328, 1988.

136. Junqueira LC, Carneiro J, Kelley RO: *Basic histology*, ed 8, Norwalk, CT, Appleton & Lange, 1995.

137. Jurell G, Jonsson CE: Increased survival of experimental skin flaps in rats following treatment with antiadrenergic drugs, *Scand J Plast Reconstr Surg* 10:169, 1976.

138. Jurell G, Kaijser L: The influence of varying pressure and duration of treatment with hyperbaric oxygen on the survival

139. of skin flaps: an experimental study, *Scand J Plast Reconstr Surg* 7:25, 1973.

139. Jurell G, Norberg K, Palmer B: Surgical denervation of the cutaneous blood vessels, *Acta Physiol Scand* 74:511, 1968.

140. Jurell G: Adrenergic nerves and the delay phenomenon, *Ann Plast Surg* 17:497, 1986.

141. Kaley G and others: *Role of prostaglandins in microcirculatory function.* In Neri GG and others, editors: *Advances in prostaglandin, thromboxane, and leukotriene research*, New York, Raven Press, 1985.

142. Kami T and others: Effects of low-power diode lasers on flap survival, *Ann Plast Surg* 14:278, 1985.

143. Kay S, Green C: The effect of a novel thromboxane synthetase inhibitor dazegrel (UK38485) on random pattern skin flaps in the rat, *Br J Plast Surg* 39:361, 1986.

144. Kennedy TJ, Pistone G, Miller SH: The effect of reserpine on microcirculatory flow in rat flaps, *Plast Reconstr Surg* 63:101, 1979.

145. Kernahan D, Zingg W, Kay C: The effects of hyperbaric oxygen on the survival of experimental skin flaps, *Plast Reconstr Surg* 36:19, 1965.

146. Kerrigan C and others: The pig as an experimental animal in plastic surgery research for the study of skin flaps, myocutaneous flaps and fasciocutaneous flaps, *Lab Animal Sci* 36:408, 1986.

147. Kerrigan C, Daniel R: Critical ischemia time and the failing skin flap, *Plast Reconstr Surg* 69:986, 1982.

148. Kerrigan C, Daniel R: Pharmacologic treatment of the failing skin flap, *Plast Reconstr Surg* 70:541, 1982.

149. Kerrigan C, Zelt R, Daniel R: Secondary critical ischemia time of experimental skin flaps, *Plast Reconstr Surg* 74:522, 1984.

150. Kerrigan C: Skin flap failure: pathophysiology, *Plast Reconstr Surg* 72:766, 1983.

151. Kiehn C, Desprez J: Effects of local hypothermia on pedicle flap tissue, *Plast Reconstr Surg* 25:349, 1960.

152. Kim YS, Im MJ, Hoopes JE: The effect of a free-radical scavenger, N-2-mercaptopropionylglycine, on the survival of skin flaps, *Ann Plast Surg* 25:18, 1990.

153. King JR, Monteiro-Riviere NA: Effects of organic solvent vehicles on the viability and morphology of isolated perfused porcine skin, *Toxicology* 69:11, 1994.

154. Kirsner RS, Eaglstein WH: The wound healing process, *Dermatol Clin* 11:629, 1993.

155. Kjartansson J, Dalsgaard C, Jonsson C: Decreased survival of experimental critical flaps in rats after sensory denervation with capsaicin, *Plast Reconstr Surg* 79:218, 1987.

156. Kleiman LA and others: The effects of carbocisplatin and radiation on skin flap survival, *Arch Otolaryngol Head Neck Surg* 118:68, 1992.

157. Klingenstrom P, Nylen B: Timing of transfer of tubed pedicles and cross flaps, *Plast Reconstr Surg* 37:1, 1966.

158. Knight K and others: Pharmacologic modification of blood flow in the rabbit microvasculature with prostacyclin and related drugs, *Plast Reconstr Surg* 75:692, 1985.

159. Knox LK and others: Nitric oxide synthase inhibitors improve skin flap survival in the rat, *Microsurgery* 15:708, 1994.

160. Koenig WJ and others: Improving acute skin-flap survival through stress conditioning using heat shock and recovery, *Plast Reconstr Surg* 90:659, 1992.

161. Komorowski-Timek E and others: Prolonged perivascular use of verapamil or lidocaine decreases skin flap necrosis, *Ann Plas Surgery* 43(3):50, 1999.

162. Kreidstein ML and others: Evidence of endothelium-dependent and endothelium-independent vasodilation in human skin flaps, *Can J Physiol Pharmacol* 70:1208, 1992.

163. Kreuger MR, Tanes DR, Mariano M: Expression of NO-synthase in cells of foreign-body and BCG-induced granulomata in mice: influence of L-NAME on the evolution of the lesion, *Immunology* 95:278, 1998.

164. Kristensen J, Wadskov S, Henriksen O: Dose-dependent effect of topical corticosteroids on blood flow in human cutaneous tissue, *Acta Derm Venereol* 58:145, 1978.

165. Kutchai HC: *Cellular membranes and transmembrane transport of solutes and water.* In Berne RM, Levy MN, editors: *Physiology,* St. Louis, Mosby, 5, 1988.

166. Landis E: Microinjection studies of capillary permeability, *Am J Physiol* 82:217, 1927.

167. Larrabee W and others: Wound tension and blood flow in skin flaps, *Ann Otol Rhinol Laryngol* 93:112–115, 1984.

168. Larrabee W: A finite element model of skin deformation, *Laryngoscope* 96(4):413–419, 1986.

169. Lasiter W, Gottschalk C: *Volume and composition of the body fluids.* In Mountcastle VB, editor: *Medical physiology,* St. Louis, CV Mosby, 1980.

170. Lawrence W and others: Prostanoid derivatives in experimental flap delay with formic acid, *Br J Plast Surg* 37:602, 1984.

171. Layton CT and others: Pharmacologic enhancement of random skin flap survival by prostaglandin E2, *Arch Otolaryngol Head Neck Surg* 120:56, 1994.

172. Leaf A: Cell swelling: a factor in ischemic tissue injury, *Circulation* 47:455, 1973.

173. Lee C, Kerrigan CL, Picard-Ami LA: Cyclophosphamide-induced neutropenia: effect on postischemic skin-flap survival, *Plast Reconstr Surg* 89:1092, 1992.

174. Lee PC and others: Impaired wound healing and angiogenesis in eNOS-deficient mice, *Am J Physiol* 277:H1600, 1999.

175. Lee RH and others: Nitric oxide expression in the healing wound: a time course study, *Surg Forum* 50:636, 1999.

176. Li X and others: Intravascular heparin protects muscle flaps from ischemia/reperfusion injury, *Microsurgery* 16:90, 1995.

177. Liston S: Nonbacterial inflammation as a means of enhancing skin flap survival, *Laryngoscope* 94:1075, 1984.

178. Lu X and others: Effect of age upon ischemia/reperfusion injury in rat muscle free flaps, *J Surg Res* 55:193, 1993.

179. Lubiatowski P and others: Enhancement of epigastric skin flap survival by adenovirus mediated VEGF gene therapy, *Ann Plast Surg* 109(6):1986–1993, 2002.

180. Macht S, Frazier W: The role of endogenous bacterial flora in skin flap survival, *Plast Reconstr Surg* 65:50, 1980.

181. Maciag T and others: An endothelial cell growth factor, *Proc Natl Acad Sci* 76:5674, 1979.

182. Macknight ADC: *Cellular response to injury.* In Staub NC, Taylor AE, editors: *Edema,* New York, Raven Press, 1984.

183. Madden JW, Peacock EE Jr: Studies on the biology of collagen in wound healing. I. rate of collagen synthesis ad deposition in cutaneous wounds of the rat, *Surgery* 64:288, 1968.

184. Maeda M and others: Extracorporeal circulation for tissue transplantation (in the case of venous flaps), *Plast Reconstr Surg* 91:113, 1993.

185. Marks M and others: Enhanced capillary blood flow in rapidly expanded random pattern flaps, *J Trauma* 26:913, 1986.

186. Martin P: Wound healing-aiming for perfect skin regeneration, *Science* 276:75, 1997.

187. Marx RE: A new concept in the treatment of osteoradionecrosis, *J Oral Maxillofac Surg* 41:351, 1983.

188. Marzella L and others: Functional and structural evaluation of the vasculature of skin flaps after ischemia and reperfusion, *Plast Reconstr Surg* 81:742, 1988.

189. Mathieu DR and others: Pedicle musculocutaneous flap transplantation: prediction of final outcome by transcutaneous oxygen measurements in hyperbaric oxygen, *Plast Reconstr Surg* 91:329, 1993.

190. May JW Jr, Chait LA, O'Brien BM: The no-reflow phenomenon in experimental free flaps, *Plast Reconstr Surg* 61:256, 1978.

191. McClain SA and others: Mesenchymal cell activation is the rate limiting step of granulation tissue induction, *Am J Path* 149:1257, 1996.

192. McCord J: Improved survival of island flaps after prolonged ischemia by perfusion with superoxide dismutase, discussion, *Plast Reconstr Surg* 77:643, 1986.

193. McCord J: Oxygen-derived free radicals in postischemic tissue injury, *N Engl J Med* 312:159, 1985.

194. McFarlane RM, DeYoung G, Henry RA: The design of a pedicle flap in the rat to study necrosis and its prevention, *Plast Reconstr Surg* 35:177, 1965.

195. Meldon JH, Garby L: The blood oxygen transport system, *Acta Med Can Suppl* 19:19, 1975.

196. Mellander S, Johansson B: Control of resistance, exchange, and capacitance functions in the peripheral circulation, *Pharmacol Rev* 20:117, 1968.

197. Mendelson B, Woods J: Effect of corticosteroids on the surviving length of skin flaps in pigs, *Br J Plast Surg* 31:293, 1978.

198. Mes L: Improving flap survival by sustained cell metabolism within ischemic cells: a study using rabbits, *Plast Reconstr Surg* 65:56, 1980.

199. Michel CC: *Fluid movements through capillary walls.* In *Handbook of physiology,* part 1 Bethesda, MD, American Physiologic Society, 4(1):375, 1984.

200. Milton S: Fallacy of the length-width ratio, *Br J Plast Surg* 57:502, 1971.

201. Moncada S, Palmer RM, Higgs EA: Nitric oxide: physiology, pathophysiology, and pharmacology, *Pharmacol Rev* 43:109, 1991.

202. Monteiro D, Santamore W, Nemir P: The influence of pentoxifylline on skin-flap survival, *Plast Reconstr Surg* 77:277, 1986.

203. Monteiro-Riviere NA and others: Development and characterization of a novel skin model for cutaneous phototoxicology, *Photodermal Photoimmunal Photomed* 10:235, 1994.

204. Moore G, Cummings C: The effect of ancrod on perfusion of myocutaneous flaps, *Arch Otolaryngol Head Neck Surg* 114:1175, 1988.

205. Moore GK, Trachy RE, Cummings C: The effect of alpha-adrenergic stimulation and blockade on perfusion of myocutaneous flaps, *Otolaryngol Head Neck Surg* 94:489, 1986.

206. Moore KL, Persaud TVN: *The developing human.* Philadelphia, WB Saunders, 1993.

207. Moran CG and others: Preservation of bone graft vascularity with the University of Wisconsin cold storage solution, *J Orthop Res* 11:840, 1993.

208. Morrison WA and others: Prefabrication of thin transferable axial-pattern skin flaps: an experimental study in rabbits, *Br J Plast Surg* 43:645, 1990.

210. Mulliken J, Im M: The etiologic role of free radicals in hematoma-induced flap necrosis—discussion, *Plast Reconstr Surg* 77:802, 1986.

211. Murphy R and others: Surgical delay and arachidonic acid metabolites: evidence for an inflammatory mechanism: an experimental study in rats, *Br J Plast Surg* 38:272, 1985.

212. Myers B: Understanding flap necrosis, *Plast Reconstr Surg* 78:813, 1986.

213. Myers MB, Cherry G: Enhancement of survival in devascularized pedicles by the use of phenoxybenzamine, *Plast Reconstr Surg* 41:254, 1968.

214. Naka Y and others: Canine heart-lung transplantation after twenty-four-hour hypothermic preservation with Belzer-UW solution, *J Heart Lung Transplant* 10:296, 1991.

215. Nakano J: *General pharmacology of prostaglandins.* In Cuthbert MF, editor: *The prostaglandins,* Philadelphia, JB Lippincott, 23, 1973.

216. Nakatsuka T and others: Effect of glucocorticoid treatment on skin capillary blood flow and viability in cutaneous and myocutaneous flaps in the pig, *Plast Reconstr Surg* 76:374, 1985.

217. Neilsen R, Parkin J: Skin flap survival: influence of infection, anemia and tubing, *Arch Otolaryngol* 102:727, 1976.

218. Neligan P and others: Pharmacologic action of isoxsuprine in cutaneous and myocutaneous flaps, *Plast Reconstr Surg* 75:363, 1985.

219. Nemiroff P and others: Effects of hyperbaric oxygen and irradiation on experimental skin flaps in rats, *Otolaryngol Head Neck Surg* 93:485, 1985.

220. Nemiroff P: Synergistic effects of Pentoxifylline and hyperbaric oxygen on skin flaps, *Arch Otolaryngol Head Neck Surg* 114:977, 1988.

221. Nissen NN and others: Vascular endothelial growth factor mediates angiogenic activity during the proliferative phase of wound healing, *Am J Pathol* 152:1445, 1998.

222. Noiri E and others: Podokinesis in endothelial cell migration: role of nitric oxide. *Am J Physiol* 247:C236, 1998.

223. Nolan J and others: The acute effects of cigarette smoke exposure on experimental skin flaps, *Plast Reconstr Surg* 75:544, 1985.

224. Nylander G and others: Reduction of postischemic edema with hyperbaric oxygen, *Plast Reconstr Surg* 76:596, 1985.

225. O'Kane S, Ferguson MW: Transforming growth factor βs and wound healing, *In J Biochem Cell Biol* 29:63, 1997.

226. Odland R and others: Reduction of tissue edema by microdialysis, *Arch Otolaryngol Head Neck Surg* 121:662, 1995.

227. Odland R and others: Use of the tunable dye laser to delay McFarlane skin flaps, *Arch Otolaryngol Head Neck Surg* 121:1158, 1995.

228. Odland R, Rice R: A comparison of tunable dye and KTP lasers in nonsurgical delay in cutaneous flaps, *Otolaryngol Head Neck Surg* 113:92, 1995.

229. Odland R, Cohen JI: Measurement of interstitial tissue compliance in skin flaps, *Arch Otolaryngol Head Neck Surg* 114:1276, 1988.

230. Ono I and others: A study on the effectiveness of a thromboxane synthetase inhibitor (OKY-046) in increasing survival length of skin flaps, *Plast Reconstr Surg* 86:1164, 1990.

231. Palmer B: Sympathetic denervation and reinnervation of cutaneous blood vessels following surgery, *Scand J Plast Reconstr Surg* 4:93, 1970.

232. Pang C and others: Assessment of the fluorescein dye test for prediction of skin flap viability in pigs, *J Surg Res* 41:173, 1986.

233. Pang C and others: Augmentation of blood flow in delayed random skin flaps in the pig: effect of length of delay period and angiogenesis, *Plast Reconstr Surg* 78:68, 1986.

234. Pang C and others: Pharmacologic manipulation of the microcirculation in cutaneous and myocutaneous flaps in pigs, *Clin Plast Surg* 12:173, 1985.

235. Pang C and others: Hemodynamics and vascular sensitivity to circulating norepinephrine in normal skin and delayed

and acute random skin flaps in the pig, *Plast Reconstr Surg* 78:75, 1986.

236. Pang C: Ischemia-induced reperfusion injury in muscle flaps: pathogenesis and major source of free radicals, *Reconstr Microsurg* 6:77, 1990.

237. Paniello R, Hayden R, Bello S: Improved survival of acute skin flaps with amino acids as free radical scavengers, *Arch Otolaryngol Head Neck Surg* 114:1400, 1988.

238. Parks, WC: Matrix metalloproteinases in repair, *Wound Rep Reg* 7:423, 1999.

239. Parsons RJ, McMaster PD: The effect of the pulse upon the formation and flow of lymph, *J Exp Med* 68:353, 1938.

240. Patterson T and others: *The effect of radiation in survival of experimental skin flaps.* In Grabb WC, Myers MB, editors: *Skin flaps,* Boston, Little, Brown, 39, 1975.

241. Pearl JM and others: Leukocyte-depleted reperfusion of transplanted human hearts prevents ultrastructural evidence of reperfusion injury, *J Surg Res* 52:298, 1992.

242. Pearl R: A unifying theory of the delay phenomenon—recovery from the hyperadrenergic state, *Ann Plast Surg* 7:102, 1981.

243. Pearl R: The delay phenomenon—why the fuss, *Ann Plast Surg* 13:307, 1984.

244. Pellitteri PK, Kennedy TL, Youn BA: The influence of intensive hyperbaric oxygen therapy on skin flap survival in a swine model, *Arch Otolaryngol Head Neck Surg* 118:1050, 1992.

245. Perdrizet GA and others: Stress conditioning, a novel approach to organ preservation, *Curr Surg* 46:23, 1989.

246. Perona BP and others: Acute difluoromethylornithine treatment increases skin flap survival in rats, *Ann Plast Surg* 25:26, 1990.

247. Perrins D: *The effect of hyperbaric oxygen on ischemic skin flaps.* In Grabb W, Myers MB, editors: *Skin flaps,* Boston, Little, Brown, 53, 1975.

248. Picard-Ami LA, Kerrigan CL: Pathophysiology of ischemic skin flaps: difference in xanthineoxidase levels between rat, pig and man, *Plast Reconstr Surg* 87:750, 1991.

249. Picard-Ami LA, MacKay A, Kerrigan CL: Effect of allopurinol on the survival of experimental pig flaps, *Plast Reconstr Surg* 89:1098, 1992.

250. Pilcher BK and others: The activity of collagenase-1 is required for keratinocyte migration on a type I collagen matrix, *J Cell Biol* 137:1445, 1997.

251. Pober JS, Cotran RS: The role of endothelial cells in inflammation, *Transplantation* 50:537, 1990.

252. Pokorny A, Bright D, Cummings C: The effects of allopurinol and superoxide dismutase in a rat model of skin flap necrosis, *Arch Otolaryngol Head Neck Surg* 115:207, 1989.

253. Price MA, Pearl RM: Multiagent pharmacotherapy to enhance skin flap survival: lack of additive effect of nitroglycerin and allopurinol, *Ann Plast Surg* 33:52, 1994.

254. Ramasastry S and others: Effect of fluosol-DA (20%) on skin flap survival in rats, *Ann Plast Surg* 15:436, 1985.

255. Rappolee DA and others: Wound macrophages express TGF-α and other growth factors in vivo: analysis by mRNA phenotyping, *Science* 241:708, 1988.

256. Rees T, Liverett D, Guy C: The effect of cigarette smoking on skin flap survival in the face lift patient, *Plast Reconstr Surg* 73:911, 1984.

257. Reichner JS and others: Molecular and metabolic evidence for the restricted expression of inducible nitric oxide synthase in healing wounds, *Am J Pathol* 154:1097, 1999.

258. Reinisch JF: The pathophysiology of skin flap circulation: the delay phenomenon, *Plast Reconstr Surg* 54:585, 1974.

259. Reneman RS and others: Muscle blood flow disturbances produced by simultaneously elevated venous pressure and total muscle pressure, *Microvasc Res* 20:307, 1980.

260. Renkin EM: *Control of microcirculation and blood-tissue exchange.* In *Handbook of physiology*, part 2, Bethesda, MD, American Physiologic Society, 4:627, 1984.

261. Reus W and others: Effect of intraarterial prostacyclin on survival of skin flaps in the pig: biphasic response, *Ann Plast Surg* 13:29, 1984.

262. Ricciardeli E and others: Acute blood flow changes in rapidly expanded and adjacent skin, *Arch Otolaryngol Head Neck Surg* 115:182, 1989.

263. Robson M, DelBeccaro E, Heggers J: The effects of prostaglandins on the dermal microcirculation after burning and the inhibition of the effect by specific pharmacological agents, *Plast Reconstr Surg* 63:781, 1979.

264. Rohrich R, Cherry G, Spira M: Enhancement of skin-flap survival using nitroglycerin ointment, *Plast Reconstr Surg* 73:943, 1984.

265. Rosen HM, Slivjak BS, McBrearty FX: Preischemic flap washout and its effect on the no-reflow phenomenon, *Plast Reconstr Surg* 76:737, 1985.

266. Ross: Platelet-derived growth factor, *Lancet* 1 (No. 8648):1179, 1989.

267. Roth A and others: Augmentation of skin flap survival by parenteral pentoxifylline, *Br J Plast Surg* 41:515, 1988.

268. Ruberg RL, Falcone RE: Effect of protein depletion the surviving length in experimental skin flaps, *Plast Reconstr Surg* 61:581, 1978.

269. Saetzler R and others: Visualization of nutritive perfusion following tourniquet ischemia in arterial pattern skin flaps: effect of vasoactive medication, *Plast Reconstr Surg* 94:652, 1994.

270. Sagi A and others: Improved survival of island flaps after prolonged ischemia by perfusion with superoxide dismutase, *Plast Reconstr Surg* 77:639, 1986.

271. Sasaki G, Pang C: Experimental evidence for involvement of prostaglandins in viability of acute skin flaps: effects on viability and mode of action, *Plast Reconstr Surg* 67:335, 1981.

272. Sasaki G, Pang C: Hemodynamics and viability of acute neurovascular island skin flaps in rats, *Plast Reconstr Surg* 65:152, 1980.

273. Sasaki G, Pang C: Pathophysiology of skin flaps raised on expanded pig skin, *Plast Reconstr Surg* 74:59, 1984.

274. Sawada Y and others: A study of topical and systemic prostaglandin E1 and survival of experimental skin flaps, *Br J Plast Surg* 46:670, 1993.

275. Sawada Y and others: The relationship between prostaglandin E1 applied area and flap survival rate, *Br J Plast Surg* 45:465, 1992.

276. Sawada Y, Hatayama I, Sone K: The effect of continuous topical application of heparin on flap survival, *Br J Plast Surg* 45:515, 1992.

277. Schaffer MR and others: Nitric oxide, an autocrine regulator of wound fibroblast synthetic function, *J Immunol* 158:2375, 1997.

278. Schaffer MR and others: Nitric oxide regulates wound healing, *J Surg Res* 63:237, 1996.

279. Schaffer MR and others: Inhibition of nitric oxide synthesis in wounds: pharmacology and effect on accumulation off collagen in wounds in mice, *Eur J Surg* 165:262, 1999.

280. Schaffer MR and others: Acute protein-calorie malnutrition impairs wound healing; a possible role of decreased nitric oxide synthesis, *J Am Col Surg* 184:37, 1997.

281. Schaffer MR and others: Diabetes-impared healing and reduced wound nitric oxide synthesis: a possible pathophysiologic correlation, *Surgery* 121:513, 1997.

282. Schmie-Schonbein GW: Capillary plugging by granulocytes and the no-reflow phenomenon in the microcirculation, *Fed Proc* 46:2397, 1987.

283. Schwarzbauer JE, Sehler JL: Fibronectin fibrilogenesis: a paradigm for extracellular matrix assembly, *Curr Opin Cell Biol* 11:622, 1999.

284. Serini G, Gabbiani G: Mechanisms of myofibroblast activity and phenotypic modulation, *Exp Cell Res* 250:273, 1999.

285. Sherman J: Normal arteriovenous anastomoses, *Medicine* 42:247, 1963.

286. Shimizu K and others: Inducible nitric oxide synthase is expressed in granuloma pyogenicum, *Br J Dermatol* 138:769, 1998.

287. Sigurdsson GH: Perioperative fluid management in microvascular surgery, *J Reconstr Microsurg* 11:57, 1995.

288. Singer AJ, and Clark RAF: Cutaneous wound Healing, *N Engl J Med*, 341:738, 1999.

289. Smith DK, Dolan RW: Effects of vasoactive topical agents on the survival of dorsal skin flaps in rats, *Otolaryngol Head Neck Surg* 121(3):220, 1999.

290. Smith RJ and others: The effect of low-energy laser on skin-flap survival in the rat and porcine animal models, *Plast Reconstr Surg* 89:306, 1992.

291. Smoot EC and others: Mechanical leech therapy to relieve venous congestion, *J Reconstr Microsurg* 11:51, 1995.

292. Southorn P, Powis D: Free radicals in medicine. I. Chemical nature and biologic reactions, *Mayo Clin Proc* 63:381, 1988.

293. Stadelmann WK, Digenis AG, Tobin GR: Physiology and healing dynamics of chronic cutaneous wounds, *Am J Surg Suppl 2A* 176:26S, 1998.

294. Stallmeyer B and others: The function of nnitric oxide in wound repair: inhibition of inducible nitric oxide-synthase severely impairs wound reepithelialization, *J Invest Dermatol* 113:1090, 1999.

295. Stepnick DW and others: Effects of tumor necrosis factor alpha and vascular permeability factor on neovascularization of the rabbit ear flap, *Arch Otolaryngol Head Neck Surg* 121:667, 1995.

296. Strock PE, Majno G: Microvascular changes in acutely ischemic rat muscle, *Surg Gynecol Obstet* 1213, 1969.

297. Su CT and others: Tissue glucose and lactate following vascular occlusion in island skin flaps, *Plast Reconstr Surg* 70:202, 1982.

298. Suzuki S and others: Effect of intravenous prostaglandin E1 on experimental flaps, *Ann Plast Surg* 19:49, 1987.

299. Suzuki S and others: Experimental study on "delay" phenomenon in relation to flap width and ischemia, *Br J Plast Surg* 41:389, 1988.

300. Tai YJ and others: The use of hyperbaric oxygen for preservation of free flaps, *Ann Plast Surg* 28:284, 1992.

301. Takahashi K, Nakanishi S, Imamura S: Direct effects of cutaneous neuropeptides on adenylyl cyclase activity and proliferation in a keratinocyte cell line: stimulation of cyclic AMP formation by CGP and VIP/PHM, and inhibition by NPY through G protein-coupled receptors, *J Invest Dermatol*, 101:646, 1993.

302. Tan C and others: Effect of hyperbaric oxygen and hyperbaric air on survival of island skin flaps, *Plast Reconstr Surg* 73:27, 1984.

303. Taylor GI and others: An anatomic review of the delay phenomenon: II. Clinical applications, *Plast Reconstr Surg* 89:408, 1992.

304. Taylor GI, Palmer JH: The vascular territories (angiosomes) of the body: Experimental study and clinical applications, *Br J Plast Surg* 40(2):113–141, 1987.

305. Thomson J, Kerrigan C: Dermofluorometry: thresholds for predicting flap survival, *Plast Reconstr Surg* 83:859, 1989.
306. Tonnesen MG, Feng X, Clark RAF: Angiogenesis in wound healing, *J Invest Dermatol Symp Proc* 5:40, 2000.
307. Toriumi D, Larrabee W: *Skin grafts and flaps.* In: Papel ID, editor: *Facial Plastic and Reconstructive Surgery* 31, 1991.
308. Trautmann A and others: Human mast cell augment fibroblast proliferation by heterotypic cell-cell contact and action of IL-4, *J Immunol* 160:5053, 1998.
309. Triana R and others: *Skin grafts and local flaps.* In Papel ID, editor: *Facial Plastic and Reconstructive Surgery* 38, 2002.
310. Tsur H, Daniller A, Strauch B: Neovascularization of skin flaps: route and timing, *Plast Reconstr Surg* 66:85, 1980.
311. Uhl E and others: Improvement of skin perfusion by subdermal injection of recombinant human basic fibroblast growth factor, *Ann Plastic Surg* 32:361, 1994.
312. Uhl E and others: Influence of ketamine and pentobarbital on microvascular perfusion in normal skin and skin flaps, *Int J Microcirc* 14:308, 1994.
313. Uhl E and others: Reduction of skin flap necrosis by transdermal application of buflomedil bound to liposomes, *Plast Reconstr Surg* 102(5):1598, 1998.
314. Ulkur E and others: Effect of hyperbaric oxygen on pedicle flaps with compromised circulation, *Microsurgery* 22:(1), 2002.
315. Um S and others: Involvement of nitric oxide in survival of random pattern skin flap, *Plast Reconstr Surg* 101:(3), 1998.
316. Waterfield MD: Epidermal growth factor and related molecules, *Lancet*, 1 (No. 8649):1243, 1989.
317. Waterhouse N and others: Observations on dermal blood flow as reflected by technetium-99m pertechnetate clearance, *Br J Plast Surg* 39:312, 1986.
318. Webster JP: Thoraco-epigastric tubed pedicles, *Surg Clin North Am* 17:145, 1937.
319. Weinberg H and others: Vascular island skin-flap tolerance to warm ischaemia: an analysis by perfusion fluorometry, *Plast Reconstr Surg* 73:949, 1984.
320. Weinberg H, Song Y, Douglas B: Enhancement of blood flow in experimental microvascular free flaps, *Microsurg* 6:121, 1985.
321. Weinberg H: Survival and blood flow evaluation of canine venous flaps—discussion, *Plast Reconstr Surg* 82:326, 1988.
322. Weinzweig N, Gonzalez M: Free tissue failure is not an all- or-none phenomenon, *Plast Reconstr Surg* 96:648, 1995.
323. Weis SJ: Tissue destruction by neutrophils, *N Engl J Med* 320:365, 1989.
324. Weisman R and others: Fluorometric assessment of skin flap viability in the rat: effect of radiation therapy, *Otolaryngol Head Neck Surg* 91:151, 1983.
325. Welch MP, Odland GF, Clark RAF: Temporal relationships of F-actin bundle formation, collagen and fibronectin matrix assembly, and fibronectin receptor expression to wound contraction, *J Cell Biol* 110:133, 1990.
326. Westin M, Heden P: Calcitonin gene-related peptide delays the no-reflow phenomenon in the rat island flap, *Ann Plast Surg* 21:329, 1988.
327. Wexler MR and others: The effect of phenoxybenzamine, phentolamine, and 6-hydroxydopamine on skin flap survival in rats, *J Surg Res* 19:83, 1975.
328. Wideman M, Tuma R, Mayorvitz H: Defining the precapillary sphincter, *Microvasc Res* 12:71, 1976.
329. Wilkins EG and others: Identification of xanthine oxidase activity following reperfusion in human tissue, *Ann Plast Surg* 31:60, 1993.
330. Witte MB, Schaffer MR, Barbul A: Phenotypic induction of nitric oxide is critical for synthetic function in wound fibroblasts, *Surg Forum* 47:703, 1996.
331. Witte MB and others: Enhancement of fibroblast collagen synthesis by nitric oxide, *Nitric Oxide* 4:572, 2000.
332. Wood MB: Discussion of Clarke H, Chen G: peripheral neovascularization of muscle and musculocutaneous flaps in the pig, *Plast Reconstr Surg* 89:109, 1992.
333. Wray R, Young V: Drug treatment and flap survival, *Plast Reconstr Surg* 73:939, 1984.
334. Yamaguchi Y, Kunihiko K: Cutaneous wound healing: an update, *J Dermatol* 28:521, 2001.
335. Yamasaki K and others: Reversal of impaired wound repair in iNOS-deficient mice by topical adenoviral-mediated iNOS gene transfer, *J Clin Invest* 101:967, 1998.
336. Young C, Hopewell W: The evaluation of an isotope clearance technique in the dermis of pig skin: a correlation of functional and morphological parameters, *Microvasc Res* 20:182, 1980.
337. Young CMA, Hopewell JW: The effects of preoperative x-irradiation on the survival and blood flow of pedicle skin flaps in the pig, *Int J Radiation Oncology Biol Phys* 9:865, 1983.
338. Zamboni WA and others: The effect of hyperbaric oxygen on reperfusion of ischemic axial skin flaps: a laser doppler analysis, *Ann Plast Surg* 23:339, 1992.
339. Zambruno G and others: Transforming growth factor-β1 modulates β1 and β5 integrin receptors and induces the de novo expression of the $\alpha v\beta$6 heterodimer in normal human keratinocytes: implications for wound healing, *J Cell Bio*, 129:853, 1995.
340. Zhang Z and others: Generation of nitric oxide by a nitrite reductase activity of xanthine oxidase: a potential pathway for nitric oxide formation in the absence of nitric oxide synthase activity, *Biochem Biophys Res Commun* 249:767, 1998.

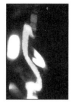

CHAPTER SIX

FREE TISSUE TRANSFER

Douglas A. Girod
Terance T. Tsue

INTRODUCTION

The expansion of knowledge, expertise, and training in the techniques of free tissue transfer since the early 1970s has redefined the standard of care in head and neck reconstructive surgery. The term *free tissue transfer* refers to the isolation of tissues (fascia, skin, fat, muscle, nerve, and bone—individually or in combination) on a supporting vascular supply with transfer to a new location in the body, using microvascular surgical techniques to revascularize the tissues in a permanent fashion. This auto-transplantation of tissues relies entirely on the anastomosis of the feeding artery and draining vein to blood vessels in the head and neck for tissue survival. Upon revascularization, the transferred tissues can then be utilized to reconstruct various complex defects of the head and neck from any etiology.

Since the first reports of free tissue transfer for reconstruction in the head and neck in early 1970s, the technique has gained widespread acceptance and growing availability. Advances in the understanding of surgical anatomy, operative microscopes, instrumentation, microsuture manufacture technology, formalized training opportunities, and unparalleled success rates have been largely responsible for this rapid growth. The additional required training (e.g., microvascular reconstructive surgery fellowships) and resources have resulted in the majority of these complex procedures being completed in larger, academic medical centers. A multidisciplinary team approach, especially for patients with neoplastic disease, is commonly employed to maximize both the oncological and reconstructive efforts. Post operative management is often labor intensive and requires additional team members to achieve maximal rehabilitative potential.

While significant additional training and resources are required to perform free tissue transfer for head and neck reconstruction, the diversity of available tis-

sues for harvest allows for the replacement of "like tissue with like tissue" in most instances with a focus on functional and cosmetic issues. Currently, more than 40 identified sites in the human body are candidates for the harvest of tissue for transfer, with new sites being added regularly.[172] It becomes the reconstructive surgeon's mandate to determine the optimal flap for free tissue transfer for each individual patient and his or her anticipated defect.

The advantages of free tissue transfer in the reconstruction of these complex defects include immediate reconstruction at the time of tumor resection (avoiding multiple, staged procedures); the transfer of well-vascularized tissue into a bed that often has salivary contamination and underlying tissue damage from earlier radiotherapy; significantly improved wound healing; immediate separation of critical compartments, including the aerodigestive tract and intracranial contents; improved ability to manage massive defects that might otherwise preclude surgical resection of tumors; and improved prospects for functional and cosmetic rehabilitation.

Specific circumstances exist in which reconstruction using free tissue transfer has become the standard of care in most communities. These include oromandibular composite defects (particularly defects involving the anterior mandibular arch)[57,199]; subtotal or total pharyngoesophageal defects;[8,52] and defects resulting from resection of recurrent carcinoma, failing organ preservation non-surgical therapy (combined chemotherapy and radiation therapy).[186] These situations have traditionally been the most challenging in head and neck reconstructive surgery and have been associated with high complication-failure rates. The introduction of free tissue transfer for reconstruction of these defects has dramatically improved the overall course for these difficult patients.

In this chapter we review the indications, patient selection, and preparation for free tissue transfer, as well as the dominant "free flaps" in use today for head and neck reconstruction. Perioperative issues, management of complications, and future directions are also discussed.

HISTORICAL PERSPECTIVES

The first clinical application of free tissue transfer was a case report by Seidenberg and others[155] as a transfer of a free jejunal segment for cervical esophageal reconstruction in 1959. This was followed by Hiebert and Cummings in 1961 who transferred and revascularized a portion of the gastric antrum for pharyngoesophageal reconstruction.[89] Other reports of the clinical application of free tissue transfer techniques began to appear in the literature in the early 1960s. The first reports of oral cavity reconstruction appearing in 1973 by Kaplan, Buncke, and Murray who utilized a free groin flap and Harii, Ohmori, and Ohmori who reported the microvascular distant transfer of a deltopectoral flap in 1974.[72,100] Panje, Bardach, and Krause at the University of Iowa are credited with being the first otolaryngologists to report the use of free tissue transfer for the reconstruction of the oral cavity in 1976.[135] Subsequent years saw rapid implementation of free tissue transfer in head and neck reconstruction by both plastic surgeons and otolaryngologists. Pioneers such as Panje, Urken, Hayden, and Sullivan worked to establish head and neck microvascular reconstructive surgery as an important part of Otolaryngology—Head and Neck Surgery as a specialty.

With the recognition of the endless possibilities afforded by free tissue transfer came the progressive study and identification of vascular supply patterns and territories that could be potential donor sites. Vascular injection studies identified axial vessels and the presence of perforating vessels passing through muscles to supply the overlying subcutaneous tissues and skin. Subsequent identification of axial vessels supplying fasciocutaneous tissues without muscular perforators followed.

Taylor, Miller, and Ham reported the first vascularized bone graft using a fibula for reconstruction of long bone injuries,[184] with Hidalgo adapting the osteocutaneous fibula flap for mandibular reconstruction in 1989.[86] Dye-injection studies proved a reliable vascular supply to the ilium from the deep circumflex iliac artery for vascularized bone transfer.[151,185] Cadaver dissections identified the vascular branch of the circumflex scapular artery to scapula allowing vascularized scapula transfer.[188] Throughout the 1980s there was a progressive development and refinement of these and other vascularized bone flaps for oromandibular reconstruction, which significantly expanded the availability of this technique.

INIDICATIONS FOR FREE TISSUE TRANSFER

Free tissue transfer is just one of many options available to the reconstructive surgeon. Well-established methods of primary closure, skin grafting, local flaps, and pedicled fasciocutaneous or musculocutaneous flaps all remain viable and necessary tools in the surgeon's armamentarium. Each patient must be evaluated individually and a multitude of factors considered when determining the ideal reconstructive method for a given situation. In the end, the advantages must outweigh the disadvantages with an emphasis on maximizing the functional and cosmetic outcome for the patient.

The indications for free tissue transfer continue to evolve with experience and as additional donor site options have emerged. The etiologies of defects that may require free tissue transfer are outlined in Table 6-1. The advantages (and disadvantages) of free tissue transfer over less sophisticated techniques have likewise become more apparent with increased experience and are outlined in Table 6-2. The tremendous versatility offered by multiple potential donor sites can test the surgeons' imagination for new reconstructive methods. The result has been a progressive evolution of new ways to tackle old problems. Certainly the driving force behind the expansion of free tissue transfer has been the potential for dramatically improved functional outcomes and a remarkable success rate in the head and neck of more than 90%.[20,77,204] In some circumstances such as the oral cavity, free tissue transfer offers a significant improvement from a functional and cosmetic standpoint compared with previously available techniques, particularly for composite defects. In other circumstances, free tissue transfer offers excellent reconstructive options where none was previously available, such as large skull base and scalp defects. Clinical situations commonly requiring free tissue transfer for reconstruction in the head and neck are outlined in Table 6-3.

As with any new surgical procedure or technique, a significant learning curve exists.[22] As a result, these procedures have been primarily available in major academic medical centers, and multiple fellowship training programs have been developed to safely convey the necessary knowledge and experience through

TABLE 6-1
ETIOLOGY OF HEAD AND NECK DEFECTS
Neoplasia
Trauma
Congenital defects
Infection-osteoradionecrosis
Secondary reconstructions

TABLE 6-2

FREE TISSUE TRANSFER IN HEAD AND NECK RECONSTRUCTION

Advantages
  Versatility in tissue (skin, muscle, bone, nerves)
  Versatility in orientation (no limitations on flap "reach" as with pedicled flaps)
  Restore shape, function, and sensation
  Single operation for complex reconstructions
  Multiple potential donor sites available
  Simultaneous resection and Flap harvest possible
  Donor sites out of field of prior treatment
  Extensive amounts of tissue available for large-massive defects
  Radiation tolerance postoperatively
  Independent blood supply for compromised tissue beds
  Improved function and cosmesis
  Dental rehabilitation possible
  High success rates (>90%) including for bony reconstruction
  Only available option for some patients
Disadvantages
  Increased technical difficulty (additional training required)
  Two operative teams (surgeons and nurses)
  Expensive instrumentation
  Longer operative times
  Post operative management more intensive
  Donor site morbidity

TABLE 6-3

DEFECTS-SITUATIONS COMMONLY REQUIRING FREE TISSUE TRANSFER

Composite defects of the oral cavity
Three-layer defects of the oral cavity (through and through)
Total or near total pharyngoesophageal defects
Extensive skull base defects
Extensive scalp defects
Massive defects not readily addressed with other techniques
Lack of other reconstructive options (failures or patient limitations)
Salvage surgery for chemoradiation failures

advanced training. From a medical center perspective, a high level of investment in personnel and equipment is necessary. Anesthesia support is critical and will be discussed later in this chapter. Additional training and experience for dedicated microsurgical operating

room nurses is advised as well. The postoperative management of patients undergoing free tissue transfer is certainly more complex and the demands on personnel are more intensive than on those who care for most head and neck surgical patients. These topics will also be discussed later. The overall cost of free tissue transfer as been examined and compared with more conventional (pedicled flap) techniques. The increased operative costs for free tissue transfer resulting from longer operating room times and instrumentation are offset by the significantly shorter lengths of hospitalization. The resulting overall cost for free tissue transfer is either comparable[196] or less[108] than the cost for pedicled flap reconstruction.

Contraindications certainly exist for free tissue transfer as well. The absolute contraindication is a patient's inability to tolerate a lengthy surgical procedure without a high risk of significant complication or death. Relative contraindications will be discussed later in this chapter when we discuss patient selection but these contraindications include patient comorbidities such as bleeding diathesis and hyper coagulopathy, metastatic carcinoma with limited patient survival potential, lack of adequate recipient vessels in the neck, and patient choice. Given the resources required for free tissue transfer, it has been suggested that this technique should be avoided in the patient who has a poor prognosis. However, studies have shown that patients in whom advanced reconstructions were avoided spend more time in the hospital during the year after surgery than those patients who underwent free tissue transfer.[22,196] Thus, from a quality of life perspective, free tissue transfer may offer more "quality time" compared with more conventional reconstructive techniques.

Donor Site Options

Although more than 40 described donor sites for free tissue transfer have been described,[172] only a handful have been found to be consistently useful in the routine reconstruction of head and neck defects. The dominant free tissue transfer flaps in use today are outlined in Table 6-4. In fact, the authors have found that the radial forearm fasciocutaneous, radial forearm osteocutaneous, and fibula osteocutaneous free flaps are utilized in more than 80% of cases of head and neck reconstruction. Disa and others have found the forearm, fibula, rectus, and jejunum flaps to account for 92% of their free flaps used for head and neck reconstruction.[53] This distribution will certainly vary based on the makeup of surgeons' practice and their preferences and experiences. Nonetheless, it is important for the reconstructive surgeon to be familiar with a full array of flaps to manage the more difficult or unusual situations.

TABLE 6-4

Free Tissue Transfer Flaps Commonly Used in Head and Neck Reconstruction

Fasciocutaneous flaps

Flap	Artery	Vein	Nerve	Reconstruction Uses
Radial forearm	Radial	Vena comitantes or cephalic	Medial and lateral antebrachial cutaneous	Oral cavity, tongue, palate, nose, face, scalp, lip, pharynx, larynx, pharyngoesophageal
Ulnar forearm	Ulnar	Vena comitantes or cephalic	Medial and lateral antebrachial cutaneous	Oral cavity, tongue, palate, nose, face, scalp, lip, pharynx, larynx, cervical esophagus
Lateral arm	Posterior radial collateral	Posterior radial collateral	Posterior cutaneous nerve of the forearm	Oral cavity, tongue, palate, pharynx
Lateral thigh	Deep femoral	Vena comitantes	Lateral femoral cutaneous nerve	Oral cavity, tongue, palate, pharynx
Scapular-parascapular	Subscapular	Subscapular	None	Oral cavity, tongue, palate, pharynx, face, lip

Muscle or myocutaneous flaps

Flap	Artery	Vein	Nerve	Reconstruction Uses
Rectus abdominus	Deep inferior epigastric	Deep inferior epigastric	Intercostals (mixed motor and sensory)	Skull base, total glossectomy
Latissimus	Subscapular	Subscapular	Thoracodorsal	Skull base, scalp

Osteocutaneous flaps

Flap	Artery	Vein	Nerve	Reconstruction Uses
Fibula	Peroneal	Peroneal	Lateral sural cutaneous	Mandible reconstruction
Radius	Radial	Vena comitantes or cephalic	Medial or lateral antebrachial cutaneous	Mandible and mid-face reconstruction
Scapula	Subscapular	Subscapular	None	Mandible and mid-face reconstruction
Iliac crest	Deep circumflex iliac	Deep circumflex iliac	None	Mandible and mid-face reconstruction

Other flaps

Flap	Artery	Vein	Nerve	Reconstruction Uses
Jejunum	Superior mesenteric branch	Superior mesenteric branch	None	Pharyngoesophageal reconstruction
Omentum	Gastroepiploic	Gastroepiploic	None	Scalp coverage
Temporal-parietal	Superficial temporal	Superficial temporal	None	Bone and cartilage coverage

While several flap options are available for most defects, the surgeon must chose one on the basis of critical characteristics such as those listed in Table 6-5. Additionally, a thorough donor site evaluation and assessment of long-term donor site morbidity must be considered. A complete discussion of each of these flaps is beyond the scope of this chapter; however, some general comments are warranted.

Soft Tissue Flaps

For many cutaneous, mucosal, and soft tissue defects in the head and neck the radial forearm fasciocutaneous free flap has proven the most versatile and reliable.* Forearm skin is available in large quantities, is

*References 39, 83, 128, 169, 170, 193, 194.

IMPORTANT CONSIDERATIONS INFLUENCING FLAP
SELECTION

Skin and soft tissue volume, bulk, and color
Pedicle length and vessel caliber
Innervation capacity (sensory-motor)
Bone quality and quantity availability
Donor site location to allow concurrent resection
    and harvest
Donor site morbidity (dysfunction, cosmetic
    deformity)

thin and pliable, and has excellent sensory capability
that is ideal for oral cavity reconstruction (Figure 6-1)
The vascular pedicle: (1) is long, (2) has a favorable
vessel caliber, (3) can easily be concurrently harvested, and (4) exhibits acceptable functional morbidity at the donor site. However, as many as 12% of
people have an incomplete superficial palmar arch
and poor communication between the deep and
superficial arches precluding the safe harvest of the
radial artery without causing hand ischemia.

The lateral arm flap is similarly thin and pliable
with sensory capability but is limited in skin quantity,
has a much shorter pedicle, and vessels of small caliber.* There is no risk of vascular compromise to the
hand, and the donor site can usually be closed primarily. The scapular and parascapular fasciocutaneous
flaps produce the largest volume of skin but are quite
bulky, have no sensory capability, and have intermediate pedicle length with large vessel caliber.[35,60,69,70,177] While the donor site may be closed
primarily, the donor site location (back) requires
patient repositioning intraoperatively, which precludes simultaneous resection and harvest.

---

*References 44, 82, 148, 179, 180, 215.

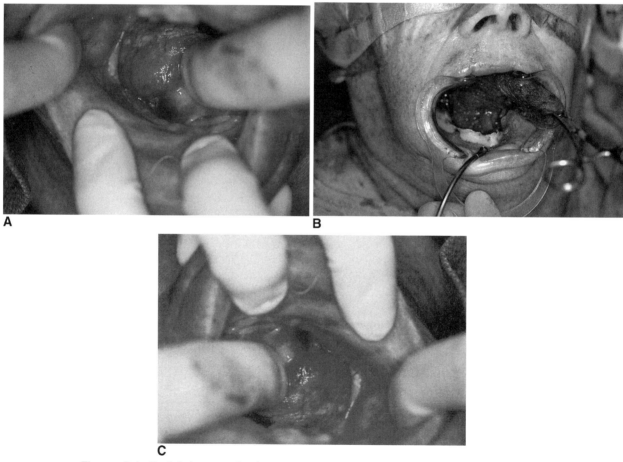

Figure 6-1. Radial forearm fasciocutaneous free flap for oral cavity reconstruction.
A, Carcinoma involving the anterior floor of the mouth and ventral oral tongue. **B,** Extensive
soft tissue defect after resection of the carcinoma. **C,** Reconstruction of the defect with a
sensate radial forearm free flap.

Muscle and Myocutaneous Flaps

Muscle and myocutaneous flaps have found a niche in the reconstruction of very large defects that require significant bulk. The most common of these defects are found at the skull base where large portions of the facial skeleton, paranasal sinuses, facial skin, and palate may be missing. The rectus abdominus flap may be harvested as a muscle or myocutaneous flap with the patient in a supine position with a long vascularized pedicle of large caliber vessels providing adequate reach to the defect site in most instances.[122,183,187,195,202] The skin of the rectus myocutaneous flap is useful for lining the nasal and oral cavities of the defect while the muscle provides the needed bulk to replace the missing facial skeleton. Donor site morbidity is minimal, although abdominal hernias may occur as a result of a weakening of the abdominal wall.

The latissimus flap may be harvested as a muscle or myocutaneous flap based off the subscapular vascular system.[32,43] Originally described as a pedicled flap, the latissimus flap has been found to be much more versatile as a single-stage, free-tissue transfer. The large amount of muscle available for harvest is very useful for very large soft tissue defects including the skull base and scalp. The subscapular system has additional versatility with the option for vascularized bone (scapula bone or rib). The vascular pedicle has large vessel caliber and a length of 6 to 10 cm, and the donor site is repaired primarily without the need for a skin graft. The major disadvantage of the latissimus flap is patient positioning for harvest. Like the scapula flaps, the patient must be placed in the lateral decubitus position, which makes simultaneous harvest with the head and neck procedure difficult or impossible. The donor site morbidity from the loss of latissimus function is well tolerated for most people. The latissimus flap has been most useful in skull base defects and larger scalp defects requiring cranial coverage (Figure 6-2).[98,195,221]

Vascularized Bone Flaps

One of the primary indications for free tissue transfer is for the reconstruction of oromandibular defects. In this setting, no other reconstructive option offers a single stage procedure with a greater than 90% success rate. Developments and refinements in microvascular reconstructive surgery are ongoing in this critical area. The choices for vascularized bone flaps also dictate the need for careful evaluation and selection. Most bone reconstructions also require some degree of soft tissue and or mucosal reconstruction.

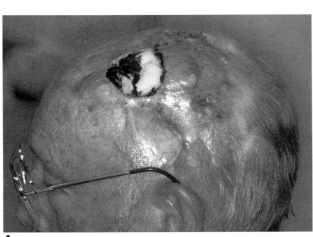

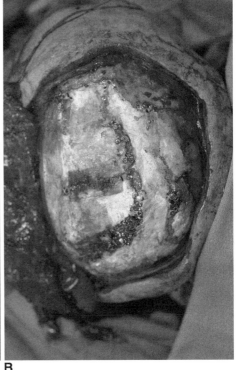

A   B

Figure 6-2. Latissimus dorsi muscle free flap to the scalp. **A,** Recurrent basal cell carcinoma after multiple surgeries and radiation therapy with involvement of underlying bone. **B,** Resection of the scalp, bone, and dura with cranioplasty using radiated rib grafts and bone cement.

Continued

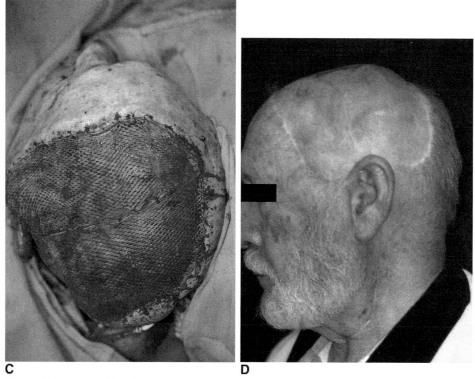

Figure 6-2, cont'd C, Latissimus dorsi muscle free flap with meshed split-thickness skin graft coverage. **D,** Long-term result of scalp reconstruction.

Therefore all aspects of the reconstruction must be evaluated and prioritized to guide flap selection. The anticipation of the length of bone required, plans for future dental implantation, soft tissue and innervation requirements, and donor site suitability and morbidity must all be considered.

Fibula Flap

The osteocutaneous fibula free flap has become the mainstay for mandibular reconstruction at most institutions (Figure 6-3).[58,78,162] The fibula is touted as the "the most donateable bone in the body" with up to 25 cm of bone available for harvest and usually has adequate

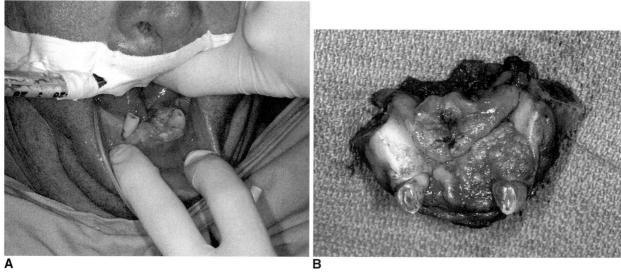

Figure 6-3. Fibula osteocutaneous free flap reconstruction of the anterior mandibular arch. **A,** Carcinoma of the anterior alveolar ridge. **B,** Resection of the anterior mandibular arch.

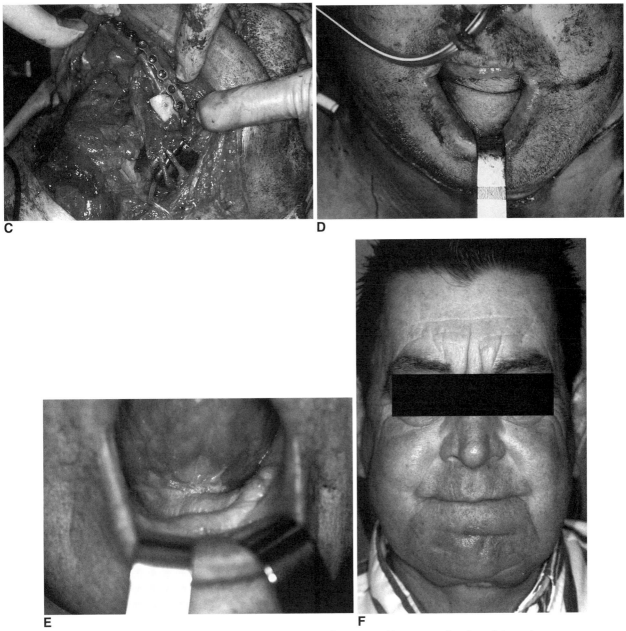

Figure 6-3, cont'd **C,** Fibula bone with osteotomies secured to a reconstruction plate replacing the missing mandible. **D,** Soft tissue repair of the oral cavity defect. **E,** One year post operative appearance of the anterior oral cavity. **F,** Frontal view one year later.

bone stock to support dental implantation.[59,126] With such lengths of bone available, the entire mandible may be reconstructed with vascularized bone if required. Multiple osteotomies may be performed to shape the fibula to reconstruct the anterior arch, body, angle, or ramus of the mandible as long as the fibular periosteum is not disrupted. The septocutaneous or musculocutaneous perforating vessels of the lower leg can be quite variable in location and quantity effecting the placement and reliability of the skin paddle.[81,211,217] The skin of the lower lateral leg is thin and pliable

with fairly large amounts of skin available and may be transferred in a sensate fashion. With smaller skin paddles, the donor defect may be closed primarily. With larger defects, a split thickness skin graft is utilized. The fibula flap is easily harvested simultaneously with the head and neck procedure.

Confirmation of three vessel flow to the distal lower extremity should be determined preoperatively to avoid vascular compromise to the foot following harvest of the peroneal artery.[107,168] The primary disadvantage of the fibula flap is the limitations of the skin paddle. Adequate skin is not available for larger soft tissue defects or most three-layer defects requiring a second flap for soft tissue repair. The somewhat unreliable nature of the presence and location of the cutaneous perforator vascular supply can usually be minimized by including a cuff of soleus muscle with the flap to include musculocutaneous perforators. If dental implants are not planned, the fibula bone results in a very broad and rounded neomandible, which is quite difficult to fit for a tissue-borne prosthesis. The donor site morbidity of the fibula flap includes prolonged pain on ambulation for some patients.[6,24,136,160,223]

Osteocutaneous Radial Forearm Flap

The radial forearm free flap (RFFF) has also been described as an osteocutaneous radial forearm free flap (OCRFFF) with harvest of a portion of the radius bone based on perforators in the intermuscular septum passing to the periosteum.[83,170,171] This significantly broadened the applicability of the already widely used forearm flap in reconstructive surgery. While seemingly the best of options with tremendous soft tissue characteristics and an option for bone harvest, the widespread acceptance of the OCRFFF has been limited by concerns about the bone quality and possible pathologic fracture of the radius bone postoperatively.

The length of radius bone that can be safely harvested without unacceptable forearm dysfunction is limited to 10 to 12 cm (Figure 6-4). To avoid pathologic fracture, most authors recommend that the thickness of the bone harvested be limited to 40% of the circumference of the radius.[123,181] This generally does not provide adequate bone stock to support endosseous dental implants.[59,126] When a segment of bone is removed from the radius, the bone is significantly weakened, especially to torsional forces. This has resulted in a postoperative pathologic radius fracture rate of up to 66% with an average of 23%.[14,26,181,194] More recently the prophylactic internal fixation of the radius bone after

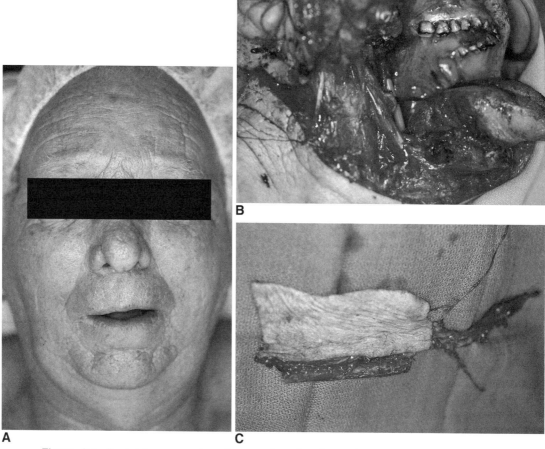

A **B** **C**

Figure 6-4. Radial forearm osteocutaneous free flap for oral cavity and lateral mandible reconstruction. **A,** Preoperative frontal view. **B,** Lateral mandibular bone defect including a larger soft tissue defect of the lateral tongue, floor of the mouth, pharynx, and palate. **C,** Harvested osteocutaneous forearm flap with skin, radius bone, vascular pedicle, and cutaneous nerves (2).

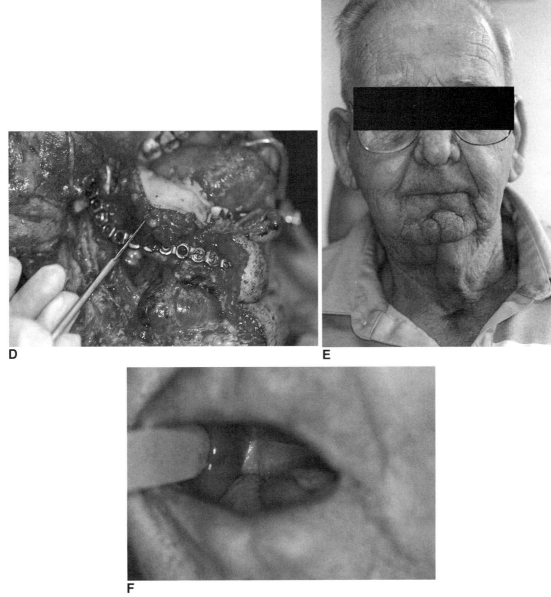

Figure 6-4, cont'd D, Closure of defect repairing mandible and soft tissue defect. **E,** Postoperative frontal view after radiation therapy. **F,** Intraoral view of the oral cavity and pharyngeal reconstruction.

OCRFFF harvest (Figure 6-5) has been shown to successfully eliminate this risk.[197,216]

Despite the limitations of bone availability with the OCRFFF, it has been used successfully for oromandibular reconstruction with fewer complications than the fasciocutaneous RFFF with plate reconstruction.[48,128,181,191] For limited mandibular defects, the radius bone is very adequate and can easily bear a tissue-borne prosthesis (denture). This has proven beneficial as many patients do no have the financial means for dental implantation, which is frequently not covered by many third-party payers. In this setting, the radius bone provides a superior contour for the support of a tissue-borne prosthesis when compared with either the fibula or scapula bone.

The OCRFFF offers the highest quality soft tissue available for oral cavity reconstruction and adequate bone for limited mandibular defects. With the risk of pathological fracture of the radius eliminated, the OCRFFF offers a very useful technique with tremendous versatility for reconstruction of the oromandibular complex.

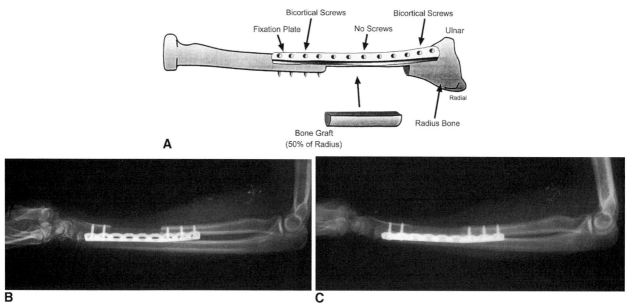

Figure 6-5. Prophylactic fixation of the radius bone after bone graft harvest. **A,** Diagram showing the harvest of the bone graft and placement of a plate spanning the defect. **B,** Post-operative radiograph of the forearm demonstrating plate fixation. **C,** One year follow-up radiograph showing significant bone formation and remodeling in the area of the defect.

Scapula Free Flap

The osteocutaneous scapula free flap remains one of the most versatile flaps available for harvest in the human body.* The subscapular arterial system offers tremendous amounts of skin, the latissimus dorsi and serratus anterior muscles and scapular bone for harvest, all supplied by one major vascular pedicle, which has both favorable length and caliber. These different tissue components each have a separate vascular branching supply allowing for almost limitless degrees of orientation in relation to each other and the recipient bed. The skin of the upper lateral back is usually quite thick with considerable subcutaneous fat resulting in significant soft tissue bulk, which can be advantageous in some reconstructive situations. This bulk will reliably remain on a long-term basis without atrophy. The skin can also be separated into scapular and parascapular skin paddles based on the transverse and descending branches of the circumflex scapular artery, respectively.[60,69,177] Unfortunately, there has been no corresponding segmental nervous supply to the skin of the region, which precludes the harvest of skin as a sensate flap. Recently, however, dorsal cutaneous rami of the T1 or T2 spinal nerves have been described, which may allow for sensate transfer of scapular cutaneous paddles.[144]

A total of 10 to 14 cm of bone is available for harvest from the lateral border of the scapula for mandibular reconstruction supplied by the periosteal branch of the circumflex scapular artery. The separation of the bony and fasciocutaneous components of the flap resulting from unique vascular supplies can be as much as 4 cm, allowing for significant versatility in hard- and soft-tissue orientation during reconstruction. Osteotomies may be safely performed for mandibular contouring as long as the periosteum is preserved. The harvested scapular bone has a thick border along the free edge of the scapula but transitions quickly to thin bone 1 to 2 cm medial to the edge. The resulting limited bone stock may not be adequate for the support of endosteal dental implants.[59,126]

The scapular osteocutaneous flap remains an optimal choice for the reconstruction of the oromandibular complex when the surgeon is faced with large complex defects, especially those involving a large surface area or with three-layer composite defects involving both the oral cavity and external soft tissues (Figure 6-6).

For extremely large defects, some surgeons have employed the scapular "mega flap," which includes scapular bone and extensive skin as described earlier in this chapter, but also the latissimus dorsi muscle or the serratus anterior muscle for additional bulk and coverage.[10,219] The muscles are based on the thoracodorsal artery and vein that branch off

---

*Refernces 35, 60, 69, 177, 178, 190.

the subscapular vessels and therefore can be harvested on the same vascular pedicle requiring only one arterial and venous anastomoses. The mega flap offers significant mobilization of the various tissue components relative to each other as a result of the branching vascular supply, providing great reconstructive versatility for the largest of defects.

The major disadvantages of the scapula flap include the bulky and insensate nature of the skin paddles and the necessity to reposition the patient several times during the operation, which adds significant time to the procedure. Long-term shoulder dysfunction can result from the harvest of the scapula osteocutaneous flap with winging of the scapula, decreased range of motion, and chronic pain. These problems can usually be minimized with careful technique and aggressive physical therapy.

Iliac Crest Flap

The iliac crest has long been a source of free bone grafts for mandibular reconstruction. A vascularized iliac crest flap harvested off the deep circumflex iliac artery (DCIA) to provide 14 to 16 cm of bone, which has a natural curvature for mandibular reconstruction. Studies have found the iliac crest provides the highest quality bone for the support of osseointegration for dental implantation of the available osteocutaneous flaps.[59,126] The cutaneous portion of the flap is both bulky and limited in mobility restricting its usefulness for large composite defects. Urken and others described the addition of the internal oblique muscle based on the ascending branch of the DCIA for mandibular reconstruction that significantly increase the versatility of the flap and provided excellent results.[201,203,205,206]

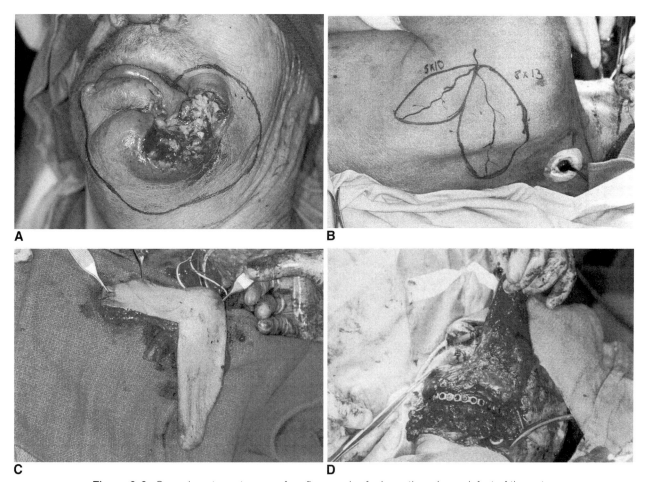

Figure 6-6. Scapula osteocutaneous free flap repair of a large three-layer defect of the anterior face and oral cavity. **A,** Larger persistent carcinoma of the lip after radiation and chemotherapy. **B,** Planned scapula flap from the left upper back with two skin paddles. **C,** Harvested scapula osteocutaneous free flap showing both skin paddles and scapula bone. **D,** Inset of the scapula flap for oral cavity and mandibular reconstruction.

Continued

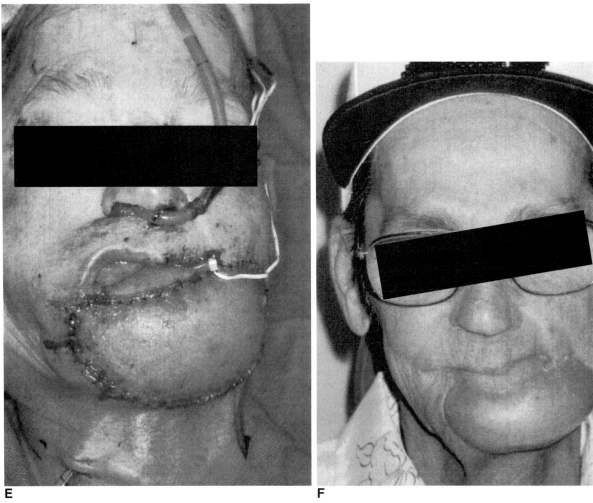

Figure 6-6, cont'd E, Post operative view of the defect repair. **F,** Six-month follow-up appearance.

Despite the high quality of the iliac bone for mandibular reconstruction, the soft tissue limitations, overall bulk, and donor site morbidity have limited the popularity of the iliac crest flap. Most surgeons will utilize this flap when the other options are precluded for reasons of peripheral vascular disease, earlier surgery or trauma, or other issues.

Dental Rehabilitation

Significant dental rehabilitation of the oral cavity after composite resection for malignancy can only be achieved with microvascular free tissue transfer of bone and soft tissue (Figure 6-7). The placement of enosseous dental implants into the replaced bone allows for the optimal rehabilitative outcome that approached that of the patient with normal dentition.[200,201] Appropriate contouring of the reconstructed oral cavity may allow the fitting of tissue borne dentures. While cosmetically acceptable, diet remains significantly affected.

Other Flaps

More unique situations that require the employment of less frequently utilized flaps always come up. Pharyngoesophageal defects have long presented one of the more challenging reconstructions in head and neck surgery. This is reflected by the first reported free tissue transfer in the head and neck described by Seidenberg and others as a transfer of a free jejunal segment for cervical esophageal reconstruction in 1959.[155] The jejunal flap may be harvested off a segmental arcade of the superior mesenteric artery for free transfer to the head and neck. As a mucus-producing tubular structure of similar size, the jejunum seems a natural replacement for the cervical esophagus. On transfer, the jejunum retains some intrinsic contractile motility, which is beneficial for swallowing (and detrimental if the jejunum is inverted on the inset) (Figure 6-8).[17,75,159,189] Through the years, experience has found the jejunum to be a fairly fragile flap that does not tol-

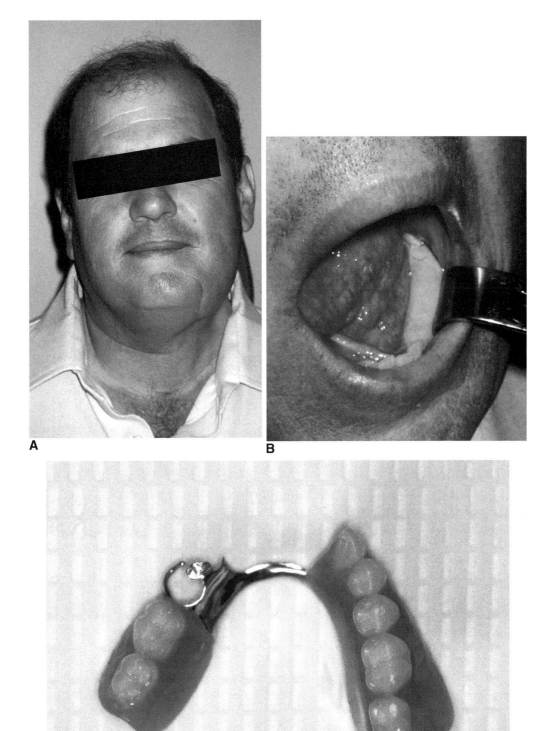

Figure 6-7. Dental rehabilitation after mandibular reconstruction. **A,** Frontal view after lateral mandibular reconstruction with fibula free flap. **B,** Intra oral appearance of intra oral reconstruction before secondary dental implant placement. **C,** Dental prosthesis for fixation with osseointegrated dental implants.

Continued

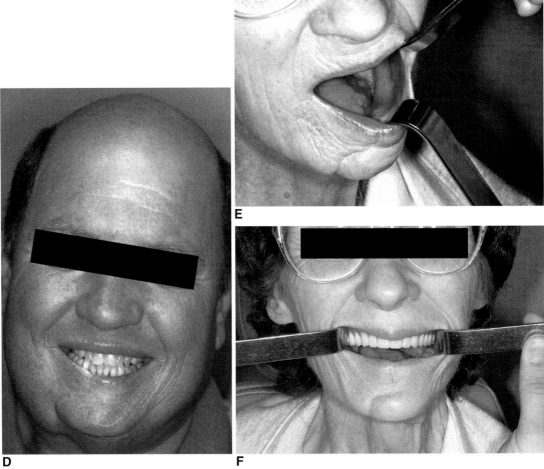

Figure 6-7, cont'd D, Patient smile with prosthesis secured in place. **E,** Intra oral reconstruction with a radial forearm osteocutaneous free flap. **F,** Patient seen in *E* with tissue-borne upper and lower dentures.

erate episodes of ischemia. The donor site morbidity of a bowel resection can be considerable. The reconstructed pharynx can successfully undergo tracheoesophageal puncture (TEP),[17,104] however this often results in a very "wet" vocal quality. As a result, most surgeons now routinely use a radial forearm fasciocutaneous free flap that is "tubed" to recreate the cervical esophagus (Figure 6-9). This results in less donor site morbidity, provides a very functional adynamic "funnel" into the thoracic esophagus, and produces a better TEP vocal quality.[50]

PATIENT EVALUATION AND PREPARATION

Despite technological advances and new options in head and neck microvascular reconstruction, the best treatment plan is still dependent initially on general patient factors. Multiple factors, other than the stage of cancer or surgical defect (i.e., comorbid conditions, overall performance status, occupational and recreational activities, and personal preferences) also

play significant roles in not only deeming a patient a safe, suitable candidate for free tissue transfer, but further dictates the possible free flap donor sites available.

The reconstructive surgeon, in consultation with the patient's other healthcare providers, needs to expeditiously address issues such as airway status, nutritional status, and uncontrolled medical conditions. Head and neck reconstructive surgery requires the input of multiple medical disciplines to maximize outcome, and this process should initiate with the surgeon's first assessment. Treatment of acute issues can occur in parallel with the reconstructive surgeon's careful evaluation.

History and Current Illness

An extensive history of symptoms gathered by the reconstructive surgeon will not only help determine the size and character of the anticipated extirpative defect that needs reconstruction, but can also yield hints to the possibility of a synchronous primary or metastatic disease. All of these factors directly influence the types of viable free flap options. Complaints of unilateral conductive hearing loss, hyponasal speech, breathy voice, ptosis, diplopia, trismus, chin numbness, otalgia, and contralateral symptoms are frequently indicators of deep or extensive disease beyond that immediately apparent.

The extent of pre-morbid and present oral cavity function is important. Not only will this hint at involved structures that need reconstruction, but dictates the possible functional goal of any reconstruction. The reconstructive functional result in terms of deglutition, taste, mastication, voice, breathing, and cosmesis generally cannot be improved beyond the pre-morbid state. In patients with compromised pre-morbid function because of neurologic disability or earlier treatments, preoperative counseling as to potential reconstructive outcome is even more crucial to provide realistic expectations.

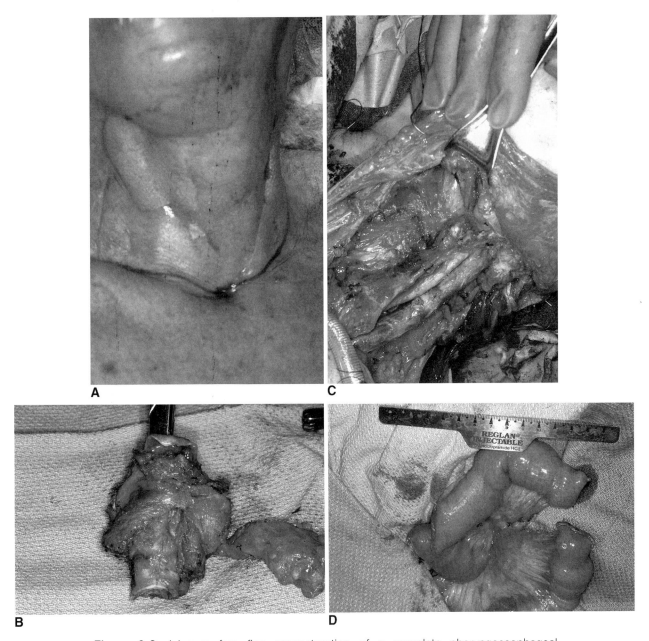

Figure 6-8. Jejunum free flap reconstruction of a complete pharyngoesophageal defect. **A,** Recurrent pharyngeal carcinoma after surgery and radiation therapy. **B,** Laryngopharyngectomy specimen with neck dissection. **C,** Surgical defect after resection. **D,** Harvest of a jejunal free flap based on a mesenteric vascular arcade.

Continued

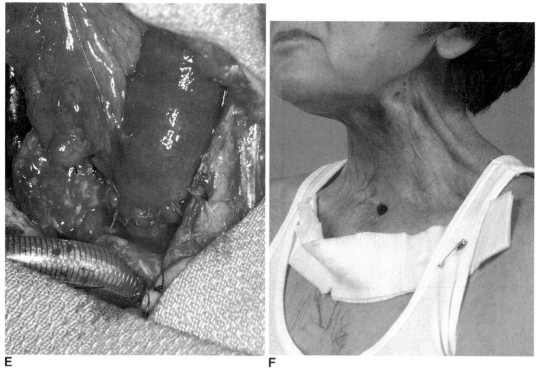

E   F

Figure 6-8, cont'd E, Repair of the pharyngeal and esophageal defect with the jejunal free flap. **F,** One-year postoperative appearance.

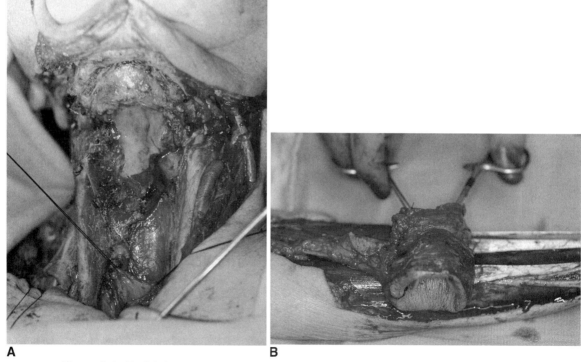

A   B

Figure 6-9. Radial forearm free flap "tubed" for reconstruction of a complete pharyngoesophageal defect. **A,** Defect after total laryngopharyngectomy for recurrent carcinoma. **B,** Forearm skin rolled onto itself creating a "tube" for pharyngoesophageal reconstruction.

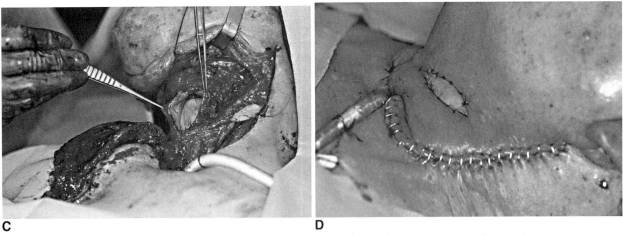

C   D

Figure 6-9, cont'd C, Inset of the "tubed" forearm skin for pharyngoesophageal reconstruction. **D,** Closure of the neck skin including a small monitoring paddle of forearm skin to allow post operative monitoring of flap vascularity.

The high incidence of smoking in microvascular patients is a result of its known carcinogenic effects. Beyond the ill effects on anesthesia and cardiopulmonary function, nicotine also causes adverse vasoconstrictive effects that can compromise flap perfusion and wound healing.[142,143] Other routes of nicotine use can also cause similar problems, and all nicotine intake should be discouraged. A history of regular alcohol usage requires aggressive perioperative withdrawal prophylaxis and nutritional supplementation. Withdrawal is associated with a higher rate of complications and flap loss.[66,214]

A history of previous radical neck dissections, neck incisions, and flaps may limit the current reconstructive options both at the recipient and donor site. Careful review of old operative reports, review of current radiographs, and discussions with previous surgeons is often necessary to supplement the patient's memory. Similarly, extensive radiotherapy can compromise recipient site vascularity and healing and cause premature vascular wall changes, but may or may not affect free flap viability.[109,153,154] Post-radiation hypothyroidism should be detected and reversed to help maximize postoperative recovery and healing. Both previous surgery and radiotherapy can cause extensive fibrosis in the operative bed, making safe isolation of needed recipient vessels and nerves very difficult if not impossible.

Donor-site specific history must also be obtained. A patient's handedness, footed ness, occupation, hobbies, and recreational activities can dictate the side or site of a free flap harvest. Previous abdominal and pelvic surgery can obviate the use of some potential free flap vascular pedicles (i.e., rectus abdominis, iliac crest). Claudication or extremity rest pain is indicative of significant peripheral vascular disease and warrants aggressive workup of extremity vascular pedicle adequacy. History of previous surgery or trauma to the donor site prompts in-depth evaluation of the donor-site anatomy. This includes work-up of both arterial and venous supplies, as well as of boney integrity.

Physical Exam

The microvascular surgeon should also perform a complete head and neck exam. Direct visualization of the neoplasm or traumatic defect, along with bimanual palpation, should complement the tumor mapping anticipated by the symptom history. This allows an educated intercourse with the extirpative surgeon in terms of the anticipated surgical defect size and potential structures to be removed (mucosa, skin—with or without bone) or exposed (brain, orbit, bone or carotid artery). A secondary survey can then focus on the anticipated fine-tuning reconstructive procedures necessary during either the primary or secondary setting to maximize both functional and aesthetic outcome. This includes status and integrity of the parotid and submandibular ducts, nasal airway, lip vermillion, oral commissure, dental occlusion, maxillary sinus, soft and hard palate, eustachian tube, facial sensation, and motor nerve function. A superinfected area of cutaneous involvement should be treated with antibiotics to help delineate infected vs neoplastically involved tissue. This can lead to a more efficient resection and also possibly improve pain, hygiene, and healing. The extent of neck disease determines not only prognosis, but the type of neck dissection.

This influences changes in neck volume, contour, and potential available recipient vessels for microvascular anastomosis. Previous facial and neck incisions and traumatic scars must be recognized since they will limit placement of future incisions.

Microvascular free tissue transfer has been used with success in the elderly. Chronologic age itself does not seem to contraindicate surgery, but the incidence of medical complications are increased after treatment.[15,21,77] Mental impairment, such as dementia, or mental illness is a very difficult situation to control in the debilitated postoperative period. Serious consideration should be given to more tolerant alternative reconstructive techniques if surgery is still considered an option. Morbid obesity may not only have an influence on perioperative recovery and healing, but may require alteration in available useful donor sites because of flap thickness and bulk.[110] These patients may also have undetected significant obstructive sleep apnea, which not only heavily influences perioperative airway management, but can be seriously exacerbated postoperatively by large, bulky, and swollen reconstructions. Additionally, the long-term treatment of this disorder must be reevaluated after surgery, and often requires prolonged tracheotomy usage.

Examination of the potential free flap donor site for scars, asymmetries, or bony deformities can often prompt a patient's memory of an old injury or surgery. Objective evaluation of the mobility, strength, and function of an extremity should confirm the patient's history. Preoperative disabilities, from previous strokes, spinal injury, or trauma, may either prompt or discourage the use of certain free flap donor sites. Non-healing sores, cold digits, loss of sensation, as well as significant distal extremity swelling are also indicators of inadequate vascularity and frequently contraindicate use of the involved extremity as a donor site. Unfortunately, most of these conditions are bilateral and usually require the use of a completely different, and often less ideal, donor site for reconstruction. Palpation of distal extremity pulses (i.e., radial, ulnar, dorsalis pedis, and posterior tibial arteries), subjective Allen's tests, and ankle-arm indexes can be reassuring, but adequacy determinations should be supplemented by formal vascular assessments in equivocal cases.[63,117,132]

Past Medical History

In all patients, special attention should be paid to preoperatively maximizing any known medical conditions. Preoperative consultation with a hospitalist can provide longitudinal medical care from before the operation to discharge with an internist who already knows the patient and initiated prophylactic care.

Patient compliance with treatment maximization is also paramount and medical noncompliance can often compromise outcomes.

Certain comorbid conditions can also affect free tissue transfer specifically, although absolute contraindicating conditions are uncommon.[5] Certain extremity vessels are known for a tendency toward advanced atherosclerotic disease in patients with peripheral vascular disease. Radial and peroneal arteries tend to be frequently affected, while the scapular arterial system remains relatively unaffected. Poor digit perfusion can be further exacerbated by donor vessel sacrifice, yielding cold intolerance or even digit necrosis. Patients with severe extremity venous or lymphatic insufficiency should also be considered for other donor sites to prevent extremity complications postoperatively. Patients with arterial vascular disease as a result of atherosclerosis or hypertension need to also be evaluated for significant concomitant cerebrovascular and cardiovascular disease. Significant carotid disease cannot only decrease the availability of adequate recipient external carotid artery branches, but intraoperative hypotension or neck extension positioning can cause perioperative strokes. Adequate cardiopulmonary reserve must be present to tolerate the often prolonged anesthesia time and intravascular fluid shifts associated with free tissue transfer operations.[38] Such comorbid disease can significantly lower the limits of resectability and reconstructability, since these procedures often require more prolonged general anesthesia and possibly even multiple trips to the operating room.

Patients who have connective tissue disorders with vasculitis are at a relatively high risk for microvascular pedicle compromise, and this should be a relative contraindication to microvascular reconstruction. Unfortunately, well controlled patients who have been aggressively treated with steroids or other immunosuppressive agents can experience poor healing or increased infectious complications.[4] Similarly, patients with hematologic disorders (i.e., von Willebrand's disease, hemophilia, lupus anticoagulant abnormality, thrombocytopenia, polycythemia vera, sickle cell disease, protein C deficiency) should also be strongly considered for non-microvascular reconstructions because of the difficulties in maintaining healthy patent anastomoses associated with pro-thrombotic and coagulopathic states.[2,11] Paraneoplastic hypercoagulability or extensive inadvertent preoperative use of anti-coagulating medicines (i.e., aspirin, nonsteroidal anti-inflammatory drugs, vitamin E) can also compromise microvascular success. Patients requiring perioperative anticoagulation because of concurrent conditions (i.e., prosthetic heart valves, deep venous thrombosis) are predisposed to compressive neck hematomas that can lead to significant blood loss, airway compromise, or flap pedicle compression.

Uncontrolled or previously undiagnosed diabetes should be aggressively treated. Diabetic wounds are known to heal slower. Necessary adjustments must be made in terms of incision line suturing and monitoring. The immunosuppressive effects of diabetes can lead to increased post-surgical infections that can cause delayed microvascular pedicle compromise. Untreated profound glucosuria can compound the already large changes in intravascular volume associated with these procedures. Secondary diabetic microvascular disease can cause poor fasciocutaneous paddle perfusion, yielding ischemic areas after harvest. Larger vessel disease not only can cause silent coronary artery disease that may not be detected preoperatively, but increase both donor and recipient vessel atherosclerosis. Poor extremity healing after harvest can lead to difficult-to-treat infections and necrosis of donor sites. Further sacrifice of extremity sensory nerves during harvest can exacerbate problems associated with diabetic peripheral neuropathy. Properly evaluated and managed diabetic patients still are suitable candidates for free tissue transfer.[46]

Laboratory and Radiologic Studies

The reconstructive surgeon should review all preoperative laboratory and radiologic exams. Abnormal liver function, platelet count, blood urea nitrogen, prothrombin, or pro thromboplastin time may lead to significant intraoperative blood loss and postoperative hematomas with possible compressive flap loss or infection. These abnormalities need to be investigated and corrected as much as possible preoperatively. Preoperative albumin, prealbumin, and leukocyte count can give an estimate of the level of malnourishment that can affect postoperative healing. Staging computed tomography (CT) and magnetic resonance imaging (MRI) scans of the head and neck region complement and confirm the history, physical exam, and endoscopic evaluation by the microvascular surgeon and help to further delineate the anticipated reconstruction needs in terms of size and structures. Magnetic resonance angiogram (MRA), CT angiography, Doppler or angiography is used in cases of potential resection for carotid artery involvement, but can also indicate the adequacy of the external carotid branches to support microvascular anastomosis.[129] At times, the patency of the transverse cervical arterial system for use as a recipient vessel can also be determined. The integrity of potential larger recipient veins in the neck can also be detected radiographically, including predicting the need for sacrifice of the internal or external jugular venous network. Need for venous angiography is rare.

Radiographic evaluation of the determined potential free flap donor sites should help supplement the physical exam in determining safe harvest. A preoperative Allen's test is crucial for maintaining adequate hand perfusion after radial or ulnar forearm free flap harvest. In cases with an equivocal subjective Allen's test, Doppler plethysmography can objectively document adequate collateral perfusion to the donor hand, allowing its safe use.[132] Additionally, other Doppler, MRA, and angiographic techniques have been used adjunctively to study donor site vasculature before harvest of extremity free flaps.[106,107,115,168] These studies can detect anatomic abnormalities, assure adequate cutaneous flap perforator supply, and document the adequacy of distal collateral arterial flow. Safe harvest with adequate distal perfusion is paramount in donor site selection. In patients with previous trauma or surgery, plain x-ray films can document adequate bony integrity and any compromising hardware.

Surgical Treatment Planning

After the initial work-up is completed, the patient is presented to the multidisciplinary Head and Neck Tumor Board to obtain a consensus on treatment options. Although, in general, the oncologic efficacy of any therapy takes preference when ranking treatment options, the Tumor Board's recommendations can also be heavily influenced by the expected postoperative functional outcome, which is somewhat dependent on the reconstructive options available. From the preoperative clinical assessment, the microvascular surgeon can generally determine which tissue types will be required to reconstruct the anticipated surgical defect. This is of course is much easier in post-traumatic defects, where loss of further tissue is unlikely. Soft tissue considerations include volume and surface area of tissue needed, need for sensory innervation, availability of and mobility from adjoining vascularized bone graft, and other characteristics such as motor, secretory, or peristaltic activity. The need to provide protected coverage of bone, large vessels, and brain parenchyma adds to the soft tissue volume needed. Bone considerations in choosing the appropriate free flap include length and caliber of bone required and character and mobility of associated soft tissue. Unfortunately, rarely is there an ideal free flap that fulfills all the reconstructive requirements perfectly. In addition, the best microvascular reconstructive option may not be available to every patient because of available expertise, previous therapy, functional or anatomic abnormality, or need for shorter anesthesia time because of medical comorbidity (shorter harvest time). Fortunately, more than one option is generally an acceptable compromise of the myriad reconstructive requirements. A priority list should be chosen with the patient, with backup donor sites always available intraoperatively. Also, other reconstructive techniques can be used in combination with free tissue transfer to maximize the overall reconstructive outcome. Whatever reconstructive technique is implemented, it should not hinder postoperative recovery with multiple surgeries, possibly delaying or preventing necessary timely adjuvant therapy. Single-stage primary reconstructions are best for meeting this goal. Post-therapeutic expectations should also be discussed in detail. These conversations should include explanation of any staged or delayed procedures anticipated to yield the maximal cosmetic and functional outcome.

This is also the time to recruit and inform family and friends for the necessary physical and emotional support that complements comprehensive medical therapy. The patient's privacy concerns should of course be respected during this process in accordance with the his or her preferences.

Efficient postoperative recovery and early in-patient discharge involves an anticipatory and multidisciplinary approach. Therapy should begin with preoperative consultation and counseling by all involved surgical colleagues (i.e., neurosurgery, ophthalmology, vascular surgery, oral surgery) and anticipated ancillary personnel (i.e., speech pathology, physical therapy, social work, prosthetician). All these experienced consultants should be familiar with the expected outcome and specific restrictions of microvascular cases so that the patient receives consistent information. The myriad preoperative appointments is best coordinated for the patient by a dedicated patient care coordinator.

Preoperative evaluation by anesthesiologists experienced in microvascular cases is paramount. Not only will this help ensure that the patient's preoperative state is maximized, this will also assure that all the necessary personnel and monitoring equipment are available at the time of surgery. An intraoperative plan can then be worked out preoperatively with the surgeon-anesthesiologist team, so that attention can be fully focused on unexpected situations.

Except in those cases where a gastric-pullup is anticipated, in patients with an expected prolonged period of enteral feedings, preoperative percutaneous or open gastrostomy tube placement is prudent. This cannot only help maximize preoperative nutritional status, but removes the postoperative necessity for a nasogastric feeding tube. Postoperative placement can be difficult and risk free flap paddle suture lines. Trans-abdominal enteral routes are generally more comfortable for the patient once healed, hidden well below clothing. These routes also decrease the incidence of sinusitis, gastroesophageal reflux, and pha-ryngeal swelling.[119] All of these factors can potentially inhibit return of postoperative deglutition. The upper endoscopy necessary for percutaneous feeding tube placement can also help detect synchronous pharyngoesophageal primaries, but has been anecdotally associated with tumor seeding. Abdominal incisions can also influence potential abdominal free flap availability and should be communicated to the endoscopist or general surgeon.

INTRAOPERATIVE MANAGEMENT

An anesthesiologist experienced in microvascular cases is essential. In such large operative cases, several certain unique factors need to be consistently considered. Although this information should be evident at the preoperative evaluation by anesthesia, the necessary available areas of the body for both the extirpative and reconstructive portions of the procedure must be well communicated. Donor extremities should be visibly marked or wrapped to prevent inadvertent blood draws or placement of intravascular catheters in potential donor vessels. The anesthesiologist should know multiple unconventional and alternate electrode and vascular access sites in order to leave all potential donor sites available. Necessary preoperative medications such as prophylactic antibiotics, steroids, and antacids should be delineated and administered.[31,165] Available blood for transfusion should be confirmed.

In the head and neck, airway considerations are frequently challenging. In the operating room, the predetermined approach to the airway is followed and close cooperation between the intubating anesthesiologist and surgeon is crucial to safe airway access. Complex, lengthy, and risky intubations, including fiberoptic intubations, can be avoided by early placement of a planned tracheostomy under local anesthesia. The patient is then positioned as the anesthesiologist continues to obtain his or her desired adequate vascular access, since further access is difficult once the case is underway. Availability of lines and electrodes is necessary during the case and the routes of these should be planned to avoid contamination of hidden sterile donor sites by the anesthesiologist. All access and monitoring equipment must be adequately fixated to the patient since changes in patient position are frequently necessary during the procedure. Adequate pressure point padding is confirmed by both surgeon and anesthesiologist. All remaining exposed nonsterile areas of the patient should be covered with a warmer and unused limbs placed in pneumatic compression devices, even if only unilaterally.

The presence of both the extirpative and reconstructive surgeon guiding the Betadine preparation of the operative patient can save a significant amount of time and trouble later in the operative day. Separate draping of both recipient and donor site operative fields is necessary to not only prevent salivary contamination, but potential donor site tumor seeding. Draping of both alternative free and pedicled flap donor sites is also performed (i.e., pectoralis major flap). Separate instrument sets for the recipient and donor sites on different operating room tables are necessary. Since most microvascular harvests occur concurrently with the extirpative surgery, two distinct scrub teams are often required. This can decrease resource utilization and overall costs.[118] Well-trained and experienced operating room personnel, especially in microvascular instrumentation and techniques, are crucial to operative efficiency and success.

Routine good anesthesia management applies to free tissue transfer surgery, as well as to other large head and neck cases.[145,164,207] Adequate blood pressure must be maintained throughout the case to provide both vital organ and flap perfusion. Hypertension can lead to excess blood loss. Hypotension should be initially treated with a decrease in the inhalation agent, which can be anti-inotropic, a vasodilator, and intravenous hydration. All vasoconstrictors should be avoided, unless the situation is life threatening, because of their intense vasospastic effect on the hypersensitive free flap pedicle.[13,68] Denervated free flaps are thought to be hypersensitive to catecholamines. Cold patient temperature can also cause peripheral vasoconstriction and increased afterload and should be avoided with the use of patient warmers, warm irrigation, and infused fluids.

Experienced anesthesiologists understand how judicious use of intravenous fluids is also crucial to operative success. Hemodilution as a result of minor blood loss and intravenous hydration, improves flap perfusion because of blood viscosity reduction and can improve flap ischemia tolerance.[51] Both crystalloid and colloid replacement has been advocated, with some colloids also having an antithrombotic advantage.[163] Fluid overload can cause pulmonary edema, but also significant intra- and postoperative edema in the head and neck and the free flap. This can impair insetting, healing, or cause pedicle compression. More than 7 liters of intravenous fluid administration is also associated with major medical complications.[77] Appropriate hydration can generally be determined by hemodynamic parameters and urine output (0.5 cc/kg/hr), but central venous monitoring may also be necessary in the patient with significant cardiac history. Too low of a hematocrit can compromise vital organ and flap oxygen delivery, and the proper level varies by individual. Packed red blood cell transfusion may be necessary, but can have anti-coagulation side

effects. The patient should be adequately ventilated and oxygenated to assist with flap perfusion, but positive end-expiratory pressure should be avoided because of its effects on venous return.

SURGICAL TECHNIQUES
Surgical Incisions

Although adequate oncologic resection is paramount in the recipient site, familiarity of the ablative team with the various needs of the anticipated free flap reconstruction is also crucial. Surgical incision planning extends beyond just the purview of the oncologic surgeon. Fortunately, frequent multiple-approach options can achieve adequate access and visualization of the surgical field. The chosen surgical approach must also eventually provide adequate visualization for adequate inset suturing of the free flap into the surgical defect. A needle holder frequently requires more maneuverable exposure than a Bovie cautery, knife, scissor, or laser. Additionally, this can be compounded by recipient site edema and initial flap bulk, which can be larger than the extirpated native tissue volume. These needs may require potential incision extension or new incisions.

Incision placement also depends on the quality of the native tissue. Previous cervicofacial incisions, traumatic incisions, skin flap elevation, prolonged steroid usage, radiation therapy, and—now more commonly—chemotherapy can all affect skin flap viability. Sub-platysmal or thicker skin flap elevations are desirable, but are often limited by oncologic considerations. Using the minimum of incisions necessary for the appropriate exposure should be attempted in all cases. Old incisions are the best initial choice, as the native vascularity is already compromised. Incisions perpendicular to or away from large vessels and the planned microvascular pedicle can decrease the exposure risk if there is incisional dehiscence. Incision breakdown often yields a poorer cosmetic result and potential large vessel, hardware, alloplast, allograft, or bony exposure. Exposure of the microvascular pedicle can result in the rapid loss of the entire reconstruction. If detected intraoperatively, the options are either providing a vascularized muscular or fascial bed underneath the compromised skin flap area or alternatively including the devascularized area as part of the extirpative defect.

Primary Recipient Site Surgery

Throughout the operation, the extirpative and microvascular surgeons must communicate freely. Frequently, both are working concurrently to minimize anesthesia time. Unanticipated areas of resection or tissue sparing and areas of potential re-resection after frozen section margin analysis should be accurately communicated to the reconstructive surgeon to allow for intraoperative adjustments. This information not only can affect free flap cutaneous paddle size, but also its shape and orientation. It's always helpful for the surgeon to mark transected nerve stumps that require subsequent re-anastomosis or cable grafting to innervated free flaps, since finding these areas at the end of the case can be frustrating. Further recipient preparation includes performing as much primary closure as possible, and trimming of jagged wound edges to facilitate the necessary even watertight closure.

In cases of osteocutaneous free flap reconstruction after segmental mandibulectomy, pre-contouring the reconstruction plate to the buccal or labial cortex is crucial for maintaining the best post-reconstruction occlusion. If there is involvement or distortion of the outer cortex of the mandible, direct plate contouring to the bone is not possible and placement of the patient into maxilla-mandibular fixation (MMF) or use of a mandibular fix bridge system (Synthes, Paoli, PA) can help maintain preoperative occlusal and joint relationships. Post-resection freehand plate contouring and fixation is difficult and suboptimal. Postoperative correction of malocclusion is possible, but difficult.[36] With the currently available low-profile locking reconstruction plates, the contoured plate can closely approximate the natural mandibular projection and contour without sacrificing durability and strength when used in conjunction with bone grafts.[84,124] These thinner reconstruction plates are usually not visible or palpable through the external skin flap, even after some subcutaneous tissue resection. The locking plate design affords less accurate contouring of the native mandible contour since it acts as an internal external-fixator device. Accurate measurement of bicortical screw length is paramount to minimizing readily palpable, and often bothersome, sharp lingual screw tips. The plate should be screw-fixated at the appropriate location along the native mandibular height such that the bone graft and overlying neo-alveolar soft tissue free flap paddle lie even with the remaining native occlusal surface. This will facilitate maintenance of the gingiva-buccal, gingiva-labial, and floor of mouth sulci to help preserve tongue mobility, oral competence and an adhesive surface area for dentures. Use of reconstruction plates to span segmental mandibular defects without the concomitant use of vascularized bone grafts can have a long-term complication rate depending on mandibular defect location and size and the type of plate used.[23,79,139,212] Depending on the size and location of the soft tissue defect, removal of the reconstruction plate before free flap inset by the microvascular surgeon may be necessary for adequate exposure to perform the paddle inset or microvascular anastomosis. Some microvascular surgeons use

miniplate fixation to attach the osteotomized vascularized bone grafts to the native mandible. This usually also requires use of MMF or a fix-bridge system to maintain proper occlusal relationships. Some miniplate placement on these flaps can occur before pedicle sacrifice at the donor site to reduce flap ischemia time.

Neck Recipient Site Surgery

Continuous inter-surgeon communication during the extirpative neck dissection or neck vessels exploration is also important. Frequently, the range of appropriate recipient vessel size needed can be estimated from the anticipated donor site. Additionally, communication of the anticipated defect location and predicted microvascular pedicle length, can guide the extirpative surgeon to save potential recipient vessels in a given area of the neck, while allowing faster dissection in non-essential areas. Gentle vessel dissection and preservation of lengthy stumps is important for maintaining multiple microvascular anastomosis options. This is important since the best pedicle geometry may not be predictable until the time of anastomosis. Although this may take extra effort and time, it usually does not compromise the adequacy of oncologic resection. Saving both the external and internal jugular veins should be attempted, although anastomotic success may be better with use of the internal jugular system.[33] All potential recipient vessels should be kept moist once exposed. Any adventitial or vessel edge dissection should be avoided at this time until the microscope is used. Similarly, anticipated resection of the proximal external carotid arterial or jugular venous systems because of neoplastic disease needs to be communicated to the reconstructive surgeon so alternative recipient vessel networks and vein grafts can be prepared.[73,125] Both can compromise anastomotic patency. Partial removal of the anterior sternocleidomastoid muscle overlying the pedicle can allow improved microvascular pedicle geometry or decrease venous pedicle compression. In cases of across-midline resections or previous ipsilateral radical neck dissections, vessels from the contralateral neck may need to be isolated and prepared. This need may prompt the extirpative surgeon to perform a full neck dissection for oncologic reasons in a borderline indication case. In most patients with previous neck dissections, adequate recipient site vessels are still available.[80] Extra-cervical recipient vessels are sometimes available, but may require a longer flap pedicle.[73] Previous anastomoses from established free flaps can also be a source of recipient vessels.[130] Reverse flow through distal ends of certain recipient arteries, such as the facial and superior thyroid arteries, is also a possibility for anastomosis in necks without normally available antegrade-flow recipient arteries.[131] In reconstructions using more than one free flap concurrently, some flaps may be sewn in series (one set of recipient vessels) rather than in parallel (two sets of recipient site vessels). The fibula and radial forearm free flaps can act as flow-through flaps and their distal pedicles may be used for additional anastomoses.

Free Flap Harvest

An experienced head and neck team can determine the approximate size of each tissue type needed from the preoperative assessment. Communication during the resection is important if these approximations fall below the actual need. Generally, many distant donor sites frequently allow harvest of the free flap by the microvascular team concurrently with the extirpative surgery. Some donor sites (i.e., scapular-parascapular, latissimus-based flaps) require repositioning for harvest and are performed after the resection, significantly increasing the overall procedure time. The separate instrument table should be set up during the extirpation and kept at a distance to remain free from oral secretion and neoplastic cell contamination.

Although certainly not mandatory, many harvests allow the use of tourniquets to minimize blood loss and potentially improving operative site visualization and harvest speed. This can hide subtle, but significant bleeders, especially along the pedicle, that should be addressed at the time of tourniquet release and reperfusion. Certainly any tourniquet time adds to the overall ischemia time of the free flap and should be meticulously monitored. Also, a time alarm should always be used with the tourniquet if used during donor site closure, since inadvertently leaving the tourniquet up under the drapes during the remaining part of the case can lead to disastrous results.

A flap that has been inset to be hidden deep beyond transoral inspection (i.e., pharyngoesophageal and skull base reconstructions) needs to have an exteriorized monitoring paddle harvested in continuity with the pedicle. At times fiberoptic visualization is possible, but often difficult. Perfusion of the monitoring paddle must reliably mimic that of the main flap paddle and this should be confirmed before final harvest.

The free flap is harvested until isolated on the intact vascular pedicle only. As soon as the arterial and venous donor vessel diameters and pedicle length are known, these are communicated to the extirpative surgeon. Gentle dissection along the pedicle with minimal bipolar cautery or hemoclip hemostasis away from the pedicle vessels is important to avoid damage. Monopolar cautery can cause vessel injury well beyond the visible changes. Some microvascular surgeons microscopically separate the artery from the sur-

rounding donor venae comitantes at this point. This conservative dissection should only be long enough to allow good pedicle anastomosis geometry, in order to minimize potential vessel damage. Copious micro-irrigation with saline or heparinized lidocaine (2% lidocaine, 100 u/ml heparin) is used to keep the vessels moist during the harvest. Once the vessels are sacrificed distally, the tourniquet is released and the free flap is perfused for as long as possible. This not only allows confirmation of good flap perfusion to all portions of the free flap, but also confirms adequate distal perfusion to the donor extremity. This also allows hemostasis of any bleeding on the free flap. Topical papaverine irrigation (30 mg/cc) is sometimes useful to enhance vasodilation and perfusion. Further hemostasis is often necessary at this point as well. The free flap paddle should be manipulated at this point as much as possible while the flap remains pedicled to its native supply (e.g., tubing, shaping, shortening, etc.). Partial closure of the donor site may also be possible at this time, with the remaining closure being done during flap anastomosis or insetting. Harvesting of any necessary vein grafts is also performed before harvest. Only when the neck recipient vessels are ready are the proximal pedicle vessels sacrificed and the free flap brought to the head and neck region. Both surgeon and anesthesiologist should note the time of harvest to indicate the beginning of flap ischemia time.

Free Flap Inset and Microvascular Anastomosis

No hard and fast rule pertains to the order of flap inset vs microvascular anastomosis. Some microvascular surgeons prefer to inset the free flap completely before performing the microvascular anastomosis to assure good pedicle geometry and adequate pedicle length, while minimizing post-anastomotic manipulation. This does lengthen the potential flap ischemia time, but can usually be performed well within most free flap tolerance limits. Some reconstructions require this initially because of the anticipated position of the pedicle, which would block safe access to perform the flap inset. Anecdotal wrapping of the finished pedicle in the drill bit during bone graft inset has occurred. Other surgeons perform the anastomosis first to minimize ischemia time, maximize exposure for the performance of the anastomoses and allow close monitoring of the flap during the remaining portion of the procedure. It is often difficult to exactly predict the amount of pedicle compression that can be attributed to flap bulk and defect swelling after flap inset. If the anastomosis is performed first, the free flap is laid in its anticipated position. Some temporary stay sutures should be placed to prevent the flap from moving or falling while under the microscope.

Extensive detail of the microvascular technique is beyond the scope of this chapter and available elsewhere.[176,182] The standard microscope used for anastomoses affords 10 to 40x magnification (250 tp 300 mm focal-length lens) with opposing binocular heads for simultaneous use by the surgeon and assistant. An attached camera with monitor can help the microvascular scrub nurse anticipate instrument needs. Some surgeons use loupe magnification (3.5 to 5.5x), especially in hospitals without an adequate microscope available.[147] Smaller vessel (smaller than 1.5 mm) anastomoses, as seen in certain free flaps and in children, may require even more magnification. A dedicated, experienced microvascular nurse is essential for operative efficiency and instrument maintenance. Meticulous and gentle handling of all instruments is paramount as the ends are easily bent and broken. Basic microvascular instrumentation includes straight and curved forceps and scissors, a microneedle holder, vessel dilators, and atraumatic single and double microvascular clamps. Micro-irrigators filled with heparinized lidocaine are useful for irrigating open vessel lumens of thrombus. Papaverine also should be available for arterial vasospasm. Nonabsorbable monofilament nylon suture (8-0 to 10-0), with various atraumatic needle sizes, is used depending on vessels size and thickness.

Gentle microsurgical technique and good pedicle geometry are the most important factors in performing the microvascular anastomosis. Good technique includes gentle vessel handling, maintenance of smooth vessel approximating edges and avoidance of suture line tension. Good vessel size match allows linear flow across a straight anastomosis. Good pedicle geometry includes smooth vessels transitions and avoidance of pedicle compression with a minimum of twisting and kinking. This also needs to be checked when the head is returned to the neutral position as this can affect pedicle geometry and jugular vein patency.[127] Adequate recipient arterial inflow should be confirmed in the chosen vessel before anastomosis, although flap arterial flow is generally more dependent on the specific flap type.[116] Good recipient vein backflow should also be confirmed before the anastomosis, but may be limited by a valve. Although the most common anastomosis is end-to-end, the end-to-side anastomosis and vein grafting techniques should also be in the microvascular surgeon's armamentarium in order to maximize pedicle geometry. This may also be necessary if the appropriate recipient vessel size is not available (i.e., a size mismatch of >3:1) or if the pedicle length is inadequate.[218]

Under the microscope, the surgeons can either sit or stand, but they must be comfortable with good arm support on the table. No jostling of the patient by anesthesia or concurrent donor site closure should occur during this time as this movement is magnified under the microscope. No hard and fast rules exist about whether the arterial or venous anastomosis should be performed first.[27] Some surgeons perform the venous anastomosis initially because it tends to be the more difficult because of wall collapse and edge infolding. On the other hand, some perform the arterial anastomosis first to reinitiate flap perfusion as soon as possible.

The end-to-end anastomotic technique is most common and technically simplest. After the recipient vessel is chosen, both vessel edges are cut sharply and smoothly to provide a clean anastomotic edge and then the vessel is gently dilated with vessel dilators. The adventitia is then sharply cleaned away from both vessel edges to beyond where the sutures penetrate the vessel wall. Care must be taken to avoid vessel wall breeches deeper than the adventitia, which is not uncommon in the preparation of the veins. Loose connective tissue should also be trimmed so that it also does not get caught in the anastomosis and act as a thrombotic agent. Both recipient and donor vessels are placed in the sliding, double-approximating vascular clamp so that the vessel edges approximate without tension. A blue background material provides good contrast for the fine suture material. Throughout the anastomosis, adequate recipient arterial inflow or donor vessel outflow should be confirmed by temporarily releasing the clamp and then re-irrigating the blood flow clear.

Multiple anastomotic techniques have been described, including bisecting and trisecting the vessel circumference with simple sutures to ensure even approximation around the entire vessel. The essence of these techniques includes placement of two or three equally spaced sutures to hold the anastomotic orientation. Penetration of any instrument into the vessel lumen should be avoided in order to minimize intimal damage. Either the outer vessel wall can be grasped or a smooth jeweler's forceps can be used intraluminally to lift the anterior vessel wall away from the posterior wall during suturing to prevent "back walling." The suture needle is inserted perpendicularly to the vessel edge at a distance one to two times the vessel wall thickness from the edge. After piercing the opposing vessel edge, three half knots are performed, taking care to make them square. One of the sutures can be cut longer to allow this to be grasped for vessel edge manipulation. Some surgeons tie each anastomotic suture as if they are thrown, while some prefer to leave them untied until half the vessel circumference sutures are placed. This latter technique allows repeated exam of the lumen to make sure no back walling has occurred. Tying these sequentially after they are all thrown can be confusing, as the loose sutures can become mixed, and usually a combination of the two techniques is most successful. After the superficial vessel half wall is sutured, the double-clamp is flipped and attention is given to closing the deep wall. Copious micro-irrigation confirms no back walling and good superficial wall anastomosis, as well as the cleaning out of any accumulated blood clots. During the venous anastomosis, irrigation can also lift the superficial wall off the deep wall. The same suture technique is used to complete the anastomosis. The interrupted suture interval can usually be larger in venous anastomosis than with arterial anastomosis because of the lower flow pressure. A continuous suture technique can also be used, but requires more experience and can narrow the vessel lumen. The clamps are then removed, downstream first, and filling across the anastomosis is observed. "Strip testing," which uses two smooth forceps under sliding compression, can confirm flow across the anastomosis, but can damage the endothelium.[138] The best confirmation is slow bright red blood flow from the flap paddle edge. Leaks can usually be repaired without further interrupting flow with simple single sutures. A Y anastomosis has been proposed to increase blood flow across the anastomosis, but is technically more difficult and not widely employed.[25]

The end-to-side anastomotic technique uses similar suturing technique. The recipient vessel is clamped both proximally and distally to the planned anastomotic site. The planned site of the arteriotomy can be grasped with a suture and stably pulled away from the recipient vessel so that the microscissors can be used to make a clean arteriotomy. This is generally not necessary for making side venotomies. The fashioned arteriotomy or venotomy needs to be slightly larger than the donor vessel to help keep the anastomosis splayed open in a "fishmouth" fashion. The donor vessel can be appropriately angled slightly to help pedicle geometry and minimize turbulence. No particular anastomotic technique is more advantageous in terms of patency.[1] Anastomotic devices have also been described and been useful for venous anastomosis. They can speed up this portion of the procedure.[47,49,222]

In some cases, vein grafts are needed, resulting in a higher complication and thrombosis rate as a result of the increased number of anastomoses. Additional vein harvest sites are necessary, usually the distal saphenous vein provides a good vessel match. Vessel size match is important for vein graft success.[74] The vein graft is always harvested longer than needed, each side branch is clipped or tied carefully and the native direction of flow marked given the potential presence of valves. The flap pedicle is then placed on a sterile

back table under the microscope. This allows a much smoother and controllable surface to perform the vein graft anastomoses. The proximal end of the vein graft (direction of flow into vein graft) is anastomosed to the donor vein, while the distal vein graft end (direction of flow out of vein graft) is anastomosed to the donor artery. This yields a U-shaped vein graft from donor artery to vein. The flap is then brought into the head and neck region. The central portion of the vein graft is then cut depending on the needed pedicle length for both donor artery and vein, followed by completion of the remaining two anastomoses.

The complete inset of the free flap involves both the soft tissue and bony portions of the free flap. It is usually necessary to perform any microscopic neural anastomoses before full inset since this will limit exposure. Reinnervated flaps can adopt sensation similar to the recipient bed sensory pattern.[112] However, even without direct neurorrhaphy, some adequate level of intraoral flap sensation is possible.[208]

Adequate hemostasis in the recipient bed is also important to minimize the risk of the formation of a microvascular compressing hematoma or later infected seroma. The bony inset is most difficult because of the close proximity of the parallel vascular pedicle, the need for monocortical screw fixation, and the frequent need for osteotomies. If a locking plate reconstruction is used, either monocortical non-locking or locking screws can be used, with non-locking screws allowing approximation of the bone grafts to the lingual surface of the reconstruction plate. Using the fewest osteotomies as possible is desirable. Necessary osteotomies of the vascularized bone graft should be done subperiosteally and wedge-shaped such that bone-to-bone approximation is maximized to facilitate bony union. Again, because of the close proximity of the vascular pedicle, extreme care must be taken during both sawing and screwing to prevent vessel injury.

Inset of the soft tissue paddle requires the gentle approximation of wound and flap edges with absorbable sutures to form a watertight seal. Meticulous soft tissue technique is important and suture lines should be under no tension. Multiple layer closures are desirable, but not always possible. Various techniques have been described to shape and contour the soft tissue paddle to mimic the resected tissue, including de epithelization, fascia rolling, and splitting the flap. These techniques can help to maximize postoperative function and aesthetics. At times, flap bulk or recipient site edema can preclude the ability to fully inset and close the soft tissue or bone portions of the free flap. Aggressive debulking can help this, but delaying both full bone screw inset and or wound closure is an option with few sequelae.

Drain Placement and Wound Closure

Drain placement at the completion of the procedure is crucial. The best type of postoperative neck drainage remains controversial. A balance between adequate drainage of all potential dead spaces and minimal interruption of any reconstructive flap pedicle must be maintained. Both passive and suction drains have been advocated.[113] A tight neck skin closure can apply significant pressure to the pedicle or a drain tube if it overlies a vascular pedicle. This can be compounded with routine postoperative swelling or compression dressings. Drains should typically be placed parallel to flap pedicles and carotid sheath contents. Drain tips should be placed away from mucosal or skin suture lines to avoid salivary or air leakage. Maintenance of internal drain position with postoperative head and neck movement can be assured by loose suturing with absorbable sutures. Additionally, the drains should be externally sutured in place to prevent inadvertent withdrawal with patient movement. Suction drains should be removed from self-suction and withdrawn carefully according to the reconstructive surgeon's parameters.

Neck incisions are generally closed in layers, but care must be taken to avoid skewering superficial pedicles during the closure. The position of a superficial pedicle should also be marked cutaneously so that postoperative Doppler monitoring may be employed if needed. This also facilitates finding the pedicle should the neck need to be re-explored.

POSTOPERATIVE MANAGEMENT

Standardized postoperative intensive care unit (ICU) orders, ward transfer orders, and clinical pathways for microvascular cases are crucial for a consistent and efficient hospital recovery.[34] As is the case during the operation, postoperative hypovolemia, hypotension, and hypothermia should be avoided. At the completion of the operation, the patient is brought to either the recovery room or ICU. By bringing the patient directly to the ICU itself, the operative team ensures that all drain and monitoring equipment are in proper working order. The operative team can also directly show the ICU nurse the microvascular paddle and monitoring sites. If a Tropicana room is required, the proper temperature can be confirmed. The patient is inspected in the ICU for compressive circumferential neck ties from a gown or tracheotomy straps, electrocardiogram wires, intravenous lines tightly overlying the neck, or improperly connected suction drains that can lead to early pedicle compromise. The proper head position to maintain pedicle geometry is also confirmed and bolstered in the ICU bed. Some microvascular surgeons prefer the patient be sedated and paralyzed for a period of time to help maintain this positioning. This must be balanced against the increased risk of pneumonia and deep venous thrombosis associated with prolonged ventilation. Postoperative monitoring of the neck incision is similar to that after any neck dissection. Fluid collections and dehiscences need to be aggressively treated since purulent collections can lead to rapid flap loss from pedicle compression or thrombosis.

Pharmacology

Successful free tissue transfer is dependent on the maintenance of blood flow through the arterial and venous microvascular anastomoses of flap vessels to the recipient vessels in the head and neck. Surgical technique is the single most important factor in patency; however, various pharmacologic therapies have been proposed in an attempt to improve on anastomotic success rates.[45] The majority of these agents have attempted to address one or more of the three common mechanisms for thrombosis—stasis, hypercoagulability, and vessel injury. Of the dozens of agents that have been tried or proposed, only three have found a role in the clinical setting—aspirin, heparin, and dextran. There remains a paucity of prospective clinical trials on which to base treatment guidelines with most surgeons relying on anecdotal experience to direct therapy.

Aspirin

Aspirin, or salicylic acid, is an antiplatelet agent that acts by acetylating cyclooxygenase and decreasing the products of arachidonic acid metabolism. These products include thromboxane, a potent platelet aggregator and vasoconstrictor, and prostacyclin, which is a potent vasodilator and inhibitor of platelet aggregation. The desired therapeutic effect for vascular surgery is a suppression of thromboxane without effect on prostacyclin. The minimal dose to achieve this effect in humans is reported to be 100 mg.[45] Higher doses will inhibit both thromboxane and prostacyclin, but do so disproportionately such that some benefit is still seen. Aspirin has been shown to reduce stroke and myocardial infarction more effectively at lower doses (81 and 325 mg). Although no microvascular surgical trials are available, aspirin has been shown to reduce graft occlusion in a range of vascular procedures if taken preoperatively or within 24 hours of surgery. Chewing is the most rapid method for anticoagulation.

Heparin

Although heparin has multiple mechanisms of action, the anticoagulation effect of heparin is largely the result of the inhibition of thrombin and subsequently, the inhibition of thrombin-induced activation of factor V and factor VIII.[45] Heparin possesses properties to prevent both platelet-induced (arterial) and coagulation-induced (venous) thrombi. In animal models, heparin infusion has been shown to be more effective than anti-platelet agents in preventing vascular occlusion.[101] Unfortunately, systemic heparin can result in significant complications (hematoma and bleeding) in the perioperative patient, which largely precludes its routine use in free flap surgery.

Topical heparin irrigation at a dose of 100 U/ml has been suggested as an alternative to systemic therapy to reduce these significant complications. Two studies have failed to show a significant benefit on flap outcome.[102,149]

Dextran

Dextran is a heterogenous polysaccharide that is synthesized by the action of the bacterium *Leuconostoc mesenteroides* on sucrose.[95] Two commercially available forms of dextran are available—dextran 40 (Rheomacrodex) and dextran 70 (Macrodex), which are named based on the average molecular weight of the polysaccharides in the preparations. Dextrans were initially used as colloids for fluid resuscitation; however, problems with potential anaphylactic reactions and effects on the coagulation system resulted in a general abandonment in this setting. It is the effects on coagulation that have been exploited in microvascular surgery. Dextrans appear to interfere with the formation of fibrin networks, increase the degradation of fibrin, decrease von Willebrand and factor VII, and expand intravascular volume.[95] Animal studies have shown improved immediate postoperative vessel patency using dextran infusion. However, Khouri and others found no improvement in flap outcome with the use of dextran in a prospective trial of pharmacologic agents.[102]

While a wide variety of regimens for the administration of dextran in the perioperative period have been advocated, two are commonly followed. Johnson and Barker recommend a 40-ml loading dose of dextran 40 before the release of clamps followed by a 25-ml/hr infusion for 5 days,[96] while Buckley, Davidson, and Das recommend 500 ml of dextran 40 before anastomosis and then 500 ml per 24-hour period for 3 days.[28] Most surgeons have used dextran in a fashion similar to these protocols.

Anaphylaxis reactions are probably rare but many surgeons suggest a test dose of 5 ml of dilute dextran before initiation of therapy. More common sequelae of dextran therapy include pulmonary edema from intravascular volume overload, especially in the elderly. Nephrotoxicity and adult respiratory distress syndrome have also been reported.

Based on 300 replants and 500 free flaps, Conrad and Adams suggest that dextran be used for digit replantation but not for routine free flap surgery, especially for patients older than 50 years of age.[45] This also remains anecdotal, and a well-designed prospective trial remains to be performed.

Summary. Aspirin, heparin, and dextran have all seen extensive use in the management of patients undergoing microvascular surgery. In the only prospective large study, no benefit was seen from any of the anticoagulant therapies in terms of flap outcome.[102] Nonetheless, many microvascular surgeons still use some form of therapy on a routine basis. Conrad and Adams have developed an algorithm based on a review of the literature and their extensive clinical experience with free flaps and replants.[45] For free flaps, they recommend a loading dose of 1.4 mg/kg of aspirin (ideally, chewed) postoperatively and then daily for 2 weeks, heparinized saline (100 U/ml) as a local irrigant during the microvascular anastomosis, and an intravenous heparin bolus intra operatively at 50 to 100 U/kg just before the release of the microvascular clamps. Given the lack of supporting data and experience with therapeutic complications, the authors prefer only intra operative heparin irrigant with or without post operative aspirin (325 mg/day post operatively or preoperatively).

Free Flap Monitoring

Close monitoring of the microvascular reconstruction is paramount, but the exact schedule and method remains controversial, and, thus, practices widely vary even within institutions. An ICU nurse experienced in the care of the microvascular patient is important to the avoidance and early detection of complications. This monitoring is supplemented by physician or electronic monitoring of the free flap. Visible flap inspection and pinprick is a reliable method that must be mastered early by all microvascular surgeons. This is the most reliable monitoring technique and should be the end-all test that determines the status of the flap. Digit palpation and Doppler monitoring of a marked superficial pedicle can supplement direct clinical flap assessment. Both these techniques have some subjectivity to them when there are early changes, and, thus, serial monitoring by the same observer is important. Later anastomotic difficulties are not subtle (as described later in this chapter).

Direct flap observation is labor intensive and can be less sensitive to early ischemic changes. Various objective monitoring methods of either pedicle blood flow or flap perfusion, both invasive and non-invasive, are being investigated with varying success. These include radioisotope scanning, color-flow Doppler, temperature and oxygen tension measurements, perfusion CT scanning, photoplethysmography and laser Doppler velocimetry.* Limitations of these methods include the cost of monitoring equipment, a wide variation of normal values with significant artifact, and the need for special expertise.

Complications and Salvage

Free flap patients are susceptible to the same systemic medical complications as any major head and neck surgery patient. All need to be aggressively treated. Local complications to the donor site are specific to each type of free flap. Familiarity with the anatomy of the donor site is paramount to recognizing complications. These range from pain, bleeding, and infection to more severe complications such as permanent sensory and motor nerve damage or even loss of the donor limb. Infections under pressure in either natural or surgically created compartments can rapidly lead to compression and thrombosis of the already compromised native extremity vascularity. Left undetected and untreated, arm or leg loss can rapidly occur. Scarring can lead to later functional and cosmetic problems that may require physical therapy or further surgery.[24] The donor site needs to be inspected with the same frequency and vigor as the recipient site.

Recipient site complications are similar to those seen with other head and neck surgery patients. Hematoma, salivary fistula, infection, and wound dehiscence can occur at any time and require rapid detection and intervention. In the radiated patient, large vessel protection is important. If these occur close to the free flap pedicle, rapid flap compromise can occur. Healthy non-irradiated vascularized tissue in the heavily irradiated recipient bed can help minimized wound complications.[186]

In the animal model, ingrowth of collateral vessels may keep an inset free flap viable, independent of the pedicle as early as 8 days.[19] Microvascular surgeons do not rely on adequate recipient bed neovascularization until 3 to 4 weeks, and probably longer in the previously irradiated patient. The bony portion of some osteocutaneous free flaps may have even longer or permanent dependence on the pedicle blood supply. Postoperative pedicle compromise should be rapidly reversed, and prolonged ischemia leads to at least partial necrosis. After approximately 12 hours of ischemia, even with reestablishment of anastomotic flow, the free flap is usually not salvageable.[120] The ischemia tolerance of the flap tissues varies by patient and tissue type, and ischemia times may be much lower than the average, with capillary perfusion changes seen as early as 10 minutes after venous pedi-

cle occlusion.[64,134,150] Arterial insufficiency is less tolerated than venous insufficiency. Most microvascular surgeons do not like ischemia times beyond a couple hours at most. Ischemic tolerance is generally less with bowel mucosa and muscle, intermediate with skin, and longest with bone. Additionally, flap compromise later in the hospital stay tends to be more difficult to reverse. Flap monitoring is usually more relaxed, resulting in a longer undetected ischemia time. Pedicle compromise is also usually caused by localized purulence, which may have a long-term effect on the pedicle and anastomotic patency.

Most free flap anastomotic ischemic complications occur within the first 48 to 72 hours. In a large series, the need for pedicle re-exploration or revision occurs approximately 8 to 9% of the time, with an overall flap loss rate of 1 to 11%.[†] Venous anastomotic thrombosis is most common, but if not remedied, both outflow and inflow will be compromised.[55,111] Early venous congestion may affect the more distal monitoring paddle, if present, before the main flap paddle, because of the proximity of the monitoring paddle to the venous anastomosis. Thus, early venous congestion changes in the monitoring paddle should be taken very seriously. Venous anastomotic thrombosis results in an increased flap turgor, rapid capillary refill with brisk bleeding of darker blood, and finally darkening and mottling of the skin paddle. Venous congestion may present with any or all of these changes, with color changes usually being a later sign. The arterial pulse can still be felt until the later stages. Arterial insufficiency presents as a profound paleness and coolness, loss of flap turgor, and absence of any capillary refill or bleeding to pinprick. Usually only a serous bubble, if anything, arises from a pinprick or cut. The superficial pedicle is no longer palpable or Dopplerable. Examination and changes in free muscle flaps are more difficult to determine than in fasciocutaneous flaps. Buried flaps again require an external monitor paddle for monitoring.[41]

Oxygen free radical injury, as well as other etiologies, contribute to flap damage from flap reperfusion after a period of ischemia.[9,30,105] Despite the injury from reperfusion, upon detection of pedicle insufficiency, rapid intervention is required to re-establish flap perfusion if the flap is to be salvaged. This may include bedside maneuvers such as suture release, drain stripping, or opening the neck incision, as the ability to get the patient to the sterile operating theater is not always immediate. Time is of the essence, especially in cases of arterial insufficiency. The patient is urgently brought back to the operating room, the neck reopened and the anastomoses explored. Not only is

---

*References 62, 65, 90, 99, 133, 152.

†References 20, 22, 77, 87, 198, 199, 204.

attention focused on reestablishing blood flow, but the inciting factor must also be corrected to prevent recurrence (e.g., evacuation of hematoma, pedicle geometry improvement, etc.). In the case of isolated venous outflow thrombosis, the venous anastomosis should be investigated and thrombectomy and thrombolysis performed. With arterial pedicle thrombosis, both anastomosis need to be taken down and revised after thrombectomy. The arterial anastomoses are then revised and thrombolysis is performed before the revision of the venous anastomosis. The timing of the release of the recipient artery vascular clamp and reestablishment of blood flow remains controversial.[192] Copious heparinized lidocaine irrigation is used throughout to help extract gross thrombus from the pedicle. Clot should be atraumatically "milked" or pulled from all arteries and veins. Fogarty catheters may also be useful. The vessels should be trimmed back to a fresh clean edge. Alternatively, new recipient vessels or vein grafts should be concurrently prepared if needed to avoid future thrombosis.

Thrombolysis is facilitated with injections of streptokinase (75,000–125,000 units/injection) or urokinase (100,000 u) using a fresh 30-gauge needle while the recipient artery is atraumatically clamped.[158] This is performed near the arterial anastomosis in case some intimal damage is caused by the penetrating needle requiring the anastomosis to be revised again. Micro catheterization of a side branch is also possible for instillation. The arterial clamp is then removed and the effluent from the donor vein collected on a sponge and discarded. This prevents systemic circulation of the agent and generalized bleeding complications. This procedure is repeated until normal venous outflow is reestablished out the donor vein. Directional massage of the flap paddle can assist this process. Once flow has been reestablished and directly observed for a period of time exiting from the donor vein, the venous anastomosis is revised. The efficacy of thrombolytic therapy remains controversial with early detection and treatment being the most important factor in flap salvage.[220] The patient is then anti-coagulated with heparin to varying degrees depending on the surgeon's preference.[91]

The use of medicinal leeches is indicated for cases of flap venous congestion in which surgical salvage has been attempted, but inadequate in reestablishing full venous outflow.[37] Prolonged leech usage has resulted in some salvage success, but requires an intense protocol. Leech use is also indicated as a temporary measure to relieve venous congestion until the patient can be brought to the operating room. This requires immediate access to medicinal leeches from the inpatient pharmacy, which may not be available in every institution. Leeches are generally available within 24 hours from a national supplier. Leeches produce both hementin and hirudin which provide local anesthesia and anticoagulation properties to the leech bite. The leech also harbors a gram-negative beta-lactamase-producing organism that requires antibiotic prophylaxis to prevent soft tissue infection and necrosis. Significant blood loss can require multiple transfusions, and wayward leeches can attach to other body areas or personnel.

Even the best salvage efforts can result in either partial or total free flap loss. A partially necrotic flap may be left to demarcate the necrotic from viable portions of the flap assuming the pedicle or major vessels are not at risk during this period. Generally, the tissues furthest from the pedicle are at highest risk. These necrotic areas should be eventually débrided down to healthy bleeding tissue. The resulting defect may be left to granulate or be replaced with other tissue depending on its size and location. Total flap necrosis should be resected in a timely fashion because of the risk of salivary contamination, infection, and disseminated intravascular coagulation. For a time the flap can act as a non-vascularized biological dressing until the patient is medically stabilized and maximized for the necessary revision surgery. The resultant defect is either reconstructed with an alternative less optimal pedicled or free flap depending on the specific patient situation.[213] One alternative with varying success after composite resection is to leave the fixated non-vascularized bone in place after loss of an osteocutaneous free flap. This then requires coverage with a healthy vascularized flap, separating the bone graft from oral contamination (i.e., pedicled pectoralis major myocutaneous flap).

Costs and Outcomes

In addition to the expertise, microvascular reconstructions require significant healthcare resources, including time, equipment, and personnel.[137] The actual costs of microvascular reconstruction are generally comparable to other techniques, with costs being more dependent on comorbidities and disease extent.[61,108,121,196]

With widespread use, further prospective evidence-based evaluation of current reconstructive techniques is warranted. As new outcome assessment tools become available, function and quality of life after microvascular reconstruction will be increasingly investigated. Focus needs to be placed on very specific anatomic areas of reconstruction rather than on a general comparison of all oral cavity, oropharyngeal, and laryngeal areas. Comparisons, mostly retrospective, with alternative forms of reconstruction, including prosthetic rehabilitation and pedicled tissue reconstruction, shows mostly improved results after microvascular reconstruction.* These investigations should also include long-term outcomes.[88] Further comparison with results after organ preservation protocols or previous reconstruction also requires further study.[18,167]

FUTURE DIRECTIONS IN FREE TISSUE TRANSFER

Enhancements to current microvascular techniques are currently being developed. Improvements in the speed of anastomoses, such as mechanical anastomotic devices, have to be matched with the equivalency of patency rates. Currently, they have been most useful with venous anastomoses, but the technique is not universally accepted by microvascular surgeons. New, less invasive, but equally successful techniques for use in all anastomoses, including the end-to-side and lumen mismatch situations need to be developed. If equally effective, these techniques may increase the overall number of centers in which microvascular reconstruction is available. Similarly, new pharmacologic agents are being investigated to assist with decreasing anastomotic thrombosis rates.[12,40]

Minimally invasive harvest techniques have been developed for some free flap donor sites, including the jejunum, gracilis, omentum, rectus abdominis, temporoparietal, and latissimus dorsi.[42,94,114,156,209] Although less scarring and potentially less donor-site morbidity results, the increased harvest times currently required can be detrimental. Multiinstitutional experience needs to be studied as these techniques become increasingly attempted before determining comparability with current harvest techniques.[54] Endoscopic harvest of saphenous vein grafts has gained some acceptance in cardiac surgery and may also be an option for the microvascular surgeon.[97]

Allograft transplantation of whole head and neck organs has gained some media attention recently. The clinical experience is very early and the necessary induced immunodeficiency certainly has serious implications for the head and neck cancer patient. Also, return of adequate native organ function still needs to be demonstrated experimentally before clinical applicability in non-oncologic reconstructions.[173]

New applications and enhancements of current techniques, as well as new donor sites, need to be developed. Discovering new indications for current free flaps should always be encouraged, including indications such as laryngoplasty and tracheal reconstruction.[16] The use of prefabricated reconstructions and hybrid alloplast, or bioengineered tissue reconstructions, is slowly gaining momentum.[7,29,71,82,175,210] Prefabricating or pre laminating an intended free flap into a more ideal reconstruction can possibly improve the overall aesthetic and functional result, but may be limited by the preparation time required, especially in oncologic patients.[3,140,141,146] A combination of free flap reconstructions with current and future alloplastic materials may provide even more expanded indications.[56,85,166] Improved aesthetic and functional outcome may be possible as new combinations are developed. These techniques should also help minimize subsequent "fine-tuning" operations that are frequently necessary to maximize overall cosmetic and functional outcomes.

REFERENCES

1. Adams WP and others: Patency of different arterial and venous end-to-side microanastomosis techniques in a rat model, *Plast Reconstr Surg* 105:156-161, 2000.
2. Aguirre A and others: Serendipitous diagnosis of protein S deficiency, *J Periodontol* 73:1197-1201, 2002.
3. Akin S: Burned ear reconstruction using a prefabricated free radial forearm flap, *J Reconstr Microsurg* 17:233-236, 2001.
4. Al Qattan MM, Bowen V: Effect of pre-existing health conditions on the results of reconstructive microvascular surgery, *Microsurgery* 14:152, 1993.
5. Alberdas JL, Shibahara T, Noma H: Histopathologic damage to vessels in head and neck microsurgery, *J Oral Maxillofac Surg* 61:191-196, 2003.
6. Anthony JP and others: Donor leg morbidity and function after fibula free flap mandible reconstruction, *Plast Reconstr Surg* 96:146-152, 1995.
7. Antohi N, Stan V, Nitescu C: One-stage reconstruction of facial paralysis associated with severe skin scar deformity, using combined flexor carpi radialis muscle and radial forearm free flap, *Microsurgery* 23:194-197, 2003.
8. Antohi N and others: Free flaps for type III complex pharyngoesophageal defects after enlarged ablative surgery for advanced cancer of larynx and hypopharynx, *Microsurgery* 23:189-193, 2003.
9. Askar I, Bozkurt M: Protective effects of immunosuppressants and steroids against ischemia-reperfusion injury in cremaster muscle flap at microcirculatory level, *Microsurgery* 22:361-366, 2002.
10. Aviv JE and others: The combined latissimus dorsi-scapular free flap in head and neck reconstruction, *Arch Otolaryngol Head Neck Surg* 117:1242-1250, 1991.
11. Ayala C, Blackwell KE: Protein C deficiency in microvascular head and neck reconstruction, *Laryngoscope* 109:259-265, 1999.
12. Azizzadeh B and others: Inhibitors of nitric oxide promote microvascular thrombosis, *Arch Facial Plast Surg* 5:31-35, 2003.
13. Banic A and others: Effects of sodium nitroprusside and phenylephrine on blood flow in free musculocutaneous flaps during general anesthesia, *Anesthesiology* 90:147-155, 1999.
14. Bardsley AF and others: Reducing morbidity in the radial forearm flap donor site, *Plast Reconstr Surg* 86:287-294, 1990.
15. Beausang ES and others: Microvascular free tissue transfer in elderly patients: the Toronto experience, *Head Neck* 25:549-553, 2003.
16. Beldholm BR and others: Reconstruction of the trachea with a tubed radial forearm free flap *J Thorac Cardiovasc Surg* 126:545-550, 2003.

---

*References 67, 76, 92, 93, 103, 157, 161, 174, 196.

17. Benazzo M and others: Voice restoration after circumferential pharyngolaryngectomy with free jejunum repair, *Eur Arch Otorhinolaryngol* 258:173-176, 2001.

18. Berthe JV and others: Do multiple consecutive head and neck reconstructions improve the patients functional outcome? *Acta Otorhinolaryngol Belg* 56:391-397, 2002.

19. Black MJM and others: How soon may the axial vessels of a surviving free flap be safely ligated: a study in pigs, *Br J Plast Surg* 31:295, 1978.

20. Blackwell KE: Unsurpassed reliability of free flaps for head and neck reconstruction, *Arch Otolaryngol Head Neck Surg* 125:295-299, 1999.

21. Blackwell KE and others: Octogenarian free flap reconstruction: complications and cost of therapy, *Otolaryngol Head Neck Surg* 126:301-306, 2002.

22. Blackwell KE, Brown MT, Gonzalez D: Overcoming the learning curve in microvascular head and neck reconstruction, *Arch Otolaryngol Head Neck Surg* 123: 1332-1335, 1997.

23. Blackwell KE, Lacombe V: The bridging lateral mandibular reconstruction plate revisited, *Arch Otolaryngol Head Neck Surg* 125:988-993, 1999.

24. Bodde EW and others: Donor-site morbidity after free vascularized autogenous fibular transfer: subjective and quantitative analyses, *Plast Reconstr Surg* 111:2237-2242, 2003.

25. Boeckx WF, De Lorenzi F, van der Hulst R: Increasing the flow output by Y-shaped microvascular anastomosis, *J Reconstr Microsurg* 18:381-386, 2002.

26. Boorman JG, Brown JA, Sykes PJ: Morbidity in the forearm flap donor arm, *Br J Plast Surg* 40:207-212, 1987.

27. Braun SA and others: The optimal sequence of microvascular repair during prolonged clamping in free flap transfer, *Plast Reconstr Surg* 111:233-241, 2003.

28. Buckley RC, Davidson SF, Das SK: The role of various antithrombotic agents in microvascular surgery *Br J Plast Surg* 47:20-23, 1994.

29. Bunaprasert T and others: Tissue engineered muscle implantation for tongue reconstruction: a preliminary report, *Laryngoscope* 113:1792-1797, 2003.

30. Carroll WR, Esclamado RM: Ischemia/reperfusion injury in microvascular surgery, *Head Neck* 22:700-713, 2000.

31. Carroll WR and others: Three-dose vs extended-course clindamycin prophylaxis for free-flap reconstruction of the head and neck, *Arch Otolaryngol Head Neck Surg* 129: 771-774, 2003.

32. Chaikhouni A and others: Latissimus dorsi free myocutaneous flap, *J Trauma* 21:398-402, 1981.

33. Chalian AA and others: Internal jugular vein versus external jugular vein anastomosis: implications for successful free tissue transfer, *Head Neck* 23:475-478, 2001.

34. Chalian AA and others: Design and impact of intraoperative pathways for head and neck resection and reconstruction, *Arch Otolaryngol Head Neck Surg* 128:892-896, 2002.

35. Chandrasekhar B, Lorant JA, Terz JJ: Parascapular free flaps for head and neck reconstruction, *Am J Surg* 160:450-453, 1990.

36. Chang YM and others: Osteotomy to treat malocclusion following reconstruction of the mandible with the free fibula flap, *Plast Reconstr Surg* 112:31-36, 2003.

37. Chepeha DB and others: Leech therapy for patients with surgically unsalvageable venous obstruction after revascularized free tissue transfer, *Arch Otolaryngol Head Neck Surg* 128:960-965, 2002.

38. Chiang S, Cohen B, Blackwell K: Myocardial infarction after microvascular head and neck reconstruction, *Laryngoscope* 112:1849-1852, 2002.

39. Chicarilli ZN, Ariyan S, Cuono CB: Free radial forearm flap versatility for the head and neck and lower extremity, *J Reconstr Microsurg* 2:221-228, 1986.

40. Ching S and others: Inhibition of microsurgical thrombosis by the platelet glycoprotein IIb/IIIa antagonist SR121566A, *Plast Reconstr Surg* 112:177-185, 2003.

41. Cho BC and others: Monitoring flap for buried free tissue transfer: its importance and reliability, *Plast Reconstr Surg* 110:1249-1258, 2002.

42. Chung KC, Cederna PS: Endoscopic harvest of temporoparietal fascial free flaps for coverage of hand wounds, *J Hand Surg [Am]* 27:525-533, 2002.

43. Civantos FJ: Latissimus dorsi microvascular flap, *Facial Plast Surg* 12:65-68, 1996.

44. Civantos FJ Jr. and others: Lateral arm microvascular flap in head and neck reconstruction, *Arch Otolaryngol Head Neck Surg* 123:830-836, 1997.

45. Conrad MH, Adams WP Jr.: Pharmacologic optimization of microsurgery in the new millennium *Plast Reconstr Surg* 108:2088-2097, 2001.

46. Cooley BC and others: The influence of diabetes on free flap transfer: I. flap survival and microvascular healing, *Ann Plast Surg* 29:58, 1992.

47. Cope C and others: Use of the vascular closure staple clip applier for microvascular anastomosis in free-flap surgery, *Plast Reconstr Surg* 106:107-110, 2000.

48. Davidson J and others: A comparison of the results following oromandibular reconstruction using a radial forearm flap with either radial bone or a reconstruction plate, *Plast Reconstr Surg* 88:201-208, 1991.

49. De Lorenzi F, van der Hulst RR, Boeckx WJ: VCS auto suture stapled microvascular anastomoses in lower leg free flaps, *Plast Reconstr Surg* 109:2023-2030, 2002.

50. Deschler DG and others: Tracheoesophageal voice following tubed free radial forearm flap reconstruction of the neopharynx, *Ann Otol Rhinol Laryngol* 103:929-936, 1994.

51. Desyatnikova S and others: Effect of anemia on the fasciocutaneous flap survival in a rat model, *Laryngoscope* 111:572-575, 2001.

52. Disa JJ and others: Microvascular reconstruction of the hypopharynx: defect classification, treatment algorithm, and functional outcome based on 165 consecutive cases, *Plast Reconstr Surg* 111:652-663, 2003.

53. Disa JJ and others: Simplifying microvascular head and neck reconstruction: a rational approach to donor site selection, *Ann Plast Surg* 47:385-389, 2001.

54. El-Shazly MM and others: Microscopic vs. endoscopic assisted harvesting and transplantation of free groin flaps: a comparative experimental study in the rat model, *Microsurgery* 22:347-351, 2002.

55. Esclamado RM, Carroll WR: The pathogenesis of vascular thrombosis and its impact in microvascular surgery, *Head Neck* 21:355-362, 1999.

56. Eufinger H, Wehmoller M: Microsurgical tissue transfer and individual computer-aided designed and manufactured prefabricated titanium implants for complex craniofacial reconstruction, *Scand J Plast Reconstr Surg Hand Surg* 36: 326-331, 2002.

57. Farwell DG, Futran ND: Oromandibular reconstruction, *Facial Plast Surg* 16:115-126, 2000.

58. Fong BP, Funk GF: Osseous free tissue transfer in head and neck reconstruction, *Facial Plast Surg* 15:45-59, 1999.

59. Frodel JL Jr. and others: Osseointegrated implants: a comparative study of bone thickness in four vascularized bone flaps, *Plast Reconstr Surg* 92:449-458, 1993.

60. Funk GF: Scapular and parascapular free flaps, *Facial Plast Surg* 12:57-63, 1996.

61. Funk GF and others: Free tissue transfer versus pedicled flap cost in head and neck cancer, *Otolaryngol Head Neck Surg* 127:205-212, 2002.

62. Futran ND and others: Green light photoplethysmography monitoring of free flaps, *Arch Otolaryngol Head Neck Surg* 126:659-662, 2000.

63. Futran ND, Stack BC Jr., Zachariah AP: Ankle-arm index as a screening examination for fibula free tissue transfer, *Ann Otol Rhinol Laryngol* 108:777-780, 1999.

64. Gabriel A and others: Effect of total venous occlusion on capillary flow and necrosis in skeletal muscle, *Plast Reconstr Surg* 108:430-433, 2001.

65. Gaggl A and others: Assessment of perfusion of facial microvascular transplants and early detection of ischemia by perfusion-CT scan, *Oral Surg Oral Med Oral Pathol Oral Radiol Endod* 94:425-431, 2002.

66. Gallivan KH, Reiter D: Acute alcohol withdrawal and free flap mandibular reconstruction outcomes, *Arch Facial Plast Surg* 3:264-266, 2001.

67. Genden EM and others: Comparison of functional and quality-of-life outcomes in patients with and without palatomaxillary reconstruction: a preliminary report, *Arch Otolaryngol Head Neck Surg* 129:775-780, 2003.

68. Godden DR and others: Catecholamine sensitivity in the rat femoral artery after microvascular anastomosis, *Microsurgery* 20:217-220, 2000.

69. Gopinath KS and others: The scapular fasciocutaneous flap: a new flap for reconstruction of the posterior neck, *Br J Plast Surg* 46:508-510, 1993.

70. Granick MS, Newton ED, Hanna DC: Scapular free flap for repair of massive lower facial composite defects, *Head Neck Surg* 8:436-441, 1986.

71. Haas F and others: Free osteocutaneous lateral arm flap: Anatomy and clinical applications, *Microsurgery* 23:87-95, 2003.

72. Harii K, Ohmori K, Ohmori S: Free deltopectoral skin flaps, *Br J Plast Surg* 24:231, 1974.

73. Harris JR and others: The thoracoacromial/cephalic vascular system for microvascular anastomoses in the vessel-depleted neck, *Arch Otolaryngol Head Neck Surg* 128:319-323, 2002.

74. Harris JR and others: Effect of diameter of microvascular interposition vein grafts on vessel patency and free flap survival in the rat model, *J Otolaryngol* 28:152-157, 1999.

75. Haughey BH: The jejunal free flap in oral cavity and pharyngeal reconstruction, *Otolaryngol Clin North Am* 27:1159-1170, 1994.

76. Haughey BH, Taylor SM, Fuller D: Fasciocutaneous flap reconstruction of the tongue and floor of mouth: outcomes and techniques, *Arch Otolaryngol Head Neck Surg* 128:1388-1395, 2002.

77. Haughey BH and others: Free flap reconstruction of the head and neck: analysis of 241 cases, *Otolaryngol Head Neck Surg* 125:10-17, 2001.

78. Haughey BH, Wilson EA: Fibula free flap, *Facial Plast Surg* 12:51-56, 1996.

79. Head C and others: Microvascular flap reconstruction of the mandible: a comparison of bone grafts and bridging plates for restoration of mandibular continuity, *Otolaryngol Head Neck Surg* 129:48-54, 2003.

80. Head C and others: Microvascular reconstruction after previous neck dissection, *Arch Otolaryngol Head Neck Surg* 128:328-331, 2002.

81. Heitmann C, Khan FN, Levin LS: Vasculature of the peroneal artery: an anatomic study focused on the perforator vessels, *J Reconstr Microsurg* 19:157-162, 2003.

82. Hennerbichler A and others: Lateral arm flap: Analysis of its anatomy and modification using a vascularized fragment of the distal humerus, *Clin Anat* 16:204-214, 2003.

83. Hentz VR and others: The radial forearm flap: a versatile source of composite tissue, *Ann Plast Surg* 19:485-498, 1987.

84. Herford AS, Ellis ER: Use of a locking reconstruction bone plate/screw system for mandibular surgery, J Oral Maxillofac Surg 56:1261-1265, 1998.

85. Heth JA and others: Free tissue transfer and local flap complications in anterior and anterolateral skull base surgery, *Head Neck* 24:901-912, 2002.

86. Hidalgo DA: Fibula free flap: a new method of mandible reconstruction, *Plast Reconstr Surg* 84:71-79, 1989.

87. Hidalgo DA and others: A review of 716 consecutive free flaps for oncologic surgical defects: refinement in donor-site selection and technique, *Plast Reconstr Surg* 102:722-734, 1998.

88. Hidalgo DA, Pusic AL: Free-flap mandibular reconstruction: a 10-year follow-up study, *Plast Reconstr Surg* 110:438-451, 2002.

89. Hiebert CA, Cumings GO: Successful replacement of the cervical esophagus by transplantation and revascularization of a free graft of gastric antrum, *Ann Surg* 154:103, 1961.

90. Hirigoyen MB, Urken ML, Weinberg H: Free flap monitoring: a review of current practice, *Microsurgery* 16:723-727, 1995.

91. Hirigoyen MB and others: Additional benefit of heparin in the thrombolytic salvage of ischemic skin flaps, *Ann Plast Surg* 35:612-619, 1995.

92. Hsiao HT and others: Swallowing function in patients who underwent hemiglossectomy: comparison of primary closure and free radial forearm flap reconstruction with videofluoroscopy, *Ann Plast Surg* 50:450-455, 2003.

93. Hsiao HT, Leu YS, Lin CC: Primary closure versus radial forearm flap reconstruction after hemiglossectomy: functional assessment of swallowing and speech, *Ann Plast Surg* 49:612-616, 2002.

94. Jackson IT, Miyawaki T: Endoscopic harvest of free temporoparietal fascial flap to improve donor-site morbidity, *Plast Reconstr Surg* 109:826, 2002.

95. Jallali N: Dextrans in microsurgery: a review, *Microsurgery* 23:78-80, 2003.

96. Johnson PC, Barker JH: Thrombosis and antithrombotic therapy in microvascular surgery, *Clin Plast Surg* 19:799, 1992.

97. Jordan WD Jr, Goldberg SP: Video-assisted endoscopic saphenous vein harvest: an evolving technique, *Semin Vasc Surg* 13:32-39, 2000.

98. Kakibuchi M and others: Functional reconstruction of maxilla with free latissimus dorsi-scapular osteomusculocutaneous flap, *Plast Reconstr Surg* 109:1238-1245, 2002.

99. Kamolz LP and others: Continuous free-flap monitoring with tissue-oxygen measurements: three-year experience, *J Reconstr Microsurg* 18:487-493, 2002.

100. Kaplan EN, Buncke HJ, Murray DE: Distant transfer of cutaneous island flaps in humans by microvascular anastomosis, *Plast Reconstr Surg* 52:301, 1973.

101. Khouri RK and others: Thrombosis of microvascular anastomoses in traumatized vessels: Firbrin versus platelets, *Plast Reconstr Surg* 86:110, 1990.

102. Khouri RK and others: A prospective study of microvascular free-flap surgery and outcome, *Plast Reconstr Surg* 102: 711-721, 1998.

103. King TW and others: Aesthetic and functional outcomes using osseous or soft tissue free flaps, *J Reconstr Microsurg* 18:365-371, 2002.

104. Kinishi M, Amatsu M, Tahara S: Further experience with tracheojejunal shunt speech after pharyngolaryngoesophagectomy, *Ann Otol Rhinol Laryngol* 110:41-44, 2001.

105. Klein MB, Chan PH, Chang J: Protective effects of superoxide dismutase against ischemia-reperfusion injury: development and application of a transgenic animal model, *Plast Reconstr Surg* 111:251-257, 2003.

106. Klein MB and others: Early experience with computed tomographic angiography in microsurgical reconstruction, *Plast Reconstr Surg* 112:498-503, 2003.

107. Klein S and others: Ankle-arm index versus angiography for the pre assessment of the fibula free flap, *Plast Reconstr Surg* 111:735-743, 2003.

108. Kroll SS and others: A comparison of resource costs for head and neck reconstruction with free and pectoralis major flaps, *Plast Reconstr Surg* 99:1282-1286, 1997.

109. Kroll SS and others: Does prior irradiation increase the risk of total or partial free-flap loss? *J Reconstr Microsurg* 14:263-268, 1998.

110. Kroll SS and others: Choice of flap and incidence of free flap success, *Plast Reconstr Surg* 98:459-463, 1996.

111. Kubo T, Yano K, Hosokawa K: Management of flaps with compromised venous outflow in head and neck microsurgical reconstruction, *Microsurgery* 22:391-395, 2002.

112. Kuriakose MA and others: Sensate radial forearm free flaps in tongue reconstruction, *Arch Otolaryngol Head Neck Surg* 127:1463-1466, 2001.

113. Lauer G and others: A clinical audit on the effect of suction drainage on microvascular anastomosis, *J Craniomaxillofac Surg* 29:298-301, 2001.

114. Lin CH, Wei FC, Lin YT: Conventional versus endoscopic free gracilis muscle harvest, *Plast Reconstr Surg* 105:89-93, 2000.

115. Lorenz RR, Esclamado R: Preoperative magnetic resonance angiography in fibular-free flap reconstruction of head and neck defects, *Head Neck* 23:844-850, 2001.

116. Lorenzetti F and others: Evaluation of blood flow in free microvascular flaps, *J Reconstr Microsurg* 17:163-167, 2001.

117. Lutz BS and others: Routine donor leg angiography before vascularized free fibula transplantation is not necessary: a prospective study in 120 clinical cases, *Plast Reconstr Surg* 103:121-127, 1999.

118. Lydiatt DD and others: The team concept in mandibular reconstruction after ablative oncologic surgery, *J Oral Maxillofac Surg* 58:607-610, 2000.

119. Mange N and others: Comparison between nasogastric tube feeding and percutaneous fluoroscopic gastrostomy in advanced head and neck cancer patients, *Eur Arch Otorhinolaryngol* 258:89-92, 2001.

120. May JW and others: The no-reflow phenomenon in experimental free flap, *Plast Reconstr Surg* 61:256, 1978.

121. McCrory AL, Magnuson JS: Free tissue transfer versus pedicled flap in head and neck reconstruction, *Laryngoscope* 112:2161-2165, 2002.

122. Meland NB and others: Experience with 80 rectus abdominis free-tissue transfers, *Plast Reconstr Surg* 83:481-487, 1989.

123. Meland NB and others: The radial forearm flap: a biomechanical study of donor-site morbidity utilizing sheep tibia, *Plast Reconstr Surg* 90:763-773, 1992.

124. Militsakh O and others: Use of 2.0 mm locking reconstruction plate system in oromandibular reconstruction, *Otolaryngol Head Neck Surg* 2003.

125. Miller MJ and others: Interposition vein grafting in head and neck reconstructive microsurgery, *J Reconstr Microsurg* 9:245-252, 1993.

126. Moscoso JF and others: Vascularized bone flaps in oromandibular reconstruction. A comparative anatomic study of bone stock from various donor sites to assess suitability for enosseous dental implants, *Arch Otolaryngol Head Neck Surg* 120:36-43, 1994.

127. Muhammad JK and others: The effect of head rotation on the diameter of the internal jugular vein: implications for free tissue transfer, *J Craniomaxillofac Surg* 29:214-218, 2001.

128. Muldowney JB and others: Oral cavity reconstruction using the free radial forearm flap, *Arch Otolaryngol Head Neck Surg* 113:1219-1224, 1987.

129. Nagler RM and others: Spiral CT angiography: an alternative vascular evaluation technique for head and neck microvascular reconstruction, *Plast Reconstr Surg* 100:1697-1702, 1997.

130. Nakayama B and others: Usefulness of a first transferred free flap vascular pedicle for secondary microvascular reconstruction in the head and neck, *Plast Reconstr Surg* 109:1246-1253, 2002.

131. Neligan PC, She-Yue H, Gullane PJ: Reverse flow as an option in microvascular recipient anastomoses, *Plast Reconstr Surg* 100:1780-1787, 1997.

132. Nuckols DA and others: Preoperative evaluation of the radial forearm free flap patient with the objective Allen's test, *Otolaryngol Head Neck Surg* 123:553-557, 2000.

133. Numata T and others: Usefulness of color Doppler sonography for assessing hemodynamics of free flaps for head and neck reconstruction, *Ann Plast Surg* 48:607-612, 2002.

134. Olivas TP and others: Timing of microcirculatory injury from ischemia reperfusion, *Plast Reconstr Surg* 107:785-788, 2001.

135. Panje WR, Bardach J, Krause CJ: Reconstruction of the oral cavity with a free flap, *Plast Reconstr Surg* 58:415-418, 1976.

136. Papadopulos NA and others: Donor site morbidity after harvest of free osteofasciocutaneous fibular flaps with an extended skin island, *Ann Plast Surg* 49:138-144, 2002.

137. Petruzzelli GJ and others: The influence of reconstructive modality on cost of care in head and neck oncologic surgery, *Arch Otolaryngol Head Neck Surg* 128:1377-1380, 2002.

138. Petry JJ, French TS, Worthan KA: The effect of the "patency-test" on arterial endothelial surface, *Plast Reconstr Surg* 77:960, 1986.

139. Poli T and others: Primary oromandibular reconstruction using free flaps and THORP plates in cancer patients: a 5-year experience, *Head Neck* 25:15-23, 2003.

140. Pribaz JJ, Fine NA: Prefabricated and prelaminated flaps for head and neck reconstruction, *Clin Plast Surg* 28:261-272, 2001.

141. Pribaz JJ and others: Prelaminated free flap reconstruction of complex central facial defects, *Plast Reconstr Surg* 104:357-367, 1999.

142. Rees TD, Liverett DM, Guy CL: The effect of cigarette smoking on skin-flap survival in the face lift patient, *Plast Reconstr Surg* 73:911-915, 1984.

143. Reus, WF, Colen LB, Straker DJ: Tobacco smoking and complications in elective microsurgery *Plast Reconstr Surg* 89:490, 1992.

144. Rhee JS and others: Intraoperative mapping of sensate flaps. Electrophysiologic techniques and neuro somal boundaries, *Arch Otolaryngol Head Neck Surg* 123:823-829, 1997.

145. Robins DW: The anaesthetic management of patients undergoing free flap transfer, *Br J Plast Surg* 36:231, 1983.

146. Rohner D and others: Treatment of severe atrophy of the maxilla with the prefabricated free vascularized fibula flap, *Clin Oral Implants Res* 13: 44-52, 2002.

147. Ross DA and others: Use of the operating microscope and loupes for head and neck free microvascular tissue transfer: a retrospective comparison, *Arch Otolaryngol Head Neck Surg* 129:189-193, 2003.

148. Ross DA and others: The extended lateral arm free flap for head and neck reconstruction: the Yale experience, *Laryngoscope* 106:14-18, 1996.

149. Rumbolo PM and others: Comparison of the influence of intralumenal irrigation solutions on free flap survival, *Microsurgery* 13:45, 1992.

150. Salgado CJ and others: Effects of late loss of arterial inflow on free flap survival, *J Reconstr Microsurg* 18:579-584, 2002.

151. Sanders R, Mayou BJ: A new vascularized bone graft transferred by microvascular anastomosis as a free flap, *Br J Surg* 66:787-788, 1979.

152. Schon R and others: Color duplex sonography for the monitoring of vascularized free bone flaps, *Otolaryngol Head Neck Surg* 129:71-76, 2003.

153. Schultze-Mosgau S and others: Vascularization in the transition area between free grafted soft tissues and pre-irradiated graft bed tissues following preoperative radiotherapy in the head and neck region, *Head Neck* 24: 42-51, 2002.

154. Schultze-Mosgau S and others: Transforming growth factor beta1 and beta2 (TGFbeta2 / TGFbeta2) profile changes in previously irradiated free flap beds, *Head Neck* 24:33-41, 2002.

155. Seidenberg B and others: Immediate reconstruction of the cervical esophagus by a revascularized isolated jejunal segment, *Ann Surg* 149:162, 1959.

156. Seify H and others: Endoscopic harvest of four muscle flaps: safe and effective techniques, *Ann Plast Surg* 48:173-179, 2002.

157. Seikaly H and others: Functional outcomes after primary oropharyngeal cancer resection and reconstruction with the radial forearm free flap, *Laryngoscope* 113:897-904, 2003.

158. Serletti JM and others: Urokinase protocol for free-flap salvage following prolonged venous thrombosis, *Plast Reconstr Surg* 102:1947-1953, 1998.

159. Shangold LM, Urken ML, Lawson W: Jejunal transplantation for pharyngoesophageal reconstruction, *Otolaryngol Clin North Am* 24:1321-1342, 1991.

160. Shindo M and others: The fibula osteocutaneous flap in head and neck reconstruction: a critical evaluation of donor site morbidity, *Arch Otolaryngol Head Neck Surg* 126:1467-1472, 2000.

161. Shpitzer T and others: The free vascularized flap and the flap plate options: comparative results of reconstruction of lateral mandibular defects, *Laryngoscope* 110:2056-2060, 2000.

162. Shpitzer T and others: The free iliac crest and fibula flaps in vascularized oromandibular reconstruction: comparison and long-term evaluation, *Head Neck* 21:639-647, 1999.

163. Sigurdsson GH: Perioperative fluid management in microvascular surgery, *J Reconstr Microsurg* 11:57-65, 1995.

164. Sigurdsson GH, Thomson D: Anaesthesia and microvascular surgery: clinical practice and research, *Eur J Anaesthesiol* 12:101-122, 1995.

165. Simons JP and others: The role of topical antibiotic prophylaxis in patients undergoing contaminated head and neck surgery with flap reconstruction, *Laryngoscope* 111:329-335, 2001.

166. Sinha UK, Zim S, Maceri D: Frontotemporal reconstruction with hydroxyapatite cement and the radial forearm free flap, *Arch Facial Plast Surg* 3:271-276, 2001.

167. Skoner JM and others: Swallowing function and tracheotomy dependence after combined-modality treatment including free tissue transfer for advanced-stage oropharyngeal cancer, *Laryngoscope* 113:1294-1298, 2003.

168. Smith RB, Thomas RD, Funk GF: Fibula free flaps: the role of angiography in patients with abnormal results on preoperative color flow Doppler studies, *Arch Otolaryngol Head Neck Surg* 129:712-715, 2003.

169. Soutar DS, McGregor IA: The radial forearm flap in intraoral reconstruction: the experience of 60 consecutive cases, *Plast Reconstr Surg* 78:1-8, 1986.

170. Soutar DS and others: The radial forearm flap: a versatile method for intra-oral reconstruction, *Br J Plast Surg* 36:1-8, 1983.

171. Soutar DS, Widdowson WP: Immediate reconstruction of the mandible using a vascularized segment of radius, *Head Neck Surg* 8:232-246, 1986.

172. Strauch B and others: *Atlas of Microvascular Surgery.* New York, Thieme, 1993.

173. Strome M and others: Laryngeal transplantation and 40-month follow-up, *N Engl J Med* 344:1676-1679, 2001.

174. Su WF and others: Functional comparison after reconstruction with a radial forearm free flap or a pectoralis major flap for cancer of the tongue, *Otolaryngol Head Neck Surg* 128:412-418, 2003.

175. Sukkar SM, Saulis AS, Dumanian GA: Radial forearm skin with flexor carpi radialis muscle: a useful composite free flap, *Ann Plast Surg* 49:486-489, 2002.

176. Sullivan MJ, Baker S, editors: *Microsurgical reconstruction of the head and neck.* New York, Churchill Livingstone, 1989.

177. Sullivan MJ, Carroll WR, Baker SR: The cutaneous scapular free flap in head and neck reconstruction, *Arch Otolaryngol Head Neck Surg* 116:600-603, 1990.

178. Sullivan MJ and others: The free scapular flap for head and neck reconstruction, *Am J Otolaryngol* 11:318-327, 1990.

179. Sullivan MJ, Carroll WR, Kuriloff DB: Lateral arm free flap in head and neck reconstruction, *Arch Otolaryngol Head Neck Surg* 118:1095-1101, 1992.

180. Summers AN, Sanger JR, Matloub HS: Lateral arm fascial flap: micro arterial anatomy and potential clinical applications, *J Reconstr Microsurg* 16:279-286, 2000.

181. Swanson E, Boyd JB, Manktelow RT: The radial forearm flap: reconstructive applications and donor-site defects in 35 consecutive patients, *Plast Reconstr Surg* 85:258-266, 1990.

182. Swartz WM, Banis JC: *Head and neck microsurgery.* Baltimore, Williams & Wilkins, 1992.

183. Taylor GI, Corlett RJ, Boyd JB: The versatile deep inferior epigastric (inferior rectus abdominis) flap, *Br J Plast Surg* 37:330-350, 1984.

184. Taylor GI, Miller GD, Ham FJ: The free vascularized bone graft. A clinical extension of microvascular techniques, *Plast Reconstr Surg* 55:533-544, 1975.

185. Taylor GI, Townsend P, Corlett R: Superiority of the deep circumflex iliac vessels as the supply for free groin flaps, *Plast Reconstr Surg* 64:595-604, 1979.

186. Teknos TN and others: Free tissue reconstruction of the hypopharynx after organ preservation therapy: analysis of wound complications, *Laryngoscope* 111:1192-1196, 2001.

187. Teknos TN and others: Microvascular free tissue transfer in reconstructing skull base defects: lessons learned, *Laryngoscope* 112:1871-1876, 2002.

188. Teot L and others: The scapular crest pedicled bone graft, *Int J Microsurg* 3:257, 1981.

189. Theile DR and others: Free jejunal interposition reconstruction after pharyngolaryngectomy: 201 consecutive cases, *Head Neck* 17:83-88, 1995.

190. Thoma A and others: The free medial scapular osteofasciocutaneous flap for head and neck reconstruction, *Br J Plast Surg* 44:477-482, 1991.

191. Thoma A and others: Oromandibular reconstruction with the radial-forearm osteocutaneous flap: experience with 60 consecutive cases, *Plast Reconstr Surg* 104:368-380, 1999.

192. Thomson JG and others: The effect of prolonged clamping and vascular stasis on the patency of arterial and venous microanastomoses, *Ann Plast Surg* 40:436-441, 1998.

193. Timmons MJ: The vascular basis of the radial forearm flap, *Plast Reconstr Surg* 77:80-92, 1986.

194. Timmons MJ and others: Complications of radial forearm flap donor sites, *Br J Plast Surg* 39:176-178, 1986.

195. Triana RJ Jr. and others: Microvascular free flap reconstructive options in patients with partial and total maxillectomy defects, *Arch Facial Plast Surg* 2:91-101, 2000.

196. Tsue TT and others: Comparison of cost and function in reconstruction of the posterior oral cavity and oropharynx. Free vs pedicled soft tissue transfer, *Arch Otolaryngol Head Neck Surg* 123:731-737, 1997.

197. Tsue TT, Girod DA: *Osteocutaneous radial forearm flap*. In Branham GEA, editor: *Otolaryngology and Facial Plastic Surgery/Reconstructive Surgery*. eMedicine.com, Inc., Omaha, Nebraska, 2001.

198. Urken ML and others: The scapular osteofasciocutaneous flap: a 12-year experience, *Arch Otolaryngol Head Neck Surg* 127:862-869, 2001.

199. Urken ML and others: Oromandibular reconstruction using microvascular composite flaps: report of 210 cases, *Arch Otolaryngol Head Neck Surg* 124:46-55, 1998.

200. Urken ML and others: Primary placement of osseointegrated implants in microvascular mandibular reconstruction, *Otolaryngol Head Neck Surg* 101:56-73, 1989.

201. Urken ML and others: Functional evaluation following microvascular oromandibular reconstruction of the oral cancer patient: a comparative study of reconstructed and non reconstructed patients, *Laryngoscope* 101:935-950, 1991.

202. Urken ML and others: The rectus abdominis free flap in head and neck reconstruction, *Arch Otolaryngol Head Neck Surg* 117:1031, 1991.

203. Urken ML and others: The internal oblique-iliac crest osteomyocutaneous free flap in oromandibular reconstruction. Report of 20 cases, *Arch Otolaryngol Head Neck Surg* 115:339-349, 1989.

204. Urken ML and others: Microvascular free flaps in head and neck reconstruction. Report of 200 cases and review of complications, *Arch Otolaryngol Head Neck Surg* 120:633-640, 1994.

205. Urken ML and others: Using the iliac crest free flap, *Plast Reconstr Surg* 85:1001-1002, 1990.

206. Urken ML and others: The internal oblique-iliac crest free flap in composite defects of the oral cavity involving bone, skin, and mucosa, *Laryngoscope* 101:257-270, 1991.

207. Vance JP, Soutar D: *General anaesthesia for microvascular surgery*. In Soutar DS, editor: *Microvascular surgery and free tissue transfer*. Boston, Little, Brown, 1993.

208. Vesper M and others: Clinical and histological results of sensory recovery after radial forearm flap transfer, *Clin Oral Investig* 6:114-118, 2002.

209. Wadsworth JT, Futran N, Eubanks TR: Laparoscopic harvest of the jejunal free flap for reconstruction of hypopharyngeal and cervical esophageal defects, *Arch Otolaryngol Head Neck Surg* 128:1384-1387, 2002.

210. Wax MK and others: The ulnar fasciocutaneous free flap in head and neck reconstruction, *Laryngoscope* 112:2155-2160, 2002.

211. Weber RA, Pederson WC: Skin paddle salvage in the fibula osteocutaneous free flap with secondary skin paddle vascular anastomosis, *J Reconstr Microsurg* 11:239-244, 1995.

212. Wei FC and others: Complications after reconstruction by plate and soft tissue free flap in composite mandibular defects and secondary salvage reconstruction with osteocutaneous flap, *Plast Reconstr Surg* 112:37-42, 2003.

213. Wei FC and others: The outcome of failed free flaps in head and neck and extremity reconstruction: what is next in the reconstructive ladder? *Plast Reconstr Surg* 108:1154-1162, 2001.

214. Weinfeld AB and others: Management of alcohol withdrawal in microvascular head and neck reconstruction, *J Reconstr Microsurg* 16:201-206, 2000.

215. Wenig BL: The lateral arm free flap for head and neck reconstruction, *Otolaryngol Head Neck Surg* 109:116-119, 1993.

216. Werle AH and others: Osteocutaneous radial forearm free flap: its use without significant donor site morbidity, *Otolaryngol Head Neck Surg* 123:711-717, 2000.

217. Winters HA, de Jongh GJ: Reliability of the proximal skin paddle of the osteocutaneous free fibula flap: a prospective clinical study, *Plast Reconstr Surg* 103:846-849, 1999.

218. Yamamoto Y and others: Superiority of end-to-side anastomosis with the internal jugular vein: the experience of 80 cases in head and neck microsurgical reconstruction, *Br J Plast Surg* 52:88-91, 1999.

219. Yamamoto Y and others: The combined flap based on a single vascular source: a clinical experience with 32 cases, *Plast Reconstr Surg* 97:1385-1390, 1996.

220. Yii NW and others: Thrombolytic therapy: what is its role in free flap salvage? *Ann Plast Surg* 46:601-604, 2001.

221. Yugueros P, Finical SJ, Johnson CH: Use of microvascular free-tissue transfer following ablative surgery of the skull base, *J Reconstr Microsurg* 16:3-6, 2000.

222. Zeebregts C and others: Clinical experience with non-penetrating vascular clips in free-flap reconstructions, *Br J Plast Surg* 55:105-110, 2002.

223. Zimmermann CE and others: Donor site morbidity after microvascular fibula transfer, *Clin Oral Investig* 5:214-219, 2001.

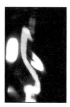

CHAPTER SEVEN

LASER SURGERY: BASIC PRINCIPLES AND SAFETY CONSIDERATIONS

Robert H. Ossoff
C. Gaelyn Garrett
Lou Reinisch

INTRODUCTION

Laser light is the brightest monochromatic (single color) light that exists today. In addition to being a standard tool in the research laboratory, the laser is currently used in communications, surveying, manufacturing, diagnostic medicine, and surgery. Supermarket bar code scanners, lecture pointers, and compact disk players bring laser technology into everyday life. The addition of lasers and the development of new lasers to the surgical armamentarium in otolaryngology offer new and exciting possibilities to improve conventional techniques and to expand the scope of otolaryngology.

This chapter reviews the principles, applications, and safety considerations associated with the use of lasers in the upper aerodigestive tract. The material presented provides a foundation for the otolaryngologist to safely and effectively apply this exciting technology in daily practice.

HISTORY OF LASERS

Laser is an acronym for *l*ight *a*mplification by the *s*timulated *e*mission of *r*adiation. Einstein[10] postulated the theoretical foundation of laser action, stimulated emission of radiation, in 1917. In his classic journal article, "Zur Quantem Theorie der Strahlung" (i.e., "The Quantum Theory of Radiation"), he discussed the interaction of atoms, ions, and molecules with electromagnetic radiation. He specifically addressed absorption and spontaneous emission of energy and proposed a third process of interaction: stimulated emission. Einstein postulated that the spontaneous emission of electromagnetic radiation from an atomic transition has an enhanced rate in the presence of similar electromagnetic radiation. This "negative absorption" is the basis of laser energy. Many attempts were made in the following years to produce stimulated emission of electromagnetic energy, but it was not until 1954 that this was suc-

cessfully accomplished. In that year, Gordon and others[18] reported their experiences with stimulated emission of radiation in the microwave range of the electromagnetic spectrum. This represented the first maser (*m*icrowave *a*mplification by the *s*timulated *e*mission of *r*adiation) and paved the way for the development of the first laser. In 1958, Schawlow and Townes[37] published "Infrared and Optical Masers," in which they discussed stimulated emission in the microwave range of the spectrum and described the desirability and principles of extending stimulated emission techniques to the infrared and optical ranges of the spectrum. Maiman[25] expanded on these theoretical writings and built the first laser in 1960. With synthetic ruby crystals, this laser produced electromagnetic radiation at a wavelength of 0.69 μm in the visible range of the spectrum. Although the laser energy produced by Maiman's ruby laser lasted less than 1 ms, it paved the way for explosive development and widespread application of this technology.

Commercial lasers were being sold for laboratory use within 1 year of being invented. Partially reacting to the recently discovered dangers of x-rays, scientists were concerned about the safety of lasers and how laser light might damage living tissue.

This concern over the safety of laser light prompted much of the early transition of the laser from the scientific laboratory to the medical clinic. In 1962, Zaret and others[51] published one of the first reports of laser light interacting with tissue. They measured the damage caused by lasers on rabbit retina and iris. In 1964, the argon (Ar) and neodymium: yttrium-aluminum-garnet (Nd:YAG) lasers were developed.[17] Excited by the ophthalmologists' progress in using the laser as a therapeutic tool, Goldman used his medical laser laboratory to look at the hazards of the laser and to consider the potential uses of the laser in medicine. Two important advances allowed the laser to be useful in otolaryngology: (1) in 1965, the carbon dioxide

(CO_2) laser was developed, and (2) in 1968, Polanyi[34] developed the articulated arm to deliver the infrared radiation from the CO_2 laser to remote targets. He combined his talents with Jako and used the articulated arm and the CO_2 laser in laryngeal surgery. Simpson and Polanyi[40] described the series of experiments and new instrumentation that made this work possible.

A laser is an electro-optical device that emits organized light (rather than the random-pattern light emitted from a light bulb) in a very narrow intense beam by a process of optical feedback and amplification. Because the explanation for this organized light involves stimulated emission, a brief review of quantum physics is necessary.

In the semi-classical picture of the atom, each proton is balanced by an electron that orbits the nucleus of the atom in one of several discrete shells or orbits. Shells correspond to specific energy levels, which are characteristic of each different atom or molecule. The smaller shells, where the electron is closer to the nucleus, have a lower energy level than the larger shells, where the electron is farther from the nucleus. Electrons of a particular atom can only orbit the nucleus at these shells or levels. Radiation of energy does not occur while the electrons remain in any of these shells.

Electrons can change their orbits, thereby changing the energy state of the atom. During excitation, an electron can make the transition from a low-energy level to a higher energy level. Excitation that comes from the electron interacting with light (a photon) is termed *absorption*. The atom always seeks its lowest energy level (i.e., the ground state). Therefore, the electron will spontaneously drop from the high-energy level back to the lowest energy level in a very short time (typically 10^{-8} sec). As the electron spontaneously drops from the higher energy level to the lower energy level, the atom must give up the energy difference. The atom emits the extra energy as a photon of light in a process termed the *spontaneous emission of radiation* (Figure 7-1).

Einstein postulated that an atom in a high-energy level could be induced to make the transition to a lower energy state even faster than the spontaneous process if it interacted with a photon of the correct energy. This process can be imagined as a photon colliding with an excited atom, resulting in two identical photons (one incident and one produced by the decay) that leave the collision. The two photons have the same frequency and energy and travel in the same direction in the spatial and temporal phase. This process, which Einstein called *stimulated emission of radiation*, is the underlying principle of laser physics (Figure 7-1).

WHAT IS A LASER?

All laser devices have an optical resonating chamber (cavity) with two mirrors. The space between these mirrors is filled with an active medium, such as Ar, Nd:YAG, or CO_2. An external energy source (e.g., an electric current) excites the active medium within the optical cavity. This excitation causes many atoms of the active medium to be raised to a higher energy state. A population inversion occurs when more than half of the atoms in the resonating chamber have reached a particular excited state. Spontaneous emission is taking place in all directions. Light (photons) emitted in the direction of the long axis of the

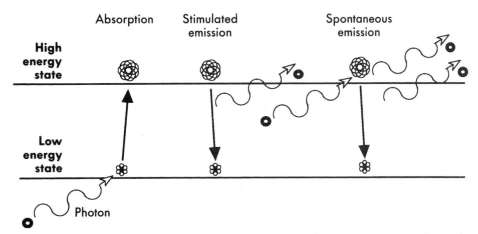

Figure 7-1. The interaction of light (a photon) with an atom. Three processes are shown: the absorption of a photon by an atom in a low-energy state, the spontaneous emission of a photon from an atom in an excited state, and the stimulated emission of a photon by a second photon of the same wavelength from an excited-state atom.

laser is retained within the optical cavity by multiple reflections off of the precisely aligned mirrors. One mirror is completely reflective, and the other is partially transmissive (Figure 7-2). Stimulated emission occurs when a photon interacts with an excited atom in the optical cavity. This yields pairs of identical photons that are of equal wavelength, frequency, and energy and are in phase with each other. This process occurs at an increasing rate with each passage of the photons through the active medium.

The mirrors serve as a positive feedback mechanism for the stimulated emission of radiation by reflecting the photons back and forth. The partially transmissive mirror emits some of the radiant energy as laser light. The radiation leaving the optical cavity through the partially transmissive mirror quickly reaches equilibrium with the pumping mechanism's rate of replenishing the population of high-energy state atoms. (In the preceding discussion, the term *atom* refers to the active material. In reality, the active material can consist of molecules, ions, atoms, semiconductors, or even free electrons in an accelerator. These other systems do not require the bound electron to be excited but may instead use different forms of excitation, including molecular vibrational excitation or the kinetic energy of an accelerated electron.)

The radiant energy emitted from the optical cavity is of the same wavelength (monochromatic), is extremely intense and unidirectional (collimated), and is temporally and spatially coherent. The term *temporal coherence* refers to the waves of light oscillating in phase over a given time; whereas *spatial coherence* means that the photons are equal and parallel across the wave front. These properties of monochromaticity, intensity, collimation, and coherence distinguish the organized radiant energy of a laser light source from the disorganized radiant energy of a light bulb or other light source (Figure 7-3).

After the laser energy exits the optical cavity through the partially transmissive mirror, the radiant energy typically passes through a lens that focuses the laser beam to a very small diameter, or spot size, ranging from 0.1–2.0 mm. When necessary, the lens system is constructed to allow the visible helium-neon aiming laser beam and the invisible CO_2 or Nd:YAG laser beam to be focused in a coplanar manner. The optical properties of each focusing lens determine the focal length or distance from the lens to the intended target tissue for focused use.

CONTROL OF THE SURGICAL LASER

With most surgical lasers, the physician can control three variables: (1) power (measured in watts); (2) spot size (measured in millimeters); and (3) exposure time (measured in seconds).

Power

Of power, spot size, and exposure time, power is the least useful variable and may be kept constant with widely varying effects, depending on the spot size and the duration of exposure. For example, the relationship between power and depth of tissue injury becomes logarithmic when the power and exposure time are kept constant and the spot size is varied.

Irradiance is a more useful measure of the intensity of the beam at the focal spot than power is because it considers the surface area of the focal spot. Specifically, irradiance is expressed (in W/cm^2) as: Irradiance = Power in the focal spot/Area of the focal spot.

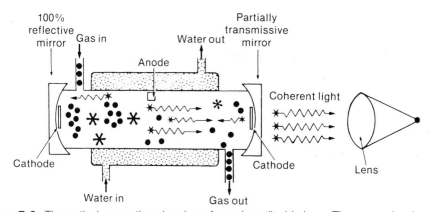

Figure 7-2. The optical resonating chamber of a carbon dioxide laser. The gas molecules are excited by an electric current. The gas is cooled by a water jacket. The two mirrors provide the optical feedback for the amplification. The emitted light is coherent, monochromatic, and collimated. The light can be focused to a small point with an external lens.

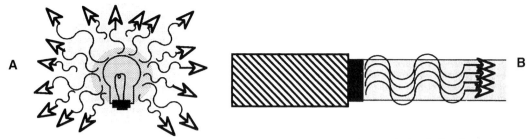

Figure 7-3. A, Light emitted from a conventional lamp. The light travels in all directions, is composed of many wavelengths, and is not coherent. **B,** Light emitted from a laser. The light travels in the same direction, it is a single wavelength, and all of the waves are in phase. The light is coherent.

Spot Size

Power and spot size are considered together, and a combination is selected to produce the appropriate irradiance. If the exposure time is kept constant, the relationship between irradiance and depth of injury is linear as the spot size is varied. Irradiance is the most important operating parameter of a surgical laser at a given wavelength. Therefore, surgeons should calculate the appropriate irradiance for each procedure to be performed. These calculations allow the surgeon to control, in a predictable manner, the tissue effects when changing from one focal length to another (e.g., from 400 mm for microlaryngeal surgery to 125 mm for hand-held surgery). Irradiance varies directly with power and inversely with surface area. This relationship of surface area to beam diameter is important when evaluating the power density because the larger the surface area, the lower the irradiance; conversely, the smaller the surface area, the higher the irradiance. Surface area (A) is expressed as:

$$A = \pi r^2 \text{ or } A = \pi d^2/4$$

where r is the beam radius and d is the beam diameter (d = 2r). Surface area and irradiance vary with the square of the beam diameter. Doubling the beam diameter (e.g., from d to 2d) increases the surface area by four times and reduces irradiance to one-fourth. Halving the beam diameter (e.g., from d to d/2) yields only one-fourth of the area and increases irradiance by a factor of four.

Current CO_2 lasers emit radiant energy with a characteristic beam intensity pattern. This beam pattern ultimately determines the depth of tissue injury and vaporization across the focal spot. Therefore, the surgeon should be aware of the characteristic beam pattern of the laser. Transverse electromagnetic mode (TEM) refers to the distribution of energy across the focal spot and determines the shape of the laser's spot. The most fundamental mode is TEM_{00}, which appears circular on cross section. The power density of the

beam follows a gaussian distribution. The greatest amount of energy is at the center of the beam and diminishes progressively toward the periphery. TEM_{01} and TEM_{11} are less fundamental modes that have a more complex distribution of energy across their focal spot, causing predictable variations in tissue vaporization depth. Additionally, their beams cannot be focused to as small a spot size as TEM_{00} lasers at the same working distance.[14]

Although simple ray diagrams normally show parallel light focused to a point, the actual situation is a bit more complicated. A lens focuses a gaussian beam to a beam waist of a finite size. This beam waist is the minimum spot diameter (d) and can be expressed as:

$$d \sim 2\lambda/D$$

where f is the focal length of the lens, λ is the wavelength of light, and D is the diameter of the laser beam incident on the lens (Figure 7-4). The beam waist occurs over a range of distances, termed the *depth of focus*, which can be expressed as:

$$\text{Depth of focus} \sim \pi d^2/2\lambda$$

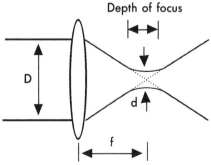

Figure 7-4. The beam waist of parallel light focused by a lens. The focal length of the lens is f and the incident beam is transverse electromagnetic mode (TEM_{00}) and has a diameter incident on the lens of 2D The beam waist has a diameter of 2d.

Depth of focus is realized when a camera is focused. With a camera, a range of objects is in focus, which can be set without carefully measuring the distance between the object and the lens. The preceding equations show that a long focal length lens leads to a large beam waist, which also translates as a large depth of focus.

The size of the laser beam on the tissue (spot size) can therefore be varied in two ways: (1) because the minimum beam diameter of the focal spot increases directly with increasing the focal length of the laser focusing lens, the surgeon can change the focal length of the lens to obtain a particular beam diameter. As the focal length decreases, a corresponding decrease occurs in the size of the focal spot. Also, the smaller the spot size is for any given power output, the greater the corresponding power density. (2) The surgeon can also vary the spot size by working in or out of focus. The minimum beam diameter and highest power concentration occur at the focal plane, where much of the precise cutting and vaporization is carried out (Figure 7-5, A). As the distance from the focal plane increases, the laser beam diverges or becomes unfocused (Figure 7-5, B). The cross-sectional area of the spot increases and thus lowers the power density for a given output. The size of the focal spot depends on the focal length of the laser lens and whether the surgeon is working in or out of focus.

Figure 7-6 shows these concepts using arbitrary ratios accurate for a current model TEM_{00} CO_2 laser. The laser lens setting (focal length) and working distance (focused/unfocused) combinations determine the size of the focal spot. The height of the various cylinders represents the amount of tissue (depth and width) vaporized after a 1-sec exposure at the three focal lengths.

Exposure Time

The surgeon can vary the amount of energy delivered to the target tissue by varying the exposure time. Fluence refers to the amount of time (measured in seconds) that a laser beam irradiates a unit area of tissue at a constant irradiance. Fluence is a measure, then, of the total amount of laser energy per unit area of exposed target tissue and is expressed (J/cm^2) as:

$$Fluence = Power\ density \times Time$$

Fluence varies directly with the length of the exposure time, which can be varied by working in the pulsed mode (duration, 0.05–0.5 sec) or in the continuous mode.

TISSUE EFFECTS

When electromagnetic energy (incident radiation) interacts with tissue, the tissue reflects, absorbs, transmits, and scatters portions of the light. The surgical interaction of this radiant energy with tissue is caused only by that portion of light that is absorbed (i.e., the incident radiation minus the sum of the reflected and transmitted portions).

The actual tissue effects produced by the radiant energy of a laser vary with the laser's wavelength. Each type of laser exhibits different characteristic biologic effects on tissue and is therefore useful for different applications. However, certain similarities exist

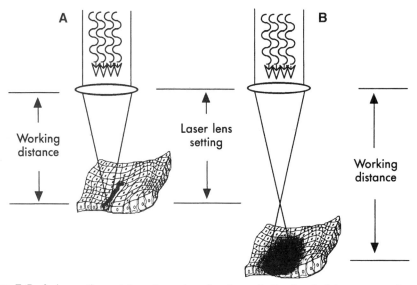

Figure 7-5. A, Laser-tissue interaction when the tissue is the focal distance away from the lens. Note the minimum beam diameter in the focal plane. **B,** Laser-tissue interaction when the tissue is not in the focal plane of the lens. The laser covers a much larger area on the tissue surface.

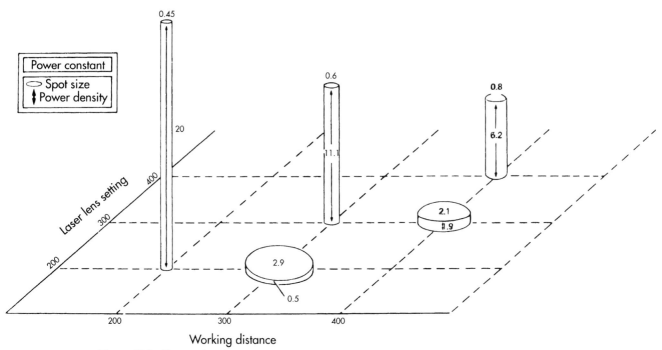

Figure 7-6. Power density versus spot size. The ratios are arbitrary for a current model carbon dioxide laser. The cylinder height represents the amount of tissue vaporized after a 1-sec exposure at the three designated focal lengths.

regarding the nature of laser light interaction with biologic tissue. The lasers used in medicine and surgery today can be ultraviolet, meaning the interactions are a complex mixture of heating and photodissociation of chemical bonds. The more commonly used lasers emit light in the visible or the infrared region of the electromagnetic spectrum, and their primary form of interaction with biologic tissue leads to heating. Therefore, if the radiant energy of a laser is to exert its effect on the target tissue, it must be absorbed by the target tissue and converted to heat (Figure 7-7). Scattering tends to spread the laser energy over a larger surface area of tissue, but it limits the penetration depth (Figure 7-8). The shorter the wavelength of light, the more it is scattered by the tissue. If the radiant energy is reflected from or transmitted through the tissue (Figures 7-9 and 7-10), no effect will occur. To select the most appropriate laser system for a particular application, the surgeon should thoroughly understand these characteristics regarding the interaction of laser light with biologic tissue.[13]

The CO_2 laser creates a characteristic wound (Figure 7-11). When the target absorbs a specific amount of radiant energy to increase its temperature to between 60°C and 65°C, protein denaturation occurs. Blanching of the tissue surface is readily visible, and the deep structural integrity of the tissue is disturbed. When the absorbed laser light heats the tissue to approximately 100°C, vaporization of intracellular

water occurs, causing vacuole formation, craters, and tissue shrinkage. Carbonization, disintegration, smoke, and gas generation with destruction of the laser-radiated tissue occurs at several hundred degrees centigrade.

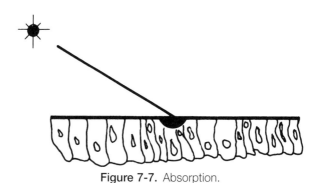

Figure 7-7. Absorption.

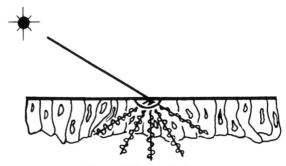

Figure 7-8. Scattering.

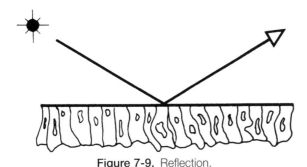

Figure 7-9. Reflection.

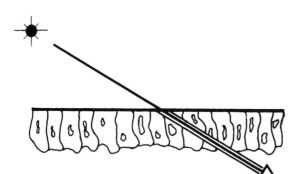

Figure 7-10. Transmission.

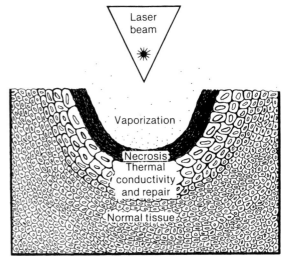

Figure 7-11. The wound created by the carbon dioxide laser, showing the representative zones of injury.

In the center of the wound is an area of tissue vaporization, where just a few flakes of carbon debris are noted. Immediately adjacent to this area is a zone of thermal necrosis (about 100 μm wide). Next is an area of thermal conductivity and repair (usually 300–500 μm wide). Small vessels, nerves, and lymphatics are sealed in the zone of thermal necrosis. The minimal operative trauma combined with the vascular seal probably account for the absence of postoperative edema characteristic of laser wounds.

Comparison animal studies have been performed on the histologic properties of healing and the tensile strength of the healing wound after laser- and scalpel-produced incisions. Several studies noted impaired wound healing with the CO_2 laser incision when compared with the scalpel-produced incision.[5,9,12,19,24] Other studies of the healing properties of laser-induced incisions concluded that laser incisions have equivalent or better healing results than surgical knife wounds.[11,29,36] Buell and Schuller[4] compared the rate of tissue repair after CO_2 laser and scalpel incisions on hogs. In this study, the tensile strength of the laser incisions was less than that of similar scalpel incisions during the first 3 weeks after surgery. After this time, the tensile strength of both wounds rapidly increased at a similar rate.

Regardless of which studies accurately depict the effects of the CO_2 laser on wound healing, the incidental, collateral thermal damage is indisputable. To minimize lateral thermal damage from thermal diffusion, the tissue should be ablated with a short laser pulse.

To understand how a pulsed laser reduces thermal diffusion, consider the analogy of filling a large bucket with a hole in the bottom. If a narrow stream of water is used to fill the bucket, the filling process will take a long time and a considerable amount of water will leak out of the hole during the filling process. Instead, if the bucket is filled in one quick dump from an even larger bucket, the water will have little time to leak out of the hole during the filling process.

This analogy can also be used to understand the ablation process. In ablation, the water represents laser energy and the filled bucket represents sufficient energy deposited in the tissue to cause ablation. The hole in the bottom of the bucket represents the thermal diffusion of heat away from the ablation site while the energy is being deposited. A low-intensity, continuous laser beam is similar to the narrow stream of water. The short-pulsed, high-peak power laser is similar to the larger bucket in that it dumps energy into the ablation site.

LASER TYPES AND APPLICATIONS

Several types of lasers are commonly used in otolaryngology. They include the Argon laser, Argon tunable dye laser, Nd:YAG laser, KTP laser, flash lamp pumped dye laser, and CO_2 laser. Many more types are in various stages of development. The potential clinical applications of these surgical lasers are determined by wavelength and the specific tissue-absorptive characteristics. Therefore, the surgeon should consider the properties of each wavelength when choosing a particular laser to achieve the surgical objective with minimal morbidity and maximal efficiency (Table 7-1).

TABLE 7-1

LASER CHOICES FOR VARIOUS LESIONS

Laser	Second-Choice Laser	Anatomic Site	Lesion	Reason
Argon		Ear	Lysis of middle ear adhesions	Optical fiber delivery, hemaglobin absorption
Argon pumped dye laser			Photodynamic therapy	Can tune the laser to maximum absorption of photosensitizer
CO_2		Glottis	Nodules	Microspot, precision
CO_2		Glottis	Polyps	Microspot, precision
CO_2		Glottis	Reinke's edema	Microspot, precision, microflap technique
CO_2		Glottis	T1 midcordal squamous cell carcinoma with no anterior commissure involvement	Excisional biopsy
CO_2	KTP	Larynx	Laryngoceles, cysts, granulomas	Coagulation, hands-off technique
CO_2		Larynx	Laryngomalacia	Aryepiglottic fold division, precision, coagulation
CO_2		Larynx	Stenoses (glottic, posterior, and subglottic)	Micro–trap door techniques
CO_2		Lingual tonsils	Recurrent tonsillitis, hypertrophy	Minimal edema with complete vaporization
CO_2		Oral cavity	Carcinoma (verrucous, superficial T1)	Less pain and edema, covers a large area
CO_2		Oral cavity	Premalignant (leukoplakia, erythroplakia)	Vaporization, excision, can cover a large area
CO_2	KTP	Glottis	Bilateral vocal cord paralysis	Laser arytenoidectomy, coagulation
CO_2	KTP	Larynx	Recurrent respiratory papilloma	Hands-off technique, less scarring, precision (although KTP may be faster)
CO_2	KTP	Larynx	Suprahyoid supraglottic T1 squamous cell carcinoma	Excision with frozen section control
CO_2	KTP	Oral cavity	Tongue T1 and limited T2 cancer	Less pain and edema, precision, coagulation
CO_2	KTP or Argon	Ear	Stapedotomy	Minimal trauma
CO_2	KTP or Nd: YAG	Oral cavity	Lymphangioma	Minimal edema, coagulation
CO_2	KTP or Nd: YAG	Oropharynx	T1 and T2 squamous cell carcinoma	Precision, coagulation, less edema, contact tip with Nd:YAG
CO_2	Nd:YAG	Nose	Turbinate hypertrophy	Coagulation, less scabbing and scarring
CO_2	Nd:YAG	Subglottis	Hemangioma	Defocused beam, shrinkage, coagulation
Flash lamp pumped dye laser			Port-wine stains	Selective photothermolysis
KTP		Nose	Polyps, concha bullosa	Debulking for visualization, coagulation
KTP	CO_2	Larynx	Obstructing squamous cell carcinoma	Debulking airway, staging, coagulation
KTP	CO_2	Oropharynx	Sleep apnea (uvulopalato-pharyngoplasty)	Coagulation

Continued

TABLE 7-1

LASER CHOICES FOR VARIOUS LESIONS—cont'd

Laser	Second-Choice Laser	Anatomic Site	Lesion	Reason
KTP	CO_2	Palatine tonsils	Recurrent tonsillitis, obstructive apnea	Coagulation ? less postoperative pain
KTP	Nd:YAG	Nose	Epistaxis	Fiber delivery, coagulation, hands-off technique
Nd:YAG	KTP	Nose	Hereditary hemorrhagic telangiectasias	Coagulation, hands-off technique
Nd:YAG	KTP or CO_2	Trachea	Obstructing malignant lesions	Debulking, coagulation, fiber delivery

CO_2, Carbon dioxide; KTP, Potassium-titanyl–phosphate; Nd:YAG, neodymium:yttrium-aluminum-garnet.

Argon (Ar) Laser

Ar lasers produce blue-green light in the visible range of the electromagnetic spectrum, with primary wavelengths of 0.488 and 0.514 μm. The radiant energy of an Ar laser may be strongly absorbed, scattered, or reflected depending on the specific biologic tissues with which it interacts. Its extinction length (i.e., the thickness of water necessary to absorb 90% of the incident radiation) in pure water is about 80 m. Therefore, the radiant energy from an Ar laser is readily transmitted through clear aqueous tissues (e.g., cornea, lens, and vitreous humor) and is absorbed and reflected to varying degrees by tissues white in color (e.g., skin, fat, and bone). Light from an Ar laser is absorbed by hemoglobin and pigmented tissues. A localized thermal reaction occurs within the target tissue, causing protein coagulation. The clinician uses this selective absorption of light from an Ar laser to photocoagulate pigmented lesions, such as port-wine stains, hemangiomas, and telangiectasis. The heat produced destroys the epidermis and upper dermis. Therefore, the surgeon should minimize the amount of laser energy delivered to the vascular cutaneous lesion to decrease the tendency of scarring in the overlying skin.

When the beam of the Ar laser is focused on a small focal spot, its power density increases sufficiently to vaporize the target tissue. This characteristic allows otologists to perform stapedotomy in patients with otosclerosis.[45] Bone, being a white tissue, reflects most of the incident radiation from an Ar laser. Therefore, to perform an Ar laser stapedotomy, it is necessary to place a drop of blood on the stapes to initiate absorption.

Argon Tunable Dye Laser

The Ar tunable dye laser works on the principle of the Ar laser. The Ar tunable dye laser makes a high-intensity beam that is focused on dye continuously circulating in a second laser optically coupled with the Ar laser. The Ar laser beam energizes the dye, causing it to emit laser energy at a longer wavelength than the pump beam. By varying the type of dye and using a tuning system, different wavelengths can be obtained. The laser energy from this dye laser can be transmitted through flexible fiberoptics and delivered through endoscopic systems or inserted directly into tumors. The major clinical use of this laser is with selective photodynamic therapy (PDT) for malignant tumors after the intravenous injection of the photosensitizer, hematoporphyrin derivative.[7]

After intravenous injection, the hematoporphyrin derivative disseminates to all of the cells of the body, rapidly moving out of normal tissue but remaining longer in neoplastic tissue. After a few days, a differential in concentration exists between the tumor cells and the normal cells. When the tumor is exposed to red light (630 nm), the dye absorbs the light, causing a photochemical reaction. Toxic oxygen radicals such as singlet oxygen are produced within the exposed cells, causing selective tissue destruction and cell death. Because healthy tissues contain less photosensitizer, a much less severe reaction or no reaction occurs. Long-term tumor control has been achieved using PDT for recurrent nasopharyngeal cancer.[23] The overall potential and the place of maximum value of this form of management remain to be established.

Neodymium: YTTRIUM-Aluminum-Garnet (Nd:YAG) Laser

Nd:YAG lasers produce light with a wavelength of 1.064 μm in the near infrared (invisible) range of the electromagnetic spectrum. Pure water weakly absorbs the radiant energy of the Nd:YAG laser. The extinction length is about 40 mm. Therefore, its radiant energy can be transmitted through clear liquids, facilitating its use in the eye or other water-filled cavities (e.g., the urinary bladder). Absorption of light from this laser is slightly color dependent, with increased absorption in darkly pigmented tissues and charred debris. In biologic tissue, strong scattering, both forward and backward, determines the effective extinction length, which is usually 2–4 mm. Backward scattering can account for up to 40% of the total amount of scattering. The zone of damage produced by the incident beam of a Nd:YAG laser produces a homogeneous zone of thermal coagulation and necrosis that may extend up to 4 mm deep and lateral from the surface, making precise control impossible.

The primary applications for the Nd:YAG laser in otolaryngology include ablation or palliation of obstructing tracheobronchial lesions, palliation of obstructing esophageal lesions, photocoagulation of vascular lesions of the head and neck, and photocoagulation of lymphatic malformations. The contact Nd:YAG laser is reportedly useful in the removal of malignant tumors in the oral cavity and oropharynx, where it is difficult to maintain a generous safety margin.[28] The Nd:YAG laser has several distinct advantages in the management of obstructing lesions of the tracheobronchial tree. Hemorrhage is the most frequent and dangerous complication associated with laser bronchoscopy, and its control is extremely important. Control of hemorrhage is more secure with this laser because of its deep penetration in tissue.

Nd:YAG laser application through an open, rigid bronchoscope allows for multiple distal suction capabilities simultaneous with laser application and rapid removal of tumor fragments and debris to prevent hypoxemia. Patients for Nd:YAG laser bronchoscopy should be selected after flexible fiberoptic bronchoscopic examination of the tracheobronchial tree and tracheal computed tomography. Patients in whom extrinsic compression of the airway can be shown should be excluded. The radiant energy from the Nd:YAG laser can be transmitted through flexible fiberoptic delivery systems, allowing its use with flexible endoscopes. In the management of patients with obstructing neoplasms of the tracheobronchial tree, it is considered safer to use a rigid ventilating bronchoscope rather than a flexible fiberoptic bronchoscope.[8] During this approach, the laser fiber is passed down the lumen of the rigid bronchoscope with a rod lens telescope and suction catheter. Other advantages of the use of the Nd:YAG laser with a rigid bronchoscope include ventilatory control of the compromised airway, palpation of the tumor–cartilage interface, use of the bronchoscope tip as a "cookie cutter," and use of the bronchoscope tip to compress a bleeding tumor bed for temporary hemostasis. The flexible fiberoptic

bronchoscope is often used through the open rigid scope to provide pulmonary toilet and more distal laser application after the major airway is secure.

This laser is an excellent surgical instrument for tissue coagulation. Vaporization and incision also can be performed with the Nd:YAG laser. When this laser is used for these functions, however, precision is lacking and tissue damage is widespread. The major disadvantage of the Nd:YAG laser is its comparatively less predictable depth of tissue penetration. This laser is used primarily to rapidly photocoagulate tumor masses in the upper- and lower-aerodigestive tract at 40- to 50-W, using 0.5- to 1-second exposures. Whenever possible, the laser beam is applied parallel to the wall of the tracheobronchial tree. The rigid tip of the bronchoscope is used mechanically to separate the devascularized tumor mass from the wall of the tracheobronchial tree.

Otolaryngologists may use the Nd:YAG laser with the CO_2 laser when performing bronchoscopic laser surgery. The effective coagulating properties of the Nd:YAG laser should augment the predictable vaporizing properties of the CO_2 laser when treating patients with obstructive tracheal and proximal endobronchial cancers, especially if an ulcerative or actively bleeding tumor is present.[32]

Carbon Dioxide (CO_2) Laser

CO_2 lasers produce light with a wavelength of 10.6 μm in the infrared (invisible) range of the electromagnetic spectrum. A second, built-in, coaxial helium-neon laser is necessary because its red light indicates the site where the invisible CO_2 laser beam will impact the target tissue. Thus, this laser acts as an aiming beam for the invisible CO_2 laser beam. The radiant energy produced by the CO_2 laser is strongly absorbed by pure, homogeneous water and by all biologic tissues high in water content. The extinction length of this wavelength is about 0.03 mm in water and in soft tissue. Reflection and scattering are negligible. Because absorption of the radiant energy produced by the CO_2 laser is independent of tissue color and because the thermal effects produced by this wavelength on adjacent nontarget tissues are minimal, the CO_2 laser has become extremely versatile in otolaryngology.

With current technology, light from the CO_2 laser cannot be transmitted through existing flexible fiberoptic endoscopes, although research and development of a suitable flexible fiber for transmission of this wavelength is being carried out internationally. At present, the radiant energy of this laser is transmitted from the optical resonating chamber to the target tissue via a series of mirrors through an articulating arm to the target tissue. The CO_2 laser can be used free-hand for macroscopic surgery, attached to the operating microscope for microscopic surgery, and adapted to an endoscopic coupler for bronchoscopic surgery. This latter application requires rigid nonfiberoptic bronchoscopes. Pattern generators coupled with a micromanipulator on the operating microscope have also been introduced to help with the surgical precision in laryngology.

The CO_2 laser is an integral instrument in all aspects of otolaryngology. The types of uses vary from endoscopic resection of malignant laryngeal tumors to the precision of laser stapedotomy, as well as to cosmetic skin treatment. The described uses are too numerous to include in this chapter, however, the CO_2 laser has found its most effective use in laryngology and bronchoesophagology.

For example, surgery for recurrent respiratory papillomatosis has advanced with the use of the laser. The increased ability to preserve normal laryngeal structures while maintaining the translaryngeal airway more than offsets the initial disappointment associated with the laser's inability to cure the disease. In a published survey, the CO_2 laser was preferred for the management of recurrent respiratory papillomatosis by 92% of the respondents.[6] In pediatric patients, surgery for webs, subglottic stenosis, capillary hemangiomas, and other space-occupying airway lesions has been significantly improved by the precision, preservation of normal tissue, and predictably minimal amount of postoperative edema associated with the judicious use of the CO_2 laser. In adults, surgery for polyps, nodules, leukoplakia, papillomas, cysts, granulomas, and other benign laryngeal conditions can be performed with the laser. Surgeons should be cautioned, however, to be aware of the associated thermal injury that can occur to surrounding normal tissues with use of the laser even at recommended settings. A study by Garrett and Reinisch showed thermal injury beyond the laser ablation crater as much as 285 μm deep into the lamina propria of canine vocal folds.[16] Fibrosis this deep into the tissue could affect the vibratory characteristics of the lamina propria.

Management of laryngotracheal stenosis is a difficult problem for the otolaryngologist. Retrospective analysis has determined that stenotic lesions appropriate for endoscopic management have two features in common[40]: (1) All lesions treated with endoscopic techniques must retain intact external cartilaginous support. (2) Lesions appropriate for endoscopic management are usually less than 1–2 cm in vertical length, yet favorable results have been reported for lesions up to 3 cm in length when endoscopic incision is combined with prolonged stenting.[39,50]

The addition of the CO_2 laser to endoscopic treatment of bilateral vocal fold immobility due to nerve injury or joint fixation allows the surgeon to perform laser cordotomy, medial arytenoidectomy, or total arytenoidectomy as needed. The precision associated with the CO_2 laser facilitates performance of this operation. Pattern generators are now available that create an incision of desired length, shape, and depth of penetration, aiding in the precision and efficiency of the operating microscope micromanipulator.

The transoral management of squamous cell carcinoma of the larynx using the CO_2 laser is an obvious extension of the application of this surgical instrument. The advantages of precision, increased hemostasis, and decreased intraoperative edema allow the surgeon to perform exquisitely accurate and relatively bloodless endoscopic surgery of the larynx.

Bronchoscopic indications for CO_2 laser surgery include management of recurrent respiratory papillomatosis or granulation tissue within the tracheobronchial tree, excision of selected subglottic or tracheal strictures, excision of bronchial adenomas, and re-establishment of the airway in patients with obstructing tracheal or endobronchial cancers. In the case of obstructing tracheal or endobronchial cancers, palliation or reduction of the patient's symptoms of airway obstruction or hemoptysis is the goal.

Potassium-Titanyl-Phosphate (KTP) Laser

The KTP laser emits light at 532 nm and is therefore comparable with the Ar laser. The scattering and absorption by skin pigments when using the KTP laser are nearly the same as the Ar laser. Yet the KTP laser light is more strongly absorbed by hemoglobin.

The KTP laser has uses in otologic, rhinologic, and laryngologic surgery. It can also be used for tonsillectomy and pigmented dermal lesions. In otology, it has been shown to be effective for initial stapes surgery, as well as for revision stapedectomy.[26] Thedinger has promoted the KTP laser for chronic ear surgery, specifically for removing hyperplastic infected mucosa, disarticulating mobile stapes suprastructure in a complete cholesteatoma removal, and removing previously inserted middle ear implants.[47] Hand-held probes also facilitate use of the KTP laser for functional endoscopic sinus surgery and other intranasal applications and for microlaryngeal applications. The optical fiber delivery of the 532-nm laser light can be manipulated through a rigid pediatric bronchoscope as small as 3 mm, facilitating lower tracheal and endobronchial lesion treatment in infants and neonates.[49]

The KTP crystal actually doubles the frequency (halves the wavelength) of an Nd:YAG laser. Therefore, with this laser, the output between the 532-nm KTP light and the 1064-nm Nd:YAG light can usually be switched.

Flash Lamp Pumped Dye Laser

The management of hemangiomas and port-wine stains with lasers has benefited from the application of the flash lamp pumped dye laser. The dye was initially selected for maximum absorption by the oxyhemoglobin at 577 nm. Tan and others showed that at 585 nm, hemoglobin absorption is maximal with minimal scattering and absorption by melanin and other pigments.[46] The light pulse is about 400 μsec long to minimize thermal diffusion in the tissue. Although dark skin types show little or no selective vascular photothermolysis with the flash lamp pumped dye laser, lighter skin types show significant results. At a threshold dose, specific vascular injury is observed without disruption of the adjacent tissue in lightly pigmented skin.

Other Lasers

In an effort to have a more controlled laser effect with less damage to adjacent tissue, several lasers in the near- to mid-infrared region have been investigated, including the erbium:YAG (Er:YAG) and the holmium:YAG (Ho:YAG). The Er:YAG emits at the infrared peak of water absorption at 2.94 μm. The extinction length in water is less than 2 μm. The laser produces very clean incisions with a minimal amount of thermal damage to the adjacent tissue. The negative aspects are: (1) The wavelength is too long to be transmitted through normal optical fibers. This gives a distinct advantage to lasers that produce light that can be transmitted through fibers. (2) More important, the thermal propagation is so short there are practically no tissue coagulation and no hemostasis. The Er:YAG laser is therefore unsuitable for use in highly vascular tissue. It has been used in dental surgery for various indications. In otolaryngology, the Er:YAG laser has been used for stapes surgery and for cutaneous applications, including rhinophyma and resurfacing for wrinkles.[2,21,30]

The Ho:YAG laser operates at 2.1 μm. This wavelength can be effectively transmitted through fibers. The extinction length in water is about 0.4 mm, which suggests that this laser light should interact with tissue in a way very similar to the CO_2 laser. The Ho:YAG has been combined with fiberoptic endoscopy for sinus surgery. The hemostasis is good, and the soft bone ablation is readily controlled. Adjacent thermal damage zones varied from 130–220 μm in a study by Stein and others.[43] The laser is as effective in sinus surgery as conventional surgical techniques with less blood loss but increased postoperative edema.[27]

PULSE STRUCTURE

As mentioned earlier in this chapter, the surgeon has three parameters to select when using a particular laser. The intensity of the laser is the least useful. The exposure time is important in that it controls the total amount of light incident on the tissue (i.e., the radiant exposure). The pulse structure of the laser light within the given exposure time is also crucial. The pulse structure is a characteristic of the active medium and the cavity configuration. It is often fixed and cannot be changed or modified by the surgeon.

Continuous Wave Lasers

Many lasers operate in a continuous wave mode. In this mode, the laser is always on. The instantaneous intensity and the average laser intensity are essentially the same. A shutter, external to the laser cavity, usually controls the exposure time, allowing the laser to operate independently of the exposure time or the frequency of exposures. This gives the most stable operation. A surgical CO_2 or Nd:YAG laser will operate in continuous wave mode at intensities of a few watts to more than 50 W.

Flash Lamp Pulsed Lasers

Certain lasers operate in a pulsed mode. Flash lamp pumped lasers can pulse from about 0.5 *m*sec to several 100 ms. The first ruby laser operated in a pulsed mode. The flash lamp used to pump the ruby crystal had a duration of about 1 ms. The laser output of this first ruby laser clearly was irregular and unstable. When observed with a fast detector and oscilloscope, the output intensity was found not to be a 1-ms long laser pulse but a series of irregular spikes. Each spike is a few microseconds long with several microseconds between the spikes. The stimulated emission in the ruby is so efficient that it quickly depletes the population inversion and the operation stops, after which the flash lamp can reestablish the population inversion and operation can resume. This process repeats until the flash lamp stops. Most of the long-pulsed lasers operate in a spiking mode.

Q-Switched Laser

The spiking of the laser output can be controlled to produce a single very short laser pulse, much shorter than the flash lamp lifetime. One technique to produce the short pulses is Q-switching, in which the laser pumping process (usually a flash lamp) builds up a large population inversion inside the laser cavity. Blocking or removing one of the mirrors prevents the laser from emitting. After a large population inversion has developed, the feedback is restored and a short intense burst of laser light depletes the accumulated population inversion, typically in 10 to 50 ns. Q-switching can be accomplished by several different methods. The most direct and earliest method is rotating the end mirror so that the light amplification by stimulated emission can occur during the short interval when the mirror is correctly aligned. Waring blender motors were often used as fast, stable motors. However, uncertain timing, lack of reliability, and vibration (not to mention the noise) led to many problems, particularly with the alignment. Electrooptic polarization rotators and acoustooptic beam deflectors are now commonly used for Q-switching.

Cavity Dumped Lasers

Cavity dumping produces slightly shorter pulses of light. In this technique, the laser is pumped and allowed to operate between completely reflecting mirrors. The light energy is trapped in the cavity until it reaches a maximum. Then one of the mirrors is "removed" from the cavity and allows all the light to leave the cavity. The laser pulse has a physical length of twice the cavity length. Thus, the duration of the laser pulse is $2\lambda c$, where λ is the length of cavity and c is the speed of light (c is about 3×10^{10} cm/sec or 1 foot/ns).

Mode Locked Lasers

Mode locking produces pulses of light as short as a few picoseconds. A Q-switched laser operates in several longitudinal modes (or slightly shifted frequencies). A fast saturable dye brings all these modes into phase. The nanosecond macropulse of light is actually a train of micropulses, each of which is several picoseconds long and repeats at about 100 MHz. These pulses can be further compressed by various techniques. The shortest laser light pulses achieved in the laboratory are less than 4 wave oscillations long (about 6 fs or 6×10^{-15} sec).

The pulsed laser dramatically changes the interaction of the light with tissue. The intensity of the laser during the pulse is extremely high (approaching 10^9 W). The high intensity and short pulse duration enable the laser light efficiently to ablate tissue before the thermal energy spreads by thermal diffusion. The pulse should be significantly shorter than the thermal diffusion time to prevent thermal diffusion from spreading damage. Typically, a tissue under laser irradiation reaches thermal equilibrium within a few milliseconds. The heat will spread over several micrometers in less than 10 μsec. Also, the transverse mode structure of the laser beam must be preserved in the short pulses to yield the small focal spot size.

SAFETY CONSIDERATIONS
Education

The laser is a precise but potentially dangerous surgical instrument that must be used with caution. Although distinct advantages are associated with the use of laser surgery in the management of certain benign and malignant diseases of the upper aerodigestive tract, these advantages must be weighed against the risks of complications. Because of these risks, the surgeon must first determine if the laser offers an advantage over conventional surgical techniques. For the surgeon to use good judgment in the selection and use of lasers in practice, prior experience in laser surgery is necessary. Therefore, some type of formal laser education program should be a prerequisite to using this technology. Most hospitals now require evidence of participation in a laser use and safety course before granting laser privileges. The surgeon who has not received training in laser surgery as a resident should attend a hands-on training course in laser surgery. Such a course should include laser biophysics, tissue interactions, safety precautions, and supervised hands-on training with laboratory animals. After completing such a course, the surgeon should practice laser surgery on cadaver or animal specimens before progressing to the more simple procedures on patients.

Hospitals that offer laser surgery should appoint a laser safety officer and set up a laser safety committee consisting of the laser safety officer, physicians using the laser, anesthesiologists, operating room nurses, a hospital administrator, and a biomedical engineer. The purpose of this committee is to develop policies and procedures for the safe use of lasers within the hospital. The safety protocols established by this committee will vary with each specialty and use of the laser. In addition, the laser safety committee should (1) make recommendations regarding the appropriate credential-certifying mechanisms required for physicians and nurses to become involved with each laser; (2) develop educational policies for surgeons, anesthesiologists, and nurses working with the laser; (3) accumulate laser patient data in cases where an investigational device was used; and (4) conduct a periodic review of all laser-related complications.

Aside from a few minor eye injuries from a laser beam exposure, most serious accidental injuries related to laser use can be traced to the ignition of surgical drapes and airway tubes.[41] Because the anesthesiologist is also concerned with the airway and because potent oxidizing gases pass through the airway in close approximation to the path of the laser beam, it is necessary to develop a team approach to the anesthetic management of the patient undergoing laser surgery of the upper aerodigestive tract. It is recommended that anesthesiologists involved with laser surgery cases attend a didactic session devoted to this subject. Finally, the operating room staff must be educated with regard to laser surgery. Attendance at an inservice workshop with exposure to clinical laser biophysics and the basic workings of the laser, as well as hands-on orientation should be the minimal requirement for nurses to participate in laser surgery.

Safety Protocol

Development of an effective laser safety protocol that stresses compliance and meticulous attention to detail by the operating room personnel (laser surgery team) is probably the most important reason this potentially dangerous surgical instrument can be used safely in treating patients with diseases of the upper aerodigestive tract.[34] Such a laser safety protocol is usually general enough to list all the major and most minor precautions necessary when laser surgery is being performed within the specialty of otolaryngology. General considerations concern provisions for protection of the eyes and skin of patients and operating room personnel and for adequate laser plume (smoke) evacuation from the operative field. Additional precautions concern the choice of anesthetic technique, the choice and protection of endotracheal tubes, and the selection of proper instruments, including bronchoscopes.

Eye Protection

Several structures of the eye are at risk. The area of injury usually depends on which structure absorbs the most radiant energy per volume of tissue. Depending on the wavelength, corneal or retinal burns, or both, are possible from acute exposure to the laser beam. The possibility for corneal or lenticular opacities (cataracts) or retinal injury exists after chronic exposure to excessive levels of laser radiation. Retinal effects occur when the laser emission wavelength occurs in the visible and near-infrared range of the electromagnetic spectrum (0.4–1.4 μm). When viewed directly or secondary to the reflection from a specular (mirror like) instrument surface, laser radiation within this wavelength range would be focused to an extremely small spot on the retina, causing serious injury. This occurs because of the focusing effects of the cornea and lens. Laser radiation in the ultraviolet (<0.4 μm) or in the infrared range of the spectrum (>1.4 μm) produces effects primarily at the cornea, although certain wavelengths also may reach the lens.[3]

To reduce the risk of ocular damage during cases involving the laser, certain precautions should be followed. Protecting the eyes of the patient, surgeon, and other operating room personnel must be addressed. The actual protective device will vary according to the wavelength of the laser used. A sign should be placed outside the operating room door warning all persons entering the room to wear protective glasses because the laser is in use. In addition, extra glasses for the specific wavelength in use should be placed on a table immediately outside the room. The doors to the operating room should remain closed during laser use.

Patients undergoing CO_2 laser surgery of the upper aerodigestive tract should have a double layer of saline-moistened eye pads placed over the eyes (Figure 7-12 *A, B*). All operating room personnel should wear protective eyeglasses with side protectors. Regular eyeglasses or contact lenses protect only the areas covered by the lens and do not provide protection from possible entry of the laser beam from the side. When working with the operating microscope and the CO_2 laser, the surgeon need not wear protective glasses. The optics of the microscope provide the necessary protection (Figure 7-13). When working with the Nd:YAG laser, all operating room personnel (and the patient) must wear wavelength-specific protective eyeglasses that are usually blue-green. Although the beam direction and point of impact may appear to be confined within the endoscope, inadvertent deflection of the beam may occur because of a faulty contact, a break in the fiber, or accidental disconnection between the fiber and endoscope. Special wavelength-specific filters are available for flexible and rigid bronchoscopes. When these filters are in place, the surgeon need not wear protective eyeglasses.[22]

When working with the Ar, KTP, or dye lasers, all personnel in the operating room, including the patient, should again wear wavelength-specific protective eyeglasses that are usually amber. When undergoing photocoagulation for selected cutaneous vascular lesions of the face, the patient usually wears protective metal eye shields rather than protective eyeglasses. Similar precautions are necessary for the visible and near-infrared wavelength lasers. The major difference is the type of eye protection that is worn.

Skin Protection

The patient's exposed skin and mucous membranes outside the surgical field should be protected by a double layer of saline-saturated surgical towels, surgical sponges, or lap pads. When microlaryngeal laser surgery is being performed, the beam might partially reflect off the proximal rim of the laryngoscope rather than go down it. Thus, saline-saturated surgical towels completely drape the patient's face. Only the proximal lumen of the laryngoscope is exposed. Great care must be exercised to keep the wet draping from drying out. It should occasionally be moistened during the procedure. Teeth in the operative field also need to be protected. Saline-saturated Telfa, surgical sponges, or specially constructed metal dental impression trays can be used. Meticulous attention is paid to the protective draping procedures at the beginning of the surgery. The same attention should be paid to the

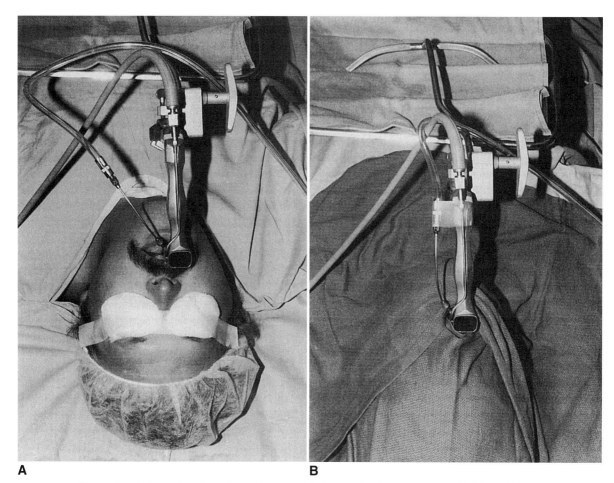

A   **B**

Figure 7-12. Patient undergoing carbon dioxide laser microlaryngoscopy with jet ventilation. **A,** Saline-moistened eye pads are secured with silk tape. The eyes are first taped closed with silk tape to prevent corneal abrasions from the eye pads. **B,** Saline-moistened towels are placed around the patient's head to cover all skin surfaces.

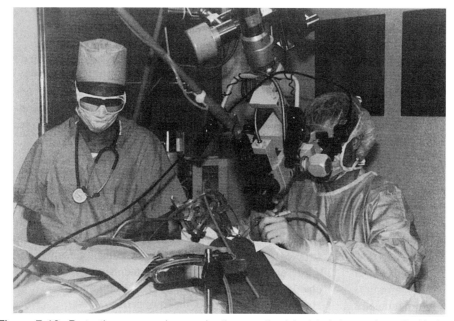

Figure 7-13. Protective eyewear is worn by the anesthesiologist during carbon dioxide laser microlaryngoscopy. The surgeon's eyes are protected by the optics of the operating microscope.

continued protection of the skin and teeth during the surgical procedure.[31]

Smoke Evacuation

Two separate suction setups should be available for all laser cases in the upper aerodigestive tract. One provides for adequate smoke and steam evacuation from the operative field; whereas the second is connected to the surgical suction tip for the aspiration of blood and mucus from the operative wound. When performing laser surgery with a closed anesthetic system, the surgeon should use constant suctioning to remove laser-induced smoke from the operating room. This helps to prevent inhalation by the patient, surgeon, and operating room personnel. When the anesthetic system is open or has jet ventilation systems, suctioning should be intermittent to maintain the forced inspiratory oxygen at a safe level. Laryngoscopes, bronchoscopes, operating platforms, mirrors, and anterior commissure and ventricle retractors with built-in smoke-evacuating channels facilitate the evacuation of smoke from the operative field. One report suggested that the smoke created by the interaction of the CO_2 laser with tissue may be mutagenic.[48] Filters in the suction lines should be used to prevent clogging by the black carbonaceous smoke debris created by the laser. Although papillomavirus and other viral particles have been detected in the laser plume, no cases of clinical transmission of diseases are documented.[1,15]

Anesthetic Considerations

Optimal anesthetic management of the patient undergoing laser surgery of the upper aerodigestive tract must include attention to the safety of the patient, the requirements of the surgeon, and the hazards of the equipment. Most patients undergo general anesthesia for upper airway endoscopy. Some laser procedures in the oral cavity and oropharynx may be performed under local anesthesia, with or without intravenous sedation. Most patients undergoing upper airway laser endoscopy, however, require general anesthesia. Any nonflammable general anesthetic is suitable. Halothane and enflurane are most often used. Because of the risk of fire associated with general endotracheal anesthesia, the inspired concentration of oxygen, a potent oxidizing gas, is important. Mixtures of helium, nitrogen, or air plus oxygen are commonly used to maintain the forced inspiratory oxygen around but not greater than 40% and to ensure that the patient is adequately oxygenated. Nitrous oxide is also a potent oxidizing gas and should not be used in the anesthetic mixture to cut the oxygen concentration. When performing laser surgery in the tracheobronchial tree through the rigid, ventilating bronchoscope, the surgeon may use 100% oxygen. In either case, intravenous supplementation with small doses of narcotics or tranquilizers is often used to shorten the emergence period after anesthesia. Jet ventilation techniques during laser surgery are effective for selected patients, such as those with subglottic stenosis. Successful use of this ventilation technique requires that the anesthesiologist be experienced in this practice.

One of the most devastating complications of laser surgery of the aerodigestive tract is endotracheal tube ignition and resulting injury to the laryngotracheal mucosa. At present, a nonflammable, universally accepted endotracheal tube for all types of laser surgery of the upper aerodigestive tract does not exist. The traditional polyvinyl endotracheal tube should not be used, either wrapped or unwrapped. It offers the least resistance to penetration by the laser beam of all the endotracheal tubes that have been tested, fire-breakdown products are toxic, and tissue destruction associated with combustion of this tube is the most severe. Endotracheal tubes for laser surgery that are wavelength specific are now available from several manufacturers and should be used at all times unless jet ventilation techniques are used.

Protection of the endotracheal tube from direct or reflected laser beam irradiation is of primary importance. If the laser beam strikes an unprotected endotracheal tube carrying oxygen, ignition of the tube could result in a catastrophic, intraluminal, blow-torch-type endotracheal tube fire. Protection should also be provided for the cuff of the endotracheal tube. Methylene blue-colored saline should be used to inflate the cuff. Saline-saturated cottonoids are then placed above the cuff in the subglottic larynx to further protect the cuff. These cottonoids require frequent moistening during the procedure. If the cuff deflates from an errant hit by the laser beam, the already saturated cottonoids turn blue to warn the surgeon of impending danger. The tube should then be removed and replaced with a new one. Use of the microlaryngeal operating platform offers further protection against potential danger. Inserted into the subglottic larynx above the level of the packed cottonoids, this unique instrument serves as a back stop to protect the cottonoids, endotracheal tube, and cuff from any direct or reflected laser beam irradiation.

Effectiveness of a Safety Protocol

Strong and Jako[46] and later Snow and others[44] warned of the possible complications associated with laser surgery of the upper aerodigestive tract, including the risks of endotracheal tube fires and tissue damage from reflection of the laser beam. In a survey of laser-related complications by Fried,[13] 49 of 152 otolaryngologists who used the laser reported 81 complications, including 28 incidents of endotracheal tube fires. Healy and others[21] reported a 0.2% complication rate in 4416 cases of CO_2 laser surgery in the upper aerodigestive tract. Ossoff[34] published an extensive view of laser-related complications experienced by 218 past registrants of hands-on laser surgery training courses that he directed. Seven surgeons experienced 8 complications and no endotracheal tube fires. The complication rate was 0.1% in more than 7200 laser surgical procedures. These papers have similar conclusions: (1) certain precautions are necessary when performing laser surgery of the upper aerodigestive tract; and (2) adherence to a rigid safety protocol allows laser surgery of the airway to be performed safely and with an extremely small risk of serious complications.

REFERENCES

1. Abramson AL, DiLorenzo TP, Steinberg BM: Is papillomavirus detectable in the plume of laser-treated laryngeal papilloma? *Arch Otolaryngol Head Neck Surg* 116:604, 1990.
2. Alster TS, Lupton JR: Erbium:YAG cutaneous laser resurfacing, *Dermatologic Clinics* 19:453, 2001.
3. American National Standards Institute: American national standard for the safe use of lasers, Z136.1, New York, American National Standards Institute, 1996.
4. Buell BR, Schuller DE: Comparison of tensile strength in CO_2 laser and scalpel skin incisions, *Arch Otolaryngol Head Neck Surg* 109:465, 1983.
5. Cochrane JPS and others: Wound healing after laser surgery: experimental study, *Br J Surg* 67:740, 1980.
6. Derkay CS: Task force on recurrent respiratory papillomas: a preliminary report, *Arch Otolaryngol Head Neck Surg* 121:1386, 1995.
7. Dougherty TJ and others: Photoradiation therapy for the treatment of malignant tumors, *Cancer Res* 38:2628, 1978.
8. Dumon JF and others: Principles for safety in application of neodymium-YAG laser in bronchology, *Chest* 86:163, 1984.
9. Durkin GE and others: Wound healing of the true vocal cord squamous epithelium after CO_2 laser ablation and cup forceps stripping, *Otolaryngol Head Neck Surg* 95:273, 1986.
10. Einstein A: Zur Quantem Theorie der Strahlung, *Phys Zeit* 18:121, 1917.
11. Finsterbush A, Rousso M, Ashur H: Healing and tensile strength of CO_2 laser incisions and scalpel wounds in rabbits, *Plast Reconstr Surg* 70:360, 1982.
12. Fisher SE and others: Comparative histological study of wound healing following CO_2 laser and conventional surgical excision of canine buccal mucosa, *Arch Oral Biol* 28:287, 1983.
13. Fried MP: A survey of the complications of laser laryngoscopy, *Arch Otolaryngol Head Neck Surg* 110:31, 1984.
14. Fuller TA: The physics of surgical lasers, *Lasers Surg Med* 1:5, 1980.
15. Garden JM and others: Papillomavirus in the vapor of carbon dioxide laser-treated verrucae, *JAMA* 259:1199, 1988.
16. Garrett CG, Reinisch L: New-generation pulsed carbon dioxide laser: comparative effects on vocal fold wound healing, *Ann Otol Rhinol Laryngol* 111:471, 2002.
17. Geusic JE, Marcos HM, Van Uitert LG: Neodymium doped yttrium-aluminum-garnet laser material, *Appl Phys Letters* 4:182, 1964.
18. Gordon JP, Zeiger HZ, Townes CH: Microwave amplification by stimulated emission, *Phys Rev* 95:282, 1954.
19. Hashimoto K and others: Laser wound healing compared with other surgical modalities, *Burns* 1:13, 1971.
20. Healy GB and others: Complications of CO_2 laser surgery of the aerodigestive tract: experience of 4416 cases, *Otolaryngol Head Neck Surg* 92:13, 1984.
21. Keck T and others: Safety of the erbium:yttrium-aluminum-garnet laser in stapes surgery in otosclerosis, *Otol Neurotol* 23:21, 2002.
22. Laser Institute of America: *Guide for the selection of laser eye protection*, Toledo, OH, Laser Institute of American, 1984.
23. Lofgren LA and others: Photodynamic therapy for recurrent nasopharyngeal cancer, *Arch Otolaryngol Head Neck Surg* 121:997, 1995.
24. Luomanen M, Meurman JH, Lehto VP: Extracellular matrix in healing CO_2 laser incision wound, *J Oral Pathol* 16:322, 1987.
25. Maiman TH: Stimulated optical radiation in ruby, *Nature* 187:493, 1960.
26. McGee TM, Diaz-Ordaz EA, Kartush JM: The role of KTP laser in revision stapedectomy, *Otolaryngol Head Neck Surg* 109:839, 1993.
27. Metson R: Holmium:YAG laser endoscopic sinus surgery: a randomized, controlled study, *Laryngoscope* 106:1, 1996.
28. Miyaguchi M, Sakai S: The contact Nd-YAG laser for oral and oropharyngeal malignant tumors, *Auris Nasus Larynx* 21:226, 1994.
29. Norris CW, Mullarry MB: Experimental skin incision made with the carbon dioxide laser, *Laryngoscope* 92:416, 1982.
30. Orenstein A and others: Treatment of rhinophyma with Er:YAG laser, *Lasers Surg Med* 29:230, 2001.
31. Ossoff RH and others: The CO_2 laser in otolaryngology-head and neck surgery: a retrospective analysis of complications, *Laryngoscope* 93:1287, 1983.
32. Ossoff RH: Bronchoscopic laser surgery: which laser when and why? *Otolaryngol Head Neck Surg* 94:378, 1986.
33. Ossoff RH: Laser safety in otolaryngology-head and neck surgery: anesthetic and educational considerations for laryngeal surgery, *Laryngoscope* 99:1, 1989.
34. Polanyi TG: Laser physics, *Otolaryngol Clin North Am* 16:753, 1983.
35. Remacle M, Lawson G, Watelet JB: Carbon dioxide laser microsurgery of benign vocal fold lesions: indications, techniques, and results in 251 patients. *Ann Otol Rhinol Laryngol* 108:156, 1999.
36. Robinson JK and others: Wound healing in porcine skin following low-output carbon dioxide laser irradiation of the incision, *Ann Plast Surg* 18:499, 1987.
37. Schawlow AL, Townes CH: Infrared and optical masers, *Physiol Rev* 112:1940, 1958.
38. Shah H and others: Benign tumors of the tracheobronchial tree. Endoscopic characteristics and role of laser resection, *Chest* 107:1744, 1995.
39. Shapshay SM, Beamis JF Jr, Dumon JF: Total cervical tracheal stenosis: treatment by laser, dilation, and stenting, *Ann Otol Rhinol Laryngol* 98:890, 1989.
40. Simpson GT, Polanyi TG: History of the carbon dioxide laser in otolaryngologic surgery, *Otolaryngol Clin North Am* 16:739, 1983.
41. Sliney DH: Laser safety, *Lasers Surg Med* 16:215, 1995.
42. Snow JC, Norton ML, Saluja TS: Fire hazard during CO_2 laser microsurgery on the larynx and trachea, *Anesth Analg* 55:146, 1976.

43. Stein E and others: Acute and chronic effects of bone ablation with a pulsed holmium laser, *Lasers Surg Med* 10:384, 1990.

44. Strong MS, Jako GJ: Laser surgery in the larynx, *Ann Otol Rhinol Larynol* 81:791, 1972.

45. Strunk CL Jr, Quinn FB Jr: Stapedectomy surgery in residency: KTP-532 laser versus argon laser, *Am J Otolaryngol* 14:113, 1993.

46. Tan OT and others: Histologic comparison of the pulsed dye laser and copper vapor laser effects on pig skin, *Lasers Surg Med* 10:551, 1990.

47. Thedinger BS: Applications of the KTP laser in chronic ear surgery, *Am J Otolaryngol* 11:79, 1990.

48. Tomita Y, Mihashi S, Nagata K: Mutagenicity of smoke condensates induced by CO_2 laser irradiation and electrocauterization, *Mutat Res* 89:145, 1981.

49. Ward RF: Treatment of tracheal and endobronchial lesions with the potassium titanyl phosphate laser, *Ann Otol Rhinol Laryngol* 101:205, 1992.

50. Whitehead E, Salam MA: Use of the carbon dioxide laser with the Montgomery T-tube in the management of extensive subglottic stenosis, *J Laryngol Otol* 106:829, 1992.

51. Zaret M and others: Biomedical experimentation with optical masers, *J Opt Soc Am* 52:607, 1962.

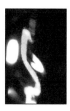

CHAPTER EIGHT

DIFFICULT AIRWAY/INTUBATION: IMPLICATIONS FOR ANESTHESIA

Lynette Mark
Seth Akst
James Michelson

OVERVIEW

Airway management is the essence of clinical anesthesiology. Complex airway management of the patient with an anticipated difficult airway/intubation or the patient with an unanticipated difficult airway/intubation is a multispecialty process that involves anesthesiologists, surgeons, pulmonologists, critical care physicians, emergency physicians, and nursing/technician staff support.

The otolaryngologist–head and neck (OLHN) surgeon with expertise in rigid laryngoscopy and bronchoscopy, flexible fiberoptic bronchoscopy, and surgical approaches to the airway is uniquely qualified to take the lead surgical role in a team approach with the anesthesiologist to safely manage difficult airway/intubation patients. The goal of airway management is simple: to provide the most expeditious form of management that has the lowest potential for injury and the greatest potential for control of the airway.[50]

The approach to the patient with a difficult airway varies, depending on whether management is elective or urgent/emergency and whether the health care setting is an operating room or a nonoperating-room environment.

This chapter presents the anesthetic component of complex airway management in a manner that OLHN surgeons can incorporate into their practice. Discussions include the following:

1. Preoperative patient evaluation by the anesthesiologist to identify a patient with a potentially difficult airway/intubation
2. Basic anesthetic techniques with specific attention to implications of anesthetics in airway management
3. Indications and limitations of airway techniques primarily used by anesthesiologist and emergency physicians

4. American Society of Anesthesiology (ASA) *Guidelines for Management of the Difficult Airway* and the role of the OLHN surgeon in using these Guidelines[3]
5. The Johns Hopkins Medical Institutions Departments of Anesthesiology and Critical Care Medicine and OLHN Airway Management Initiative
6. Establishing an Airway Management Service at your institution
7. Mechanisms for communicating patient airway information to other health care providers and patients
8. Case presentations focused on the use of the ASA Difficult Airway Algorithm
9. Case presentations focused on catastrophic events and the role of the OLHN surgeon

The focus of this chapter is on clinical airway algorithms and the decisions that must be made by the anesthesiologist together with the OLHN surgeon to safely provide anesthesia and airway management for their patient or for a non-OLHN patient seen by them in joint consultation for airway management. In-depth discussions about the pharmacology and physiology of anesthesiology are beyond the scope of this chapter but can be found in any of numerous authoritative textbooks of anesthesiology.[38,49]

DIFFICULT AIRWAY/INTUBATION: A MULTISPECIALITY PROBLEM

Complex airway management is a multifaceted problem involving health care providers in a variety of clinical settings. The consequences of failed airway maintenance, endotracheal intubation, or both, can be devastating to the patient, the practitioner, and the health care system. Critical issues include identification of difficult airway/intubation patients, mobilization of physician and support staff, mobilization of airway management equipment, preparation of the patient, implementation of appropriate airway algorithms, documentation of airway management techniques, dissemination of critical airway information to future health care providers, and quality improvement/medicolegal considerations.

Patient Identification

Controversy regarding predictors and definitions of "difficult" exists both intraspecialty and interspecialty, dependent and independent of practitioner skill, related to specific techniques and complicated by changing patient pathophysiology.[7] Some patients may be anticipated to be difficult to intubate on the basis of a history of difficulty intubation or clinical predictors of difficult intubation. The *ASA Practice Guidelines for Management of the Difficult Airway*[3] reviews some of the historical or physical examination findings possibly suggestive of a difficult intubation. Some of these predictors of anticipated difficulty with conventional direct laryngoscopy (MAC/Miller) include a large overbite, large tongue, narrow mouth opening, or short chin. Various prediction models, such as correlation with Mallampati oral view I to IV to the Cormack and Lehand laryngoscopic view grades I to IV have been proposed, but none offer 100% sensitivity for prediction of a difficult airway (Figures 8-1 to 8-4).[29] Historically, anesthesiology literature cites an incidence of 1% to 3% for unanticipated difficult airway/intubation in patients undergoing general endotracheal anesthesia.[3,30,54] The airway management technique used to define "difficult" in this literature was conventional rigid laryngoscopy (Macintosh or Miller blades).

Despite advances in airway management techniques and refinement of difficulty predictors, the

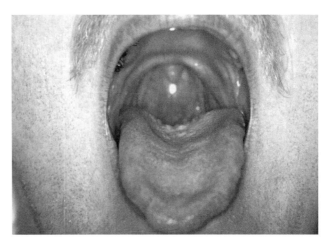

Figure 8-2. Anesthesia resident with thick neck, 5'8", 95 kg, viewed by colleagues as "anticipated difficult" airway. Mallampati class I oral view. Airway algorithm for elective surgery: mask ventilation easy; direct laryngoscopy times one with MAC No. 4 with full grade I laryngoscopic view. To view this image in color, please go to *www.ototext.com* or the Electronic Image Collection CD, bound into your copy of Cummings Otolaryngology—Head and Neck Surgery, 4th edition.

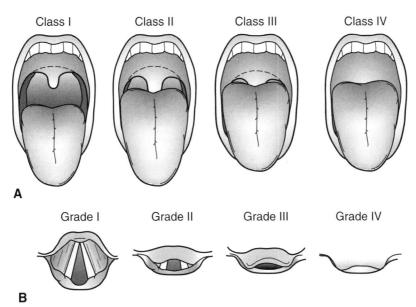

Class I   Class II   Class III   Class IV

A

Grade I   Grade II   Grade III   Grade IV

B

Figure 8-1. Mallampati, Cormach, and Lehand **A,** oral and **B,** laryngoscopic views. To view this image in color, please go to *www.ototext.com* or the Electronic Image Collection CD, bound into your copy of Cummings Otolaryngology—Head and Neck Surgery, 4th edition.

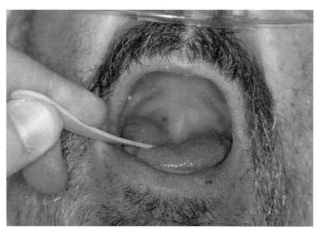

Figure 8-3. Patient evaluated to have a Mallampati class II airway with a tongue blade and anticipated easy intubation with conventional laryngoscopy. Airway algorithm for elective surgery: mask ventilation easy; unsuccessful direct laryngoscopy with MAC No. 3/4 Miller No. 2/3 times 4; successful asleep oral fiberoptic intubation with No. 7.0 ETT with view of complete glottic opening. To view this image in color, please go to *www.ototext.com* or the Electronic Image Collection CD, bound into your copy of Cummings Otolaryngology—Head and Neck Surgery, 4th edition.

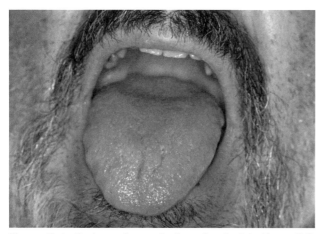

Figure 8-4. Postoperative evaluation of patient in Figure 8-3. Note that without the tongue blade, the patient has a Mallampati class 4 airway and should have been considered to be anticipated difficult intubation with conventional laryngoscopy. To view this image in color, please go to *www.ototext.com* or the Electronic Image Collection CD, bound into your copy of Cummings Otolaryngology—Head and Neck Surgery, 4th edition.

cited 1% to 3% incidence of unanticipated difficulty has not changed and is still defined by conventional laryngoscopy.[12,30,46,53] In an institution with approximately 25,000 general endotracheal anesthetic procedures annually, there are potentially 250 to 750 unanticipated difficult airway/intubations per year.

Assuming that a full-time practicing anesthesiologist would encounter one unanticipated difficult airway/intubation per year, then, based on ASA membership (which represents 90% of practicing anesthesiologists) there are potentially 30,000 to 90,000 unanticipated difficult airway/intubations annually in the United States. However, these numbers may underestimate the true incidence, because anesthesiologists may not recall the more common near misses as vividly they recall the smaller number of actual difficult airway/intubations in which the outcome was suboptimal. On a national and international level, the scope of this problem and its impact on patients, practitioners, and the health care system is sufficient to warrant vigorous efforts to identify solutions.

In addition to those patients who have unanticipated difficult airway/intubations on initial presentation, there are cohorts of patients who have anticipated complex airway management; these patients can be successfully managed by a variety of innovative and specialty-specific techniques. Some of these techniques (laryngeal mask airway [LMA][10] and Combitube)[18] are readily available, require minimal practitioner education or training, and are inexpensive; other techniques (fiberoptic bronchoscope, surgical airway, specialized rigid laryngoscopes, and fluoroscopic-assisted intubation) are available primarily in specialty centers, may require extensive practitioner skill, and may be relatively expensive. For patients who have undergone head and neck surgery and have visible or hidden implants (laryngeal stents, thyroplasties, etc.), specific considerations for airway management may be unknown to future providers (e.g., thyroplasty patients might require smaller endotracheal tubes than anticipated), thus compromising patient safety and increasing practitioner risk for adverse events.

Successful future management of previously unanticipated difficult airway/intubation patients depends on identification of those patients, and documentation and dissemination of information detailing successful and unsuccessful airway management techniques and primary difficulties encountered. These patients then become anticipated difficult airway/intubations, and the availability of this information promotes quality of care.

Consequences of Difficult Airway Management

The consequences of difficult airway/intubation (with or without an adverse outcome) may be as unsettling as the event itself. The patient may perceive this as a threat to future anesthetic safety or may lack understanding as to the significance of the difficulty. There may be practitioner-perceived threat to professional security. The impact of complex airway management–related events in direct and indirect costs to the health care system is far reaching.

Three studies specifically demonstrated the consequences of difficult airway/intubation management on liability exposure.[2,11,31] An analysis of approximately 5000 claims filed in the Maryland legal system over a 15-year period in which one or more anesthesiologists were named as defendants revealed that insertion of an endotracheal tube was the sixth most common medical procedure leading to a liability claim. Most of these claims also included other members of the operating room team (e.g., otolaryngologists, general surgeons, nurse anesthetists, orthopedic surgeons, plastic surgeons, cardiac surgeons, dentists, or nurses) as defendants. One claim (in 1994) resulted in a jury award of $5 million.[40] In a 1992 loss analysis study conducted by the Physicians Insurers Association of America (PIAA), files from 43 physician-owned malpractice insurance companies (representing approximately 2000 anesthesiologists nationally) ranked "intubation problems" as the third most prevalent misadventure (behind "tooth injury" and "no medical misadventures"). The average paid indemnity for 175 of 339 files was $196,958.[40] The ASA Committee on Professional Liability closed claims study found that respiratory events were the most common cause of brain damage and death during anesthesia, with difficult intubation being the likeliest category for risk reduction. The median payment for respiratory claims was $200,000.[2]

To put these statistics in perspective, the following must be considered.

1. The number of malpractice claims reported represents only a small fraction (one eighth) of all adverse outcomes,[40] with one malpractice claim filed for every 7.5 patient injuries from difficult airway/intubation events and adverse outcomes.[40]
2. Claims may often be aborted by good physician–patient communication.
3. Claims are often initiated against physicians because of poor communication and inadequate records.[27]

Routine Anesthetic Care of the Patient with the Nondifficult Airway

Before discussing management of the difficult airway, this section will discuss the routine provision of anesthesia to provide a framework for the discussion that follows. The three main tasks of the anesthesiology team are: to keep the patient safe; to keep the patient comfortable; and to provide for good operating conditions during the preoperative, intraoperative, and immediate postoperative periods. The component qualities of an anesthetic are loss of consciousness, amnesia, analgesia, and muscle relaxation/

paralysis. Anesthesia can be general, regional, or local; general anesthesia is provided for most head and neck surgeries, thus the need for airway management.

For a routine patient receiving a general anesthetic, the anesthetic "take-off" will follow after a thorough preoperative history and physical. The patient will then be brought into the operating room and positioned supine. Standard monitors will be placed, as described later in this section. Preoxygenation will occur with 100% inspired oxygen to denitrogenate the patient's functional residual capacity. At that point anesthesia will be induced, and the airway will be managed appropriately. After intubation or other airway control, invasive monitors or additional intravenous access may be placed, and then the surgery is allowed to commence.

Advances in Monitoring

As a previous section made clear, there are serious legal and financial consequences of failed airway management. Fortunately, adverse outcomes related to poor airway management have decreased in frequency with the standardization of anesthetic monitoring. The American Society of Anesthesiology Standards for Basic Anesthetic Monitoring statement was first released in 1986 and further amended in 1998.[48] These standards call for continual evaluation of the patient's oxygenation, ventilation, circulation, and temperature during all administered anesthetics. Practically speaking, the standard mandates continuous oxygen analysis of the anesthetic circuit, pulse oximetry, end-tidal capnometry, tidal volume measurement, electrocardiography, and temperature, as well as intermittent (no less frequent than every 5 minutes) measurement of arterial blood pressure and heart rate. In addition, the routine use of the neuromuscular blockade (NMB) monitor (also called the "twitch" monitor) to assess degree of muscle paralysis and return of muscle strength after pharmacological reversal of paralyzing agents significantly contributed to improved patient safety. Compared with earlier eras, this document made the important leap of elevating pulse oximetry and capnometry to standards of care, thus allowing more rapid, accurate recognition of oxygen desaturation and rapid recognition of previously unrecognized esophageal intubation.

The consequences of this change were staggering. Respiratory system adverse events (including airway mishaps) accounted for 36% of claims in the ASA Closed Claims Project data set for the 1970s, but this percentage decreased to 14% of claims in the 1990s after implementation of the routine use of capnometry and pulse oximetry.[27] Claims related to death or brain injury likewise had a similar drop in the percentage that was attributable to respiratory adverse outcomes. Caused in part by continuous pulse oximetry and capnometry, anesthesiology has been a leader in the patient safety movement in the past decade.

Standard Anesthetic Pharmacology

This section will provide a brief introduction to the array of drugs used by anesthesiologists to facilitate anesthesia and maintain control of the airway. An in-depth discussion of these agents is not within the scope of this chapter; however, certain features of these drugs that are particularly applicable to airway management will be highlighted.

Induction Agents and Volatile Anesthetics

In most adult patients, a peripheral intravenous line is started preoperatively to administer fluid and drugs. Therefore, most adult patients receive an intravenous induction of anesthesia. The most commonly used intravenous induction agents are thiopental, propofol, etomidate, and ketamine. Each of the intravenous induction agents has the advantage of quick onset, producing unconsciousness within 1 to 2 minutes when given in standard induction doses. Of note, thiopental and propofol are both associated with negative inotropic effects and a related drop in blood pressure when used for induction of general anesthesia. Etomidate's effects are considered to be more hemodynamically stable, but this drug has the drawbacks of potential adrenal suppression and myoclonic activity. Thiopental, propofol, and etomidate all produce apnea along with unconsciousness. In contrast to the other three agents, ketamine is notable for not producing apnea with administration. The maintenance of spontaneous ventilation with ketamine is an important consideration in the management of patients with potentially difficult airways and other subsets of patients presenting for surgery. In addition, ketamine has the advantage of being able to be given intramuscularly in patients without intravenous access. The major disadvantages of ketamine include emergence delirium and the sympathomimetic effects of the drug, and thus can cause tachycardia and hypertension, which limit its role in the treatment of patients with cardiovascular disease. In addition, ketamine also produces exaggerated secretions, and an antisialogue such as glycopyrrolate should be coadministered if the airway is not secured immediately after induction.

For most adults, the volatile anesthetic agents (such as halothane, isoflurane, sevoflurane, and desflurane) are used for maintenance of anesthesia rather than induction. Their role in induction of anesthesia is limited by slower onset of activity and patient inability to tolerate the scent of the anesthetic gas. However, in pediatric anesthesia, where most patients are intolerant of intravenous placement before coming to the operating room, "mask inductions" with volatile agents is very common. Sevoflurane is typically the agent used for mask induction, because it is considered less noxious than the other agents. All of the volatile agents have the significant advantage of maintaining spontaneous respiration while producing unconsciousness.

Adjuncts to Induction: Sedatives and Opioids

Benzodiazepines are also commonly given in the immediate preoperative period for their anxiolytic and amnestic effects. Midazolam is the most commonly used benzodiazepine, because it has onset of activity in 2 to 4 minutes. In larger doses, benzodiazepines can also be used as induction agents themselves. In sedative doses, the benzodiazepines do not typically produce significant respiratory depression. However, in combination with opioids, the respiratory depression can be synergistic. Furthermore, the response to benzodiazepines can be idiosyncratic, and a sedative dose can produce unconsciousness and apnea in sensitive patients.

Opioids are used intraoperatively to provide analgesia and a balanced anesthetic. When given as part of anesthetic induction, they are useful in blunting the sympathetic response to laryngoscopy and intubation. They also have a role during sedation of patients, because they can produce a sense of well-being, with decreased responsiveness to noxious stimuli. Commonly used opioids are fentanyl, sufentanil, remifentanil, morphine, and hydromorphone. Opioids produce a dose-dependent central respiratory depression with increased P_{aco2} and diminished respiratory drive. This respiratory depression can often be offset in the awake patient by asking them to consciously breathe deeply. However, the combination of opioids with benzodiazepines can result in a patient with central apnea who is unresponsive to instructions to breathe. Both opioids and benzodiazepines can be antagonized at the receptor level by naloxone and flumazenil, respectively.

Lidocaine is sometimes used as adjunct during anesthetic induction, although not in doses large enough to be an induction agent itself. Propofol can cause venous irritation during administration, and pretreatment with lidocaine into the same vein may decrease patient discomfort. In addition, lidocaine does have its own anesthetic effects and may decrease sympathetic response to laryngoscopy and intubation. Doses are kept to 1 to 1.5 mg/kg to avoid potential toxicity of local anesthetics, which will be described later.

Paralytic Agents

Paralysis of the patient eases endotracheal intubation by relaxing the jaw and stopping vocal cord motion. Furthermore, paralysis is often necessary for the surgical procedure itself. There are two classes of paralytics, depolarizing agents and nondepolarizing neuromuscular blockers.

The depolarizing agent used in the United States is succinylcholine. Succinylcholine acts at the acetylcholine receptor in the neuromuscular junction, activating the receptor but then occupying it and therefore prolonging the refractory period before the muscle can contract again. The drug eventually diffuses away from the receptor and is metabolized and deactivated by pseudocholinesterase. Succinylcholine does produce fasciculation of the muscle, which can cause postoperative myalgia. In addition, the original opening of the receptor causes potassium efflux from the muscle, which raises the serum potassium transiently by approximately 0.5 mEq/L. This increase in potassium is exaggerated in patients with up-regulated amounts of acetylcholine receptors, such as after differentiation caused by stroke or other central nervous system injury. In patients with already elevated serum potassium levels, succinylcholine can precipitate ventricular dysrhythmias.

The major advantage of succinylcholine is its very fast onset of action. Paralysis sufficient for endotracheal intubation can be reliably produced within 45 to 60 seconds. Another advantage is its short duration of action, because clinical paralysis usually dissipates within 5 minutes of an intubating dose. It has been thought that this quick return of strength would allow resumption of spontaneous respirations if positive-pressure ventilation were not successful. However, a recent study shows that deleterious oxygen desaturation may occur before resumption of spontaneous respirations.[59] In addition, the small percentage of patients who are pseudocholinesterase deficient will have prolonged paralysis after administration of succinylcholine. Vigilant use of the NMB monitor has led to increased diagnosis of patients with atypical cholinesterase activity, which varies with the population but is cited to be 1:2800 in the general population in the United States, with a 1:1 male/female ratio.[41] Confirmatory blood laboratory diagnosis is made by determining the patient's dibucaine number.[41] Succinylcholine has also been identified as the most common muscle relaxant trigger for malignant hyperthermia (MH).[28] Primary contraindications for the use of succinylcholine include known or suspected MH, increased intracranial pressure, increased intraocular pressure, and elevated potassium. Although not contraindicated in patients with pseudocholinesterase deficiency, administration should be monitored with the NMB monitor to verify full return of strength before extubation.

The other group of paralytics is the nondepolarizing neuromuscular blockers. These drugs work in the neuromuscular junction by preventing the binding of acetylcholine to its receptor and subsequent muscle contraction. There are many different nondepolarizing agents, clinically distinct because of their different times of onset, durations of action, and different routes of metabolism. None of these agents work as quickly as succinylcholine. In the patient in whom there is a contradiction to the use of succinylcholine, the nondepolarizer of choice for rapid sequence intubation is rocuronium, which has an onset of action between 60 and 75 seconds. However, when given in doses sufficient for intubating conditions, the effects of rocuronium persist for 30 to 40 minutes (and cannot be pharmacologically reversed for 20–30 minutes), which can be a major problem if the initial attempt(s) to intubate the trachea is/are unsuccessful. Establishment of mask ventilation is then essential, and although the risk of aspiration is now greater, there are no other options available to the practitioner.

Local Anesthetics

Local anesthetics are discussed here because of their use surgically as an adjunct for analgesia, and also because of their use for topical and regional anesthesia of the airway in awake patients. Lidocaine and bupivacaine are the most commonly used local anesthetics for local infiltration or nerve blocks at our institution. The surgeon must be aware of the maximum dose allowable, given the risk of local anesthetic toxicity, manifested first by central nervous depression and seizures, followed by cardiovascular dysrhythmias and potentially ventricular fibrillation. The maximum dose of lidocaine is 5 mg/kg, and up to 7 mg/kg can be given safely if epinephrine is used in the solution to slow uptake through subcutaneous tissues into the central circulation. A 2% lidocaine solution contains 20 mg/mL of lidocaine, so a 70-kg patient should receive no more than 17.5 mL of this solution. The effects of intravenous lidocaine administered during induction are additive to the amount of lidocaine absorbed from local infiltration, topical application, or regional block, so communication between the anesthesiology and surgical teams is crucial to avoid potentially toxic overdoses. The maximum dose of bupivacaine is 2 to 3 mg/kg, with the upper end of the range reflecting the addition of epinephrine to the solution during local infiltration. As a word of caution, toxic effects are seen with much lower doses of local anesthetics administered directly into the circulation, so careful aspiration must be done before injection of these drugs during infiltration or regional blocks. Injection into the carotid artery during extraoral glossopharyngeal block can produce immediate seizures and loss of consciousness.

Cocaine is also used for topicalization of the airway during head and neck surgery. The advantage of cocaine applied to the nasal mucosa is its vasoconstrictive properties in addition to its anesthetic properties. However, the side effects of cocaine include tachycardia and hypertension, which can be particularly deleterious in patients with coronary artery or other cardiovascular disease. The addition of phenylephrine to lidocaine jelly offers similar vasoconstrictive properties with fewer risks than cocaine. In addition, cocaine has significant addictive properties, so its use by operating room personnel must be intensively monitored.

Antihypertensives

Airway management in the last decade has been radically advanced by the increased understanding of the pathophysiology of ischemia and the judicious perioperative use of antihypertensives for patients at increased risk of ischemic events. Intraoperative hypertension and tachycardia can be a direct response to agents used in topicalization of the airway for awake airway management techniques, specifically cocaine, epinephrine in lidocaine mixtures, and phenylephrine in lidocaine mixtures. In the asleep patient, translaryngeal intubation of the trachea stimulates laryngeal and tracheal receptors, resulting in marked increase in the elaboration of sympathomimetic amines. This sympathetic stimulation results in tachycardia and a rise in blood pressure. In normotensive patients, this rise is approximately 20 to 25 mmHg; it is much greater in hypertensive patients. This increase in blood pressure results from vasoconstriction, owing to unopposed alpha stimulation in hypertensive patients taking β-blocking agents.[58]

The most commonly used antihypertensives for intraoperative control of hypertension and tachycardia related to airway management include the β-blockers esmolol and metoprolol, and the α- and β-blocker labetalol. Most blood pressure and heart rate changes occur about 15 seconds after the start of direct laryngoscopy and become maximal after 30 to 45 seconds. Esmolol is especially effective in blunting these responses because of its almost immediate onset of action, ease in titration, and short action of duration with half-life of 9 minutes. Labetalol is comparable in attenuating hemodynamic effects, but is less immediate in onset of action, and has a half-life of 5 hours.[58]

Standard Induction vs Rapid Sequence Induction

After the patient with an expected routine airway is monitored and anesthesia is induced, the next step is appropriate management of the airway.

An important question to ask before this point is whether the patient is at risk for aspiration of gastric contents into the airway, an event that can be potentially catastrophic. The patient's risk of aspiration of gastric contents will help determine whether the patient should be managed with rapid-sequence induction (RSI) and intubation or with a nonrapid sequence of events. The increased risk of aspiration is due to the presence of gastric contents and is the reason anesthesiologists are concerned about the length of time patients have been without food or drink before surgery. The ASA has published guidelines for preoperative fasting that are based on the time required for gastric emptying in healthy patients.[44] As surgeons, your familiarity with these guidelines can prevent the delay or cancellation of elective surgery.

The summary of fasting recommendations is 2 hours for clear liquids, 4 hours for breast milk, and 6 hours for other food or beverage, including infant formula and milk. In patients with delayed gastric emptying, such as diabetic gastroparesis, further fasting may be necessary for reduced risk of aspiration. In addition to adherence to fasting guidelines, pharmacological agents given preoperatively may reduce risk of aspiration and include clear antacids (30 mL of 0.3 M sodium citrate), anticholinergic agents (atropine or glycopyrrolate), metoclopramide (to stimulate gastric emptying and to increase lower esophageal sphincter tone), and H_2-receptor antagonists (cimetidine or ranitidine) to decrease further secretion of additional acid.

In patients without increased risk of aspiration, a controlled and stepwise approach is taken with induction and intubation. After monitoring and preoxygenation, general anesthesia is induced. Once the patient is unconscious, positive-pressure mask ventilation is performed. Only after successful mask ventilation is established is a paralyzing agent given. This stepwise approach to the airway increases patient safety because, even if intubation cannot be performed successfully, it is known that the patient can be mask ventilated and oxygenated while the paralytic wears off or alternative intubation techniques are readied. The ability to ventilate a patient is more crucial than the ability to intubate a patient, and bag-valve-mask ventilation is a lifesaving skill that every anesthesiologist must master. After successful mask ventilation, the paralytic is given, and intubation is performed after the paralytic takes effect.

RSI and intubation are done for patients with an increased risk of aspiration, such as a patient with a full stomach or a patient with a significant history of gastroesophageal reflux. During an RSI technique, mask ventilation is not done, because it can fill the stomach with air and increase the risk of aspiration even further. Instead, the paralytic agent is given immediately after the induction agent. Cricoid pressure is held throughout, and the patient is not ventilated for the time it takes the paralysis to take effect.

Proper preoxygenation allows most apneic patients to maintain oxygen saturation during this minute. The patient is intubated once paralysis is achieved, usually by means of direct laryngoscopy. After confirmation of proper endotracheal tube placement by end-tidal CO_2 and auscultation of bilateral breath sounds, the endotracheal tube cuff is inflated, and cricoid pressure can be released.

The risk of an RSI is that intubation may not be successful and the ability to mask ventilate the patient has not been previously established. The most dangerous result of failed RSI could be a paralyzed patient who cannot be ventilated or intubated (see Case 8).

Therefore, the stepwise approach to the induction of anesthesia and establishment of mask ventilation before paralysis is the safer and preferred technique for a patient without increased risk of aspiration and without an expected difficult airway. The stepwise approach for a patient with risk for aspiration and with an expected difficult airway requiring general anesthesia is awake vs RSI, with immediate backup in the event failed intubation.

DIFFICULT AIRWAY/INTUBATION: ADVANCES IN AIRWAY DEVICES AND TECHNIQUES

In parallel with organizational responses to difficult airway management, individual practitioners responded with inventions of new airway devices and with innovative combinations of existing techniques. In Table 8-4, a brief review of many of these devices is presented, with identification of primary use by anesthesiology and of OLHN. For a more in-depth discussion of the devices and appropriate techniques, the reader is referred to *Airway Management, Principles and Practice*[6] and references identified in Table 8-4.

To appreciate the scope and magnitude of these efforts, consider that in the early 1990s, most anesthesiologists in the United States had the following airway management techniques: awake blind nasal, awake nasal fiberoptic intubation, and awake and asleep conventional laryngoscopy. Select difficult patients would undergo spontaneous ventilation "breathe-down" inductions without paralysis to facilitate optimal conditions for the OLHN surgeon to attempt to secure the patient's airway with either

rigid laryngoscopy or bronchoscopy. Complications of this technique included laryngospasm, aspiration, lost airway because of inability to maintain spontaneous ventilation and/or difficult positive pressure mask ventilation, and inability to intubate by the OLHN surgeon.

In the early 1990s, OLHN surgeons had the following airway management techniques: awake and asleep surgical airway, awake fiberoptic bronchoscopy, and asleep rigid laryngoscopy and bronchoscopy.

Indisputably, the most significant invention in the recent history of airway management was the LMA.[10] Although introduced into the United States in the early 1990s as an alternative to elective face mask ventilation in general anesthetics not requiring intubation, the value of the LMA as a rescue device for the most devastating situation "cannot intubate/cannot ventilate" quickly became realized. In the 1993 ASA *Practice Guidelines for Management of the Difficult Airway*, the LMA was the airway device that routed the Difficult Airway Algorithm into the significant branch points.[3] In the 2002 amended Guidelines, the LMA was promoted as a first choice device for cannot-ventilate rescue options.[22,42]

In the past decade, for elective difficult airway management, the "family" of LMAs (Classic, ProSeal, Flexible, and Fastrach)[12] has had a major impact on the decision branches with the Difficult Airway Algorithm. Specifically, many practitioners decide that if they can mask the patient with an LMA, definitive placement of an endotracheal tube (ETT) can be achieved with either fiberoptic bronchoscopy or ETT tube exchanger assistance. Backup plans, however, must be in place, because these techniques can be difficult and unsuccessful, as described in Case 7.

Table 8-4 briefly presents many of the advances in airway management devices discussed previously and throughout this chapter. References, including links to more comprehensive web sites, are provided for additional information. Cases 1 to 10 span 10 years of experiences with difficult airway patients and advancements of airway management techniques.

THE JOHNS HOPKINS DEPARTMENTS OF ANESTHESIOLOGY/CRITICAL CARE MEDICINE AND OTOLARYNGOLOGY–HEAD AND NECK SURGICAL AIRWAY MANAGEMENT INITIATIVE AND FORMATION OF A HOSPITAL-WIDE AIRWAY SERVICE

The following section briefly outlines ongoing efforts of the Departments of Anesthesiology/Critical Care Medicine and Otolaryngology—Head and Neck Surgery Airway Management Initiative and formation of a hospital-wide Airway Service. Airway Service protocols and forms are provided in the appendix to assist the

TABLE 8-1

DIFFICULT AIRWAY/INTUBATION: ADVANCES IN AIRWAY DEVICES

Technique	Visualization	Site	Awake/sleep	Contradictions	Olhn	Anes	Comments	References
Face mask	none	oral	both	Full stomach	–	+	Nasal/oral airways to optimize; headstrap to optimize	
Laryngeal mask airway (LMA)	none	oral	both	Full stomach	–	+	New variants include intubating LMA, LMA flexible, LMA ProSeal	www.lmana.com, Figure 8-11
Blind nasal	none	nasal	both	Nasal pathology, coagulation status	–	+		
Digital	none	oral	both	Limited jaw opening	–	+		
Lighted stylet	none	oral nasal	both	Nasal or laryngeal pathology, large neck/mass	–	+	Requires tansillumination at sternal notch	Interactive Airway IDevice Tutorials: www.anest.ufl.edu[24]
Conventional Laryngoscopy	direct	oral	both	Limited jaw opening	–	+	Macintosh/Miller Blades	
Endotracheal tube guides (Eschmann, Frova, Arndt, Aintree)	direct or none	oral nasal	both		+	+	Adjunct to conventional and rigid laryngoscopy intubation with LMA, and extubation techniques	www.cookgroup.com
Rigid laryngoscopy (Hollinger/Dedo)	direct	oral	both	Limited jaw opening	+	–	Hollinger is difficult airway scope	

Technique	Vision	Route				Limitations/Notes	Comments	Reference
Rigid bronchoscopy	direct	oral	both	+	–	Limited jaw opening		
Fiberoptic bronchoscopy	direct	both	both	–	+	Blood or secretions		
Rigid fiberoptic laryngoscope (Bullard, Upsher, Wu)	indirect	oral	both	–	+	Blood or secretions	Combination of fiberoptic and conventional laryngoscopy	Figure 8-12[9]
Retrograde intubation	indirect	neck	both	+	+			www.cookgroup.com
Percutaneous cricothyrotomy	indirect	neck	both	+	+	Neck pathology, technique	OLHN assisted with FOB/direct visualization	
Cricothyrotomy	direct	neck	both	+	–	Neck pathology, technique		
Tracheotomy	direct	neck	both	+	–	Neck pathology, technique		
Transtracheal jet ventilation		oral / neck	both	+	+	Via angiocath, attachement to rigid laryngoscope, ventilating EET changers		gasnet.med.yale.edu/airway/opt12.htm
Combitube	indirect	oral	both	–	?	Limited jaw opening	AHA guidelines for prehospital management; Interactive frame face with Combitube	Figure 8-13[19,22]

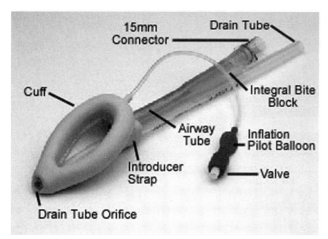

Figure 8-5. Demonstration of LMA use. (Courtesy of LMA, North America Inc.). To view this image in color, please go to *www.ototext.com* or the Electronic Image Collection CD, bound into your copy of Cummings Otolaryngology—Head and Neck Surgery, 4th edition.

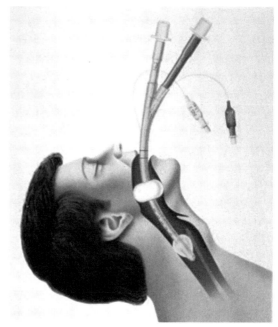

Figure 8-7. Diagram of usage of a Combitube. To view this image in color, please go to *www.ototext.com* or the Electronic Image Collection CD, bound into your copy of Cummings Otolaryngology—Head and Neck Surgery, 4th edition.

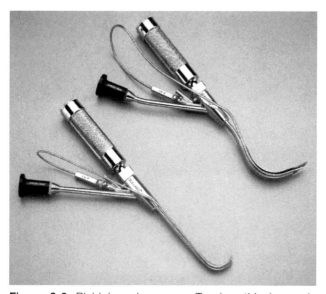

Figure 8-6. Rigid bronchoscopes. To view this image in color, please go to *www.ototext.com* or the Electronic Image Collection CD, bound into your copy of Cummings Otolaryngology—Head and Neck Surgery, 4th edition.

reader in the establishment of an Airway Service at the reader's institution.

Conceptual Framework

The Johns Hopkins Medical Institutions Departments of Anesthesiology/Critical Care and Otolaryngology—Head and Neck Surgery responded to the release of the ASA Guidelines by developing an Airway Management Initiative that has evolved over the past 10 years into the present-day Airway Management Service, education program, and hospital-wide difficult airway

management response system. For the first 6 years, both departments provided financial support. However, in 1999, the Legal Department issued the following statement regarding the Airway Management Initiative and multidisciplinary Airway Service that resulted in full financial support by The Johns Hopkins Medical Institutions:

The institution will be well served by supporting a coordinated team approach dealing with patients with difficult airways. Being able to call upon such a team would assist us in preventing claims and would help with management of claims that do arise because of the assurance of excellence of care and good documentation.

We were fortunate enough to have a lawsuit dismissed in which we allegedly did not render appropriate care for a patient with a difficult airway. The dismissal was a direct result of involvement of members of the multidisciplinary airway service team and their review of the case and their expert opinions.

With appropriate funding and education about the multidisciplinary airway service team, we may have been able to avoid an incident that led us to settling a case last year in which a patient's compromised airway led to an arrest and her death.

Based on even these two examples, it will be prudent for the Hospital to fund the multi-disciplinary airway service and to make sure that it remains functional. We would also need to make sure that the medical staff is aware of the existence and expertise of the service as well.[26]

Multispecialty Service and Joint Clinical Faculty Appointment

To facilitate familiarity between faculty from each department and to support the academic careers of individuals, joint faculty appointments were/are awarded to physicians interested in becoming active members of the Airway Management Service. At any given time, there are two to three members from each department with such appointments. These individuals have the primary responsibility for teaching other faculty, residents, nursing, and support staff within an organized educational program that includes a month-long elective for senior anesthesiology residents (Airway Elective, initiated 1993, see Appendix B). They are the physicians who provide consultation electively and urgently for patients requiring difficult airway management. They are encouraged to be members of Society of Airway Management (SAM) and to participate in the annual meeting.

Preoperative Evaluation and Identification of "Airway Alert"

Approximately 50% of patients seen for surgery are evaluated in our Preoperative Evaluation Center (PEC) several days or weeks before their scheduled procedure by the PEC staff, which consists of an attending anesthesiologist, anesthesiology resident, and nurse practitioner. The PEC anesthesiologist identifies the difficult airway/intubation patient on the basis of prior documented history, physical examination, or specific surgical needs. If consultation with an otolaryngologist or other specialist is needed to facilitate airway management, this is arranged. On the basis of the PEC staff evaluation, the patient is identified as an "Airway Alert" on the Preanesthesia Assessment Form (Appendix C) and entered into the hospital's operating room scheduling system (ORSCIS) with "Airway Alert" identified in the free text field associated with the surgical procedure. Whenever possible, an anesthesia attending is identified who will be available for assistance with airway management on the day of surgery and who has experience with the specific condition or airway difficulty the patient has and the recommended technique. However, the designated anesthesiologist and surgeon caring for the patient during the surgical procedure determine the final airway management plan. When appropriate, postoperative intensive care unit beds are requested to facilitate extubation management. The PEC anesthesiologist, and Airway Service members if consulted, discuss with the patient overall concerns and probable airway management plans A, B, and C. Discussions include

any potential for the procedure to be aborted if issues arise during airway management that are not appropriately planned for. Written informed consent is obtained, including for elective tracheotomy if considered part of the airway management plans. For select patients, recommendations are made for enrollment into Medic Alert.

Before surgery, the anesthesiologist reviews the Preanesthesia Assessment Form to specifically identify the following information: surgical procedure, airway requirements (nasal/oral ETT, jaw wired at end of procedure, tracheotomy as part of procedure, etc.), patient's yes/no response to the presence of gastroesophageal reflux/hiatal hernia (to assess aspiration risk and potential for awake vs RSI technique), previous anesthesia experiences/airway difficulties, height and weight, and attempted-standardized airway examination (oral excursion in fingerbreadths [scale of 1 to 4], temporomandibular distance in fingerbreadths [scale of 1 to 4], upper and lower dentition [normal, dentures, caps, decayed], Mallampati I to IV, neck extension/flexion [scale of normal to decreased by 1 to 2]). The final patient interview and examination are conducted, and the anesthesiologist and surgeon (with assistance from Airway Service, as requested) formulate their actual plans A, B, and C.

Formulation of Intraoperative and Postoperative Plans A, B, and C

Members of the Airway Service are familiar with the ASA difficult airway/intubation algorithm and our institutional experience with rigid laryngoscopy as a primary otolaryngology technique within the ASA algorithm.

The first question the Service asks is, "What is the surgical expectation at the end of the procedure?" Specific answers need to be provided for questions about if and at what stage of the procedure the patient might have a tracheotomy done, if the jaw will be wired closed, whether direct manipulation of the airway will result in edema or significant bleeding, whether positioning could cause airway edema, what will total fluid management entail, and what other considerations might suggest continued intubation at the end of the procedure. For these patients, precise extubation strategies are planned to include the location of extubation (intensive care unit vs returning to the operating room for extubation) and physicians, staff, and equipment resources that must be available.

Next, the Service explores the concept of "difficult." Although the ASA attempts to distinguish between difficult mask and difficult intubation, when the patient does not have a documented prior airway history and is assessed to be difficult for either mask or intubation, considerations for awake intubation techniques are discussed. Obvious limitations to awake techniques are severe mental status issues (intoxication, noncooperative, mental retardation, etc.), severe respiratory/hemodynamic compromise, and unstable trauma. In our experience, patient refusal of an awake intubation has rarely been an issue, primarily because of the positive approach to awake intubation taken by the anesthesiologist during the discussion with the patient.

The next question the Service asks is, "Should the intubation be awake, oral, nasal, or surgical?" followed by, "What is the surgical preference for the ETT (cuffed or uncuffed, smaller-than-expected size, right-angle endotracheal (RAE) or nasal RAE tube, reinforced, laser, double lumen, microlaryngeal, or other specialty ETT)?"

Finally, the Service addresses the issue of the patient's surgical attending airway management expertise and comfort with specific airway management techniques. Specifically, if the situation deteriorates and an emergency surgical airway becomes necessary, who will do it: the patient's surgical attending or OLHN member of the Airway Service?

On the basis of this knowledge, plans A, B, and C are developed by the Service and communicated to the surgeon, patient, and nursing and support staff. Modifications to the plans are made jointly, as needed, before the initiation of any airway management.

Operating Room Preparation

In the early years of the Airway Management Initiative, the Airway Service had as resources four designated OLHN operating rooms (in a single operating room suite) and a small work room to house and clean airway equipment. As the Airway Service expanded coverage to non-OLHN patient consultations in multiple operating room suites within the institution, and responded to emergency responses in nonoperating room locations, the need for duplicate central locations and numerous mobile sites became apparent. In addition, the standard airway equipment in each operating room was expanded and upgraded to facilitate more efficient operating room preparation for both elective and emergency airway management.

Equipment: Standard Anesthesia Equipment and Airway Service Resources

Standard anesthesia equipment in all adult anesthetizing locations includes the following airway management equipment: Eschmann stylet; LMA sizes 3, 4, and 5; conventional laryngoscopes (MAC No. 2, 3, and 4; Miller No. 2 and 3); Sanders jet ventilator; and AMBU bag.

Airway Service resources include a wall poster listing contact numbers for the surgical airway support individuals who are in the hospital daily (elective and on call), the airway equipment specialist support staff contact numbers (Appendix D), and a copy of the Johns Hopkins Adult Airway Management Card (Appendix E). There is specific identification of which services are available and when (24 hours a day, electively, or emergently). The Airway Management Card includes the following information: the contents of the anesthesia fiberoptic cart, the contents of the adult emergency airway cart, information on local anesthesia toxicity, techniques for topical anesthesia, airway blocks, techniques for fiberoptic intubation, information on size issues with the LMA, techniques for changing from LMA to ETT, techniques for changing from a double-lumen ET to a single-lumen ETT, information about size issues with the light wand, lung isolation techniques, techniques for jet ventilation and cricothyrotomy, and information about airway fires, surgical airways, challenging situations, and difficult airway telephone numbers.

Carts: Anesthesia Fiberoptic Cart and Adult Emergency Airway Cart

Two airway carts were created to address specific airway management situations: the Anesthesia Fiberoptic Cart and the Adult Emergency Airway Cart. Both are available with and without a monitor. Both carts include airway alert wristbands and information on how to enroll patients in the in-hospital registry, enter an airway note into the Electronic Patient Record (EPR), and enroll into Medic Alert. The complete contents for each cart are listed on the Adult Airway Management Card.

The Anesthesia Fiberoptic Cart is specifically set up for elective fiberoptic intubations or for fiberoptic verification of double-lumen ETT placement. It has both an LF 1/2 Olympus (3.5/4.0 mm) bronchoscope and adult bronchoscope, Olympus (5.0/6.0 mm) assorted airway management equipment, and topical anesthesia supplies (Figure 8-14). This cart is specifically designed to be used by anesthesiologists in the operating room.

The Adult Emergency Airway Cart is specifically set up for elective procedures in the operating room in which the following techniques are part of the airway management plan and for which the otolaryngologist has primary involvement: fiberoptic bronchoscopy, rigid laryngoscopy, rigid bronchoscopy, jet ventilation, surgical airway (Figure 8-14). Adult Emergency Airway Carts are also located in all intensive care units and the Emergency Department. To note, monitors are included with these carts.

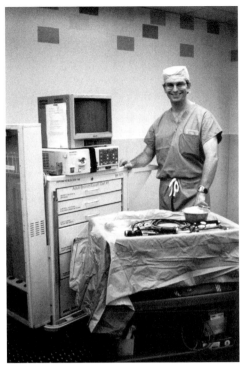

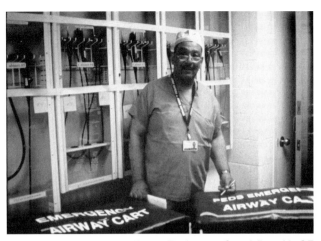

Figure 8-9. M. Witcher, Airway Equipment Specialist with OR Adult Emergency Airway Cart. To view this image in color, please go to *www.ototext.com* or the Electronic Image Collection CD, bound into your copy of Cummings Otolaryngology—Head and Neck Surgery, 4th edition.

Figure 8-8. Adult emergency airway cart with monitor, adult emergency airway cart without monitor for OR use. S. Akst, M.D., with laminated pocket card. JH Adult Airway Management. To view this image in color, please go to *www.ototext.com* or the Electronic Image Collection CD, bound into your copy of Cummings Otolaryngology—Head and Neck Surgery, 4th edition.

For an emergency in the operating room, our otolaryngologists prefer to use the Adult Emergency Airway Cart (Figure 8-15) without the monitor and organized on a single flat-surface cart without numerous drawers. It has the same equipment as the preceding Adult Emergency Airway Cart, but the critical equipment, rigid laryngoscopes and adult fiberoptic bronchoscope, is already assembled for immediate use.

Staff: Anesthesiologist, Specialty Nursing Staff, Surgical Technologists, and Airway Equipment Specialist

For years, anesthesiologists were taught to believe that all aspects of airway management were the responsibility of the anesthesiologist, without specified assistance from nursing or support staff. At the Johns Hopkins Medical Institutions, it was the practice of otolaryngologists and pulmonologists to schedule patients with complex airway pathology to have a diagnostic fiberoptic bronchoscopy in the operating room, with monitored sedation by an anesthesiologist. It became increasingly apparent that successful management of these patients required a team of four

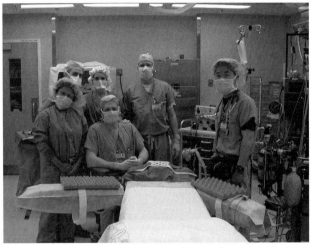

Figure 8-10. Members of Airway Service (from left to right): N. Gorsuch, RN, OLHN, resident; E. Waldman, MD; K. Deweese, RN; G. Ruff, Surgical Technician, OLHN Fellow; J. Schindler, MD, Anesthesia resident; D. Pennington, MD. To view this image in color, please go to *www.ototext.com* or the Electronic Image Collection CD, bound into your copy of Cummings Otolaryngology—Head and Neck Surgery, 4th edition.

professionals: an anesthesiologist to monitor and provide sedation, a surgeon or pulmonologist to perform the bronchoscopy, a nurse to assist with the bronchoscopy, and an equipment specialist to set up the equipment. We found that if any one of the team members failed to perform these duties, the patient's airway management was compromised. We realized that it was not reasonable to expect that an anesthesiologist (or other physician with airway expertise) working alone could provide all the components of complex airway management in a timely, and successful, manner. In cases in which the OLHN surgeon was not immediately required, the Airway Service provided an additional anesthesiologist to provide patient monitoring and sedation while the airway management was being accomplished by the Airway Service and/or operating room anesthesiologist facile with complex airway management. The goals were successful airway management, patient safety, patient satisfaction, and efficient use of operating room resources.

The Airway Service currently has support staff from the Departments of Anesthesiology/Critical Care, Surgery, and Nursing, including specialty operating room nurses,[47] airway equipment specialists, certified surgical technologists (CST), and critical care technicians (Figure 8-16). Their primary responsibilities are to assist physicians in difficult airway management, maintain and upgrade airway equipment, and ensure that the organizational process of a functional airway team is maintained. They are also responsible for the educational of other operating room staff, specifically as to their roles in airway emergencies. Examples of checklists, job descriptions, and educational in-services provided for these staff are included in Appendices F and G (online).

Operating Room Setup

There are three standard operating room bed positions that we use, depending on the surgeon, anesthesiologist, and procedure to be performed. These are: (1) the classic position with the patient's head in alignment with the anesthesiologist; (2) the patient's head rotated 90 degrees from the anesthesiologist; and (3) the patient's head rotated 180 degrees from the anesthesiologist. Decisions regarding positioning are determined by specific operating room equipment issues, the choice of airway algorithm, and the comfort of the anesthesiologist and/or support anesthesia staff (such as staff is needed) with having the patient's head rotated away from the classic position and the anesthesia machine. For example, if the clinical algorithm has plan A as conventional laryngoscopy and plan B as rigid laryngoscopy and the anesthesia team includes an attending and resident, an optimal position to facilitate the rigid laryngoscopy set up is with the patient's head/operating room table rotated 90 degrees from the classic position (Figure 8-17). One member of the anesthesia team has the designated role of monitoring the anesthesia, while the other member is responsible for the airway; the otolaryngologist and nurse are set up to immediately assist, if required.

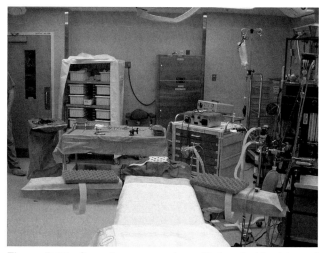

Figure 8-11. Operating room setup with head of bed turned 90 degrees from anesthesiologist area and OLHN rigid laryngoscopes setup. To view this image in color, please go to *www.ototext.com* or the Electronic Image Collection CD, bound into your copy of Cummings Otolaryngology—Head and Neck Surgery, 4th edition.

Advanced Monitoring in the Operating Room and Postoperative Considerations

In efforts to optimize the surgical positioning, as described previously, careful planning of advanced monitoring—specifically arterial and central venous monitoring—must be communicated between the anesthesia and surgery teams. In procedures in which the positioning involves both patient's arms tucked by the sides and the bed rotated 180 degrees from the anesthesiologist, placement of a radial, dorsal pedal, or femoral arterial catheter facilitates more precise management of blood pressure and ability to easily obtain laboratory values as required. Considerations for central venous access include limitations of adequate peripheral venous access (either difficult peripheral venous access or request by surgeon not to access the patient's arms for flap procedures), potential for large blood loss, or patient cardiac issues that suggest monitoring of central venous pressures for optimal management. Communication with the surgical staff facilitates placement of internal/external jugular, subclavian, or femoral venous cannulation. Specific indications for use of pulmonary artery catheters and/or invasive cardiac pacing catheters can be limited by surgical request for femoral venous only and must be carefully considered for relative risk/benefit and issues of difficulty with successful placement from the femoral venous site.

Difficult airway management includes algorithms for difficult extubation management.[14] Specific considerations include when, where, and how to extubate, and the safe disposition of the patient postoperatively.

Preoperative discussions between anesthesiologists, surgeons, and patients should always include the extubation strategy. Issues can occur in the event that a relief anesthesia teams takes over the patient's care, but extubation strategies are not clearly communicated by the original team. In an attempt to avoid the potential for adverse airway events, it is our practice to clearly communicate the entire airway management plan to the operating room nursing, recovery, and intensive care unit staff when possible. When a team decision is made to extubate a complex airway patient, techniques to optimize successful extubation include the following: (1) elevation of the head to at least 45 degrees; (2) careful suctioning of the trachea and oropharynx; (3) nebulizations with bronchodilators; (4) suctioning of the stomach and administration of an antiemetic drug; (5) verification of the reversal of muscle relaxants; (6) verification of appropriate respiratory parameters (head lift of 5 seconds, tidal volume approximately 10 mL/kg, negative inspiratory effort of –20 mmHg, oxygenation of >90%, appropriate level of CO_2); (7) appropriate volume status (nonedematous); (8) hemodynamic stability, (9) and normal laboratory values, if indicated. Considerations for extubation over an Eschmann or ventilating ETT changer, the use of heliox,[15,40] or a "trial extubation" should be clearly communicated to all appropriate physician, nursing, and technician support staff. Emergency airway equipment should be immediately available. The final algorithm for a potentially difficult extubation poses the question, "Who does the emergency tracheotomy?" If the answer is uncertain and the appropriate physicians are not immediately available, it might be prudent to leave the patient intubated and transport to the recovery room or to an intensive care unit.

Extubation Locations

In The Johns Hopkins Medical Institutions, extubations of known difficult airway/intubation patients are done in the recovery room or intensive care units but treated as if they were in the operating room in that the patient must be optimized for a successful extubation, emergency airway equipment must be immediately available and/or set up, a physician who can do a surgical airway must be present, and a physician must be present who can monitor the patient and administer anesthesia or resuscitation medications, if needed. Depending on the complexity of the airway management, some patients are returned to the operating room for extubation and airway management as required.

Nursing Critical Pathway for Difficult Airway/Intubation Patients

Once the care of the patient is transferred to the recovery room or intensive care unit, the patient is entered into a nursing critical pathway, a key element of which is education and Medic Alert enrollment of the patient with a difficult airway/intubation. The pathway prompts nursing personnel to specifically query difficult airway/intubation preoperatively and again on arrival in the recovery room (Appendix H). If difficult airway/intubation is present, the pathway initiates implementation of a specific protocol that includes in-hospital identification, patient-family teaching, enrollment into the in-hospital registry, and a quality improvement system.

In-Hospital Difficult Airway/Intubation Alert Wristbands and Chart Labels

Difficult airway/intubation patient identification also includes a green identification wristband and a patient chart airway alert label (Figure 8-18). This facilitates transition from a temporary in-hospital registry to the permanent Medic Alert Registry (Figure 8-19). Similar in appearance to an allergy alert wristband, the green difficult airway/intubation wristband provides continued patient identification and safety during hospitalization. The Joint Committee on Clinical Investigations at The Johns Hopkins Medical Institutions issued a waiver on the need to obtain written informed consent before placing green wristbands on identified patients with a difficult airway/intubation. Health care personnel and patients recognize that the tremendous implications to patient safety outweigh the concern for breach of confidentiality, as already modeled in existing in-hospital allergy alert temporary wristbands and out-of-hospital permanent medical alert bracelets.[32]

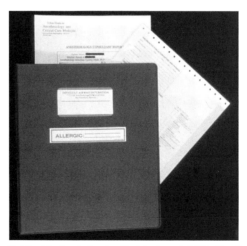

Figure 8-12. Medical chart with label and ACR. To view this image in color, please go to *www.ototext.com* or the Electronic Image Collection CD, bound into your copy of Cummings Otolaryngology—Head and Neck Surgery, 4th edition.

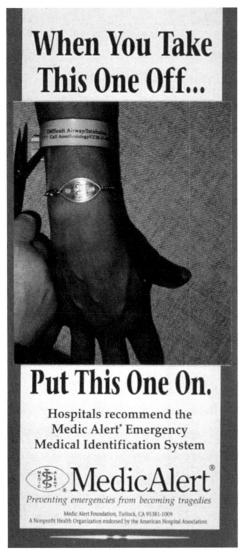

Figure 8-13. Transition from in-hospital airway registry to Medic Alert Foundation. To view this image in color, please go to *www.ototext.com* or the Electronic Image Collection CD, bound into your copy of Cummings Otolaryngology—Head and Neck Surgery, 4th edition.

Education

The educational component of the Airway Initiative and Airway Service is divided into directed efforts toward family and patient, physicians and health care providers within the institution, administrators of The Johns Hopkins Medical Institutions, and health care providers at large.

Patient and Family

At numerous times during a patient's hospitalization, effective communication with the patient and family is accomplished in preoperative consultation, immediately preoperatively, during the procedure (as requested), immediately postoperatively, and during the postoperative course. Discharge follow-up consists of a letter from the Department of Anesthesiology (Appendix I) with an enclosed brochure for enrollment into Medic Alert, as previously discussed with the patient.

Physicians

Physicians at The Johns Hopkins Medical Institutions are invited to participate in the Airway Rotation as appropriate. During this rotation, in addition to exposure to airway devices identified in the ASA Difficult Airway Guidelines, senior anesthesia residents receive training in the elective use of the OLHN Hollinger and Dedo rigid laryngoscopes. Before elective use in the operating room, the anesthesia resident completes an in-service and mannequin practice under OLHN attending guidance. The series of photographs (Figures 8-20 through 8-29) are presented to show the ease in which successful elective rigid laryngoscopy can be taught. The narrations accompanying the photographs summarize the airway management of a patient scheduled for a suspension microlaryngoscopy (SML) and biopsy of a vocal cord lesion. On initial airway evaluation, the patient had a known history of easy intubation with conventional laryngoscopy and no contraindications to this airway management plan. The airway management plan—asleep mask ventilation and direct laryngoscopy with OLHN rigid laryngoscopes—is an acceptable standard of care. The "teaching" aspect to this case was that the senior anesthesia resident was the physician designated to manage the patient's airway as described earlier under direct supervision of an attending OLHN

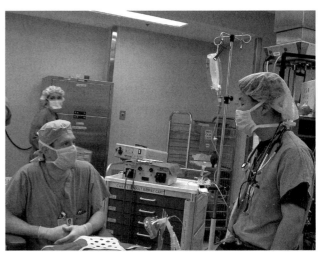

Figure 8-14. Final discussions regarding airway management. To view this image in color, please go to *www.ototext.com* or the Electronic Image Collection CD, bound into your copy of Cummings Otolaryngology—Head and Neck Surgery, 4th edition.

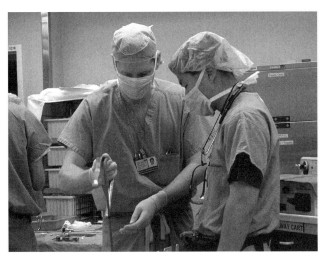

Figure 8-15. Teaching fine points with the Hollinger rigid laryngoscope. To view this image in color, please go to *www.ototext.com* or the Electronic Image Collection CD, bound into your copy of Cummings Otolaryngology—Head and Neck Surgery, 4th edition.

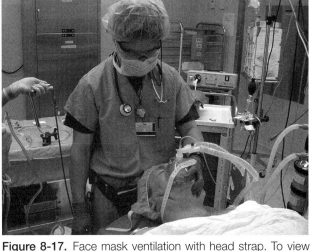

Figure 8-17. Face mask ventilation with head strap. To view this image in color, please go to *www.ototext.com* or the Electronic Image Collection CD, bound into your copy of Cummings Otolaryngology—Head and Neck Surgery, 4th edition.

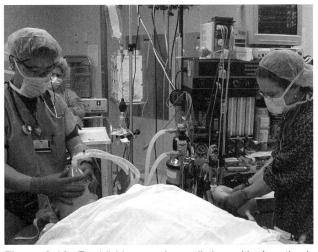

Figure 8-16. Establishing mask ventilation with Anesthesia Attending L. Mark, M.D. To view this image in color, please go to *www.ototext.com* or the Electronic Image Collection CD, bound into your copy of Cummings Otolaryngology—Head and Neck Surgery, 4th edition.

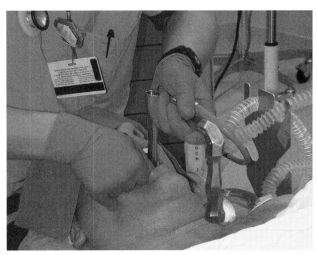

Figure 8-18. Placement of the Hollinger with tooth guard. To view this image in color, please go to *www.ototext.com* or the Electronic Image Collection CD, bound into your copy of Cummings Otolaryngology—Head and Neck Surgery, 4th edition.

surgeon and attending anesthesiologist. The patient was successfully mask ventilated and intubated with a Hollinger rigid laryngoscope/Eschmann/ETT technique. There were no associated morbidities with this procedure.

Physicians are also invited to attend monthly Airway Management Multidisciplinary Case Conferences, attend quarterly mandatory Risk Management Seminars in which airway events are highlighted, and participate in monthly equipment workshops and optional cadaver laboratories. Arrangements can be made to observe

airway management in the operating room, intensive care units, or Emergency Department as appropriate.

Institutional Systems Approach

All operating room personnel participate in yearly disaster drills in which difficult airway management is highlighted and protocols are reviewed. The use of simulation has been a component of the educational program for the past 4 years, with acute airway management being the most recent component. Effective education in difficult airway management

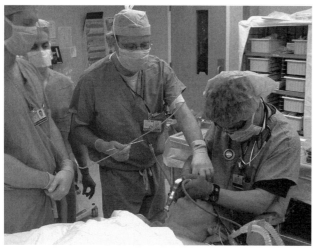

Figure 8-19. Viewing the glottic opening. To view this image in color, please go to *www.ototext.com* or the Electronic Image Collection CD, bound into your copy of Cummings Otolaryngology—Head and Neck Surgery, 4th edition.

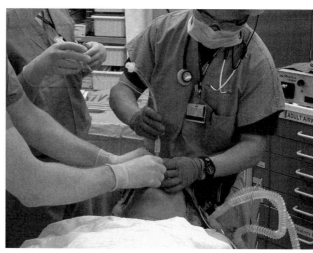

Figure 8-21. Advancing the ETT over the Eschmann stylet. To view this image in color, please go to *www.ototext.com* or the Electronic Image Collection CD, bound into your copy of Cummings Otolaryngology—Head and Neck Surgery, 4th edition.

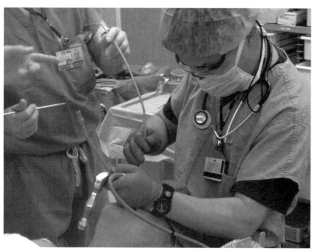

Figure 8-20. Placement of the Eschmann stylet through the Hollinger into the glottic opening. To view this image in color, please go to *www.ototext.com* or the Electronic Image Collection CD, bound into your copy of Cummings Otolaryngology—Head and Neck Surgery, 4th edition.

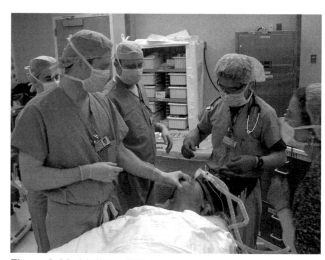

Figure 8-22. Verifying ETT position with $ETCO_2$ and auscultation and assessing for soft tissue trauma. To view this image in color, please go to *www.ototext.com* or the Electronic Image Collection CD, bound into your copy of Cummings Otolaryngology—Head and Neck Surgery, 4th edition.

encompasses much more than simple task training. The high-level components of learning difficult airway management skills include: (1) task training (different techniques of airway management); (2) decision making (learning to recognize and react appropriately to an evolving critical situation); and (3) team building (who needs to be present and what their roles are). Classically, this process has taken place in the setting of delivering patient care, under conditions that may not be particularly conducive to education.

Ongoing Education and CME: Workshops, Role of Simulator, and SAM Annual Meeting

Ongoing education includes a series of annual workshops organized by the Airway Service and offered to all members of the medical institution. They include cadaver surgical airway techniques; mannequin rigid laryngoscopy, fiberoptic bronchoscopy, light wands and a variety of other specialty scopes; and mannequin percutaneous cricothyrotomy and jet ventilation. All are case-based to facilitate discussion and are staffed by at least one attending anesthesiologist, otolaryn-

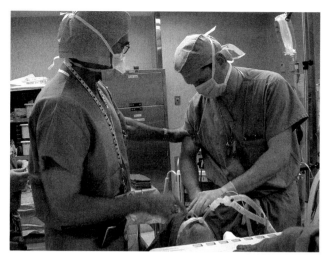

Figure 8-23. Mentorship from OLHN Attending C. W. Cummings, M.D. To view this image in color, please go to *www.ototext.com* or the Electronic Image Collection CD, bound into your copy of Cummings Otolaryngology—Head and Neck Surgery, 4th edition.

gologist, nursing specialist, and airway equipment specialist.

In recent years, technology has been developed that can realistically simulate a myriad of critical airway scenarios by use of computerized mannequins. Depending on the verisimilitude required, such mannequins can cost between $30,000 and $300,000, with operating costs ranging from negligible to $60,000 per year. Despite the apparent high cost, the use of simulation in airway management education ultimately should be cost-effective with respect to the improved outcomes that would be expected from better-educated clinicians.

The implementation of simulation is occurring in the context of the "competency-based" education movement that is underway in medical education as a whole. The advantages of simulation over the classical methods of patient-based education are fourfold. First, by using simulation, the trainees can get unlimited experience in critical airway situations that are not very common, thereby having an opportunity to practice and improve their skills until a level of proficiency is achieved. Every time an adverse outcome results, the student can review it, learn from it, and hit the reset button to revive the mannequin to try again. Second, the mannequin is programmed to respond to the interventions of the student, whether correct or not. In either case, the student is forced to reassess the situation and make alternative plans. This decision-making process is essential to learn if one is to be capable of managing the difficult airway. The entire process is recorded and compared with instructor-developed objective

standards, which permits focused learning. Third, critical airway management is a team game and requires an understanding of the roles of each team member. This is easily simulated using the mannequins while in an environment that is less pressured than if a real critical airway event was taking place. This facilitates better communication between team members, so that everyone has a common understanding of the overall process. Last, the use of simulation ensures that all the clinicians have educational exposure to a set of clinical situations that are standardized with respect to the specific conditions and the specific learning objectives to be achieved. This is not possible in the patient-based educational model (Figure 8-30).

Individuals interested in participating in a formal CME, multidisciplinary, comprehensive, airway course, compete with simulatory technology are encouraged to attend the annual SAM Meeting.

DIFFICULT AIRWAY/INTUBATION: DOCUMENTATION AND DISSEMINATION OF CRITICAL AIRWAY INFORMATION TO PATIENTS

Written documentation of airway events is institution-specific and specialty variable. No standardized, uniform, readily available document exists to precisely record airway events and summarizes salient issues.

Issues with Conveying Information Verbally to Difficult Airway/Intubation Patients

When complex airway management patients are discharged, information about critical airway events may be inadvertently not communicated or miscommunicated. Verbal communication of difficult airway

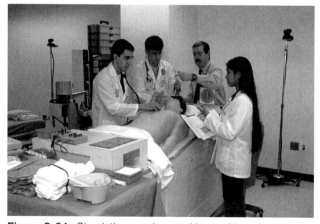

Figure 8-24. Simulation can be used in teaching airway management to medical students (shown), as well as residents, fellows, and paramedical personnel. To view this image in color, please go to *www.ototext.com* or the Electronic Image Collection CD, bound into your copy of Cummings Otolaryngology—Head and Neck Surgery, 4th edition.

information by the provider to the patient is unreliable. Communication may be hindered by patient intubation, sedation, or both. The patient may be expeditiously discharged from the health care facility or discharged by personnel other than primary health care provider before airway events have been fully communicated. Miscommunication may arise because of the patient's lack of medical knowledge or because of overriding anxiety related to the medical condition. In addition, providers may underrepresent the severity of difficulty, attempting to allay the patient's anxiety or because they themselves fear liability exposure. Written communication of difficult airway/intubation information by the provider to the patient may be a more effective strategy, but the patient may fail to accurately and comprehensively convey this information to future health care providers. Patients may lose the anesthesiologist's letter or memo or fail to give a copy of it to their primary care provider. Then, in an emergency situation, the information will most likely be inaccessible.

When difficult airway/intubation patients reenter the health care system electively or emergently, they may relate vague verbal histories, deny any difficult airway/intubation history, or be physically unable to communicate.

Issues with Obtaining Information from Previous Medical Records

Attempts to retrieve prior anesthesia records and documentation should be initiated but may be unsuccessful because of time constraints or unavailability. Even when available, written documentation may be incomplete and difficult for other health care providers to decipher. These situations create confusion as to the exact nature of the airway difficulty encountered and airway management used, thus potentially delaying or compromising patient care.

Even when written documentation is complete and adequate, the information is contained in the patient's original medical record. Subsequent elective or emergent retrieval of records by future health care providers, who are separated by geography or time from the original event, may prove to be untimely or impossible.

The Electronic Patient Record: Airway Notes and Anesthesiology Consultant Report

Building the electronic patient record (EPR) at Johns Hopkins, we developed and implemented two templates (Appendix G) that can be used by the anesthesiologist for either dictating or typing a note on a patient with a difficult airway/intubation. The first template, the Airway Note, is a brief, free-text dictated entry that specifically summarizes airway manage-

ment. The second, more complete template, the Anesthesiology Consultant Report (ACR), is a one-page to two-page summary that includes airway information in addition to more comprehensive anesthesia concerns.[32] Templates are included in Appendix K.[35,39]

"Difficult Airway/Intubation" is placed as a "problem" in the patient's PAM (problem, allergy, medication) list in the overview of the medical record, so that subsequent health care providers will be aware of this specific issue. Because many providers may not read the specific notes on a patient, this PAM alert, similar to an allergy alert, is immediately highlighted whenever the medical record is accessed.

As electronic anesthesia intraoperative records begin to appear in hospitals, it is imperative that they be integrated into the hospital EPR, so that the anesthesiologist only needs to enter relevant difficult airway/intubation information one time. Finally, to close the loop from the surgical side, all surgeons, particularly OLHN surgeons who understand the nuances of difficult airway management, should be encouraged to include in their operative dictation an accurate description of whatever difficult or unanticipated airway events occurred.

Finally, a letter regarding the airway management (Appendix I) is sent from the Department of Anesthesiology to the patient, along with a brochure for enrollment into the Medic Alert Foundation.

Medic Alert Foundation

Medic Alert Foundation is a 501(c)3 nonprofit organization that has more than 40 years of experience with information exchange. Its stated mission is to protect and save lives by disseminating critical patient information immediately and accurately while maintaining patient confidentiality and privacy. This service is provided by a three-part system: a 24-hour emergency response center, a visible alert emblem worn by the patient (Figure 8-5), and a wallet card (Figure 8-6). By 2000, Medic Alert had expanded its system to include a fax alert. Medic Alert reliably tracks patients and updates their medical information. An initial enrollment fee (the costs of which depends on the type of metal selected for the emblem) is waived for patients who are unable to pay if enrollment is accompanied by a letter from the health care provider. Patients are contacted yearly to update medical information, and a nominal annual fee is requested. In 1979, Medic Alert Foundation was endorsed by the ASA House of Delegates. For years anesthesiologists had recognized the value of the Medic Alert emergency response system for patients with malignant hyperthermia (INDEX ZERO hotline) and had enrolled patients with difficult intubation/airways in a nonuniform way. In 1992, the Anesthesia Advisory Council recommended the cre-

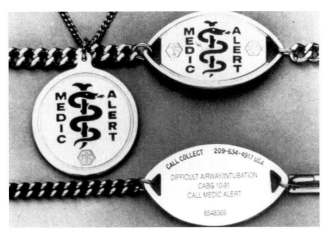

Figure 8-25. *Clockwise from left*, The Medic Alert emblem as a necklace, the Medic Alert emblem as a bracelet, and the reverse side of the Medic Alert emblem, which shows the Medic Alert collect phone number (accessible nationally and internationally without charge to the caller), the Difficult Airway/Intubation Registry designation, and the patient's unique identification number for the Medic Alert system. To view this image in color, please go to *www.ototext.com* or the Electronic Image Collection CD, bound into your copy of Cummings Otolaryngology—Head and Neck Surgery, 4th edition.

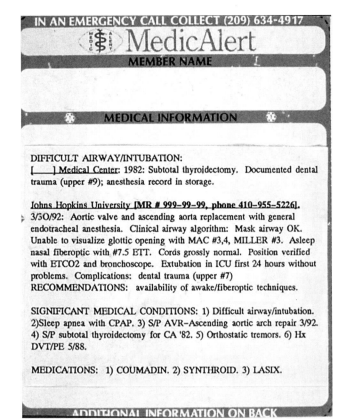

Figure 8-26. The Medic Alert wallet card with Airway Registry information. To view this image in color, please go to *www.ototext.com* or the Electronic Image Collection CD, bound into your copy of Cummings Otolaryngology—Head and Neck Surgery, 4th edition.

ation of the National Difficult Airway/Intubation Registry within the Medic Alert Foundation.[35,36] The establishment of the National Difficult Airway/Intubation Registry within Medic Alert promoted a standardization of terminology and an expanded database specifically for airway patients (Figure 8-7).

To create the National Airway/Intubation Registry, the Medic Alert Foundation system, which already included a 24-hour computerized emergency response center (with telephone access nationally and internationally without charge to the caller), wallet card, and visible alert emblem, was expanded to accommodate a more extensive database and a fax service for hard copy.

Components of the Difficult Airway Registry

The core of the Registry is the Medic Alert emergency response service, which includes a 24-hour emergency response center with phone and fax capability, visible alert emblem, and wallet card. The Medic Alert phone number (209-634-4917) is imprinted on the visible alert emblem. Callers are instructed to call collect. This phone number is accessible both nationally and internationally, unlike an 800 number, which cannot be accessed outside the United States.

For the purposes of the Difficulty Airway/Intubation Registry, the basic Medic Alert service was expanded to include the following components.

Specialized enrollment brochure. Enrollment in the Registry was facilitated by a brochure specifically designed to address the concerns of health care providers and patients (Figure 8-8). Although the brochure is no longer distributed by Medic Alert, the information panels can provide practitioners and patients with information about frequently asked questions about difficult airway management and are included in this chapter to facilitate perioperative discussion with patients.

- Health care provider information panel (Figure 8-9).
- Patient information panel (Figure 8-10).
- Medic Alert service.
- Legal statement.
- Enrollment section.

Information requested for the enrollment section includes patient demographics, emergency contacts, medical information to be engraved on the visible alert emblem, and other emergency medical information. Specific registry information supplied by the practitioner includes hospital name, medical record number, surgical procedure, date of procedure, clinical anesthesia profile, nature of difficulty encountered, reason(s) for difficulty, successful and

5. TO BE FILLED OUT BY PRACTITIONER (Patient should proceed to question 6): Not placed on Medic Alert computer record until validated by physician.

1. _____

| HOSPITAL NAME | MEDICAL RECORD # (Very important) |

2. Clinical profile: ❏ Anesthesiologist ❏ CRNA ❏ Otolaryngologist ❏ ED

   Other_____

   ASA Classification ❏ I ❏ II ❏ III ❏ IV ❏ V ❏ E

   HT_____ Wt/kg _____

   Site: ❏ OR ❏ Non-OR ❏ Ward ❏ ED Other _____

   Monitors utilized: ❏ Capnography ❏ Oximetry Other_____

3. The difficult airway was: ❏ anticipated ❏ unanticipated

4. If anticipated, how was the difficulty discovered?

   ❏ airway history by patient/family interview ❏ physical exam

   ❏ documentation in medical record ❏ diagnostic tests/consultations

   Specify_____

5. What type of difficult airway was encountered?

   ❏ mask/ventilation ❏ intubation ❏ extubation Other_____

6. The difficulty encountered was primarily:

   ❏ small mouth ❏ tongue ❏ dentition ❏ ant/superior larynx

   ❏ limited jaw opening/mobility ❏ limited neck extension ❏ C-spine stability

   ❏ distorted anatomy ❏ infection ❏ pregnancy Other_____

7. Visualization (check all that apply)

   ❏ complete glottic opening ❏ partial glottic opening ❏ arytenoids ❏ tip of epiglottis

| PROCEDURE | ___/___/___ Mo Day Year |

8. What equipment/techniques were successful in airway management? (circle all that apply)

   awake • asleep • nasal • oral • blind nasal • laryngeal mask • MAC #1 2 3 4 • MILLER #1 2 3 4 • fiberoptic • intubation guide • retrograde • lightwand • jet ventilation • cricothyrotomy • existing trach/surgical airway • percutaneous crico/trach • bougie • Combitube • tracheotomy • specialized laryngoscope, blade & size (specify)_____

   endotracheal tube & size (specify) _____

   Other & size (specify)_____

9. What equipment/techniques were unsuccessful in airway management? (circle all that apply)

   awake • asleep • nasal • oral • blind nasal • laryngeal mask • MAC #1 2 3 4 • MILLER #1 2 3 4 • fiberoptic • intubation guide • retrograde • lightwand • jet ventilation • cricothyrotomy • existing trach/surgical airway • percutaneous crico/trach • bougie • Combitube • tracheotomy • specialized laryngoscope, blade & size (specify) _____

   endotracheal tube & size (specify) _____

   Other & size (specify)_____

10. What was the outcome? ❏ no adverse outcomes ❏ cancel procedure

    ❏ dental trauma ❏ soft tissue/nasal trauma ❏ laryngeal trauma ❏ desaturation

    ❏ vocal chord trauma ❏ tracheal trauma ❏ cardiovascular compromise ❏ aspiration

    Other _____

Specify clinically applied algorithm, number of attempts and pertinent findings._____

_____

Recommendations for colleagues:_____

Physician or Anesthestist's Signature _____ Print Name/Phone #_____

Include on Wallet Card? ❏ Yes ❏ No

Figure 8-27. Airway management database section of the Medic Alert National Airway/Intubation Registry enrollment form. It can be scanned and faxed to facilitate rapid dissemination of critical airway information. Although this database section is no longer distributed by Medic Alert Foundation, practitioners may include any/all of this information in the patient's medical information section of the current Medic Alert enrollment form.

unsuccessful techniques, best visualization of airway anatomy, clinically applied algorithm, and clinical outcome. The section of the brochure that contains information by the practitioner is scannable and able to be faxed. The enrolling health care provider's signature authenticates the information provided; however, anonymity is honored if requested. Select information from this database is compiled in paragraph form, printed on the patient's wallet card, and sent by fax when requested. With the exception of specific airway requirements (such as those caused by tracheal surgery, stenosis, or other conditions requiring specific sizes of endotracheal tubes), recommendations for future airway management are *not* printed on the wallet card, thereby avoiding conflicts with other practitioners' choices of future airway management techniques. Clinical outcome information from the original health care provider is confidential, collected for research purposes only, and is not disseminated to the patient or future health care providers.

Patient signature. Informed consent must be obtained for enrollment.

Practitioner security. Practitioner security is increased by the Registry in two ways: (1) by improving provider–patient communication; and (2) by documenting and disseminating critical airway information to future health care providers.

Malpractice claims are often initiated because of poor communication.[27] Enrollment in the Registry gives providers an opportunity to inform patients of their airway difficulties and adverse events while offering a way to protect patients from airway difficulties in the future. A survey showed that, despite experiencing adverse outcomes (cancellation of surgery, dental trauma, soft tissue trauma, desaturation, cardiovascular compromise, and cricothyrotomy or tracheostomy), 100% of Registry patients were satisfied with enrollment in the Registry and had a sense of comfort that future health care providers would understand the significance of their difficult airway/intubation and the concept of Medic Alert.[13] Even after a difficult experience, patients favorably responded to their anesthesiologists' knowledgeable presentation of organized efforts to register their problem and reduce the risk of recurrence. Enrollment in the Registry, as documented in patients' charts, is a

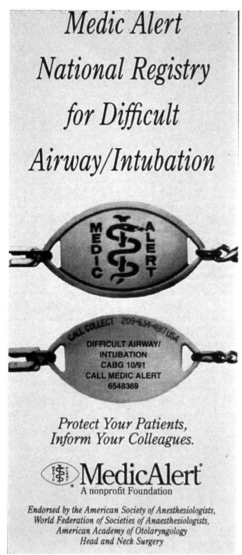

Figure 8-28. The cover of the Medic Alert National Difficult Airway/Intubation Registry enrollment brochure. To view this image in color, please go to *www.ototext.com* or the Electronic Image Collection CD, bound into your copy of Cummings Otolaryngology—Head and Neck Surgery, 4th edition.

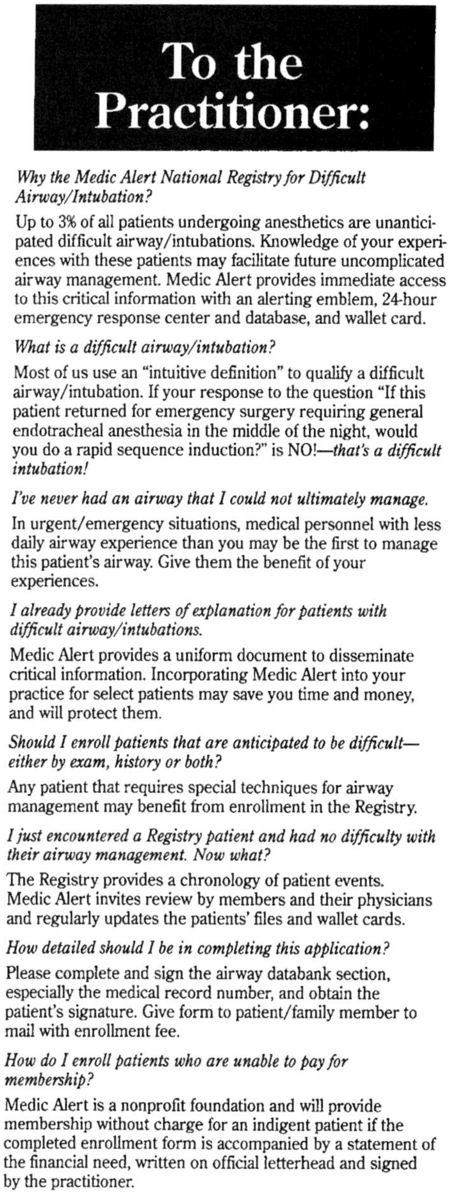

positive reflection on the providers' concern for future patient safety.

Malpractice claims are often initiated because of poor documentation.[23] At present, the intraoperative anesthesia record does not provide information in a standardized, easily readable form and is not readily accessible to providers to use during future episodes of care. In contrast, information from the Registry is standardized and detailed and can be obtained by telephone or fax within 5 minutes of the request. Not only is this information readily available, but it is also important to note that for more than 40 years there have been no claims against Medic Alert for breach of confidentiality or dissemination of incorrect medical

To the Practitioner:

Why the Medic Alert National Registry for Difficult Airway/Intubation?

Up to 3% of all patients undergoing anesthetics are unanticipated difficult airway/intubations. Knowledge of your experiences with these patients may facilitate future uncomplicated airway management. Medic Alert provides immediate access to this critical information with an alerting emblem, 24-hour emergency response center and database, and wallet card.

What is a difficult airway/intubation?

Most of us use an "intuitive definition" to qualify a difficult airway/intubation. If your response to the question "If this patient returned for emergency surgery requiring general endotracheal anesthesia in the middle of the night, would you do a rapid sequence induction?" is NO!—*that's a difficult intubation!*

I've never had an airway that I could not ultimately manage.

In urgent/emergency situations, medical personnel with less daily airway experience than you may be the first to manage this patient's airway. Give them the benefit of your experiences.

I already provide letters of explanation for patients with difficult airway/intubations.

Medic Alert provides a uniform document to disseminate critical information. Incorporating Medic Alert into your practice for select patients may save you time and money, and will protect them.

Should I enroll patients that are anticipated to be difficult—either by exam, history or both?

Any patient that requires special techniques for airway management may benefit from enrollment in the Registry.

I just encountered a Registry patient and had no difficulty with their airway management. Now what?

The Registry provides a chronology of patient events. Medic Alert invites review by members and their physicians and regularly updates the patients' files and wallet cards.

How detailed should I be in completing this application?

Please complete and sign the airway databank section, especially the medical record number, and obtain the patient's signature. Give form to patient/family member to mail with enrollment fee.

How do I enroll patients who are unable to pay for membership?

Medic Alert is a nonprofit foundation and will provide membership without charge for an indigent patient if the completed enrollment form is accompanied by a statement of the financial need, written on official letterhead and signed by the practitioner.

Figure 8-29. Health provider information panel, Medic Alert National Registry for Difficult Airway/Intubation. Note: although no longer distributed by Medic Alert, the information presented may facilitate positive communication with patients who might benefit from enrollment into Medic Alert.

information. When patients sign the informed consent for enrollment in Medic Alert, they are agreeing to a confidential exchange of physician-verified medical information.

Cost savings. The cost of initial enrollment in the Registry is justified by future savings realized by the patient and provider or institution. A preliminary study of selective patient charges for anesthesia preparation time (i.e., anesthesiologist's professional fee, anesthesia resident's charge, drug and supply charges,

To the Patient:

What Is Difficult Airway/Intubation?

During general anesthesia, a specially trained professional assists your breathing. For a majority of patients, this is easily done by placing a mask over your nose and mouth, inserting a breathing tube into your windpipe or both. Individual differences in jaw structure, mouth opening and dentition, and neck movement might make some patients more difficult to manage than others.

If a physician can anticipate or is alerted to previous airway difficulty, they can implement special techniques that are safe and comfortable.

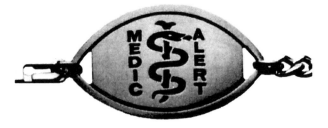

How Can Medic Alert Help?

Medic Alert can provide readily available information regarding your history with difficult airway/intubation, in future elective and emergency medical situations. This is important, particularly in emergency situations, when someone other than your primary physician is involved in providing you with emergency health care. The Medic Alert emblem will immediately alert the health care provider to vital information that is critical to your safety.

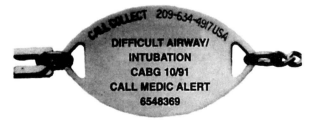

How Can I Enroll In Medic Alert?

If your physician experienced airway difficulty and feels you should be enrolled in the Medic Alert program, he/she will provide information on this form about your airway management.

You must provide personal data and other significant medical conditions. When completed, please sign form and mail with enrollment fee.

Figure 8-30. Patient information panel. See note on Figure 8-9.

and operating room time charges) was done for all 690 patients undergoing coronary artery bypass graft (CABG) surgery as the first procedure of the day at The Johns Hopkins Medical Institutions during a 10-month period. Of these patients, 684 had no airway difficulty (control group), and 6 had difficult airway/intubations and were subsequently enrolled in the Medic Alert National Difficult Airway/Intubation Registry. Results of the survey showed that the mean selective patient charge for anesthesia preparation time for the Registry group was $1578.24; this represented a 59% increase over the control group mean selective patient charge of $990.71.[33] Knowledge of difficulties previously encountered and techniques used can promote the cost-effective use of equipment and operating room time for difficult airway/intubation patients.

Anticipation and preparation for a difficult airway/intubation patient, as identified by the Registry, may decrease the incidence of cancellations, adverse outcomes, and malpractice claims. Even one settlement can cost the provider or institution significantly more than the time, effort, and cost of enrolling many patients in the Registry.

Characteristics of Registry Patients. Between 1992 and 1994, more than 250 adult and pediatric patients throughout the United States were enrolled in the Medic Alert National Difficult Airway/Intubation Registry. Approximately 50% were in ASA classes I to II, and 50% were in ASA classes III to IV. Enrolled patients required general anesthesia, had difficulty, and/or did not require airway management at the time of enrollment but had a documented history of prior airway management. Patients were enrolled from private and academic institutions, outpatient surgical centers, and by self-referral. In a preliminary report of 111 of these patients, a variety of airway techniques were used, and adverse outcomes were reported[20,35,33] (Tables 8-1 to 8-3). To ensure patient safety, providers encouraged these patients to enroll when there were

TABLE 8-2	
CHARACTERISTICS OF PATIENTS ENROLLED IN THE MEDIC ALERT NATIONAL DIFFICULT AIRWAY/INTUBATION REGISTRY	
Characteristic	**Cases* (%)**
Adult (age > 18 years)	99
Emergency	1
ASA classes I and II	54
ASA classes III and IV	46
ASA class V	0
Anticipated difficult	44
Unanticipated difficult	56
Difficult mask airway	10
Difficult intubation	97

*n = 111
ASA, American Society of Anesthesiologists.

TABLE 8-3

AIRWAY MANAGEMENT TECHNIQUES USED FOR PATIENTS IN THE MEDIC ALERT NATIONAL DIFFICULT AIRWAY/INTUBATION REGISTRY

| | OUTCOME | |
Technique	Successful (n = 110)	Unsuccessful (n = 200)
Conventional laryngoscopy	20	170
Fiberoptic bronchoscopy	66	13
Lighted stylet	1	1
Surgical airway	11	3
Specialized others	12	13

TABLE 8-4

ADVERSE OUTCOMES FOR PATIENTS IN THE MEDIC ALERT NATIONAL DIFFICULT AIRWAY/INTUBATION REGISTRY

Type	Frequency (n = 31)
Cancellation	9
Dental trauma	3
Desaturation	7
Soft tissue or nasal trauma	8
Tracheal trauma	3
Cardiovascular compromise	2
Other	7

minor or major adverse outcomes, despite concerns of liability exposure.

DIFFICULT AIRWAY/INTUBATION: FUTURE DIRECTIONS FOR NATIONAL ELECTRONIC PATIENT RECORDS AND SHARED HOSPITAL AIRWAY REGISTRIES

Interest has been high for several years in the concept of a national EPR. In 1991, the Institute of Medicine set a goal of 10 years for widespread use of the computerized patient record. In January 1994, the Computer-Based Patient Record Institute, Inc. announced that it would seek major funding to finalize the development of standards for health care informatics. It seems inevitable, given the current interest and effort by government and private sectors, that a national EPR will become a reality. However, because of the complexity and scope of the issues involved, the time frame for accomplishing this goal remains far from certain. The objectives of the National Airway/Intubation Registry are in agreement with those organizations supporting development of the EPR. The Medic Alert system (with its centralized and computerized database of medical information accessible by telephone or fax within 5 minutes and with Internet access in development) already embodies many of the concepts of the EPR (see Appendix L for contact information). Proposals are being developed to allow electronic data transfers while accommodating patient confidentiality and medical records security through appropriate documentation and encryption techniques. Once these safety mechanisms are in place, automated queries of the Registry will become possible, obviating the need for telephone calls that interrupt the flow of patient evaluation in busy outpatient practices. As the electronic computerized patient record becomes more common in preanesthetic evaluation,[21] such automated queries of the Registry will become commonplace. Future developments could include supplementary photodocumentation. As development of the electronic patient record continues, Medic Alert's goals and information format will easily mesh with the infrastructure of an emerging electronic patient record. Although Medic Alert is not defined as a "Covered Entity" under HIPAA regulations,[36] it follows rigid patient information privacy standards that are consistent with the HIPAA rules. The data contained in their database of patient information are kept confidential, being shared only with medical providers in the course of caring for the patient. Medic Alert also complies with principles that govern the retention, collection, and safeguarding of data as defined by the European Union SafeHarbor framework.[57]

CLINICAL PRACTICES: CASE PRESENTATIONS OF DIFFICULT AIRWAY/INTUBATION PATIENTS
Case 1: Consultation with the Airway Service for Future Airway Management

The patient was a 25-year-old woman who was seen in consultation for future airway management for elective surgery or in the event of an emergency. She had been referred for airway management consultation by her sister, a nurse. By profession, she was a law student. Her medical history was significant for hemangioma of the tongue. She was status post numerous embolizations as a child and young adult with increasingly difficult airway management. The last incident, 5 years prior, was one in which the anesthesia team was unable to nasally or orally intubate her trachea, and the procedure was canceled. She was now contemplating uterine surgery for fibroids and wanted to understand all the options she had for airway management.

On physical examination, she was 5'6" and weighed 58 kg. Her facial structures appeared normal until she opened her mouth. Her mouth opening was three fingerbreadths, and her entire oral cavity was filled with the hemangioma, which had caused her upper and lower teeth to protrude outward. On nasal examination, there was extension into her nasopharynx. Her neck had normal range of motion; her thyroid was within normal limits and her trachea mobile. Her speech was remarkable for distinct thickness and slurring of some words.

After an in-depth discussion between the anesthesiologist and otolaryngologist, a joint recommendation was made for an awake tracheotomy in the event of required general anesthesia or for regional anesthesia (if appropriate), with the immediate availability of a surgeon capable of doing a tracheotomy in the event that regional anesthesia failed or the situation became an airway emergency.

Discussion

1. Despite major advances in airway techniques, anesthetic agents, and monitoring, there remain instances when an elective tracheotomy is the airway management technique of choice. The consultation facilitated a discussion that addressed risks and benefits and allayed the patient's fears regarding the uncomfortableness and permanence of a tracheotomy.
2. The patient requested enrollment into Medic Alert. She had an active lifestyle and was very realistic about the potential for an adverse outcome related to her airway if she were unable to communicate the consultant's recommendation of an awake/urgent tracheotomy.

Case 2: Anticipated from Physical Examination: Awake Nasal Intubation

The patient was a 66-year-old woman who was seen in the operating room for a direct laryngoscopy with biopsy. She had the specific designation of "Airway Alert: Awake Intubation" from the Preoperative Evaluation Center (PEC). The otolaryngologist had followed her case for 3 years with a diagnosis of a left vocal cord polyp, which had greatly enlarged over the previous 6 months. Her chief complaint was respiratory difficulty. Flexible laryngoscopy in the otolaryngology clinic confirmed the presence of a ball-valving pedunculated polyp originating near the anterior commissure of the vocal fold. On expiration, the polyp blocked her airway when it bulged into the oral pharynx. Medical history was significant for morbid obesity (5′2″, 162 kg), asthma, emphysema, diabetes, obstructive sleep apnea, and gastroesophageal reflux disease.

The surgeon communicated with the anesthesiologist the request for an awake intubation with a direct

visualization technique, citing the possibility of dislodging the large polyp into the trachea as a significant risk factor during airway management. In addition, a small (6.0-mm cuffed) ETT was requested. With these comorbidities identified, including difficulty lying supine, the plan was to proceed with an awake nasal fiberoptic intubation with the patient positioned in the sitting position.

The patient was brought to the operating room and positioned in the sitting position. She received minimal sedation with glycopyrrolate, midazolam, and fentanyl. She was topicalized with nebulized lidocaine, and her nasal cavity was progressively dilated to pass a 6.0-mm cuffed ETT with a fiberoptic bronchoscope, as visualized with a monitor. The lesion was seen to prolapse into the airway on expiration. During expiration, the ETT was passed through the cords to approximately 1 to 2 cm above the carina. After confirmation by capnography, general anesthesia was induced and the patient placed supine. Adequate visualization of the cords could not be achieved with the Dedo laryngoscope. A Hollinger scope was introduced, and full exposure of the cords was obtained. The patient underwent a suspension microlaryngoscopy and the polyp was removed first in large pieces and then several smaller pieces, until there was a smaller area where the pedicle remained. Hemostasis was achieved with cocaine-soaked pledgets. The patient's airway management was returned to the anesthesiologist. She was placed in the head-up position, awakened, and extubated without incident.

Discussion

1. Operating room management of this patient was assigned to members of the Airway Service who had a high level of comfort and expertise with the fiberoptic bronchoscope. The basic setup included the elective FOB cart with monitor and elective OLHN suspension table with Dedo and Hollinger laryngoscopes.
2. The operating room anesthesia team consisted of attending and resident members. The attending was designated to sedate and monitor the patient, whereas the resident worked with the OLHN surgeons to topicalize and secure the airway with the fiberoptic bronchoscope.
3. Knowing that the glottic opening was not easily visualized with the Dedo laryngoscope is significant for future airway management and supports the teaching that, of the two scopes, the Hollinger laryngoscope is the more difficult airway rigid laryngoscope of choice for the OLHN surgeon.

Case 3: Anticipated from Surgical Procedure: Three Staged Surgeries for Temporomandibular Joint (TMJ) Surgery; Three Airway Management Algorithms

The patient was a 23-year-old woman who was scheduled for TMJ surgery. On physical examination, she was 5′4″ and weighed 59 kg. Her mouth opening was limited to 2 mm. Nasal passages were clear, and neck anatomy was normal. The surgeon requested a nasal intubation for the procedure. The anesthesia team evaluated her and suggested an awake nasal intubation, which was accomplished without incident.

The patient returned to the operating room 6 months later for the second stage of her TMJ surgery. On physical examination, she now had a mouth opening of 3 cm. The surgeon requested a nasal ETT for the procedure. The anesthesia team now suggested an asleep Magill forceps–assisted nasal intubation with conventional laryngoscopy. This was accomplished without incident.

The patient returned to the operating room 2 months later for the final stage of her TMJ surgery. The surgeon no longer requested a nasal intubation for the patient. The anesthesia team suggested asleep conventional laryngoscopy, which was accomplished without incident.

Discussion

1. This case illustrates the concept that, for each patient, the airway algorithm used is on the basis of these concepts: full stomach (yes/no), oral or nasal intubation (or neck/surgical), and awake or asleep intubation. For each surgical procedure, there were a number of airway techniques that might have been successful. In each case, the anesthesia team chose a technique that they had expertise with, that suited the surgical needs, and that was agreed on with the patient. There were no adverse events.
2. EPR documentation for this patient included detailed notes describing a progression of steps from the patient being an airway alert to easy conventional laryngoscopy. The significance of this is that, to date, most first response airway management in elective and emergent situations in the operating room (and in nonoperating locations) continues to be conventional laryngoscopy with MAC and Miller laryngoscopes. For this patient, because of the surgery, she progressed from being considered an anticipated difficult intubation patient to becoming a patient in whom airway management was easily facilitated with conventional laryngoscopy.

Case 4: Anticipated Difficult Intubation and Extubation: Trismus vs Fused TMJ

The patient was a 35-year-old woman, who was transferred from another hospital for evaluation of trismus and biopsy of an oral lesion. Her medical history was significant for medical evacuation from Asia with complaints of malaise, fever, jaw pain, and increasing trismus. There was no definitive diagnosis.

On physical examination, she was 5′5″ and weighed 52 kg. She appeared to be clenching her jaw shut and was unable to open it for examination, citing pain as the reason. There was slight swelling of her mandible. Nasal passages were clear. The thyroid and neck were normal.

The otolaryngologist suggested asleep conventional laryngoscopy would be sufficient and thought that the trismus would be released with muscle paralysis. The anesthesiologist was concerned about the diagnosis of trismus and the fact that the patient had never had a general anesthetic that required endotracheal intubation (and no proven record of easy intubation with conventional laryngoscopy). They agreed to proceed with an awake nasal fiberoptic intubation, with a consent for tracheotomy if needed.

The patient was brought into the operating room. She received minimal sedation and was topicalized for an awake nasal intubation in the sitting position. A 6.5-mm cuffed ETT was placed with the fiberoptic bronchoscope without incident. The glottis and vocal cords were grossly normal. The patient was placed supine and induced for general anesthesia. An intubating dose of succinylcholine was given, and complete paralysis was verified with a neuroblockade monitor. All attempts to open her mouth were unsuccessful because of bilateral TMJ pathology/limitation in opening. The biopsy was completed, and a nasogastric tube previously advanced into her stomach was removed. An antiemetic was given, and she was awakened in the sitting position. She was extubated while awake over an Eschmann stylet, which was removed a few minutes later without incident. She was taken to the recovery room with the Adult Emergency Airway Cart at her side. She was given an airway alert bracelet and an airway alert was dictated into EPR.

Discussion

1. The diagnosis of trismus presents practitioners with at least two major challenges: (1) distinguishing between masseter muscle spasm/pain and TMJ limited opening; and (2) having multiple airway techniques immediately available, and limited by (1). Although asleep techniques may have been successful, there was enough uncertainty as to the patient's diagnosis in

this case to warrant an awake technique. Other awake options included blind nasal, nasal lighted stylet, or a surgical airway.

2. Succinylcholine, which has the most profound and immediate onset of paralysis of the neuromuscular agents, was used as a diagnostic agent to distinguish between trismus and TMJ limitations. The neuromuscular blockade monitor was essential to validate paralysis.

3. The extubation was a critical part of this airway management plan. Postoperative nausea in the setting of residual anesthesia can place patients at increased risk of aspiration, especially when there are TMJ limitations and the patient cannot be effectively suctioned. There must be meticulous attention in this area. The Eschmann stylet, and other ventilating ETT tube changers, has a significant role in the extubation of such difficult airway/intubation patient[14]; however, its use is not without complications. The immediate availability of an airway cart and a physician with expertise in performing the surgical airway technique were critical to the safe management of this patient.

Case 5: Anticipated Difficult Intubation: Asleep Oral Intubation

A 77-year-old man was admitted to the emergency department with pulmonary edema. As the staff were preparing to electively/urgently intubate him for respiratory failure, he informed them that he was a Medic Alert member and that he was a difficult airway/intubation (as identified during prior cardiac surgery at the same institution). The staff paged the Airway Service and mobilized the Adult Airway Emergency Cart, which was located in the emergency department. In addition, they attempted to retrieve his EPR medical record and his old paper medical record. His surgery had been in 1993, but the EPR was not available until 1995. The old paper record was in off-site storage.

He had been enrolled in the Medic Alert Airway Registry, and his specific airway algorithm had been entered in his Medic Alert record. Medic Alert was contacted, and they immediately faxed his Airway Registry information.

Medical Information

Diabetes, coronary artery bypass graft. Call Medic Alert. Difficult Airway/Intubation. Information was anesthesiologist-reported at The Johns Hopkins Hospital, Baltimore, MD. Phone 410-955-5226. Medical record file ######. Procedure: Re-do CABG, date ##/93. Clinical airway algorithm: Unanticipated. Successful mask airway. Unsuccessful asleep direct laryngoscopy with MAC No. 3, Miller No. 3 (×4) with

visualization of arytenoids. Successful asleep oral fiberoptic intubation with 8.0-mm cuffed ETT. Primary difficulty encountered: Long epiglottis. Recommendation: Availability of awake and fiberoptic techniques.

The Airway Service made a decision to induce general anesthesia, "validate" that he was a difficult airway/intubation with conventional laryngoscopy, and then proceed to rigid laryngoscopy if necessary. He was induced, and mask ventilation was established. Direct laryngoscopy with a MAC No. 4 did not reveal the glottic opening. The otolaryngologist successfully intubated the patient with the Hollinger laryngoscope, Eschmann stylette, and 8.0-mm ETT. The procedure took less than 5 minutes, and there were no adverse outcomes.

Discussion

1. As of 2003, Medic Alert continues to play a significant role in the immediate availability of critical information. This case confirmed what preliminary data from the Medic Alert Registry suggested: anticipation of a difficult airway/intubation results in fewer techniques used and a lower incidence of adverse outcomes.[16,27,34] After intubation, an airway note was entered into the EPR.

2. The mobilization of the Airway Service and the Adult Emergency Airway Cart (complete with the rigid laryngoscopes) in the emergency department has significantly and positively impacted difficult airway management there. In the ideal medical community, all specialties involved with airway management would be facile with all airway techniques, including fiberoptic bronchoscopy, rigid laryngoscopy, and surgical airway. The emergency medicine literature approaches difficult airway management in a way that is similar to the ASA but without a good understanding of the role of the otolaryngologist in nonsurgical airway management. When The Johns Hopkins Medical Institutions made the commitment to fund the Airway Management Service and equipment in both operating rooms and nonoperating locations (intensive care units and emergency department), it was on the condition that an otolaryngologist would be called when the equipment was used to ensure physician expertise. Because of the size of our OLHN residency program, we are able have senior residents, experienced with difficult airway management, available for the Airway Service 24 hours a day, 7 days a week. Although there was initial resistance to shared airway management in the Emergency Department and intensive care

units, with time and experience, the culture has changed and the Airway Service functions well in all locations.

3. There were numerous algorithms that could have been successfully implemented, including awake techniques. In this case, the anesthesiologist "just wanted to make sure that conventional laryngoscopy had been unsuccessful" and, after the patient's evaluation, felt confident that mask ventilation could be established without difficulty. The surgeon felt confident of his ability to secure the airway with the Hollinger laryngoscope. Backup plans were made, and short-acting agents given in case they were incorrect and the patient needed to be awakened.

Case 6: Unanticipated Difficult Intubation, Difficult Mask Ventilation with LMA, Can Wake Up

The patient is a 41-year-old woman who was brought to the operating room to undergo a laparoscopic cholecystectomy. She was evaluated and found to be a candidate for general endotracheal anesthesia. She underwent an intravenous induction with sodium pentothal. There was an immediate inability to mask ventilate the patient. An oral airway was placed and two-handed bag/mask ventilation was attempted. The patient desaturated to the low 80s, and stat anesthesia was called. The patient remained hemodynamically stable throughout. A No. 4 LMA was placed with some difficulty, and ventilation was established. The patient's oxygen saturation returned to the low 90s, and she made efforts to breathe spontaneously. The surgical attending was present throughout the airway management, and a joint decision was made to wake the patient up, remove the LMA, and observe the patient overnight.

The patient was brought back to the operating the following day and underwent an awake nasal fiberoptic intubation without incident. She was extubated awake at the completion of the procedure without problems.

The anesthesiologist dictated a note in the EPR regarding both airway management events and entered the phrase "Difficult endotracheal intubation" in the patient's overview Problems, Allergies, Medications (PAM) list. The surgeon dictated in the operative report in the EPR that the patient was induced with general anesthesia and *easily* orally intubated by the anesthesia staff.

Discussion

1. This was a case of difficult mask ventilation in which the LMA proved invaluable as a "bail out" device. The return of spontaneous respirations was the deciding point for the operating room

physicians with respect to continuing with definitive airway management (fiberoptic by way of the LMA, change to intubating LMA, conventional laryngoscopy, rigid laryngoscopy, among other techniques) or aborting the procedure. No attempts at direct laryngoscopy were made because a muscle relaxant had not been given, and mouth opening would not have been optimized. Therefore, it was never ascertained whether conventional laryngoscopy would have been easy or difficult. Many patients are, in fact, difficult to mask ventilate but easy to intubate with conventional laryngoscopy. The overall incidence of difficult-to-mask ventilate vs difficult-to-ventilate patients is uncertain, but is cited as 1 in 10,000.[7] The decision to return another day allowed the surgeon and anesthesiologist to regroup and reassess their airway management plan and assure themselves that the patient had not had an adverse event related to the first experience.

2. Controversy exists among anesthesiologists as to the value of "verifying" easy direct laryngoscopy with conventional blades after an airway has already been secured (while awake or asleep) with a nonconventional technique. Although some think that viewing the ETT in the glottic opening with the MAC/Miller blade indicates that ETT placement would have be easy, others disagree. They comment that the ETT is facilitating this view of the glottic opening with the MAC/Miller blade and that this laryngeal view is not indicative of what the laryngeal view would be like without it.

3. The importance of clear and correct documentation cannot be overemphasized. Until it becomes standard to have anesthesia documentation within electronic medical records, surgeons should be encouraged to briefly document the airway management of their patient in their dictated operative note. In the meantime, the issues of how to avoid the discrepancy of the anesthesiologist documenting "difficult airway" while the surgeon dictates "easy to intubate" in the operative report can only be addressed by precise communication between surgeons and anesthesiologists.

Case 7: Unanticipated Difficult Intubation, Maskable, Cannot Wake Up Because of Long-Acting Paralysis

The patient was a 60-year-old man who was brought to the operating room for a left radical neck dissection. A stat page was initiated for members of the Airway Service and the Adult Emergency Airway Cart 45 minutes after the induction of anesthesia. On arrival in the operating room, the anesthesiologist communicated that the patient was stable hemodynamically but that the airway was not secured. A No. 4 LMA was in place, and the patient was being easily oxygenated and ventilated. The attending plastic surgeon was not present.

In brief discussion, the operating room anesthesia team communicated to members of the Airway Service what events had transpired and where they were in their airway algorithm decisions. The operating room anesthesia team had evaluated the patient and had decided that the patient was a candidate for conventional laryngoscopy with general anesthesia. Induction had been without incident, with an easy mask airway. A long-acting muscle relaxant had been administered. When conventional laryngoscopy was unsuccessful, a No. 4 LMA had been placed without incident. Fiberoptic bronchoscopy with an Aintree catheter through the LMA[56] was unsuccessful for visualization of the glottic opening, and after numerous attempts, they decided to stop before there was trauma to the glottis. The OLHN surgeon inquired about awakening the patient and was told that, with the paralysis, it would be at least 20 minutes. Laryngoscopy with the Holinger by the OLHN surgeon revealed the glottic opening. An Eschmann stylet was placed, and 7.0-mm cuffed ETT was advanced without incident, and the position was confirmed with capnography. There were no adverse events related to airway management. The attending surgeon arrived at the operating room suite, was informed of the airway events, and thanked the operating room anesthesia team and the Airway Service.

Discussion

1. As anesthesiologists become more facile with a variety of airway techniques and there are smoother transitions from plan A to plan B to plan C for successful airway management, surgical colleagues need to be reminded of their role in airway management at induction, extubation, and if an urgency/emergency arises during the case (specifically during regional or sedation anesthesia). In our institution, it is standard practice for the OLHN surgeon to be present at induction and extubation. It is not the practice of other surgical specialties, however, to be present in the operating room for induction and extubation. When a stat airway emergency arises in non-OLHN operating rooms, we have an otolaryngologist available for assistance. Our backup for the hospital-wide Airway Service is the in-house senior otolaryngology resident, with attending consultation as requested.

2. Choice of anesthesia, specifically long-acting muscle relaxants, can mandate definitive airway management rather than the return to spontaneous ventilation.

3. In the hands of an experienced practitioner, the Hollinger laryngoscope has a significant role in the management of difficult airway/intubations, as detailed in *The ASA Difficult Airway Management Algorithm.*[3]

Case 8: Unanticipated Difficult Intubation, Failed RSI, Respiratory Compromise

The patient was a 50-year-old man who was seen in the operating room for a lumbar laminectomy. On physical examination, he was 6′2″ and weighed 98 kg. He had a Mallampati II oral view, good mouth opening, and poor dentition. He had good neck range of motion. He had significant esophageal reflux, which was not well controlled. Medical history was significant for prior nasal surgery 1 year earlier with general anesthesia. The patient denied any history of difficult intubation. The anesthesiologist planned to proceed with general endotracheal anesthesia with a RSI.

The patient was brought to the operating room, monitors were applied, and the patient was preoxygenated with 100% oxygen for 5 minutes. With cricoid pressure applied, he was induced with sodium pentothal and succinylcholine. After verification of full paralysis, direct laryngoscopy with a MAC No. 4 was performed. There was visualization of the tip of the epiglottis only, and a Miller No. 3 was tried next, still with cricoid pressure. The glottis was not visualized, and the patient acutely desaturated into the low 70s. Mask ventilation with cricoid pressure was attempted, but failed. The anesthesiologist called a stat page and requested that the surgeon perform an emergency cricothyrotomy. The code cart and Adult Airway Emergency Cart were brought into the room by nursing staff and set up. The surgeon responded that he had not done one in years, at which time the anesthesiologist attempted to establish jet ventilation with an 18-gauge angiocatheter in the cricothyroid membrane. The patient was in cardiovascular and respiratory collapse, and cardiopulmonary resuscitation was initiated. Jet ventilation resulted in significant neck and face subcutaneous emphysema bilaterally. The anesthesiologist requested a scalpel and performed a cricothyrotomy and inserted a 5-mm cuffed ETT into the trachea. The Airway Service otolaryngologist arrived and assessed the situation. The patient was stable hemodynamically, and an arterial blood gas revealed normal acid/base status, with a CO_2 of 40 mmHg and oxygen of 395 torr. He was, however, bleeding significantly from the cricothyrotomy site, and the ETT cuff was nonfunctional. In addition, the patient had marked subcutaneous emphysema. The otolaryngologist planned for emergent direct laryngoscopy with intubation orally, wound exploration, and possible revision of the tracheotomy.

The pharynx was examined with Dedo and Hollinger laryngoscopes. The trachea was examined, and an Eschmann stylet was placed, followed by intubation with a 7.5-mm cuffed ETT. The damaged ETT was removed from the cricothyrotomy site. The neck was prepared and draped in the standard fashion. The neck wound was explored, and hemostasis was achieved. The site of initial surgical airway was confirmed to be a cricothyrotomy. Given the size of the patient among other considerations, the otolaryngologist decided that the cricothyrotomy could be left as the definitive airway, given the anticipated short time frame required for a surgical airway. A No. 8 Shiley tracheostomy tube was then placed as the ETT was withdrawn from the mouth. The position was confirmed with end tidal CO_2. The patient was transferred to the intensive care unit in stable condition.

On postoperative day 2, the patient was decannulated without incident. He was recommended for and enrolled in the Medic Alert Difficult Airway/Intubation Registry. As was the practice for patients entered in the Registry, attempts to obtain all prior anesthesia/airway history were initiated. The patient authorized release of his medical record from his prior surgery at a neighboring institution, which clearly documented that he had been a difficult intubation then. When questioned about his knowledge and/or understanding of this, he replied that he had been informed by his anesthesiologist then but did not want the anesthesiologists here to "worry." He acknowledged the fact that during the preoperative interview, the anesthesiologist here had extensively questioned him about his prior anesthesia/surgery history.

Discussion

1. The issue of "Who does the emergency surgical airway?" was not effectively communicated before the induction of general anesthesia. Although anesthesiologists assume that most surgeons are facile with surgical airways, this is not always the reality in an emergency situation. Although the introduction of percutaneous cricothyrotomy[51] into anesthesiologists' difficult airway algorithms was thought to address this issue, there are many complications related to its emergency use.[45] This has reinforced the prospective identification of a physician with expertise in surgical airways in the operating room and/or the ability to stat page/mobilize such a physician to the patient's bedside in the event of an emergency.

2. Complications of jet ventilation include catheter kinks and subcutaneous emphysema.[43] On the basis of this experience, a swivel adaptor was attached to all jet ventilators (Figure 8-31), and physicians were educated regarding the potential complications of jet ventilation. In addition, after a risk management conference, the role of jet ventilation in emergency airway management was recommended to be limited to be used as a bridge to emergent cricothyrotomy and to be performed by the most qualified person available.

3. Precise documentation of this airway event, retrieval of medical records from the other institution, and patient-consented enrollment into the Medic Alert Difficult Airway/Intubation Registry supported the fact that the patient knew/had prior knowledge that he was/had been a difficulty airway/intubation. This documentation played a critical role in the dismissal of litigation.

4. This was a landmark case for The Johns Hopkins Airway Management Initiative and facilitated hospital recognition of and financial support for the multidisciplinary Airway Service.

Case 9: Known Difficult Intubation Patient: Consequences of Failed Regional Anesthesia

The patient is a 41-year-old woman, who was seen in the operating room for a revision of a urinary diversion. Medical history was significant for numerous urologic procedures for chronic symptoms involving

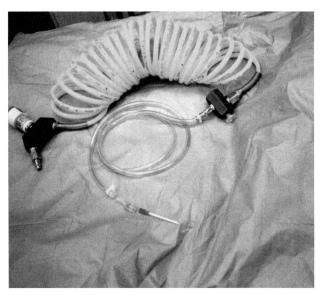

Figure 8-31. Jet ventilator with swivel adaptor to prevent catheter kinking. See Case 8. To view this image in color, please go to *www.ototext.com* or the Electronic Image Collection CD, bound into your copy of Cummings Otolaryngology—Head and Neck Surgery, 4th edition.

her bladder. Anesthesia history was significant for numerous regional anesthetics. The previous procedure, attempted with spinal anesthesia, was complicated by hypotension and loss of consciousness. Resuscitation then included successful mask ventilation. Direct laryngoscopy and intubation with conventional MAC/Miller laryngoscopes was unsuccessful. The patient was able to resume spontaneous ventilation, the procedure was completed, and the patient was taken to the intensive care unit for overnight observation. Of note, on physical examination, the patient was 5′4″ and weighed 72 kg. She had a Mallampati class 3 oral view, normal thyromental distance, and normal neck flexion/extension. She had full caps across her top teeth and decreased mouth opening of two fingerbreadths. She had no history of gastroesophageal reflux disease.

For this procedure, the anesthesiologist planned epidural anesthesia and sedation and the patient gave consent for such. The airway management plan in the operating room included the presence of the anesthesia fiberoptic cart with an LFI bronchoscope.[1] The patient was brought to the operating room and had an epidural placed without incident. Sedation was initiated, and a vancomycin infusion to be titrated over an hour was started. Immediately after an abdominal incision, the patient suddenly expressed that she was feeling quite ill. She seemed to demonstrate an anaphylactic reaction consisting of hypotension, bradycardia, facial swelling, and loss of consciousness. Mask ventilation was difficult because of her clenched jaw, and the anesthesiologist administered an intubating dose of succinylcholine, placed an oral airway, and established mask ventilation. Direct laryngoscopy ×3 with MAC and Miller laryngoscopes failed to visualize the glottic opening, and mask ventilation was reestablished. Initial attempts at nasal intubation with the LFI bronchoscope were unsuccessful because of edema and secretions. With her continued hemodynamic decline and lack of a secured airway, a stat page was initiated. In addition to the code cart and additional anesthesia support, the Adult Emergency Airway Cart and members of the Airway Service arrived for assistance. By this time, the succinylcholine had metabolized, and the patient had resumed spontaneous ventilation but was not awake. The otolaryngologist proceeded with an asleep spontaneously ventilating nasal fiberoptic intubation with an adult bronchoscope (Olympus 5.0/6.0 mm) from the Adult Emergency Airway Cart. This was accomplished with some difficulty because of the significant airway edema. The patient's airway was secured with a 7.0-mm cuffed ETT, without additional airway morbidity. The patient was hemodynamically stabilized, the procedure was aborted, and the patient was brought to the intensive care unit for further management.

Discussion

1. This is a case of regional vs general anesthesia for a patient with a known difficult airway/intubation. Many anesthesiologists would argue that regional anesthesia was appropriate, given the location of the surgical procedure.[1] The airway equipment brought into the operating room for backup was less than optimal in the face of the unanticipated anaphylactic reaction with significant swelling and secretions. It was, however, consistent with the ASA Guidelines equipment recommendation for availability of a fiberoptic bronchoscope. For many anesthesia departments, the LFI-size bronchoscope serves the dual purpose of facilitating elective fiberoptic intubations and verifying proper positioning of a double-lumen endotracheal tube, at half the cost of an adult bronchoscope. Unfortunately, the Olympus (4.0 mm) LFI has limited optics and a suboptimal suction port compared with the adult bronchoscope. Of historical note is the fact that this event occurred when the LMA was not immediately available in all anesthetizing locations.

2. The otolaryngologist assessed that, given the patient's oral examination, as well as the presence of swelling, airway trauma, secretions, and a moderately difficult mask airway, the first choice would be an attempt with spontaneously ventilating fiberoptic bronchoscopy with an adult bronchoscope. The Hollinger laryngoscope might have been successful with optimum positioning and repeated doses of drugs to maintain full paralysis. However, if unsuccessful, the patient's ability to ventilate might have been severely compromised.

3. The authors strongly advocate for immediate availability of appropriate airway management equipment and support staff for any patient with a difficult airway/intubation receiving regional anesthesia throughout the entire operative period.[1,43]

Case 10: Reality Health Care 2003: "Fast Track Evaluation"
Preoperative Evaluation and Airway Management of a Patient with Prader-Willie Syndrome

The patient was a 35-year-old man with history of Prader-Willie syndrome who was seen in the operating room for repair of a large ventral hernia with mesh placement.

The surgeon had identified the patient as an "Airway Alert" in the ORSCIS system when the procedure had been posted 2 weeks before the date of surgery. For patient reasons, the patient had missed his PEC Consultation 1 week before surgery and had come to the operating room on the morning of surgery for evaluation by both the Airway Service *and* surgery. The anesthesiologist assigned to the patient was a member of the Airway Service and had contacted the Airway Service otolaryngologist the night before surgery for consultation and assistance the next morning, if required, on the basis of the EPR chart review of the patient's history. This was communicated to the attending surgeon so that delays/rescheduling could be anticipated if required.

The patient's medical history was significant for gastric bypass surgery 7 years earlier and a cholecystectomy 2 years after that. Airway management for the bypass procedure was significant for an emergency tracheotomy at the time of induction of anesthesia. Airway management for the cholecystectomy was reported to be a fiberoptic intubation, but the patient did not remember specific details (oral vs nasal). Anesthesia records were not available. Additional medical history was significant for seizure disorder, gastroesophageal reflux, moderate obstructive sleep apnea, asthma, and renal insufficiency. In addition, the patient reported an "allergic reaction" to anesthesia but was unable to provide any additional information. Medical records were immediately unavailable.

On physical examination, he was 4'11" and weighed 117 kg (a weight 50 kg less than at the time of his bypass surgery). Neurologically, he was quick-witted with a good memory. He had a small, very thin nose that was partially obstructed bilaterally. His mouth opening was limited to two fingerbreaths, his tongue large, and was a Mallampati class 4 oral view. He had full dentition. He had limited neck extension and a tracheotomy scar 4 cm below the sternal notch. He was unable to lie flat, and slept at night sitting in a chair. He was noncompliant with continuous positive airway pressure.

Operating room setup on the morning of anticipated surgery, before his arrival to the hospital for preparation for surgery, and first-time evaluation by the Airway Service included a request for specialty Airway Service nursing and Airway Equipment Specialist. Operating room equipment requests included mobilization of the Anesthesia Fiberoptic Cart with adult and pediatric bronchoscopes, Adult Emergency Cart, and tracheotomy tray. The setup for topicalization of the airway included a facemask and oral nebulizers, lidocaine for both airway blocks and topical localization, and cocaine. Medications for sedation included midazolam, fentanyl, and propofol.

After a thorough preoperative evaluation by the Airway Service, the patient, parents, and general surgeon were presented with the following airway management algorithm: minimal sedation and topicalization; nasopharyngoscopy to assess potential for nasal vs oral intubation; awake nasal fiberoptic intubation; awake vs oral fiberoptic intubation; asleep suspension microlaryngoscopy with Hollinger scope and Eschmann. Awaken if necessary, with elective or urgent tracheotomy as required.

Informed consent was obtained for tracheotomy, elective or urgent, as required. The extubation algorithm and location was deferred, pending operating room findings. The general surgeon was informed that this would delay surgery by approximately 1 hour and agreed to the plan.

The patient was brought into the operating room. Minimal sedation and topicalization of the airway was initiated. Nasal topicalization was difficult, and the nasopharyngoscopy revealed left nasal synechia. The right nares were adequately topicalized and dilated and an adult bronchoscope facilitated placement of a 6.0-mm cuffed ETT. The larynx was grossly normal. The dimple from the prior tracheotomy was visualized and the ETT advanced to a position 3 cm above the carina without incident. Position was confirmed with end tidal CO_2, and general anesthesia was induced. The patient was paralyzed and muscle relaxation verified. Suspension microlaryngoscopy with the Hollinger revealed the entire glottic opening without difficulty. Direct laryngoscopy with Macintosh and Miller blades did not reveal the complete glottic opening. The time for evaluation and intubation was 1 hour. An arterial catheter and central venous catheter were placed, and the surgery was completed without incident and lasted 6 hours. The extubation algorithm included overnight intubation and stabilization. When extubation criteria were met, the patient would be extubated in the intensive care unit, awake, and in the sitting position. The otolaryngologist and Adult Airway Cart would be at the bedside, along with a physician who would monitor the patient and administer anesthetics. In the event of failed extubation, immediate induction of general anesthesia with complete paralysis would be initiated and the airway secured with the Hollinger scope and Eschmann stylette. Tracheotomy would be the immediate backup plan. The patient was taken sedated and intubated to the intensive care unit for observation. The extubation strategy was communicated to the intensive care unit staff, general surgeon, and family.

The patient remained intubated for 48 hours secondary to surgical issues. The patient was evaluated for and met extubation criteria, as defined by intensive care unit protocols, with clinical support of the intensive care unit attending physician staff. The Airway Service otolaryngologist and anesthesiologist, along with the Adult Emergency Airway Cart, were at the patient's bedside in the intensive care unit. The patient was extubated without incident.

Discussion

1. The optimal evaluation of this patient would have been to be seen by members of the Airway Service before the day of surgery, as had been originally planned by the attending surgeon. Because of the patient's unexpected hospital admission the week before, this was not done. During the PEC evaluation, prior anesthesia records would have been obtained, and a formal consultation with the otolaryngologist would have been requested. Although in reality this was accomplished on the morning of surgery, additional operating room time was not requested, and resources were not mobilized ahead of schedule. Clearly, had our Airway Service with resources not been established, there would have been a high probability for cancellation on the morning of surgery because of this lack of appropriate resources in an operating room efficient manner.
2. The intraoperative suspension microlaryngoscopy with the Hollinger laryngoscope was critical to deciding on the extubation algorithm and which airway resources and members of the Airway Service were required to be at the patient's bedside for extubation.
3. Documentation in the EPR and communication with the family was key in the successful management of this complicated patient. The patient was recommended for enrollment into Medic Alert.[43]

CLINICAL PRACTICES: CASE PRESENTATIONS OF CATASTROPHIC EVENTS IN THE OPERATING ROOM AND THE ROLE OF THE OLHN SURGEON

Unexpected catastrophic patient events not involving airway management may occur in any operating room that the otolaryngologist–head and neck surgeon, and any surgeon, must be aware of and be prepared to assist the anesthesiologist in the management of these patients. These include fire in the airway, postobstructive pulmonary edema, pneumothorax, anaphylaxis, malignant hypothermia (MH), and undiagnosed pheochromocytoma.

Over the past 15 years at The Johns Hopkins Medical Institutions, the following catastrophic events have occurred in the OLHN operating rooms. These events happened to OLHN patients and were not related to difficult airway management. Although the responsibility of resuscitation of the patient lies primarily with the anesthesiologist, the OLHN surgeon can be recruited by the anesthesiologist to assist. In each case, the OLHN surgeon played a critical role in the ultimate survival of the patient. In some cases, other surgical specialties were also called stat to the operating room to assist with the resuscitation. Briefly presented are the actual scenarios, with references cited for more in-depth details of management and discussion as desired. These cases have all been discussed at combined Anesthesiology and OLHN Performance Improvement Conferences as part of the Airway Management Team Initiative. Each time, the specific question posed was: "What skills should OLHN surgeons obtain and maintain to assist the anesthesiologist in the unexpected catastrophic event?" Specific recommendations for OLHN surgeons were made in an attempt to answer this question and to facilitate their participation in the resuscitation of their patients.

Case A: Fire in the Airway

The patient was a 65-year-old woman, who was seen in the operating room for a composite bilateral neck dissection, percutaneous endoscopic gastrostomy (PEG), and tracheotomy. The initial airway management was uneventful with general anesthesia and conventional laryngoscopy. During the creation of the tracheotomy, the plastic surgeon requested that the anesthesiologist lower the inspired oxygen concentration and be prepared to withdraw the ETT in anticipation of entering the trachea. As the anesthesiologist was focusing his attention on these tasks, the surgeon used the electrocautery to enter the trachea. There was an immediate burst of flames. The anesthesiologist immediately removed the ETT tube from the patient's mouth, and the surgeon drenched the surgical site with saline. Once there was no evidence of continued fire, mask ventilation was reestablished with 100% O_2 and the patient reintubated. The procedure was terminated, and patient was taken, intubated, to the intensive care unit. An otolaryngology consult was requested.

Discussion

1. The best treatment for fire in the airway is prevention. For there to be a fire, there must be a source of oxygen and a source of combustion. In this case, both were present. Although many consider the ETT to be the only source of combustion in the airway, crusted secretions in a nonintubated patient can also be a nidus for fire. Although lowering the FiO_2 and avoiding N_2O may decrease the severity of a fire, it will not prevent

one. In addition, the patient might not be able to tolerate the lower FiO_2. Therefore, the absolute caveat for the surgeon is to *not* enter the trachea with the electrocautery. The absolute caveat for the anesthesiologist is to maintain vigilance at the moment of entry into the trachea and maintain communication with the surgeon as to the status of the patient.

2. In the event of an airway fire, the following steps should be taken:

- Stop the flow of O_2 to the ETT.
- Remove the ETT tube.
- Flood the field with fluids, if appropriate.
- Mask ventilate with 100% O_2.
- Reintubate as soon as possible.
- Consider positive end-expiratory pressure (PEEP), continued ventilatory support, and high-dose steroids.
- Call for immediate consultation with an otolaryngologist to evaluate the extent of the airway burn.

Case B: Postobstructive Pulmonary Edema[24]

A 42-year-old woman was brought to the operating room for bilateral ethmoidectomies and revision septoplasty. She was 5'2" and weighed 90 kg. On physical examination, the patient had limited neck extension, a small mouth, a jaw opening of 2 cm, and a limited oral view (Mallampati class 4). Medical history was significant for unanticipated difficult airway management years earlier, consisting of urgent asleep fiberoptic bronchoscopy and intubation of the trachea. Subsequent surgeries requiring general endotracheal intubation were managed by awake fiberoptic bronchoscopy without complications.

Six months earlier, a surgical procedure had been attempted at an outpatient center with local anesthesia and intravenous sedation. The patient had become apneic early in the procedure, and mask ventilation was difficult to establish and maintain. Shortly after the reestablishment of spontaneous ventilation, she showed persistent desaturation to the high 80s. The procedure was aborted. In the recovery room, the patient complained of chest discomfort and continued to have oxygen saturations <90%, despite application of a nonrebreathing face mask. She was transferred to an inpatient hospital and admitted to the intensive care unit for stabilization. Further diagnostic evaluation included an echocardiogram and thallium stress test, neither of which showed evidence of cardiac disease. The chest x-ray was consistent with pulmonary edema. No diagnosis was made regarding the initial operating room event of apnea and desaturation. No physician communicated to the patient "what had happened."

In reviewing the entire medical record before this procedure, the anesthesia team made a presumptive diagnosis of postobstructive pulmonary edema, secondary to apnea and airway obstruction during sedation. The anesthesia team planned an awake oral fiberoptic intubation of the trachea. The patient arrived in the operating room accompanied by the surgeon, who promptly explained to everyone that the easiest and safest choice was local anesthesia with intravenous sedation. The anesthesiologist requested that the surgeon discuss privately the issues related to this patient's prior airway management and potential for similar adverse events related to sedation and potential for airway obstruction. The surgeon insisted that he would be more vigilant with the use of local anesthesia and that the patient was very "motivated" to stay awake and avoid general anesthesia. Reluctantly, the anesthesiologist agreed but requested that the surgeon identify phases of the surgery that could be interrupted in the event that semielective airway management and the initiation of general anesthesia could be facilitated. The procedure was completed with local anesthesia and minimal sedation but was difficult for the surgeon, anesthesiologist, and patient. The patient complained about severe headaches and nausea with the local anesthesia; the surgeon complained that the patient was "restless" and needed more sedation. There were no adverse events; however, the anesthesiologist communicated to the surgeon that in the advent of additional sinus surgery, the patient would be a candidate for general endotracheal anesthesia. The surgeon agreed.

Discussion

1. Postobstructive pulmonary edema, also referred to as negative pressure pulmonary edema, has been described in a variety of circumstances.[5,52] The incidence of pulmonary edema associated with airway obstruction has been estimated at 12% and 11% in pediatric and adult populations, respectively, requiring active airway intervention for acute upper airway obstruction of varying etiology.[5,52] Although the cause is not clear, the common denominator is hypoxia associated with airway obstruction. Negative intrapleural pressure is the primary pathologic event and develops against a closed glottis with catecholamine activation.[52] This promotes translocation of blood from the systemic to the pulmonary circulation, which further increases pulmonary microvascular pressures. With the relief of the obstruction, either with a surgical airway or oral/nasal ETT, the pulmonary edema becomes evident but can be delayed for some time after the episode of obstruction. Prompt recognition and treatment

are essential and include reintubation/surgical airway, oxygenation, PEEP, and diuretics as indicated.

2. Populations of patients at increased risk for postobstructive pulmonary edema include those with unanticipated difficult mask ventilation/intubation; obstructive sleep apnea; acute upper airway obstruction secondary to croup, epiglottis, tumor; unanticipated difficult extubation with obstruction to mask ventilation.

3. The diagnosis is many times made by exclusion of other etiologies of pulmonary edema and/or myocardial ischemia, as was the case here. This diagnosis was not fully appreciated by the attending surgeon or patient. Appropriate airway management would have been either minimal sedation or general ETT anesthesia at the beginning of the procedure.

Case C: Rule Out Tension Pneumothorax vs Anaphylactic Reaction

A 24-year-old man was seen in consultation for surgical resection of a malignant juvenile sarcoma of the neck of the parotid gland, inferotemporal fossa, and parapharyngeal space. Of note, he was a Jehovah's Witness and came for his preoperative evaluation with his Jehovah's Witness advisor. He was 6'2" and weighed 100 kg. On physical examination, the patient had normal neck extension, good jaw opening, and Mallampati class 1 oral view. The tumor did not seem to compromise his airway. Airway management was planned to be conventional asleep laryngoscopy. Monitoring was to include arterial and central venous catheters because of the potential for significant blood loss.

The patient was brought to the operating room for radical parotidectomy and neck dissection with an inferotemporal preauricular approach to the parapharyngeal space with dislocation of the mandible and dissection and mobilization of the carotid artery.

He was preoxygenated after placement of routine monitors. Induction was uneventful, conventional laryngoscopy was performed, and endotracheal intubation was confirmed with capnography. A radial artery catheter was placed without difficulty. During difficult placement of the right internal jugular catheter, the patient was noted to acutely desaturate to the high 80s with end tidal CO_2 present. Hemodynamically, he became tachycardic to the 140s and hypotensive with a mean arterial pressure of <30 mmHg. Coincidental to the placement of the central venous catheter was the placement of a Foley catheter. Antibiotics had not been given. The presumptive diagnosis was tension pneumothorax. The central venous catheter placement was abandoned,

and the surgeon was requested to place a right chest tube. This was done without incident; however, the patient's hemodynamic and respiratory parameters continued to acutely decline. Cardiopulmonary resuscitation was initiated. Sterile prep drapes were removed from the patient, and he was noted to have massive angioedema of his lips and hives over his entire body. The presumptive diagnosis was now severe anaphylactic response to latex.

The resuscitation was massive and involved near-complete removal of all latex-containing objects that were in contact with the patient. A "latex-free" emergency supply cart was brought into the operating room to facilitate this. A femoral central venous catheter was placed, with the physician wearing latex-free gloves. Pharmacological resuscitation included systemic steroids, antihistamines, H_2-blockers, bronchodilators, epinephrine, and norepinephrine. Blood samples were taken for laboratory analysis.

The procedure was aborted, and the patient was taken to the intensive care unit on significant amounts of vasopressor support. Postoperative discussion with the family confirmed that the patient had extreme sensitivity to latex gloves but had not wanted us to "worry" about it in light of the other issues related to this surgery (JW status).

The patient was extubated 48 hours later and enrolled into Medic Alert Foundation.

Discussion

1. Many patients come to the operating room and request that no blood products be transfused to them during their hospital course. Although some make this request because of religious convictions (Jehovah's Witness in particular), others feel as strongly and present to the practitioner an advanced directive that explicitly requests that no blood products be transfused to them during their hospital course. This patient presented for surgery in 1997. Avoidance of donor-blood transfusions was limited to selective use of recombinant erythropoietin and blood salvage (noncancer surgeries), nonblood volume expanders, and meticulous surgical technique. By 2003, more comprehensive practices for these patients had been initiated. These practices may include recombinant erythropoietin and iron (2–4 weeks ahead of surgical date), topical hemostatic agents, tissue adhesives, and nonblood volume expanders. In addition, there are minimally invasive surgery and blood conservation techniques that can be offered and include hemodilution and blood salvage, minimally invasive surgical techniques, and meticulous surgical technique. Our current practice is to refer patients to our Advanced

Transfusion Practices (ATP) Clinical Center for evaluation and management.[4]

2. Rule out tension pneumothorax was the obvious first choice in the differential diagnosis, because this patient was acutely respiratory decompensating, with desaturation, increased peak airway pressures, and diminished breath sounds in the right side of the chest. In addition, the timing of the decompensation was directly linked to difficult right internal jugular venous cannulation. In this case, unfortunately, the surgeons wore latex gloves as they placed the right chest tube, which undoubtedly worsened the patient's hemodynamic response.

3. Rule out latex anaphylaxis has increasingly become the number one differential diagnosis when faced with acute respiratory and cardiovascular compromise that appears anaphylactic in presentation. In August 1997, the Food and Drug Administration (FDA) received incident reports of more that 2300 allergic reactions involving latex-containing medical products, including 225 cases of anaphylactic reactions, 53 cardiac arrests, and 17 deaths. Latex is the inciting factor in at least 10% of anaphylactic reactions that have been reported during anesthesia.[8]

This case was a hallmark case for our institution, and we requested immediate consultation with Dr. Robert Brown, a colleague and senior member of the ASA Task Force on Latex Sensitivity.[8] It was cited as the pinnacle case in ongoing efforts by the JHH Latex Task Force to convert the hospital to a "latex safe" one. The reader is referred to the referenced Web site[55] for a more comprehensive discussion and identification of latex free medical devices.

Case D: Rule out MH

A 20-year-old patient was brought to the operating room for removal of an acoustic neuroma. He had undergone a prior uncomplicated anesthetic as a child. He had no family history of problems with anesthesia. Two hours into the procedure, he was noted to have myoglobinuria. Laboratory examination revealed a normal state of acidosis and electrolytes. He was hemodynamically stable with a normal temperature. The anesthesiologist was concerned, alerted the surgeon, and discontinued the inhalational agents. A total intravenous anesthetic was administered. Of note, the muscle relaxant succinylcholine had not been administered with the induction of anesthesia. Within the hour, the patient was noted to have increasingly elevated end tidal CO_2 levels that would not correct with hyperventilation. Laboratory analysis now revealed hyperkalemia with a mixed respiratory and metabolic acidosis. Hemodynamically, the patient was tachycardic and tachypneic. A presumptive diagnosis of MH was made, and the procedure was terminated. Dantrolene was administered as part of the total resuscitation.

Discussion

1. MH, first described in 1960 by Denborough and Lorell, is a clinical syndrome of markedly accelerated metabolic state characterized by fever, tachycardia, tachypnea, cyanosis, and hypercarbia. The clinical presentation occurs when triggering agents are used in the anesthetic management of susceptible patients. *A patient with a history of uncomplicated anesthesia can be triggered by subsequent anesthetics.* Although no anesthetic is completely safe, the anesthetic agents best avoided include the inhalational agents and muscle relaxants. Although MH is a heterogeneous polygenic disorder, most cases are nonfamilial. The best-accepted theory of pathophysiology identifies a defect in the excitation-contraction coupling of calcium to the sarcolemma in the muscle.[28]

2. Treatment includes immediate notification to the surgeon, discontinuation of any potential triggering agents, administration of dantrolene, and cardiovascular support of the patient. Temperature increases can be a late sign, and meticulous measurement of temperature and appropriate treatment are critical. In this case, the first sign was myoglobinuria, which alerted the anesthesiologist to the potential for an MH trigger. His immediate initiation of treatment plans was critical in the successful resuscitation of this patient.

3. The Malignant Hyperthermia Association of the United States (MHAUS) has a 24-hour hotline (1-800-644-9737) for management of an acute event.[37] In addition, nonemergency requests for information regarding preoperative management, or referral to MH Biopsy Centers, is available either by phone or the Internet. Treatment protocols and contact information are found in Figure 8-32.

Case E: Rule Out Pheochromocytoma

A 63-year-old patient was brought to the operating room for resection of a parotid tumor. The patient had a history of stress-related palpitations for which he was treated with a β-blocker and followed by a cardiologist. Airway examination was unremarkable. The anesthetic plan was standard monitors, general anesthesia, and conventional laryngoscopy.

During induction and before laryngoscopy, the patient became acutely hypertensive with a wide

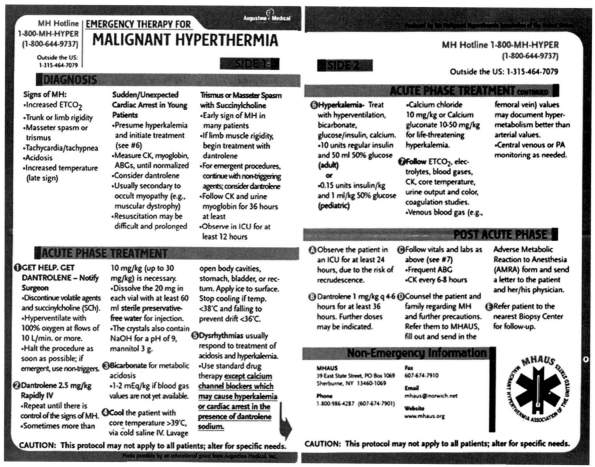

Figure 8-32. Emergency Therapy for Malignant Hyperthermia, side 1 and 2, Augustine Medical. To view this image in color, please go to *www.ototext.com* or the Electronic Image Collection CD, bound into your copy of Cummings Otolaryngology—Head and Neck Surgery, 4th edition.

complex ventricular arrhythmia that immediately converted into a supraventricular tachycardia. He was treated with a β-blocker and antihypertensive medication and intubated without incident. The anesthesiologist stabilized his hemodynamics and made a decision with the surgeon to abort the procedure and wake up the patient. This was easily done, because short-acting induction agents and paralysis had been chosen. He was wakened, extubated, and transferred to the coronary care unit for evaluation. The presumptive diagnosis was primary cardiac event vs rule out pheochromocytoma. Evaluation was negative for both. The presumptive diagnosis was sensitivity to one of the anesthetic agents and/or preoperative anxiety.

The patient returned to the operating room 4 months later for the same procedure. The anesthesia team chose to premedicate him with anxiolytics, use different induction agents, and place an arterial catheter after induction. The patient was induced, mask ventilation was established, and an interme-

diate-acting, cardiac-stable paralytic drug was administered. He became acutely hypertensive with a supraventricular tachycardia, which was immediately broken with a β-blocker. The airway was secured without incident; however, the patient continued to deteriorate hemodynamically. A stat was called, and a massive resuscitation was initiated. The patient was ultimately stabilized with the use of a variety of antiarrhythmics and vasopressors. Intraoperative monitoring included a pulmonary artery catheter, transesophageal echocardiography, and a ZOLL pacing defibrillator. Intraoperative consultations with cardiology, electrophysiology, cardiac surgery, and intensivists were obtained. The patient was transferred to the intensive care unit and discharged from the hospital a week later without adverse sequelae.

Intensive evaluation revealed an extramedullary pheochromocytoma. He was treated 1 to 2 months before surgery with α- and β-blockers and underwent uneventful resection of his pheochromocytoma.

Discussion

1. Pheochromocytomas are catecholamine-secreting tumors of neuroendocrine tissue. Although they are usually located in the adrenal medullae or sympathetic paraganglia, up to 10% of these are located elsewhere and can be difficult to find. Although pheochromocytomas only account for 0.1% of cases of hypertension, when first identified unexpectedly under general anesthesia, the physiologic effects of released catecholamines can be catastrophic and life threatening.[25]

2. Diagnosis of pheochromocytoma can be made by urinary catecholamines, plasma catecholamine concentrations, and clonidine suppression of norepinephrine secretion. Localization of the tumor can be made with computed tomography, with or without ^{131}I-labeled metaiodobenzyl guanidine (MIBG), arteriography and selective adrenal venous catheterization and sampling, and magnetic resonance imaging (MRI). In this case, after both aborted anesthetics, the blood and urine laboratory values were nondiagnostic. Because of the magnitude of the physiologic response by the patient to what was considered routine anesthesia, numerous adrenal venous samples on different occasions were obtained, and a diagnosis of pheochromocytoma was ultimately made.

3. The peak incidence of pheochromocytomas occur in the third to fifth decades, in both genders, with approximately 5% of cases inherited as part of the neoplastic syndrome, *adenomatosis (MEA)*. Although this patient does not have known MEA, practitioners must be vigilant in the evaluation of patients in risk populations for MEA, specifically to diagnose pheochromocytoma *before* the diagnosis is made under general anesthesia.[25]

The preceding cases were selected to reinforce the concept that when unexpected catastrophic events occur, successful resuscitation may depend on the active participation of all members of the health care team. The medical community has in place numerous courses and certifications that OLHN surgeons, and all physicians, might consider completing that would provide the practitioner with state-of-the-art knowledge and skill sets necessary to allow them to assist in acute resuscitations. These courses and certifications include the following.

1. Basic Life Support (BLS) and advanced cardiac life support (ACLS) certification
2. Consider advanced trauma life support (ATLS) certification, depending on the scope of practice (central line access, chest tube)
3. Automatic external defibrillator (AED) training
4. Simulation Center: Airway management, resuscitation, crisis management
5. World Wide Web online resources

CONCLUSION

Difficult airway management, anticipated or unanticipated, is multidisciplinary. Although there is an obvious interactive role for the OLHN surgeon and the anesthesiologist in the "airway" of the ABCs of patient management, successful management depends on joint preoperative evaluation, precise discussions of airway plans, and discussion of immediate plans of action in the event of failed airway management or patient compromise for nonairway issues.

Effective communications, verbal and written, regarding critical airway information is essential to the future safety of patients and facilitates efficient and appropriate future airway management. Practitioners are encouraged to incorporate any/all of the documents presented in this chapter into their practice. Enrollment into Medic Alert should be encouraged for all patients who might benefit from the immediate identification of critical medical information (difficult airway, anaphylaxis, etc.).

Development of an institutional Airway Service can be significant in the delivery of quality patient care. Familiarity with medical, societal, and institutional airway algorithms is a key in the success of an Airway Service.

Finally, all physicians must remain current in basic and advanced resuscitation protocols if they are to actively practice in environments that administer sedation or general anesthesia to patients, because unexpected catastrophic events cannot be predicted and occur when one least expects them or is in adequately prepared to immediately respond to the emergency.

ACKNOWLEDGMENTS

We wish to acknowledge Mr. Matthew Logan for photodocumentation presented in this chapter and Ms. Susan Turley for her assistance with medical editing.

REFERENCES

1. Akst S, Mark L. *Should regional or general anesthesia be used for cases in which the patient has an anticipated difficult airway?* In Fleisher LA, editor: *Evidence-based practice*, Philadelphia, 2004, Elsevier Science.
2. American Society of Anesthesiologists Committee on Professional Liability: Preliminary study of closed claims, *ASA Newsletter* 52:8, 1988.
3. American Society of Anesthesiologists Task Force on Guidelines for Management of the Difficult Airway: Practice guidelines for management of the difficult airway, *Anesthesiology* 78:597, 1993. *www.asahq.org.*

4. The ATP Center, Johns Hopkins Hospital, 600 North Wolfe Street, Baltimore, MD. Phone: 877-474-8558. *www.atpcenter.org.*

5. Bainton CR: *Complications of managing the airway.* In Benumof JL, editor: *Airway management: principles and practice,* St Louis, 1996, Mosby–Year Book, p 886.

6. Benumof JL, editor: *Airway management: principles and practice,* St. Louis, 1996, Mosby-Year Book.

7. Benumof JL: Management of the difficult adult airway, *Anesthesiology* 75:1087, 1991.

8. Berry AJ, Task Force on Latex Sensitivity. Natural rubber latex allergy: considerations for anesthesiologists, *ASA Physician Booklet,* 2001.

9. Bjoraker-DG: The Bullard intubating laryngoscopes, *Anesth Rev* 17:640, 1990.

10. Brain AIJ: The laryngeal mask: a new concept in airway management, *Br J Anaesth* 55: 801, 1983. *www.lmana.org.*

11. Caplan RA: Anesthetic liability: what it is and what it isn't. In *1992 Review Course Lectures.* Cleveland, 1994, International Anesthesia Research Society.

12. Caplan RA and others: Adverse respiratory events in anesthesia: a closed claims analysis, *Anesthesiology* 72:828, 1990.

13. Cherian M and others: *The National Medic Alert Difficult Airway/Intubation Registry: patient safety and patient satisfaction* [abstract], Presented at the Annual Meeting of the American Society of Anesthesiologists, San Francisco, October 1994.

14. Cooper RM: Safe extubation, *Anesth Clin North Am* 13:683, 1995.

15. Fleming MD and others: Effect of helium and oxygen on airflow in a narrowed airway, *Arch Surg* 127:956, 1992.

16. Foley L and others: Computerized in-hospital immediate access difficult airway/ intubation registry [abstract], *Anesthesiology* 83:A1124, 1995.

17. Foley L and others: Effect of difficult airway (DA) registry on subsequent airway management: experience in the first two years of the DA registry [abstract], *Anesthesiology* 89: A1220, 1998.

18. Frass M and others: Evaluation of esophageal tracheal Combitube in cardiopulmonary resuscitation, *Crit Care Med* 15:609, 1987.

19. Frass M and others: Ventilation with the esophageal tracheal Combitube in cardiopulmonary resuscitation. Promptness and effectiveness, *Chest* 83:781, 1988.

20. Gibby GL, Mark L, Drake J: *Effectiveness of Teleforms scan based input tool for difficult airway registry: preliminary results* [abstract], Presented at the Annual Meeting of the Society for Technology in Anesthesia, 1995.

21. Gibby GL and others: Development of problem categories for computerized preanesthesia evaluation of outpatients [abstract], *J Clin Monit* 8:156,1992.

22. Hagberg CA: Current concepts in the management of the difficult airway, *ASA Annual Refresher Course Lectures,* 1, 2001.

23. How to avoid small complaints about quality of care [editorial], *Maryland BPQA (Maryland Board of Physician Quality Assurance) Newsletter* 1(4):1, 1993.

24. Hung-OR, Stewart-RD. Lightwand intubation: I. A new lightwand device, *Can J Anaesth* 42:820, 1995.

25. Kerr GE. *Pheochromocytoma.* In Yao F-S F, Artusio JF, Jr. editors: *Anesthesiology. Problem-oriented patient management,* ed 4, Philadelphia, 1998, Lippincott Williams & Wilkins, p 584.

26. Kidwell R: Correspondence to Airway Service, 1999.

27. Kidwell R: Personal Communication with Lynette Mark, July17, 1994.

28. Lee LA, Domnino KB: The Closed Claims Project: has it influenced anesthetic outcome and practice, *Anesthesiol Clin North Am* 20:247, 2002.

29. Malhotra V: *Malignant hyperthermia.* In Yao F-S F, Artusio JF, Jr, editors: *Anesthesiology. problem-oriented patient management,* ed 4, Philadelphia, 1998, Lippincott Williams & Wilkins, p 878.

30. Mallampati SR: *Recognition of the difficult airway.* In Benumof JL, editor: *Airway management: principles and practice,* St. Louis, 1996, Mosby-Year Book, p126.

31. Mallampati SR and others: A clinical sign to predict difficult intubation: a prospective study, *Can Anaesth Soc J* 32:429, 1985.

32. Mark L, Drake J: Professional liability and patient safety: the Medic Alert National Difficult Airway/Intubation Registry, *Anesthesiology Alert* 3:1, 1994.

33. Mark L and others: The difficult airway: mechanisms for effective dissemination of critical information, *J Clin Anesth* 4:247, 1992.

34. Mark L and others: *Practice guidelines to clinical practices: Medic Alert Difficult Airway/Intubation Registry* [abstract], Presented at the Annual Meeting of the American Society of Anesthesiologists, 1994.

35. Mark L and others: *The Medic Alert National Difficult Airway/Intubation Registry: technology that pays for itself* [abstract], Presented at the Annual Meeting of the Society for Technology in Anesthesia, 1995.

36. Mark L and others: *Effective dissemination of critical airway information: The Medic Alert National Difficult Airway/Intubation Registry.* In Benumof JL, editor: *Airway management: principles and practice,* St Louis, 1996, Mosby-Year Book, p 931.

37. Medic Alert Foundation International, 2323 Colorado Avenue, Turlock, California 95382. Phone: 888-633-4298. Non-USA phone: 209-668-3333. *www.medicalert.*

38. MHAUA, 39 East Street, P.O.Box 1069, Shelburne, New York. 13460-1069. Phone 800-986-4287. *www.mhaus.org.*

39. Miller RD, editor: *Anesthesia,* ed 6, New York, 2004, Churchill Livingstone. In press.

40. Morlock L: Personal communication with Lynette Mark, July 17, 1994.

41. Norton ML, editor: *Atlas of the difficult airway,* ed 2, St Louis, 1996, Mosby.

42. Pashayan AG and others: The helium protocol for laryngotracheal operations with CO_2 laser: a retrospective review of 523 cases, *Anesthesiology* 68:801, 1988.

43. Poznak AV: *Prolonged apnea.* In Yao F-S F, Artusio JF, Jr, editor: *Anesthesiology. Problem-oriented patient management,* ed 4, Philadelphia, 1998, Lippincott Williams & Wilkins, p 891.

44. *Practice guidelines for management of the difficult airway,* Approved 1992; last amended 2002. *www.asahq.org/publicationsAndSerices/practiceparam.htm*

45. Practice Guidelines for Management of the Difficult Airway: an updated report by the American Society of Anesthesiologists Task Force on Management of the Difficult Airway, *Anesthesiology* 98:1269, 2003.

46. *Practice guidelines for preoperative fasting and the use of pharmacologic agents to reduce the risk of pulmonary aspiration: application to health patients undergoing elective procedures,* American Society of Anesthesiology, 1999. *www.asahq.org.*

47. Richtsmeier WJ, Eisele DW, MacMurray A: Transtracheal ventilation with crash cart equipment, *Otolaryngol Head Neck Surg* 102:191, 1990.

48. Rose DK, Cohen MM: The airway problem and predictors in 18,500 patients, *Can J Anaesth* 41:372, 1994.

49. Society of Otorhinolaryngology and Head-Neck Nursing, Inc., 116 Canal Street, Suite A, New Smyrna Beach, Florida 32168. *www.sohn.org.*

50. *Standards for basic anesthetic monitoring*, American Society of Anesthesiology, 1998. *www.asahq.org.*

51. Stoelting RK: *Pharmacology and physiology in anesthetic practice*, Philadelphia, 1998, Lippincott Williams & Wilkins.

52. Weymuller EA Jr: *Acute airway management* In Cummings CW, editor: *Otolaryngology head & neck surgery*, ed 3, St Louis, 1998, Mosby–Year Book.

53. Weymuller EA Jr and others: Management of difficult airway problems with percutaneous transtracheal ventilation, *Ann Otol Rhinol Laryngol* 96:34, 1987.

54. White DK: *Medical central resource: negative pressure pulmonary edema, Grand Rounds Presentation*, Brigham & Woman's Hospital, Boston, MA, 1997, Harvard.

55. Williamson JA and others: Difficult intubation: an analysis of 2000 incident reports, *Anaesth Intensive Care* 21:602, 1993.

56. Wilson ME and others: Predicting difficult intubation, *Br J Anaesth* 61:211, 1988.

57. *www.asahq/pulicationsAndServices/latexallergy.html.*

58. *www.cookcriticalcare.com.*

59. *www.export.cov/safeharbor/.*

60. Yao F-S F. *Hypertension*. In Yao F-S F, Artusio JF Jr, editors: *Anesthesiology. Problem-oriented patient management,* ed 4, Philadelphia, 1998, Lippincott Williams & Wilkins, p 316.

61. Yao F-S F, Artusio, Jr JF, editors: *Anesthesiology. Problem-oriented patient management*, ed 4, Philadelphia, 1998, Lippincott Williams & Wilkins.

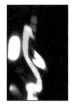

CHAPTER NINE

ALLERGY AND IMMUNOLOGY OF THE UPPER AIRWAY

Fuad M. Baroody
Robert M. Naclerio

INTRODUCTION

The importance of the immune system in health and disease has long been recognized. Not only does the immune system—with its diverse collection of pathogenic mechanisms—protect the organism from infectious microbes, but it also avoids responses that produce damage of self tissues. This basic property of the immune system relies on detecting structural features of the pathogens that are distinct from host cells. This host-pathogen discrimination is essential to eliminate the pathogen without excessive damage to self tissues.

The immune system is divided into the innate and adaptive systems. The adaptive immune system distinguishes itself from the innate system by the following features: specificity of antigen recognition, diversity of the antigen receptor repertoire, rapid clonal expansion, adaptiveness to the changing environment, and immunological memory. This chapter reviews the immune system and its various components and discusses the pathophysiology of immunoglobulin E (IgE)-mediated allergic rhinitis.

INNATE AND ADAPTIVE IMMUNITY

Broadly defined, the innate immune system includes all aspects of the host defense mechanisms that are encoded in the germ-line genes of the host. These include barrier mechanisms, such as epithelial cell layers that express tight cell-cell contact, the secreted mucus layer that overlays the epithelium, and the epithelial cilia that sweep away this mucus layer, permitting it to be constantly refreshed after it has been contaminated with inhaled or ingested particles. The innate response also includes soluble proteins and small bioactive molecules that are either constitutively present in biological fluids (such as the complement proteins and defensins)[83,280] or released from activated cells (including cytokines, chemokines, lipid mediators of inflammation, and bioactive amines and enzymes that also contribute to tissue inflammation). Activated phagocytes (including neutrophils, monocytes, and macrophages) are also part of the innate immune system.

The skin is the most effective first line of defense of the innate immune system. Most infectious organisms cannot penetrate intact skin. Mucosal surfaces of the upper airway, on the other hand, are less resistant than the skin and are thus more frequent portals for offending pathogens. The innate immune system reduces that vulnerability by the presence of various physical and biochemical factors. A good example is the enzyme lysozyme, which is distributed widely in secretions and can split the cell walls of most bacteria. If an offending organism penetrates this first line of defense, bone marrow-derived phagocytic cells attempt to engulf and destroy it. Last, the innate immune system includes cell surface receptors that bind molecular patterns expressed on the surfaces of invading microbes.

Unlike the innate mechanisms of defense, the adaptive immune system manifests exquisite specificity for its target antigens. Adaptive responses are based primarily on the antigen-specific receptors expressed on the surfaces of T- and B-lymphocytes. These antigen-specific receptors of the adaptive immune response are assembled by somatic rearrangement of germ line gene elements to form intact T-cell receptor (TCR) and B-cell antigen receptor genes. The assembly of antigen receptors from a collection of a few hundred germ line-encoded gene elements permits the formation of millions of different antigen receptors, each with a potentially unique specificity for a different antigen.

Because the recognition molecules used by the innate system are expressed broadly on a large number of cells, this system is poised to act rapidly after an invading pathogen is encountered. The second set of responses constitutes the adaptive immune response. Because the adaptive system is composed of small numbers of cells with specificity for any individual pathogen, the responding cells must proliferate after encountering the pathogen to attain sufficient numbers to mount an effective response against the microbe. Thus the adaptive response generally expresses itself temporally after the innate response in host defense. A key feature of the adaptive system is that it produces long-lived cells that persist in an apparently dormant state, but can re-express effector functions rapidly after repeated encounter with an antigen. This provides the adaptive response with immune memory, permitting it to contribute to a more effective host response against specific pathogens when they are encountered a second time, even decades after the initial sensitizing encounter.

The innate and adaptive immune systems are often described as contrasting separate arms of the immune response because they are fundamentally different in their mechanisms of action. However, they usually act together with the innate response representing the first line of host defense and the adaptive response becoming prominent after several days, as antigen specific B and T cells have undergone clonal expansion. Thus, the two systems act synergistically to provide a concerted immune response, the end result of which is to eliminate and control the invading pathogen.

SELF AND NONSELF

The essence of specific immunity is the ability to discriminate at the molecular level between self and nonself. This ability allows the immune system to attack and destroy potentially harmful microorganisms without simultaneously destroying the person infected by these agents, a process also known as self-tolerance. Failure of self-tolerance underlies the broad class of autoimmune diseases. This crucial function is mediated by the molecules determined by the human leukocyte antigen (HLA) complex. Initial study of the HLA system focused on the role of these antigens in determining the success of organ and tissue transplantation. The HLA complex and its homologues in other species were thus termed the *major histocompatibility complex* (MHC). In humans, the MHC occupies about 4000 Kilo Daltons (KD) of deoxyribonucleic acid (DNA) on the short arm of chromosome 6 and contains many genes that encode molecules for various functions. Among these molecules, a group of glycoproteins belonging to the immunoglobulin supergene family are present on the cell surface and play a major role in allowing the immune system to distinguish between self and nonself. These are MHC class I molecules (HLA-A, -B, and -C) and class II molecules (HLA-DR, -DQ, and -DP).

MHC class I molecules are present on the surface of most nucleated somatic cells. They are responsible for presenting endogenous antigens to cytotoxic T cells, allowing the recognition and elimination of virus-infected cells and cells containing autoantibodies. A class I molecule and an antigenic (e.g., viral) peptide are recognized as a complex by the TCR. When cytotoxic T-lymphocyte precursors recognize the combination of a particular foreign peptide and a particular class I molecule on a sensitizing cell, they proliferate and differentiate to become mature cytotoxic T-lymphocytes (CD8+). These mature lymphocytes recognize and kill only target cells that bear the same class I molecule and the same viral peptide as were present on the sensitizing cells. Cytotoxic T-lymphocyte killing is peptide-specific (lymphocytes will not lyse a target cell bearing the same class I molecule infected with a different virus). Cytotoxic T-lymphocyte killing is also class I restricted (lymphocytes will not lyse a cell bearing a different class I molecule infected with the same virus).

In contrast to class I molecules, MHC class II molecules are expressed primarily on immunocompetent antigen-presenting cells (APC), including macrophages, monocytes, dendritic cells, and B lymphocytes. Class II molecules can be up-regulated by interferon (IFN)-γ, permitting these cells to present antigens to CD4+ cells at sites of inflammation. Class II molecules allow binding of peptides of 10 to 25 amino acids, and the bound peptide and the class II molecule constitute the ligand for the receptor on a CD4+ T lymphocyte (T-helper cell). Thus, just as class I molecules restrict the recognition of peptides by CD8+ T cells, class II molecules restrict the recognition of peptides by CD4+ T cells. Therefore, class II molecules are necessary for the presentation of exogenous antigen to T-helper cells.

CELLS OF THE IMMUNE SYSTEM

The human immune system consists of dispersed organs (spleen, thymus, lymph nodes) and of cells capable of moving from the bone marrow to the blood and the lymphatic system. An intact immune response includes contributions from many subsets of leukocytes. The different leukocyte subsets can be discriminated morphologically through the use of conventional histologic stains and, more accurately, by surface phenotype as defined by monoclonal antibody binding to registered differentiation antigens. These differentiation antigens are assigned cluster of differentiation (CD) numbers and updates are issued by the International Workshop on Human Leukocyte Differentiation Antigens (published at *http://www. ncbi.nlm.nih.gov/prow*).

The pluripotent stem cells, which are derived from the yolk sac and ultimately reside in the bone marrow, are the progenitor cells from which all cells of the immune system are derived (Figure 9-1). These pluripotent stem cells give rise to lymphoid and myeloid stem cells. Lymphoid stem cells differentiate further into the three major populations: T cells, B cells, and natural killer (NK) cells. T cells are defined by their cell surface expression of the TCR, a transmembrane heterodimeric protein that binds processed antigen displayed by antigen processing cells (APC). B cells are phenotypically defined by their expression of the B cell receptor for antigen, membrane bound Ig. NK cells are defined morphologically as large granular lymphocytes. They are distinguished by their lack of either TCR or surface Ig. They recognize their virus-infected or tumor cell targets through the use of a complex collection of activating and inhibitory cell surface receptors.[172] Lymphocytes represent about 25% of leukocytes in the peripheral blood. The relative contribution of each subtype to this percentage is as follows: T lymphocytes, 80%; B lymphocytes, 10%; NK large granular lymphocytes, 10%.

Myeloid stem cells give rise to different forms of granulocytes, megakaryocytes and platelets, and erythrocytes. Cells of the granulocyte lineage that play prominent immune roles include neutrophils, monocytes, eosinophils, basophils, and mast cells. Differentiation of the myeloid stem cell occurs in the bone marrow, as does the development of B lymphocytes and NK lymphocytes. In contrast, T-cell progenitors leave the bone marrow and migrate to the thymus, where they differentiate into mature T lymphocytes.

Differentiation of lymphoid and myeloid stem cells is dependent on their interaction through their surface receptors with soluble ligands (cytokines) or surface ligands (cell interaction molecules). Therefore,

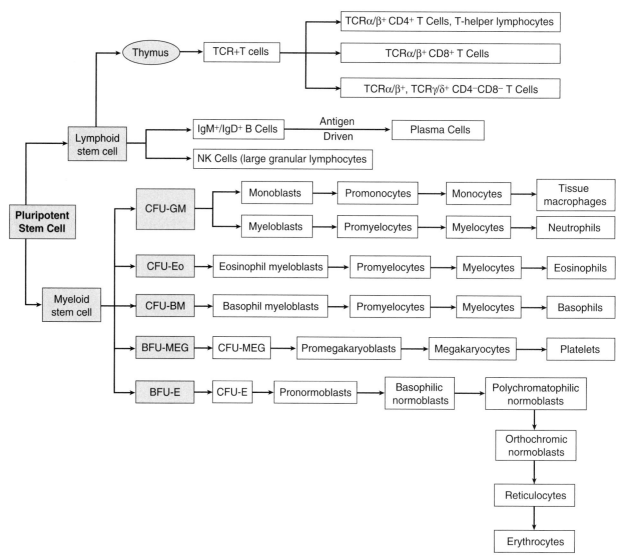

Figure 9-1. The development of the various cells that are important in the immune response from their pluripotent stem cell origin to their final stages of maturation.

proliferation and differentiation along one of the myeloid or lymphoid lineages are controlled (1) through the spatially and temporally regulated exposure of these stem cells to different ligands or factors and (2) through the differential expression of receptors on the stem cells. Cytokines have pleiotropic effects on the development of lymphoid and myeloid cells, affecting growth and maintenance of pluripotent stem cells and development and differentiation of specific lineages. Stromal cells within the bone marrow and thymus also regulate cell growth and differentiation by releasing cytokines, such as IL-4, IL-6, IL-7, IL-11, granulocyte-macrophage colony-stimulating factor (GM-CSF), and others.[70] They also participate in cell-cell interactions with progenitors through engagement of cell-surface molecules that provide additional regulatory stimuli and participate in the development of the intercellular matrix (e.g., collagen, fibronectin).[70,284]

T Cells

Lymphoid stem cells leave the bone marrow and reach the thymus gland via the bloodstream. At this stage of development, these cells lack surface antigens that make up the TCR complex and mature T-cell markers (e.g., CD4, CD8) associated with specific effector functions. The major class of T cells is defined by its surface expression of the αβ T-cell receptor. This recognizes peptide antigens presented in a complex with class I or II MHC proteins. Each individual T cell bears antigen receptors of a single specificity. A repertoire of T cells that can protect against the large number of microbial pathogens must contain a large number of cells encoding a huge array of discrete TCRs. These receptors are somatically assembled from variable, diverse, and joining gene elements to generate mature $V_\alpha J_\alpha$ chains and $V_\beta D_\beta J_\beta$ chains.[6]

The assembly of these gene elements is initiated by the lymphoid-specific recombinase-activating gene 1 (RAG1) and RAG2 proteins that cleave the DNA near the V, D, and J segments. The gene segments are rejoined by a collection of DNA repair enzymes including DNA-dependent protein kinase, DNA ligase IV, and Artemis.[97] The action of these recombinase enzymes results in the V, D, and J gene elements assembling in an apparently random process, so they often produce nonfunctional genes.

Selection of cells carrying functional TCR genes occurs in the thymus.[169] The thymus contains three compartments. The first, the subcapsular zone, is where the bone marrow–derived prothymocytes begin to differentiate, proliferate, and rearrange their TCR β chains. The cells then move to the thymic cortex where the α chain gene elements rearrange, potentially forming a functional, mature αβ TCR. In the cor-

tex, cells test whether their receptors have sufficient affinity for self MHC molecules to permit them to ultimately recognize antigen-MHC complexes. This involves interactions between the developing lymphocyte and the specialized cortical epithelium.[259] If a lymphocyte fails this positive selection, it undergoes apoptosis and is cleared by thymic macrophages. Finally, in the thymic medulla, cells are screened for potential autoreactivity. Self-reactive cells are removed by apoptosis, and cells that have survived this negative selection are exported to the circulation. Fewer than 5% of the developing T cells survive positive and negative selection.

Approximately 90% to 95% of circulating T cells use the αβ TCR. The other 5 to 10% use an alternate heterodimeric TCR composed of γ and δ chains. The γ and δ chains assemble by RAG1/RAG2-mediated rearrangement of V, D, and J elements. A portion of the γδ T cells are generated in the thymus, with a major fraction generated in an extra thymic compartment, resulting in cells that largely populate the gastrointestinal (GI) tract.[166]

The antigen-specific α and β chains of the TCR associate with invariant accessory chains that serve to transduce signals when the TCR binds to antigen-MHC complexes.[203] These accessory chains make up the CD3 complex. Interaction of the TCR/CD3 complex with antigenic peptide presented in an HLA molecule provides only a partial signal for cellular activation. Full activation requires the additional participation of a costimulatory molecule, such as CD28 on the T cell and CD80 or CD86 on the antigen presenting cell.[150] Interaction of peptide-MHC with the TCR without a costimulator can lead to an anergic state of prolonged T-cell nonresponsiveness.[106]

During their progress through the thymus, αβ T cells differentiate into discrete subpopulations, each with defined repertoires of effector functions. The major subsets are defined by their selective surface expression of CD4 or CD8. In the thymus, most developing T cells follow a developmental program in the cortex, where they first express neither CD4 nor CD8 (double negative), and then express both CD4 and CD8 (double positive).[262] Double positive cells are tested by positive selection in the thymic cortex. Those that are selected on class I MHC molecules become CD4−CD8+, and those that are selected on class II MHC molecules become CD4+CD8−. The cells then move to the thymic medulla for negative selection and export to the periphery. Thus, CD4+ cells recognize antigen in the context of MHC class II molecules, whereas CD8+ cells recognize antigen presented by class I molecules. CD4 and CD8 T cells remain restricted by the MHC antigen for the duration of their life span.

In the blood and secondary lymphoid organs, 60% to 70% of T cells are CD4+CD8− (CD4+), and 30% to 40% are CD4−CD8+ (CD8+). CD4+ cells are generally designated *helper cells* and work to activate both humoral immune responses (B-cell help) and cellular responses (delayed-type hypersensitivity responses). CD8+ cells show a major cytotoxic activity against cells infected with intracellular microbes and against tumor cells. They also contain regulatory cells that down-regulate immune responses, *suppressor cells*. An important class of down-regulatory cells is characterized as CD4+CD25+, which secrete the immunoregulatory cytokines transforming growth factor (TGF)-β and IL-10.[235] Approximately 5% to 10% of T cells in the peripheral circulation, lymph nodes, and spleen are CD4−CD8−. Some of these cells use αβ TCRs and others use γδ TCRs. Double negative cells do not recognize antigen in the context of MHC class I or II. Some of these cells recognize antigen in the class I-related protein CD1 that is adapted to presentation of glycolipid components of mycobacteria and other microbes.[102] A subset of double negative γδ T cells recognizes the MHC class I-related chain (MIC).[278]

Both CD4+ and CD8+ T cells differentiate into functionally distinct subsets after exposure to antigen. This is best described for the transition of CD4+ T cells from naïve to effector populations.[1] Resting naïve CD4+ T cells (designated T-helper cells, Th) release almost no cytokines. Early after stimulation by antigen and APC, the Th cells begin to produce IL-2 and are designated Th0. As the Th cells continue to respond to the activating signal, they progress toward polar extremes of differentiation designated TH1 and TH, depending on the nature of the cytokines present at the site of activation.[177] IL-12 produced by macrophages or NK cells induces differentiation towards TH, and IL-4 produced by NK1.1+ T cells or mast cells induce differentiation towards TH2. TH1 cells produce IL-2, IFN-γ, and lymphotoxin; whereas TH cells produce IL-4, IL-5, IL-9, IL-10, IL-13, and granulocyte-macrophage colony stimulating factor (GMCSF). In most immune responses, Th cells show a combination of TH1 and TH2 features; however, after prolonged immunization, the response can become dominantly TH1-like or TH2-like. Generally, TH1 cells support cell-mediated immune responses and play a critical role in the defense against intracellular pathogens, such as viruses *Mycobacteria* and *Listeria*, whereas TH2 cells are critical in the responses induced by extracellular pathogens-antigens such as parasites, bacteria, and allergens. CD8+ cells also can manifest type 1 and type 2 cytokine responses, in which case the cells are designated T cytotoxic cell type 1 (Tc1) and Tc2.[254] Recent progress with immunization to different types of adjuvants demonstrates the feasibility of reprogramming allergic TH2-type responses in atopic patients to nonallergic TH1-type responses, thereby potentially altering the course of allergic disease.[240]

B Cells

B cells constitute approximately 15% of peripheral blood leukocytes. They are defined by their production of immunoglobulins (Ig). B cells differentiate from hematopoietic stem cells in the bone marrow. It is here that their antigen receptors (surface Ig) are assembled from genetic building blocks in a RAG1/RAG2-mediated process similar to that used for the production of functional TCR.[29] Differentiation of stem cells to the B lineage depends on bone marrow stromal cells that produce IL-7. The developing B cells follow a program of differential surface antigen expression and sequential heavy and light chain gene rearrangement. Naïve B cells express IgM and IgD on their cell surfaces.[18] As B cells mature under the influence of helper T cells, T-cell–derived cytokines induce isotype switching. IL-1 and IL-2 promote B-cell activation and growth,[94,210] IL-10 causes switching to IgG1 and IgG3. IL-4 and IL-13 cause switching to IgE, and transforming growth factor-β causes switching to IgA. IFN-γ, or some other undefined product of TH1 cells, appears to induce switching to IgG2.

At the same time that B cells undergo isotype switching, an active process produces mutations, apparently randomly, in the antigen-binding portions of the heavy and light chains. If these mutations result in loss of affinity for the antigen, the cell loses important receptor-mediated growth signals and dies. If, however, the mutations result in increased affinity for the antigen, the cell producing that antibody has a proliferative advantage in response to antigen and grows to dominate the pool of responding cells. Somatic mutation and clonal expansion of mutated cells occurs in the germinal centers of secondary lymphoid tissues.

Large Granular Lymphocytes

Large granular lymphocytes are the third major subtype of lymphocytes and are referred to as *natural killer cells*. These cells are usually larger than typical lymphocytes and display less nuclear material and more cytoplasm. They possess electron-dense, peroxidase-negative granules and a well-developed Golgi apparatus. These cells lack rearranged Ig or TCR genes and therefore do not express surface Ig or the TCR complex. NK cells provide nonspecific cytotoxic activity toward virally infected cells and tumor cells. They can also mediate antibody-dependent cellular cytotoxicity (ADCC) by activation through their IgG Fc receptors and the subsequent production of cytokines such as IFN-γ, which can affect the proliferation and differentiation of other cell types. Resting NK cells can be induced to proliferate and can be activated by IL-2 derived from antigen-activated T cells.[103]

Monocytes and Macrophages

Monocytes and macrophages arise from colony-forming unit-granulocyte-macrophage (CFU-GM) progenitors, which differentiate into monoblasts, promonocytes, and monocytes. Monocytes account for about 10% of circulating leukocytes. Several cytokines—including stem cell factor (SCF), IL-3, IL-6, IL-11, and GM-CSF—promote the development of myeloid-lineage cells from CD34+ stem cells, predominantly in the early stages of differentiation. The macrophage colony-stimulating factor (MCSF) acts at the later stages of development and induces maturation of macrophages.[114] Mature monocytes leave the bone marrow and circulate in the bloodstream until they enter tissues, where they develop into macrophages. These cells include Langerhans cells in the epidermis, Kupffer cells in the liver, microglial cells in the central nervous system, and the broad class of dendritic cells that are present in most tissues of the body and concentrated in the secondary lymphoid tissues. All of these cells express both class I and class II MHC molecules that are used to permit recognition of processed antigen by the TCR on T cells. Dendritic cells appear to be the most potent APC, but macrophages, Langerhans cells, and Kupffer cells are also prominent APCs.

Like neutrophils, monocytes and macrophages are also highly phagocytic for microbes and particles that have been marked for clearance by binding Ig, complement, or both. Phagocytosis is facilitated by opsonization, which coats foreign material with antibodies. After phagocytosis, an intracellular vacuole forms around the foreign material and lysosomal enzymes released into the vacuole destroy the foreign invader. These cells appear to be mobilized shortly after neutrophils and they persist for long periods at sites of chronic inflammation and infection. They use production of nitric oxide as a major mechanism for killing microbial pathogens and produce large amounts of cytokines, such as IL-12 and INF-γ, giving them a regulatory role in adaptive immune responses.[260]

Neutrophils

Neutrophils arise from CFU-GM progenitor cells that give rise to myeloblasts, which differentiate into promyelocytes, myelocytes, and finally, mature neutrophils. After maturation in the bone marrow, neutrophils circulate in the peripheral blood, where they account for 60% to 65% of leukocytes. As for monocytes, SCF, IL-3, IL-6, IL-11, and GM-CSF promote the growth and development of neutrophil precursors. Other cytokines that exhibit more specific effects on neutrophils include granulocyte colony-stimulating factor (G-CSF), which induces maturation of neutrophil precursors into neutrophils.[167] IL-4 also enhances neutrophil differentiation induced by G-CSF. Neutrophils produce large quantities of oxygen species that are cytotoxic to bacterial pathogens and enzymes that appear to participate in tissue remodeling and repair after injury. They accumulate in large quantities at sites of bacterial infection and tissue injury and possess prominent phagocytic capabilities that permit them to sequester microbes and particulate antigens internally where they can be destroyed and degraded. Thus, they play a major role in the clearance of microbial pathogens and repair of tissue injury.[58] More recently, however, neutrophils have been recognized to produce substantial amounts of the cytokines tumor necrosis factor (TNF) and IL-12, as well as certain chemokines. This supports an additional immunoregulatory role of these cells.

Eosinophils

Eosinophils are derived from colony-forming unit-eosinophil (CFU-Eo), a progenitor that differentiates into an eosinophilic myeloblast, promyelocyte, myelocyte, and finally a mature eosinophil. Eosinophils comprise 2% to 5% of circulating leukocytes and are readily recognized by their prominent cytoplasmic granules that contain toxic molecules and enzymes that are particularly active against helminthes and other parasites.[3] GM-CSF and IL-3 promote eosinophil growth and differentiation.[271] The production of eosinophils from the bone marrow and their survival in peripheral tissues are enhanced by the cytokine IL-5, which maintains their viability through inhibition of apoptosis.[245]

Eosinophils are prominent cells in most allergic responses.[139] Eosinophils possess several surface markers and receptors involved in differentiation, recruitment into tissues, activation, and synthesis and release of their multiple mediators. Receptors for immunoglobulins include those for IgG, IgE, and IgA. The receptor for IgG on eosinophils is principally the low-affinity FcγRII (CD32). Eosinophils also have three potential receptors for IgE. They may express the high-affinity IgE receptor FcεRI, as well as FcεRII, the low-affinity IgE receptor CD23, found on lymphocytes, monocytes and other cells.[101] Eosinophil expression of IgE receptors is notable because IgE levels and eosinophil numbers frequently increase concomitantly in helminth parasitic infections and in allergic diseases.

Eosinophils express FcαRI (CD89), which binds secretory IgA more potently than do other forms of IgA.

Engagement of FcαRI triggers eosinophil release of granule proteins.[178] With the characteristic localization of eosinophils to mucosal surfaces of the respiratory, gastrointestinal, and genitourinary tracts, this IgA receptor enables eosinophils to engage secretory IgA present at these mucosal sites.

Eosinophils have receptors for complement components, including C1q (CR1), C3b/C4b (CR1), iC3b (CR3), C3a, and C5a. Both C3a and C5a are eosinophil chemoattractants and stimulate oxygen radical production by eosinophils. Eosinophils potentially express several receptors for chemokines. CCR1 is a receptor for MIP-1α, MCP-3, and regulated on activation, normal T cell expressed and secreted (RANTES); CCR3 is a receptor for eotaxin, eotaxin-2, eotaxin-3, MCP-3, and RANTES.[220]

Mature eosinophils, like their immature precursors, express functional heterodimeric receptors for the three cytokines—GM-CSF, IL-3, and IL-5—that promote eosinophilopoiesis and stimulate the functioning of mature eosinophils. Eosinophils also have receptors for a broad range of other cytokines including IL-1α, IL-2, IL-4, IFN-γ, IFN-α, TNF-α, SCF, and IL-16. Receptors are also expressed on eosinophils for several lipid mediators including platelet activating factor (PAF) and leukotriene B4 (LTB4), which are chemoattractants for eosinophils and stimulate eosinophil degranulation and respiratory burst activity. Eosinophils also have receptors for prostaglandin E2 and for cysteinyl leukotrienes.

The eosinophil's cationic granule proteins have been studied extensively; they include major basic protein (MBP), eosinophil peroxidase (EPO), eosinophil cationic protein (ECP), and eosinophil-derived neurotoxin (EDN). Another prominent protein of the eosinophil is the Charcot-Leyden crystal (CLC) protein, which constitutes an estimated 7% to 10% of total cellular protein, possesses lysophospholipase activity, and forms the distinctive hexagonal bipyramidal crystals that are the hallmark of eosinophil-associated inflammation.

MBP is present in eosinophils and basophils (at much lower concentrations than in eosinophils), and mast cells may acquire MBP by endocytosis and vesicular uptake. MBP is a potent cytotoxin and helminth toxin in vitro. MBP can kill bacteria and many types of normal and neoplastic mammalian cells, stimulate histamine release from basophils and mast cells, activate neutrophils and platelets, and augment superoxide generation by alveolar macrophages. It can also induce bronchoconstriction and transient airway hyperreactivity when instilled into the monkey trachea.[3]

As with MBP and ECP, EPO is highly cationic and exerts some cytotoxic effects on parasites and mam-malian cells in the absence of hydrogen peroxide. However, EPO is highly effective in combination with hydrogen peroxide and a halide cofactor (iodide, bromide, or chloride) from which EPO catalyzes the production of the toxic hypohalous acid. In the presence of these compounds, EPO is highly toxic to various unicellular, multicellular, and other targets, including viruses, mycoplasma, bacteria, fungi, and parasites.

ECP, similar to MBP, has marked toxicity for helminth parasites, blood hemoflagellates, bacteria, and mammalian cells and tissues. Purified ECP has been used in several studies in which respiratory epithelial damage (epithelial stripping, mucus plugging), similar to that in severe asthmatics, has been reproduced.

EDN induces a syndrome of muscle rigidity, ataxia, eventual paralysis, widespread loss of Purkinje's cells, and spongiform degeneration of the white matter of the cerebellum, brainstem, and spinal cord when injected intrathecally or intracerebrally into experimental rabbits or guinea pigs. Unlike the other eosinophil granule cationic proteins, EDN is a poor cationic toxin, with only limited toxicity for helminths and mammalian cells at very high concentrations. In allergic conditions, eosinophils may play a dual role. They can suppress the local tissue response to inflammatory mediators involved in IgE-mediated hypersensitivity reactions by inactivating histamine, platelet-activating factor, and heparin. On the other hand, eosinophils can augment destruction by the toxic effects of the products they release on degranulation. The balance between these two seemingly contradictory functions of eosinophils in IgE-mediated reactions is still under investigation.

Basophils and Mast Cells

Basophils mature from a progenitor colony-forming unit-basophil mast cell (CFU-BM) into basophilic myeloblasts, promyelocytes, myelocytes, and then mature basophils. Mast cells are thought to develop from the same progenitor, but less is known about their specific stages of development. IL-3 and SCF induce the most consistent effects on human basophil and mast cell growth and differentiation. These cytokines act synergistically to induce basophil and mast cell development from CD34+ progenitor cells.[132] SCF induces functional maturation of human mast cells. Nerve growth factor and GM-CSF[257] affect basophil growth IL-5 enhances basophil differentiation.[67] Basophils and mast cells are morphologically similar and both exhibit cell surface expression of high-affinity receptors for IgE (FcεRI), which makes them key initiators of immediate hypersensitivity responses and the host response to helminthic parasites, releasing histamine and other preformed mediators from their granules and producing important quantities of lipid mediators that stimulate tissue inflammation, edema, and smooth muscle contraction. Recent studies have shown that in addition to this role, mast cells also play prominent roles in the host response to bacterial infections.[2]

Platelets and Erythrocytes

Platelets and erythrocytes are derived from stem cell progenitors, which in turn differentiate into burst-forming units-megakaryocytes (BFU-MEG) in the case of platelets and into burst-forming units-erythroid (BFU-E) in the case of erythrocytes. BFU-MEG then differentiate into CFU-MEG, promegakaryoblasts, megakaryocytes, and platelets. IL-1, IL-3, GM-CSF, IL-6, and IL-11 affect the growth and differentiation of platelets.[186,243,249] The erythrocyte precursor BFU-E differentiates into colony-forming unit-erythroid (CFU-E), pronormoblasts, basophilic normoblasts, polychromatophilic normoblasts, orthochromic normoblasts, reticulocytes, and erythrocytes. Cytokines important in the various stages of erythrocyte differentiation and development include GM-CSF, SCF, IL-9, and erythropoietin.[80]

LYMPHOID ORGANS

The primary lymphoid organs, sites where lymphocytes differentiate and mature from stem cells into effector cells, include the thymus and bone marrow. The secondary lymphoid organs are sites where mature lymphocytes reside and immune responses are generated. A major challenge for the immune system of a naïve subject is to bring together rare antigen-specific B cells, rare antigen-specific T cells, and antigen-charged antigen presenting cells. The primary role of the secondary lymphoid tissues is to facilitate these interactions. The secondary lymphoid organs are divided into the systemic immune system, which includes the spleen and lymph nodes, and the mucosal immune system, which includes the tonsils, Peyer's patches, scattered lymphoid follicles, intraepithelial lymphocytes, and the lamina propria of mucosal tissues. The spleen protects the body from antigens in the bloodstream, whereas lymph nodes respond to antigens delivered through lymphatics draining the skin and deeper tissues. The secondary lymphoid organs, specifically lymph nodes and the mucosal immune system, are of particular interest to otolaryngologists.

Lymph Nodes

Lymph nodes occur as chains or groups. They are oval structures with a hilus where blood vessels enter and leave the nodes and a surrounding fibrous capsule.

After entering the node, blood vessels and nerves branch within the fibrous trabeculae that traverse the node to its various parts. Beneath the lymph node capsule, a sinus receives afferent lymphatic vessels from the structures that drain into the lymph nodes. These vessels carry antigen-processing cells and foreign antigens that are subsequently transported into the substance of the lymph node. Lymph nodes are divided into two major regions, the cortex and the medulla.

The cortex contains numerous primary and secondary lymphoid follicles in which B cells predominate. Primary follicles, consisting of a mantle zone without germinal centers, contain resting B cells expressing surface IgM or IgD and CD23. In addition to an outer mantle zone, secondary follicles contain inner germinal centers, which form in response to antigen stimulation. Immunoglobulin class switch, affinity maturation through somatic mutation, and development of memory B cells occur within germinal centers. CD4+ T cells are also found in these centers and play a key role in the B-cell responses (described earlier) through interactions between CD40 (expressed on the B cell) and the ligand for CD40 (CD, present on activated CD4+ cells). The paracortical region of the lymph node cortex surrounds the lymphoid follicles and contains mostly T cells (both CD4+ and CD8+) and some macrophages, dendritic cells, and B cells (accessory cells). The accessory cells present peptide antigens in association with MHC molecules to the TCR on T cells, resulting in their activation.

The medulla, the region at the center of the lymph node, is divided into medullary cords surrounded by medullary sinuses that drain into the hilus. Medullary cords contain B cells, T cells, macrophages, and many plasma cells. These cells are joined by B and T cells that migrate from the cortex to the medulla. Efferent lymphatic vessels leave the hilus carrying antibodies and mature B and T cells that migrate to other tissues and act as memory cells during subsequent immune exposure. The lymphatic system eventually drains into the thoracic duct and into the circulation, therefore allowing lymphocytes to circulate throughout the body.

Mucosal Immune System

Mucosal surfaces and skin encounter the environment and possess an immune system capable of responding to pathogens and foreign antigens. The mucosal immune system is composed of the organized mucosal immune system (including tonsils, Peyer's patches, and isolated lymphoid follicles) and the diffuse mucosal immune system (including intraepithelial lymphocytes and lamina propria).

Tonsils

Three lymphoid structures surround the entrance to the throat: the adenoids, the palatine tonsils, and the lingual tonsils. These structures reach full development in childhood and begin to involute around puberty. The palatine tonsils are surrounded by a poorly organized capsule, except at the pharyngeal surface, which is covered with stratified squamous epithelium. Trabeculae extend from the capsule and divide the tonsils into lobules. Blood vessels and nerves enter through the capsule and extend within the trabeculae. The tonsillar surface is covered by pits, which open into crypts that branch down within the tissue of the tonsil, maximizing the surface area exposed to the pharynx. Each lobule contains numerous lymphoid follicles with germinal centers that predominantly contain B cells[89]; the lymphoid tissue that surrounds the follicles contains T cells, macrophages, dendritic cells, and B cells. These structures are strategically located at sites of entry of airborne particles through the nose (adenoids) and at sites of food particle entry (tonsils). The structures filter unwanted organisms and antigens and function as a mucosal immune barrier.

Peyer's Patches and Lymphoid Follicles

Peyer's patches are aggregates of lymphoid follicles within the mucosa of the jejunum and ileum, with most in the terminal ileum. The full development of this component of the mucosal immune system, including the formation of follicles containing germinal centers, occurs several weeks after birth; their number increases until puberty and then decreases.

Lymphoid follicles, another component of the mucosal immune system with structures similar to follicles of a Peyer's patch, are scattered throughout the gastrointestinal, respiratory, and genitourinary tract mucosa. These lymphoid organs facilitate antigen presentation from the intestinal lumen to T and B cells. Unlike the epithelium of the gastrointestinal tract, the epithelium overlying Peyer's patches and isolated lymphoid follicles lacks villi and contains few goblet cells.

Antigen uptake occurs in this epithelium by specialized epithelial cells (M cells) through pinocytosis. The epithelium also expresses MHC class II antigens (with the exception of M cells) but not the immunoglobulin receptor required for secretion of IgA. The subepithelial region contains many T cells (including CD4+ cells). Beneath this region is the dome, which contains many T cells, macrophages, dendritic cells, and B cells. Antigens, pinocytosed by M cells, are transported to the dome region, where they are presented to T cells by macrophages and dendritic cells.

Follicles lie beneath the dome region and contain mantle zones with predominantly resting B cells, most of which express IgM and IgD on their surface. Most Peyer's patch follicles have germinal centers containing activated B cells, dendritic cells, CD4+ T cells, and macrophages. An interfollicular region contains many CD4+ and CD8+ T cells, dendritic cells, macrophages, and some B cells.

Intraepithelial Lymphocytes

Intraepithelial lymphocytes are found at the basal surface of the epithelium and are interdigitated with epithelial cells. Initially, they were considered to be lamina propria cells that invaded the epithelial layer. However, it is now clear that they are phenotypically and probably functionally distinct from lamina propria cells. Most are T cells (CD8+ or CD4− CD8−), and although most express the TCR$\alpha\beta$, some express the TCR$\gamma\delta$, further setting them apart from other lymphoid sites. The function of intraepithelial lymphocytes is not understood, but studies have shown their capacity to generate cytotoxic activity.[99,147]

Lamina Propria

The lamina propria, located beneath the epithelium, is a loosely structured tissue populated by various groups of cells. One of the key functions of this tissue is the secretion of IgA antibody from the many IgA plasma cells.[122] IgA is transported from the lamina propria to the epithelium and is then secreted into the lumen. The lamina propria also contains many CD4+ and CD8+ T lymphocytes in a ratio of about 2:1. In contrast to intraepithelial lymphocytes, most lamina propria T cells express the TCR-$\alpha\beta$. Other effector cells of the lamina propria include IgG B cells, macrophages, dendritic cells, eosinophils, mast cells, and neutrophils.

ANTIGEN PRESENTATION

Antigen presentation is carried out by specialized cells referred to as antigen-presenting cells (APC), a diverse group of leukocytes including monocytes, macrophages, dendritic cells, and B cells. These cells are found primarily in the solid lymphoid organs and the skin. APC express high levels of class II MHC molecules and possess the capacity to internalize, process, and present foreign antigens in the MHC groove.

Follicular dendritic cells are specialized APC in the B-cell areas of lymph nodes and the spleen and are important in the generation and maintenance of memory B cells by trapping antigen-antibody complexes. Peripheral tissue dendritic cells engulf and process antigen, leave the tissues, then go home to T-cell areas in draining lymph nodes or the spleen. The predominant APC of the skin are Langerhans cells, which are found in the epidermis and deliver antigens entering the skin to the effector cells of the lymph nodes. In the lymph nodes, these APC can directly present processed antigens to resting T cells to induce their proliferation and differentiation. Monocytes-macrophages exist as monocytes in blood and as macrophages (a more differentiated form) in various tissues, such as the lungs, liver, and brain. In addition to phagocytic and cytotoxic functions, these cells have receptors for various cytokines (IL-4, IFN-γ), which can regulate their function. Activated macrophages are also a major source of several cytokines (IFN, IL-1, TNF), complement proteins, and prostaglandins.[215] All APC have MHC class II surface molecules.

Foreign or self proteins undergo hydrolytic cleavage within the APC and become oligopeptides, which are then loaded onto antigen-binding grooves of MHC molecules before expression at the cell surface (Figure 9-2). Class I molecules usually bind peptides that are 8 to 10 amino acids long and are derived from proteins synthesized intracellularly (e.g., tumor antigens and viruses), whereas class II molecules bind peptides that are 14 to 22 amino acids long and are derived from proteins synthesized extracellularly (e.g., non replicating vaccines and extracellular bacteria). Lipids and lipid derivatives are processed in a manner similar to extracellular proteins in endosomes, combined with CD1 (an MHC-like molecule) and presented to double-negative or CD8 T cells frequently bearing $\gamma\delta$ receptors.

In addition to the mechanism of presentation of oligopeptide antigens to lymphocytes via MHC molecules, T cells can recognize haptens, which are covalently or noncovalently complexed with peptides residing in the MHC-binding groove. Another exception is the presentation of super antigens, which are about 30 kD proteins produced by a broad spectrum of microbes ranging from retroviruses to bacteria. These antigens do not undergo processing to oligopeptides but bind intact to class II MHC molecules and the TCR outside the antigen-binding grooves. They can activate more T cells than conventional peptide antigens.

CELL-MEDIATED IMMUNE RESPONSES

Initial lymphocyte activation is a two-step event. The first activation signal is provided by antigens. As already discussed, the antigens that stimulate T cells are limited to oligopeptides (or haptens attached to peptides) that reside within the antigen-binding groove of a self MHC molecule. TCRs do not bind antigen in solution. B cells, on the other hand, can be stimulated by antigens in solution or fixed to a solid matrix. The second signal necessary for T-cell activation is provided by accessory molecules expressed on the surface of the APC for stimulation of T cells, or on the surface of a T-helper cell for activation of B lymphocytes. The growth and differentiation of T cells and B cells also require stimulation with one or more cytokines, which are secreted by activated T cells and APC.

T lymphocytes expressing the TCR-$\alpha\beta$ are divided into two major subpopulations based on the class of the MHC molecule that their TCR recognizes. T cells expressing CD4, or T-helper (TH) cells, recognize antigen bound to class II MHC molecules; T cells expressing CD8, or T-suppressor

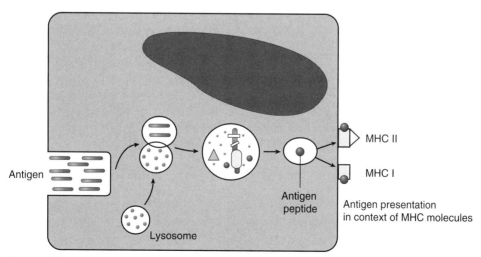

Figure 9-2. Antigen processing and presentation. Antigen undergoes hydrolytic cleavage within antigen-presenting cells, and the resultant oligopeptides are loaded on antigen-binding grooves of major histocompatibility complex molecules and expressed at the cell surface.

cells, recognize antigen bound to MHC class I molecules. CD8+ T cells are commonly cytotoxic T-lymphocytes (CTL) and are important effectors of the cell-mediated immune response. The ratio of CD4 to CD8 cells in peripheral blood is usually 2:1, but may vary considerably.

CD4+ T Cells

After recognizing antigens presented by MHC class II molecules, CD4+ cells become activated to secrete IL-2, partly in response to monocyte-derived IL-1 and partly in response to autocrine stimulation by IL-2 as part of a positive feedback loop (Figure 9-3). Activated

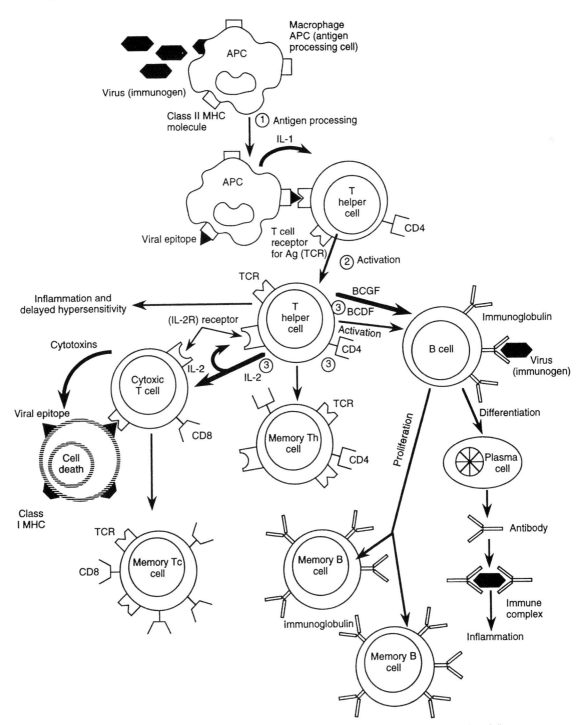

Figure 9-3. Summary of the cell-mediated immune response showing the events that follow exposure to an immunogen and the role of the T-helper cell in orchestrating these events. (From Stites DP, Terr AI, editors: *Basic and clinical immunology*, ed 7. Norwalk, CT, Appleton & Lange, 1991.)

CD4+ cells interact with other CD4+ or CD8+ cells by secreting IL-2, and with B cells by secreting B-cell growth and differentiation factors (IL-2, IL-4, IL-6). Thus, CD4+ cells augment immune responses by stimulating B cells sensitized by antigen, and by stimulating CD8+ cells sensitized by binding of antigen in the context of MHC class I molecules. The activities of these CD4+ cells are largely mediated via the secretion of cytokines, which are small protein hormones that control the growth and differentiation of cells in the microenvironment.

The pattern of cytokine secretion of TH cells allows further subdivision into TH-1 and TH-2 cells.[177] TH-1 cells elaborate inflammatory cytokines involved in effector functions of cell-mediated immunity, such as IL-2 and IFN-γ, whereas TH-2 cells elaborate cytokines such as IL-4 and IL-13, which control and regulate antibody responses. Some CD4+ cells, capable of secreting both TH1 and TH2 cytokines, are designated TH-0 cells and are precursors to TH-1 and TH-2 cells. Differentiation into TH-1 vs TH-2 cells is regulated by positive feedback loops promoted primarily by IL-12 and IL-4, respectively.[229] Cytokines produced by activated T cells can down-regulate, as well as initiate or amplify, immune responses. Cytokines with such activity include IL-10 (produced by both T cells and B cells) and transforming growth factor-β (TGF-β). The functions of IL-10 in vivo are thought to include both suppression of the production of proinflammatory cytokines and enhancement of IgM and IgA synthesis. TGF-β is produced by virtually all cells and expresses a broad array of biological activities, including the promotion of wound healing and the suppression of both humoral and cell-mediated immune responses.

In addition to their central role in initiating and regulating immune responses, CD4+ T lymphocytes are important effectors of cell-mediated immunity by virtue of the cytokines that they elaborate. These cytokines, particularly IFN-γ, are essential contributors to the generation of chronic inflammatory responses characterized by mononuclear cellular infiltration and activated macrophages. Furthermore, CD4+ cells can contribute to the cellular immune response by functioning as cytotoxic effectors, directly as CTL or by secreting cytotoxic cytokines such as TNF-β.

In addition to orchestrating the immune response by secreting various cytokines and contributing to T-lymphocyte cytotoxic activities, the characteristic inflammatory reaction induced by CD4+ T lymphocytes is delayed-type hypersensitivity (DTH). DTH is elicited by challenge with antigen in immune, sensitized persons. The typical example is the cutaneous reaction to challenge with the purified protein derivative (PPD) of *Mycobacterium tuberculosis* in previously infected or vaccinated persons. Clinically, DTH is manifested by local erythema and induration 24 to 48 hours after challenge. Microscopically, the lesion shows perivascular accumulations of leukocytes (initially neutrophils, later lymphocytes and activated macrophages), edema, and fibrin deposition. Chronic DTH reactions result in the formation of granulomas (nodular collections of macrophages and lymphocytes) and possibly fibrosis as a result of the cytokines produced by macrophages, which stimulate fibroblast proliferation and collagen synthesis.

DTH involves reactions by various immune system components. A sensitized person has activated and memory T lymphocytes specific for the immunizing antigen. A subsequent antigen challenge induces local inflammation and the release of cytokines that stimulate the expression of intercellular adhesion molecule (ICAM)-1 and vascular cell adhesion molecule (VCAM)-1 on vascular endothelium. These molecules bind activated and memory T lymphocytes, which express a high level of ligands that interact with ICAM-1—lymphocyte function antigen (LFA-1) and VCAM-1 [very late antigen (VLA-4)]. These interactions lead to tissue accumulation of T lymphocytes, which are presented with the antigen by APC in the context of MHC molecules (in the case of a PPD-DTH reaction, the T lymphocytes are CD4+ and the MHC molecules are class II). Recognition of antigen by the T lymphocytes leads to an increase in the affinity of T-cell LFA-1 and VLA-4 for their specific ligands. For example, VLA-4 binds to fibronectin in the extracellular matrix and therefore promotes the retention of antigen-stimulated T cells in the extravascular tissue.

Activated T cells also secrete cytokines. The most important cytokines in DTH are IFN-γ (a potent activator of macrophages) and TNF, which increases the expression of leukocyte adhesion molecules on endothelium and initiates recruitment of leukocytes (neutrophils and monocytes) to the site. IL-2 is also secreted by activated T cells and stimulates the proliferation of T cells. As discussed earlier in this chapter, these cytokines are produced by the TH-1 cells. The recruited inflammatory leukocytes and the resident activated tissue macrophages then phagocytose the antigen and secrete various substances with microbicidal activity (reactive oxygen intermediates, lysosomal enzymes), which also contribute to tissue injury. DTH is seen in various clinical situations, such as in the skin lesions of contact sensitivity to chemicals, in infections with certain microbes (*M. tuberculosis*), in some fungal and parasitic infections,[130] and in certain autoimmune diseases.[55,282]

Another type of inflammation that occurs in some T-cell–mediated immune responses is characterized by the accumulation of eosinophils and is caused by the activation of TH-2 cells. These secrete IL-4 and IL-5, which promote the recruitment and survival of eosinophils in tissue sites of inflammation. Allergic reactions are a good example of this process. The pathophysiology of allergic rhinitis is discussed later in this chapter.

CD8+ T Cells and Cytotoxicity

The best understood function of CD8+ cells is that of cytotoxic effectors (CTL). Their function as suppressors of the immune response is more controversial, and the mechanism of this activity is not very well understood; in some instances, it is thought to be mediated by the production of nonspecific inhibitory cytokines. Although CD4+ and CD8+ lymphocytes can both act as cytotoxic effectors, the CD8+ population has a higher frequency of cytotoxic effectors than the CD4+ population.

The initial event in the destruction of target cells by cytotoxic effectors involves contact with the target cell membrane components. When the cytotoxic effector is a CD8+ cell (as is most often the case), the foreign peptide is recognized by a class I MHC molecule on the target cell. Transmembrane signaling then occurs. The adhesion between the two cells is strengthened, and conjugation takes place. This nonspecific adhesion between the two cells is achieved by the binding of LFA-1 on the cytotoxic effectors to ICAM-1 on the target cells, when available, and CD2 on the cytotoxic effectors to LFA-3 on the target cells. A lethal hit is then delivered by the cytotoxic effector to the target cell by exocytosis of cytotoxic effectors granules into the junctional region between effector and target. These granules contain perforins, which are proteins that create pores within the target cell membrane, making it permeable. Granzymes and other proteases and granule mediators released from the cytotoxic effector can then enter the target cell and affect internal disintegration. After delivering a lethal hit to a target cell, the cytotoxic effector still contains additional granules and can immediately recycle to engage and lyse additional target cells. Because of an unidentified property of their plasma membranes, cytotoxic effectors are resistant to lysis by their own exocytoses granules.

Another pathway for cytotoxic cell function involves the cell-surface molecule Fas, which is a member of the TNF receptor-nerve growth factor receptor-CD40 superfamily and mediates apoptosis.[123] Binding of the cell-surface Fas molecule on a target cell to the Fas ligand on the cytotoxic effector leads to apoptosis of the target cell. Fas-mediated cytotoxicity is thought to play a role in the negative selection process in T-cell development; however, the role of

this pathway for cytolysis in various infectious diseases has not been defined. Another mechanism for the induction of cytotoxicity, which is thought to play a key role in many inflammatory processes, involves the secretion of cytolytic cytokines by cytotoxic effectors (e.g., TNF).

CTL exert cell contact-dependent cytotoxic functions through the mechanisms mentioned. The perforin-dependent pathway of cytotoxicity is largely responsible for cell-mediated clearance of infectious viruses (e.g., cytomegalovirus, Epstein-Barr virus, hepatitis B and C, human immunodeficiency virus-1, influenza A and B, measles, mumps, respiratory syncytial virus, rubella, and vaccinia) and certain intracellular bacterial infections, and for the rejection of allogenic tissue grafts and tumors. The Fas antigen-ligand pathway of cytotoxicity appears to be important in the elimination of T cells during differentiation and tolerance induction.

HUMORAL IMMUNE RESPONSE
T-Cell Dependent and T-Cell Independent B-Cell Responses

Humoral immunity consists of responses that are T-cell dependent (TD) and T-cell independent. *T-cell independent B-cell responses* occur with large antigens that have repeating antigenic determinants, such as carbohydrates, which constitute the capsule and cell wall components of bacteria. This T-cell response represents a major protective role against bacterial pathogens such as *S. pneumoniae*. These pathogens bridge immunoglobulins on the B-cell surface, causing activation and the subsequent secretion of antibodies, primarily of the IgM class. Antibodies to *S. pneumoniae* mediate the opsonization of bacteria by binding to the bacterial cell surface, thereby targeting them for destruction by Fc receptor-bearing macrophages. Young children and the elderly, who generally respond poorly to T-cell independent antigens, are at increased risk for these bacterial infections. Protective immunity against *Haemophilus influenzae* and meningococcal infections is also mediated by T-cell independent B-cell responses.

In *T-cell-dependent B-cell responses*, antigens that activate T cells, as well as B cells, establish Ig responses in which T cells provide help for the B cells to mature. This maturation includes both induction of isotype switching, in which the T cell cytokines control the isotype of Ig produced, and activation of somatic mutation. The cellular interactions underlying T-cell help are driven by the specific antigen and take advantage of the ability of B cells to serve as APCs. Membrane IgM and membrane IgD are capable of capturing antigen and mediating presentation. A special advantage of B-cell antigen presentation is that very low concentrations of antigen can be captured by membrane immunoglobulins bearing the appropriate specificity and targeted within the cell for presentation to T cells.[143] B cells that capture their cognate antigen through their membrane Ig can internalize the antigen, proteolytically degrade it, and associate it with class II MHC molecules. The antigen is then presented on the cell surface in the B cell's class II HLA proteins. Uptake of antigen induces increased class II expression and expression of CD80 and CD86. T cells activated by this combination of costimulator and antigen-class II complex on the B cell then signal reciprocally to the B cell through the interaction of the T cell CD40 ligand (CD40L) with B cell CD40. Signaling through CD40 is essential for induction of isotype switching. An additional interaction between B and T cells also occurs, namely the cross-linking of CD28, a costimulatory molecule on the T-helper cell surface, to its counter receptor on the B cell, B7/BB1 (CD80). This interaction results in enhanced T-cell proliferation and lymphokine production.[154]

Multiple lymphokines are produced by TH cells and encounter B cells that have been rendered responsive to the growth and differentiating effects of these lymphokines via the actions of CD40. Among these cytokines, IL-4 and IL-10 are important growth factors, especially for CD40-triggered B cells. IL-4 also mediates the production of IgE and IgG4 from CD40-activated B cells[125]; and IL-10 is an important factor regulating the production of IgG and IgA.[64] TGF-β induces the switching of B cells to IgA production, and multiple other cytokines (IL-1, IL-2, IL-3, IL-6, IFN-γ, TNF-α) have modulating roles in the magnitude of B-cell responses.[63] Isotype switching and somatic mutations are strongly associated with the development of B-cell memory. Memory responses, defined as the rapid induction of high levels of high affinity antibody after secondary antigen challenge, are characterized by the production of IgG, IgA, and IgE antibodies, and by somatic mutations in the antigen-binding domains of the heavy and light chains of these antibodies. The development of B cell memory is critical to the success of vaccination against pathogens and perpetuates the pathology of many autoimmune and allergic syndromes.

Antibody-Dependent Cellular Cytotoxicity

Antibody-dependent cellular cytotoxicity (ADCC) can lead to the destruction of invading foreign organisms (bacteria and helminths), virus-infected cells, or tumor cells. In the process of destruction of invading organisms, ADCC involves the targeting of effector cells to these organisms by antibodies. The antibody's variable regions provide specificity for the organism,

whereas the antibody's constant region focuses effector cells to the site via various Fc receptors. In ADCC directed against altered self cells, the process involves the reaction of antibodies with cell-surface receptors producing antibody-coated target cells for reaction with NK cells that secondarily destroy these altered self cells. The process occurs via binding of the antibody to FcγRIII receptor (CD16) on NK cells.

Immunoglobulins

The antibodies (immunoglobulins) secreted by activated B cells are glycoproteins composed of polypeptide (82%–96%) and carbohydrate (4%–18%). They account for approximately 20% of the total plasma proteins and, on serum electrophoresis, migrate to the γ-globulin and β-globulin zones. Ig molecules are composed of two identical 50 kDa heavy chains and two identical 25 kDa κ or λ light chains (Figure 9-4). The amino terminal portions of the heavy and light chains vary in amino acid sequence from one antibody molecule to another. These variable portions are designated V_H and V_κ or V_λ, respectively. The juxtaposition of one V_H segment and one V_κ or V_λ segment creates the antigen-binding portion of the Ig molecule. The variable regions of both the heavy and light chains contain three subregions that are highly variable between different antibody molecules. These hypervariable sequences are brought together in the Ig protein to form the antigen-binding domain of the molecule. Thus, each Ig molecule has two identical antigen-binding sites. The carboxyl terminal portions of the heavy and light chains are constant in each subclass of antibody. The heavy-chain constant regions pair to form the Fc domain of the molecule that is

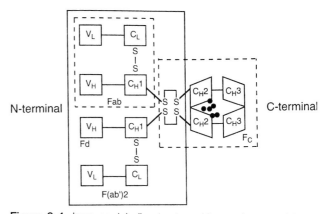

Figure 9-4. Immunoglobulin structure. Human immunoglobulin G1 is a representative example of immunoglobulin structure. H=heavy chains, L=light chains, V=variable regions, C=constant regions. *Dark circles* represent carbohydrate residues between the C_H2 domains. (From Wright A, Shin SU, Morrison SL: Genetically engineered antibodies: progress and prospects, *Crit Rev Immunol* 12:125, 1992, Copyright CRC Press.)

responsible for most of the effector functions of the Ig molecule, including binding to Fc receptors and activating complement. The genes encoding the κ and λ light chains are encoded on chromosomes 2 and 22, respectively. The complex heavy-chain locus is encoded on chromosome 14. The light-chain and heavy-chain loci are each composed of a series of V (variable) gene elements, followed by several D (diversity) segments (for the heavy chain gene only), some J (joining) segments, and C (constant region) exons. The constant regions of both the κ and λ light-chain genes are encoded as single exons. In contrast, the heavy-chain gene contains exons that encode nine different constant regions that are used to produce the different classes and subclasses of Ig.

The isotype of a heavy or light chain is defined by the constant region antigenic determinants that are defined by the particular constant region gene of that isotype. All isotypes are present in a healthy person. Because there are nine known separate heavy-chain, constant region genes, there are nine heavy-chain isotypes that define the class and subclass of the antibody molecule. These are designated $\gamma 1$, $\gamma 2$, $\gamma 3$, $\gamma 4$, μ, $\alpha 1$, $\alpha 2$, δ, and ε, and the corresponding immunoglobulin isotypes (class or subclass) are IgG1, IgG2, IgG3, IgG4, IgM, IgA1, IgA2, IgD, and IgE. Monomers consist of a single immunoglobulin molecule (e.g., IgG), whereas polymers have multiple basic units (e.g., IgM has five basic units and dimeric IgA has two units). The polymerization of these immunoglobulins is facilitated by the presence of a small glycopeptide with an unusually high content of aspartic acid, known as the J chain.

Immunoglobulin G

IgG constitutes approximately 75% of the total serum immunoglobulins and consists of four subclasses (IgG1, IgG2, IgG3, IgG4). It is a monomer with a molecular weight of 150,000 D. IgG1, IgG3, and, to a lesser extent, IgG2 can bind and fix complement. Specific Fc receptors for IgG are present on monocytes, macrophages, and neutrophils. IgG is usually bound to the Fc receptor before binding with antigen. Because of these interactions with antigen and phagocytic cells, IgG functions as an opsonin that facilitates phagocytosis. The Fc receptors for IgG include FcγRI on monocytes and macrophages, FcγRII on most hematopoietic cells except erythrocytes, and FcγRIII on NK cells, eosinophils, neutrophils, and macrophages. Interaction of IgG with NK cells can generate ADCC, which is one mechanism of lymphocyte-mediated killing of bacteria, virus-infected cells, and tumor cells. In general, the IgG antibody response to soluble protein antigens involves the IgG1 and IgG3 subclasses, whereas polysaccharide antigens elicit primarily IgG2 antibodies. IgG is the immunoglobulin

primarily involved in secondary or recall immune responses, and is the only immunoglobulin that can cross the placenta and protect the neonate. IgG can fix complement, leading to neutralization, opsonization, bacteriolysis, agglutination, and hemolysis.

Immunoglobulin M

IgM constitutes approximately 10% of serum immunoglobulins. IgM normally exists as a pentamer of five IgM subunits linked by disulfide bonds and J chains with a molecular weight of 900,000 D. It is the major immunoglobulin (along with IgD) expressed on the surface of B cells. Membrane IgM functions as the earliest antigen receptor on B cells. Antigen binding results in B-cell activation and differentiation, leading to pentameric IgM secretion. Because pentameric IgM contains 10 antibody-binding sites, binding avidity is greatly enhanced. IgM predominates in the early humoral response, and levels then decline rapidly and are replaced by IgG of the same specificity. IgM is the most efficient complement fixing antibody, which, similar to IgG, increases its array of biologic activities.

Immunoglobulin A

IgA constitutes 15% of the total serum immunoglobulins and exists in both monomeric and polymeric forms (the IgA dimer is a single J chain joined to two IgA monomeric subunits). Each immunoglobulin molecule has a molecular weight of 160,000 D. Humans produce more IgA than any other immunoglobulin class, and the major role of this immunoglobulin is mucosal immunity. Monomeric IgA is synthesized by plasma cells located in the interstitial space of exocrine glands. These monomers combine with the J chain, which is also synthesized by IgA plasma cells, to form IgA2-J dimers. These dimers are too large to cross the tight junctions of the exocrine gland epithelium. They are transported across the epithelium by an active secretory component-dependent mechanism.[138] The secretory component is synthesized by epithelial cells and is located at the basolateral surface of epithelial cells, which are exposed to locally produced IgA dimers. The secretory component specifically binds to the J chain of IgA dimers, and the resultant, noncovalently associated secretory component-IgA dimer complex is endocytosed into intracellular vesicles and transported across epithelial cells to the apical plasma membrane. During transport, IgA dimer covalently links to the secretory component by a disulfide bond, and the newly formed complex of IgA dimer and secretory component is referred to as *secretory IgA*. Finally, secretory IgA cleaves from the membrane-anchoring domain of the membrane secretory component and is subsequently released into exocrine secretions by exocytosis. Secretory IgA appears to be derived from locally produced IgA, not intravascular IgA.[65]

IgA is the predominant immunoglobulin in external secretions and provides the primary defense mechanism against local mucosal infections. The main function of IgA is to neutralize foreign substances and prevent their systemic access.

Immunoglobulin E

IgE comprises only 0.004% of the total serum immunoglobulins and normally exists as a monomer with a molecular weight of 200,000 D. IgE-specific Fc receptors exist on mast cells and basophils, neutrophils, eosinophils, macrophages, and platelets. Cross-bridging of IgE molecules on the surface of mast cells and basophils by antigen triggers mediator release from mast cells and basophils. These mediators—the most notable being histamine—are responsible for allergic reactions. In addition to mediating immediate hypersensitivity reactions, IgE can mediate antibody-mediated cellular cytotoxicity.

Immunoglobulin D

IgD constitutes 0.2% of the total serum immunoglobulins and exists as a monomer with a molecular weight of 180,000 D. The primary function of IgD appears to be that of a membrane-bound antigen receptor on the B-cell surface.

INNATE IMMUNE SYSTEM

The adaptive T- and B-cell immune responses detailed earlier in this chapter provide important protection for the host and permit the development of immune memory. Mutations in elements of the innate immune response, however, demonstrate that innate immune effectors are critical for effective host defense. In addition to local defenses at mucosal surfaces, such as mucus and mucociliary transport, the effectors of innate immunity include toll-like receptors (TLRs), antimicrobial peptides, phagocytic cells, natural killer cells, and complement.

Toll-Like Receptors

Toll was first identified in *Drosophila*. Host defense in *Drosophila* is mediated in part by the Toll family of receptors that lead to induction of antimicrobial peptides on activation and the elimination of the foreign invader. An important advance in our understanding of innate immunity to microbial pathogens was the identification of a human homolog of *Drosophila* Toll.

Mammalian TLR family members are transmembrane proteins containing repeated leucine-rich motifs in their extracellular portions. Mammalian TLR proteins contain a cytoplasmic portion that is homologous to the IL-1 receptor, and can therefore trigger intracellular signaling pathways. Substantial evidence now supports a role for mammalian TLRs in innate immunity. TLRs are pattern recognition receptors that recognize pathogen-associated molecular patterns present on a variety of bacteria and fungi. TLRs are also expressed at the interface with the environment where the host must defend against microbes. The activation of TLRs induces expression of costimulatory molecules and the release of cytokines that instruct the adaptive immune response. Finally, TLRs directly activate host defense mechanisms that directly combat the foreign invader or contribute to tissue injury.[170]

TLR Expression and Distribution

TLRs were initially found to be expressed in all lymphoid tissue but are most highly expressed in peripheral blood leukocytes. Expression of TLR mRNA has been found in monocytes, B cells, T cells, and dendritic cells.[5,180] The expression of TLRs on cells of the monocyte-macrophage lineage is consistent with the role of TLRs in modulating inflammatory responses via cytokine release. Because these cells migrate into sites that interface with the environment, the location of TLR-expressing cells would be situated to defend against invading microbes. The regulation of TLR expression is critical to their role in host defense, yet few factors have been identified that modulate their expression. IL-4 acts to down-regulate TLR expression, suggesting that TH2 adaptive responses might inhibit TLR activation.[242]

Activators of the Different TLRs

Lipopolysaccharides (LPS) of gram-negative bacteria seem to generate responses mediated via the TLR4 receptor. Mice with naturally occurring mutations in the TLR4 gene are hyporesponsive to LPS[208] and studies in knockout mice demonstrate that TLR4 mediates the response to LPS.[250] Microbial lipoproteins and lipopeptides have been shown to activate cells in a TLR2-dependent manner[52] and the ability of lipoproteins to activate TLRs was further corroborated using the TLR2 gene knockout mouse, which does not respond to lipoproteins. Lipoproteins have been found extensively in both gram-positive and gram-negative bacteria, as well as spirochetes. Mammalian TLR9 mediates the immune response to a specific pattern in bacterial DNA, an unmethylated cytidine-phosphate-guanosine (CpG) dinucleotide with appropriate flanking regions. These CpG-DNA sequences are 20-fold more common in microbial than mammalian DNA; thus, mammalian TLR9 is more likely to be activated by bacterial than mammalian DNA. Hemmi and others showed that immune cells from mice in which the TLR9 gene had been selectively inactivated did not proliferate or release cytokines in response to CpG DNA.[113] Human TLR9 confers responsiveness to bacterial DNA via species-specific CpG motif recognition.[30] Mammalian TLR5 has been shown to mediate the response to flagellin, a component of bacterial flagella.[111] Mammalian TLR3 mediates the response to double-stranded RNA, a molecular pattern expressed by many viruses during infection.[9] Activation of TLR3 induced IFN-α and IFN-β, cytokines important for antiviral responses.

TLRs and the Adaptive Immune Response

Critical proinflammatory and immunomodulatory cytokines such as IL-1, IL-6, IL-8, IL-10, IL-12, and TNF-α have been shown to be induced after activation of TLRs by microbial ligands.[170] Activation of TLRs on dendritic cells triggers their maturation, leading to cell surface changes that enhance antigen presentation, thus promoting the ability of these cells to present antigen to T cells and generate TH1 responses critical for cell-mediated immunity. Therefore, activation of TLRs as part of the innate response can influence and modulate the adaptive T-cell response.

TLR and the Host

Similar to the *Drosophila*, mammalian TLRs have been shown to play a prominent role in directly activating host defense mechanisms. For example, activation of TLR2 by microbial lipoproteins induces activation of the inducible nitric oxide synthase promoter that leads to the production of nitric oxide, a known antimicrobial agent.[52] In *Drosophila*, activation of Toll leads to the NF-κB–dependent induction of a variety of antimicrobial peptides.[116] In a similar fashion, it has been shown that LPS induces β-defensin-2 in tracheobronchial epithelium, suggesting similar pathways in humans.[32] The activation of TLRs can also be detrimental, causing tissue injury. The administration of LPS to mice can result in septic shock, a feature that is dependent on TLR4,[208] and microbial lipoproteins induce features of apoptosis via TLR2.[10] Thus, microbial lipoproteins have the ability to induce both TLR-dependent activation of host defense and tissue pathology. This might be one way for the immune system to activate host defenses and then down-regulate the response from causing tissue injury by apoptosis.

Antimicrobial Peptides

The existence of antimicrobial peptides (AMPs) has been known for several decades, but only recently has it been recognized that their function is essential to the mammalian immune response. They participate primarily in the innate immune system and are used as a first-line immune defense by many organisms including plants, bacteria, insects, and vertebrates. AMPs directly kill a broad spectrum of microbes, including gram-positive and gram-negative bacteria, fungi, and certain viruses. In addition, these peptides interact with the host itself, triggering events that complement their role as antibiotics. AMPs can be divided into several categories on the basis of their structures, but most of them maintain certain common structural features, including a cationic charge and the ability to interact with bacterial membranes through hydrophobic amino acids. Two major families of AMPs have been characterized in mammals: defensins and cathelicidins.

Cathelicidins

These peptides are related by a similar "Cathelin precursor" domain. They are characterized by an N-terminal signal peptide, a highly conserved pro sequence, and a structurally variable cationic peptide at the C-terminus. The pro sequence is very similar to that of Cathelin, a protein originally isolated from porcine neutrophils as an inhibitor of cathepsin L (hence the term: cathe-L-in).[217] To date, cathelicidins have been found only in mammals; the only human cathelicidin, LL-37 or hCAP-18, was isolated from human bone marrow.[4] LL-37 has a broad spectrum of antimicrobial activity and acts as a chemoattractant for mast cells.[188] Thus, this AMP has the potential to participate in the innate immune response both by killing bacteria and by recruiting a cellular immune response.

Defensins

Defensins are a broadly dispersed family of gene-encoded antibiotics that typically are 28 to 44 amino acids long and contain 6 to 8 cysteine residues that form characteristic intramolecular disulfide bridges. They exhibit antimicrobial activity against bacteria, fungi, and enveloped viruses.[92,148] Defensins are classified into three distinct families: the α-defensins, the β-defensins, and the θ-defensins.

α-defensins. These are 29 to 35 amino acids in length. Human neutrophils express a number of distinct defensins.[110] To date, six α-defensins have been identified. Of these six, four are known as α-defensins 1, 2, 3, and 4 (also referred to as *human neutrophil peptides* HNP 1 through 4). The other two α-defensins, known as human defensins 5 and 6 (HD-5, HD-6), are abundantly expressed in Paneth's cells of the small intestinal crypts[126,230] and in epithelial cells of the female urogenital tract.[211] HNPs 1 through 4 are localized in azurophilic granules of neutrophils and contribute to the oxygen-independent killing of phagocytosed microorganisms. Furthermore, HNPs 1 through 3 can increase the expression of TNF-α and IL-1 in human monocytes that have been activated by *Staphylococcus aureus,* or reduce expression of VCAM-1 in human umbilical vein endothelial cells activated by TNF-α.[57]

β-defensins. In human beings, four types of β-defensins have been identified thus far; they are referred to as human β-defensins (HBDs) 1 through 4. They have a broad spectrum of antimicrobial activity, bind to CCR6, and are chemotactic for immature dendritic cells and memory T cells.[279] HBD-2 can also promote histamine release and prostaglandin D_2 production in mast cells, suggesting a role in allergic reactions.[189,33] Thus, the defensins, like the cathelicidins can contribute to the immune response by both killing bacteria and influencing the cellular innate and adaptive immune response.

θ-defensins. θ-defensins have been isolated from rhesus monkey neutrophils but no data about the presence of these molecules in different tissues are currently available.

Tissue Distribution of AMPs

Human cathelicidin LL-37 expression has been observed in epidermal keratinocytes under inflammatory conditions such as psoriasis and contact dermatitis[85] and it is increased in the epidermis after injury.[69] HBD-2 and 3 have also been demonstrated in lesional keratinocytes of psoriatic patients.[108] HBD-1 and 2 have been seen in ductal epithelia of sweat glands and in hair follicles under normal conditions.[86]

A likely scenario for the role in AMPs in skin defense is as follows: under resting conditions, sites of potential entry of bacteria, such as follicular structures, produce small amounts of AMPs that likely provide a chemical barrier to infection where a physical one is absent. After injury, the skin reacts rapidly by increased production of AMPs from the epithelium and deposition of AMPs from degranulation of recruited neutrophils. The chemotactic activity of both LL-37 and HBD-2 might further amplify the process by stimulating additional leukocyte recruitment. All of the β-defensins are present in the respiratory system. These are expressed at various levels in the epithelia of the trachea and lung, as well as in the serous cells of the submucosal glands.[109,93,283] Cathelicidins are also present in the conducting airway epithelium, pulmonary epithelium, and submucosal glands.[16] Recent investigations have also documented these peptides in the nose and paranasal sinuses in health and disease. Human β-defensin-1 mRNA has been detected by RT-PCR in

inferior turbinate tissues from normal individuals and was localized to epithelial cells and glandular epithelium by in-situ hybridization.[145] This antimicrobial peptide is found in inferior turbinate and polyp tissue of patients with chronic sinusitis and is not up-regulated in these disease conditions compared to turbinate tissues obtained from normal individuals.[146] mRNA for HBD-2, however, is found only in tissues obtained from chronic sinusitis patients but not normal controls, as is expression of α-defensins 1, 2 and 3.[146] Thus, some of these peptides are constitutively expressed in the nasal mucosa and some are up-regulated in chronic sinusitis, which is probably a reflection of activation of the innate immune system in the disease process.

The importance of these peptides has also been demonstrated in animal studies, such as those showing that mice deficient in β-defensins 1 demonstrate decreased ability to clear *Haemophilus influenzae* instilled into their lungs,[173] and the ones showing that increased delivery of LL-37 to the mouse airway resulted in decreased bacterial load and mortality after challenge with *Pseudomonas aeruginosa* or *Escherichia coli.*[17]

Complement System

The complement system is an important effector of both the innate and adaptive immune responses. It consists of more than 25 plasma and cell surface proteins that are sequentially activated and can interact with each other, with antibodies, and with cell membranes. These interactions mediate functions such as immune adherence, phagocytosis, chemotaxis, and cytolysis. Complement system proteins comprise about 15% of the globulin fraction of plasma and circulate as inactive molecules. Complement activation centers around cleavage of C3, which can be achieved by classic, alternative, or lectin pathways (Figure 9-5).

The classic pathway comprises C1, C4, and C2. C1, in turn, consists of C1q, C1r, and C1s. Antigen-antibody complexes (containing IgG1, IgG2, IgG3, or IgM) provide the activating signal for the classic pathway of complement activation. Sequential activation of complement components C1, C4, and C2 produces the C3 convertase enzyme that then cleaves C3 into C3a and C3b. At this point, the classic and alternative pathways merge. The alternative pathway is activated in the absence of specific antigen-antibody complexes by microbial structures that neutralize inhibitors of spontaneous complement activation. In this pathway, C3 interacts with factors B and D to generate the alternative pathway C3 convertase, which also cleaves C3 to C3a and C3b. The third pathway of complement activation, the lectin pathway, is triggered by microbial cell wall components containing mannans.[91] The interaction of mannan-containing

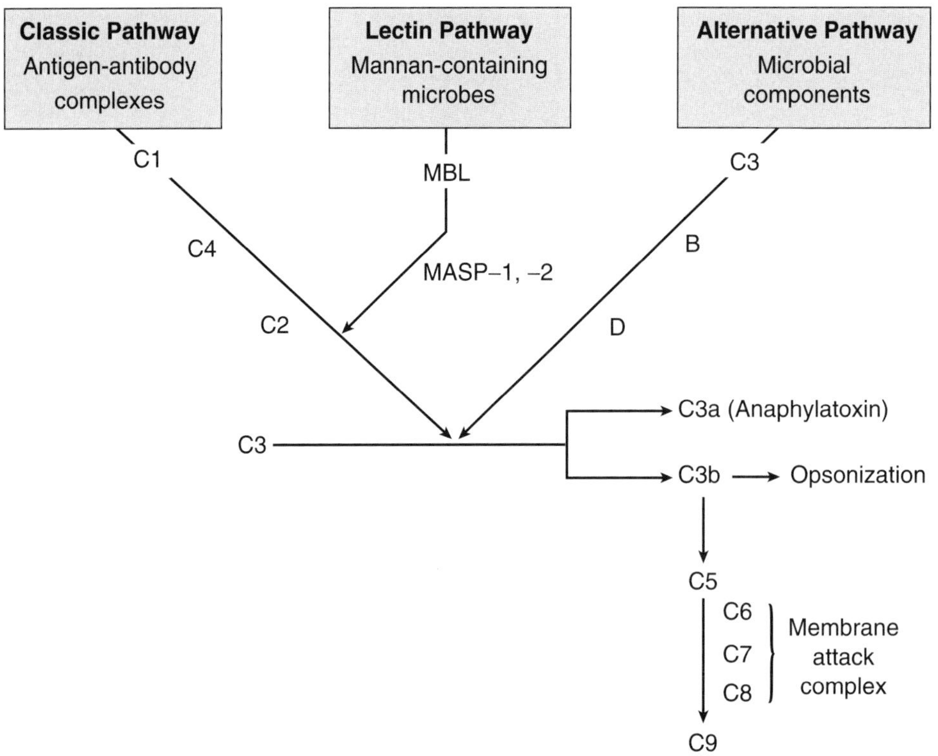

Figure 9-5. Complement system. The three pathways of the complement system are illustrated. Please refer to the text for a description of the functions of the complement system.

microbes with plasma mannan-binding lectin (MBL) activates the zymogenic plasma proteases MBL-associated serine proteases 1 and 2 (MASP-1, MASP-2). These form a protease analogous to the activated C1 of the classical pathway that then goes on to activate C4, C2, and the remainder of the pathway leading to C3 convertase.

Cleavage of C3 results in the release of the small C3a fragment—a potent anaphylatoxin that induces mast cell degranulation, creates edema, and recruits phagocytic cells—and the larger C3b fragment, which covalently attaches to the activating antigen, marking it for destruction. C3b serves both as a site for attack of the complement membrane attack complex (MAC), a self-assembling pore-forming complex of the plasma uproteins C5, C6, C7, C8, and C9 that kills targets by osmotic lysis, and as an opsonin, enhancing phagocytosis by its binding to complement receptors on the surfaces of neutrophils and macrophages.[155] The effector mechanism of complement is potent and recruits intense local inflammation; its importance is underscored by the phenotypes of inherited deficiencies of individual components. For example, deficiencies of components of the MAC lead to increased susceptibility to *Neisseria* infections, deficiency of C3 results in life-threatening susceptibility to pyogenic infections,

often fatal during childhood, deficiency of C4 or C2 causes a lupus-like immune complex disease, and deficiency of the serum inhibitor of C1 leads to episodic mast cell-independent episodes of angioedema.

Natural Killer Cell Cytotoxicity

The ability of CD4+ and CD8+ T cells to recognize only peptides presented by self MHC molecules is termed *MHC restriction*, and cytolytic activity mediated by these cells is known as *MHC-restricted cytotoxicity*. In contrast to these two cell types, NK cells (large granular lymphocytes) are capable of cytotoxic activity that is not restricted to recognition of target cells that display MHC molecules. This process is termed *unrestricted toxicity*.

NK cells are distinct from T cells or B cells and can manufacture and release various cytokines, including IFN-γ, TNF-α, and GM-CSF. These cells express a unique pattern of surface molecules not usually expressed on other lymphocytes, including CD16 (FcγRIII), a receptor for the Fc portion of immunoglobulin, and CD56, an adhesion molecule that is also expressed on neural cells.[142,184,202,256] In addition, they express CD2, which is also expressed on T cells.[184] NK cells are present in the peripheral circulation and in the spleen, lungs, and liver.[43,270] They are not found in lymph nodes and do not recirculate through the thoracic duct lymph. The cytotoxic mechanisms of NK cells appear to be similar to those of CTL, including perforin-mediated destruction of cells, receptor-induced apoptosis, and release of cytokines such as TNF-β. NK cells have no antigen-specific receptors. Their cytotoxic activity is inhibited by encounter with self-MHC molecules through inhibitory receptors on their surface that recognize class I. They thus kill self cells that have down-regulated class I molecules expression. This is important in host defense, as several viruses have developed mechanisms to down-regulate class I expression in infected cells as a strategy to avoid CD8+ cell killing. NK cells can destroy target cells by antibody-dependent cell-mediated cytotoxicity. They have prominent antitumor effects and are potent killers of virally infected cells.[53]

Cytokines

Cytokines are a diverse group of small, secreted protein mediators that mediate interactions among different effector cells. Each cytokine may have multiple activities on different cell types, and several cytokines often have related functions. They can also have synergistic or antagonistic activities and can inhibit or induce the synthesis of other cytokines. Cytokines can be grouped by structure into three families: the hematopoietins, the interferons, and the TNF family. Others are unassigned a family grouping. These different cytokines, their principal cell sources, and their main effects in humans are summarized in Table 9-1.

Chemokines

The chemokines are a superfamily of low-molecular weight, secreted, heparin-binding molecules that serve as potent chemoattractants for cells of the immune system. More than 50 chemokines are currently recognized and they are characterized by the presence of three or four conserved cysteine residues. They can be divided into four families, based on the positioning of the N-terminal cysteine residues. The CXC family is characterized by the separation of the first two cysteines by a variable amino acid. In the CC family, the cysteine residues are adjacent to each other. The

TABLE 9-1

TYPES OF CYTOKINES

Cytokine	Cell Sources	Predominant Effects
Hematopoietin family		
Epo (erythropoietin)	Kidney cells, hepatocytes	Stimulates erythroid progenitors
IL-2	T cells	T-cell proliferation
IL-3	T cells, thymic epithelial cells	Synergistic action in early hematopoiesis
IL-4	T cells, mast cells	B-cell activation, IgE switch, suppresses TH1 cells
IL-5	T cells, mast cells	Eosinophil growth and differentiation
IL-6	T cells, macrophages, endothelial cells	T- and B-cell growth and differentiation, acute phase protein production, fever
IL-7	Non-T cells	Growth of pre-B cells and pre-T cells
IL-9	T cells	Mast cell–enhancing activity, stimulates TH2
IL-11	Stromal fibroblasts	Synergistic action with IL-3 and IL-4 in hematopoiesis
IL-13	T cells	B-cell growth and differentiation, IgE switch, inhibits macrophage inflammatory cytokine production and TH1 cells
G-CSF	Fibroblasts and monocytes	Stimulates neutrophil development and differentiation
IL-15	Many non-T cells	Stimulates growth of intestinal epithelium, T cells, and NK cells
GM-CSF	Macrophages, T cells	Stimulates growth and differentiation of myelomonocytic lineage cells, particularly dendritic cells
OSM	T cells, macrophages	Stimulates Kaposi's sarcoma cells, inhibits melanoma growth
LIF	Bone marrow stroma, fibroblasts	Maintains embryonic stem cells, like IL-6, IL-11, OSM

Continued

TABLE 9-1

TYPES OF CYTOKINES—cont'd

Cytokine	Cell Sources	Predominant Effects
Interferon Family		
IFN-γ	T cells, NK cells	Macrophage activation, increased expression of MHC molecules and antigen presenting components, Ig class switching, suppresses TH2
IFN-α	Leukocytes	Antiviral, increased MHC class I expression
IFN-β	Fibroblasts	Antiviral, increased MHC class I expression
TNF Family		
TNF-α	Macrophages, NK cells, T cells	Local inflammation, endothelial activation
TNF-β	T cells, B cells	Killing, endothelial activation
LT-β	T cells, B cells	Lymph node development
CD40 ligand	T cells, mast cells	B-cell activation, class switching
Fas ligand	T cells	Apoptosis, Ca-independent cytotoxicity
CD27 ligand	T cells	Stimulates T cell proliferation
CD30 ligand	T cells	Stimulates T and B cell proliferation
4-1BBL	T cells	Co-stimulates T and B cells
Trail	T cells, monocytes	Apoptosis of activated T cells and tumor cells
OPG-L	Osteoblasts, T cells	Stimulates osteoclasts and bone resorption
Unassigned Cytokines		
TGF-β	Chondrocytes, monocytes, T cells	Inhibits cell growth, anti-inflammatory, induces IgA secretion by B cells
IL-1α	Macrophages, epithelial cells	Fever, T-cell, and macrophage activation
IL-1β	Macrophages, epithelial cells	Fever, T-cell and macrophage activation
IL-1 RA	Monocytes, macrophages, neutrophils, hepatocytes	Natural IL-1 function antagonist
IL-10	T cells, macrophages, EBV-transformed B cells	Potent suppressant of macrophage functions
IL-12	B cells, macrophages	Activates NK cells, induces CD4 T-cell differentiation to TH1-like cells
MIF	T cells, pituitary cells	Inhibits macrophage migration, stimulates macrophage activation, induces steroid resistance
IL-16	T cells, mast cells, eosinophils	Chemoattractant for CD4 T cells, monocytes, and eosinophils, antiapoptotic for IL-2-stimulated T cells
IL-17	CD4 memory cells	Induces cytokine production by epithelial and endothelial cells, and fibroblasts
IL-18	Activated macrophages and Kupffer cells	Induces IFN-γ production by T cells and NK cells, favors TH1 induction and later TH2 responses

majority of these chemokines are contained in these two families. Chemokines of the C family lack the first and third cysteine, containing a single cysteine residue in the conserved position. Members of the CX3C have the two N-terminal cysteine residues separated by three variable amino acids. The C and CX3C families are small, with one or fewer members per family. Table 9-2 lists the new systematic name of these chemokines, as well as their common names and their target cells.

Phagocytes

The phagocytic system consists of circulating and fixed cells. Monocytes and granulocytes circulate, whereas Kupffer's cells, macrophages, and brain microglial cells remain fixed. Migration of phagocytic cells can occur

TABLE 9-2

Types of Chemokines

Systematic Name	Common Name-Ligand	Target Cell(s)
CXC Family		
CXCL1	GROα/MGSAα	Neutrophil
CXCL2	GROβ/MGSAβ	Neutrophil
CXCL3	GROǵ/MGSAǵ	Neutrophil
CXCL4	PF4	Fibroblast
CXCL5	ENA-78	Neutrophil
CXCL6	GCP-2	Neutrophil
CXCL7	NAP-2	Neutrophil
CXCL8	IL-8	Neutrophil, basophil, T cell
CXCL9	Mig	Activated T cell
CXCL10	IP-10	Activated T cell
CXCL11	I-TAC	Activated T cell
CXCL12	SDF-1a/b	CD34+ bone marrow cell, T cell, dendritic cell, B cell, activated CD4 cell
CXCL13	BCA-1	Naïve B cell, activated CD4 cell
CXCL14	BRAK-boekine	
CXCL15	Unknown	
CXCL16	Unknown	T cell, NK T cell
CC Family		
CCL1	I-309	Neutrophil, T cell
CCL2	MCP-1/MCAF/TDCF	T cell, monocyte, basophil
CCL3	MIP-1α/LD78α	Monocyte, macrophage, T cell, NK cell, basophil
CCL3L1	LD78β	
CCL4	MIP-1β	Monocyte, macrophage, T cell, NK cell, basophil
CCL5	RANTES	Monocyte, macrophage, T cell, NK cell, basophil, eosinophil, dendritic cell
CCL6	Unknown	
CCL7	MCP-3	T cell, Monocyte, eosinophil, basophil, dendritic cell
CCL8	MCP-2	T cell, monocyte, eosinophil, basophil
CCL9/10	Unknown	
CCL11	Eotaxin	Eosinophil
CCL12	Unknown	
CCL13	MCP-4	T cell, monocyte, eosinophil, basophil, dendritic cell
CCL14	HCC-1	Monocyte
CCL15	HCC-2/Lkn-1/MIP-1δ	T cell, monocyte, dendritic cell
CCL16	HCC-4/LEC/LCC-1	Monocyte
CCL17	TARC	T cell, immature dendritic cell, T cell, thymocyte
CCL18	DC-CK1/PARC/AMAC-1	Naïve T cell, T cell
CCL19	MIP-3b/ELC/exodus-3	Naïve T cell, mature dendritic cell, B cell
CCL20	MIP-3a/LARC/exodus-1	T cell, bone marrow dendritic cell
CCL21	6Ckine/SLC/exodus-2	Naïve T cell, B cell
CCL22	MDC/STCP-1	Immature dendritic cell, T cell
CCL23	MPIF-1/CKβ8/CKβ8-1	Monocyte, T cell
CCL24	Eotaxin-2/MPIF-2	Eosinophil, basophil
CCL25	TECK	Macrophage, thymocyte, dendritic cell
CCL26	Eotaxin-3	
CCL27	CTACK/ILC	T cell
CCL28	MEC	T cell, eosinophil

Continued

TABLE 9-2

TYPES OF CHEMOKINES—cont'd

Systematic Name	Common Name-Ligand	Target Cell(s)
C and CXC3C Families		
XCL1	Lymphotactin/SCM1α/ATAC	T cell, NK cell
XCL2	SCM-1β	
CXC3C Family		
CXC3CL1	Fracktalkine	T cell, monocyte

GRO, growth related oncogene; MGSA, melanoma growth stimulatory activity; PF, platelet factor; ENA, epithelial neutrophil activating; GCP, granulocyte chemotactic protein; NAP, neutrophil-activating peptide; Mig, monokine-induced by IFN-γ; IP, IFN-γ inducible protein; I-TAC, IFN-inducible T-cell α chemoattractant; SDF-1, stromal cell-derived factor 1; BCA, B-cell attracting chemokine; BRAK, breast and kidney-expressed chemokine; SCM, single C motif; ATAC, activation-induced; chemokine-related molecule; I-309, a nameless human chemokine; MCP, monocyte chemoattractant protein; MCAF, monocyte chemotactic and activating factor; TDCF, tumor-derived chemotactic factor; MIP, macrophage inflammatory protein; LD78, macrophage inflammatory protein −1; RANTES, regulated upon activation; normal T cell expressed and secreted; HCC, human CC chemokine; Lkn, leukotactin; LEC, liver-expressed chemokine; TARC, thymus- and activation-regulated chemokine; DC-CK1, dendritic cell-derived CC chemokine; PARC, pulmonary and activation-regulated chemokine; AMAC, alternative macrophage activation-associated CC chemokine; ELC, EBL-1 ligand chemokine; LARC, liver- and activation-regulated chemokine; SLC, secondary lymphoid tissue chemokine; MDC, macrophage-derived chemokine; STCP, stimulated T-cell chemoattractant protein; MPIF, myeloid progenitor inhibitory factor; CK, chemokine; TECK, thymus-expressed chemokine; CTACK, cutaneous T cell-activating chemokine; ILC, IL-11 receptor alpha-locus chemokine; MEC, mucosae-associated epithelial chemokine.

randomly or in response to a directed signal, a process known as *chemotaxis*. Substances with chemotactic properties include complement and bacterial products. Once attracted to a particular site, phagocytes engulf foreign material. Phagocytic cells use a variety of Fc receptors and complement receptors to enhance uptake of particles that have been marked by the adaptive and innate immune systems for destruction. Phagocytosis is facilitated by opsonization, which coats foreign material with antibodies. After phagocytosis, an intracellular vacuole forms around the foreign material and lysosomal enzymes released into the vacuole destroy the foreign invader.

IMMUNOPATHOLOGY

The two major effector arms of the adaptive immune response are humoral and cellular. In the defense against infections, antibodies are operative against bacteria or bacterial products; cell-mediated immunity operates primarily against viral, fungal, and mycotic infections. With few exceptions, antibody-mediated immune mechanisms work best when directed to extracellular infections, whereas cell-mediated immunity is effective against intracellular infections. The killing effects of immune reactions are extremely efficient, and when specifically directed, can eliminate many organisms quickly. However, these same immune mechanisms may cause host-tissue destruction and therefore lead to disease states.

This destructive effect of immune reactions is termed *allergy* or *hypersensitivity* and is considered an immunopathologic reaction.

For several years, these reactions were divided into four types according to the Gell and Coombs classification proposed in 1963[96]: type I, immediate hypersensitivity (IgE mediated); type II, cytotoxic reactions (IgG, IgM mediated); type III, immune complex reactions (IgG, IgM complex mediated); and type IV, delayed hypersensitivity reactions (T-cell mediated). The division of these immune reactions into neat categories, although easy to comprehend, is oversimplified. For example, allergic reactions are classified as IgE-mediated, type I immunopathologic responses but involve all components of the immune system.

Type I Mast Cell–Mediated Reactions

Possibly as a remnant of host defense mechanisms to parasites,[234,273] the immediate hypersensitivity reaction uses the release of mast cell or basophil mediators to create immediate and delayed (4–8 hours) responses to sensitizing allergens. These reactions can be IgE-dependent (anaphylactic) or IgE-independent (anaphylactoid). In anaphylaxis, allergen-specific IgE antibody attaches to IgE receptors on mast cells. On reexposure to allergen, a clinical reaction is initiated, such as anaphylaxis to penicillins. An example of an IgE-independent reaction is sensitivity to iodide contrast media.

Type II Antibody–Mediated Reactions

Type II antibody (non-IgE)–mediated immune reactions involve IgG and IgM antibodies binding to antigens on the surface of target cells (e.g., erythrocytes, neutrophils, platelets, and epithelial cells of glandular or mucosal surfaces) or to antigens on tissues such as basement membranes. The sensitizing antigens in these cases can be natural cell-surface antigens, modified cell-surface antigens, or haptens attached to cell surfaces. This interaction between IgG and IgM antibodies and cell-surface antigens leads to destruction of these cells by one of three mechanisms: opsonization, complement activation, and cell lysis and ADCC. These mechanisms afford protection against infections and eradication of malignant cells, but can also damage self antigens in various tissues.

One example occurs when penicillin binds to the surfaces of erythrocytes, creating a nonself antigen composed of penicillin-modified erythrocyte cell surfaces.[205] Antipenicilloyl antibodies, initially IgM and later IgG, fix to these surfaces and concomitantly activate complement, leading to the lysis of the cell by penetration of the terminal hydrophobic complement components, C7 to C9. Clinically, this condition is known as penicillin-induced autoimmune hemolytic anemia.

Type III Immune Complex–Mediated Reactions

Type III reactions are similar to type II reactions in that they involve antibody-mediated inflammation. However, in type III reactions, the antibody and its antigen form low-solubility immune complexes, which are deposited in normal tissues and precipitate an immune response. These immune complexes are usually deposited around the basement membranes of vessels with a high plasma outflow. They activate complement and set off an inflammatory response characterized primarily by neutrophil influx, which inflicts tissue injury. Knowledge of this immunologic disease became widespread in the early 1900s, when physicians began using immune animal sera, usually equine sera, to treat bacterial infections, which led to serious illness and even death of the treated subjects.[135] Immune complexes of antibody (IgM or IgG) and antigen, activated complement components, and neutrophil chemotaxis are important participants in this hypersensitivity reaction, which is better known as *serum sickness*. Immune complex vasculitis in the skin can also occur in a series of clinical conditions, such as systemic lupus erythematosus, rheumatoid arthritis, drug reactions, and infections.

Type IV Cell–Mediated Reactions

This category of the classic hypersensitivity reactions is caused by antibody-independent mechanisms involving T cells or NK cells. These reactions are the pathologic variants of a normal T-cell–mediated immune response in which the T-cell response to an environmental antigen becomes exaggerated. The typical type IV immune response is the delayed hypersensitivity reaction caused by sensitized T cells, in particular the CD4+ (helper) cell population. A clinical example of such a reaction is the cutaneous reaction to challenge with the PPD of *M. tuberculosis* in previously infected or vaccinated patients.

Although the focus is on delayed hypersensitivity reactions involving the skin and sensitizing antigens, other reactions involving other organ systems and target antigens are known. Examples of such reactions are the T-cell infiltration of tumor beds and the T-cell infiltration of blood vessels and alveoli in chronic asthma. Some type IV hypersensitivity responses are also mediated by CD8+ T cells and NK cells. In contrast to the neutrophilic infiltration of the tissues in type III reactions, the cell infiltrate in type IV reactions is dominated by lymphocytes, monocytes, and macrophages.

HYGIENE HYPOTHESIS

Epidemiologic data provide strong evidence of a steady rise in the incidence of allergic (asthma,[277] rhinitis,[258] and atopic dermatitis[275]) and autoimmune diseases (multiple sclerosis,[209] insulin-dependent diabetes mellitus,[81] and Crohn's disease[248]) in developed countries since the beginning of the 1970s. Concomitantly, an obvious decrease in the incidence of many infectious diseases in developed countries has occurred as a result of antibiotics, vaccination, or more simply improved hygiene and better socioeconomic conditions. A hypothesis has thus emerged that the decrease in infectious diseases is causally linked to the increase in the incidence of allergic and autoimmune diseases, the "hygiene hypothesis." This is not a new concept as Leibowitz and others, suggested in 1966[149] that the risk of multiple sclerosis is increased among persons who spent their childhood in a home with a high level of sanitation. Almost 20 years later, Strachan observed that the risk of allergic rhinitis was inversely linked to birth order and the size of the family.[246] He proposed that infections within households in early childhood have a role in preventing allergic rhinitis.

The geographical distribution of allergic and autoimmune diseases in the world also shows interesting patterns. The incidence of disease decreases from north to south in the Northern Hemisphere and reciprocally from south to north in the Southern Hemisphere. Under diagnosis of allergic and autoimmune diseases in underdeveloped countries could explain these geographical differences, but this is not likely. Although this explanation might be proposed for allergic rhinitis and atopic dermatitis, relatively benign diseases, it is not likely to apply to type I diabetes and multiple sclerosis, which lead to significant symptoms and are not likely to go undiagnosed. Environment seems to play an important role in this gradient. This is well illustrated by the fact that the rate of development of type I diabetes among the children of Pakistanis who migrated to the United Kingdom is the same as the rate among nonimmigrants in that country and about 10 times as high as the incidence of type I diabetes in Pakistan.[41,244] An obvious factor in the north-south gradient is socioeconomic differences. Several studies have found a lower frequency of immunologic diseases in populations with a low socioeconomic status. Some infections have been found to be distributed according to a south-north gradient in European countries that mirrors the gradient for autoimmune diseases. Low socioeconomic levels and high temperatures, two common features of southern countries, may predispose to infections in a number of ways: less stringent control of microbial contamination of water and food, an increased risk of bacterial proliferation with higher ambient temperatures, and poorer housing conditions may all affect the risk of contamination between persons.

When infections are an incriminating factor, they often occur in childhood. In Yorkshire, a case-control study demonstrated an inverse correlation between the incidence of type I diabetes and the degree of social mixing, including day-care attendance and the number of infections that occur before 1 year of age.[165] Furthermore, young children with older brothers and sisters at home and those who attend a day-care center during the first 6 months of life subsequently have a lower incidence of asthma[15] and type I diabetes[165] than children who do not attend a day-care center and have no older siblings.

The administration of antibiotics to children has been suspected to increase the risk of asthma and allergy. Droste and others observed that the use of antibiotics in the first year of life increased the risk of asthma or other allergic diseases in children with a genetic predisposition to atopy.[71] Antibiotics might act by decreasing the number of infections or by modifying intestinal flora.

Differences in disease incidence between urban and suburban dwellers have been observed, and factors other than air pollution have been implicated. In 1999, Braun-Fahrländer and colleagues found that children whose parents were farmers and who lived on the farm were less likely to become allergic than children from the same rural region who were not raised on a farm.[47] Another study confirmed these findings and showed that allergies were less frequent when the children were exposed early and for a prolonged period to farm animals and cow's milk.[216] An inverse correlation between endotoxin levels in bedding and the incidence of atopic diseases among children living in rural areas was also found, suggesting that a subject's environmental exposure to endotoxin may have a crucial role in the development of tolerance to ubiquitous allergens found in natural environments.[48]

Animal studies support the above epidemiologic observations, because autoimmune diseases in susceptible strains of mice or rats develop earlier and at a higher rate among animals bred in a specific pathogen-free environment than among animals bred in a conventional environment. The same has been observed relating to allergic diseases. Administration of *Mycobacterium bovis* and *M. vaccae* can attenuate the late-phase response, airway hyperresponsiveness, and bronchoalveolar lavage eosinophilia in a mouse model of bronchial asthma.[120]

Several mechanisms might explain these relationships. The development of most autoimmune diseases depends on the TH1 cytokines IL-2 and IFN-γ, whereas the development of allergic diseases requires the TH2 cytokines IL-4 and IL-5. Initial reports that suggested an inverse relationship between the incidence of autoimmune and allergic diseases[253] led to speculation that the reciprocal down-regulation of TH1 cytokines by TH2 cytokines, and the reverse, might account for these observations. However more recent evidence supports an association between the incidence of allergic and autoimmune diseases.[131,238] These observations would fit with the concept of common mechanisms underlying infection-mediated protection against autoimmunity and allergy.

Another potential mechanism involves regulatory T cells and cytokines. The decrease in antigenic stimulation related to the decreased frequency of childhood infections has resulted in a decrease in the levels of regulatory cytokines, specifically IL-10, and possible transforming growth factor-β (TGF-β). CD25$^+$ T cells and other regulatory T cells produce these two cytokines which, in turn, act to down-regulate both TH1 and TH2-mediated responses. Data from humans and animal models tend to support the concept that infectious agents stimulate the production of regulatory cells whose effects extend beyond the responses to the invading microbe.[11,269] IL-10 and TGF-β, which may be produced by CD25$^+$ and other regulatory T cells,[105] can inhibit both TH1 and TH2 responses, and thus are plausible candidates as mediators of the inverse relationship between infections on the one hand and allergic and autoimmune diseases on the other.

Another hypothesized mechanism relates to stimulation of the innate immune system by viruses and bacteria and their components (such as endotoxin), which may be important in the ontogeny of the normal immune system. This is likely to be mediated by TLRs, which are receptors for various bacterial components. When TLRs bind to bacterial ligands, they stimulate mononuclear cells to produce cytokines, some of which could down-regulate allergic and autoimmune responses.

Another interesting observation relates to the presence of pets in the house and the risk of asthma. Farm animals have not been common in big European and American cities, but domestic pets are extremely common. They are a prolific source of allergen, and sensitization to these allergens is strongly associated with asthma.[158] Reports from Europe suggest that the presence of a cat in the home decreases the risk of sensitization to cat allergens.[218] Because of studies that suggest that the same effect occurs in countries where domestic animals are equally common in the homes of families with a history of asthma as in the homes of families without such history, the initially proposed explanation that this effect could be secondary to decisions by families with allergic disease not to have pets is unlikely. Ownby, Johnson, and Peterson strengthened these initial observations.[196] They report that children in a birth cohort raised in a house with two or more dogs or cats in the first year of life have not only less allergic sensitization to dog and cat as determined by skin prick tests and allergen specific IgE levels, but also less sensitization to allergens in general at age 6 to 7 years. Because domestic animals can be a source of endotoxin, this finding suggests the possibility that the effects of pets as described by Ownby, Johnson, and Peterson in the United States could be comparable to that of cows and farm animals in Europe. Mechanisms similar to those discussed earlier in this chapter involving regulatory T cells and inhibitory cytokines are being investigated to explain these findings.

Therefore, the interesting relationships between infections and immune mediated diseases, such as allergic and autoimmune diseases, and between early exposure to some allergens and the lowered risk of future allergic sensitization, potentially create new therapeutic strategies. The challenge will be to elucidate the responsible immune mechanisms involved and to determine the extent of exposure that will ensure safety and the desired outcome—the development of healthy children with a very low risk of allergic and autoimmune disease.

PATHOPHYSIOLOGY OF ALLERGIC RHINITIS

Allergic rhinitis, defined as a clinical hypersensitivity of the nasal mucosa to foreign substances mediated through IgE antibodies, affects millions of Americans and is encountered frequently by the otolaryngologist. This IgE-dependent disease involves more than a mast cell-mediated reaction. The pathophysiologic events involve interactions of the multiple components of the immune response.

Sensitization and Immunoglobulin E Production

During the initial stage of the disease, low-dose exposure leads to the production of specific IgE antibodies. Antigen that is deposited on the nasal mucosa is engulfed by APC (macrophages, dendritic cells, Langerhans cells) and partially degraded within their phagolysosomes. Portions of the antigen are then exteriorized on the surfaces of APC and are recognized by T-helper cells and class II MHC molecules. IL-1-activated T-helper cells then secrete cytokines, which promote the growth and differentiation of other cells involved in the immune response.

TH2 CD4+ cells are thought to be an important contributor to allergic reactions. They secrete the cytokines IL-4 and IL-5. IL-4 promotes B-cell isotype switching to the production of IgE.[66] Increased production of IL-4 by peripheral blood mononuclear cells has been associated with high serum IgE levels[95] whereas IFN-γ (secreted by TH1 cells) has the opposite effect.[198] The importance of TH2 cells and IL-4 is further supported by the preferential release of TH2 cytokines from allergen-specific T-cell clones of atopic donors.[197] Durham and others, using *in situ* hybridization, found the message for IL-4 in nasal biopsy specimens of patients with allergic rhinitis 24 hours after provocation with an allergen.[73]

Antigen-specific IgE then attaches to high-affinity receptors on mast cells and basophils and to low-affinity receptors on other cells, thereby sensitizing the nasal mucosa. On subsequent exposure to the offending allergen, the IgE antibodies on the surface of these cells serve as receptors for the antigen molecules. Cross-linking of adjacent IgE molecules on mast cells leads to the release of inflammatory mediators that stimulate nerves, glands, and blood vessels to cause the clinical manifestations of the disease, namely sneezing, pruritus, rhinorrhea, and nasal obstruction. These events are known as the early allergic response.

Early Response to Antigen

Within minutes after exposure of an allergic patient to antigen, an inflammatory response occurs. The patient first senses tingling and pruritus, followed by sneezing, rhinorrhea, and, last, nasal congestion. These subjective feelings correlate with physiologic changes that are measured after antigen provocation, such as increases in nasal secretions and nasal airway resistance (NAR).[22] In addition to these physiologic changes, increases are noted in the levels of mediators such as histamine,[183] kinins, tryptase,[56] prostaglandin D_2 (PGD_2),[31] leukotriene C_4 (LTC_4),[62] leukotriene B_4 (LTB_4),[84] MBP,[28] and platelet-activating factor (PAF).[168] Histamine and tryptase are found in mast cell granules, and their detection in nasal secretions after antigen provocation provides support for mast cell degranulation during the nasal allergic reaction. PGD_2, a newly synthesized mediator of the cyclooxygenase pathway, is also secreted by mast cells. Direct evidence for the role of nasal mast cells in the immediate allergic reaction was provided by Gomez and others, who biopsied the nasal mucosa in allergic patients 20 minutes after provocation with antigen and found them degranulated.[98]

Neuronal Contribution

Sneezing and itching during the early response to allergen provocation involve the nervous system. Konno and Togawa[137] and others[25,213] showed the importance of neural reflexes in patients with allergic rhinitis when stimulation of one nasal cavity with histamine led to bilateral nasal secretions. Unilateral intranasal challenge with antigen in patients with allergic rhinitis led to an increase in sneezes, rhinorrhea, nasal secretions, histamine, NAR,[24] and PGD_2[214,265] on the side of challenge. Contralateral to the challenge, rhinorrhea, secretion weights, and PGD_2 increased significantly.[265] The contralateral secretory response was rich in the glandular markers lactoferrin and lysozyme[214] and was inhibited by atropine, an anticholinergic,[25] suggesting that the efferent limb was cholinergically mediated. The muscarinic receptors that mediate the actions of acetylcholine in the nasal mucosa have been characterized pharmacologically in human inferior turbinates.[192] These studies showed the presence of muscarinic (M_1) and M_3 receptor subtypes with 45% of the total receptors being M_1. High densities of M_1 and M_3 receptors coexisted in submucosal glands; M_3 receptors predominated in vessels, and M_2 receptors were not found.

Several neuropeptides—in addition to sympathetic and parasympathetic nerves and their transmitters—are found in the nasal mucosa. These neuropeptides are secreted by unmyelinated nociceptive C fibers [tachykinins, calcitonin gene-related peptide (CGRP), neurokinin (NKA), gastrin-releasing peptide], parasympathetic nerve endings [vasoactive intestinal peptide (VIP), peptide histidine methionine], and sympathetic nerve endings (neuropeptide Y). Substance P (SP), a member of the tachykinin family, is often found as a CO transmitter with NKA and CGRP; it has been found in high density in arterial vessels and, to some extent, in veins, gland acini,

and epithelium.[19] Several studies support the concept that neuronal mechanisms mediated by these peptides amplify the inflammatory allergic reaction. Nasal provocation with neuropeptide Y, a 36-amino acid peptide co-localized with norepinephrine in sympathetic fibers, increases the expression of ICAM-1.[247] Nasal challenge with SP induces few changes in healthy patients, but leads to a modest increase in vascular permeability, NAR, and eosinophil and neutrophil chemotaxis in rhinitics.[51,226] In an in vitro study, Okamoto and others incubated nasal biopsy specimens of patients with perennial rhinitis and nonallergic rhinitis with SP or mite allergen.[191] SP and allergen challenge resulted in significant increases in mRNA for IL-1β, IL-2, IL-3, IL-4, IL-5, IL-6, TNF-α, and IFN-γ in nasal biopsy specimens of allergic patients. These increases were blocked by an SP antagonist. Because these cytokines are important in allergic reactions, this study supports the importance of SP as a proinflammatory neuropeptide. VIP stimulates serous cell secretion,[20] dilates nasal vessels,[159] and regulates mucociliary clearance in dogs.[185]

Mosimann and others challenged allergic rhinitis patients with histamine and antigen and measured levels of neuropeptides in recovered nasal washes.[176] Only VIP increased above baseline after histamine challenge; levels of SP, CGRP, and VIP increased significantly immediately after antigen challenge and returned to baseline within 2 hours. In patients who experienced a late reaction, only SP increased slightly.

These experiments suggest that neuropeptides are released in vivo in humans after allergen challenge and might be partly responsible for symptoms of the allergic reaction. Furthermore, the recovery of VIP after histamine challenge suggests that histamine-induced cholinergic reflexes induce the release of VIP.

Repetitive application of capsaicin, the essence of chili peppers, releases SP and CGRP from sensory nerves and initiates both central and axonal reflexes.[118] Capsaicin causes a burning sensation and profuse bilateral rhinorrhea when applied to one side of the nasal cavity, and repeated administration causes tachyphylaxis.[27,204] Unlike its effects in rodents, the capsaicin-induced nasal secretory response in humans is glandular and not caused by increased vascular permeability.[207] Capsaicin challenge caused significant increases in leukocyte counts from the pre-challenge baseline at 10 minutes, 30 minutes, and 4 hours after challenge, with no difference between rhinitic and healthy subjects.[206] The rise in the number of inflammatory cells represented significant increases in neutrophils, eosinophils, and mononuclear cells, supporting a nonspecific inflammatory effect of sensory nerve activation.

The neuropeptide-depleting property of capsaicin decreased symptoms of nonallergic chronic rhinitis.[140] Lacroix and others showed that the decrease in symptoms of these patients correlated with a significant decrease in CGRP in the nasal mucosa.[140] Furthermore, capsaicin desensitization reduces sneezing in response to antigen and histamine challenges.[136] Therefore, several experimental findings point to the importance of the participation of neurogenic elements to the allergic response, including the presence of nasonasal reflexes after nasal antigen provocation, the presence of neuropeptides in nasal tissues and their recovery in nasal secretions after antigen challenge, the ability of these peptides to produce symptoms and inflammatory responses similar to those obtained after exposure to antigen, and finally, the clinical efficacy of capsaicin, which depletes the stores of these substances. More specific delineation of the role of each of these substances awaits the development of specific antagonists.

The early reaction to allergen challenge with the release of mast cell mediators results in increased symptoms. However, these changes are measured in minutes, in contrast to clinical disease in which symptoms last for hours after exposure to allergen. Furthermore, other discrepancies exist between the early reaction and clinical disease, such as the chronic inflammation and hyperresponsiveness seen in allergic patients during the allergy season, and the lack of inhibition of the early response by systemic corticosteroids that are effective in the treatment of allergic rhinitis. Therefore, the early response does not mimic all aspects of clinical disease, and investigations have evaluated the events that occur hours after antigen exposure.

Late Response to Antigen

Hours after antigen challenge, some patients experience a recurrence of symptoms, most notably nasal congestion. This is termed the *late response*. Several investigators have documented elevations in NAR 4 to 10 hours after antigen challenge, with a peak around 6 hours and resolution by 24 hours.[75,201] After nasal challenge with antigen, the early rise in mediators as part of the early reaction was followed by a recurrence of symptoms and increases in the levels of histamine, tosyl-L-arginine methyl ester (TAME)-esterase, and kinins, but not PGD_2.[181] Other mediators, including eosinophil products, have also been detected.[28] The peak and pattern of mediator production during the late phase varied among patients.

Levels of nitric oxide (NO) have been detected in exhaled air during nasal and oral breathing in patients with seasonal allergic rhinitis and in healthy subjects.[163] Concentrations of nasally exhaled NO were significantly higher in the allergic patients than in the healthy subjects, suggesting a role for this mediator in the pathophysiology of allergic rhinitis. Nitric oxide is synthesized from L-arginine in various cell types by the action of NO synthases, including the constitutive forms of nitric oxide synthase in vascular endothelial cells (type III nitric oxide synthase) and neurons (type I nitric oxide synthase) and the inducible form (type II nitric oxide synthase) induced by cytokines in macrophages, neutrophils, mast cells, smooth muscle cells, and fibroblasts. NO has vasodilatory and antimicrobial properties, and its increased production in the nose could contribute to nasal obstruction and plasma protein extravasation in allergic disease.

Type III nitric oxide synthase immunoreactivity and mRNA were observed in endothelial cells, surface epithelium, and submucosal glands; type II nitric oxide synthase immunoreactivity was less intense and was observed in surface epithelium, vascular endothelial and smooth muscle cells, submucosal glands, and inflammatory cells, and mRNA for type II nitric oxide synthase was localized mainly to inflammatory cells.[88] Type II nitric oxide synthase immunoreactivity was more intense in the specimens with more severe inflammatory changes and correlated with the extent of inflammation. Bacci and others reported on the presence of neuronal nitric oxide synthase immunoreactivity in mast cell granules in biopsy specimens of normal nasal mucosa from four patients undergoing rhinoplasties.[13] These studies support the presence of nitric oxide synthase in the nasal mucosa and suggest a possible role for NO in the pathophysiology of nasal diseases, including allergic rhinitis.

To investigate the role of the neuronal contribution to the late nasal allergic reaction, levels of histamine in nasal secretions were measured hourly, for 10 hours, after allergen provocations from the site of challenge and from the contralateral nostril.[264] Histamine release occurred at the site of challenge during the early response and hours after allergen provocation. On the contralateral side of challenge, histamine production showed no significant increase during the early phase but significant increase in histamine (compared with challenge in healthy subjects) during the late phase. In another group of subjects, an influx of basophils to the contralateral nasal cavity occurred 24 hours after provocation with allergen but not after control challenge. These studies suggest a neuronal contribution to the late inflammatory response.

Cellular Events

Along with the physiologic changes and inflammatory mediator production that occur hours after antigen provocation, inflammatory cellular influx occurs in the nasal mucosa and in recovered nasal secretions after experimental provocation and in seasonally exposed patients. A slight initial increase in eosinophils in nasal secretions occurred within 1 to 2 hours of challenge and was followed by a peak 6 to 8 hours later.[26] MBP, a mediator secreted by eosinophils, was also recovered in nasal lavages hours after antigen provocation, and its levels correlated with the number of eosinophils, suggesting that these cells influx into nasal secretions and release inflammatory mediators.[28] Juliusson and others observed a rapid and significant increase in the number of eosinophils in allergic patients as early as 2 hours after challenge in the lavage specimens and 4 hours after challenge in the brush samples.[127] The percentage of activated eosinophils in brush samples increased and reached a peak 8 hours after provocation, and the basal values of eosinophils correlated significantly with symptoms of congestion, sneezing, and rhinorrhea observed after challenge.[127] To examine changes in eosinophil numbers and activation status during natural exposure, Bentley and others performed nasal biopsies in allergic patients during the pollen season and reported significant seasonal increases in total MBP and activated (EG2[+]) eosinophils in the submucosa of these patients compared with preseasonal eosinophil numbers or from nonallergic subjects.[35]

Lim and others obtained nasal lavages and inferior turbinate biopsy specimens before and 24 hours after challenging allergic patients with allergen.[152] Similar to findings reported by other investigators, the number of eosinophils and polymorphonuclear cells in nasal lavages and the number of eosinophils and mononuclear cells in the nasal mucosa were significantly increased. The predominant cell types in nasal secretions were polymorphonuclear cells and eosinophils, whereas mononuclear cells predominated in the nasal mucosa, suggesting that nasal secretions and the nasal mucosa are two separate compartments with different inflammatory cellular predominance during allergic inflammation.

Basophils constitute 1% of the recovered cells. Their number correlates significantly with levels of histamine recovered in nasal secretions during the late-phase response (r = 0.72, $P < .0001$), suggesting that these cells are the source of the late rise in histamine.[26]

Similar cellular changes have been observed during seasonal exposure of allergic patients, lending credibility to the observations after experimental allergen challenge. In separately conducted studies, Bryan and Bryan[54] and Okuda and Ohtsuka[193] observed basophilic cells in nasal secretions during seasonal exposure of allergic patients to pollen. In contrast to nasal secretions, which represent the most superficial compartment of the nasal mucosa, examination of nasal mucosal scrapings[190,194] or biopsy specimens,[79,194]

which sample deeper layers, showed that most metachromatic cells in these compartments were mast cells. The mast cells were divided into two subpopulations, one located in the epithelium and the other located deeper, in the lamina propria.[195] Enerback, Pipkorn, and Granerus showed a seasonal increase in mast cells on the surface of the nasal epithelium after 4 or 5 days of exposure to pollen.[79] Because the overall number of mast cells in the nasal mucosa remained unchanged, they suggested that seasonal exposure led to migration of mast cells from the deeper layers of the lamina propria to the epithelium. Bentley and others reported a similar significant increase in intraepithelial tryptase-positive mast cells in nasal biopsy specimens of allergic patients during the pollen season.[35] The consensus of most authors is that basophils predominate in nasal secretions, whereas mast cells are more abundant in the epithelium and lamina propria of allergic patients exposed to antigen either experimentally or naturally.

Eosinophils and mast cells, which are most frequently associated with allergic reactions, occur in the nasal submucosa, but most cells in this location are mononuclear cells (lymphocytes and monocytes). Varney and others showed that numbers of CD4[+] (T-helper) lymphocytes and CD25[+] cells were significantly increased after antigen challenge compared to challenge with the diluent.[261] The number of CD25[+] cells correlated positively with the numbers of CD3[+] and CD4[+] cells, suggesting that CD25[+] cells were activated lymphocytes. In support of these observations, Hamid and others showed that 60% to 100% of CD25[+] cells identified in the nasal mucosa 24 hours after antigen challenge were also CD3[+].[107] Unlike changes after antigen provocation, there were no significant increases in CD45[+], CD3[+], CD4[+], CD8[+], CD25[+], CD68[+] cells, or neutrophils in the nasal submucosa during the season.[35] This might be related to the lower dose of antigen to which allergic patients are exposed during the season compared with the amount during experimental provocation or related to the site of the nasal biopsy and the placement of allergen.

Another important cell type detected in the nasal mucosa of allergic patients are Langerhans cells, which are large mononuclear dendritic cells that are important in antigen presentation. Fokkens and others showed that the numbers of intraepithelial CD1[+] (Langerhans cells) cells in healthy subjects and grass-allergic patients before and after the pollen season were not different, but the numbers of intraepithelial CD1[+] cells were significantly increased during the allergy season compared with the other time points and nonallergic subjects.[82] In another study involving patients with perennial allergic rhinitis, the same investigators showed a significant decrease in

Langerhans cells in the epithelium after 3 months of treatment with fluticasone propionate.[117] These studies support the importance of Langerhans cells in the allergic reaction and suggest that they are not constitutively more numerous in patients with allergic rhinitis but are more likely to be up-regulated upon exposure to allergen.

Detection of Cytokines in Nasal Secretions and Cells After Allergen Provocation

In addition to the different preformed and newly generated inflammatory mediators secreted by mast cells and other inflammatory cells during the allergic reaction, cytokines have been identified in the nasal mucosa and in nasal secretions of allergic patients during natural exposure and allergen provocation.

Sim and others challenged allergic patients with diluent, followed by increasing doses of allergen, until a symptomatic response was obtained.[236] Compared with the diluent challenges, there were significant increases in the levels of IL-1β during the early- and late-phase responses, and of GM-CSF and IL-6 during the late-phase response, in all patients. In five of eight patients studied, there were significant elevations of IL-5 during the early- and late-phase responses. Levels of IL-2 or IL-4 were not detectable after challenge. Levels of IL-1β correlated with symptom scores during the early and late reactions, and levels of GM-CSF and IL-6 correlated with symptoms during the late response. In a similar study, the same investigators studied the effect of premedication with intranasal corticosteroids.[237] In addition to duplicating their findings with IL-1β and GM-CSF, they showed significant increases in levels of macrophage inflammatory protein-1α during the early and late responses and IL-8 and RANTES during the late response. Pretreatment with intranasal corticosteroids significantly inhibited the rise in the levels of all the cytokines and chemokines measured.

Using nasal lavage to sample nasal secretions after allergen challenge, Gosset and others detected significant elevations in levels of IL-1α and IL-6 in patients with dual early and late responses.[100] Bachert, Wagenmann, and Hauser also measured significant increases in levels of IL-1β and TNF within 2 hours after challenge in nasal lavage specimens, and increases in levels of IL-6 and IL-8, 6 to 8 hours after challenge.[14] They detected significantly elevated baseline levels of IL-1β, IL-6, and IL-8 in patients with seasonal allergic rhinitis compared with those of healthy subjects. Similar increases in levels of IL-1β and GM-CSF were detected by Linden and others in nasal lavage specimens from allergic patients shortly after challenge with antigen.[153] Finally, Saengpanich and others have demonstrated significant increases in lev-

els of IL-5, TNFα, and soluble ICAM-1 in nasal lavages obtained 24 hours after allergen challenge when compared with baseline.[221]

In nasal biopsies, Bradding and others detected significantly more IL-4$^+$ cells in the nasal mucosa of perennial rhinitis patients compared with healthy subjects.[45,46] These investigators also showed that 78 to 100% of the IL-4$^+$ cells contained mast cell tryptase. Immunoreactivity for IL-5, IL-6, and IL-8 was present in most biopsy specimens from perennial rhinitis patients and healthy subjects. No significant differences existed between the two populations in the number of cytokine-positive cells. Most IL5$^+$ cells were mast cells, with some eosinophils. Most IL-6$^+$ cells were mast cells, and IL-8 was localized to the cytoplasm of epithelial cells.[45] No cytokine reactivity was localized to CD3$^+$ or CD4$^+$ cells. These data suggest that IL-4, IL-5, and IL-6 are localized to mast cells in the nasal mucosa of patients with perennial allergic rhinitis. The investigators attribute the lack of localization of any of the cytokines to T lymphocytes to the fact that cytokines generated by activated T cells are rapidly transported from the cell, and do not accumulate in sufficient concentrations to be detected by their technique. They hypothesize that mast cells provide the initial burst of IL-4, which enhances other cells (e.g., T lymphocytes) to continue secreting this and other cytokines, thus perpetuating the inflammatory allergic reaction. The same investigators showed that pretreatment with intranasal corticosteroids suppressed the seasonal increases in epithelial eosinophils, submucosal eosinophils, and epithelial mast cells and also led to a significant suppression of IL-4$^+$ cells in the nasal submucosa, without significant effects on the number of IL-5 and IL-6 immunoreactive cells.[44]

Durham and others found that biopsy samples after allergen challenge showed significant increases in cells bearing mRNA for IL-3, IL-4, IL-5, and GM-CSF, but not for IL-2 or IFN-γ compared with biopsies obtained after a sham challenge of allergic individuals.[73] Activated eosinophils (EG2$^+$) increased significantly after allergen challenge and correlated positively with mRNA expression for IL-5, IL-4, GM-CSF, IL-3, and IL-2 but not for IFN-γ. The strongest correlation was with IL-5 (r = 0.9, P < .0001), and the weakest correlations were with IL-3 (r = 0.63, P = .05) and IL-2 (r = 0.65, P = .04). Ying and others showed that most IL-5 mRNA$^+$ cells were also CD3$^+$ (83%), and the rest were positive for tryptase (16.4%).[281] These findings suggest that T lymphocytes are a major contributor to IL-5 in nasal allergic reactions. The same investigators also studied the effects of therapeutic intervention with intranasal corticosteroids and immunotherapy on the expression of mRNA for the different cytokines in the nasal mucosa. Pretreatment with fluticasone propionate before allergen challenge and subsequent biopsy resulted in significant inhibition of nasal symptoms and inhibition of an allergen-induced increase in cells expressing mRNA for IL-4 but not for IL-5.[164] Pretreatment with intranasal corticosteroids also significantly inhibited allergen-induced increases in submucosal IL-2 receptor-bearing cells (CD25[+]) and activated eosinophils (EG2[+]). Immunotherapy, in addition to inhibiting cellular influx into the nasal mucosa, also induced a TH-1 cell response, with a significant increase in cells expressing mRNA for IFN-γ.[74]

The various techniques of cytokine detection all support the importance of these proteins in the allergic reaction in vivo. Difficulty measuring some cytokines in nasal secretions, most notably IL-4 and IL-5, might be related to the lack of sensitivity of available assays. The cytokine profile observed after allergen provocation supports the involvement of TH2 cells in the allergic reaction. Because IL-5 promotes the differentiation,[59] vascular adhesion,[268] and in vitro survival of eosinophils[157] and enhances histamine release from basophils,[115] and because IL-4 is a mast cell growth factor[222] and promotes the switching of B cells to the production of IgE,[198] TH2-like T cells are thought to be particularly important in allergic disease.

Adhesion Molecules and Cellular Recruitment

Cellular trafficking is integral to human immune response because it allows cells to be selectively recruited from the bloodstream into sites of tissue inflammation. Cellular recruitment into sites of allergic reactions is an example of such trafficking.

Numerous inflammatory cells are present in the nasal mucosa and in nasal secretions of allergic patients during allergen exposure but not in healthy subjects. Mechanisms should therefore exist for the migration and accumulation of these effector cells during allergic inflammation. Recruitment of cells such as eosinophils and activated T lymphocytes are mediated, in part, by interactions between adhesion molecules on the cells themselves and those on vascular endothelial cells, with cytokines playing various regulating roles in these interactions.

The molecules responsible for adhesion on leukocytes belong to different families, such as the integrin family, which consists of molecules with three α chains (CD11a, b, or c) and a common β2 chain (CD18, β2 integrin), which can combine noncovalently to form LFA-1, Mac-1, and p150,95, respectively.[8] Another set of adhesion proteins present on leukocytes possesses a different common β subunit, β1 (CD29), and at least seven α chains and comprises the VLA antigen family.[112] Another leukocyte adhesion protein, L-selectin, belongs to the selectin adhesion molecule family and allows attachment to endothelium under conditions of shear stress caused by blood flow.[37] Adhesion molecules on the vascular endothelial cell surface include ICAM-1 (CD54), ICAM-2, E-selectin, P-selectin (GMP-140, CD62), and VCAM-1.[241] Receptor-counter-receptor pairs for adhesion molecules include LFA-1 with ICAM-1 and ICAM-2, Mac-1 with ICAM-1, VLA-4 with VCAM-1, the carbohydrate structure sialyl-Lewis X with E-selectin and P-selectin, and the recently identified structure GlyCAM-1 for L-selectin.[8,37]

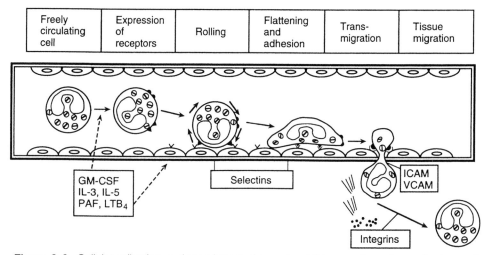

Figure 9-6. Cellular adhesion and recruitment. An eosinophil is seen from the early stage of free circulation, on to rolling, adhesion to the vascular endothelium, transendothelial migration, and, finally, tissue migration. In the case of the eosinophil, these events are regulated and mediated by multiple cytokines and adhesion molecules. (From Mygind N and others, editors: *Essential allergy*, ed 2, Oxford, Blackwell Scientific Publications, 1996.)

It is currently thought that a series of events occurs during the migration of circulating leukocytes into tissues (Figure 9-6). The cells initially undergo reversible margination and can be seen rolling along the endothelial surface on intravital microscopy.[241] These changes are mediated by interactions between carbohydrates and selectins. Leukocyte activation occurs next, presumably as a result of exposure to chemoattractants or other activating factors released by endothelial cells or by nearby tissue-dwelling cells. Leukocyte activation is associated with changes in affinity and expression of adhesion molecules on the leukocyte surface. Leukocytes also may be activated directly by their interaction with adhesion molecules on activated endothelial cells.[156] Activated leukocytes then attach to endothelial cells and migrate across the endothelium into the extravascular space. These events are mediated by one or more members of the integrin, selectin, and immunoglobulin families of adhesion molecules. Furthermore, it is likely that the preferential recruitment of leukocytes involves multiple steps, such as leukocyte activation, vascular endothelial cell expression of adhesion molecules, adhesion of leukocytes to vascular endothelium, transendothelial migration, chemotaxis, and localized survival within the tissues. Multiple cytokines and other factors are important in up-regulating adhesion molecules on circulating leukocytes and vascular endothelium and are crucial in chemotaxis and leukocyte survival within the tissues.

Because the eosinophil consistently increases in tissues and in secretions of patients with allergic rhinitis, in vitro and in vivo evidence helps elucidate the mechanism of selective eosinophil recruitment into inflammatory sites. Exposure of endothelial cells to IL-1 or TNF induces endothelial expression of ICAM-1, E-selectin, and VCAM-1 and enhances adhesion of eosinophils, basophils, and neutrophils.[36,39,141,228] Blocking antibodies to VCAM-1 were extremely effective in inhibiting eosinophil adherence and, to a lesser degree, basophil adherence but had no effect on neutrophil adherence, suggesting that eosinophils and basophils, in contrast to neutrophils, recognize VCAM-1.[40] Consistent with these observations were the findings that neutrophils did not express VLA-4, the counter ligand for VCAM-1, whereas eosinophils and basophils did[40,68,267,272]; the antibodies to VLA-4 inhibited eosinophil but not neutrophil adhesion.[68,267] These studies show that the VLA-4 and VCAM-1 interaction may be important in eosinophil recruitment, and they raise the possibility that conditions leading to selective VCAM-1 expression on endothelial cells result in the preferential adherence of eosinophils. The cytokine IL-4 induces VCAM-1 expression selectively in endothelial cells,[255] and incubation of endothelial cells with IL-4 induced eosinophil and basophil adherence with no effect on the adherence of neutrophils.[227] Much of this adherence was inhibited by addition of anti-VCAM-1 or anti-VLA-4 blocking antibodies.[227] These findings were consistent with the observations in vivo that mice transgenic for IL-4 developed eosinophilic inflammatory lesions[251] and that mice injected with a tumor cell line producing IL-4 form an intense eosinophilic infiltrate at the site of the tumor.[252] Therefore, IL-4-induced VCAM-1 expression is probably important in inflammatory responses; however, its interaction with VLA-4 cannot, by itself, explain selective eosinophil recruitment because VLA-4 is also expressed on other cell types, including lymphocytes and monocytes.

After adhering to vascular endothelial cells, eosinophils leave the circulation and enter local inflammatory sites by migrating across the endothelium. Similar to the findings with adhesion to endothelial cells, exposing endothelial monolayers to IL-1 or TNF induced the expression of E-selectin, ICAM-1, and VCAM-1, and increased transendothelial migration of neutrophils[160,174] and eosinophils.[78,175] For eosinophils, transendothelial migration through IL-1-activated endothelium was inhibited almost completely by antibodies to CD18 ($\beta 2$ integrin), whereas CD29 ($\beta 1$ integrin, one of the chains of VLA antigens) antibody had essentially no effect.[78] A combination of antibodies against ICAM-1, E-selectin, and VCAM-1 was more effective than anti-ICAM-1 alone in inhibiting eosinophil transmigration.[77] These data suggest that transendothelial migration of eosinophils is mediated by adhesion molecules on the eosinophils and the vascular endothelium, and that the mechanisms of adhesion may be different from those of transmigration.

In addition to cytokines and chemoattractants that can affect the function and expression of leukocyte and endothelial adhesion molecules, another family of mediators, the chemokines, plays a role. One of these chemokines, IL-8, is released by epithelial cells and appears to be necessary for transendothelial migration of neutrophils.[121] Another member of this family, RANTES, selectively promotes chemotaxis of memory T lymphocytes, monocytes,[225] and eosinophils.[7,76,128,219] In the transendothelial migration assay, RANTES stimulates eosinophil migration but has no effect on neutrophils. In contrast to previous studies in which anti-$\beta 2$ integrin antibody almost completely inhibited eosinophil transendothelial migration, a combination of anti-$\beta 2$ and anti-VLA-4 antibodies was required for complete inhibition of RANTES-induced transmigration across activated endothelium.[76] Corroborating the importance of these chemokines in allergic reactions is the fact that RANTES, macrophage inflammatory protein-1α, and IL-8 have been detected in nasal lavages after allergen provocation.[237] IL-8 protein has also been localized to the nasal mucosa of patients with perennial allergic rhinitis and to the nasal mucosa of healthy subjects.[45]

Clear evidence shows that endothelial activation occurs during allergic rhinitis in vivo. Montefort and others found enhanced expression of ICAM-1 and VCAM-1, but not E-selectin, in the mucosa of allergic patients.[171] Lee and others found significant up-regulation in the expression of VCAM-1 in the biopsy specimens of allergic patients obtained 24 hours after antigen challenge.[144] Concomitantly, the number of eosinophils significantly increased 24 hours after allergen challenge in the allergic patients. These studies of adhesion molecules in vivo suggest that these molecules, along with their counter ligands on circulating leukocytes, have an important role in cellular recruitment to allergic inflammatory sites. Further studies are needed for better definition of the role of these adhesion mechanisms in allergic rhinitis and for determination of whether interfering with the process of adhesion will modify the course and severity of the disease.

Hyperresponsiveness

One of the hallmarks of allergic rhinitis is the hyperresponsiveness of allergic patients to specific stimuli, such as antigen (a phenomenon known as *priming*) and nonspecific stimuli.

Specific Hyperresponsiveness

Many allergic patients report worsening symptoms as the allergy season progresses, despite unchanged or decreased pollen counts. This phenomenon is probably caused by a shift in the threshold of responsiveness. Connell found that the dose of pollen necessary to create symptoms decreased more than fivefold by the fourth day of consecutive antigen challenges.[60] Wachs and others challenged asymptomatic allergic patients with increasing doses of antigen on consecutive days.[263] When the patients were challenged 24 hours after earlier exposure, they had significantly more sneezes in response to provocation, and the threshold for the initiation of sneezes decreased. The dose necessary to initiate sneezing during the priming response was reduced to about 100 grains of ragweed extract, a dose easily inhaled during a brief period of the pollen season. This is in comparison with 10,000 grains needed to initiate sneezing during a challenge out of season. Concomitant with the priming response observed for sneezes, significantly higher levels of histamine and kinins were present in nasal lavage samples compared with the levels in the initial challenge. An increase in the number of total cells, neutrophils,

eosinophils, and basophils was present in nasal lavages on the days when priming occurred than on the initial challenge day. These observations suggest that mechanisms of priming involve cellular infiltration, increased mediator production, and possible increased end-organ responsiveness. Influxing inflammatory cells are hypothesized to alter the mucosal penetration of antigen and to provide additional targets for antigen stimulation and increased generation of inflammatory mediators, which would, in turn, encounter more responsive end organs, thus leading to the exaggerated response noted after repeated antigen exposure.

Nonspecific Hyperresponsiveness

Increased reactivity to irritant stimuli is often reported by allergic patients. This phenomenon has been studied by observation of the nasal response to nonantigenic nasal secretagogues, such as histamine and the cholinergic agonist methacholine. Patients challenged with antigen, followed 24 hours later by a histamine challenge, showed increased sensitivity to histamine compared with a baseline histamine challenge.[266] This increased responsiveness to histamine plateaued and was reversible. Other investigators confirmed the increased responsiveness to histamine 24 hours after antigen challenge and inhibited this phenomenon by pretreatment with topical corticosteroids.[12,23] The number of eosinophils 24 hours after antigen challenge correlated with the magnitude of reactivity to histamine and inhibition by topical corticosteroids was accompanied by an inhibition of the increase of eosinophils in nasal secretions.[23]

To examine the effect of seasonal exposure on nasal responsiveness to histamine, Majchel and others challenged allergic patients with histamine before, at the peak of, near the end of, and 2 weeks after the ragweed pollen season and monitored the response by symptoms and markers of vascular permeability in recovered nasal lavage specimens.[161] They observed a significant increase in all monitored parameters at the peak of the pollen season. These symptoms returned to baseline with the disappearance of pollen. However, the increase above baseline at the peak of the season was not significant for any of the parameters measured, suggesting that increased reactivity to histamine with seasonal exposure represents a change in baseline rather than an increased sensitivity to histamine itself. This change in baseline reactivity was inhibited in patients undergoing immunotherapy.

Similar studies show nasal hyperresponsiveness to the cholinomimetic agonist methacholine. Druce and others showed significantly more responsiveness in atopic vs non-atopic patients.[72] Borum showed that patients with perennial rhinitis had a significantly more pronounced methacholine-induced secretory response than did healthy subjects.[42] Klementsson and others also measured the secretory response to methacholine before and after antigen challenge of allergic patients out of season and observed significant increases over baseline in methacholine-induced secretions at 2, 4, 6, 8, 10, and 24 hours after antigen challenge.[133] Although the numbers of eosinophils in nasal secretions increased significantly after antigen challenge, their numbers did not correlate with the increase in nonspecific hyperresponsiveness to methacholine. The same investigators also showed increased responsiveness to methacholine and a significant increase in eosinophils in nasal brushings during a weak pollen season. Both were inhibited significantly by pretreatment with budesonide.[134] Again, number of eosinophils did not correlate with the degree of secretory responsiveness. These observations suggest that the allergen-induced increase in nonspecific responsiveness to methacholine is a complex phenomenon that is not solely dependent on eosinophil influx into the nasal mucosa.

In allergic patients during the allergy season, the hyperresponsiveness caused by nonspecific irritants probably reflects complex interactions among inflammatory cellular influx, epithelial injury, and increased end-organ responsiveness caused by exposure to antigen.

The pathophysiologic mechanisms in allergic rhinitis can be synthesized in the following scenario (Figure 9-7): sensitization of the nasal mucosa to a certain allergen entails multiple interactions among APC cells, T lymphocytes, and B cells that lead to the production of antigen-specific IgE antibodies, which then localize to mast cells and basophils. Subsequent exposure leads to cross-linking of specific IgE receptors on mast cells and their resultant degranulation, with the release of a host of inflammatory mediators that are, in large part, responsible for allergic nasal symptoms. Other proinflammatory substances are also generated after antigen exposure, most prominent are eosinophil products and cytokines. Cytokines are thought to be generated in part by lymphocytes, which are abundant in resting and stimulated nasal

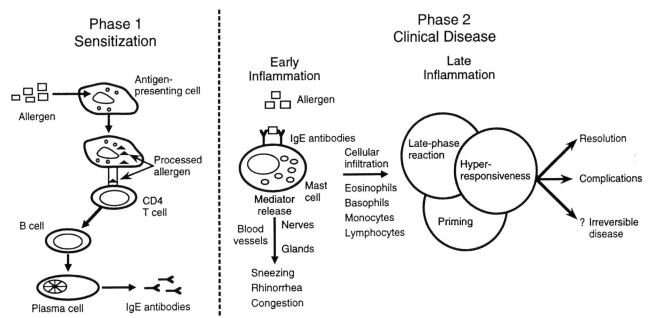

Figure 9-7. Pathophysiology of allergic rhinitis. The first stage of development of allergic rhinitis involves antigen processing and the production of specific immunoglobulin E (IgE) antibodies, which attach to mast cells, basophils, and other inflammatory cells. On subsequent exposure to the same allergen, IgE receptors on the surface of mast cells are cross-linked, leading to the degranulation of these cells and the release of preformed and newly synthesized mediators that are responsible for symptoms of the disease. Recruitment of inflammatory cells to the nasal mucosa also occurs, as does a resultant state of chronic inflammation with a heightened state of reactivity to specific and nonspecific stimuli, a hallmark of allergic nasal disease. In addition to the early and late inflammatory responses, exposure to allergen leads to a secondary immune response with increased production of specific IgE and a perpetuation of the state of susceptibility to allergen. (From Naclerio RM: Allergic rhinitis, *N Engl J Med* 325:860, 1991.)

mucosa. Recent evidence also points to an important role for mast cells in the storage and probable production and secretion of cytokines. Cytokines will up-regulate adhesion molecules on the vascular endothelium, and possibly on marginating leukocytes, and lead to the migration of these inflammatory cells into the site of tissue inflammation. Various cytokines will also promote the chemotaxis and survival of these recruited inflammatory cells and lead to a secondary immune response by virtue of their capability to promote IgE synthesis by B cells. Also important is the nervous system, which amplifies the allergic reaction by central and peripheral reflexes that result in changes at sites distant from those of antigen deposition. These changes lower the threshold of mucosal responsiveness to various specific and nonspecific stimuli, making allergic patients more responsive to stimuli to which they are exposed every day.

Interaction Between the Nose and Other Organs

Allergic rhinitis and asthma are both inflammatory diseases of the upper and lower airways, respectively, and are often comorbid conditions.[151] Asthma has been diagnosed in 21% to 58% of patients with allergic rhinitis,[179,199] and of patients with asthma, 28% to 92% have also been diagnosed with allergic rhinitis.[104,162] When allergic rhinitis and asthma coexist, allergic rhinitis may exacerbate asthma, and, conversely, treating nasal symptoms in these patients has had positive effects on their asthma status.[223,274,276] Nasal allergen challenge in subjects with both allergic rhinitis and asthma has worsened underlying asthma by increasing bronchial hyperresponsiveness and producing lower airway symptoms.[61,90]

To study the effects of nasal allergic inflammation on the lower airways, Braunstahl and others performed a nasal allergen challenge in allergic subjects out of season and monitored inflammation in both the nose and lungs by obtaining nasal and bronchial biopsies.[50] The number of eosinophils and expression of adhesion molecules increased not only in the challenged nose but also in the unchallenged lungs, suggesting that the inflammation triggered at the site of the allergen challenge (the nose) led to the inflammatory reaction in the lungs. In similar experiments, the same group has shown that bronchial challenge with allergen induces a nasal inflammatory reaction.[49]

Another disease that often coexists with allergic rhinitis is rhinosinusitis. Allergy is a known contributing factor to both acute and chronic rhinosinusitis,* and the relationship between allergic rhinitis

*References 38, 124, 212, 224, 232, 233, 239.

and rhinosinusitis has long been recognized and supported by the finding of a higher frequency of allergy in patients with rhinosinusitis.[212,224] In adults, up to 54% of those with chronic rhinosinusitis had symptoms of allergic rhinitis.[34] Similarly, a high concordance (25–75%) of these disorders was found in children.[87] Conversely, there is a high prevalence of sinus disease in patients with allergic rhinitis. Abnormal sinus radiographs occur in more than 50% of adults and children with perennial allergic rhinitis.[212,233] Acute rhinosinusitis occurs often during allergen seasons, and allergy is a frequently described factor complicating the failure of rhinosinusitis treatment.[129,231] During the pollen season, CT scans showed that 60% of sensitive adult subjects had sinus mucosal abnormalities.[182] In atopic patients, the allergic status may influence the severity of rhinosinusitis. A significant relationship was found between the severity of chronic rhinosinusitis and markers of allergy including eosinophilia and specific IgE to inhalant allergens.[119,187]

A pathophysiologic link between allergic rhinitis and sinusitis was demonstrated when, after nasal allergen challenge, sinus radiographs showed opacification accompanied by clinical symptoms, including maxillary sinus pressure, acute headache, and, sometimes, otalgia. After nasal allergen provocation in patients with chronic maxillary rhinosinusitis, 78% of those who developed positive nasal responses demonstrated radiographic changes (mucosal edema or opacification) of the maxillary sinuses 120 minutes after allergen challenge.[200] In other studies, we have seen a demonstrated influx of eosinophils into the maxillary sinus after nasal challenge of allergic subjects.[21] The mechanisms of these observations linking the nose, lung, and paranasal sinuses in allergic diseases are not well understood, but they raise the hypothesis that exposure of any sensitized upper or lower airway mucosa to allergen might lead to a systemic inflammatory response that manifests itself in other body organs. Another possible explanation for these findings and the close relationship between allergic rhinitis, asthma, and rhinosinusitis is the existence of nasopulmonary or nasosinal reflexes that contribute to the close relationship between these diseases. A combination of both of these mechanisms might also be responsible.

This overview of the immune system examines its different components, which include innate and adaptive immunity, the complement system, and the various phagocytic cells functioning in concert to protect the body from foreign invaders. When the immune system behaves in a misdirected fashion, however, disease states develop from the injurious effects of this powerful system.

REFERENCES

1. Abbas AK, Murphy KM, Sher A: Functional diversity of helper T lymphocytes, *Nature* 383:787, 1996.
2. Abraham SN, Malaviya R: Mast cells in infection and immunity, *Infect Immun* 65:3501, 1997.
3. Ackerman SJ: *Eosinophils: biologic and clinical aspects in allergy and inflammation.* In Rich RR and others, editors: *Clinical immunology: principles and practice,* vol 1, St Louis, Mosby-Year Book, 1996.
4. Agerberth B and others: FALL-39, a putative human peptide antibiotic, is cysteine-free and expressed in bone marrow and testis, *Proc Natl Acad Sci USA* 92:195, 1995.
5. Akashi S and others: Cutting edge: cell surface expression and lipopolysaccharide signaling via the toll-like receptor 4-MD-2 complex on mouse peritoneal macrophages, *J Immunol* 164:3471, 2000.
6. Alam R, Gorska M: Lymphocytes, *J Allergy Clin Immunol* 111:S476, 2003.
7. Alam R and others: RANTES is a chemotactic and activating factor for human eosinophils, *J Immunol* 150:3442, 1993.
8. Albelda SM, Buck CA: Integrins and other cell adhesion molecules, *FASEB J* 4:2868, 1990.
9. Alexopoulou L and others: Recognition of double stranded RNA and activation of NF-κB by Toll-like receptor 3, *Nature* 413:732, 2001.
10. Aliprantis AO and others: Cell activation and apoptosis by bacterial lipoproteins through Toll-like receptor-2, *Science* 285:736, 1999.
11. al-Sabbagh A and others: Antigen-driven tissue-specific suppression following oral tolerance: orally administered myelin basic protein suppresses proteolipid protein-induced experimental autoimmune encephalomyelitis in the SJL mouse, *Eur J Immunol* 24:2104, 1994.
12. Andersson M, Andersson P, Pipkorn U: Allergen-induced specific and non-specific nasal reactions: reciprocal relationship and inhibition by topical glucocortico-steroids, *Acta Otolaryngol (Stockh)* 107:270, 1989.
13. Bacci S and others: Localization of nitric oxide synthase immunoreactivity in mast cells of human nasal mucosa, *Histochemistry* 102:89, 1994.
14. Bachert C, Wagenmann M, Hauser U: Proinflammatory cytokines: measurement in nasal secretion and induction of adhesion receptor expression, *Int Arch Allergy Immunol* 107:106, 1995.
15. Ball TM and others: Siblings, day-care attendance, and the risk of asthma and wheezing during childhood, *N Engl J Med* 343:538, 2000.
16. Bals R and others: The peptide antibiotic LL-37/hCAP-18 is expressed in epithelia of the human lung where it has broad antimicrobial activity at the airway surface, *Proc Natl Acad Sci USA* 95:9541, 1998.
17. Bals R and others: Augmentation of innate host defense by expression of a cathelicidin antimicrobial peptide, *Infect Immun* 67:6084, 1999.
18. Banchereau J, Rousset F: Human B lymphocytes: phenotype, proliferation, and differentiation, *Adv Immunol* 52:125, 1992.
19. Baraniuk JN and others: Substance P and neurokinin A in human nasal mucosa, *Am J Respir Cell Mol Biol* 4:228, 1991.
20. Baraniuk JN and others: Vasoactive intestinal peptide (VIP) in human nasal mucosa, *J Clin Invest* 86:825, 1990.
21. Baroody FM and others: Influx of eosinophils into the maxillary sinus after nasal challenge with allergen, *J Allergy Clin Immunol* 105:S70, 2000 (abstract).
22. Baroody FM and others: Relationship between histamine and physiologic changes during the early response to nasal antigen provocation, *J Appl Physiol* 86:659, 1999.
23. Baroody FM and others: Intranasal beclomethasone inhibits antigen-induced nasal hyperresponsiveness to histamine, *J Allergy Clin Immunol* 90:373, 1992.
24. Baroody FM and others: Physiologic responses and histamine release after nasal antigen challenge: effect of atropine, *Am J Respir Crit Care Med* 149:1457, 1994.
25. Baroody FM, Wagenmann M, Naclerio RM: A comparison of the secretory response of the nasal mucosa to histamine and methacholine, *J Appl Physiol* 74:2661, 1993.
26. Bascom R and others: Basophil influx occurs after nasal antigen challenge: effects of topical corticosteroid pretreatment, *J Allergy Clin Immunol* 81:580, 1988.
27. Bascom R, Kagey-Sobotka A, Proud D: Effect of intranasal capsaicin on symptoms and mediator release, *J Pharmacol Exp Ther* 259:1323, 1991.
28. Bascom R and others: Major basic protein and eosinophil-derived neurotoxin concentrations in nasal lavage fluid after antigen challenge: effect of systemic corticosteroids and relationship to eosinophil influx, *J Allergy Clin Immunol* 84:338, 1989.
29. Bassing CH, Swat W, Alt FW: The mechanism and regulation of chromosomal V(D)J recombination, *Cell* 109:S45, 2002.
30. Bauer S and others: Human TLR9 confers responsiveness to bacterial DNA via species-specific CpG motif recognition, *Proc Natl Acad Sci USA* 98:9237, 2001.
31. Baumgarten CR and others: Influx of kininogens into nasal secretions following antigen challenge of allergic individuals, *J Clin Invest* 76:191, 1985.
32. Becker MN and others: CD14-dependent lipopolysaccharide-induced β-defensin-2 expression in human tracheobronchial epithelium, *J Biol Chem* 275:29731, 2000.
33. Befus AD and others: Neutrophil defensins induce histamine secretion from mast cells: mechanisms of action, *J Immunol* 163:947, 1999.
34. Benninger M: Rhinitis, sinusitis and their relationships to allergies, *Am J Rhinol* 6:37, 1992.
35. Bentley AM and others: Immunohistology of the nasal mucosa in seasonal allergic rhinitis: increase in activated eosinophils and epithelial mast cells, *J Allergy Clin Immunol* 89:877, 1992.
36. Bevilacqua MP and others: Interleukin 1 acts on cultured human vascular endothelium to increase the adhesion of polymorphonuclear leukocytes, monocytes and related leukocytic cell lines, *J Clin Invest* 76:2003, 1985.
37. Bevilacqua MP, Nelson RM: Selectins, *J Clin Invest* 91:379, 1993.
38. Binder E and others: Clinical findings in patients with allergic rhinitis, *Rhinology* 22:250, 1984.
39. Bochner BS and others: Adherence of human basophils to cultured umbilical vein vascular endothelial cells, *J Clin Invest* 81:1355, 1988.
40. Bochner BS and others: Adhesion of human basophils, eosinophils, and neutrophils to interleukin 1-activated human vascular endothelial cells: contribution of endothelial cell adhesion molecules, *J Exp Med* 173:1553, 1991.
41. Bodansky HJ and others: Evidence for an environmental effect in the aetiology of insulin dependent diabetes in a transmigratory population, *BMJ* 304:1020, 1992.
42. Borum P: Nasal methacholine challenge: a test for the measurement of nasal reactivity, *J Allergy Clin Immunol* 63:253, 1979.
43. Bouwens L, Wisse E: Pit cells in the liver, *Liver* 12:3, 1992.

44. Bradding P and others: Cytokine immunoreactivity in seasonal rhinitis: regulation by a topical corticosteroid, *Am J Respir Crit Care Med* 151:1900, 1995.

45. Bradding P and others: Immunolocalization of cytokines in the nasal mucosa of normal and perennial rhinitic subjects: the mast cell as a source of IL-4, IL-5, and IL-6 in human allergic mucosal inflammation, *J Immunol* 151:3853, 1993.

46. Bradding P and others: Interleukin 4 is localized to and released by human mast cells, *J Exp Med* 176:1381, 1992.

47. Braun-Fahrländer C and others: Prevalence of hay fever and allergic sensitization in farmer's children and their peers living in the same rural community, *Clin Exp Allergy* 29:28, 1999.

48. Braun-Fahrländer C and others: Environmental exposure to endotoxin and its relation to asthma in school-age children, *N Engl J Med* 347:869, 2002.

49. Braunstahl GJ and others: Segmental bronchial provocation induces nasal inflammation in allergic rhinitis patients, *Am J Respir Crit Care Med* 161:2051, 2000.

50. Braunstahl GJ and others: Nasal allergen provocation induces adhesion molecule expression and tissue eosinophilia in upper and lower airways, *J Allergy Clin Immunol* 107:469, 2001.

51. Braunstein G and others: Clinical and inflammatory responses to exogenous tachykinins in allergic rhinitis, *Am Rev Respir Dis* 144:630, 1991.

52. Brightbill HD and others: Host defense mechanisms triggered by microbial lipoproteins through toll-like receptors, *Science* 285:732, 1999.

53. Brown MG and others: Vital involvement of a natural killer cell activation receptor in resistance to viral infections, *Science* 292:934, 2001.

54. Bryan WTK, Bryan MP: Significance of mast cells in nasal secretions, *Trans Am Acad Ophthalmol Otolaryngol* 63:613, 1959.

55. Castano L, Eisenbarth GS: Type-I diabetes: a chronic autoimmune disease of human, mouse, and rat, *Annu Rev Immunol* 8:647, 1990.

56. Castells M, Schwartz LB: Tryptase levels in nasal lavage fluid as an indicator of the early allergic reaction, *J Allergy Clin Immunol* 82:348, 1988.

57. Chaly YV and others: Neutrophil alpha-defensin human neutrophil peptide modulates cytokine production in human monocytes and adhesion molecule expression in endothelial cells, *Eur Cytokine Netw* 11:257, 2000.

58. Chertov O and others: Leukocyte granule proteins mobilize innate host defenses and adaptive immune responses, *Immunol Rev* 177:68, 2000.

59. Clutterbuck EJ, Hirst EMA, Sanderson CJ: Human interleukin-5 (IL-5) regulates the production of eosinophils in human bone marrow cultures: comparison and interaction with IL-1, IL-3, IL-6 and GM-CSF, *Blood* 73:1504, 1989.

60. Connell JT: Quantitative intranasal pollen challenge: III. The priming effect in allergic rhinitis, *J Allergy* 43:33, 1969.

61. Corren J, Adinoff AD, Irvin CG: Changes in bronchial responsiveness following nasal provocation with allergen, *J Allergy Clin Immunol* 89:611, 1992.

62. Creticos PS and others: Peptide leukotriene release after antigen challenge in patients sensitive to ragweed, *N Engl J Med* 310:1626, 1984.

63. DeFrance T, Banchereau J: *Role of cytokines in the ontogeny, activation and proliferation of B lymphocytes*. London, Academic Press, 1990.

64. DeFrance T and others: Interleukin 10 and transforming growth factor beta cooperate to induce anti-CD40-activated naive human B cells to secrete immunoglobulin A, *J Exp Med* 175:671, 1992.

65. Delacroix DL and others: Selective transport of polymeric immunoglobulin A in bile, *J Clin Invest* 70:230, 1982.

66. Del Prete G and others: IL-4 is an essential co-factor for the IgE synthesis induced in vitro by human T cell clones and their supernatants, *J Immunol* 140:4193, 1988.

67. Denburg JA, Silver JE, Abrams JS: Interleukin-5 is a human basophilopoietin: induction of histamine content and basophilic differentiation of HL-60 cells and of peripheral blood basophil-eosinophil progenitors, *Blood* 77:1462, 1991.

68. Dobrina A and others: Mechanisms of eosinophil adherence to cultured vascular endothelial cells: eosinophils bind to the cytokine-induced endothelial ligand vascular cell adhesion molecule-1 via the very late activation antigen-4 integrin receptor, *J Clin Invest* 88:20, 1991.

69. Dorschner RA and others: Cutaneous injury induces the release of cathelicidin antimicrobial peptides active against group A Streptococcus, *J Invest Dermatol* 117:91, 2001.

70. Dorshkind K: Regulation of hemopoiesis by bone marrow stromal cells and their products, *Annu Rev Immunol* 8:111, 1990.

71. Droste JHJ and others: Does the use of antibiotics in early childhood increase the risk of asthma and allergic disease? *Clin Exp Allergy* 30:1547, 2000.

72. Druce HM and others: Cholinergic nasal hyperreactivity in atopic subjects, *J Allergy Clin Immunol* 76:445, 1985.

73. Durham SR and others: Cytokine messenger RNA expression for IL-3, IL-4, IL-5, and granulocyte/macrophage-colony-stimulating factor in the nasal mucosa after local allergen provocation: relationship to tissue eosinophilia, *J Immunol* 148:2390, 1992.

74. Durham SR, Kay AB, Hamid Q: Changes in allergic inflammation associated with successful immunotherapy, *Int Arch Allergy Immunol* 107:282, 1995.

75. Dvoracek JE and others: Induction of nasal late-phase reactions by insufflation of ragweed-pollen extract, *J Allergy Clin Immunol* 73:363, 1984.

76. Ebisawa M and others: Eosinophil transendothelial migration induced by cytokines: III. Effect of the chemokine RANTES, *J Immunol* 153:2153, 1994.

77. Ebisawa M and others: Eosinophil transendothelial migration induced by cytokines: II. Potentiation of eosinophil transendothelial migration by eosinophil-active cytokines, *J Immunol* 152:4590, 1994.

78. Ebisawa M and others: Eosinophil transendothelial migration induced by cytokines: I. Role of endothelial and eosinophil adhesion molecules in IL-1 b-induced transendothelial migration, *J Immunol* 149:4021, 1992.

79. Enerback L, Pipkorn U, Granerus G: Intraepithelial migration of nasal mucosal mast cells in hay fever, *Int Arch Allergy Appl Immunol* 80:44, 1986.

80. Erickson N, Quesenberry PJ: Regulation of erythropoiesis: the role of growth factors, *Med Clin North Am* 76:745, 1992.

81. EURODIAB ACE Study Group: Variation and trends in incidence of childhood diabetes in Europe, *Lancet* 355:873, 2000.

82. Fokkens WJ and others: Fluctuation of the number of CD-1 (T6)-positive dendritic cells, presumably Langerhans cells, in the nasal mucosa of patients with an isolated grass-pollen allergy before, during, and after the grass-pollen season, *J Allergy Clin Immunol* 84:39, 1989.

83. Frank MM, Fries LF: The role of complement in inflammation and phagocytosis, *Immunol Today* 12:322, 1991.

84. Freeland H and others: Leukotriene B$_4$ as a mediator of early and late reactions to antigen in humans: the effect of systemic glucocorticoid treatment in vivo, *J Allergy Clin Immunol* 83:634, 1989.

85. Frohm M and others: The expression of the gene coding for the antibacterial peptide LL-37 is induced in human keratinocytes during inflammatory disorders, *J Biol Chem* 272:15258, 1997.

86. Fulton C and others: Expression of natural peptide antibiotics in human skin, *Lancet* 350:1750, 1997.

87. Furukawa CT: The role of allergy in sinusitis in children, *J Allergy Clin Immunol* 90:515, 1992.

88. Furukawa K and others: Expression of nitric oxide synthase in the human nasal mucosa, *Am J Respir Crit Care Med* 153:847, 1996.

89. Gadol N, Peacock MA, Ault KA: Antigenic phenotype and functional characterization of human tonsil B cells, *Blood* 71:1048, 1988.

90. Gaga M and others: Eosinophils are a feature of upper and lower airway pathology in non-atopic asthma, irrespective of the presence of rhinitis, *Clin Exp Allergy* 30:663, 2000.

91. Gal P, Ambrus G: Structure and function of complement activating enzyme complexes: C1 and MBL-MASPs, *Curr Protein Pept Sci* 2:43, 2001.

92. Ganz T and others: Defensins. Natural peptide antibiotics of human neutrophils, *J Clin Invest* 76:1427, 1985.

93. Garcia JR and others: Human beta-defensin 4: a novel inducible peptide with a specific salt-sensitive spectrum of antimicrobial activity, *FASEB J* 15:1819, 2001.

94. Gascan H and others: Human B cell clones can be induced to proliferate and to switch to IgE and IgG4 synthesis by interleukin 4 and a signal provided by activated CD4+ T cell clones, *J Exp Med* 173:747, 1991.

95. Gascan H and others: Regulation of human IgE synthesis, *Clin Exp Allergy* 21:162, 1991.

96. Gell PGH, Coombs RRA: *Clinical aspects of immunology.* Oxford, Blackwell, 1963.

97. Gellert M: V(D)J recombination: rag proteins, repair factors, and regulation, *Annu Rev Biochem* 71:101, 2002.

98. Gomez E and others: Direct in vivo evidence for mast cell degranulation during allergen-induced reactions in man, *J Allergy Clin Immunol* 78:637, 1986.

99. Goodman T, Lefrancois L: Intraepithelial lymphocytes: anatomical site, not T cell receptor form, dictates phenotype and function, *J Exp Med* 170:1569, 1989.

100. Gosset P and others: Interleukin-6 and interleukin-1 alpha production is associated with antigen-induced late nasal response, *J Allergy Clin Immunol* 92:878, 1993.

101. Gounni AS and others: High affinity IgE receptor on eosinophils is involved in defense against parasites, *Nature* 367:183, 1994.

102. Grant EP and others: Molecular recognition of lipid antigens by T cell receptors, *J Exp Med* 189:195, 1999.

103. Gray JD, Horwitz DA: Lymphocytes expressing type 3 receptors proliferate in response to interleukin 2 and are the precursors of lymphokine-activated killer cells, *J Clin Invest* 81:1247, 1988.

104. Greisner WA, Settipane RJ, Settipane GA: Co-existence of asthma and allergic rhinitis: a 23-year follow-up study of college students, *Allergy Asthma Proc* 19:185, 1998.

105. Groux H and others: A CD4+ T-cell subset inhibits antigen-specific T-cell responses and prevents colitis, *Nature* 389:737, 1997.

106. Guerder S, Flavell RA: Costimulation in tolerance and autoimmunity, *Int Rev Immunol* 13:135, 1995.

107. Hamid Q and others: Co-expression of CD25 and CD3 in atopic allergy and asthma, *Immunology* 75:659, 1992.

108. Harder J and others: A peptide antibiotic from human skin, *Nature* 387:861, 1997.

109. Harder J and others: Isolation and characterization of human beta-defensin-3, a novel human inducible peptide antibiotic, *J Biol Chem* 276:5707, 2001.

110. Harwig SS, Ganz T, Lehrer RI: Neutrophil defensins: purification, characterization, and antimicrobial testing, *Methods Enzymol* 236:160, 1994.

111. Hayashi F and others: The innate immune response to bacterial flagellin is mediated by Toll-like receptor 5, *Nature* 410:1099, 2001.

112. Hemler ME: VLA proteins in the integrin family: structures, functions, and their role on leukocytes, *Annu Rev Immunol* 8:365, 1990.

113. Hemmi H and others: A Toll-like receptor that recognizes bacterial DNA, *Nature* 408:740, 2000.

114. Heyworth CM and others: Stem cell factor directly stimulates the development of enriched granulocyte-macrophage colony-forming cells and promotes the effects of other colony stimulating factors, *Blood* 80:2230, 1992.

115. Hirai K and others: Enhancement of human basophil histamine release by interleukin 5, *J Exp Med* 172:1525, 1990.

116. Hoffmann JA and others: Phylogenetic perspectives in innate immunity, *Science* 284:1313, 1999.

117. Holm AF and others: Effect of 3 months' nasal steroid therapy on nasal T cells and Langerhans cells in patients suffering from allergic rhinitis, *Allergy* 50:204, 1995.

118. Holzer P: Capsaicin: cellular targets, mechanisms of action, and selectivity for thin sensory neurons, *Pharmacol Rev* 43:143, 1991.

119. Hoover GE and others: Chronic sinusitis: risk factors for extensive disease, *J Allergy Clin Immunol* 100:185, 1997.

120. Hopfenspirger MT and others: Mycobacterial antigens attenuate late phase response, airway hyperresponsiveness, and bronchoalveolar lavage eosinophilia in a mouse model of bronchial asthma, *Int Immunopharmacol* 1:1743, 2001.

121. Huber AR and others: Regulation of transendothelial neutrophil migration by endogenous interleukin-8, *Science* 254:99, 1991.

122. Husband AJ, Gowans JL: The origin and antigen-dependent distribution of IgA-containing cells in the intestine, *J Exp Med* 148:1146, 1978.

123. Itoh N and others: The polypeptide encoded by the cDNA for human cell surface antigen Fas can mediate apoptosis, *Cell* 66:233, 1991.

124. Iwens P, Clement PA: Sinusitis in allergic patients, *Rhinology* 32:67, 1994.

125. Jabara HH and others: CD40 and IgE: synergism between anti-CD40 monoclonal antibody and interleukin 4 in the induction of IgE synthesis by highly purified human B cells, *J Exp Med* 172:1861, 1990.

126. Jones DE, Bevins CL: Defensin-6 mRNA in human Paneth cells: implications for antimicrobial peptides in host defense of the human bowel, *FEBS Lett* 315:187, 1993.

127. Juliusson S and others: Mast cells and eosinophils in the allergic mucosal response to allergen challenge: changes in distribution and signs of activation in relation to symptoms, *J Allergy Clin Immunol* 90:898, 1992.

128. Kameyoshi Y and others: Cytokine RANTES released by thrombin-stimulated platelets is a potent attractant for human eosinophils, *J Exp Med* 176:587, 1992.

129. Karlsson G, Holmburg K: Does allergic rhinitis predispose to sinusitis? *Acta Otolaryngol Suppl* 515:26, 1994.

130. Kaufmann SHE: Immunity to intracellular bacteria, *Annu Rev Immunol* 11:129, 1993.

131. Kero J and others: Could TH1 and TH2 diseases coexist? Evaluation of asthma incidence in children with coeliac disease, type 1 diabetes, or rheumatoid arthritis: a register study, *J Allergy Clin Immunol* 108:781, 2001.

132. Kirshenbaum AS and others: Effect of IL-3 and stem cell factor on the appearance of human basophils and mast cells from CD34+ pluripotent progenitor cells, *J Immunol* 148:772, 1992.

133. Klementsson H and others: Changes in non-specific nasal reactivity and eosinophil influx and activation after allergen challenge, *Clin Exp Allergy* 20:539, 1990.

134. Klementsson H and others: Eosinophils, secretory responsiveness and glucocorticoid-induced effects on the nasal mucosa during a weak pollen season, *Clin Exp Allergy* 21:705, 1991.

135. Kojis FG: Serum sickness and anaphylaxis: analysis of 6,211 patients treated with horse serum for various infections, *Am J Dis Child* 64:93, 1942.

136. Kokumai S and others: Effect of capsaicin as a neuropeptide-releasing substance on sneezing reflex in a type 1 allergic animal model, *Int Arch Allergy Immunol* 98:256, 1992.

137. Konno A, Togawa K: Role of the vidian nerve in nasal allergy, *Ann Otol Rhinol Laryngol* 88:258, 1979.

138. Kuhn LC, Kraehenbuhl JP: Role of secretory component, a secreted glycoprotein, in the specific uptake of IgA dimer by epithelial cells, *J Biol Chem* 254:11072, 1979.

139. Lacy P, Moqbel R: Immune effector functions of eosinophils in allergic airway inflammation, *Curr Opin Allergy Clin Immunol* 1:79, 2001.

140. Lacroix JS and others: Improvement of symptoms of non-allergic chronic rhinitis by local treatment with capsaicin, *Clin Exp Allergy* 21:595, 1991.

141. Lamas AM, Mulroney CR, Schleimer RP: Studies on the adhesive interaction between human eosinophils and cultured vascular endothelial cells, *J Immunol* 140:1500, 1988.

142. Lanier LL and others: The relationship of CD16 (Leu-11) and Leu-19 (NKH-1) antigen expression on human peripheral blood NK cells and cytotoxic T lymphocytes, *J Immunol* 136:4480, 1986.

143. Lanzavecchia A: Antigen-specific interaction between T and B cells, *Nature* 314:537, 1985.

144. Lee BJ and others: Upregulation of vascular cell adhesion molecule-1 (VCAM-1) after nasal allergen (Ag) challenge, *J Allergy Clin Immunol* 94:1006, 1994.

145. Lee SH and others: Expression of human beta-defensin 1 mRNA in human nasal mucosa, *Acta Otolaryngol* 120:58, 2000.

146. Lee SH and others: Antimicrobial defensin peptides of the human nasal mucosa, *Ann Otol Rhinol Laryngol* 111:135, 2002.

147. Lefrancois L, Goodman T: In vivo modulation of cytolytic activity and Thy-1 expression in TCR γδ intraepithelial lymphocytes, *Science* 243:1716, 1989.

148. Lehrer RI and others: Direct inactivation of viruses by MCP-1 and MCP-2, natural peptide antibiotics from rabbit leukocytes, *J Virol* 54:467, 1985.

149. Leibowitz U and others: Epidemiological study of multiple sclerosis in Israel. II. Multiple sclerosis and level of sanitation, *J Neurol Neurosurg Psychiatry* 29:60, 1966.

150. Lenschow DJ, Walunas TL, Bluestone JA: CD28/B7 system of T cell costimulation, *Annu Rev Immunol* 14:233, 1996.

151. Leynaert B and others: Perennial rhinitis: An independent risk factor for asthma in nonatopic subjects: results from the European Community Respiratory Health Survey, *J Allergy Clin Immunol* 104:301, 1999.

152. Lim MC, Taylor RM, Naclerio RM: The histology of allergic rhinitis and its comparison to nasal lavage, *Am J Respir Crit Care Med* 151:136, 1995.

153. Linden M and others: Nasal cytokines in common cold and allergic rhinitis, *Clin Exp Allergy* 25:166, 1995.

154. Linsley PS and others: Binding of the B cell activation antigen B7 to CD28 costimulates T cell proliferation and interleukin 2 mRNA accumulation, *J Exp Med* 173:721, 1991.

155. Liszewski MK and others: Control of the complement system, *Adv Immunol* 61:201, 1996.

156. Lo SK and others: Endothelial-leukocyte adhesion molecule-1 stimulates the adhesive activity of leukocyte integrin CR3 (CD11b/CD18, Mac-1, alpha$_m$ beta$_2$) on human neutrophils, *J Exp Med* 173:1493, 1991.

157. Lopez AF and others: Recombinant human interleukin 5 is a selective activator of human eosinophil function, *J Exp Med* 167:219, 1988.

158. Luczynska CM and others: Airborne concentrations and particle size distribution of allergen derived from domestic cats (Felis domesticus): measurements using cascade impactor, liquid impinger and a two site monoclonal antibody assay for Fel d 1, *Am Rev Respir Dis* 141:361, 1990.

159. Lung MA, Widdicombe JG: Lung reflexes and nasal vascular resistance in the anesthetized dog, *J Physiol* 386:465, 1987.

160. Luscinskas FW and others: Cytokine-activated human endothelial monolayers support enhanced neutrophil transmigration via a mechanism involving both endothelial-leukocyte adhesion molecule-1 and intracellular adhesion molecule-1, *J Immunol* 146:1617, 1991.

161. Majchel AM and others: The nasal response to histamine challenge: effect of the pollen season and immunotherapy, *J Allergy Clin Immunol* 90:85, 1992.

162. Malo JL and others: Prevalence and intensity of rhinoconjunctivitis in subjects with occupational asthma, *Eur Respir J* 10:1513, 1997.

163. Martin U and others: Increased levels of exhaled nitric oxide during nasal and oral breathing in subjects with seasonal rhinitis, *J Allergy Clin Immunol* 97:768, 1996.

164. Masuyama K and others: Topical glucocorticosteroid (fluticasone propionate) inhibits cells expressing cytokine mRNA for interleukin-4 in the nasal mucosa in allergen-induced rhinitis, *Immunology* 82:192, 1994.

165. McKinney PA and others: Early social mixing and childhood type 1 diabetes mellitus: a case-control study in Yorkshire, UK, *Diabet Med* 17:236, 2000.

166. McVay LD, Carding SR: Generation of human gamma delta T-cell repertoires, *Crit Rev Immunol* 19:431, 1999.

167. Mendoza JF and others: Evidence that G-CSF is a fibroblast growth factor that induces granulocytes to increase phagocytosis and to present a mature morphology, and that macrophages secrete 45-kd molecules with these activities as well as with G-CSF like activity, *Exp Hematol* 18:903, 1990.

168. Miadonna A and others: Evidence of PAF-acether metabolic pathway activation in antigen challenge of upper respiratory airways, *Am Rev Respir Dis* 140:142, 1989.

169. Miller JF: The discovery of thymus function and of thymus-derived lymphocytes, *Immunol Rev* 185:7, 2002.

170. Modlin RL: Mammalian Toll-like receptors, *Ann Allergy Asthma Immunol* 88:543, 2002.

171. Montefort S and others: The expression of leukocyte-endothelial adhesion molecules is increased in perennial allergic rhinitis, *Am J Respir Cell Mol Biol* 7:393, 1992.

172. Moretta L and others: Surface receptors that regulate the NK cell function: beyond the NK cell scope, *Curr Top Microbiol Immunol* 266:11, 2002.

173. Moser C and others: Beta-defensin 1 contributes to pulmonary innate immunity in mice, *Infect Immun* 70:3068, 2002.

174. Moser R and others: Interleukin 1 and tumor necrosis factor stimulate human vascular endothelial cells to promote transendothelial neutrophil passage, *J Clin Invest* 83:444, 1989.

175. Moser R and others: Migration of primed human eosinophils across cytokine-activated endothelial cell monolayers, *Blood* 79:2937, 1992.

176. Mosimann BL and others: Substance P, calcitonin gene-related peptide, and vasoactive intestinal peptide increase in nasal secretions after allergen challenge in atopic patients, *J Allergy Clin Immunol* 92:95, 1993.

177. Mosmamn TR, Coffman RL: TH1 and TH2 cells: different patterns of lymphokine secretion lead to different functional properties, *Annu Rev Immunol* 7:145, 1989.

178. Motegi Y, Kita H: Interaction with secretory component stimulates effector functions of human eosinophils, but not of neutrophils, *J Immunol* 161:4340, 1998.

179. Mullarkey MF, Hill JS, Webb DR: Allergic and nonallergic rhinitis: their characterization with attention to the meaning of nasal eosinophilia, *J Allergy Clin Immunol* 65:122, 1980.

180. Muzio M and others: Differential expression and regulation of toll-like receptors (TLR) in human leukocytes: selective expression of TLR3 in dendritic cells, *J Immunol* 164:5998, 2000.

181. Naclerio RM and others: Inflammatory mediators in late antigen-induced rhinitis, *N Engl J Med* 313:65, 1985.

182. Naclerio RM, DeTineo ML, Baroody FM: Ragweed allergic rhinitis and the paranasal sinuses: a computed tomographic study, *Arch Otolaryngol Head Neck Surg* 123:193, 1997.

183. Naclerio RM and others: Mediator release after airway challenge with antigen, *Am Rev Respir Dis* 128:597, 1983.

184. Nagler A and others: Comparative studies of human FcRIII-positive and negative natural killer cells, *J Immunol* 143:3183, 1989.

185. Nathanson I, Widdicombe JG, Barnes PJ: Effect of vasoactive intestinal peptide on ion transport across dog tracheal epithelium, *J Appl Physiol* 55:1844, 1983.

186. Neben TY and others: Recombinant human interleukin-11 stimulates megakaryocytopoiesis and increases peripheral platelets in normal and splenectomized mice, *Blood* 81:901, 1993.

187. Newman LJ and others: Chronic sinusitis: relationship of computed tomography findings to allergy, asthma, and eosinophilia, *JAMA* 271:363, 1994.

188. Niyonsaba F and others: A cathelicidin family of human antibacterial peptide LL-37 induces mast cell chemotaxis, *Immunology* 106:20, 2002.

189. Niyonsaba F: Evaluation of the effects of peptide antibiotics human beta-defensins-1/-2 and LL-37 on histamine release and prostaglandin D(2) production from mast cells, *Eur J Immunol* 31:1066, 2001.

190. Ohtsuka H: Heterogeneity of metachromatic cells in the human nose: significance of mucosal mast cells, *J Allergy Clin Immunol* 76:695, 1985.

191. Okamoto Y and others: Cytokine expression after the topical administration of substance P to human nasal mucosa: the role of substance P in nasal allergy, *J Immunol* 151:4391, 1993.

192. Okayama M and others: Muscarinic receptor subtypes in human nasal mucosa: characterization, autoradiographic

193. Okuda M, Ohtsuka H: Basophilic cells in allergic nasal secretions, *Arch Otorhinolaryngol* 214:283, 1977.

194. Okuda M, Ohtsuka H, Kawabori S: Basophil leukocytes and mast cells in the nose, *Eur J Respir Dis Suppl* 64:7, 1983.

195. Okuda M and others: Ultrastructural heterogeneity of the basophilic cells in the allergic nasal mucosa, *Ann Allergy* 154:152, 1985.

196. Ownby DR, Johnson CC, Peterson EL: Exposure to dogs and cats in the first year of life and risk of allergic sensitivity at 6 to 7 years of age, *JAMA* 288:963, 2002.

197. Parronchi P and others: Allergen and bacterial antigen-specific T cell clones established from atopic donors show a different profile of cytokine production, *Proc Natl Acad Sci USA* 88:4538, 1991.

198. Parronchi P and others: IL-4 and IFN (alpha and gamma) exert opposite regulatory effects on the development of cytolytic potential by T_{H1} or T_{H2} human T cell clones, *J Immunol* 149:2977, 1992.

199. Pedersen PA, Weeke ER: Asthma and allergic rhinitis in the same patients, *Allergy* 38:25, 1983.

200. Pelikan Z, Pelikan-Filipek M: Role of nasal allergy in chronic maxillary sinusitis-diagnostic value of nasal challenge with allergen, *J Allergy Clin Immunol* 86:484, 1990.

201. Pelikan Z: Late and delayed responses of the nasal mucosa to allergen challenge, *Ann Allergy* 41:37, 1978.

202. Perussia B, London L, Trinchieri G: Phenotypic characteristics of human natural killer cells, *Biomed Pharmacother* 39:13, 1985.

203. Peterson EJ and others: Adaptor proteins in lymphocyte antigen-receptor signaling, *Curr Opin Immunol* 10:337, 1998.

204. Petersson G and others: Capsaicin evokes secretion of nasal fluid and depletes substance P and calcitonin-gene related peptide from the nasal mucosa in the rat, *Br J Pharmacol* 98:930, 1989.

205. Petz LD, Branch DR: *Drug induced immune hemolytic anemia*. In Chaplin H, editor: *Methods in hematology*, vol 12. New York, Churchill Livingstone, 1985.

206. Philip G, Sanico AM, Togias A: Inflammatory cellular influx follows capsaicin nasal challenge, *Am J Respir Crit Care Med* 153:1222, 1996.

207. Philip G and others: The human nasal response to capsaicin, *J Allergy Clin Immunol* 94:1035, 1994.

208. Poltorak A and others: Defective LPS signaling in C3H/HeJ and C57BL/10ScCr mice: mutations in Tlr4 gene, *Science* 282:2085, 1998.

209. Poser S and others: Increasing incidence of multiple sclerosis in South Lower Saxony, Germany, *Neuroepidemiology* 8:207, 1989.

210. Punnonen J and others: Interleukin 13 induces interleukin 4-independent IgG4 and IgE synthesis and CD23 expression by human B cells, *Proc Natl Acad Sci USA* 90:3730, 1993.

211. Quayle AJ and others: Gene expression, immunolocalization, and secretion of human defensin-5 in human female reproductive tract, *Am J Pathol* 152:1247, 1998.

212. Rachelefsky GS and others: Sinus disease in children with respiratory allergy, *J Allergy Clin Immunol* 61:310, 1978.

213. Raphael GD and others: Pathophysiology of rhinitis: II. Assessment of the sources of protein in histamine-induced nasal secretions, *Am Rev Respir Dis* 139:791, 1989.

214. Raphael GD and others: The pathophysiology of rhinitis: V. Sources of protein in allergen-induced nasal secretions, *J Allergy Clin Immunol* 88:33, 1991.

215. Rappolee DA, Werb A: *Macrophage-derived growth factors.* In Russell SW, Gordon S, editors: *Macrophage biology and activation.* Berlin, Springer-Verlag, 1992.

216. Riedler J and others: Exposure to farming in early life and development of asthma and allergy: a cross-sectional survey, *Lancet* 358:1129, 2001.

217. Ritonja A and others: Primary structure of a new cysteine proteinase inhibitor from pig leukocytes, *FEBS Lett* 255:211, 1989.

218. Roost HP and others: Role of current and childhood exposure to cat and atopic sensitization: European Community Respiratory Health Survey, *J Allergy Clin Immunol* 104:941, 1999.

219. Rot A and others: RANTES and macrophage inflammatory protein 1 alpha induce the migration and activation of normal human eosinophil granulocytes, *J Exp Med* 176:1489, 1992.

220. Sabroe I and others: Differential regulation of eosinophil chemokine signaling via CCR3 and non-CCR3 pathways, *J Immunol* 162:2946, 1999.

221. Saengpanich S and others: Effects of Intranasal Azelastine on the Response to Nasal Allergen Challenge, *Laryngoscope* 112:47, 2002.

222. Saito H and others: Selective differentiation and proliferation of hematopoietic cells induced by recombinant human interleukins, *Proc Natl Acad Sci USA* 85:2288, 1988.

223. Sarti W, Gomes-Monteiro LA, Machado CSM: The treatment of allergic rhinitis improves the recovery from asthma and upper respiratory infections, *Sao Paulo Medical Journal/RPM* 113:968, 1995.

224. Savolainen S: Allergy in patients with acute maxillary sinusitis, *Allergy* 44:116, 1989.

225. Schall TJ and others: Selective attraction of monocytes and T lymphocytes of the memory phenotype by cytokine RANTES, *Nature* 347:669, 1990.

226. Schierhorn K and others: Substance-P-induced histamine release from human nasal mucosa in vitro, *Int Arch Allergy Immunol* 107:109, 1995.

227. Schleimer RP and others: IL-4 induces adherence of human eosinophils and basophils but not neutrophils to endothelium: association with expression of VCAM-1, *J Immunol* 148:1086, 1992.

228. Schleimer RP, Rutledge BK: Cultured human vascular endothelial cells acquire adhesiveness for leukocytes following stimulation with interleukin-1, endotoxin, and tumor promoting phorbol esters, *J Immunol* 136:649, 1986.

229. Seder RA, Paul WE: Acquisition of lymphokine-producing phenotype by CD4+ T cells, *Annu Rev Immunol* 12:635, 1994.

230. Selsted ME and others: Enteric defensins: antibiotic peptide components of intestinal host defense, *J Cell Biol* 118:929, 1992.

231. Settipane RA: Complications of allergic rhinitis, *Allergy Asthma Proc* 20:209, 1999.

232. Shapiro GG and others: Immunologic defects in patients with refractory sinusitis, *Pediatrics* 87:311, 1991.

233. Shapiro GG: Role of allergy in sinusitis, *Pediatr Infect Dis* 4:S55, 1985.

234. Sher A, Ottesen E: *Immunoparasitology.* In Samter M and others, editors: *Immunological diseases,* ed 4. Boston, Little, Brown, 1988.

235. Shevach EM: CD4+ CD25+ suppressor T cells: more questions than answers, *Nat Rev Immunol* 2:389, 2002.

236. Sim TC and others: Proinflammatory cytokines in nasal secretions of allergic subjects after antigen challenge, *Am J Respir Crit Care Med* 149:339, 1994.

237. Sim TC and others: Secretion of chemokines and other cytokines in allergen-induced nasal responses: inhibition by topical steroid treatment, *Am J Respir Crit Care Med* 152:927, 1995.

238. Simpson CR and others: Coincidence of immune-mediated diseases driven by Th1 and Th2 subsets suggests a common aetiology: a population-based study using computerized general practice data, *Clin Exp Allergy* 32:37, 2002.

239. Spector SL: The role of allergy in sinusitis in adults, *J Allergy Clin Immunol* 90:518, 1992.

240. Spiegelberg HL, Raz E: DNA-based approaches to the treatment of allergies, *Curr Opin Mol Ther* 4:64, 2002.

241. Springer TA: Adhesion receptors of the immune system, *Nature* 346:425, 1990.

242. Staege H, Schaffner A, Schneemann M: Human toll-like receptors 2 and 4 are targets for deactivation of mononuclear phagocytes by interleukin-4, *Immunol Lett* 71:1, 2000.

243. Stahl CP and others: Differential effects of sequential, simultaneous, and single agent interleukin-3 and granulocyte-macrophage colony-stimulating factor on megakaryocyte maturation and platelet response in primates, *Blood* 80:2479, 1992.

244. Staines A and others: Incidence of insulin dependent diabetes mellitus in Karachi, Pakistan, *Arch Dis Child* 76:121, 1997.

245. Stern M and others: Apoptosis in human eosinophils: programmed cell death in the eosinophil leads to phagocytosis by macrophages and is modulated by IL-5, *J Immunol* 148:3543, 1992.

246. Strachan DP: Hay fever, hygiene, and household size, *BMJ* 299:1259, 1989.

247. Sung CP, Arleth AJ, Feverstein GZ: Neuropeptide Y upregulates the adhesiveness of human endothelial cells for leukocytes, *Clin Res* 68:314, 1991.

248. Swarbrick ET, Farrokhyar F, Irvine EJ: A critical review of epidemiological studies in inflammatory bowel disease, *Scand J Gastroenterol* 36:2, 2001.

249. Takahashi T and others: Megakaryocyte potentiating activity of IL-1, IL-6 and GM-CSF as evaluated by their action on in vitro human megakaryocytic colonies, *Br J Haematol* 78:480, 1991.

250. Takeuchi O and others: Differential roles of TLR2 and TLR4 in recognition of gram-negative and gram-positive bacterial cell wall components, *Immunity* 11:443, 1999.

251. Tepper RI and others: IL-4 induces allergic-like inflammatory disease and alters T cell development in transgenic mice, *Cell* 62:457, 1990.

252. Tepper RI, Pattengale PK, Leder P: Murine interleukin-4 displays potent anti-tumor activity in vivo, *Cell* 57:503, 1989.

253. The EURODIAB Substudy 2 Study Group: Decreased prevalence of atopic diseases in children with diabetes, *J Pediatr* 137:470, 2000.

254. Thomas MJ and others: T cytotoxic 1 and T cytotoxic 2 CD8 T cells both inhibit IgE responses, *Int Arch Allergy Immunol* 124:187, 2001.

255. Thornhill MH, Kyan-Aung U, Haskard DO: IL-4 increases human endothelial cell adhesiveness for T cells but not for neutrophils, *J Immunol* 144:3060, 1990.

256. Timonen T, Ortaldo JR, Herberman RB: Characteristics of human large granular lymphocytes and relationship to natural killer and NK cells, *J Exp Med* 153:569, 1981.

257. Tsuda T and others: Synergistic effects of nerve growth factor and granulocyte-macrophage colony-stimulating factor on human basophilic cell differentiation, *Blood* 77:971, 1991.

258. Upton MN and others: Intergenerational 20 year trends in the prevalence of asthma and hay fever in adults: the Midspan family study surveys of parents and offspring, *BMJ* 321:88, 2000.

259. Van Ewijk W: T-cell differentiation is influenced by thymic microenvironments, *Annu Rev Immunol* 9:591, 1991.

260. van Rooijen N and others: Macrophages in host defense mechanisms, *Curr Top Microbiol Immunol* 210:159, 1996.

261. Varney VA and others: Immunohistology of the nasal mucosa following allergen-induced rhinitis, *Am Rev Respir Dis* 146:170, 1992.

262. Von Boehmer H and others: The expression of CD4 and CD8 accessory molecules on mature T cells is not random but correlates with the specificity of the alpha beta receptor for antigen, *Immunol Rev* 109:143, 1989.

263. Wachs M and others: Observations on the pathogenesis of nasal priming, *J Allergy Clin Immunol* 84:492, 1989.

264. Wagenmann M and others: Bilateral increases in histamine after unilateral nasal allergen challenge, *Am J Respir Crit Care Med* 155:426, 1997.

265. Wagenmann M and others: Unilateral nasal allergen challenge leads to bilateral release of prostaglandin D$_2$, *Clin Exp Allergy* 26:371, 1996.

266. Walden SM and others: Antigen-provoked increase in histamine reactivity: observations on mechanisms, *Am Rev Respir Dis* 143:642, 1991.

267. Walsh GM and others: Human eosinophil, but not neutrophil, adherence to IL-1 stimulated human umbilical vascular endothelial cells is a 4b1 (very late antigen-4) dependent, *J Immunol* 146:3419, 1991.

268. Walsh GM and others: IL-5 enhances the in vitro adhesion of human eosinophils, but not neutrophils, in a leukocyte integrin (CD11/18)-dependent manner, *Immunology* 71:258, 1990.

269. Weiner HL and others: Oral tolerance: immunologic mechanisms and treatment of animal and human organ-specific autoimmune diseases by oral administration of autoantigens, *Annu Rev Immunol* 12:809, 1994.

270. Weissler JC and others: Natural killer cell function in human lung is compartmentalized, *Am Rev Respir Dis* 135:941, 1987.

271. Weller PF: Cytokine regulation of eosinophil function, *Clin Immunol Immunopathol* 62:S55, 1992.

272. Weller PF and others: Human eosinophil adherence to vascular endothelium mediated by binding to vascular cell adhesion molecule-1 and endothelial leukocyte adhesion molecule-1, *Proc Natl Acad Sci U S A* 88:7430, 1991.

273. Weller PF: The immunobiology of eosinophils, *N Engl J Med* 324:1110, 1991.

274. Welsh PW and others: Efficacy of beclomethasone nasal solution, flunisolide, and cromolyn in relieving symptoms of ragweed allergy, *Mayo Clin Proc* 62:125, 1987.

275. Williams HC: Is the prevalence of atopic dermatitis increasing? *Clin Exp Dermatol* 17:385, 1992.

276. Wilson AM and others: Antiasthmatic effects of mediator blockade versus topical corticosteroids in allergic rhinitis and asthma, *Am J Respir Crit Care Med* 162:1297, 2000.

277. Woolcock AJ, Peat JK: Evidence for the increase in asthma worldwide, *CIBA Found Symp* 206:122, 1997.

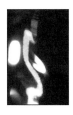

CHAPTER TEN

HEAD AND NECK MANIFESTATIONS OF HUMAN IMMUNODEFICIENCY VIRUS INFECTION

Steven D. Pletcher
Andrew N. Goldberg

INTRODUCTION

The human immunodeficiency virus (HIV) infects and debilitates lymphocytes and macrophages leading to progressive immune compromise. This decline in immune function leaves the patient susceptible to a myriad of pathologic conditions including opportunistic infections and neoplasms, culminating in the acquired immunodeficiency syndrome (AIDS). Much of this pathology can manifest in the head and neck, and thus otolaryngologists should be familiar with the disease and its multiple manifestations.

Anecdotal reports of unusual infections and idiopathic immune deficiency, primarily in homosexual men, began in the early 1980s[216] and rapidly grew into the epidemic now known as AIDS. Since this time, AIDS has been responsible for nearly 500,000 deaths in the United States alone, and close to 1 million Americans are believed to be living with HIV with an estimated 40,000 new infections per year.[44] Although staggering, these national statistics are dwarfed by worldwide statistics. An estimated 42 million people are currently living with HIV infections; 5 million people acquired the virus in 2001 alone.[134]

Transmission of HIV occurs through body fluids and tissues. Virus from an infected patient can inoculate the bloodstream of a potential patient through a breach in the skin or mucosa or via intravenous infusion. Modes of transmission include sexual intercourse (homosexual or heterosexual), the sharing of needles by intravenous drug users, perinatal transmission from mother to child, and, rarely, transfusion of contaminated blood products or accidental exposure in health care workers. Men who have sex with men represent just over 40% of all new cases of HIV infection in the United States with heterosexual intercourse and injection drug use leading to one third and one quarter of new infections, respectively.[44]

Biology and Immunology

HIV is a retrovirus on the Lentivirus subfamily. This group is named for the slow progression of disease in affected individuals and was discovered and initially studied in Icelandic sheep. These viruses establish chronic infections with a long incubation time and slow progression of disease. Viruses in the Lentivirus family typically infect cells involved in immune modulation—in the case of HIV, primarily CD4 T cells and macrophages. HIV is composed of a nucleocapsid core containing two identical genomic RNA strands of approximately 10,000 nucleotides, structural proteins, and a membrane envelope.

The virus life cycle begins when the virus binds to the CD4 receptor, a surface protein on the T-helper subset of T lymphocytes that is also expressed on macrophages. Fusion of the viral and cell membranes allows entry of the viral core into the cell. The reverse transcriptase enzyme, a protein carried by the virus that allows transcription of ribonucleic acid (RNA) into deoxyribonucleic acid (DNA; a reversal of normal transcription) then mediates transcription of the viral RNA genome into viral DNA. Viral integrase, another viral protein, then facilitates incorporation of the viral DNA into the host genome. The viral DNA is then transcribed into multiple RNA copies by the host cell. This newly created RNA can have several fates; it may be spliced and translated into viral proteins or it may remain intact as a future viral genome. Translation of some viral RNA sequences results in protein precursors or multiple proteins bound together. These precursors undergo proteolytic processing by a viral protease that liberates the functional viral proteins. These proteases are required for viral infectivity. After replication of the viral genome and proteins, the new viruses bud from the infected cell and proceed to infect new cells.

Based on the rate of turnover of infected cells, it is estimated that nearly 1 billion infectious events per day occur in patients with active HIV infection.[275] This results in massive requirements for RNA and DNA transcription. The viral DNA polymerase is error prone, incorporating one mismatched nucleotide per genome per round of transcription. This, combined with the amount of replication that occurs, establishes a vast pool of genetic diversity.[176,209] Selection of the least immunogenic and most pathogenic strains of the virus leads to an increased virulence of the virus within the same host.[100,233] The development of vast genetic diversity also gives the virus an advantage in the development of drug resistance and provides a critical barrier to vaccine development.

As the virus infects and damages helper T cells, both humoral and cell-mediated immunity are impaired. This results in increased vulnerability to infection and neoplasm. HIV infection has also been associated with abnormal immune regulation resulting in increased atopy and autoimmune disease. Macrophage function may be impaired because of direct infection or a lack of T-cell stimulation. This results in impaired chemotaxis and phagocytosis with increased vulnerability to infections such as candidiasis and toxoplasmosis. A lack of T-cell stimulation of B cells results in decreased immunoglobulin production and a vulnerability to encapsulated organisms such as *Streptococcus pneumoniae* and other bacteria.[74,100,179] These problems are compounded by impaired neutrophil function. Iatrogenic neutropenia may also result from medications used to treat HIV infections such as zidovudine, ganciclovir, and antineoplastic chemotherapy.[60]

Natural History

When left untreated, HIV infection causes gradual debilitation of the immune system resulting, over a period of years, in profound immunocompromise and AIDS. Patients with AIDS are susceptible to multiple infections and neoplastic conditions. Morbidity can also result from neurotropism and the ability of HIV to cause neurologic and neurotologic dysfunction.

Advances in understanding of HIV biology has allowed for the production of medications targeting the reverse transcriptase and protease enzymes critical to the viral life cycle. Combinations of these protease inhibitors and reverse transcriptase inhibitors are used to create highly active antiretroviral therapy (HAART). The use of this drug "cocktail" has led to an estimated three-fold decrease in mortality and a six-fold decrease in opportunistic infection in HIV patients with a CD4 count of less than 100.[206] As the use of HAART increases, more will be known regarding the long-term prognosis of patients treated with this regimen.

Medications used in HAART therapy can be broadly divided into three categories: nucleoside reverse transcriptase inhibitors (NRTIs), nonnucleoside reverse transcriptase inhibitors (NNRTIs), and protease inhibitors (PIs). Many patients will ultimately experience at least one treatment failure. Because the initial regimen affects choices available for subsequent regimens, clinicians typically avoid using initial regimens that involve medications from all three classes.[316]

The proper timing for the initiation of HAART remains controversial. Recent cohort data demonstrate the importance of initiating HAART before a patient's CD4 count drops below 200/µL.[123,271] In patients with a CD4 count above 350/µL, risk of 3-year clinical progression is low, and additional concerns about the impact of antiretroviral regimens on quality of life, risk of serious adverse drug effects, and limitations on future treatment options may outweigh the benefits of durable viral suppression.[316] The initiation of therapy should also be considered in patients with a viral load above 50,000 to 100,000 copies/mL regardless of CD4 count.[68]

The complex dosing regimens involved in multidrug HAART treatment is a key cause of the virologic failure of antiretroviral treatments.[59] A recent study found a doubling of viral load for every 10% decrement from complete adherence.[11] The viral load response in prisoners with directly observed treatment has been noted to be significantly greater (85% to 100% vs 50% to 80%) than that of patients treated with comparable regimens in an outpatient research clinic.[77,270] Strategic treatment interruptions or "drug holidays" have been considered and reviewed.[114,170] With the paucity of controlled studies and the potential risks, strategic treatment interruptions are not recommended for current clinical practice.[316]

The differential diagnosis of any lesion in an HIV-infected patient depends on the patient's immune status. This is most accurately ascertained through the laboratory values of CD4 count and HIV viral load. CD4 counts have been used as indicators of disease stage in HIV-positive patients for nearly two decades. The likelihood of developing specific opportunistic infections is closely related to CD4 count. The use of CD4 count in the era of HAART is less clear because it is unproven whether CD4 nadir or current CD4 count best correlates with risk of opportunistic infection. HIV viral load is a good predictor of disease progression, even independent of CD4 count.[118,184] HIV viral load also represents a strong surrogate marker for the clinical benefit of treatment.[125,200] HIV-positive patients should be evaluated in the context of their evolving immune status, thus knowledge of the patient's CD4 count, viral load, and treatment status is critical.

Diagnosis and Classification

HIV infection is diagnosed when anti-HIV antibodies are detected in the serum by enzyme-linked immunosorbent assay (ELISA) and Western blot. Persistent antibodies against HIV typically occur within 3 months of infection. The Centers for Disease Control and Prevention (CDC) classification for HIV is based on the clinical manifestations of disease and the patient's CD4 count. These classifications assist in assessing the level of immune compromise and the corresponding risk for development of opportunistic infection or neoplasm. Three clinical categories have been identified: (A) asymptomatic HIV infection, persistent generalized lymphadenopathy (PGL), or acute HIV infection (a mononucleosis-type syndrome); (B) symptomatic conditions such as oral thrush, oral hairy leukoplakia, and fungal sinusitis that are attributed to HIV infection but do not fall into category A or C; (C) AIDS (Box 10-1). Patients in each category can be further stratified according to their CD4+ counts: (1) 500 or more cells/μL, (2) 200 to 499 cells/μL, (3) fewer than 200 cells/μL. The lowest accurate CD4+ count, not the most recent, has been used for classification purposes. AIDS is diagnosed for any patient in category C or 3.

CERVICAL ADENOPATHY IN THE SETTING OF HIV INFECTION

An otolaryngologist is often consulted to evaluate cervical adenopathy in HIV-infected patients. Ideopathic follicular hyperplasia is the most common cause of cervical adenopathy in this patient population and is clinically evident in 12% to 45% of HIV-positive patients.[26] In the background of hyperplastic adenopathy, however, cases of infectious and neoplastic etiology exist, including *Mycobacterium tuberculosis, Pneumocystis carinii,* lymphoma, Kaposi's sarcoma (KS), and other processes that also occur in the general population[157] (Box 10-2). Differentiating among these processes remains challenging yet critical to the appropriate management of lymphadenopathy in the setting of HIV infection. The tendencies for multiple pathologic processes to coexist in HIV-infected patients and the poor sensitivity of many clinical findings and tests often make it necessary to perform microbiologic and histologic evaluations of lymph node tissue.

BOX 10-1
CONDITIONS THAT DEFINE AIDS

Candidiasis, pulmonary or esophageal
Cervical cancer, invasive
Coccidioidomycosis, disseminated or extrapulmonary
Cryptococcosis, extrapulmonary
Cryptosporidiosis, chronic intestinal (>1 month)
Cytomegalovirus disease (liver, spleen, and nodes excluded)
Cytomegalovirus retinitis
Encephalopathy, human immunodeficiency virus–related
Herpes simplex, chronic ulcers (>1 month), pulmonary or esophageal
Histoplasmosis, disseminated or extrapulmonary
Isosporiasis, chronic intestinal (>1 month)
Kaposi's sarcoma
Non-Hodgkin's lymphoma
Mycobacterium avium complex, *Mycobacterium kansasii,* or other species, disseminated or extrapulmonary
Mycobacterium tuberculosis, any site
Pneumocystis carinii pneumonia
Pneumonia, recurrent
Progressive multifocal leukoencephalopathy
Salmonella septicemia, recurrent
Toxoplasmosis of brain
Wasting syndrome caused by human immunodeficiency virus
CD4+ T-helper lymphocyte count less than 200 cells/μL

(Taken from Centers for Disease Control: *MMWR Morb Mortal Wkly Rep* 41:1, 1992.)

BOX 10-2
DIFFERENTIAL DIAGNOSIS OF LYMPHADENOPATHY IN HIV INFECTION

Infectious
Mycobacterial lymphadenitis: tuberculous* and atypical organisms[†]
Pneumocystis lymphadenitis*
Pneumocystis thyroiditis*
Viral lymphadenitis: cytomegalovirus, Epstein-Barr virus
Toxoplasma lymphadenitis
Bacterial lymphadenitis or abscess secondary to oropharyngeal infection
Cat-scratch disease

Neoplastic
Lymphoma
    Non-Hodgkin's[†]
    Hodgkin's disease
Metastatic Kaposi's sarcoma[†]
Metastatic carcinoma
Metastatic melanoma
Salivary gland tumors
Thyroid tumors

Idiopathic
Persistent generalized lymphadenopathy*
Lymphoepithelial cysts of the parotid gland*

---

*Incidence is significantly increased in human immunodeficiency virus infection.
[†]Incidence is significantly increased in acquired immunodeficiency syndrome.

Persistent Generalized Lymphadenopathy

PGL is a common early symptom of HIV infection and a common cause of cervical adenopathy. PGL is defined as lymphadenopathy without an identifiable infectious or neoplastic etiology, which involves two or more extrainguinal sites for at least 3 months, in a patient at risk for or confirmed to be HIV infected.[14,37,58]

The neck is the third most common site of PGL after the axillary and inguinal regions. Within the neck, cervical adenopathy occurs in the posterior triangle (85%), the preauricular and postauricular regions (51%, 47%), the anterior triangle (37%), and the occipital region (30%).[3] Enlarged nodes are usually asymptomatic, but when bulky they sometimes elicit pain. Associated lymphoid hyperplasia in the pharynx may be present and has been implicated in the pathogenesis of middle ear effusions.

Three histologic patterns occur in PGL lymph nodes: (1) follicular hyperplasia—follicles increase in number and size and the mantle zones are either irregular (fragmented) or intact (nonfragmented); (2) follicular involution—follicles are small and mantle zones are absent, whereas germinal centers are either inactive or scarred; and (3) lymphoid depletion—the node is infiltrated by immunoblasts and plasma cells, follicles are absent, and microvascular proliferation is significant.[14,37,58]

As HIV infection approaches end-stage AIDS, the lymph node architecture degenerates from one histologic type to another. Of patients with follicular hyperplasia, 77% progress to follicular involution and lymphoid depletion.[46] It has been proposed that lymph node architecture is of prognostic value in HIV infection because the incidence of constitutional symptoms and opportunistic infections is increased and the life expectancy for patients who progress through these histologic stages is decreased.[2,38,46,162] Proposed mechanisms for this histologic progression include direct cytopathic effects of HIV or similar effects by other viruses, including Epstein Barr virus (EBV), cytomegalovirus (CMV), or herpesviruses.

Evaluation of Cervical Lymphadenopathy in HIV-Positive Patients

In an HIV-infected patient, cervical lymphadenopathy due to pathologic processes that pose a health risk to the patient, such as tuberculosis (TB), lymphoma, and metastatic carcinoma, must be differentiated from PGL. The diagnostic work-up of cervical lymphadenopathy starts with a thorough history and physical examination. The clinician should question the patient about risk factors for infectious causes of cervical adenopathy, including contact with cats and dogs and exposure to TB, as well as risk factors for head and neck malignancy, including tobacco and alcohol use. An enlarged lymph node is more likely to be pathologic when certain local and constitutional features are found on history and physical examination. Fine-needle aspiration (FNA) should be the initial method of pathologic sampling for suspicious nodes.

Although constitutional symptoms by themselves are not a specific indicator of infection or malignancy, the presence of such symptoms without a known cause warrants further investigation. Cervical lymphadenopathy caused by granulomatous disease and lymphoma in HIV infection is associated with weight loss in 33%, night sweats in 50% and fever in 67% of cases.[2,162] However, PGL is also associated with a relatively high incidence of weight loss (24%), night sweats (35%), and fever (47%) caused by other HIV-related processes.

The distribution, size, and mobility of neck nodes may suggest infectious or malignant etiology. Cervical lymphadenopathy that is greater than 2 cm, unilateral, painful, deep, or asymmetric is suspicious for pathology, specifically granulomatous disease or lymphoma.[251] Tender adenopathy is more likely to be secondary to bacterial infections, including TB, whereas nontender enlarging neck nodes may result from malignancy.[38] A thorough head and neck examination should include a search for potential primary sites of infection or malignancy.

The patient's immune status, as indicated by the history of opportunistic infection, CD4+ count, and viral load, may help narrow the differential diagnosis of cervical adenopathy. Lymphoma or mycobacterial infection are more likely to be present when the CD4+ count is less than 100 cells/mL or a history of AIDS is present, whereas PGL is more likely when the CD4+ count is greater than 500 cells/mL. The CD4+ count alone, however, is not sufficient for excluding malignancy or infection.[21,231]

The purified protein derivative (PPD) or tuberculin skin test may facilitate the diagnosis of mycobacterial lymphadenitis. In the setting of advanced HIV infection and immune compromise, however, the patient can become anergic, resulting in a low sensitivity of the PPD test. The criterion for a positive result in an HIV-infected patient is a skin reaction greater than 5 mm in diameter, rather than 10 mm as in the general population.

The effect of HAART on cervical disease in HIV-positive patients is largely unknown. Both KS and non-Hodgkin's lymphoma have significantly decreased in prevalence after the introduction of HAART.[8] Some reports suggest that initiation of therapy involving a protease inhibitor in patients with a low CD4+ count and subclinical mycobacterial infection may result in a significant immune response with suppurative lymphadenopathy and fever.[28,223]

Tissue Sampling in HIV-Positive Patients

FNA should be the initial method of tissue sampling in most cases of suspicious cervical lymphadenopathy in HIV-infected patients. If possible, a cell block should be created from the sample, and the sample should be sent for cytology, flow cytometry, and culture and stains for aerobic and anaerobic bacteria, mycobacteria, and fungi. In a study of 655 aspirates, FNA provided a definitive diagnosis in more than half of the patients and directed further clinical investigation in another 30%; 20% of the initial samples were inadequate for pathologic evaluation.[70] Reactive or benign changes consistent with PGL were found in 37% of patients with suspected or confirmed malignancy in 13%. Inflammation was found in 30%, more than half of which had identifiable organisms on stain, culture, or both.[70] The addition of culture for all specimens was found to be a valuable adjunct.

The diagnostic yield of FNA is increased with multiple passes of the needle while suction is applied to the plunger. The presence of a cytopathologist or a technician is beneficial for two reasons: preparation of the specimen for cytology can be properly and judiciously carried out, and the adequacy of the aspirate for diagnosis can be determined and FNA repeated if necessary. Ultrasound guidance increases the diagnostic yield in nodes that are difficult to palpate. Sensitivities as high as 95% have been reported for the diagnosis of lymphoma in HIV-positive patients.[274] The overall sensitivity and specificity of FNA in HIV-positive cervical adenopathy has not been clearly defined and likely is operator dependent. Sampling errors, improper preparation of cytopathology slides, and misinterpretation of the cytologic features can cause false-negative results.

An FNA diagnosis of follicular hyperplasia should be correlated with the clinical picture and should not, by itself, absolve the clinician's suspicion of lymphoma. The decision to perform a diagnostic open biopsy should be driven by a suspicion of malignancy or infection in the setting of a negative or inconclusive FNA.[57] Conditions that would favor proceeding with an open biopsy in the setting of an FNA that does not demonstrate neoplasm or infection include nodes greater than 2 cm and growing; onset is associated with a low CD4+ count; asymmetric, unilateral, or localized lymphadenopathy; constitutional symptoms of unknown origin; mediastinal adenopathy; or hepatosplenomegaly. Open biopsy of suspected metastatic carcinoma should be avoided and, if possible, the diagnosis should be made by FNA. When metastatic carcinoma is diagnosed, a thorough examination of the upper aerodigestive tract in search of a primary tumor should be performed with the patient under general anesthesia.

Because lymphoma is always a concern, if possible, a cell block should be obtained from the FNA specimen. This allows for further diagnostic evaluation such as flow cytometry to clearly differentiate reactive tissue from lymphoma and determine the class of lymphoma, which may have treatment implications. In patients with lymphoma diagnosed via FNA but without adequate specimen for histologic typing, an open biopsy should be considered. Fresh biopsy specimens should be sent directly to the pathologist, who should be informed of the possibility of lymphoma.

HIV-ASSOCIATED HEAD AND NECK NEOPLASMS

Increased cancer risk is associated with most types of immune deficiency. This has been previously noted in patients with congenital immune disorders and those being treated with immune suppressants after organ transplantation. Malignancies such as non-Hodgkin's lymphoma (NHL) and KS have a strong correlation with advanced HIV infection, so much so that they have been designated as *AIDS-defining illnesses*. The relationship between HIV and other head and neck malignancies is less clear. Although squamous cell carcinomas appear to have a more virulent course in HIV-infected patients, there is no clear increase in the prevalence of squamous cell carcinoma among HIV-positive patients.

Non-Hodgkin's Lymphoma
Epidemiology and Presentation

AIDS-related lymphoma occurs in 3% to 10% of HIV-positive patients.[247] In 1997, this malignancy was the AIDS-defining illness in an estimated 5% of all AIDS cases in the United States.[53,254] The risk of developing NHL steadily rises in conjunction with the duration of HIV infection and the associated immune suppression. The incidence of NHL among homosexual men has been shown to increase from 0.8% 3 years after seroconversion to 2.6% after 8 years of HIV infection.[221] The majority of HIV-positive patients who develop NHL have a CD4+ count lower than 200 cells/μL, and as many as 32% of patients have been previously diagnosed with AIDS. Thus, a high index of suspicion for lymphoma must be maintained for patients with low CD4 counts.

Despite the predilection for relative immune suppression, NHL may occur in the setting of relative immune competence and thus can not be ruled out based on a high CD4+ count or low viral load. Burkitt's lymphoma, in particular, has been noted to occur in patients with a relatively high CD4+ count.[21,231] Interestingly, although the introduction of HAART has lowered the incidence of NHL in HIV-positive patients, HAART has had less of an impact on the incidence of NHL than on that of KS. Whereas the incidence of KS has dropped by more than two thirds since the introduction of HAART, the incidence of NHL remains more than 50% of what it was before the introduction of HAART.[8]

There has been some suggestion that homosexual, bisexual, and hemophiliac patients have a greater risk of developing HIV-related NHL than Intravenous Drug Use (IVDU) patients.[21] This has been used as an argument for an infectious role in the pathogenesis of HIV-related NHL. EBV has been identified in 40% to 60% of HIV-associated NHL.[106,107,247] EBV has also been implicated in the loss of function of the tumor suppressor p53, which could result in an increased propensity for malignancy.[41] Although it is tempting to conclude that HIV-associated NHL is caused by EBV infection, this appears to be premature. Certainly a large proportion of HIV-associated NHL is found in patients free of EBV. Also, the prevalence of other cancers (e.g., nasopharyngeal cancer) known to be linked to EBV has not shown any increase in patients with HIV infection.[182] Although EBV may play a role in the oncogenesis of some HIV-associated NHL, a clear causal relationship seems unlikely.

Localized nodal disease is uncommon in HIV-associated NHL. The presence of extranodal disease (68% to 80%) is nearly double that of non–HIV-associated NHL.[42,139,159] A predilection for the head and neck region is also noted, with 50% to 60% of cases involving the head and neck. Extranodal head and neck sites include the oral cavity, sinonasal region, pharynx, nasopharynx, orbit, parotid gland, larynx, and the central nervous system (CNS).[79,135,235,295] In a series involving 58 HIV-positive patients with head and neck lymphomas, 26 of the disorders occurred in the neck, 13 in the CNS, seven in the mandible, six in the paranasal sinuses, three in the larynx, two in the oropharynx, and one in the orbit.[76] Other sites of extranodal disease include the gastrointestinal (GI) tract, bone marrow, and liver. Nodal disease predominates in the neck with frequent involvement of the submandibular, jugulodigastric, and supraclavicular regions.[252]

NHL of the head and neck often presents as a growing mass. Constitutional symptoms are frequently present with fever, night sweats, and unintentional weight loss (greater than 10% of body mass) present in 82% of patients.[160] Initial symptoms are dependent on the location of disease. Sinonasal disease may present with epistaxis, nasal obstruction, proptosis, and oral extension.[217,252] NHL of the oral cavity most commonly affects the gingiva and palate and can manifest as a persistent sore, an enlarging mass, or loose teeth. Hoarseness, respiratory symptoms, and dysphagia may indicate laryngeal or pharyngeal disease. Nasopharyngeal lymphoma may present with nasal obstruction and serous otitis media. Because of the close association, patients newly diagnosed with NHL should be screened for HIV infection.

Diagnosis

The diagnosis of lymphoma in HIV-positive patients begins with a high index of suspicion, particularly for patients with a low CD4+ count. Multiple common manifestations of HIV disease such as peripheral generalized lymphadenopathy and benign oral ulcerations can mimic the findings for patients with lymphoma. The combination of rapid enlargement and constitutional symptoms is particularly concerning for NHL. In a series of 28 patients with head and neck NHL excluding CNS involvement, a mean diagnostic delay of 2 months was noted.[43] The diagnosis of lymphoma can be made with FNA. Although histologic type can be determined from a cell block after aspiration, this might not be performed and some pathologists prefer larger tissue specimens for diagnosis and determination of histologic type. Thus, open biopsies may be considered for patients with NHL. The prognosis and management depend on the presence of extranodal disease; thus a thorough investigation of the CNS, mediastinum, and abdomen should be performed with magnetic resonance imaging (MRI), or computed tomography (CT) if MRI is not available. A bone scan and bone marrow biopsy can also be useful in the staging process. Lumbar puncture is recommended because up to 60% of patients may have asymptomatic leptomeningeal lymphoma.[242]

Prognosis and Treatment

The prognosis of NHL in HIV-positive patients is significantly worse than that of the general population. Ninety-five percent of HIV-associated NHLs are of B-cell origin, with high-grade tumors (60%) and medium-grade tumors (33%) making up the vast majority. This is in stark contrast to the 10% to 15% reported rate of high-grade NHLs in the HIV-negative population.[159,222] The most common types in HIV-infected patients are B-immunoblastic, small non-cleaved Burkitt's, non-Burkitt's, and diffuse large cell lymphomas.

The advanced stage and grade of NHL in HIV-positive patients combined with the relative state of immune suppression result in rapid progression of disease. The susceptibility of HIV-positive patients to opportunistic infections is exacerbated by the chemotherapeutic treatments for NHL, resulting in a high rate of morbidity and mortality. Factors predictive of a short life expectancy (on the order of months) include extranodal involvement, a previous AIDS diagnosis, a

Karnofsky performance status less than 70%, and a CD4+ count less than 200 cells/μL.[43,160] The histologic type does not appear to be predictive of outcome. NHL confined to the cervical nodes has an improved response to therapy with an associated survival that is longer than that of extranodal disease of the paranasal sinus, mandible, and other extranodal sites.[76] Primary CNS lymphoma has perhaps the poorest prognosis because of its tendency to recur and association with profound immune suppression.[159]

HIV-related NHL is typically treated with multiagent chemotherapy. The therapy must balance the need to eradicate the neoplasm with the risk of further immune suppression. Although investigations continue, the introduction of HAART appears to lower the incidence of HIV-related NHL and increase survival when used in conjunction with multiagent chemotherapy.[277,284] This improvement in survival may be related to a decreased incidence of opportunistic infection because the cause of death in patients with AIDS-associated NHL is relatively evenly divided between progression of lymphoma and opportunistic infection.[140] Radiotherapy has a role for patients with localized disease or symptomatic lesions.

No effective therapy for relapsed or refractory disease in HIV-positive patients has been demonstrated. Patients with NHL without HIV infection are treated with high-dose therapy with stem-cell support. This approach has not been adopted in HIV-positive patients for fear of increasing opportunistic infection and toxicity. It is unclear whether high-dose therapy will have a role in patients whose HIV disease is well controlled with HAART.

Kaposi's Sarcoma

KS is a mesenchymal cell tumor involving blood and lymphatic vessels. The classic form of KS occurs in the lower extremities of elderly men of Mediterranean or Ashkenazic Jewish descent. An endemic variety of KS present in Africa occurs in black men aged 25 to 40 and children aged 2 to 13 years.[298,318] Epidemic KS most commonly occurs in patients who are immunocompromised, specifically those with AIDS, but it has also been noted in organ transplant recipients being treated with immunosuppressive medications. Specific indications for the treatment of KS include cosmetically disfiguring lesions, symptomatic oral lesions, symptomatic visceral lesions, or pain or edema associated with lymphadenopathy or extensive cutaneous disease.

In 1989, KS was the primary AIDS-defining illness in 15% of all reported AIDS cases in U.S. residents.[22] The overall risk of KS in patients with AIDS was estimated to be 20,000 times that of the general population and more than 300 times that of other immunosuppressed patients. A striking difference was also noted among subpopulations of AIDS patients. The risk for acquiring AIDS-KS was reported to be as low as 1% for patients who acquired HIV via blood transfusion. Patients who contracted the virus through homosexual intercourse were found to have a 21% risk of developing AIDS-KS. Women who acquired HIV from heterosexual contact with bisexual men as opposed to intravenous drug users were at an increased risk for AIDS-KS. These epidemiologic disparities led to suspicion of an infectious component to AIDS-KS.[22]

In 1994, a newly recognized human herpesvirus (HHV-8) was identified within KS lesions.[48] The virus was noted within endothelial spindle cells[269] in all types of KS: classic, endemic, and AIDS-KS.[243] The seropositive rates for KS were also consistent with the epidemiology of AIDS-KS; specifically, gay men had the highest seropositive rates.[143] Finally, the virus was found in the peripheral blood mononuclear cells in many patients with KS, frequently preceding the development of KS in patients with AIDS.[309] This array of evidence has led to the general acceptance that HHV-8 plays a causative role in the development of KS.

The modes of transmission of HHV-8 are yet to be fully elucidated. The high prevalence of HHV-8 seropositivity among homosexual men in the United States suggests that sex between men may be an important route of transmission. In South African populations, however, the correlation between seropositivity and number of sexual partners is not strong.[257] Also, the presence of KS in children in sub-Saharan Africa even before the arrival of HIV suggests mother-to-child transmission.[31] However, this does not explain the increase in prevalence of HHV-8 infection throughout childhood, suggesting a role for child-to-child nonsexual transmission.[7,215]

Compared with the classic form of KS, AIDS-KS is more aggressive and less responsive to therapy. Most patients (90%) have multiple lesions, and visceral disease is more common in AIDS-KS. Treatment is complicated by the increased susceptibility for developing opportunistic infection. KS is associated with a shortened life expectancy, although most patients die from opportunistic infection or lymphoma, not KS per se.[45]

KS occurs in the head and neck in as many as 63% of cases.[255] Frequently involved sites include the skin, oral mucosa, and lymph nodes. Cutaneous and mucosal KS occur at roughly equal rates. Cutaneous disease presents as multicentric purple or red macular lesions that are neither tender nor blanching. These frequently coalesce and progress to violaceous, nodular lesions (Figure 10-1). They are usually asymptomatic but can become pruritic and aesthetically displeasing.

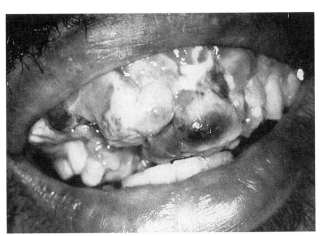

Figure 10-1. Nodular Kaposi's sarcoma of the gingiva and palate. Given the ulcerated and fungating appearance, the differential diagnosis includes non-Hodgkin's lymphoma and squamous cell carcinoma. (Courtesy of Dr. Russel Corio.)

Mucosal KS commonly occurs in the oral cavity. The oral cavity has been found to be the initial KS presentation site for up to 20% of patients.[97] The hard palate and gingiva are the most frequently affected sites.[75] Mucosal KS is more likely to be symptomatic than cutaneous disease with pain, ulceration, and bleeding. Loose teeth can impair mastication, and patients with pharyngeal or laryngeal disease may present with dysphagia or stridor.[210] Oral KS is also associated with a lower CD4+ count than cutaneous disease.[94]

Depending on its location, visceral KS can be asymptomatic or rapidly fatal. Postmortem studies suggest that more than 25% of AIDS-KS patients have visceral lesions.[116] These most commonly involve the GI tract, liver, spleen, and lungs. GI disease is often asymptomatic whereas pulmonary KS is severely debilitating and rapidly fatal if left untreated.[158] Presenting symptoms include dyspnea without fever, which may be accompanied by hemoptysis. The contrasting scans seen in pulmonary KS with thallium and technetium-99m studies can be helpful in differentiating pulmonary KS from other pulmonary processes such as lymphoma and infection, which are typically gallium avid.[294]

Otolaryngologists may encounter patients with KS of the larynx. KS of the larynx generally presents in a manner similar to that of other tumors in this location, with hoarseness, airway obstruction, cough, and dyspnea.[98] If diagnosis and treatment proceed appropriately, acute airway obstruction may be avoided. Treatment, local if the disease is isolated or systemic with multicentric disease, is recommended to avoid progression to airway compromise.[98]

Once the diagnosis of KS is suspected, biopsy should be performed for pathologic confirmation. The histopathology of KS is characterized by proliferation of slit-like vascular channels, extravasated erythrocytes, and spindle-cell proliferation (Figure 10-2). Three histologic forms have been reported: spindle cell, anaplastic, and mixed-cell, the last of which is the most common in AIDS-KS. Early lesions may be mimicked by bacillary angiomatosis or cat-scratch fever. The presence of pleomorphic bacilli on Warthin-Starry silver stain helps distinguish bacillary angiomatosis. The identification of HHV-8 DNA can help distinguish KS from other vascular lesions.[131] If

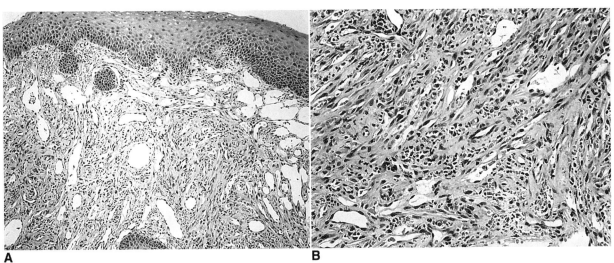

A   **B**

Figure 10-2. Mucosal Kaposi's sarcoma. **A,** Photomicrograph of submucosal Kaposi's sarcoma showing slit-like vascular channels and scattered extravasation of erythrocytes (×100). **B,** Higher-power photomicrograph of the same lesion showing characteristic spindle cell proliferation (×200).

KS is identified in a patient without a known history of HIV infection, an HIV test is warranted.

At the initial evaluation of a patient with KS, a complete skin examination and oral cavity examination should be performed. A normal examination in these areas does not ensure the absence of KS because clinically significant visceral lesions may present in the absence of mucocutaneous disease. If unexplained GI or pulmonary symptoms are present, endoscopy should be performed. The classic appearance of small, submucosal vascular nodules establishes the diagnosis of visceral KS. Endobronchial biopsy can result in significant hemorrhage and is discouraged. The constitutional symptoms of fevers, night sweats, and weight loss should be recorded as well as the immunologic status including CD4+ count and viral load.

Treatment of AIDS-KS can be divided into local and systemic therapies. Despite multiple therapeutic options, treatment is palliative; no curative therapy exists. KS may follow an indolent course not requiring therapeutic intervention or may have a rapidly progressive course leading to patient demise.[280] The treatment regimen, therefore, must be tailored to the patient's specific symptoms. The prognosis is generally related to factors other than tumor burden. The AIDS Clinical Trial Group has thus devised a staging system for KS, taking into account immune status, functional status, and tumor burden[152,153] (Box 10-3). Specific indications for treatment include cosmetically disfiguring lesions, symptomatic oral lesions, symptomatic visceral lesions, or pain or edema associated with lymphadenopathy or extensive cutaneous disease.

Local therapies include alitretinoin topical gel, local radiation, intralesional chemotherapy injection, cryotherapy, laser therapy, and surgical excision. Alitretinoin gel has a 35% to 50% local response rate with toxicity limited to local skin reaction.[300] Radiation has a local response rate of 90% when treated with less than 20 Gy.[145] Good clinical response has been described using 15 Gy in 10 divided doses.[23] The low overall dose and small fractions improve tolerance. If a complete response is not obtained, therapy can proceed to 24 or 30 Gy. Patients with AIDS-KS demonstrate increased susceptibility to radiation toxicity (including mucositis) and weight loss when compared with other AIDS patients. Intraoral lesions are particularly sensitive to radiation morbidity.[98] Intralesional injections of vinblastine or vincristine have reported response rates of 70% to 90% but are associated with significant pain and dyschromic scarring.[30,33] Cryotherapy using liquid nitrogen has a similar reported response rate. Hypopigmentation and local KS recurrence, however, are common after cryotherapy.[279] Laser therapy can be effective in temporary local control, but KS often returns within months.[281] Surgical excision has been used for local control but is also associated with a high rate of local recurrence.[280]

Intensification of HAART has been proposed as a primary systemic treatment modality for AIDS-KS. HAART has resulted in a clear decline in the incidence of AIDS-KS. The mechanism may be a combination of anti-HIV effects resulting in improved immune status and direct antiviral potency against HHV-8.[249] Anecdotally, AIDS-KS has been described to respond well to HAART.[1,195] The use of HAART has also been demonstrated to increase the time to KS recurrence nearly three-fold.[32] And although this data is encouraging, HAART alone remains limited as a treatment for KS by poor patient compliance and viral resistance.[116]

Chemotherapy is largely reserved for visceral disease. The most common chemotherapeutic agents include vincristine, vinblastine, bleomycin, anthracycline, and paclitaxel. These medications may be useful for patients with rapidly progressive or symptomatic visceral disease, however their use is severely hampered by the increased propensity of HIV-positive patients to develop opportunistic infections.[161] Liposomal anthracyclines used as single-agent therapy have demonstrated improved duration of response and overall survival when compared with traditional multiagent chemotherapy.[90,199,272] These medications are now considered first-line therapy for the treatment of advanced AIDS-KS.

Pathogenesis-based therapies have been designed to target HHV infection and the cytokine and growth factor milieu associated with KS proliferation. These therapies include antiangiogenic compounds such as thalidomide and IM-862, retinoids, and antiviral medications such as ganciclovir, cidofovir, and foscarnet. These medications remain in the experimental stages and can be combined with intensification of

---

BOX 10-3

STAGING SYSTEM FOR PATIENTS WITH KAPOSI'S SARCOMA

Stage	Characteristics
I	No history of opportunistic infections, no constitutional symptoms, CD4+ greater than 300 cells/μL
II	No history of opportunistic infections, no constitutional symptoms, CD4+ less than 300 cells/μL
III	No history of opportunistic infections, constitutional symptoms
IV	History of prior or coexistent opportunistic infections (median survival, 7 months)

HAART therapy. Interferon alpha was the first approved treatment for AIDS-KS and has demonstrated antiviral, antiangiogenic, and immunomodulatory effects. Its use has been limited by toxicities including malaise, fatigue, myalgia, and bone marrow suppression.[161]

Hodgkin's Lymphoma

Hodgkin's lymphoma (HL) has been identified as the most common type of non–AIDS-defining tumor.[80,96] The risk of HL is approximately 10-fold in HIV+ patients compared with the general population.[83,108] Along with an increased prevalence, HIV-HL is associated with a more aggressive clinical course with noncontiguous spread and frequent involvement of the bone marrow and liver.[293] HL occurs in patients with a wide range of immune function. Approximately 20% of HIV-HL occurs in patients who carry a diagnosis of AIDS and a wide range of CD4+ counts are found among HIV-HL patients.[248]

The histology of HIV-associated HL is distinct from that of the general population: HIV-positive patients more frequently develop the aggressive mixed cellularity and lymphodepleted subtypes in comparison to the predominance of nodular lymphocytic subtypes in the general population.[226] Also, an 80% to 100% association with EBV has been reported for HIV-HL[65] in comparison to a 40% rate of EBV positivity in non–HIV-associated HL.[119] Complete response to chemotherapy and overall survival are far below that expected for non–HIV-associated HL.[72,292]

HIV-HL frequently presents as a mass in the head and neck region associated with fever, night sweats, and weight loss. On histologic diagnosis, staging work-up should include brain, thoracic, and abdominal imaging and a bone marrow biopsy. Evaluation of the patient's immune status with CD4+ count and viral load testing should also be performed.

The treatment of HIV-HL consists of combination chemotherapy and antiretroviral therapy. Patients treated with HAART in combination with chemotherapy have shown improved response to therapy, longer disease-free survival, and longer overall survival compared with patients treated with combination chemotherapy alone.[228] The estimated 2-year survival was 45% in patients treated with chemotherapy alone vs 62% in those treated with combined HAART and chemotherapy.[86]

Cutaneous Neoplasms

Basal cell carcinoma (BCC) and melanoma may be occurring at an increasing rate in the HIV-positive population.[169,301] BCC is second behind KS as the most common skin malignancy in HIV-positive patients with a prevalence of 1.8%.[263] Melanoma is still quite uncommon. Both tumors occur in the setting of relative immune compromise but rarely in conjunction with AIDS. These tumors may become more prevalent in the era of HAART as more patients live with the relative immunocompromise of HIV infection.

Despite similar risk factors of fair skin and sun exposure, the distribution and histology of BCC lesions varies between the HIV-positive and general populations. Thirty percent of BCCs occur in the head and neck region in HIV-positive patients compared with 85% in the general population. The infiltrative subtype of BCC is significantly more common in the HIV-positive population.[203] BCC in HIV-positive patients is often multicentric and may metastasize.[258] Because of the locally aggressive nature of BCC in this population, Mohs surgery is the treatment of choice.[124]

Melanoma also has more aggressive features in the setting of HIV infection. The thickness of the skin lesion has an inverse relationship to CD4+ count. Shorter disease-free and overall survival have also been demonstrated in HIV-positive patients with melanoma.[230] The aggressive course of cutaneous malignancy in HIV-positive patients requires a low threshold for biopsy of suspicious skin lesions in these patients.

Squamous Cell Carcinoma

To date, no clear evidence exists that squamous cell carcinoma (SCC) is significantly more common in HIV-positive patients. These patients, however, do experience a more virulent clinical course than the general population. HIV-positive patients tend to present at an earlier age with more advanced disease than their HIV-negative counterparts. Singh and others[256] noted that HIV-positive patients presented with a median of stage IV disease and T3 staging at the primary site—significantly more advanced disease than the median stage III and T2 staging in the general population. As expected, the 1- and 2-year survival rates for HIV-positive patients were also significantly less: 57% and 32%, respectively, compared with 74% and 59% in the general population. With the advent of effective antiretroviral therapy HIV-positive patients are living longer, which may increase the incidence of SCC in these patients.

The high rate of tobacco and alcohol use among HIV-positive patients with SCC suggests a similar pathogenesis to that of the general population. Some studies, however, suggest that human papillomavirus (HPV) may play a role in the development of SCC, specifically in the tonsil.[92] Theoretically, HIV-related immunocompromise could lead to an increased infection rate of oncogenic virus, resulting in an accelerated disease course in younger patients.[78,232] HIV-associated SCC also appears to have a predilection for the larynx, which is also a favored site for HPV infection as demonstrated by papillomas in the larynx.[84,232,256]

The diagnosis of SCC can be delayed by the prolonged management of presumed benign disease.[78] The myriad of oral cavity and oropharyngeal lesions in HIV-positive patients makes surveillance for malignant disease quite challenging. A high level of suspicion and a low threshold for biopsy, particularly in patients with a history of tobacco and alcohol use, should be maintained to avoid diagnostic delay.

Treatment of HIV-positive patients with SCC may be quite challenging. Although surgical intervention is an important option, patients with advanced disease often require combined therapy. The use of chemotherapy in patients with advanced HIV disease may put these patients at significant risk for opportunistic infection. The use of radiation therapy can be limited by the increased toxicity of radiation in HIV-positive patients.[145]

Lymphoepithelial Cysts of the Parotid Gland

HIV-positive patients have a higher incidence of benign and malignant parotid masses. The increase in benign and malignant lymphoproliferative disorders involving the lymphatic tissue of the parotid gland accounts for this difference because salivary tumors of the parotid gland are not known to have an increased propensity for occurrence in HIV-positive patients.[266] Among children with HIV infection, 30% have bilateral parotid enlargement as a result of lymphocytic infiltration of the gland parenchyma. This is often associated with pulmonary lymphoid hyperplasia.[238,315] In patients with AIDS, parotid gland enlargement can result from an AIDS-related malignancy such as NHL or metastatic KS.[128,191] The majority of parotid gland enlargement in HIV-positive patients, however, is the result of a benign cystic lymphoproliferative process known as *benign lymphoepithelial cyst* (BLC). This type of lesion is associated with ductal metaplasia of the parotid gland and typically occurs in a setting of relative immune competence. These lesions are almost always associated with progressive generalized lymphadenopathy.[260,268,289]

Cystic lymphoepithelial disease of the parotid gland produces persistent, nontender parotid enlargement. These lesions have varying proportions of cystic and solid components[239,267] and although only unilateral clinical disease may be evident, radiologic evaluation nearly always reveals bilateral changes.[264] The differential diagnosis of cystic parotid lesions includes Sjögren's syndrome, cystic Warthin's tumor, and branchial cleft cysts. Bilateral cystic Warthin's tumors may be differentiated radiologically from BLC based on the presence of focal nodularity in Warthin's tumors and the associated generalized lymphadenopathy of BLC.[264] HIV-associated BLC should be considered in the differential diagnosis of all cystic parotid masses.

The histology of HIV-associated BLC is similar to that of parotid enlargement associated with Sjögren's syndrome.[129] The histologic similarities of BLC and Sjögren's syndrome combined with the finding of xeophthalmia and xerostomia in selected patients with BLC suggests that HIV infection may trigger an autoimmune process responsible for some cases of HIV-associated parotid gland enlargement.[150,264] An exuberant lymphoid hyperplasia replaces the parotid parenchyma. Germinal centers, epimyothelial islands representing metaplasia of ductal epithelium, and cystic ductal dilatation (Figure 10-3) differentiate BLC from lymphoma.[260]

The evaluation of an HIV-positive patient who presents with a parotid mass should begin with a thorough history focusing on the time of onset and rate of growth of the mass as well as any symptoms associated with the mass, such as pain. Constitutional symptoms such as weight loss, fever, and night sweats should be investigated, and if present, should alert the physician to the possibility of lymphoma or TB. The physical examination should focus on the common features of BLCs—the myoepithelial parotid gland should be examined for bilateral masses, and the neck should be examined for PGL. The examiner should look for evidence of malignancy such as induration, fixation, or facial nerve dysfunction.

FNA can be useful in the diagnosis of parotid masses. Unilateral masses or masses suspicious for malignancy should undergo FNA. A study of 99 parotid FNAs in HIV-positive patients found 75% to be consistent with BLCs, 14% were infectious/inflammatory, and 6% were neoplastic. Of the neoplastic lesions, all were malignant; there were three NHLs,

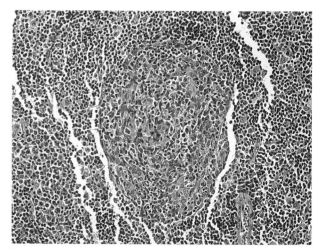

Figure 10-3. Photomicrograph of a benign lymphoepithelial cyst island resulting from squamous metaplasia of the ductal epithelium in human immunodeficiency virus–related cystic lymphoepithelial disease of the parotid gland (×200).

one multiple myeloma, one metastatic adenocarcinoma from the lung, and direct extension from a cutaneous BCC. In 6% of patients the FNA was nondiagnostic.[50] The authors report no false-positive or false-negative diagnosis, although previously published reports of FNAs of the parotid gland in the general population have not demonstrated a high false-negative rate.[10,320] Aspiration can also be useful for the relief of symptoms in larger cysts, although the lesions invariably recur. Initial aspirates should be sent for cytologic and microbiologic evaluation.

A variety of treatment options exist for patients with BLCs. For minimally symptomatic patients without significant cosmetic deformity, observation alone represents the best option. Low-dose radiation treatment results in a reduction in the size of the lesion greater than 50%. This improvement, however, typically lasts less than 10 months.[15] Some patients are treated with repeated needle aspirations, although the repetitive nature of this treatment is suboptimal. Needle aspiration combined with doxycycline sclerotherapy can result in significant size decrease.[172] A 1-mg/mL doxycycline solution has been used, injecting 1 to 2 mL through an angiocath after cyst aspiration. Most patients are left with residual fibrotic masses, and some elect for parotidectomy after sclerosis treatment. The long-term results of this treatment are unknown.[172]

HIV-associated BLC typically does not require parotidectomy. Parotidectomy may be considered in those rare cases of BLCs that undergo rapid size change, are disfiguring, or have significant pressure symptoms. Other indications for parotidectomy include FNA cytology suggestive of neoplasm or unilateral masses with a significant solid component or features worrisome for malignancy.

SINONASAL INFECTION

Symptoms of sinonasal disease are among the most common complaints of HIV-positive patients. Nearly 70% of this population will experience an episode of acute sinusitis, and 58% of these patients will develop either recurrent acute or chronic sinusitis.[49,95,121,237] These findings are tempered by a recent cross-sectional study comparing the subjective symptomatology of patients presenting to an HIV clinic (n = 203) with those presenting to a nearby general clinic (n = 100). Although sinonasal symptoms were the most frequent head and neck symptoms reported among HIV-positive patients, the rate of sinonasal symptoms in the past 6 months was nearly identical for the two groups, 66% and 67% for the HIV-positive and general medicine patients, respectively. Among those patients with sinonasal symptoms, 54% and 61%, respectively, reported an episode of bacterial

sinusitis in the past 6 months. No significant difference was noted in subjective severity of disease between the two groups.[218]

Among HIV-positive patients with sinusitis, the maxillary and ethmoid sinuses are most frequently involved.[319] Sphenoid infection, however has been noted to occur in 57% of patients with sinusitis, which is nearly twice the overall incidence among patients with sinusitis.[9] Symptoms of acute or chronic sinusitis in HIV-positive patients are similar to those of the general population. These include fever, facial pain or pressure, nasal congestion, and mucopurulent nasal discharge and postnasal drainage. Often patients with chronic sinusitis are relatively asymptomatic, reporting only congestion and nasal discharge. Some patients initially present with pulmonary complaints, such as bronchospasm or infection, resulting from postnasal drainage.

Three pathogenic mechanisms have been proposed as contributing to the high incidence of sinusitis in HIV-positive patients. First, impaired systemic and local immunity due to HIV infection leaves the host susceptible to infection. Second, decreased mucociliary clearance times have been noted in patients with HIV infection.[188] This decreased transit time can result in stasis of secretions and increased susceptibility to sinonasal infection, or it may reflect damage to the nasal microenvironment from repeated infection resulting in decreased transport time. Finally, increased atopy has been noted in up to 87% of HIV-positive patients, manifesting as new or increased allergic symptoms (e.g., allergic rhinitis, drug allergies, and asthma).[240] This increased atopy has been attributed to polyclonal B-cell activation with increased immunoglobulin production, including immunoglobulin E.[278] Attempts to directly correlate sinusitis with atopic disease in HIV-positive patients, however, have been unsuccessful.[85]

The clinical characteristics of sinusitis are closely linked to the clinical stage of HIV infection. Acute sinusitis is more likely to resolve with standard medical management in patients with a CD4+ count of greater than 200. Patients with a CD4+ count below 200 typically have more extensive disease and a greater propensity to develop chronic sinusitis.[95,218,237] The more aggressive pathogens such as *Aspergillus* and *Pseudomonas* species are also seen in a greater propensity in patients with a CD4+ count of less than 200/μL.[117,126,202]

The spectrum of bacteria implicated in HIV-associated sinusitis is broader than that of sinusitis in the general population. The most commonly cultured organisms are *Streptococcus pneumoniae, Streptococcus viridans,* coagulase-negative staphylococci, *Staphylococcus aureus,* and *Haemophilus influenzae.*[189] Unusual organisms cultured from HIV-infected patients include *Cryptococcus neoformans,*[51] *Legionella pneumophila,*[245] *Acanthamoeba,*[229,282] *Mycobacterium kansasii,* and CMV.[290] CMV may act as a primary cause of erosive sinusitis or as a cofactor in the pathogenesis of bacterial or fungal sinusitis via local effects on mucosa and systemic effect of neutrophil dysfunction.[290,312,317] CMV sinusitis has been reported as the presenting symptom for HIV infection.[136]

Pseudomonas aeruginosa and fungi such as *Aspergillus* organisms and mucormycosis are particularly important pathogens in HIV-related sinusitis because these organisms have the potential to cause the most clinically severe disease. *P. aeruginosa* species is rarely the primary pathogen in sinusitis in the general population, but it has been noted to cause severe infections in HIV-positive patients. Depressed humoral immunity combined with neutrophil dysfunction likely contribute to the susceptibility of HIV-positive patients. The chronic use of antibiotic prophylaxis for the prevention of opportunistic infection may change the microbiologic environment, predisposing such patients to the development of *Pseudomonas* infections. *Pseudomonas* sinusitis typically occurs in patients with AIDS and low CD4+ counts (<50/μL) and may be associated with *Pseudomonas* bacteremia and orbital complications in up to 50% of infections.[117,202]

Invasive fungal sinusitis most commonly occurs in late-stage AIDS. In a review of the literature on fungal sinusitis in HIV-positive patients, the median CD4+ count was 8 at the time of diagnosis.[126] *Aspergillus fumigatus* is the most common fungal pathogen in HIV sinusitis, although *Candida albicans,*[52] *Rhizopus arrhizus,*[27] and others have been reported. Neutrophils and macrophages form the primary defense against *Aspergillus* infection. Neutropenia and neutrophil dysfunction caused by HIV infection or medications have been identified as risk factors for invasive pulmonary and sinonasal aspergillosis.[60,187]

Invasive fungal sinusitis is a life-threatening condition, and early diagnosis and treatment are paramount. Histopathology combined with culture and stains is the most effective diagnostic approach for fungal sinusitis. A low (<50) CD4+ count, unilateral symptoms (e.g., facial paresthesias, swelling, and pain), and fever refractory to broad-spectrum antibiotics all suggest invasive fungal sinusitis. Proptosis along with cranial nerve findings, such as decreased extraocular motions or vision, suggest orbital involvement. Meningismus and mental status changes are late-stage symptoms suggestive of intracranial spread.

The endoscopic findings in patients with nasal aspergillosis range from pale, ischemic mucosa to well-circumscribed necrotic plaques. Perforations of the nasal septum and hard palate may be present. Fungal infection may be accompanied by suppuration, causing confusion with bacterial sinusitis.[187] Unilateral disease such as edema of the sinonasal mucosa with or without bony erosion on CT scan (Figure 10-4) should lead to suspicion of fungal sinusitis or a neoplasm. Any suspicious lesions should undergo biopsy with silver staining, histopatholgy, and culture. Drainage from the middle meatus should also be collected and sent for bacterial and fungal culture. Diagnostic antral lavage should be considered in all HIV-positive patients with persistent sinusitis. A lack of fungal elements on antral tap does not rule out fungal sinusitis.[187]

An MRI may help differentiate fungal from bacterial sinusitis. Whereas the T1 image is isointense in both infections, the T2 images should be low intensity for the fungal disease and high intensity for bacterial disease. MRI scan of the orbits and skull base may be useful in determining the invasion outside of the paranasal sinuses.

Fungal sinusitis can extend via thrombophlebitic or hematologic spread and thus may enter into the orbit or intracranially without histologic evidence of mucosal invasion.[171] Thus, in the clinical scenario consistent with fungal sinusitis and fungal elements identified on silver stain or culture, treatment of fungal sinusitis should begin regardless of the histologic confirmation of invasion. The angiocentric invasion pattern of *Aspergillus* may allow extension of disease into the orbit or intracranially without evidence of bony destruction on imaging study.

Management of Sinusitis in HIV-Positive Patients

The goals of management of sinusitis in HIV-positive patients include swift treatment of bacterial sinusitis and early identification of fungal sinusitis or neoplasm. The initial evaluation should include nasal endoscopy to identify mucosal or structural abnormalities. Endoscopy-guided cultures should be obtained if discharge from the middle meatus or sphenoethmoidal recess is identified. Any mucosal lesions should be biopsied under endoscopic guidance with samples sent for histopathologic and microbiologic evaluation. CT scans may be useful in patients with headache or fever without a source to look for evidence of sinus disease and for patients refractory to antibiotic therapy. Patients with findings of physical examination that elicit concern regarding complications of sinusitis should also undergo CT or MRI imaging. A low threshold for imaging patients with low CD4+ counts is advised.

Antral lavage is another useful tool in the evaluation and management of HIV-positive patients with

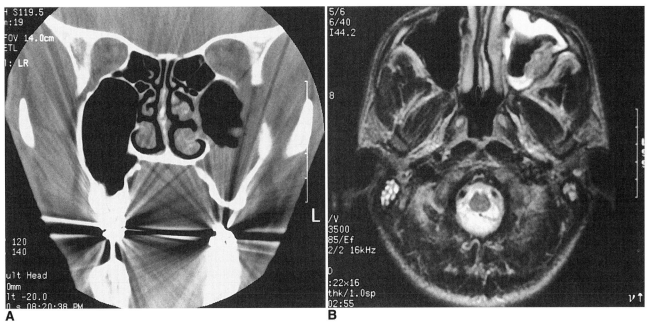

Figure 10-4. Computed tomography and magnetic resonance imaging of *Aspergillus* sinusitis. **A,** Coronal computed tomography of the paranasal sinuses shows left maxillary sinusitis with erosion of the superior lateral bony wall. **B,** T2-weighted axial magnetic resonance imaging of the same case shows thickened left maxillary sinus mucosa with a hyperintense signal consistent with inflammation and a transmural process of the lateral wall with a hypointense signal corresponding to the region of bone destruction on computed tomography. Differential diagnosis includes invasive fungal disease, lymphoma, and squamous cell carcinoma.

sinusitis. All patients with a diagnosis of AIDS should be considered for diagnostic lavage at the time of presentation with bacterial, fungal, and viral cultures. Antral lavage also has some therapeutic value.[95]

Initial medical management consists of broad-spectrum antibiotics, decongestants, and mucolytics. Antibiotics should have good coverage of *Streptococcus* sp., *Staphylococcus* sp., and *H. influenzae.* Amoxicillin/pot clavulana (Augmentin) or cefuroxime represent good first-line choices for HIV-positive patients. Decongestants and high-dose guaifenesin enhance sinus drainage and provide symptomatic improvement.[304] Patients should be closely observed, and if fever or local symptoms persist after 10 days of therapy, antibiotic coverage should be expanded to include *Pseudomonas* sp. and antral lavage should be considered. Surgical drainage should be considered in patients who remain refractory to antibiotic therapy.

Patients with a rapidly progressive course or toxic presentation should undergo early imaging and aggressive treatment, including parenteral antibiotics and possible surgical intervention. As culture and biopsy results become available, the antibiotic coverage may be narrowed. Antibiotics should be administered for a total of 4 to 6 weeks.[109]

Patients who grow pseudomonas organisms on their cultures should be treated aggressively with multidrug therapy and surgical drainage. Double antibiotic therapy is recommended for patients with pseudomonal infection and has been shown to decrease mortality in HIV-positive patients with pseudomonal sepsis by nearly 50% when compared with single-drug therapy.[120,186] An antipseudomonal penicillin or cephalosporin combined with an aminoglycoside is standard therapy. A fluoroquinolone may be substituted but should be avoided if the patient has a history of frequent prior fluoroquinolone use because this can lead to resistance. *Pseudomonas* cultures in patients who have taken frequent or chronic ciprofloxacin regimens have demonstrated resistance to this medication.[117,202] Such patients should be closely monitored for the development of sepsis or regional complications including orbital involvement or cavernous sinus thrombosis.

Fungal sinusitis should be suspected when fever or other symptoms persist despite antral lavage and broad-spectrum antibiotics. Histopathology combined with culture and stains is the most effective diagnostic approach for fungal sinusitis. Sinusotomy and débridement should be pursued to establish drainage and obtain mucosa and sinus contents for histopathologic and microbiologic evaluation. Surgical intervention is particularly important for patients with low CD4+ counts or other evidence of immunosuppression such as neutropenia or chronic corticosteroid therapy. Endoscopic or external approaches may be used depending on the surgeon's preference. Fresh frozen section should be performed on suspicious mucosal lesions to allow rapid diagnosis and timely débridement.

HIV-positive patients with a diagnosis of invasive fungal sinusitis require immediate, aggressive treatment. As with all immunocompromised patients with invasive fungal sinusitis, the ideal treatment involves three components: systemic antifungal therapy, débridement of infected tissue, and restoration of immune function. Initiation of HAART should be considered in an attempt to improve the underlying immune status. High-dose, broad-spectrum antifungal medication such as amphotericin B should be administered intravenously in all cases with a clinical picture compatible with invasive sinusitis in which *Aspergillus* or *Rhizopus* species have been identified, regardless of evidence of invasion. Liposomal amphotericin,[296] triazoles,[213] and new echinocandin lipopeptides such as caspofungin[105] represent alternative medical therapy for patients with poor renal function.

Surgical débridement of involved tissue is important to minimize fungal load because medical therapy alone is typically insufficient. The severity of infection and the level of immune impairment should be considered when planning surgical intervention. Sinusotomy alone is insufficient; as much as possible, involved tissue should be débrided.[91] Endoscopic approaches may suffice for limited disease; however, transfacial approaches may be required in the setting of extensive disease, and this may require maxillectomy, orbital exenteration, or craniofacial resection for optimal disease control. Intraoperative frozen sections may assist in defining the extent of resection by determining the boundaries of angioinvasion. Aggressive surgery must be considered in the context of the patient's overall condition and prognosis.

In patients with only moderate impairment of the immune system, fungal sinusitis can be managed without en bloc resection of all infected tissue. Endoscopic débridement of grossly involved tissue combined with amphotericin B may suffice in patients who have not progressed to AIDS and do not have other immunosuppressive factors.[27] Repeat débridements may be required. Granulocyte-macrophage colony-stimulating factor has been used in these patients in an effort to improve outcomes with this conservative surgical approach, though the attempts have been without proven benefit.[175] Careful follow-up and a low threshold for en bloc resection are required in such patients if fungal disease persists.

HIV-positive patients with chronic sinusitis are also candidates for surgical intervention. Friedman and others[82] found that endoscopic sinus surgery in HIV-positive patients with chronic sinusitis resulted in symptomatic improvement in 75% of patients with limited follow-up. This was comparable to their results in the general population. This effect was found to be independent of CD4+ count and led the authors to suggest the same treatment algorithm for chronic sinusitis in patients regardless of HIV status.[82] These findings were bolstered by Murphy and colleagues[193] who showed a significant decrease in the symptoms of sinusitis and increased quality of life in HIV-positive patients with chronic sinusitis after endoscopic sinus surgery. Follow-up time in this study was also limited.

OTOLOGIC AND NEUROTOLOGIC MANIFESTATIONS OF HIV INFECTION

The incidence of otologic symptoms in patients with HIV has been reported to be as high as 56%.[25] Hearing loss, otalgia, and otorrhea are the most common presenting symptoms,[148] with sensorineural hearing loss (SNHL), otitis externa (OE), acute otitis media (AOM), and serous otitis media (SOM) being the most common otologic diagnoses in the HIV-infected population.

Human Immunodeficiency Virus–Related Diseases of the Outer and Middle Ear

The risk of OE and malignant OE is increased in patients with AIDS.[305] As in the general population, *P. aeruginosa* is the primary causative agent of both disease entities. The susceptibility of the HIV-infected patient to *P. aeruginosa* is heightened by a combination of impaired humoral immunity, neutrophil function, and complement activation.[144] The pathogenesis of OE is further facilitated by the breakdown of the local cutaneous barrier in the external auditory canal (EAC) resulting from dermatologic lesions (e.g., eczema, seborrhea) and self-induced trauma caused by pruritus. OE may progress to necrotization and malignant OE if not managed aggressively and in a timely fashion. Therapy should consist of frequent cleaning of the EAC by the clinician and topical instillation of drops with adequate pseudomonal coverage, with the duration of treatment dependent on the patient's response to these measures. Oral antibiotics, particularly fluoroquinolones, should be considered as a possible treatment for severely immunocompromised patients or when early auricular perichondritis is present. Temporal bone osteomyelitis should be suspected when otalgia, swelling, and otorrhea persist despite therapy or when there is onset of facial nerve paralysis or other cranial nerve dysfunction.

Early diagnosis and management of skull base osteomyelitis is essential because this is a life-threatening condition, especially in patients with low CD4+ counts and neutropenia.[305] Otoscopy often reveals granulation tissue at the bony cartilaginous junction of the EAC. The diagnosis is confirmed by increased uptake of technetium-99 by the temporal bone on a bone scan. A CT scan may show erosion of the EAC bone. EAC debris should be cultured and stained for bacteria, fungi, acid-fast bacilli, and *Pneumocystis* sp. Management of malignant OE consists of 6 weeks of broad-spectrum intravenous antibiotics with adequate coverage against *P. aeruginosa.* An antipseudomonal penicillin or third-generation cephalosporin given with an aminoglycoside is standard therapy, although combinations containing quinolones can also be used. Serial gallium-67 bone scans help monitor the response to therapy.

Eustachian tube obstruction caused by adenoidal hypertrophy or sinonasal disease is prevalent in HIV-infected children and adults. It is therefore not surprising that OM commonly occurs in the HIV-infected population, particularly in children.[110,313] SOM and conductive hearing loss are more prevalent in adults and older children, whereas AOM frequently occurs in young children.[13,61] The frequency of recurrent AOM increases as immune function deteriorates. During the first 3 years of life, HIV-infected children with CD4+ counts less than 1500 cells/mL have up to twice the incidence of AOM as children with CD4+ counts greater than 1500 cells/mL in the first 3 years of life.[13] The bacteriology of acute OM parallels that in non–HIV-infected patients, with *S. pneumoniae, H. influenzae,* group A *Streptococcus,* and *Moraxella catarrhalis* predominating.[155,177,250] An exception to this is a severely immunocompromised child, in whom *S. aureus* causes OM at a significantly higher rate. Therefore, initial therapy for acute OM is the same as that for non–HIV-infected patients. However, in a severely immunocompromised child, antibiotic coverage should be expanded to include *S. aureus.* If OM persists, tympanocentesis should be considered to guide therapy by culture and sensitivity results.

The role of tympanostomy tube placement and adenoidectomy in the management of recurrent OM and persistent SOM is poorly established in HIV-infected patients. As with non–HIV-infected patients, the placement of tympanostomy tubes can result in chronic otorrhea or persistent tympanic membrane perforation. It is unclear whether these adverse scenarios are seen more frequently in HIV-positive patients. The severity of hearing loss and morbidity associated with OM should be taken into account when deciding whether to place tympanostomy tubes.

HIV-positive patients who progress to develop chronic OM, cholesteatoma, or persistent tympanic membrane perforations should be evaluated for surgical intervention. Kohan and Giacchi[146] found no adverse events in HIV-positive patients undergoing elective otologic surgery. Patients undergoing emergent surgery for complications of OM or OE, however, had severe immune compromise and a poor prognosis. Advances in the treatment of HIV infection have resulted in HIV-positive patients living longer with relatively less immune compromise. The improved overall prognosis of HIV-positive patients can lead to an increase in chronic ear disease and suggests that HIV-positive patients have more potential benefit from chronic ear surgery.

Petrous apicitis, cranial neuropathies (VII and VIII), temporal bone osteomyelitis, and intracranial sepsis are uncommon complications of OM that are more likely to occur in the setting of advanced immunocompromise.[166] Patients with suppurative OM refractory to antibiotics should undergo early tympanocentesis for culture and special stains, and granulation tissue, polyps, and other masses should be carefully biopsied to rule out neoplasms and atypical infections. *A. fumigatus* and *P. carinii* are examples of organisms that cause otomastoiditis refractory to standard antibiotic therapy.

Otomastoiditis and OE caused by *P. carinii* usually occur in the absence of pulmonary disease.[34,88,148,303] Patients with pneumocystis otomastoiditis commonly present with unilateral otalgia, otorrhea, hearing loss, and a polypoid mass on otoscopy. CT of the temporal bones reveals bony sclerosis without erosions and opacification of the middle ear and mastoid air spaces.

A persistent aural polyp accompanied by signs and symptoms of OM despite otic drops and systemic antibiotics should undergo biopsy for histopathology and special stains. Silver stains should be requested and may reveal *P. carinii* organisms surrounded by a foamy granular exudate. *P. carinii* otitis is resolved with recovery of hearing using oral trimethoprim-sulfamethoxazole (15 mg/kg/day trimethoprim) in three to four divided doses for 10 to 14 days.[34] Other regimens have been used successfully, including trimethoprim and dapsone[88] and pentamidine.[207] The route of transmission of *P. carinii* to the temporal bone is not clear. Retrograde spread from the nasopharynx through the eustachian tube and hematogenous spread have been proposed.

Invasive Aspergillosis of the External and Middle Ear

A. fumigatus infection of the EAC may be superficial in the relatively immunocompetent HIV-infected patient, causing a chronic OE. However, in severely immunocompromised patients, invasive aspergillus infection of the temporal bone can cause malignant OE and otomastoiditis with skull base and intracranial extension.[227] Risk factors for invasive aspergillosis of the temporal bone include a low CD4+ count, AIDS diagnosis, neutropenia, corticosteroid therapy, antineoplastic therapy, and prolonged antibiotic therapy.

Invasive OE caused by *A. fumigatus* presents with otalgia, otorrhea, and hearing loss. Otoscopy usually reveals white debris in the EAC, which may be mistaken for cholesteatoma. Facial nerve weakness indicates bone invasion, which can often be confirmed by the presence of bony erosion on temporal bone CT.

Otomastoiditis caused by *A. fumigatus* can start in the middle ear space or extend from the EAC.[111] Invasive disease results in destruction of ossicles, erosion of the facial canal with nerve invasion, and destruction of dural plates with possible extension to the dural sinuses and other intracranial structures.[273] Patients often have a history of worsening otalgia, otorrhea, and hearing loss despite antibiotic therapy.[173] Vertigo indicates labyrinthine invasion by aspergillus organisms, whereas meningismus and mental status changes indicate intracranial extension. Otoscopy often reveals a pale tympanic membrane with enlarging single or multiple perforations. The middle ear mucosa may be pale or necrotic, and white fungal debris resembling cholesteatoma may also be seen.

There should be a high index of suspicion for the presence of invasive aspergilli of the temporal bone, particularly in the patients with AIDS who have persistent OE or OM and new cranial nerve findings. Otorrhea should be routinely cultured and stained for bacterial and fungal organisms and for pneumocystis. If the TM is intact, tympanocentesis should be performed when antibiotic therapy is ineffective. If aspergillus organisms are identified on stain or culture, invasive disease can be implied by the presence of bone erosion on CT. The presence of fungal invasion in a mucosal biopsy from the middle ear is diagnostic for *Aspergillus* otomastoiditis. MRI of the skull base should be performed if extensive mastoid disease or dural plate erosion is present on CT; special attention should be given to lateral sinus blood flow and other clues of intracranial extension.

OE and OM caused by invasive *A. fumigatus* require prompt surgical and drug therapy.[273] High-dose amphotericin B should be started immediately. As much aspergillus-infected tissue as possible should be removed to slow down extension of disease to vital structures and to facilitate the ameliorating effects of drug therapy and host immunity. In the case of OE caused by invasive *Aspergillus*, infected soft tissue and bone of the EAC should be débrided. Limited disease can be addressed by a transcanal approach, but a

transmastoid approach with removal of the canal wall will provide more complete débridement and less risk to the facial nerve. Otomastoiditis should be managed with a radical mastoidectomy if middle ear contents and mastoid air cells are to be removed. The management of the facial nerve in these cases is controversial because invasion of the nerve by aspergillus organisms is not easily proved without biopsy. When the facial nerve is paralyzed and gross evidence of invasion and necrosis is present, the nerve should be resected and grafted when appropriate.

The absence of tissue invasion on histopathology and the absence of bone erosion on CT do not rule out the diagnosis of invasive *Aspergillus* of the temporal bone. The clinician should maintain a high index of suspicion for invasive aspergillosis in HIV-infected patients with severe immunocompromise, despite the absence of these findings. Therefore, patients with early *Aspergillus* infection can first be treated with topical clotrimazole and seen up to several times per week for frequent cleaning of EAC debris. If symptoms persist or cranial nerve deficits occur, surgery and amphotericin B should be considered after biopsies are taken and CT studies repeated.

Cranial Nerve and Central Nervous System Effects

Neurologic disorders are a common manifestation of HIV infection resulting from the neurotropic and immunosuppressive properties of the virus. As many as 40% of HIV-infected adults have clinical signs of neurologic disease, and 70% to 80% show neuropathologic abnormalities at autopsy.[69,164] Peripheral neuropathy composes 5% to 20% of all neurologic complications in HIV infection.[208] Among patients with AIDS, 2% to 3% develop cranial neuropathies. The most commonly affected are the facial, trigeminal, optic, and cochleovestibular nerves.[69,288]

Neuropathy associated with early-stage HIV infection exhibits a tendency for motor nerve involvement, whereas sensory nerves are more likely to be affected in later stages.[208] Neuropathies associated with HIV seroconversion and asymptomatic HIV infection tend to result from autoimmune demyelination as demonstrated by common pathologic findings and electrophysiologic correlates.[69,166,208] An autoimmune etiology is supported by the presence of increased titers of circulating antibodies against peripheral nerve antigens, subperineural deposition of immunoglobulin M, and improvement in nerve function with plasmapheresis. Neuropathies associated with symptomatic HIV infection and AIDS are characterized by distal symmetric polyneuropathy and axonal degeneration. A similar pattern of neuropathy selectively affects cranial nerves in the form of a mononeuritis multiplex resulting in a transient mononeuropathy or progressive sensorimotor polyneuropathy.[55] Axonal degeneration induced by necrotizing vasculitis may be the underlying pathologic process.

In later stages of HIV infection, cranial nerve dysfunction is often associated with CNS disease.[164,262] AIDS dementia (subacute encephalitis) is the most common neurologic manifestation of HIV infection and is sometimes associated with focal motor deficits. Aseptic meningitis is thought to be a less fulminant form of subacute encephalitis, occurring in less-immunocompromised patients and occasionally associated with dysfunction of cranial nerves V, VII, and VIII. Progressive multifocal leukoencephalopathy (PML) is a demyelinating disease of the CNS associated with papovavirus infection. In PML, there is progressive deterioration of mentation and other neurologic functions, including cranial nerve weakness. *Toxoplasma gondii* infection of the brain produces large areas of coagulation necrosis. The resulting mass lesion causes altered levels of consciousness and focal deficits, including cranial nerve dysfunction. Toxoplasmosis is definitively diagnosed by brain biopsy but is usually diagnosed presumptively by the presence of an enhancing lesion on MRI or CT and a clinical and radiographic response to empiric management with pyrimethamine and either sulfadiazine or clindamycin. Cranial nerve deficits are rare complications of primary CNS lymphomas, occurring at a rate of 8% to 15%.[155,164] Other neurologic complications of HIV infection include cryptococcal meningitis, which is associated with cranial neuropathies in the presence of increased intracranial pressure, tuberculous meningitis, and toxic neuropathy caused by therapy with didanosine, zalcitabine, stavudine, and other agents.[89] Diagnosis of cranial neuropathies can be complicated by the presence of multiple concurrent pathologic processes of the CNS and the peripheral nervous system.

Sensorineural Hearing Loss

Various degrees of SNHL can be found in as many as 49% of HIV-infected patients. Vestibular symptoms, however, are relatively uncommon.[155,225] Audiometry most commonly demonstrates a high-frequency SNHL.[12,104,155,283] Cochleovestibular dysfunction increases with the duration of HIV infection.[12,25,113] The pure-tone average gradually increases as the T-cell ratio falls in an AIDS patient, possibly because of an accumulation of insults to the CNS by opportunistic diseases or from HIV itself.[25,149,164] The differential diagnosis of SNHL in an HIV-infected patient is influenced by the level of immunocompromise. Peripheral auditory pathology caused by drug-induced ototoxicity and otosyphilis and by idiopathic processes may

produce SNHL at any stage in HIV infection, whereas central causes of hearing loss are more likely to occur in later stages of the disease (Box 10-4).

Progressive central auditory dysfunction appears to be a common cause of SNHL associated with HIV infection and is shown by the results of auditory brainstem response testing. Auditory brainstem response testing of asymptomatic HIV-infected patients commonly shows a delayed and poorly defined wave V, suggesting auditory brainstem conduction abnormalities.[12,25,234,261,307] These auditory brainstem response abnormalities occur in early HIV infection, often preceding the onset of symptoms of hearing loss or elevation of hearing thresholds.[81,115] The central auditory pathway in the upper brainstem is dysfunctional in earlier stages of HIV infection as indicated by prolonged I-V and III-V intervals, whereas the lower brainstem is affected in advanced HIV infection as indicated by a prolonged I-III interval.[205] Positive stapedial reflex decay, increased interaural time delay, and the absence of recruitment are common findings in HIV-related SNHL, supporting retrocochlear pathology.[81] Central auditory processing can also be impaired in the absence of auditory brainstem response abnormalities because of HIV-related cortical pathology and dementia.[12]

The causes of central auditory pathology include the direct effects of HIV and the secondary effects of immunosuppression. Early demyelination of the central auditory tract is suggested by prolonged wave latencies when faster click rates are used in auditory

---

BOX 10-4

DIFFERENTIAL DIAGNOSIS OF SENSORINEURAL HEARING LOSS IN HIV INFECTION

Otosyphilis
Cryptococcal meningitis*
Central nervous system toxoplasmosis*
Mycobacterial meningitis*
Central effects of HIV infection
   Aseptic meningitis
   Autoimmune demyelination of the cochlear nerve
   Subacute encephalitis*
Progressive multifocal leukoencephalopathy*
Hodgkin's lymphoma
Non-Hodgkin's lymphoma of the brain and meninges*
Mass lesions of the cerebellopontine angle/internal
   auditory canal and petrous apex
Ototoxic medications
   Cerebrovascular accident
   Ideopathic

---

*Associated with late HIV infection, including acquired immunodeficiency syndrome.

brainstem response studies of asymptomatic HIV-infected subjects.[12,81] The progressive demyelination of the central auditory pathway may be a direct effect of HIV on neuroglia as part of the pathogenesis of subacute encephalitis.[208] Multiple cranial nerve abnormalities, including deafness, may also result from central demyelination associated with PML of the brainstem.[154] Opportunistic diseases including CNS toxoplasmosis, TB meningitis, cryptococcal meningitis, and NHL may also cause SNHL in a patient with AIDS.

The labyrinth is not as common a site of HIV-related pathology as is the central auditory system. Few abnormal findings are present on temporal bone histopathology,[47] even on specimens from which viruses have been cultured.[57] Sudden deafness and vestibular hypofunction have occurred in association with acute HIV infection and aseptic meningitis, possibly as a result of a viral labyrinthitis or cochleovestibular neuropathy.[104] The ototoxic effects of new antiretroviral drugs and the long-term effects of various drug combinations are not well established. Medications that have potential ototoxic effects when used for long periods of time include acyclovir, aminoglycosides, amphotericin B, azidothymidine, flucytosine, pentamidine, azithromycin, and trimethoprim-sulfamethoxazole.[5,147,299] Chemotherapy and radiotherapy for the management of malignancy can also lead to ototoxicity and hearing loss. Syphilis and cryptococcal meningitis are manageable causes of temporal bone pathology and SNHL, which can cause significant morbidity in HIV-infected patients if they are not discovered and managed in a timely fashion.

Otosyphilis. HIV is most frequently contracted through sexual contact, accounting for a high coincidence of other sexually transmitted diseases, including syphilis.[259] Otosyphilis should be suspected in any HIV-infected patient who presents with cochleovestibular complaints. In turn, HIV infection should be suspected in all patients diagnosed with syphilis. Hearing loss resulting from syphilis is often bilateral, can be progressive or fluctuate, or can have a sudden onset.[56,168,311] Tinnitus, aural fullness, and disequilibrium occasionally occur. The audiometric curve often shows a low-frequency hearing loss in association with diminished speech discrimination scores.

The diagnosis of otosyphilis is based on history and serologic testing. The fluorescent treponemal antibody absorption (FTA-ABS) test and microhemagglutination-*Treponema pallidum* (MHA-TP) test are treponeme-specific serologic tests with results that remain positive for life, even after eradication of the infection. The Venereal Disease Research Laboratory (VDRL) test or rapid plasmin reagin (RPR) indicate active infection when results are positive along with the FTA-ABS or MHA-TP. However, the VDRL (or RPR) can be negative in primary and tertiary disease. Although a useful screening tool in low-risk populations, VDRL (or RPR) is not sufficiently sensitive to the study of high-risk groups. In the HIV-infected population, as many as 63% of patients have a history of syphilis.[220] In this population, a positive FTA-ABS and cochleovestibular abnormalities are strongly predictive of otosyphilis.[220] These patients should undergo therapy for otosyphilis even if the VDRL is negative.

Progression of primary syphilis to otosyphilis and neurosyphilis is accelerated in HIV-positive patients, even after appropriate management.[259] The interval between primary infection and onset of otosyphilis appears to be shortened to 2 to 5 years in HIV infection compared with 15 to 30 years in the general population. Viable treponemes have been found in perilymph[311] and in temporal bone tissue[174] of patients clinically cured of syphilis. Smith and Canalis[259] hypothesized that residual treponemes, which remain dormant in the temporal bone, are reactivated as cell-mediated immunity deteriorates because of HIV infection. Otosyphilis should therefore be suspected in an HIV-infected patient with cochleovestibular abnormalities and a previous history of treated syphilis because labyrinthine disease may result from reactivation, reinfection, or persistent treponemal infection.

The mainstay of management of otosyphilis is penicillin and corticosteroids. Use of corticosteroids in an HIV-infected patient may be associated with a risk of further immunocompromise, leading to infectious complications. Corticosteroid therapy should be of short duration and be given in close consultation with the patient's primary care provider. Higher than usual doses of penicillin and longer management times have been suggested for the treatment of otosyphilis because organisms tend to persist in the temporal bone. A more aggressive management regimen may be especially necessary in HIV-infected patients who cannot take corticosteroids. These patients will not benefit from the proposed salutary effects of corticosteroids on endarteritis, which increase vessel patency for improved delivery of antibiotics to the temporal bone.[56,259] Smith and Canalis[259] propose a 3-week course of up to 24 million units/day of penicillin G in HIV-infected patients.

Sensorineural Hearing Loss Caused by Cryptococcal Meningitis. Cryptoccal meningitis is an opportunistic infection by the fungus *Cryptococcus neoformans* and is considered an AIDS-defining illness. Before the introduction of HAART, opportunistic infections with *C. neoformans* have been reported to occur in as many as 5% of HIV-positive persons, with meningitis as the most common infection.[54] Since the introduction of HAART, the incidence has decreased by approximately one half.[138] Cryptococcal meningitis is associated with severe immunocompromise and rarely occurs when the CD4+ count is greater than 100 cells/mL. Permanent SNHL occurs in as many as 27% of patients with non–HIV-related cryptococcal meningitis[165] (Box 10-5). Deafness may be sudden or rapidly progressive, and it is often bilateral.[180] Audiometry, including discrimination scores and auditory brainstem response studies, demonstrate predominantly retrocochlear pathology.[113,180] Cryptococcal meningitis can also be associated with facial nerve weakness and dysequilibrium, which usually occurs after the onset of hearing loss.[155,180]

Temporal bone histopathology supports the retrocochlear audiometric features of cryptococcus-induced hearing loss. *C. neoformans* causes extensive invasion and destruction of the fibers and spiral ganglion of the cochlear nerve. Relative sparing of cochlear structures and vestibular nerves occurs in most cases of cryptococcal meningitis, except in fulminant infections.[113,127,154,181] Less prominent involvement of the vestibular nerve on temporal bone histopathology is seen, consistent with the clinical picture of relative sparing of the vestibular system.[113,180]

The diagnosis of cryptococcal meningitis may be delayed because of its sometimes indolent course. The most common presenting symptoms are frontal headache (71%), cranial nerve abnormalities (66%), disorientation (52%), and nausea and vomiting (50%).[165,180] Meningeal signs and fever may be found in one half of patients. However, patients with cryptococcal meningitis may only complain of sudden hearing loss.[181] Hearing loss is the most common cranial nerve manifestation, followed by abnormal papillary reflexes, extraocular muscle paralysis, facial nerve paralysis, and blurred vision. Intracranial hypertension is thought to be the primary cause of visual and extraocular abnormalities associated with cryptococcal meningitis.[133,142]

If SNHL resulting from cryptococcal meningitis is misdiagnosed as idiopathic sudden hearing loss or autoimmune inner ear disease, management with corticosteroids places the patient at risk of developing fulminant life-threatening cryptococcal infection. Sudden and rapidly progressive hearing loss in an immunocompromised HIV-infected patient should therefore include serum cryptococcal antigen and a lumbar puncture before corticosteroid therapy is considered. The cerebrospinal fluid (CSF) abnormalities that are most commonly associated with cryptococcal meningitis are an elevated cell count (may be normal in severe cases), an increased protein level, and a high opening pressure.[165] The diagnosis is made by the detection of cryptococcal antigen and by the identification of *C. neoformans* on culture. Visualization of the encapsulated budding yeast using India ink is a quick and easy but less sensitive test. The current standard therapy is at least 2 weeks of amphotericin B (0.7 mg/kg/day) with or without 5-fluorocytosine, followed by high-dose fluconazole (at least 400 mg/day) for approximately 6 weeks, and then life-long suppression therapy with fluconazole (200 mg/day).[310] Persistent intracranial hypertension may require serial lumbar punctures, acetazolamide, or ventricular-peritoneal shunt placement.[133]

Evaluation of Sensorineural Hearing Loss

The first priority in the evaluation of SNHL in a patient with HIV infection is to rule out potentially life-threatening disease. A thorough history should include a description of the rate of progression of hearing loss and the presence of dysequilibrium, other neurologic symptoms, headache, fever, or neck stiffness. A complete list of all medications should be obtained and ototoxic drugs discontinued if medically feasible. A complete head and neck and neurologic examination should be performed. An audiometric evaluation should include a pure tone audiogram, stapedial reflex testing, and speech discrimination scores. Electronystagmography is useful in the evaluation of dysequilibrium to assess peripheral function. Laboratory studies, including VDRL, FTA-ABS, serum cryptococcus antigen, antinuclear antibodies, erythrocyte sedimentation rate (ESR), and rheumatoid factor (RF) titers should be routine in the evaluation of patients with SNHL. If SNHL is accompanied by headache, fever, meningeal signs, or other neurologic abnormalities, head CT or MRI should be followed by lumbar puncture. Patients with advanced immunocompromise and progressive or sudden SNHL should also undergo brain imaging followed by CSF examination.

BOX 10-5

CRYPTOCOCCAL MENINGITIS AND SENSORINEURAL HEARING LOSS (SNHL)

Associated with low CD4+ counts (<100 cells/μL)

Common presenting symptoms: frontal headache, cranial nerve abnormalities, disorientation

Sudden or rapidly progressive SNHL may be the only symptom

Rule out cryptococcal meningitis by lumbar puncture before treating with corticosteroids for sudden SNHL

Cryptococcal antigen and fungal, mycobacterial, and bacterial cultures should be performed. CSF should also be examined for cytology, VDRL and cell count, protein, and glucose. MRI of the cerebellopontine angle with gadolinium should be considered in patients with asymmetric hearing loss and an otherwise negative workup to rule out acoustic neuromas or other lesions of this region. Auditory brainstem response abnormalities are common in the HIV-infected population, rendering this test insensitive for the detection of cochlear nerve pathology caused by mass lesions in the cerebellopontine angle and internal auditory canal.

Management of hearing loss in the HIV-infected population should focus on the underlying cause. As mentioned above, indiscriminate administration of corticosteroids in the setting of HIV infection is risky. There may be multiple causes of hearing loss during the course of HIV infection. As a result, the clinician should be prepared to repeat the evaluation in search for new causes of SNHL in cases of sudden and rapid deterioration of residual hearing. Finally, auditory rehabilitation with hearing aids has an important role in maintaining the quality of life in an otherwise disabling and isolating disease.

Facial Nerve Paralysis

Unilateral and bilateral idiopathic facial nerve paralyses occur with a 100-fold greater frequency in the HIV-infected population: 4.1%[244] vs about 0.04% in the general population. Isolated facial nerve paralysis more commonly occurs in early-stage HIV infection,[16,18,35] whereas facial nerve paralysis in patients with AIDS may be accompanied by other cranial neuropathies and neurologic abnormalities.[288] For patients with early-stage isolated facial nerve paralysis, recovery appears to be more common than persistent palsy, although the literature in this area is sparse.[151] The differential diagnosis for facial nerve paralysis in HIV-positive patients is quite broad and includes infectious, neoplastic, and autoimmune etiologies (Box 10-6).

Facial nerve palsy may be one of several neurologic abnormalities resulting from AIDS-related CNS disease.[17,155,163] Lalwani and Sooy[155] reported that facial nerve paralysis was present in 7.2% of AIDS patients with neurologic disease. Facial nerve paralysis occurred in 30% of patients with toxoplasmosis, 22% of patients with AIDS encephalopathy, 13% of patients with CNS lymphoma, and 8.7% of patients with cryptococcal meningitis.[155] Facial nerve paralysis may also be one of several neurologic deficits caused by progressive multifocal leukoencephalopathy, the progressive demyelinating disease of the CNS.[17,156,167] There is strong evidence that on crossing the blood-brain

---

BOX 10-6

DIFFERENTIAL DIAGNOSIS OF FACIAL NERVE PARALYSIS IN HIV INFECTION

Isolated Facial Nerve Paralysis
Geniculate ganglionitis
  Herpes zoster
  Herpes simplex, cytomegalovirus, Epstein-Barr virus, or HIV
Neuritis
  HIV
  Autoimmune demyelination
  Mononeuritis
Malignant otitis externa
Complicated otomastoiditis
Space-occupying lesion of cerebellopontine angle/internal auditory canal
Malignancy of parotid gland or temporal bone
Ideopathic

Facial Nerve Paralysis Associated with other Neurologic Abnormalities
Effects of HIV infection
  Autoimmune demyelination
  Mononeuritis multiplex
  Subacute encephalitis
Central nervous system infections
  Toxoplasmosis
  Cryptococcal meningitis
  Progressive multifocal leukoencephalopathy
  Mycobacterial meningitis
Central nervous system neoplasms
  Non-Hodgkin's lymphoma
  Metastatic Kaposi's sarcoma
Skull base neoplasm
Cerebrovascular accident

---

barrier, HIV incites a host-mediated autoimmune demyelination of cranial nerves similar to Guillain-Barré syndrome.[3,55] Increased immunoglobulins and lymphocyte pleocytosis in the CSF often occurs in association with facial nerve and other cranial neuropathies, supporting an autoimmune etiology in some cases of cranial polyneuropathy.[16,89]

Isolated facial nerve paralysis may be the first symptom of HIV infection occurring in association with the acute infection or thereafter.[17,314] An exception to this is Ramsey-Hunt syndrome, which occurs more frequently in the setting of impaired cell-mediated immunity in later stages of HIV infection. When associated with acute HIV infection, transient facial nerve paralysis precedes seroconversion by 4 to 6 weeks,[308] complicating the early diagnosis of HIV in patients who present with facial nerve palsy. Aseptic meningitis is commonly associated with facial nerve paralysis in this setting.[151,214] A flu-like illness marked by fever, myalgia, lymphadenopathy, diarrhea, and a rash usually precedes the onset of facial palsy by 3 weeks.[196,244]

The pathogenesis of isolated facial nerve weakness in HIV infection is similar to that in the general population but is likely to be influenced by the neurotropic effects of HIV and the increased susceptibility of the host to other infectious agents (see Box 10-6). Nerve conduction measurements using magnetic stimulation reveal normal function of the intracranial portion of the nerve and its cortical and bulbar connections.[236] However, the intratemporal portion of the nerve shows abnormal conduction properties and clinical evidence of complete axonotmesis in most cases. This is supported by MRI findings of increased enhancement of the facial nerve in the labyrinthine portion of the fallopian canal, especially in the perigeniculate region.[67,241]

The underlying mechanisms of HIV-related isolated facial nerve paralysis therefore appear to be similar to those of Bell's palsy and herpes zoster oticus. Inflammation of the nerve leads to intraneural edema and nerve compression at the meatal foramen and the narrow labyrinthine segment of the canal. A viscous cycle of nerve ischemia is followed by further swelling and compression, resulting in progression from neuropraxia to axonotmesis and degeneration. The viral agents that produce facial nerve dysfunction are ambiguous.[198] Inciting events leading to this cascade are likely to occur in the geniculate ganglion where herpes simplex[285] or herpes zoster[16,190] may be reactivated in the immunocompromised patient, or there may be primary infection by CMV, EBV, or HIV. Zoster oticus is a relatively infrequent cause of facial nerve paralysis in association with HIV infection. However, when it occurs in a patient diagnosed with or at risk for HIV infection, it is a predictor of deteriorating immune function and impending AIDS.[183] The prevalence of HIV infection among patients with idiopathic facial nerve paralysis is disproportionately high in endemic populations of Africa, accounting for 25% of cases in Kenya[6] and 69% of cases in Central Africa.[16] This variation in the prevalence of HIV-related facial nerve paralysis in different parts of the world suggests that either different endemic organisms are involved or there are several strains of the same organism with different neurotropic properties. HIV strains, for instance, are known to differ in their neurotropism.[163]

The often reported association among acute HIV infection, aseptic meningitis, and acute facial paralysis supports a direct role by HIV in some cases.[244,288] HIV may directly infect the geniculate ganglion or Schwann cells. Alternatively, inflammation associated with autoimmune demyelination of the nerve in response to infection of the CNS by HIV can result

in facial nerve compression in the narrow segments of the fallopian canal. Etiologic agents thought to be involved in the pathogenesis of Bell's palsy in the general population (e.g., herpes simplex)[36,192] may infect the geniculate ganglion, or latent infection may be reactivated at an increased rate in the HIV-infected population.

Evaluation and Management

The work-up of facial nerve weakness may provide the initial diagnosis of HIV infection. Belec and others[18] reported that 15 of 16 patients with HIV-related facial palsy were diagnosed with HIV in the course of their evaluation for facial weakness. However, because HIV-related facial nerve paralysis can occur before HIV seroconversion and the symptom onset of HIV infection, the true diagnosis can be easily missed.[151] Facial nerve paralysis has a high predictive value for HIV infection in populations with high rates of seroconversion.[6,18] HIV serology should therefore be included in the routine evaluation of facial nerve paralysis, especially in patients with high-risk behavior. The clinician's suspicion for HIV infection should be further increased by the presence of bilateral facial nerve paralysis, a recent flu-like illness, and Ramsay Hunt syndrome with disseminated herpes zoster. Because the onset of facial weakness may precede HIV seroconversion, negative HIV test results in patients at risk for HIV infection should be followed by a repeat test in 6 weeks.[151]

Evaluation of facial nerve paralysis in HIV-infected patients should include a search for potentially life-threatening and treatable causes, such as malignant OE, temporal bone and parotid tumors, cryptococcal meningitis, and toxoplasmosis or NHL of the CNS. The history should include an account of other symptoms associated with facial nerve paralysis, including neurologic symptoms, headache, meningismus, and fever. A recent history of a flu-like illness may indicate acute HIV infection. The physical examination should include a complete neurologic examination. Otoscopy should be routinely performed to rule out middle ear and EAC pathology. Vesicles in the concha and EAC, especially when associated with otalgia, are diagnostic of zoster oticus. The parotid glands should be palpated for masses. Audiometry should be routinely performed as part of the cranial nerve evaluation. Blood should be tested for cryptococcal antigen, VDRL, FTA-ABS, ESR, and antinuclear antibodies.

Subsequent tests should be directed by the level of immunocompromise, results of the neurologic evaluation, and time course of the facial paralysis. The presence of other neurologic abnormalities along with facial nerve dysfunction, especially in the setting of AIDS, should raise the clinician's suspicion of an intracranial process. A brain MRI should be performed in search for toxoplasmosis, NHL, and PML.[164,262] A lumbar puncture should be performed and CSF sent for cell counts; glucose; protein; VDRL; cryptococcal antigen; immunoglobulin panel to evaluate for demyelinating process; fungal, viral, and bacterial cultures; and cytology for lymphoma. Unfortunately, lymphomatous meningitis is not always detected with the use of brain imaging or CSF cytology. Serial CSF cytology may have to be performed in the setting of persistent or progressive cranial polyneuropathy and other neurologic findings. In patients with a history of systemic NHL, a presumptive diagnosis of CNS lymphoma can be made and empiric management of the brain with radiotherapy considered.[262] Isolated and idiopathic facial nerve palsy in an asymptomatic and relatively immunocompetent HIV-infected patient may be followed clinically, similar to Bell's palsy in the general population. The absence of improvement in facial function by 4 to 6 weeks should lead to MRI or CT of the brain, temporal bones, and parotid glands to rule out pathology in these locations, followed by examination of the CSF.

HIV-infected patients with facial nerve paralysis, especially those with bilateral disease, are at increased risk for exposure keratitis because of poor eye closure. When eye closure is insufficient to protect the cornea, artificial tears should be used throughout the day, and a moisture chamber should be placed over each involved eye at bedtime. Frequent oral rinses and effective dental hygiene should be instituted to protect against periodontal disease, which may be exacerbated by loss of oral competence and oral dryness.

Medical therapy may be beneficial in some cases of HIV-related facial nerve paralysis, whereas other cases resolve spontaneously. Zidovudine has been proposed for early HIV-related paralysis, but there are no well-controlled studies to demonstrate efficacy. Corticosteroids, which are used in the management of Bell's palsy in immunocompetent patients, may increase the risks of life-threatening infection in HIV-infected patients. However, in early HIV infection, especially in cases of bilateral facial paralysis, a short course of corticosteroids should be given because the risks of management are outweighed by the possible ophthalmologic and dental complications of the neuropathy. High-dose acyclovir may be beneficial in HIV-infected patients with an idiopathic facial palsy, although this has not been systematically studied.[154] Plasmapheresis may be considered for patients who are significantly disabled by multiple cranial nerve deficits resulting from autoimmune demyelination similar to Guillain-Barré syndrome and in whom corticosteroid therapy is too risky.[164] The role of surgical decompression of the entrapped facial nerve in HIV

infection is unknown. However, the potential benefit of improved nerve recovery should be weighed against the risks of craniotomy in the presence of immunocompromise.

The literature on the quality of facial nerve recovery in HIV infection is sparse. Complete recovery is more commonly reported than is incomplete recovery. The duration of weakness ranges from days to months and tends to be shorter and associated with a better outcome in early HIV infection.[151]

ORAL MANIFESTATIONS OF HIV INFECTION

Oral lesions occur in almost all patients during the course of HIV infection.[62] The most commonly encountered oral manifestations include candidiasis, oral hairy leukoplakia (OHL), KS, periodontal and gingival infections, aphthous ulcers, herpes simplex stomatitis, and xerostomia (Box 10-7). The presence of one or more of these oral lesions in a patient who is at risk for HIV infection is highly predictive for HIV seroconversion.[185] KS and NHL are the most prevalent malignancies occurring in the oral cavity and pharynx. However, as the longevity of patients with AIDS increases, so does their risk of developing other malignancies. The clinician should be prepared to handle this increasing challenge (1) by being familiar with the oral lesions that commonly occur in this patient population, (2) by performing biopsies of all lesions that are suspicious or that do not respond to a short course of empiric therapy, and (3) by not assuming that multiple concurrent lesions have the same pathogenesis.

Oral Candidiasis

Candidal infection is the most common oral manifestation of HIV infection. Oral candidiasis occurs in 70% to 90% of patients with symptomatic HIV infection

---

BOX 10-7

DIFFERENTIAL DIAGNOSIS OF ORAL LESIONS IN HIV INFECTION

Oral candidiasis
Oral hairy leukoplakia
Herpes stomatitis
Gingival and periodontal disease
   Acute necrotizing ulcerative gingivitis*
   Necrotizing stomatitis
Aphthous ulcers
Bacillary angiomatosis*
Squamous cell carcinoma*
Leukoplakia
Non-Hodgkin's lymphoma*
Kaposi's sarcoma

*May be associated with bone erosion.

and AIDS.[253] Oral candidiasis appears to be presenting in increasingly advanced stages of HIV infection according to a report by Glick and others,[94] who demonstrated a mean CD4+ count of 149.5 cells/mL at diagnosis. These patients have a poorer than average prognosis and progress rapidly to AIDS.

Candidal infection of the oral mucosa can take four forms[101]: (1) Pseudo-membranous candidiasis presents as a smooth white or cottage cheese–like plaques that can occur on any mucosal surface. When the plaque is wiped off, an erythematous and bleeding base remains. (2) Atrophic candidiasis presents as zones of hyperemia and tenderness on the dorsum of the tongue or the hard palate. (3) Hyperplastic candidiasis most commonly involves the buccal mucosa to produce raised white plaques that cannot be scraped off. The differential diagnosis of this lesion includes leukoplakia, carcinoma in situ, and OHL. Diagnosis is made by biopsy or potassium hydroxide preparation, which reveals hyphae and yeast. (4) Angular cheilitis presents as tender and erythematous fissures and ulcers at the oral commissure (Figure 10-5).

Candidal infection can be diagnosed based on the resolution of these lesions with empiric anticandidal therapy. A more definitive diagnosis can be made through the use of a potassium hydroxide preparation or Gram's stain of a scraping or by periodic acid-Schiff stain of a biopsy specimen. Topical therapy is effective for oral candidiasis in early HIV infection. Nystatin solution (200,000 to 400,000 units five times/day) or clotrimazole (10 mg five times/day) are commonly used. Angular cheilitis can be managed with topical antifungal creams, such as nystatin, clotrimazole, or ketoconazole. Oral candidiasis can also be effectively managed with systemic therapy, including ketoconazole (200 mg/day) or fluconazole (50 mg/day). A combination of topical and systemic therapy should be used in patients in severe immunocompromise.

Oral Hairy Leukoplakia

OHL is a white lesion with a corrugated and shaggy surface; it most frequently occurs on the lateral surface of the tongue. OHL affects 17% to 25% of HIV-positive patients with AIDS and was initially thought to be pathognomonic for HIV infection.[94,253] Several case reports, however, have demonstrated OHL in immunosuppressed transplant patients.[102,276] OHL appears to result from a local opportunistic infection by EBV.[103] Its presence in an otherwise asymptomatic patient is a strong indicator of a diagnosis of HIV infection and moderate to severe immunosuppression. In one series, the mean CD4+ count of patients with OHL was 143 cells/mL.[94] OHL indicates a poor prognosis for progression to AIDS.[101] The presence of

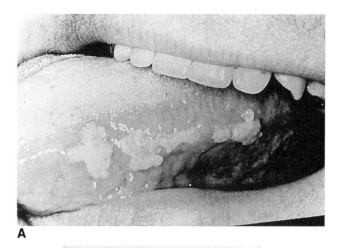

A

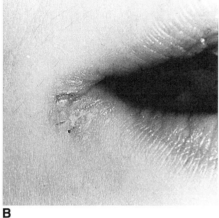

B

Figure 10-5. Pseudomembranous candidiasis and angular cheilitis. **A,** Pseudomembranous candidiasis of the lateral surface of the tongue. These smooth white plaques are easily scraped from the mucosa, leaving an erythematous and bleeding base. **B,** Angular cheilitis characterized by tender ulcers and fissures of the oral commissure as a result of candidal infection. (Courtesy of Dr. Steven Ashman.)

OHL has been demonstrated to have prognostic value for HIV disease progression. In a study controlling for CD4+ count, the presence of OHL increased the rate of developing AIDS in 6 months nearly two-fold.[141]

When an oral lesion persists despite a short course of anticandidal therapy, a biopsy is indicated to rule out a malignant or premalignant lesion. The differential diagnosis of OHL includes leukoplakia, carcinoma in situ, hypertrophic candidiasis, and lichen planus. OHL is diagnosed on biopsy by the presence of hyperkeratosis, acanthosis, clear or "balloon" cells in the upper spinous cell layer with minimal inflammation, and the presence of EBV in the basal epithelial cells[101] (Figure 10-6). Once the diagnosis is made, further management is rarely needed because OHL is asymptomatic and does not undergo malignant transformation. No single medication has been consistently successful in producing a remission of OHL. Occasional

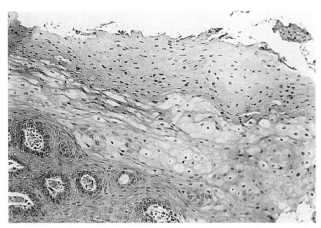

Figure 10-6. Photomicrograph of oral hairy leukoplakia. Characteristic hyperparakeratosis is present, as is a layer of "balloon cells" in the upper spinous cell layer. (Courtesy of Dr. Russel Corio.)

success has been reported with the use of acyclovir, zidovudine, and sulfa drugs, but the recurrence rate is high.[24,101]

Herpes Simplex Stomatitis

Infections of the oral cavity by herpes simplex virus (HSV) increase in all stages of HIV infection. The overall incidence is 5%, whereas in late-stage HIV infection it is 9% to 29%.[94,253] Herpetic lesions are particularly persistent when the CD4+ count is less than 100 cells/mL. Herpes labialis is the most common manifestation of herpes simplex infection of the oral cavity. When they occur in the HIV-infected patient, these "fever blisters" are generally larger and more numerous, persist longer, and recur more frequently than in the general population. Intraoral infection by herpes simplex usually affects the keratinized and attached mucosa of the hard palate and gingiva and the dorsum of the tongue. The characteristic appearance is that of small round ulcers without an erythematous halo. Multiple ulcers can produce significant discomfort with mastication and swallowing, threatening nutrition. HSV infection in an HIV-infected patient is likely to be prolonged and less localized than in the general population.

Herpes simplex infection can be diagnosed by culturing the virus from vesicles or by showing HSV in cells scraped from the base of the lesion using monoclonal anti-HSV antibodies (Tzanck test). As soon as vesicles consistent with HSV infection appear, topical acyclovir therapy should be instituted five times/ day for 5 days. In a severely immunocompromised patient or in a patient with a generalized vesicular rash, topical therapy should be combined with systemic therapy for 5 days, with acyclovir at 200 mg five times/day.[101]

Gingivitis and Periodontal Disease

Infection of the gingiva and periodontal structures in an HIV-infected patient can produce a spectrum of pathology ranging from gingivitis to necrotizing stomatitis. Despite good oral hygiene and timely therapy, gingivitis and periodontal disease commonly recur in HIV-infected patients. Gingivitis presents as a red line at the free gingival margin, and the gums bleed with minimal trauma.[101] Periodontitis results from the extension of infection to the peridontium and resorption of alveolar bone, resulting in loosening and loss of teeth and deep dental pain.

A rapidly progressive and necrotizing form of gingivitis is known as *acute necrotizing ulcerative gingivitis* (ANUG). Gingivitis progresses to ANUG within 4 weeks, resulting in the necrosis of gingival tissue and alveolar bone.[101] Symptoms include deep jaw pain, bleeding, halitosis, and loose teeth. The tissue above the interdental papillae is typically yellow-grey and bleeds easily. Acute necrotizing periodontitis is a progression of ANUG resulting from extensive soft tissue destruction and the exposure of bone with significant bone destruction and sequestration.[99] Gram-negative anaerobes appear to play an important role in the pathogenesis of ANUG and necrotizing stomatitis.

The risk of progression from gingivitis to periodontitis and then to ANUG increases as immune function deteriorates and the CD4+ count falls. Drinkard et al[66] observed good periodontal health for a cohort of 106 HIV-positive patients who had not yet progressed to AIDS, whereas Glick et al[94] found a 6.3% prevalence of ANUG in a population of 750 patients with advanced HIV infection as evidenced by a mean CD4+ count of 32 cells/mm^3.

The differential diagnosis of a destructive process that involves the soft tissue and bone of the alveolar crests includes lymphoma, SCC, KS, bacillary angiomatosis, fungal infection, and mycobacterial infection. The presence of bone destruction out of proportion with the soft tissue changes is more likely to be caused by bacillary angiomatosis than ANUG.[93] Tissue should be sent for histopathology and microbiology. Periodontal consultation should be requested for appropriate and expeditious management of periodontal disease.

The mainstay of therapy for HIV-related gingivitis and periodontitis includes dental plaque removal and oral rinses with 10% povidone-iodine with 0.1% to 0.2% chlorhexidine gluconate.[101] Management of ANUG and necrotizing stomatitis includes a combination of local care and systemic antianaerobic drug therapy. The necrotic tissue should be débrided, the teeth scaled, and parenteral antibiotic therapy with clindamycin or metronidazole (Flagyl) instituted.

Aphthous Ulcers

Aphthous ulcers are of three types, all of which affect unattached oral mucosa. Herpetiform ulcers are smaller than 0.2 mm in diameter and are self-limited. Minor aphthous ulcers are well-circumscribed, painful ulcers less than 6 mm in diameter with an erythematous halo. In HIV-infected patients, ulcers frequently coalesce to form larger lesions lasting about 2 weeks.

Major aphthous ulcers (Sutton's disease) are larger than 6 mm in diameter (Figure 10-7). They are painful, persist for weeks, and threaten nutritional intake. They are difficult to grossly differentiate from malignancy. The incidence of major aphthous ulcers is as high as 14% in association with HIV infection.[253] Glick and others[94] have shown that major aphthous ulcers are highly predictive of a CD4+ count less than 200 cells/mL presenting in patients with a mean CD4+ count of 33.7 cells/mL.

Management should focus on ruling out malignancy, providing symptomatic relief, and monitoring nutritional status. The edge of the ulcer should be biopsied and submitted for histopathology to rule out lymphoma and SCC. The size, chronicity, and exquisite tenderness of major aphthous ulcers mandate close monitoring of body weight and the provision of liquid nutritional supplements. Aphthous ulcers are treated with topical corticosteroids, such as triamcinolone or flucinonide and applied up to six times per day.[101] Other topical preparations include tetracycline (250 mg per 5 mL) used as a mouth wash four times/day for 4 days, or chlorhexidine 0.1% to 0.2% twice per day for 7 days. The prudent use of systemic corticosteroids may be necessary in major aphthous ulcers.

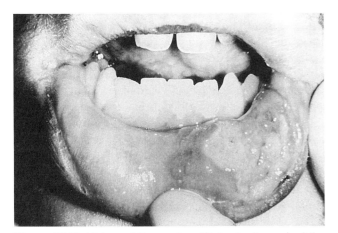

Figure 10-7. Major aphthous ulcer (Sutton's disease) of the lower lip. This lesion is indistinguishable from lymphoma or squamous cell carcinoma and should undergo biopsy. (Courtesy of Dr. Steven Ashman.)

Xerostomia

Xerostomia is a complaint of 7% to 14% HIV-infected patients.[94,253] Some cases are iatrogenically induced by the use of antidepressants and other drugs, whereas others are caused by chronic mouth breathing resulting from sinonasal disease or adenoidal hypertrophy. HIV-related xerostomia is associated with parotid enlargement in 33% of cases possibly because of autoimmune or infectious disease of the salivary glands. The incidence of dental caries is increased, and deglutition is often impaired. Salivary substitutes, frequent saline rinses, and sialogogues help alleviate these problems. Dental caries can be prevented with fluoride.

Oral Manifestations of HIV in the Era of HAART

A significant decline in the frequency of oral lesions in HIV-positive patients has occurred since the introduction of HAART. These findings likely represent earlier detection and improved overall medical care of HIV-positive patients, increased use of prophylactic medications to prevent opportunistic infection,[194] and perhaps most importantly the availability of potent antiretroviral therapy.[71,297] Reports of the prevalence of oral lesions show a 47% to 74% prevalence before the introduction of HAART and a 29% to 38% prevalence afterward.[63,211,224] Candidiasis and OHL rates have been significantly reduced from 51% to 17%[64] and from 30% to 16%,[224] respectively. In patients who receive HAART, the presence of these lesions might indicate failure of antiretroviral treatment.[73] Other oral lesions such as KS, aphtous ulcers, and oral herpes have also shown a decline since the introduction of HAART.[224]

OCCUPATIONAL EXPOSURE TO HIV INFECTION

With nearly 1 million HIV-positive patients in the United States and the prevalence of otolaryngologic complaints among these patients, most otolaryngologists will treat HIV-positive patients at some point in their careers. In addition to blood, HIV has been isolated from bodily fluids commonly encountered by the otolaryngologist including middle ear effusion, tears, and saliva.[265] An understanding of the risks of occupational transmission as well as precautions that may minimize such transmission is essential.

Risks of Transmission

As of December 2001, voluntary reports of 57 documented cases of HIV seroconversion among U.S. health care personnel temporally related to occupational exposure to HIV had been reported.[122,291] An additional 138 infections among health care personnel were considered to be possible cases of occupational HIV transmission. Percutaneous injuries, specifically those from hollow-bore needles, represent the most common mechanism of occupational HIV transmission. The CDC estimates that 380,000 needle-stick injuries occur in hospitals each year, with 61% of these injuries occurring with hollow-bore devices.[201] Pooled prospective data suggest an average risk of HIV transmission of 0.3% for needle sticks and 0.09% after mucous membrane exposure.[291] The risk of transmission from fluid other than blood or transmission through non-intact skin is too low to be estimated in prospective studies. Although occupational HIV infection has been attributed to suture needles among surgical personnel, suture needles have not been implicated as a source of transmission in prospective studies.

Multiple factors suggesting increased risk of transmission have been identified. Exposures involving hollow-bore needles, devices that contain visible blood, devices previously used for vein or artery insertion, deep injury to the health care provider, or exposures from source patients who die within 2 months after exposure all increase the risk of occupational transmission.[40] All of these factors suggest that the quantitative viral inoculum is an important factor in transmission. Although a low plasma HIV RNA titer indicates a lower inoculum and suggests decreased risk of transmission of disease, these tests do not account for cell-associated HIV. Transmission from source patients with undetectable viral loads have been reported.[291]

Many occupational exposures occur in patients whose HIV status is unknown. Using current enzyme immunoassays, the interval between onset of viremia and detection of HIV antibody is a few days at most.[39] Thus, in the case of a negative test result in a source patient who is without HIV risk factors or clinical evidence of acute HIV infection, the risk of HIV transmission is assumed to be zero.

Prevention of Transmission and Postexposure Prophylaxis

Prevention of blood exposure through the use of safe practices, barrier precautions, safe-needle devices and other innovations is the best way to prevent infection with HIV and other bloodborne pathogens.[197,291] Unfortunately, universal precaution compliance among physicians has been reported as low as 16%.[112] For otolaryngologists, independent risk factors for occupational exposure include operations lasting longer than 3 hours and head and neck cases.[20] Inexperienced surgeons, particularly interns and residents, are more likely to suffer sharp injuries.[137] Simple strategies such as using double gloves, eye protection, impermeable gowns, and special techniques for passing sharp objects have all been suggested to minimize exposure risk.

Despite such precautions, needle sticks and mucosal exposures will continue. To minimize the risk of disease transmission in such instances, postexposure prophylaxis (PEP) has been proposed. The pathogenesis of HIV infection suggests a window of opportunity in which antiretroviral therapy may prevent infection.[87] Animal models have demonstrated the benefits of PEP and have also demonstrated the importance of minimizing the time between viral inoculum and initiation of prophylaxis.[29,178,204,286,287]

PEP typically consists of multiple antiretroviral medications taken for 4 weeks. Treatment may be discontinued if the source patient subsequently tests negative for HIV infection and does not demonstrate any evidence of acute HIV infection. Current recommendations for needle sticks are based on risk stratification of the exposure and the HIV status of the source patient. For health care workers who sustain high-risk injuries including large-bore hollow-needle sticks, injury with visibly bloody devices, deep puncture wounds, or injury from a needle previously used in an artery or vein from an HIV-positive patient, an expanded, three-drug prophylaxis is recommended. For health care workers who sustain low-risk exposures including solid-needle, superficial injures, the treatment recommendation depends on the source patient's HIV status. For HIV-positive but asymptomatic source patients with a viral load less than 1500, the basic two-drug prophylaxis is recommended. If the source patient is symptomatic for HIV infection including the viral prodrome, has AIDS, or has a viral load greater than 1500, the expanded, three-drug regimen is recommended. For patients whose HIV status is unknown, prophylaxis is generally not warranted, regardless of exposure risk, unless the source patient has HIV risk factors, in which case the two-drug regimen is recommended.[291]

Protection after PEP is not complete. In the United States and abroad, more than 20 cases of occupational transmission occurring despite the use of PEP have been reported.* Some of these cases included patients who received multiple drug regimens. A retrospective, case-controlled study using zidovudine alone for PEP suggested an 81% reduction in the risk of HIV transmission.[39] Postexposure regimens that include three drugs are more likely to result in adverse events and early discontinuation of treatment than are two-drug regimens.[302] Viral resistance has been suggested as a mechanism for PEP failure. In a study of 41 occupational exposures to HIV, virus from the source patient was found to have a 39% rate of mutations associated with resistance to reverse transcriptase inhibitors

---

*References 19, 132, 212, 219, 291, 306.

and a 10% rate of mutations associated with protease inhibitor resistance. Unfortunately, clinical data and current laboratory techniques do not allow for accurate, timely analysis of viral resistance, and thus two or more antiviral drugs are typically used for prophylaxis after an occupational exposure.[87]

PEP has been associated with significant adverse effects. One half of health care personnel taking PEP report adverse effects and one third discontinue PEP as a result.[302] Minor adverse effects such as GI discomfort are the most common. Severe effects such as hepatitis, pancytopenia, impairment or extraocular muscles, and nephrolithiasis have been reported. Nevirapine in particular has been associated with multiple severe adverse effects and is no longer recommended for prophylaxis.[4,246]

SUMMARY

The emergence of HIV has dramatically changed the landscape of medicine both in the United States and throughout the world. In virtually all fields of medicine, the management of HIV-positive patients has proved challenging. A clear understanding of the basic pathophysiology of HIV infection combined with the common manifestations in the ear, nose, throat, oral cavity, and neck will allow otolaryngologists to effectively evaluate and manage HIV-positive patients.

REFERENCES

1. Aboulafia DM: Regression of acquired immunodeficiency syndrome-related pulmonary Kaposi's sarcoma after highly active antiretroviral therapy, *Mayo Clin Proc* 73:439, 1998.
2. Abrams DI: AIDS-related lymphadenopathy: the role of biopsy, *J Clin Oncol* 4:126, 1986.
3. Abrams DI and others: Persistent diffuse lymphadenopathy in homosexual men: endpoint or prodrome, *Ann Intern Med* 100:801, 1984.
4. Adverse effects associated with the use of nevirapine in HIV postexposure prophylaxis for 2 health care workers, *JAMA* 284:2722, 2000.
5. AHFS, McEvoy GK, editor: *Drug information*. Bethesda, Md, American Society of Health-Systems Pharmacists, Inc, 1996.
6. Amayo EO, Kwasa TO: HIV and acute peripheral facial nerve palsy, *East Afr Med J* 68:948, 1991.
7. Andreoni M and others: Primary human herpesvirus 8 in immunocompetent children, *JAMA* 287:1295, 2002.
8. Appleby P and others: International collaboration on HIV and cancer: highly active antiretroviral therapy and incidence of cancer in human immunodeficiency virus–infected adults, *J Natl Cancer Inst* 92:1823, 2000.
9. Armstrong M and others: Radiographic imaging of sinusitis in HIV infection, *Otolaryngol Head Neck Surg* 108:36, 1993.
10. Atula T and others: Fine-needle aspiration biopsy in the diagnosis of parotid gland lesions: evaluation of 438 biopsies, *Diagn Cytopathol* 15:185, 1996.
11. Bangsberg DR and others: Adherence to protease inhibitors, HIV-1 viral load, and development of drug resistance in an inigent population, *AIDS* 14:357, 2000.
12. Bankaitis AE, Keith RW: Audiological changes associated with HIV infection, *Ear Nose Throat J* 74:353, 1995.

13. Barnett E and others: Otitis media in children born to human immunodeficiency virus–infected mothers, *Pediatr Infect Dis J* 11:360, 1992.
14. Baroni CD, Uccini S: The lymphadenopathy of HIV infection, *Am J Clin Pathol* 99:397, 1993.
15. Beitler and others: Low-dose radiotherapy for multicystic benign lymphoepithelial lesions of the parotid gland in HIV-positive patients: long-term results, *Head Neck* 17:35, 1995.
16. Belec L and others: Peripheral facial nerve palsy related to HIV infection: relationship with the immunological status and the HIV staging in Central Africa, *Cent Afr J Med* 37:88, 1991.
17. Belec L and others: Peripheral facial paralysis and HIV infection: report of four African cases and review of the literature, *J Neurol* 236:411, 1989.
18. Belec L and others: Peripheral facial paralysis indicating HIV infection, *Lancet* 2:1421, 1988.
19. Beltrami EM and others: *HIV transmission after an occupational exposure despite postexposure prophylaxis with a combination drug regimen [abstract]. In Program and abstracts of the 4th Decennial International Conference on Nosocomial and Healthcare-Associated Infections: in conjunction with the 10th annual meeting of SHEA, Atlanta March 5-9, 2000.* Atlanta, 2000, Centers for Disease Control and Prevention, p 125.
20. Benninger MS and others: Intraoperative infectious disease exposure to otolaryngology operating room personnel, *Laryngoscope* 101:1276, 1991.
21. Beral V and others: AIDS-associated non-Hodgkins lymphoma, *Lancet* 337:805, 1991.
22. Beral V and others: Kaposi's sarcoma among persons with AIDS: a sexually transmitted infection? *Lancet* 335:123, 1990.
23. Berson and others: Radiation therapy for AIDS-related Kaposi's sarcoma, *Int J Radiat Oncol Biol Phys* 19:569-575, 1990.
24. Birchall M, Murphy S: *HIV infection and AIDS.* Edinburgh, Scotland, Churchill Livingstone, 1992.
25. Birchall MA and others: Auditory function in patients infected with the human immunodeficiency virus, *Clin Otolaryngol* 17:117, 1992.
26. Birchall MA and others: Changing patterns of HIV infection in otolaryngology, *Clin Otolaryngol* 19:473, 1994.
27. Blatt SP and others: Rhinocerebral zygomycosis in a patient with AIDS [letter], *J Infect Dis* 164:215, 1991.
28. Bloom DC and others: Head and neck manifestations of mycobacterium avium complex disease as a consequence of return of immunocompetency in AIDS, *Otolaryngol Head Neck Surg* 125:668, 2001.
29. Bottinger D and others: Prevention of simian immunodeficiency virus, SIVsm, or HIV-2 infection in cynomolgus monkeys by pre- and post-exposure administration of BEA-005, *AIDS* 11:157, 1997.
30. Boudreaux AA and others: Intralesional cinblastine for cutaneous Kaposi's sarcoma associated with acquired immunodeficiency syndrome, *J Am Acad Dermatol* 28:68, 1993.
31. Bourboulia D and others: Serologic evidence for mother-to-child transmission of Kaposi sarcoma-associated herpesvirus infection, *JAMA* 280:31, 1998.
32. Bower M and others: Highly active anti-retroviral therapy prolongs time to treatment failure in Kaposi's sarcoma, *AIDS* 13:2105, 1999.
33. Brambilla L and others: Intralesional chemotherapy for Kaposi's sarcoma, *Dermatologica* 169:150, 1984.

34. Breda SD and others: Pneumocystis carinii in the temporal bone as a primary manifestation of the acquired immunodeficiency syndrome, *Ann Otol Rhinol Laryngol* 97:427, 1988.

35. Brown MM and others: Bell's palsy and HIV infection, *J Neurol Neurosurg Psychiatry* 51:425, 1988.

36. Burgess R and others: Polymerase chain reaction amplification of herpes simplex viral DNA from the geniculate ganglion of a patient with Bell's palsy, *Ann Otol Rhinol Laryngol* 103:775, 1994.

37. Burke AP and others: Systemic lymphadenopathic histology in human immunodeficiency virus-1 seropositive drug addicts without apparent acquired immunodeficiency syndrome, *Hum Pathol* 25:248, 1994.

38. Burton F and others: Open cervical node biopsy in HIV-positive patients, *Otolaryngol Head Neck Surg* 107:367, 1992.

39. Busch M and others: Time course of detection of viral and serologic markers preceding human immunodeficiency virus type 1 seroconversion: implications for screening of blood and tissue donations, *Transfusion* 35:91, 1995.

40. Caardo DM and others: A case-control study of HIV seroconversion in health care workers after percutaneous exposure, *N Engl J Med* 337:1485, 1997.

41. Calzolari A and others: Epstein-Barr virus infection and p53 expression in HIV-related oral large B cell lymphoma, *Head Neck* 21:454-460, 1999.

42. Carbone A and others: A clinicopathologic stidy of lymphoid neoplama associated with human immunodeficiency virus infection in Italy, *Cancer* 68:842, 1991.

43. Carbone A and others: Head and neck lymphomas associated with human immunodeficiency virus infection, *Arch Otolaryngol Head Neck Surg* 121:210, 1995.

44. Centers for Disease Control and Prevention: HIV/AIDS update 2003.

45. Chachoua and others: Prognostic factors and staging classification of patients with epidemic Kaposi's sarcoma, *J Clin Oncol* 7:774, 1989.

46. Chadburn A and others: Progressive lymph node histology and its prognostic value in patients with acquired immunodeficiency syndrome and AIDS-related complex, *Hum Pathol* 20:579, 1989.

47. Chandrasekhar SS, Siverls V, Sekhar HK: Histopathologic and ultrastructural changes in the temporal bones of HIV-infected human adults, *Am J Otol* 13:207, 1991.

48. Chang Y and others: Identification of herpes virus-like DNA sequences in AIDS-associated Kaposi's sarcoma, *Science* 255:1865, 1994.

49. Cheung S, Lee K, Cha I: Orbitocerebral complications of pseudomonas sinusitis, *Laryngoscope* 102:1385-1389, 1992.

50. Chhieng DC and others: Utility of fine-needle aspiration in the diagnosis of salivary gland lesions in patients infected with human immunodeficiency virus, *Diagn Cytopathol* 21:260-264, 1999.

51. Choi SS and others: Cryptococcal sinusitis: a case report and review of the literature, *Otolaryngol Head Neck Surg* 99:414, 1988.

52. Colmenero C and others: Successfully treated Candida sinusitis in an AIDS patient, *J Craniomaxillofacial Surg* 18:175, 1990.

53. Cote TR and others: Non-Hodgkin's lymphoma among people with AIDS: incidence, presentation, and public health burden: AIDS/Cancer study group, *Int J Cancer* 73:645, 1997.

54. Currie BP, Casadevall A: Estimation of the prevalence of cryptococcal infection among patients infected with the human immunodeficiency virus in New York City, *Clin Infect Dis* 19:1029-1033, 1994.

55. Dalakas MC, Pezeshkpour GH: Neuromuscular diseases associated with human immunodeficiency virus infection, *Ann Neurol* 23:S38, 1988.

56. Darmstadt GL, Harris JP: Luetic hearing loss: clinical presentation, diagnosis and treatment, *Am J Otolaryngol* 10:410, 1989.

57. Davidson BJ and others: Lymphadenopathy in the HIV-seropositive patient, *Ear Nose Throat J* 69:478, 1990.

58. Davis JM and others: Lymph node biopsy in patients with human immunodeficiency virus infection, *Arch Surg* 123:1349; 1988.

59. Deeks SG: Determinants of virological response to antiretroviral therapy, *Cin Infec Dis* 30(Suppl 2):S177, 2000.

60. Denning DW and others: Pulmonary aspergillosis in the acquired immunodeficiency syndrome, *N Engl J Med* 324:654, 1991.

61. Desai S: Seropositivity, adenoid hypertrophy, and secretory otitis media in adults: a recognized clinical entity, *Otolaryngol Head Neck Surg* 107:755, 1992.

62. Dichtel W: *Oral manifestations of human immunodeficiency virus infection.* In Tami TA, editor: *Otolaryngologic manifestations of the acquired immunodeficiency syndrome.* Philadelphia, 1992, WB Saunders.

63. Diz-Dios P and others: Changing prevalence of human immunodeficiency virus-associated oral lesions [letter], *Oral Surg Oral Med Oral Pathol Oral Radiol Endod* 90:403, 2000.

64. Diz-Dios P and others: Frequency of oral candidiasis in HIV-infected patients on protease inhibitor therapy, *Oral Surg Oral Med Oral Pathol Oral Radiol Endod* 87:437, 1999.

65. Dolcetti R and others: Pahtogenic and histogenetic features of HIV-associated Hodgkin's disease, *Eur J Cancer* 37:1276, 2001.

66. Drinkard CR and others: Periodontal status of individuals in early stages of human immunodeficiency virus infection, *Community Dent Oral Epidemiol* 19:281, 1991.

67. Durham TM and others: Facial nerve paralysis related to HIV disease: case report and dental considerations, *Oral Surg Oral Med Oral Pathol* 75:37, 1993.

68. Egger M: *Prognosis of HIV-1 infected drug naïve patients starting potent antiretroviral therapy.* From *41st Interscience Conferece on Antimicrobial Agents and Chemotherapy,* December 16-19, 2001, Chicago, Ill, Abstract LB-18.

69. Elder GA, Sever JL: AIDS and neurological disorders: an overview, *Ann Neurol* 23:S4, 1988.

70. Ellison E, Lapuerta P, Martin SE: Fine needle aspiration (FNA) in HIV+ patients: results from a series of 655 aspirates, *Cytopathology* 9:222, 1998.

71. Eron JJ: HIV-1 protease inhibitors, *Clin Inect Dis* 30(Suppl 2): S160, 2000.

72. Errante D and others: Hodgkin's disease in patients with HIV infection and in the general population: comparison of clinicopathological features and survival, *Ann Oncol* 5(Suppl 2):S37, 1994.

73. Eyeson JD and others: Oral manifestations of an HIV positive cohort in the era of highly active anti-retroviral therapy (HAART) in south London, *J Oral Pathol Med* 31:169, 2002.

74. Fauci AS: The human immunodeficiency virus: infectivity and mechanisms of pathogenesis, *Science* 239:617, 1988.

75. Ficarro G and others: Kaposi's sarcoma of the oral cavity: a study of 134 patients with a review of the pathogenesis, epidemiology, clinical aspects, and treatment, *Oral Surg Oral Med Oral Pathol* 66:543, 1988.

76. Finn DG: Lymphoma of the head and neck and acquired immunodeficiency syndrome: clinical investigation and immunohistochemical study, *Laryngoscope* 105(Suppl 68):1, 1995.

77. Fischl M and others: *Impact of directly observed therapy on outcomes in HIV clinical treials.* From *7th Conference on Retroviruses and Opportunistic infections,* January 30-February 2, 2000, San Francisco, California, Abstract 71.

78. Flaitz CM and others: Intraoral squamous cell carcinoma in human immunodeficiency virus infection: a clincopathologic study, *Oral Surg Oral Med Oral Pathol* 80:55, 1994.

79. Franceschi S, Dal Maso L, La Vecchjia C: Advances in the epidemiology of HIV-associated hon-Hodgkin's lymphoma and other lymphoid neoplasms, *Int J Cancer* 83:481, 1999.

80. Franceschi S and others: Risk of cancer other than Kaposi's sarcoma and non-Hodgkin's lymphoma in persons with AIDS in Italy, *Br J Cancer* 78:966, 1998.

81. Frank Y, Pahwa S: Serial brainstem auditory evoked responses in infants and children with AIDS, *Clin Electroencephalogr* 24:160, 1993.

82. Friedman M and others: Endoscopic sinus surgery in patients infected with HIV, *Laryngoscope* 110:1613, 2000.

83. Frisch M and others: AIDS-Cancer Match Registry Study Group. Association of cancer with AIDS-related immunosuppression in adults, *JAMA* 285:1736, 2001.

84. Gachupin-Garcia A and others: Population-based study of malignancies and HIV infection among injection drug users in a New York City methadone treatment program, 1985-1991, *AIDS* 6:843, 1992.

85. Garcia-Rodiguez J and others: Rhinosinusitis and atopy in patients infected with HIV, *Laryngoscope* 109:939-944, 1999.

86. Gerard L and others: Improved survival in HIV-related Hodgkin's lymphoma since the introduction of highly active antiretroviral therapy, *AIDS* 17:81; 2003.

87. Gerberding JL: Occupational exposure to HIV in health care settings, *N Engl J Med* 348:826, 2003.

88. Gherman CR and others: *Pneumocystis carinii* otitis media and mastoiditis as the initial manifestation of the acquired immunodeficiency syndrome, *Am J Med* 85:250, 1988.

89. Ghika-Schmid F and others: Diversite de l'atteinte neuromusculaire de 47 patients infectes par le virus de l'immunodeficience humaine, *Schweiz Med Wochenschr* 124:791, 1994.

90. Gill PS and others: Randomized phase III trial of liposomal daunorubicin (DaunoXome) versus doxorubicin, bleomycin, vincreistine (ABV) in AIDS-related Kaposi's sarcoma, *J Clin Oncol* 14:2353, 1996.

91. Gillespie MB, O'Maley BW: An algorithmic approach to the diagnosis and management of invasive fungal rhinosinusitis in the immunocompromised patient, *Otolaryngol Clin North Am* 33:323, 2000.

92. Gillison ML, Shah KV: Human papillomavirus-associated head and neck squamous cell carcinoma: mounting evidence for an etiologic role for human papillomavirus in a subset of head and neck cancers, *Curr Opin Oncolog* 13:183, 2001.

93. Glick M, Cleveland D: Oral mucosal bacillary epithelioid angiomatosis in a patient with AIDS associated with rapid alveolar bone loss: case report, *J Oral Pathol Med* 22:235, 1993.

94. Glick M and others: Oral manifestations associated with HIV-related disease as markers for immune suppression and AIDS, *Oral Surg Oral Med Oral Pathol* 77:344, 1994.

95. Godofsky E and others: Sinusitis in the HIV infected patients: a clinical and radiologic review, *Am J Med* 93:163-169, 1992.

96. Goedert JJ: The epidemiology of acquired immunodeficiency syndrome malignancies, *Semin Oncol* 27:390, 2000.

97. Goldberg AN: Kaposi's sarcoma of the head and neck in acquired immunodeficiency syndrome, *Am J Otolaryngol* 14:5, 1993.

98. Goldberg AN and others: Management of Kaposi's Sarcoma of the larynx in acquired immunodeficiency syndrome, *Trans Am Broncho Esophagol Assoc* 27–32, 1994.

99. Grbic JT, Lamster IB: Oral manifestations of HIV infection, *AIDS Patient Care STDs* 11:19, 1997.

100. Greenberg P: *Immunopathogenesis of HIV infection.* In Corey L, editor: *AIDS: problems and prospects.* New York, 1993, WW Norton.

101. Greenspan D and others: *AIDS and the mouth.* Copenhagen, Denmark, Munksgaard, 1990.

102. Greenspan D and others: Oral hairy leukoplkakia in an HIV-negative renal transplant recipient, *J Oral Pathol Med* 18:32, 1989.

103. Greenspan J and others: Replication of Epstein-Barr virus within the epithelial cells of oral hairy leukoplakia: an AIDS-associated lesion, *N Engl J Med* 313:1564, 1985.

104. Grimaldi LME and others: Bilateral eighth cranial nerve neuropathy in human immunodeficiency virus infection, *J Neurol* 240:363, 1993.

105. Groll AH, Walsh TJ: Caspofungin: pharmacology, safety and therapeutic potential in superficial and invasive fungal infections, *Expert Opin Investig Drugs* 10:1545, 2001.

106. Grulich AE: AIDS-associated non-Hodgkin's lymphoma in the era of highly active antiretroviral therapy, *J Acquir Immune Defic Syndr* 21(Suppl. 1):S27, 1999.

107. Grulich AE: Cancer risk in persons with HIV/AIDS in the era of combination antiretroviral therapy, *The AIDS Reader* 10:341-346, 2000.

108. Grulich AE: Update: cancer risk in persons with HIV? AIDS in the era of combination antiretroviral therapy, *AIDS Read* 10:341, 2000.

109. Gurney TA, Lee KC, Murr AH: Contemporary issues in rhinosinusitis and HIV infection, *Curr Opin Otolaryngol Head Neck Surg* 11:45, 2003.

110. Hadfield P and others: The ENT manifestations of HIV infection in children, *Clin Otolaryngol* 21:30, 1996.

111. Hall P, Farrior J: Aspergillus mastoiditis, *Otolaryngol Head Neck Surg* 108:167, 1993.

112. Hammond JS and others: HIV, trauma, and infection control: universal precautions are universally ignored, *J Trauma* 30:555, 1990.

113. Harada T and others: Temporal bone histopathology in deafness due to cryptococcal meningitis, *Ann Otol* 88:630, 1979.

114. Haubrich RH: Structured treatment interruptions, *Top HIV Med* 8:9, 2000.

115. Hausler R and others: Neuro-otological manifestations in different stages of HIV infection, *Acta Otolaryngol (Stockh)* 481:S515, 1991.

116. Hengge UR and others: Update od Kaposi's sarcoma and other HHV8 associated diseases. Part 1: epidemiology, environmental predispositions, clinical manifestations, and therapy, *Lancet Infect Dis* 2:281, 2002.

117. Hern JD and others: ENT manifestations of Pseudomonas aeruginosa infection in HIV and AIDS, *Int J Clin Pract* 52:141, 1998.

118. Hernard DR and others: Natural history of HIV-1 cell-free viremia, *JAMA* 275:554, 1995.

119. Herndier BG and others: High prevalence of Epstein-Barr virus in the Reed-Sternberg cells of HIV-associated Hodgkin's disease, *Am J Pathol* 142:1073-1079, 1993.

120. Hilf M and others: Antibiotic therapy for *Pseudomonas aeruginosa* bacteraemia: outcome correlations in a prospective study of 200 patients, *Am J Med* 87:540, 1989.
121. Hinni M, McCaffrey T, Kasperbauer J: Early mucosal changes in experimental sinusitis, *Otolaryngol Head Neck Surg* 107:537-548, 1992.
122. *HIV/AIDS surveillance report,* vol 12, no 1. Atlanta, Centers for Disease Control and Prevention, 2000, p 24.
123. Hoggs RS and others: Rates of disease progression by baseline CD4 cell count and viral load after initiating triple drug therapy, *JAMA* 286:2568, 2001.
124. Hruza GJ, Snow SN: Basal cell carcinoma in a patient with acquired immune deficiency syndrome: treatment with Mohs micrographic surgery fixed-tissue technique, *J Dermatol Surg Oncol* 15:545, 1989.
125. Hughes MD and others: Monitoring plasma HIV-1 RNA levels in addition to CD4+ lymphocyte count improves assessment of antiretroviral therapeutic response, *Ann Intern Med* 126:929-938, 1997.
126. Hunt SM and others: Invasive fungal sinusitis in the acquired immunodeficiency syndrome, *Otolaryngol Clin N Am* 33:335, 2000.
127. Igarashi M and others: Temporal bone findings in Cryptococcal meningitis, *Arch Otolaryngol* 101:577, 1975.
128. Ioachim HL, Ryan JR, Blaugrund SM: Salivary gland lymph nodes: the site of lymphadenopathies and lymphomas associated with human immunodeficiency virus infection, *Arch Pathol Lab Med* 112:1224, 1988.
129. Istecu S: Diffuse infiltrative lymphocytosis syndrome in human immunodeficiency virus infection: a Sjogren's-like disease, *Rheum Dis Clin North Am* 17:99, 1991.
130. Jaffe HW: The laboratory diagnosis of syphilis, *Ann Intern Med* 83:846, 1975.
131. Jin J and others: Detection of Kaposi's sarcoma-associated herpesvirus-like DNA sequence in vascular lesions: a reliable diagnostic marker for Kaposi's sarcoma, *Am J Clin Pathol* 105:360, 1996.
132. Jochimsen EM: Failures of zidovudine postesposure prophylaxis, *Am J Med* 102(Suppl 5B):52, 1997.
133. Johnston S and others: Raised intracranial pressure and visual complications in AIDS patients with cryptococcal meningitis, *J Infect* 24:185, 1992.
134. Joint United Nations Program on HIV/AIDS: AIDS Epidemic Update. December 2002.
135. Jordan RC and others: Oral lymphoma in HIV infection, *Oral Diseases* 3:S135, 1997.
136. Jutte A and others: CMV sinusitis as the initial manifestation of AIDS, *HIV Med* 1:123, 2000.
137. Kantu and others: Safety awareness for the otolaryngologist caring for the IV-positive patient, *Laryngoscope* 106:982, 1996.
138. Kaplan JE and others: Epidemiology of human immunodeficiency virus associated opportunistic infections in the United States in the era of highly active antiretroviral therapy, *Clin Infect Dis* 30:S5-S14, 2000.
139. Kaplan LD and others: AIDS-associated non-Hodgkin's lymphoma in San Francisco, *JAMA* 261:719, 1989.
140. Kaplan LD and others: Low-dose compared with standard dose m-BACOD chemotherapy for non-Hodgkin's lymphoma associated with human immunodeficiency virus infection. National Institute of Allergy and Infectious Disease AIDS Clinical Trials Group, *N Engl J Med* 336:1641, 1997.
141. Katz MH and others: Progression to AIDS in HIV-infected homosexual and bisexual men with hairly leukoplakia and oral candidiasis, *AIDS* 6:95, 1992.
142. Keane J: Intermittent third nerve palsy with cryptococcal meningitis, *J Clin Neuroophthalmol* 13:124, 1993.
143. Kedes DH and others: The seroepidemiology of human herpesvirus 8 (Kaposi's sarcoma-associated herpesvirus): distribution of infection in KS risk groups and evidence for sexual transmission, *Nat Med* 2:918, 1996.
144. Kielhofner M and others: Life-threatening *Pseudomonas aeruginosa* infections in patients with human immunodeficiency virus, *Clin Infect Dis* 14:403, 1992.
145. Kirova YM and others: Radiotherapy in the management of epidemic Kaposi's sarcoma: a retrospective study of 643 cases, *Radiother Oncol* 46:19, 1998.
146. Kohan D, Giacchi R: Otologic surgery in patients with HIV and AIDS, *Otolaryngol Head Neck Surg* 121:355, 1999.
147. Kohan D and others: Otologic disease in AIDS patients: CT correlation, *Laryngoscope* 100:1326, 1990.
148. Kohan D and others: Otologic disease in patients with acquired immunodeficiency syndrome, *Ann Otol Rhinol Laryngol* 97:636, 1988.
149. Koralnik IJ and others: A controlled study of early neurologic abnormalities in men with asymptomatic human immunodeficiency virus infection, *N Engl J Med* 323:864, 1990.
150. Kordossis T and others: Prevalence of Sjogren's-like syndrome in a cohort of HIV-1–positive patients: descriptive pathology and immunopathology, *Br J Rheumatol* 37:691, 1998.
151. Krasner CG, Cohen SH: Bilateral Bell's palsy and aseptic meningitis in a patient with acute human immunodeficiency virus seroconversion, *West J Med* 159:604, 1993.
152. Krown SE, Metroka C, Wernz JC: Kaposi's sarcoma and the acquired immunodeficiency syndrome: a proposal for a uniform evaluation, response and staging criteria, *J Clin Oncol* 7:1201, 1989.
153. Krown SE and others: AIDS related Kaposi's sarcoma: prospective validation of the AIDS Clinical Trials Group staging classification, *J Clin Oncol* 15:3085, 1997.
154. Kwartler JA and others: Sudden hearing loss due to AIDS-related cryptococcal meningitis: a temporal bone study, *Otolaryngol Head Neck Surg* 104:265, 1991.
155. Lalwani AK, Sooy CD: Otologic and neurotologic manifestations of acquired immunodeficiency syndrome, *Otolaryngol Clin North Am* 25:1183, 1992.
156. Langford-Kuntz A and and others: Impairment of cranio-facial nerves due to AIDS, *Int J Oral Maxillofac Surg* 17:227, 1988.
157. Lee K, Cheung S: Evaluation of the neck mass in human immunodeficiency virus–infected patients, *Otolaryngol Clin North Am* 25:1287, 1992.
158. Lee VW and others: Pulmonary Kaposi sarcoma in patients with AIDS: scintigraphic diagnosis with sequential thalliwm and gallium scanning, *Radiology* 180:409, 1991.
159. Levine AM: Acquired immunodeficiency syndrome-related lymphoma, *Blood* 80:8, 1992.
160. Levine AM: Epidemiology, clinical characteristics, and management of AIDS-related lymphoma, *Hematol Oncol Clin North Am* 5:331, 1991.
161. Levine AM, Tulpule A: Clinical aspects and management of AIDS-related Kaposi's sarcoma, *Eur J Cancer* 37:1288, 2001.
162. Levine AM and others: Results of initial lymph node biopsy in homosexual men with generalized lymphadenopathy, *J Clin Oncol* 4:165, 1986.
163. Levy JA: *The retroviruses and pathogenesis of HIV infection.* In Corey L, editor: *AIDS: problems and prospects.* New York, 1993, WW Norton & Co.
164. Levy RM and others: Neurological manifestations of the acquired immunodeficiency syndrome (AIDS): experience at UCSF and review of the literature, *J Neurosurg* 62:475, 1985.

165. Lewis JL, Rabinovich S: The wide spectrum of cryptococcal infections, *Am J Med* 53:315, 1972.

166. Linstrom CJ and others: Otologic neurotologic manifestations of HIV-related disease, *Otolaryngol Head Neck Surg* 108:680, 1993.

167. Lipton RB and others: Progressive multifocal leukoencephalopathy of the posterior fossa in an AIDS patient: clinical, radiographic and evoked potential findings, *Eur Neurol* 28:285, 1988.

168. Little JP and others: Otosyphilis in a patient with human immunodeficiency virus: internal auditory canal gumma, *Otolaryngol Head Neck Surg* 112:488, 1995.

169. Lobo DV, Chu P, Greckin RC, and others: Nonmelanoma skin cancers and infection with the human immunodeficiency virus, *Arch Dermatol* 128:623, 1992.

170. Lori F, Lisziewicz J: Structured treatment interruptions for the management of HIV infection, *JAMA* 286:2981, 2001.

171. Lortholary O and others: Invasive aspergillosis in patients with acquired immunodeficiency syndrome: a report of 33 cases, *Am J Med* 95:177, 1993.

172. Lustig LR and others: Doxycycline sclerosis of benign lymphoepithelial cysts in patients infected with HIV, *Laryngoscope* 108:1199-1205, 1998.

173. Lyos A and others: Invasive aspergillosis of the temporal bone: an unusual manifestation of acquired immunodeficiency syndrome, *Am J Otol* 14:444, 1993.

174. Mack LW and others: Temporal bone treponemes, *Arch Otolaryngol Head Neck Surg* 90:37, 1969.

175. Manfredi R and others: Recombinant human granulocyte-macrophages colony-stimulating factor (RHUGM-CSF) in leukopenic patients with advanced HIV disease, *J Chemother* 8:214, 1996.

176. Mansky LM, Temin HM: Lower in vivo mutation rate of human immunodeficiency virus type 1 than that predicted from the fidelity of purified reverse transcriptase, *J Virol* 69:5087-5094; 1995.

177. Marchisio P and others: Etiology of acute otitis media in human immunodeficiency virus–infected children, *Pediatr Infect Dis J* 15:58, 1996.

178. Martin LN and others: Effects of initiation of 3'azido,3'-deoxythymidine (zidovudine) treatment at different times after infection of rhesus monkeys with simian immunodeficiency virus, *J Infect Dis* 168:825, 1993.

179. Mascart-Lemone F and others: Differential effect of human immunodeficiency virus infection on the IgA and IgG antibody responses to pneumococcal vaccine, *J Infect Dis* 172:1253, 1995.

180. Maslan MJ and others: Cryptococcal meningitis: presentation as sudden deafness, *Am J Otol* 6:435, 1985.

181. McGill TJI: Mycotic infection of the temporal bone, *Arch Otolaryngol Head Neck Surg* 104:140, 1978.

182. Melbye M and others: Nasopharyngeal carcinoma: an EBV-associated tumour not significantly influenced by HIV-induced immunosuppression: The AIDS/Cancer Working Group, *Br J Cancer* 73:995, 1996.

183. Melbye M and others: Risk of AIDS after herpes zoster, *Lancet* 1:728, 1987.

184. Mellors JW and others: Plasma viral load and CD4+ lymphocytes as prognostic markers of HIV-1 infection, *Ann Intern Med* 124:946, 1997.

185. Melnick S and others: Oral mucosal lesions: association with the presence of antibodies to the human immunodeficiency virus, *Oral Surg Oral Med Oral Pathol* 68:37, 1989.

186. Mendelson MH, Gurtman A, Szabo S, and others: *Pseudomonas aeruginosa* bacteraemia in patients with AIDS, *Clin Infect Dis* 18:886, 1994.

187. Meyer RD and others: Fungal sinusitis in patients with AIDS: report of 4 cases and review of the literature, *Medicine* 73:69, 1994.

188. Milgrim L, Rubin J, Small C: Mucociliary clearance abnormalities in the HIV-infected patient, *Laryngoscope* 105:1202-1208, 1995.

189. Milgrim L and others: Sinusitis in human immunodeficiency virus infection: typical and atypical organisms, *J Otolaryngol* 23:450, 1994.

190. Mishell JH, Applebaum EL: Ramsey-Hunt syndrome in a patient with HIV infection, *Otolaryngol Head Neck Surg* 102:177, 1990.

191. Mukherjee A and others: Kaposi's sarcoma of the parotid gland in acquired immunodeficiency syndrome, *Am Surg* 64:259, 1998.

192. Mulkens P and others: Acute facial paralysis: a virological study, *Clin Otolaryngol* 5:305, 1980.

193. Murphy C, Davidson TM, Jellison W: Sinonasal disease and olfactory impairment in HIV disease: endoscopic sinus surgery and outcome measures, *Laryngoscope* 110:1707, 2000.

194. Murphy EL and others: Highly active antiretroviral therapy decreases mortality and morbidity in patients with advanced HIV disease, *Ann Intern Med* 135:17, 2001.

195. Murphy M and others: Regression of AIDS-related Kaposi's sarcoma following treatment with an HIV-1 protease inhibitor, *AIDS* 11:262, 1997.

196. Murr AH, Benecke JE: Association of facial paralysis with HIV positivity, *Am J Otol* 12:450, 1991.

197. *NIOSH alert: preventing needlestick injuries in health care settings* (DHHS publication no.(NIOSH) 2000-108). Cincinnati, Ohio, National Institute for Occupational Safety and Health, November 1999.

198. Niparko J: *The acute facial palsies.* In Jackler RK, Brackman D, editors: *Neurotology.* 1994, St Louis, Mosby.

199. Northfelt DW and others: Pegylated liposomal doxorubicin versus doxorubicin, bleomycin, vincristine in the treatment of AIDS-related Kaposi's sarcoma, *J Clin Oncol* 17:683, 1998.

200. Obrien WA and others: Changes in plasma HIV RNA levels and CD4+ lymphocyte counts and the risk of progression to AIDS, *N Engl J Med* 334:426-431, 1996.

201. *Occupational safety: selected cost and benefit implications of needlestick prevention devices for hospitals* (GAO-01-60R). Washington, D.C., General Accounting Office, Nov. 17, 2000.

202. O'Donnel JG, Sorbello AF, Condolci, DV: Pseudomonal sinusitis in AIDS, *Clin Infect Dis* 16:404, 1993.

203. Oram Y and others: Histologic patterns of basal cell carcinoma based upon patient immunostatus, *Dermatol Surg* 21:611, 1995.

204. Otton RA and others: Efficacy of postexposure prophylaxis after intravaginal exposure of pig-tailed macaques to a human-derived retrovirus (human immunodeficiency virus type 2), *J Virol* 74:9771, 2000.

205. Pagano MA and others: Brain-stem auditory evoked potentials in human immunodeficiency virus–seropositive patients with and without acquired immunodeficiency syndrome, *Arch Neurol* 49:166, 1992.

206. Palella F and others: Declining morbidity and mortality among patients with advanced human immunodeficiency virus infection, *N Engl J Med* 338:853, 1998.

207. Park S and others: Pneumocystis carinii infection in the middle ear, *Arch Otolaryngol Head Neck Surg* 118:269, 1992.

208. Parry GJ: Peripheral neuropathies associated with human immunodeficiency virus infection, *Ann Neurol* 23:S49, 1988.

209. Pathak VK and others. Broad spectrum of in vivo forward mutations, hypermutations, and mutational hotspots in a retroviral shuttle vector after a single replication cycle: substitutions, frameshifts, and hypermutations, *Proc Natl Acad Sci USA* 87:6019; 1990.

210. Patow C and others: Pharyngeal obstruction by Kaposi's sarcoma in a homosexual male with acquired immune deficiency syndrome, *Otolaryngol Head Neck Surg* 92:713, 1984.

211. Patton LL and others: Changing prevalence of oral manifestations of human immunodeficiency virus in the era of protease inhibitor therapy, *Oral Surg Oral Med Oral Pathol Oral Radiol Endod* 89:299, 2000.

212. Perdue B and others: *HIV-1 transmission by a needlestick injury despite rapid initiation of four-drug prophylaxis [abstract]. In Program and abstracts of the 6th Conference on Retroviruses and Opportunistic Infections, Chicago, January 31-February 4, 1999.* Chicago, 1999, Foundation for Retrovirology and Human Health, p 107.

213. Perea S, Patterson TF: Invasive Aspergillus infections in hematologic malignancy patients, *Semin Resp Infect* 17:99, 2002.

214. Piette AM and others: Acute neuropathy coincident with seroconversion for anti-LAV/HTLV-III, *Lancet* 1:852, 1986.

215. Plancoulaine S and others: Herpesvirus 8 transmission from mother to child and between siblings in an endemic population, *Lancet* 356:1063, 2000.

216. Pneumocystis pneumonia: Los Angeles, *MMWR Morb Mortal Wkly Rep* 30:250-252, 1981.

217. Pomilla PV and others: Sinonasal non-Hodgkin's lymphoma in patients infected with human immunodeficiency virus: report of three cases and review, *Clin Infect Dis* 21:137, 1995.

218. Porter J and others: Prevalence of sinonasal symptoms in patients with HIV infection, *Am J Rhinol* 13:203-308, 1999.

219. Pratt RD and others: Virologic characterization of primary human immunodeficiency virus type 1 infection in a health care worker following needlestick injury, *J Infect Dis* 172:851, 1995.

220. Quinn TC and others: Serologic and immunologic studies in patients with AIDS in North America and Africa, *JAMA* 257:2617, 1987.

221. Rabkin CS, Goedert JJ: Risks of non-Hodgkin lymphoma and Kaposi's sarcoma in homosexual men, *Lancet* 336:248, 1990.

222. Rabkin CS and others: Increasing incidence of cancers associated with the human immunodeficiency virus epidemic, *Int J Cancer* 47:692, 1991.

223. Race E and others: Focal mycobacterial lymphadenitis following initiation of protease-inhibitor therapy in patients with advanced HIV-1 disease, *Lancet* 351:252, 1998.

224. Ramirez-Amador V and others: The changing clinical spectrum of human immunodeficiency virus (HIV)-related oral lesions in 1,000 consecutive patients: a 12-year study in a referral center in Mexico, *Medicine* 82:39, 2003.

225. Rarey KE: Otologic pathophysiology in patients with human immunodeficiency virus, *Am J Otolaryngol* 11:366, 1990.

226. Ree HJ and others: Human immunodeficiency virus-associated Hodgkin's disease: clinicopathologic study of 24 cases and preponderance of mixed cellularity type characterized by the occurrence of fibrohistiocytoid stromal cells, *Cancer* 67:1614, 1991.

227. Reiss P and others: Invasive external otitis caused by *Aspergillus fumigatus* in two patients with AIDS, *AIDS* 5:605, 1991.

228. Ribera JM and others: Prognostic impact of highly active antiretroviral therapy in HIV-related Hodgkin's disease, *AIDS* 16:1973, 2002.

229. Rivera MA, Padhya TA: Acanthamoeba: a rare primary cause of rhinosinusitis, *Laryngoscope* 112:1201, 2002.

230. Rodrigues LK and others: Altered clinical course of malignant melanoma in HIV-positive patients, *Arch Dermatol* 138:765, 2002.

231. Roithman S and others: AIDS-associated non-Hodgkin's lymphoma, *Lancet* 338:884, 1991.

232. Roland JT and others: Squamous Cell Carcinoma in HIV-positive patients under the age of 45, *Laryngoscope* 103:509, 1993.

233. Rosenberg ZF, Fauci AS: The immunopathogenesis of HIV infection, *Adv Immunol* 47:377, 1989.

234. Rosenhall U and others: Otoneurological abnormalities in asymptomatic HIV-seropositive patients, *Acta Neurol Scand* 79:140, 1989.

235. Rosenstiel DB, Carroll WR, Listinsky CM: MALT lymphoma presenting as a cystic salivary gland mass, *Head Neck* 23:254-258, 2001.

236. Rosler KM and others: Electrophysiological characteristics of lesions in facial palsies of different etiologies: a study using electrical and magnetic stimulation techniques, *Electroencephalogr Clin Neurophysiol* 97:355, 1995.

237. Rubin J, Honigsberg R: Sinusitis in patients with acquired immune deficiency syndrome, *Ear Nose Throat J* 69:460-463, 1990.

238. Rubinstein A: *Pediatric AIDS.* In Lockhart JD and others, editors: *Current Problems in Pediatrics.* Chicago 1986, Mosby.

239. Ryan JR and others: Acquired immune deficiency syndrome–related lymphadnopathies presenting as salivary gland lymph nodes, *Arch Otolaryngol* 111:554, 1985.

240. Sample S and others: Elevated serum IgE antibodies to environmental allergens in HIV-seropositive male homosexuals, *J Allergy Clin Immunol* 86:876, 1990.

241. Sartoretti-Schefer S and others: Idiopathic, herpetic, and HIV-associated facial nerve palsies: abnormal MR enhancement patterns, *AJNR Am J Neuroradiol* 15:479, 1994.

242. Schurmann D and others: Intensive treatment of AIDS-related non-Hodgkin's lymphomas with the MACOP-B protocol, *Eur J Haemotol* 54:73, 1995.

243. Schalling M and others: A role for a new herpes virus (KSHV) in different forms of Kaposi's sarcoma, *Nat Med* 1:707, 1995.

244. Schielke E and others: Peripheral facial nerve palsy associated with HIV infection, *Lancet* 1:553, 1989.

245. Schlanger G and others: Sinusitis caused y legionella pneumophilia in a patient with acquired immune deficiency syndrome. A, *J Med* 77:957; 1984.

246. Serious adverse events attributed to nevirapine regimens for postexposure prophylaxis after HIV exposures: worldwide, 1997-2000, *MMWR Morb Mortal Wkly Rep* 49:1153-1156, 2001.

247. Serraino D and others: Cancer incidence in a cohort of human immunodeficiency virus seroconverters, *Cancer* 79:1004, 1997.

248. Serrano M and others: Hodgkin's disease in patients with antibodies to human immunodeficiency virus, *Cancer* 65:2248, 1990.

249. Sgadari C and others: HIV protease inhibitors are potent anti-angiogeneic molecules and promote regression of Kaposi sarcoma, *Nat Med* 8:225, 2002.

250. Shapiro NL, Novelli N: Otitis media in children with vertically-acquired HIV infection: the Great Ormond Street Hospital experience, *Int J Pediatr Otorhinolaryngol* 45:69, 1998.

251. Shapiro AL, Pincus RL: Fine-needle aspiration of diffuse cervical lymphadenopathy, *Otolaryngol Head Neck Surg* 105:419, 1991.

252. Shapiro AL and others: Head and neck lymphoma in patients with the acquired immune deficiency syndrome, *Otolaryngol Head Neck Surg* 106:258, 1992.

253. Silverman S and others: Oral findings in people with or at risk for AIDS: a study of 375 homosexual males, *J Am Dent Assoc* 112:187, 1986.

254. Singh B and others: Head and neck manifestations of hon-Hodgkin's lymphoma in human immunodeficiency virus–infected patients, *Am J Otolaryngol* 21:10, 2000.

255. Singh B and others: Kaposi's sarcoma of the head and neck in patients with acquired immunodeficiency syndrome, *Otolaryngol Dead Neck Surg* 111:618, 1994.

256. Singh B and others: Upper Aerodigestive tract squamous cell carcinoma: the human immunodeficiency virus connection, *Arch Otolaryngol Head Neck Surg* 122:639, 1996.

257. Sitas F and others: Antibodies against human herpesvirus 8 in black South African patients with cancer, *N Engl J Med* 340:1863, 1999.

258. Sitz KV and others: Metastatic basal cell carcinoma in acquired immunodeficiency syndrome-related complex, *JAMA* 257:340, 1987.

259. Smith ME, Canalis RF: Otologic manifestations of AIDS: the otosyphilis connection, *Laryngoscope* 99:365, 1989.

260. Smith FB and others: Benign lymphoepithelial lesions of the parotid gland in intravenous drug-users, *Arch Pathol Lab Med* 112:742, 1988.

261. Smith T and others: Clinical and electrophysiological studies of human immunodeficiency virus-seropositive men without AIDS, *Ann Neurol* 23:295, 1988.

262. Snider WD and others: Neurological complications of acquired immune deficiency syndrome: analysis of 50 patients, *Ann Neurol* 14:403, 1983.

263. Smith KJ and others: Cutaneous neoplasm in the military population of HIV-1 positive patients, *J Am Acad Dermatol* 19:400, 1993.

264. Som PM and others: Nodal inclusion cysts of the parotid gland and parapharyngeal space: a discussion of lymphoepithelial, AIDS-related paroted, and branchial cysts, cystic Warthin's tumors, and cysts in Sjogren's syndrome, *Laryngoscope* 105:1122, 1995.

265. Sooy CD, Geberding JL, Kaplan MJ: The risk of otolaryngologists who treat patients with AIDS virus infection: report of an in-process study, *Laryngoscope* 97:430, 1987.

266. Sperling NM, Lin PT: Parotid disease associated with human immunodeficiency virus infection, *Ear Nose Throat J* 69:475, 1990.

267. Sperling NM and others: Parotid disease associated with human immunodeficiency virus infection, *Ear Nose Throat J* 69:475, 1990.

268. Staskus KA and others: Kaposi's sarcoma-associated herpesvirus gene expression in endothelial (spindle) tumor cells, *J Virol* 71:715, 1997.

269. Stenzel MS and others: Enhancing adherence to HAART, *AIDS Read* 111:317, 2001.

270. Sterling TR and others: *CD4+ lymphocyte level is better than HIV-1 plasma viral load in determining when to initiate HAART.* From *8th Conference on Retroviruses and Opportunistic Infections*, February 4-8, 2001, Chicago, Ill, Abstract 519.

271. Stewart S and others: Randomized comparative trial of pegylated liposomal doxorubicin versus bleomycin and vincristine in the treatment of AIDS-related Kaposi's sarcoma, *J Clin Oncol* 16:683, 1998.

272. Strauss M, Fine E: Aspergillus otomastoiditis in acquired immunodeficiency syndrome, *Am J Otol* 12:49, 1991.

273. Strigle SM and others: The use of fine needle aspiration cytology in the management of human immunodeficiency virus–related non-Hodgkin's lymphoma and Hodgkin's disease, *J Acquir Defic Syndr* 6:1329, 1993.

274. Swanstorm R, Wehbie R: *Biology of HIV infection.* In Holmes KK and others, editors: *Sexually Transmitted Diseases.* New York, 1999, McGraw-Hill.

275. Syrganen S and others: Oral hairy leukoplakia is not a specific sign of HIV infection but related to suppression in general, *J Oral Pathol Med* 18:28, 1989.

276. Tam HK and others: Effect of highly active antiretroviral therapy on survival among HIV-infected men with Kaposi sarcoma or non-Hodgkin lymphoma, *Int J Cancer* 98:916, 2002.

277. Tami TA: The management of sinusitis in patients infected with the human immunodeficiency virus (HIV), *Ear Nose Throat J* 74:360, 1995.

278. Tappero JW and others: Cryotherapy for cutaneous Kaposi's sarcoma associated with AIDS: a phase II trial, *J AIDS* 4:839, 1991.

279. Tappero JW and others: Kaposi's sarcoma: epidemiology, pathogenesis, histology, clinical spectrum, staging criteria, and therapy, *J Am Acad Dermatol* 28:371, 1993.

280. Tappero JW and others: Pulsed-dye laser therapy for cutaneous Kaposi's sarcoma associated with acquired immunodeficiency syndrome, *J Am Acad Dermatol* 28:188, 1992.

281. Teknos TN and others: Acanthamoeba rhinosinusitis: characterization, diagnosis, and treatment, *Am J Rhinology* 14:387, 2000.

282. Timon CI, Walsh MA: Sudden sensorineural hearing loss as a presentation of HIV infection, *J Laryngol Otol* 103:1071, 1989.

283. Tirelli U, Bernardi D: Inpact of HAART on the clinical management of AIDS-related cancers, *Eur J Cancer* 37:1320, 2001.

284. Toma E and others: Herpes simplex type 2 pericarditis and bilateral facial palsy in a petine with AIDS, *J Infect Dis* 160:553, 1989.

285. Tsai C-C and others: Effectiveness of postinoculation (R)-9 (2-phosphonylmethoxypropyl) adenine treatment for prevention of persistent simian immunodeficiency virus SIVmne infection depends critically on timing of initiation and duration of treatment, *J Virol* 72:4265-4273, 1998.

286. Tsai C-C and others: Prevention of SIV infection in macaques by (R)-9(2-phosphonylmethoxypropyl) adenine, *Science* 270:1197, 1995.

287. Uldry PA, Regli F: Paralysie faciale peripherique isolee et recidivante dans l'infection a human immunodeficiency virus (HIV), *Schweiz Med Wochenschr* 118:1029, 1988.

288. Ulirsch RC, Jaffe ES: Sjogren's syndrome–like illness associated with acquired immunodeficiency syndrome–related complex, *Hum Pathol* 18:1063, 1987.

289. Upadhyay S and others: Bacteriology of sinusitis in human immunodeficiency virus–positive patients: implications for management, *Laryngoscope* 105:1058, 1995.

290. Updated U.S. Public Health Service guidelines for the management of occupational exposure to HBV, HCV, and HIV and recommendations for post-exposure prophylaxis, *MMWR Morb Mortal Wkly Rep* 50(RR-11):1-52, 2001.

291. Urba WJ, Longo DL: Hodgkin's disease, *N Engl J Med* 326:678, 1992.

292. Vaccher E, Spina M, Tirelli U: Clinical aspects and management of Hodgkin's disease and other tumours in HIV individuals, *Eur J Cancer* 37:1306, 2001.

293. Vanarthos WJ and others: Diagnostic uses of nuclear medicine in AIDS, *Radiographics* 12:731, 1992.

294. Vazquez-Pinero T and others: HIV associated oral pleomorphic B-cell malignant lymphoma, *Oral Surg Oral Med Oral Pathol Oral Radiol Endod* 84:142, 1997.

295. Viscoli C, Castagnola E: Emerging fungal pathogens, drug resistance and the role of lipid formulations of amphotericin B in the treatment of fungal infections in cancer patients: a review, *Int J Infect Dis* 3:109-118, 1998-99.

296. Volberding PA: Advances in the medical management of patients with HIV-1 infection: an overview, *AIDS* 13: S1, 1999.

297. Wabinga HR and others: Trends in cancer incidence in Kyadondo county, Uganda, 1960-1997, *Br J Cancer* 82:1585, 2000.

298. Wallace M and others: Ototoxicity with azithromycin, *Lancet* 343:241, 1994.

299. Walmsley S and others: Treatment of AIDS-related cutaneous Kaposi's sarcoma with topical alitretinoin (9-cis-retinoic) gel, *J AIDS* 22:235, 1999.

300. Wang CY and others: Skin cancers associated with acquired immunodeficiency syndrome, *Mayo Clin Proc* 70:755, 1995.

301. Wang SA and others: Experience of healthcare workers taking postexposure prophylaxis after occupational HIV exposures: findings of the HIV Postexposure Prophylaxis Registry, *Infect Control Hosp Epidemiol* 21:780, 2000.

302. Wasserman L, Haghighi P: Otic and ophthalmic pneumocystosis in acquired immunodeficiency syndrome, *Arch Pathol Lab Med* 116:500, 1992.

303. Wawrose SF and others: The role of guaifenesin in the treatment of sinonasal disease in patients infected with the human immunodeficiency virus (HIV), *Laryngoscope* 102:1225, 1992.

304. Weinroth S and others: Malignant otitis externa in AIDS patients: case report and review of the literature, *Ear Nose Throat J* 7:772, 1994.

305. Weisburd G and others: *HIV seroconversion after a work place accident and treated with zidovudine [abstract].* In *Abstracts of the XI International Conference on AIDS.* Vancouver, B.C., July 7-12, 1996, p 460.

306. Welkoborosky H-J, Lowitzsch K: Auditory brain stem responses in patients with human immunotropic virus infection of different stages, *Ear Hear* 13:55, 1992.

307. Weschler AF, Ho DD: Bilateral Bell's palsy at the time of HIV seroconversion, *Neurology* 39:747, 1989.

308. Whitby D and others: Detection of Kaposi's sarcoma associated herpesvirus in peripheral blood of HIV-infected individuals and progression to Kaposi's sarcoma, *Lancet* 346:799, 1995.

309. White M, Armstrong D: Cryptococcus, *Infect Dis Clin North Am* 8:383, 1994.

310. Wiet RJ, Milko DA: Isolation of the spirochetes in the perilymph despite prior antisyphilitic therapy, *Arch Otolaryngol Head Neck Surg* 101:104, 1975.

311. Williams JD and others: Cytomegalovirus sinusitis in a patient with acquired immune deficiency syndrome, *Otolarygol Head Neck Surg* 112:750, 1995.

312. Williams MA: Head and neck findings in pediatric acquired immune deficiency syndrome, *Laryngoscope* 97:713, 1987.

313. Wiselka MJ and others: Acute infection with human immunodeficiency virus associated with facial nerve palsy and neuralgia, *J Infect* 15:189, 1987.

314. Wiselka MJ and others: Head and neck findings in acquired immune deficiency syndrome, *Laryngoscope* 97:713, 1987.

315. Yeni PG and others: Antiretroviral treatment for adult HIV infection in 2002: updated recommendations of the International AIDS Society-USA Panel, *JAMA* 288:222-235, 2002.

316. Yourtee E and others: Neutrophil response and function during acute cytomegalovirus infection in guinea pigs, *Infect Immunol* 36:11, 1982.

317. Ziegler JL, Katongole-Mbidde E: Kaposi's sarcoma in childhood: an analysis of 100 cases from Uganda and relationship to HIV infection, *Int J Cancer* 65:200, 1996.

318. Zurlo JJ and others: Sinusitis in HIV-1 infection, *Am J Med* 93:157, 1992.

319. Zurrida S and others: Fine needle aspiration of parotid masses, *Cancer* 72:2306, 1993.

CHAPTER ELEVEN

SPECIAL CONSIDERATIONS IN MANAGING GERIATRIC PATIENTS

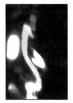

Matthew L. Kashima
W. Jarrard Goodwin, Jr.
Thomas Balkany
Roy R. Casiano

INTRODUCTION

The social and economic significance of the graying of America has received a great deal of attention in recent times. Numerous articles and editorials in the literature document the projected rate of growth of the geriatric population and how it will affect the practice of medicine. Together, geriatricians and other specialists in geriatric medicine and surgery are developing a system of care that keeps elderly adults healthier, more functional, and more independent at older ages than was previously possible. Otolaryngologists have taken up the challenge of describing and treating problems involving the senescent ear, nose, and throat, especially disorders involving communication. However, otolaryngologists are more familiar with the relationship of pathophysiology to disease than with the relationship of the disease to the elderly.[33] In our role as communication specialists, otolaryngologists are a key resource for helping the elderly to avoid isolation.

MAGNITUDE

In 1900, only 4% of the United States population lived to age 65; since then, this number has increased significantly. By 1960, the proportion had increased to 9%. In 1994, it was 12.6%. Recent estimates indicate that, by 2030, more than 20% of the population will be more than 65 years old. The proportion of the population over the age of 65 is not only increasing, but it is increasing at an accelerating pace. This population has expanded so much that it is now often divided into the "young old" and the "old old" (85 years old or older). The old old is the fastest-growing subgroup of the population: currently, there are 3.5 million people who are 85 years old and older, and it is anticipated that this subgroup will represent 7 million people by 2020 and double to 14 million people by 2040.[79] The truth is that the growth of this subgroup of the population represents more than a demographic change; the old old as a group use the healthcare system more than younger groups. In 1989, the segment of the population that was 65 years old and older accounted for more than 29% of medical expenditures, although they made up only 11% of the population.[33] The expected growth of the geriatric population portends a significant impact on society's social, economic, medical, and ethical needs and obligations.

Demographic changes in population will be important, as will the changes in the social support systems. The old age dependency ratio is a measurement used to summarize the relationship between the elderly and the young in a population. This number is obtained by dividing the population that is 65 years old and older by the working population (individuals between the ages of 18 and 64). Currently there are approximately 5 supporting individuals for every elderly person. By 2050, this number is expected to drop to 2.5.[79] Although this is a crude number, it is nevertheless informative of the changing demographics of our population.

Ratios within the population also demonstrate the rapidly expanding population over the age of 85. With this increase in the old old, we now can see larger group of elderly caring for their parents. In 1990, there were 31 persons 85 years old or older for every 100 persons between the ages of 65 and 69. By 2010, this number is expected to reach 52, and, by 2050, the number is expected to reach 109.[79] It is easy to see how this increase in the old old population will tax society at large and how the young old could be affected as primary caregivers.

Although disability and disease are greatest in the elderly population, not everyone over age 65 is ill or disabled. Forty-five percent of elderly surveyed reported their health as excellent or very good as opposed to 24% reporting fair or poor health. That being said, limitations in activities of daily living are seen in the elderly population and increase with age. Fifty-three percent of people over the age of 85 report functional limitations[38]; these limitations can result in an increase in the dependence of the elderly.

Aging is not well understood, but there are various theories about its mechanism. Aging can be viewed as the maturation of an organism from birth through death through a series of "natural causes," as a result of genetically programmed changes, or as a result of insults to the organism over time. As research continues to investigate aging, some of these fundamental questions will be answered. In the meantime, however, we will all need to learn how to best care for the aging patient.

BASIC PRINCIPLES OF GERIATRIC MEDICINE

Irvine[31] defined six basic principles that are useful in the care of elderly patients. Clinical decisions in this patient group tend to be complex, and these fundamentals are worthy of review and emphasis.

1. *Coexistence of multiple diseases:* The unitary disease hypothesis usually does not apply. As people age, they accumulate medical diagnoses, both major and minor. These comorbidities can have an impact on the presentation and response to therapy in the elderly. Signs and symptoms are more likely to be the result of several medical problems.
2. *Unique spectrum of illness:* In addition to many of the diseases seen in their younger counterparts, the elderly tend to suffer certain diseases that occur only in old age. This includes a wide range of degenerative disorders and certain cancers.
3. *Unusual presentation of illness:* Typical symptoms, such as fever and pain, are often absent, and nonspecific symptoms, such as anorexia or falling, may herald a serious underlying disorder.
4. *Proper role of the aging process:* Differentiating treatable disease from the natural aging process may be difficult, particularly in the area of degenerative diseases. Most geriatric specialists believe that patients and families have a tendency to overrate the role of aging. As a result, they experience unnecessary suffering and dysfunction; specific disease processes should be sought and treated whenever possible.
5. *Underreporting of health problems:* Patients and families often fail to report symptoms commonly relegated to old age.
6. *Function-based treatment goals:* Improving a patient's quality of life may shift therapeutic goals toward maximizing function and independence, possibly at the expense of potential for cure.

Medical care provided to the elderly serves several purposes. Treatment can be directed at specific acute disease processes, and the goal of this therapy can be curative or paliative. Health care interaction can be directed toward chronic conditions related to the aging process, such as presbycusis. Treatment can be directed toward reversing these conditions, preventing further disability, or educating patients about their condition. Providing preventive encounters is an important function of all health care practitioners. Otolaryngologists should take advantage of opportunities during patient encounters to educate patients about activities that they are involved in that have implications regarding their future health.

The goal of therapy, whether palliative or curative, must be explicitly discussed with patients and their familes to ensure that everyone is on the same page and considering the patient's global state of health.[38] Difficulties can arise when there is a difference in goals between a patient and his or her adult children or when the patient's or family's expectations are unrealistic. As the population ages, society may be forced to make some of these decisions as an increasing population competes for limited resources. Additionally, the financial burden that this population places on society will need to be addressed.

ACCESS TO MEDICAL CARE

A decreased level of strength and confidence may limit the ability of the elderly to visit a physician's office or the hospital, especially in the absence of strong family or community support. Social support systems often function better for acute and more serious problems; therefore, the well-known benefits of early detection and treatment may be lost. The high cost of modern health care may also create a relative barrier.

Society and physicians share a responsibility for providing care to all segments of the population, and a point can be made for making allowances for the elderly. Physicians remain the most effective patient advocates, despite the increasing role of other parties.

An additional barrier to care may be difficulty in obtaining accurate data from this population. The elderly have a relatively high incidence of memory impairment and cognitive dysfunction, which can significantly affect the ability of the practitioner to obtain an accurate history.[33] Even the presence of involved caregivers (e.g., adult children) may not be enough to provide complete and historic data regarding exposures and pediatric, surgical, and medical health histories.

DIAGNOSTIC TESTING

Because of the general principles mentioned previously, diagnosis may be the most challenging aspect of medical care in the elderly population; the focus should be on identifying treatable diseases and symptoms. A good deal of judgment is required to separate specific illness from the adverse (but natural) effects of aging, and it is usually not appropriate to attribute symptoms to aging unless other causes have been ruled out.

Invasive diagnostic procedures are relatively contraindicated when functional reserve is poor. Fortunately, modern diagnostic techniques—especially in imaging—have limited the need for invasive procedures.

TREATMENT
Medical Therapy

The proper use of medications is particularly important in the elderly. Indeed, one study showed that adverse effects of medication were the most common cause of symptoms that were confused with senile dementia.[43] Adverse effects of medication are also among the most common causes of hospital admissions in the elderly. According to Avon and Gurwitz,[2] any symptom in an elderly patient may be a drug side effect until proved otherwise. Up to 60% of elderly patients hospitalized for major surgical procedures suffer acute delerium or confusion.[38] It is well known that sensitivity to drugs increases with advancing age, but the reasons for this are not completely clear. There is some evidence that drug metabolism by the liver and clearance by the kidney both decline as one ages, but this does not explain the entire phenomenon. Drug receptors at the cellular level actually seem to increase in sensitivity. Drug interactions can be prevented by carefully evaluating existing drug therapy before starting any new medicines; this is especially important in the geriatric population, because most elderly patients are taking several drugs (both over the counter and prescription) at any given time.

Finally, use of some medications by the elderly should be completely avoided because of the known high incidence of side effects. A good example is sympathomimetic decongestants in elderly men, which frequently cause urinary retention.

Surgery

The decision to operate is never made lightly, and this is particularly true for the elderly patient. The physiologic changes that occur with aging affect the body's ability to respond to insults. Thus, wounds in the elderly heal slower; this is a result of retarded fibroplasia and decreased ability to remodel collagen. Santos and Gelperin[73] reported an overall mortality rate of 4.9% (8% for major surgery and 0.9% for minor procedures) in 1286 operations performed on patients that were more than 70 years old. Similarly, Seymour and Pringle[77] encountered life-threatening complications in 18.6% of 258 elderly surgical patients, of whom 5.8% died. Complications and mortality were more common after emergency procedures. Inactive patients (those who left their home less than twice weekly during the month before surgery) fared poorly and had a particularly high incidence of respiratory and cardiac complications.

THE AGING EAR

The normal process of aging affects all parts of the ear, but the greatest clinical impact is on cochlear and vestibular function. Presbycusis, which is the loss of hearing that is associated with aging, is the most common type of auditory dysfunction and is thought to be due to a series of insults over time, including age-related degeneration, noise exposure, and diseases of the ear. It is greatly affected by genetic background, diet, and systemic disease. Vestibular symptoms are present in more than half of elderly persons. Because balance depends on input from the ears, eyes, and peripheral sensory systems—all of which degenerate over time—impaired function in any of these systems contributes to vestibular complaints.

The pinna is commonly involved in actinic disorders, especially basal and squamous cell carcinoma. Sun protection and frequent inspection are important. The external auditory canal suffers a decrease in cerumen production due to degeneration of cerumen glands and a reduction in the total number of glands. This may lead to a drier cerumen that is less protective of the underlying skin and may result in a higher incidence of impaction and infection. Ceruminosis can be exacerbated by an increase in hair at the external auditory meatus. The skin also undergoes atrophy, which results in itching, fragility, and subsequent self-induced lacerations. The use of topical emollients has been recommended for difficult cases.

Mild middle ear histologic changes may be caused by the inflammatory effects of degenerative arthritis on arthrodial joints (incudomalleolar and incudostapedial). Histopathologic correlates may include hyalinization or calcification of the joint capsules and calcification of the articular cartilage. Little or no conductive hearing loss has been associated with these conditions.

Presbycusis, which is the auditory dysfunction associated with the aging process, is a generic term used to include several forms of the degeneration of hearing. This very common disorder, which affects up to 40% of the geriatric population,[38] may have a devastating effect on older individuals by reducing their ability to communicate, thereby jeopardizing autonomy and limiting opportunities of being an active member of society. With the growth of the aged population, presbycusis has become a great challenge to the otologist. The secondary effects of sensory deprivation include changes in perception, changes in personality (especially introversion), social disengagement, and socioeconomic considerations.[17]

Prevalence of Presbycusis

Accurate estimates of the prevalence of presbycusis in particular (and sensorineural hearing loss in general) are not available. However, survey data demonstrate that the estimated number of hearing-impaired people in the United States is 20,732,000, which is 8.8% of all Americans.[11] The tendency is for hearing-impaired people to underreport their hearing loss, so the numbers may be higher.

The specific causes of presbycusis are speculative at this time, but they are likely a combination of the effects of years of function; exposure to noise, chemicals, and so forth; and genetically programmed biologic degeneration. There is direct evidence of a gradual loss of cells of most organ systems that accompanies the aging process. This decrease in normal weight, cell count, and other cellular components is found in all aging organisms. Remaining cells may be larger, and total body mass may change only slightly changed during aging due to an increase in adipose tissue.

Physiologic changes include decreased oxygen use, reduced circulation, intracellular accumulation of lipofuscin and other substances, and extracellular deposition of cholesterol lipids.

Aging may also be seen as a degenerating genetic cellular system. Genetic damage may be a result of random deterioration as well as programmed deterioration. In the former, somatic cell genes undergo the inactivation of deoxyribonucleic acid at an irregular rate that accumulates throughout life. In the latter, there is selective activation and repression of genes during ontogeny of the cell.[87]

It is clear that morphologic changes in human beings (as well as animal models) regularly demonstrate the age-related loss of inner and outer hair cells and supporting cells, primarily from the basal turns of the cochlea. Outer hair cells decrease more than inner hair cells. Age-related loss of eighth nerve fibers has been reported to be as high as 20% in old rats.[25] Age-related changes may occur as high as the superior olivary complex in the brainstem.

Nixon,[61] in 1962, and previously Glorig and Davis[19] showed high-frequency conductive hearing losses attributed to stiffness and laxity of the joints in the aging middle ear. They also proposed the concept of an inner ear conductive hearing loss due to stiffness of the cochlear partition.

Gacek and Schuknecht[17] defined four histopathologic types of presbycusis: (1) sensory, which is char-

acterized by hair cell loss; (2) neural, which is associated with the loss of spiral ganglion cells and axons; (3) metabolic, which is characterized by strial atrophy; and (4) mechanical or conductive.

Sensory Presbycusis

The audiometric findings in this type of presbycusis include an abrupt, steep, and high-frequency sensorineural loss with slow symmetric bilateral progression, usually beginning during middle age. Pathologic lesions are limited to the first few millimeters of the basal turn of the cochlea. There is flattening and atrophy of the organ of Corti due to the loss of hair cells and supporting cells. There is also an accumulation of lipofuscin, which is the aging pigment.

Neural Presbycusis

Audiometric findings include gradual hearing loss with a moderate slope toward the high frequencies; however, these is a disproportionately severe decrease in speech discrimination. This difficulty with speech discrimination makes hearing loss refractory to amplification in many cases. Atrophy of the spiral ganglion and nerves of the osseous spiral lamina occur mainly in the basal turn of the cochlea. The organ of Corti is largely intact, as opposed to what is found in sensory presbycusis.

Strial Presbycusis (Metabolic Presbycusis)

The hearing loss associated with strial presbycusis is flat sensory loss beginning during the third through sixth decades and progressing slowly. Speech discrimination is generally good, and no recruitment is present. This condition is often familial, and patients do well with amplification. The characteristic pathologic findings are that atrophy of the stria vascularis is either patchy in the basal and apical turns or diffuse. The organ of Corti and spiral ganglion cells are usually unaffected.

Inner Ear Conductive Presbycusis

Both inner ear conductive presbycusis and atrophy of the spiral ligament cause bilateral symmetric sensorineural loss, with an upward slope toward the high frequency and preserved speech discrimination. No anatomic correlates with conductive sensorineural hearing loss are known, but it is hypothesized that the functional loss is due to stiffness of the basilar membrane, which correlates with its anatomic shape. The histopathologic pattern of atrophy of the spiral ligament includes different degrees of pathologic changes that are progressive through the patient's life; it is most noticeable in the apical turn and least in the basal turn. Cystic degeneration may cause detachment of the organ of Corti from the lateral cochlear wall, thereby resulting in hearing loss.

Proposed Etiologies
Vascular

Circulatory disorders have long been proposed as the cause of hearing loss in aging persons. However, there is insufficient histopathologic evidence of this etiology for confirmation. The relationship between high-frequency sensorineural hearing loss and the degree of cerebral atherosclerosis has been used to support this theory; unfortunately, both may be independent but age related. Atherosclerotic disease of renal vessels and inner-ear vessels has also been related to age. In 1959, Johnson and Hawkins[34] demonstrated the progressive involution of the human cochlear vasculature from the fetus and newborn through the aged. They noted that, during the first decade of life, the radiating arterioles and outer spiral vessels in the basal coil attain adult size. Devascularization of capillaries and arterioles was subsequently found in the spiral ligament that is associated with aging. They found a similarity between the degeneration of inner ear vessels with analogous changes in the retina due to microangiopathy,[22] and they demonstrated that the plugging of vascular canals by bony tissue is a generalized phenomenon that is related to aging. They felt that the plugging of vascular canals was one of the major causes of presbycusis.

Diabetic Presbycusis

Diabetic angiopathy is thought to be a specific entity. In this disorder, disseminated proliferation and hypertrophy of the intimal endothelium of arterials, capillaries, and venules occurs and causes significant narrowing of the lumen; there is also the precipitation of lipids and other substances in the vascular wall. In addition, arteriolosclerosis is thought to be more common and more extensive in patients with diabetes. However, clinical audiologic and pathologic studies of the correlation between diabetes and presbycusis are conflicting and contradictory. The great variability of incidence of hearing loss in diabetics is thought to be due to poor design in previously performed studies. In well-controlled studies, no correlation between sensorineural hearing loss and diabetes was found.

Noise

Noise is thought to be a common cause of presbycusis. It is clear that a direct correlation exists between noise-induced inner ear damage and the frequency, intensity, and duration of noise exposure. However, some may effectively argue that noise exposure causes hearing loss at any age and is not true presbycusis.

Noise-induced hearing loss may arise from mechanical damage, metabolic exhaustion, or vascular changes. Mechanical damage is seen in cochleas that have been exposed to high-intensity or impulse noise of short duration. There may be detachment of the organ of Corti from the basal membrane. Metabolic exhaustion is characterized by changes of intracellular ultrastructure, thereby indicating the depletion of enzymes and metabolites in overstimulated sensory cells. Noise has clearly been shown to cause ischemic changes of the inner ear. Capillaries below the basilar membrane have been noted histologically to undergo spasmodic changes. In addition, edema of endothelial cells impairs blood flow to the spiral ligament and stria vascularis. Sludging and aggregation of erythrocytes with increased blood viscosity secondary to decreased capillary flow also occurs.

Metabolic Etiologies

In Rosen's studies of Finnish patients on long-term controlled diets,[71] the reduction of saturated fat resulted in a significant lowering of serum cholesterol and an improvement in auditory threshold testing. Subsequent studies demonstrated that hypolipoproteinemia is the correlate to Rosen's clinical epidemiologic studies and is related to presbycusis as well as obesity, atherosclerosis, and coronary artery disease.

Genetic Considerations

Diagnosis of genetic sensorineural hearing loss—especially when of adult onset and without external abnormalities—is extremely difficult, but it should be considered. The diagnosis of these disorders relies primarily on the history given by the patient and on the audiometric configuration that is characteristic. The typical hearing loss is a basin-shaped curve with good discrimination and no recruitment. Over the years, this pattern may change to a gradual or abrupt slope. Pathologically, the most prominent feature in this disorder is atrophy of the stria vascularis, which is parallel to Schuknecht's strial atrophy category.

Hearing and Dementias

Recent studies of the cochlea in temporal bones from patients with confirmed Alzheimer's disease showed a lack of degeneration in the cochlea, which is typical of Alzheimer's patients. This finding is distinguished from findings in the peripheral olfactory and visual systems, which show the typical neurofibrillary tangles and neuritic plaques.[82]

Conversely, a possible relationship between central auditory dysfunction was found in the Framingham follow-up study of 1662 subjects. However, that study is weakened by the absence of objective testing in competing message tests.[18]

Treatment

Regardless of the mechanism or etiology of hearing loss in the elderly, its impact on quality of life can be quite significant. Hearing loss can be related to social withdrawal in the elderly as a result of frustration and inability to communicate. This impaired ability to communicate can have wide-ranging health effects, because it can affect communication between a patient and his or her health care provider, thereby leading to missed diagnoses.[38.]

Unfortunately, the term *presbycusis* is somewhat vague, and specific signs and symptoms should be identified to clarify its definition. Classic presbycusis includes bilaterally symmetric sensorineural hearing loss in the absence of other etiologies. Although dietary measures over the long term may be effective in reducing the progression of hearing loss in certain aging patients, further data are necessary before this treatment modality is clinically accepted. Amplification remains the mainstay of treatment for presbycusis.

Cochlear Implantation in the Elderly

Severe to profound sensorineural deafness in the elderly is most often due to an underlying pathologic process, such as Ménière's disease or otosclerosis in combination with presbycusis; the latter does not produce this degree of hearing impairment on its own. One of the authors of this chapter performed cochlear implantation on patients who were up to 85 years old, with good results. Mean audiologic test scores increase significantly following implantation and are comparable with results achieved by younger recipients. In addition, the isolation of aging and the loss of known companionship (e.g., spouse and close friends) is greatly compounded by the social effects of severe to profound hearing loss. Elderly cochlear implant recipients are among the most satisfied due to their renewed ability to communicate, socialize, and, in most cases, use the telephone. The latter is especially important for a patient's confidence, because they know that they will be able to obtain emergency help, if needed. Complications have not been experienced, but they may be expected to be somewhat higher in elderly patients with intercurrent cardiac or respiratory disorders.

PRESBYSTASIS

Presbystasis, which is the disequilibrium of aging, is a group of disorders that affect the mobility of a large number of elderly persons. Due to the degeneration of the vestibular, proprioceptive, and visual senses, the ability to walk and drive can be reduced to the point of incapacitation; lessening spatial-orientation abilities contribute to this as well. Loss of balance is the most common manifestation of vestibular dysfunction in elderly persons.

Although attempts have been made to categorize the dysequilibrium of aging as a single specific entity, a large number of vestibular disorders are seen in elderly patients. These include vascular disease, Ménière's disease, benign positional vertigo, and adaptation deficits. Input from the vestibular, visual, proprioceptive, and other systems can be thought of as providing input into a common central processor that, in turn, controls posture and eye movement.

Disorders of these sensory organ systems have traditionally been treated by otolaryngologists, neurologists, and ophthalmologists, depending on the organ system causing the most obvious dysfunction. However, development of the unifying discipline of neurotology has led to an integrated approach to, evaluation of, and care for elderly persons with dysequilibrium. Otolaryngologists must be aware of other causes of disequilibrium or dizziness, because a variety of organ systems may contribute to these difficulties, including vestibular, ocular, proprioceptive, musculoskeletal, central processing, and neuromotor; systemic diseases and side effects from medications may be causes as well.[38]

The National Health Interview Survey supplement on aging[23] showed that more than 18% of persons 65 years old and older and more than 25% of those more than 75 years old had a falling incident in 1985. These falls are not without consequences: 2% result in hip fractures, up to 10% result in serious injury, and 50% result in at least a minor injury, such as a laceration. Moreover, individuals who have fallen tend to fear repeat events and restrict their activities.[38] Fifteen to 23% of the individuals that fell reported doing so because they were dizzy. Thirty-four percent of those between 65 and 74 years old felt that ". . . dizziness prevents you from doing things you otherwise could do."[23] Extrapolating these figures to the population of the United States, 12.5 million people more than 65 years old note that dizziness represents a serious impairment of their normal activities.

In a 1981 study of outpatient medical care, dizziness was the most common presenting complaint for patients who were more than 75 years old.[39] Dizziness was a presenting complaint in 38 of 1000 patient visits. In a Finnish longitudinal study of geriatric outpatients,[62] dizziness occurred in 81% of men and 91% of women. The most significant complications of presbystasis are falls and hip fractures. More than 200,000 hip fractures occur annually among Americans that are more than 65 years old. The direct mortality due to hip fractures is more than 15%, and morbidity often includes permanent failure to ambulate. Of course, other disorders that affect this population play important roles, including the use of psychotropic medication, abnormalities in blood pressure, leg-muscle weakness, and loss of coordination. It is believed that the failure of one of the previously mentioned organ systems can be compensated for; however, with multisystem failure, increasingly severe deficits occur.

Pathology

Age-related degeneration has been noted in hair cells, neurons, and supporting structures of the peripheral vestibular system.[3n] Hair cell loss has been found in the semicircular canals, the utricle, and the saccule. This degeneration is most noted in the central area of the cristae, whereas macular degeneration is more diffuse. Degeneration of the saccule may be greater than that of the macula. A decrease in the total number of peripheral vestibular neurons—as well as a decrease in the size of myelinated nerve fibers—has been described in patients that are more than 65 years old. Degenerative changes also occur in otoconia of the human maculae, deformities of the vestibular end organs, and degeneration of the synaptic structures of afferent dendrites.[57] These degenerative changes are considered to be the vestibular equivalent of presbycusis. Unlike presbycusis, however, asymmetric loss of vestibular function can result in incapacitation. Degenerative changes of the vestibular nuclei and cerebellum have also been reported.

Diagnostic Methods

The use of objective tests to identify the etiologic basis of presbystasis is essential. Vestibular function studies described elsewhere in this chapter are applicable in the elderly. Avoidance of a "trash basket" diagnosis of presbystasis and continuing clinical research into etiologic diagnosis are essential.

A wide variety of findings have been noted and have indicated both peripheral and central vestibular abnormalities. Studies normalizing electronystagmography, platform posturography, and sinusoidal harmonic acceleration in the elderly are ongoing.

In cases of presbystasis arising in the peripheral labyrinth, generalized hypofunction is often found. Symmetric maximum slow-phase velocity responses to warm and cool caloric stimulation of less than 10°C per second per irrigation is empirically used by the authors of this chapter to identify this condition.

In cases of peripheral hypofunction, the use of vestibular nerve suppressants may be contraindicated. Such treatment further reduces the already reduced vestibular input, thereby resulting in further incapacitation.

Treatment

Nonvestibular causes of presbystasis need to be identified and treated specifically. Examples include postural hypotension associated with antihypertensive medications, endocrine imbalances, malnutrition, and cardiovascular insufficiency.

Because of the adaptive control feedback mechanism in this complex system, treatment modalities have been developed to allow for compensation. This adaptive control system alters afferent signals from the various receptors at both visual-vestibular interfaces as well as proprioceptive-vestibular interfaces. Control circuits are affected by disturbances in the general condition of the patient, the availability of the neurotransmitter, and in pathologic disorders.[30] Other feedback loops help control visual tracking and postural adjustment in response to motion. Cognitive controls also exist and contribute primarily in the areas of spatial orientation, the hallucination of motion, and the development of athletic skills.

Vestibular habituation training is a more recent treatment modality that offers promise for presbystasis. These "exercises" are based on feedback control initiated by the habituation effect. Mechanisms of adaptation and compensation are stimulated through repeated elicitation of minor degrees of vertigo.

Other goals of vestibular exercise programs include the improvement of visual following when the head is stationary, gaze stability during head movement, and visual-vestibular interactions during head movement and general balance. These exercises are designed to incorporate visual and proprioceptive experiences with vestibular cues.

The twin goals of these exercises are the reestablishment of balance and the reduction of the symptoms of dizziness and disorientation. In many cases, consultation and therapy with a physical or occupational therapist trained in vestibular compensation exercises can be extremely helpful.

Another important consideration that must be stressed to the patient is the prevention of falls. Precautions include the use of night lights (especially en route to the bathroom), the removal of throw rugs, the avoidance of stairs, and the use of ambulatory assistance devices when necessary.

THE AGING NOSE

Nasal structure and physiology are affected directly by the aging process and by a multitude of indirect factors that are commonly seen in the elderly. Also, many elderly people become accustomed to living with a dysfunctional nose due to trauma, infection, or allergy. These individuals may complain only when nasal dysfunction interferes with sleep, eating, breathing, or sensation (smell and taste). Some medications used commonly by the elderly (e.g., diuretics, antihypertensives) may desiccate the nose. Decongestants and antihistamines make secretions thicker and worsen postnasal drip. In addition, a number of disease processes associated with aging can affect the nose.

Mucoepithelial Changes

Studies have shown that there is no definite relationship between age and the type of nasal epithelium.[27] Neither age nor smoking has been related to a reduction in ciliated cells. Other unknown factors may influence change in the viscoelastic properties of the nasal mucus and therefore predispose the elderly to nasal crusting.[42]

The effect of age on mucociliary transport is modest. Mucociliary transport rates are not significantly different between young adults and middle-aged adults or between middle-aged adults and the elderly. However, significant differences exist between younger adults and the elderly.[72]

Olfactory Changes

There are many studies that have researched age-related changes in taste and smell. Most of these studies have shown that olfactory thresholds for a wide range of odorants progressively decrease with age.* The process seems to begin earlier in men; this is probably due to a combination of a loss of receptors and neurons, with alterations in neurotransmitters and central pathways.[74] There is also a decrease in olfactory epithelium, with increased degenerative changes and loss of olfactory bulb fibers.[49,63,83]

Changes in Nasal Appearance and Intranasal Examination

There is a significant increase in the nasolabial angle and a decrease in the height:length ratio of the nose with age. This may be due to the lengthening of the upper lip, resorption of premaxillary fat, resorption of the malar and alveolar ridge, and changes in dentition that are caused by the degenerative process of aging. The decreased height:length ratio accentuates the drooping of the nose as it ages. Weakening of the lower lateral cartilage and the caudal septum, along with the loss of elasticity in the enveloping skin, contributes to the descent of the aged nose tip.

Abnormalities of the nasopharynx are not common in older subjects. This may reflect increased atrophy of the lymphatic structures and a diminished secretory capacity of mucus-secreting glands.

*References 12–15, 41, 53, 58, 59, 84.

Common Symptoms

The most common nasal complaints in the elderly are nasal drainage, postnasal drip, sneezing, coughing, olfactory loss, and gustatory rhinitis.[16] Other symptoms, such as nasal obstruction, epistaxis, and sinus pain, have not been shown to significantly increase with age. It is felt that nasal discharge and postnasal drip among the elderly may be explained by the loss of autonomic control. Gustatory rhinitis, which is nasal discharge that is stimulated by eating, similarly may be caused by overactivation of the autonomic control of the mucoserous and Bowman's glands initiated by the sight of food or the act of eating.

There is a general increase in nasal resistance with age, despite the lack of subjective symptoms of nasal obstruction. This may be explained by the fact that many older patients believe that some nasal obstruction is normal and hence not worth mentioning. However, the elderly often notice that nasal airflow is subjectively less with exertion. Studies of sinusitis have shown that this condition is more frequently bilateral and severe in children.[30] By contrast, the frequency of nasal polyps increases with advancing years.[76]

Treatment

As is the case with younger age groups, medical or surgical treatment of rhinologic problems in the elderly requires an accurate diagnosis to select appropriate treatment. Humidification is generally helpful. Topical and systemic decongestants should be avoided, because they may aggravate dryness and mucosal atrophy. Underlying osteomeatal blockage due to allergies or infection may be addressed; this may involve treatment in a multidisciplinary setting by the pulmonologist, allergist, otolaryngologist, and other specialists. The treatment of associated medical conditions may be helpful. Medications that desiccate the nose should be avoided unless there are no other alternatives. In patients with vasomotor or gustatory rhinitis, anticholinergics such as ipratropium bromide spray may be effective.

Surgical reconstruction is aimed at reconstituting support for the upper lateral cartilage and elevating the drooping nasal tip.[65] The removal of turbinate mucosa should be avoided, especially when excessive dryness is already a factor. Vidian neurectomy may be indicated in select cases.

THE AGING VOICE AND THE UPPER AERODIGESTIVE TRACT

The phonatory organ is comprised of the resonator (larynx), the articulators (supraglottic structures), and the compressors (lungs).[88] Age-related changes in any one or all of these structures can have a direct impact on voice quality and general comfort level (Table 11-1). Furthermore, older people are often exposed to a wide array of environmental and medicinal irritants (indirect factors) that compound the problem (Table 11-2). Elderly patients may also suffer from a host of medical conditions that are common as one progresses in age and that may affect vocal quality.[5,48,67-69,95] Diseases including cancer, vocal fold paralysis, Parkinson's disease, amyotrophic lateral sclerosis, benign essential tremor, diabetes, and other endocrine dysfunctions must be excluded (see Tables 11-1 and 11-2). Additionally, the frequent occurrence of depression and sensorineural hearing loss can lead to a hyperfunctional voice and muscular tension dysphonia, and the adverse effect of long-term tobacco smoking on voice is also well recognized. Therefore, treatment of geriatric patients with vocal problems must be directed not only at maximizing the efficiency of the aging phonatory organ through appropriate voice therapy or surgery but also at treatment of the underlying medical, neurologic, or psychiatric disorder.

Histologic Changes

Laryngeal tissues change a good deal before alterations in the voice are detected. Histologic changes seen within the aging larynx appear to occur with approximately equal frequency in both sexes but at a different rate. Histologic examination suggests that the yellowish discoloration seen clinically represents fat degeneration or keratosis of the mucous membrane. Vocal fold atrophy is thought to represent the laryngeal manifestation of senescent changes in muscle and mucous membranes. There is general thinning,

TABLE 11-1

COMMON FACTORS WITH A DIRECT EFFECT ON VOCAL QUALITY

Factors	Effect on Vocal Quality
Laryngeal muscle atrophy/fibrosis	Effect on glottic gap and vocal fold thickness, resulting in increased air loss and abnormal acoustics
Cricoarytenoid joint changes	
Mucosal atrophy	Increased chance for injury, pain, and guarding, which affect articulation
Salivary gland atrophy	Decreased lubrication, dry mouth, and secondary dental problems
Alveolar bone resorption	Increased chance for injury, pain, and guarding, which affect articulation
Dental/gingival loss	
Temporomandibular joint disease	
Lower respiratory tract changes	Decreased chest elasticity, abdominal tone, and breath support, which result in decreased vital capacity, vocal fatigue, and decreased volume

TABLE 11-2

COMMON FACTORS WITH AN INDIRECT EFFECT ON VOCAL QUALITY

Factors	Effect on Vocal Quality
Hearing loss	Vocal misuse
Anxiety/depression	
Dehydrants: alcohol, antihistamines, decongestants, diuretics, megadoses of vitamin C, antidepressants, antihypertensives	Reduced lubrication/altered secretions
Surgery/disease processes: prior intubation, laryngeal surgery or disease, oral/pharyngeal surgery or disease, nasal/sinus surgery or disease, superior/recurrent laryngeal injury, dental/temporomandibular joint surgery or disease, abdominal/thoracic surgery or disease, limb surgery or disease	Changes in phonation, resonance, and articulation; reduced pulmonary support/altered posture
Mucosal irritants: allergies, smoking, gastroesophageal reflux, pollution	Direct effect on mucous membranes/altered secretions
Endocrine dysfunction: hypothyroidism, hormonal therapy	Mucosal/soft tissue alterations, vocal fold edema
Abrupt weight change	Multifactorial

decreased fiber density, fatty degeneration of the laryngeal muscles, and a decrease in fragmentation of elastic fibers in the submucosa.[20] Decreased fiber density is also seen in the laryngeal ligaments and the conus elasticus.

Progressive calcification of the laryngeal cartilages is also observed.[66] Calcification and ossification begins during the early 20s and is essentially completed by the sixth decade. Small islands of cartilage remain in the central portion of the thyroid cartilage of men; there is preservation of cartilage in the upper portion in women. The cricoid may be almost completely ossified. The arytenoid undergoes ossification of the body and muscular process, with the apex remaining cartilaginous (Figure 11-1, *A* and *B*). There

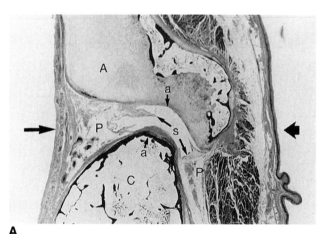

A

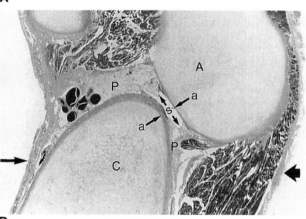

B

Figure 11-1. A, Young cricoarytenoid joint (patient is 29 years old). *A,* Arytenoid; *C,* cricoid; *a,* articular surface; *S,* synovium; *P,* periarticular soft tissues; *fat arrow,* hypopharyngeal epithelium; *thin arrow,* subglottic respiratory epithelium. (Hematoxylin-eosin; ×3.) **B,** Old cricoarytenoid joint (patient is 69 years old). *A,* Arytenoid; *C,* cricoid; *a,* articular surface; *S,* synovium; *P,* periarticular soft tissues; *fat arrow,* hypopharyngeal epithelium; *thin arrow,* subglottic respiratory epithelium. Note increased calcification and muscle atrophy. (Hematoxylin-eosin; ×3.)

seems to be some controversy regarding whether the vocalis process ossifies.[37] This ossification represents the creation of a true haversian system with lamella, osteocytes, and fat marrow. In general, the onset of ossification is later and less extensive in women, and the entire process is quite variable among individuals. Age-related changes may occur in the cricoarytenoid joint as well.[47]

Laryngoscopic Appearance

Laryngoscopic characteristics of the aging larynx include a yellowish or dark grayish discoloration of the vocal fold, edema, and vocal fold atrophy. This results in bowing of the vocal fold edges, incomplete glottic closure, and visibility of the ventricle. The prominence of the contour of the vocal process leads to the typical "arrowhead configuration" of the glottis that is seen so often in the senescent larynx.[29,89] Atrophy of the vocal folds occurs in 67% of men and 27% of women.[29]

Acoustic Changes

Dsyphonia is present in at least 10% of the elderly. Although variable, the senescent voice is typically stereotyped as being tremulous, weak, hoarse, and altered in pitch. Overall, jitter (cycle-to-cycle frequency variation) continues to be significantly greater in the aging population as compared with younger age groups, particularly in men.[4] Aging of the larynx is also associated with a slowing in the opening quotient of the vocal folds, which further adversely affects vocal quality.[56] In men, fundamental frequency levels progressively decrease from 20 to 40 years of age and then increase from 60 through 80 years of age.[28] Vocal fold edema, which is seen in some women, is thought to be due to general endocrine changes that occur after menopause. The latter, along with the lowering of laryngeal position that occurs in women that are more than 60 years old, results in marked lowering of the fundamental frequency and roughness courses of the voice.[55] The aging woman also tends to read with larger intonation ranges and a greater number of inflections and younger adults.[9]

The aging process results in significant changes within the mucosa of the oral cavity, salivary glands, teeth, mandible, maxilla, temporomandibular joint, and taste buds. In combination or individually, oral dryness, soft tissue atrophy, decreased mandibular excursion, and temporomandibular joint disease can significantly affect the voice by altering its resident characteristics. The acoustic characteristics of women's voices show a significant lowering of the frequency of the first formant (f1) with advancing age, which suggests age-related changes in the vocal tract and mentions or positions of speech structures.

Mucosal Changes

The epithelium of the mouth becomes atrophic, especially in the prickle cell layer. Parakeratosis and hyperkeratosis may be present, particularly in areas of denture use. Histologically, there is thinning of the tunica propria and blunting of the rete pegs; decreases in capillaries, water content, hyaluronic acid, and collagen content; and an increase in ground substance. In combination with small vessel disease (e.g., arteriosclerosis), these changes make oral tissues more prone to injury,[60] prolonged wound healing, and contribute to the shiny smooth appearance of the senescent oral mucosa. Guarding as a result of oral trauma may adversely affect the voice by modifying the way one articulates and projects speech sounds.

Glandular Changes

Normal physiologic changes that occur in the salivary glands of the elderly are the principal cause of dry mouth syndrome, which is one of the most common complaints of this population.[51,75] Secretory rates diminish and salivary viscosity increases in these patients. Submandibular gland parenchymal volume decreases as a result of a reduction in acinar tissue, whereas ducts enlarge. There is also an increase in focal chronic inflammatory changes resulting from hyalinization of the asini and an increase in salivary duct adhesions and obstructions. The end result is a loss of one quarter of the active secretory parenchymal volume and its replacement by connective tissue and fat.[75] Because adequate lubrication is essential for the production of sound in the phonatory apparatus, the presence of dry mouth should be recognized and treated.

The loss of taste in the elderly can be attributed to two factors. One factor may be a reduction in salivation; the other is a reduction in the number of taste buds, which occurs normally during the aging process.[24] Many elderly patients complain of a metallic or salty taste and decreased levels of sensitivity to sweet, bitter, and sour foods. These problems, combined with decreased salivation, result in poor tissue repair in periodontal and mucosal tissues. Subsequent difficulties with dentures and an increase in dental caries in remaining teeth may arise.

Dental/Mandibular Changes

As one ages, there is resorption of mandibular and maxillary alveolar bone (the mandibular bone, to a greater degree), thereby leading to a loss in the vertical dimension of the face and a "purse-string" appearance of the mouth. Histologically, the aging mandible often displays signs of osteoporosis in the form of cortical thinning and loss of the coarse trabeculation patterns. In the edentulous maxilla, osteoporosis is extensive, especially in women. A diminution in regenerative capacity occurs, along with the presence of osteogenesis. Bone resorption and the diminution of connective tissue around the nerves allow the neurovascular surface to be more easily damaged. Common complaints are paresthesia or pain due to irritation of the mental nerve by ill-fitting dentures and a burning sensation of the hard palate. As in other areas of the oral cavity, these connective tissue changes contribute to a reduction in the repair capacity after injury. As far as teeth are concerned, a secondary dentin (calcified dentin) replaces most of the dental pulp. The cementum shows continued deposition and calcification throughout life. Apical migration of gingival tissue leads to a gradual exposure of the tooth root. These processes make individuals prone to periapical infection and periodontal disease. Any changes in the bony architecture of the maxilla or mandible may adversely affect the voice by affecting the resonance characteristics of speech sounds. The absence of teeth, the use of ill-fitting dentures, oral or dental pain, and paresthesias may further affect certain speech sounds, particularly those involving tongue-to-lip, palate, or teeth apposition. The ability to produce clear plosive (p, t, k, b, d, and g) and fricative (s, z, f, v, sh, ph, and th) sounds may therefore be affected.

The temporomandibular joint may also be affected by the aging process. There is a loss of elasticity and hardening of the articular disc and capsular ligament, a thinning of the articular disc, fibrosis of the articular space, and a flattening of the articular surfaces. Complaints such as joint clicking, dislocation, subluxation, and fracture of the articular head (with subsequent decrease in mouth opening) may indirectly affect the voice, again by altering resonance characteristics and the projection of speech sounds. Speaking with a tight oral aperture narrows resonance of sound within the oral cavity; it may further result in laryngeal elevation, which increases tension in the vocal tract.

The effects of aging on pulmonary function are significant. Pulmonary perfusion, forced expiratory volume, forced vital capacity, elastic recoil, and dynamic pulmonary compliance decrease significantly with age.[7,36,40,46,66] There is a ventilation perfusion mismatch, an increase in alveolar dead space, an increase in the alveoloarterial gradient for oxygen delivery, a loss of alveolar surface area, and a change in the pulmonary circulation.[1,86] Calcification of the tracheal cartilage increases with age, and respiratory neural outflow decreases.[8] Body weight commonly increases with age, which increases the demand on the respiratory system. In addition, age causes changes in the musculature of the lower respiratory tract that affect the function of the chest wall, abdomen, and diaphragm. Older men have been found to require more intrasentence breaths, which is felt to be related to decreased vital capacity.[80] All of these changes can result in inadequate breath support and excessively harsh glottal closure. Over time, this can fatigue the laryngeal apparatus and result in secondary muscular tension dysphonia.

For the most part, treatment of presbyphonia is directed at controlling the underlying medical illness and maximizing the efficiency of the phonatory apparatus. This typically involves a multidisciplinary approach involving the expertise of a speech pathologist, otolaryngologist, pulmonologist, neurologist, psychiatrist, oral surgeon, and a generalist. Treatment for gastric acid reflux and attention to proper hydration and other general vocal hygiene measures are important. Maximizing pulmonary efficiency in patients with underlying pulmonary disease is a necessity. General conditioning may be quite helpful in motivated patients. Symptomatic dryness can be addressed with the judicious use of sialogogues, salivary substitutes, and expectorants. Other specific medical illnesses discussed above must be addressed, when present.

Surgical procedures have been devised in an attempt to adjust vocal pitch as well as strengthen the voice of patients with flaccid or bowed vocal folds.[44] Isshiki[32] advocates a type 4 thyroplasty for this problem. Others have advocated similar advancement of the anterior commissure to adjust vocal cord tension through an anterior commissure laryngoplasty.[92] Short-term success with these procedures has been achieved, with improvement in loudness and clarity and a decrease in breathiness and air escape. Surgery is recommended only after the more conservative measures addressed above fail to achieve the results required by the patient.

PRESBYPHAGIA

Dysphagia is relatively common in the elderly. It has been estimated that 50% of patients in nursing homes have a swallowing impairment[91]; this has contributed to the supposition that swallowing deficits may reflect normal age-related changes. Granieri[21] suggests that the effects of aging on swallowing can be divided into primary, secondary, and tertiary categories.

Primary effects of aging on swallowing include physiologic and structural changes in the oral cavity, pharyngeal, and laryngeal structures. Detailed information regarding these changes is emerging in the literature.[45,70,78,85,90] These age-related changes provide the context for potential changes in swallowing physiology but generally do not result in clinically significant dysphagia. Secondary factors include a plethora of general medical and neurologic conditions and side effects from the use of pharmacologic agents, which is more common in the elderly. Included secondary factors are head and neck cancers and their treatments and the general deconditioning associated with illness and reduced mobility that can result in oropharyngeal swallowing deficits. Tertiary aspects involve those changes that can result from social, environmental, and psychologic factors.

Diagnostic Testing

When swallowing disorders are suspected in the elderly, a complete oropharyngeal and esophageal swallowing evaluation is warranted because of the increased incidence of concomitant problems in both areas. A careful history and physical examination should allow the clinician to distinguish between the two major categories of swallowing impairment: difficulty initiating swallowing and obstruction.[10] Because speech, voice, and swallowing problems are often the first signs of degenerative neurologic or neuromuscular disease, the physical examination should include both head and neck and neurologic evaluations.

Radiographic assessment is considered the gold standard for dysphagia assessment. The modified barium swallow (MBS), which is a videofluoroscopic swallowing study of the head and neck, provides critical physiologic information (i.e., bolus transit from the mouth to the cervical esophagus), swallow transitions, and biomechanics of the swallow that are necessary for treatment. The procedure also provides valuable information about the timing and etiology of aspiration and the effectiveness of rehabilitative strategies. The esophagus can be evaluated by routine barium swallow after the MBS procedure. If the study reveals structural or motility disorders, endoscopy and manometric examination are the next diagnostic steps.

Flexible endoscopic evaluation of swallowing is an adjunctive assessment tool to the MBS. Visualization of the pharyngeal-laryngeal mechanism provides symptomatic information about the swallow (i.e., aspiration and pharyngeal residue). This type of endoscopic evaluation is also a valuable biofeedback tool for airway closure maneuvers.

Treatment

Proper treatment of swallowing disorders in the elderly requires management by the multidisciplinary team and is contingent on correct diagnosis. Treatment may be medical or surgical, but it is more often rehabilitative. Rehabilitative treatment strategies that will improve the safety and efficiency of the swallow are identified during the radiographic procedure and based on the nature of the patient's disorder. Many swallowing rehabilitation techniques require the application of voluntary control to disordered aspects of swallow physiology. However, a number of treatment strategies require little patient cognition or cooperation by the elderly individual. General treatment strategies may include postural techniques, swallowing therapy strategies (e.g., supraglottic swallow, Mendelsohn maneuver), increased sensory input, volume changes, and changes in diet or food consistency.[50] If nonoral feeding is required, reevaluation at regular intervals should be conducted to determine progress in recovery and the optimal time to reinitiate oral intake.

Dysphagia in the elderly represents a fairly common and challenging clinical problem. Limited evidence indicates that normal aging has generally minor effects on the swallowing mechanism and that significant dysphagia is more typically the result of secondary or tertiary processes. An understanding of normal swallowing in older individuals and a comprehensive diagnostic assessment will facilitate proper diagnosis and management.

Facial Fractures

The facial skeleton undergoes changes with aging; the most prominent change is resorption of the alveolar bone in the maxilla and mandible. This problem is magnified in edentulous patients, in whom up to 50% of the mandibular height may be lost. The bone of the facial skeleton becomes brittle, and decreased metabolic activity in the bone makes healing times prolonged. Resoption of bone and its fragility can make placing fixation plates difficult. Planing for repairing facial fractures in the elderly must take these facts into account to ensure the best possible outcome.

HEAD AND NECK ONCOLOGY

More than one half of all cancer patients are more than 65 years old at the time of original diagnosis;[94] the mean age of patients who have squamous cell carcinoma of the upper aerodigestive tract is 60 years. Indeed, aging seems to be a primary cause of cancer. Although the vast majority of cancer patients are more than 65 years old, they represent a minority of participants in clinical trials.[26]

Etiology

Environmental exposure to carcinogens—most notably tobacco and alcohol—is an important cause of these cancers. The occurrence of cancer in advanced age is probably related to the duration of carcinogen exposure and to immune senescence. Immune dysfunction associated with aging is complex and involves several components of the immune system. Wolf[94] suggests that the most important deficit may be in antigen-specific T-cell cytotoxic function. Interestingly, autoimmune diseases also are more common with advancing age and may facilitate tumor progression.

Treatment

Elderly patients tolerate the treatment of early localized cancer well, but age becomes a significant factor in the management of advanced cancer. Combined treatment with surgery and radiation therapy has improved local control rates in patients with advanced cancer, but elderly patients tolerate multimodality therapy poorly and may never fully recover from treatments.

Elderly patients generally tolerate major head and neck cancer surgery well. Morgan and others[54] reviewed 1773 patients undergoing major head and neck operations under general anesthesia. Of the 810 patients between the ages of 65 and 95 years, 3.5% died, and 32% suffered nonlethal complications. By contrast, only 8 of 863 patients between the ages of 35 and 65 years died (0.8%), and the complication rate was 21%. The differences in mortality and complication rates are both significant, but a mortality rate of 3.5% in those more than 65 years old does not seem prohibitive. In a more recent study, McGuirt[52] found that patients who were more than 80 years old had a similar prognosis to that of patients between 65 and 80 years old; complications were more common with advancing age. Johnson, Rabuzzi, and Tucker[35] studied patients who were undergoing composite resection and compared several factors found in patients who were more than 65 years old with those in a younger cohort. The older patients fared at least as well with regard to complications, mortality, and rehabilitation. Nevertheless, the authors' clinical experience suggests that the rehabilitation of speech and swallowing dysfunction after such surgery is more challenging with increasing age. The authors have found percutaneous endoscopic gastrostomy particularly valuable in elderly patients undergoing the resection of large portions of the tongue and pharynx without laryngectomy.

Thyroid disease is common in the geriatric population, and thyroid cancer behaves more aggressively in older patients.[81] Undifferentiated carcinoma is more common, and recurrence and metastasis occur more frequently in the elderly, even with well-differentiated thyroid cancer. The mainstay of management for well-differentiated thyroid cancer is surgery, but multimodality therapy that includes radioactive iodine is commonly advised in older patients, especially those who have follicular cancer. Bliss and colleagues[6] investigated thyroid surgery in patients that were more than 50 years old. They found no difference in morbidity or mortality when comparing patients 50 to 60 years old with patients 61 to 70 years old and with patients that were more than 70 years old.

Regardless of pathology, before advising a major surgical procedure, careful consideration is given to the patient's motivation as evidenced by his or her current level of function. An active 80-year-old patient with good muscle tone may be a better surgical candidate than a sedentary 65-year-old patient with poor functional residual capacity. A comprehensive preoperative evaluation needs to be completed in all surgical candidates. Current trends in health care are to minimize inpatient care and shorten postoperative admissions. Although this may be feasible for young, healthy adults, the goal of short-stay admissions for the elderly may not be realistic; this needs to be taken into account when planning treatments for geriatric patients.[26]

Preoperative teaching is important for all patients and their families, and selected patients may benefit from a two-week course of nutritional and physical therapy aimed primarily at improving cardiorespiratory function. Patients should understand that they will need to participate in the recovery process, which may last several months; a substantial portion of this time will not be spent in an acute care setting. Patients should understand that recovery may entail a period of rehabilitation at a rehabilitation facility or a subacute care facility; placement in one of these facilities is not to be construed by the patient or his or her family as an adverse event or failure of treatment.

CONCLUSION

Otolaryngologists and all healthcare providers are faced with an aging population. Although the spectrum of disease is likely to remain constant for practitioners, the makeup of individual practices may reflect this change in demographics. To prepare for this change, we must continue to expand our knowledge base of the disease processes that affect the elderly and our ability to treat this population. Future research will also need to include this group.

REFERENCES

1. Anthonisen NR and others: Airway closure as a function of age, *Respir Physiol* 8:58, 1969/1970.
2. Avon J, Gurwitz J: *Principles of pharmacology.* In Cassel CK, Riesenberg DE, Sorensen LB, editors: *Geriatric medicine,* ed. 2, New York, 1990, Springer-Verlag, pp 66–77.
3. Babin RW, Harker LA: The vestibular system in the elderly, *Otolaryngol Clin North Am* 15:2, 1982.
4. Benjamin BJ: Frequency variability in the aged voice, *J Gerontol* 36:722, 1981.
5. Biever DM, Bless DM: Vibratory characteristics of the vocal folds in young adult and geriatric women, *J Voice* 3:120, 1989.
6. Bliss R and others: Age is no contraindication to thyroid surgery, *Age Aging* 28:363, 1999.
7. Bosisio E and others: Mean transit time forced expiratory volume and age in healthy male smokers and non-smokers, *Respiration* 49:23, 1986.
8. Bradsetter RD, Kazemi H: Aging and the respiratory system, *Med Clin North Am* 67:419, 1983.
9. Brown WS, Morris RJ, Michel JF: Vocal jitter in young adult and aged female voices, *J Voice* 3:113, 1989.
10. Castell DO: *Eating and swallowing disorders.* In Hazzard WR and others, editors: *Principles of Geriatric medicine and gerontology, ed. 2,* New York, 1990, McGraw-Hill, pp 1155–1160.
11. Dawson DA, Adams PF: Current estimates from the health interview survey, United States, 1986, *Vital Health Statistics,* Series 10, no. 164, Hyattsville, Md, National Center for Health Statistics, 1987. U.S. Department of Health and Human Services publication PHS 87.
12. Deems DA, Doty RL: Age-related changes in the phenyl ethylalcohol odor detection threshold, *Trans Pa Acad Ophthalmol Otolaryngol* 39:646, 1987.
13. Doty RL: *Age-related alterations in taste and smell function.* In Goldstein JC, Kashima HK, Koopman CF Jr, editors: *Geriatric otolaryngology,* Toronto, 1989, Decker, pp 97–104.
14. Doty RL, Reyes P, Gregor T: Presence of both odor identification and detection deficits in Alzeheimer's disease, *Brain Res Bull* 18:597, 1982.
15. Doty RL and others: Smell identification ability: changes with age, *Science* 226:1441, 1984.
16. Edelstein DR: Aging of the normal nose in adults, *Laryngoscope* 106:1, 1996.
17. Gacek RR, Schuknecht HF: Pathology of presbycusis, *Int Audiol* 8:199, 1969.
18. Gates GA and others: Central auditory dysfunction, cognitive dysfunction, and dementia in older people, *Arch Otolaryngol Head Neck Surg* 122:161, 1996.
19. Glorig A, Davis H: Age noise and hearing loss, *Ann Oral Rhinol Laryngol* 70:556, 1961.
20. Gracco C, Kahane JC: Age-related changes in the vestibular folds of the human larynx: a histomorphometric study, *J Voice* 3:204, 1989.
21. Granieri E: Nutrition and the older adult, *Dysphagia* 4:196, 1990.
22. Gussan R: Plugging of the vascular channels in the otic capsule, *Ann Otol Rhinol Laryngol* 78:1306, 1969.
23. Havlik RJ: Aging in the eighties: impaired senses for sound and light in persons aged 65 years and over: preliminary data from the Supplement on Aging to the National Health Interview Survey: United States; January-June 1984, *Vital Health Statistics,* Hyattsville, Md, National Center for Health Statistics, 1986, p 125. U.S. Department of Health and Human Services publication PHS 86-1250.
24. Hermel J and others: Taste sensation in aging man, *J Oral Med* 25:39, 1970.
25. Hoeffding V, Feldman ML: Changes with advanced age in the morphology of the rat auditory nerve, *Soc Neurosci Abstr* 1987:13, 1259.
26. Hoekstra HJ: Cancer surgery in the elderly, *Eur J Cancer* 37(Suppl 7):S235, 2001.
27. Hollender AR: Histopathology of the nasal mucosa of older persons, *Arch Otolaryngol Head Neck Surg* 40:92, 1994.
28. Hollien H, Shipp T: Speaking fundamental frequency and chronologic I age in males, *J Speech Hear Res* 15:155, 1972.
29. Honjo I, Isshiki N: Laryngoscopic and voice characteristic of aged persons, *Arch Otolaryngol* 106:149, 1980.
30. Honrubia V: Vestibular function in the elderly, *Ear Nose Throat J* 68:904, 1989.
31. Irvine PW: *Patterns of disease: the challenge of multiple illnesses.* In Cassel CK, Riesenberg DE, Sorensen LB, editors: *Geriatric medicine, ed. 2,* New York, 1990, Springer-Verlag, pp 96–101.

32. Isshiki N and others: Thyroplasty as a new phonosurgical technique, *Acta Otolaryngol* 78:451, 1974.

33. Johns M and others: Goals and mechanisms for training otolaryngologists in the area of geriatric medicine, *Otolaryngol Head Neck Surg* 100:4, 1989.

34. Johnson LG, Hawkins JE: Vascular changes in the human inner ear associated with aging, *Ann Otol* 81:364, 1972.

35. Johnson JT, Rabuzzi DD, Tucker HM: Composite resection in the elderly: a well-tolerated procedure, *Laryngoscope* 87:1509, 1977.

36. Jordanoglou J and others: Effective time of the forced expiratory spirogram in health and airways obstruction, *Thorax* 34:187, 1979.

37. Kahane JC: *A survey of age related changes in the connective tissues in the human adult larynx.* In Bless DM, Abbs JH, editors: *Vocal cord physiology,* San Diego, 1983, College-Hill Press.

38. Katz PR and others: *Geriatrics syllabus for specialists.* New York, The American Geriatrics Society, 2002.

39. Keil CH, Smith MC: Office based ambulatory care for patients 75 years and over: National Ambulatory Medical Care Survey, 1980, *Vital Health Statistics,* no. 110, Hyattsville, Md, National Center for Health Statistics, 1985. U.S. Department of Health and Human Services publication PHS 85.

40. Knudson RJ and others: Changes in the normal maximal expiratory flow-volume curve with growth and aging, *Am Rev Respir Dis* 127:725, 1983.

41. Krmpotic-Nemanic J: Presbycusis presbystatis and presbyosmia as consequences of the analogous biological process, *Acta Otolaryngol (Stockh)* 67:217, 1969.

42. Kushnick SD and others: A scanning electron microscopic study of smoking and age-related changes in human nasal epithelium, *Am J Rhinol* 6:185, 1992.

43. Larson EB and others: Adverse drug reactions associated with global cognitive impairment in elderly persons, *Ann Intern Med* 107:169, 1987.

44. LeJeeune FE, Guice CE, Samuels PM: Early experiences with vocal ligament tightening, *Am Otol Rhinol Laryngol* 92:475, 1983.

45. Levine R, Robbins J, Maser A: Periventricular white changes in oropharyngeal swallowing in normal individuals, *Dysphagia* 7:142, 1992.

46. Levitzky MG: Effects of aging on the respiratory system, *Physiologist* 27:102, 1984.

47. Linvell SE, Fisher HB: Acoustic characteristics of women's voices with advanced age, *J Gerontol* 40:324, 1985.

48. Liss JM, Weisner G, Rosenbek JC: Selected acoustic characteristics of speech production in very old males, *J Gerontology* 45:35, 1990.

49. Liss L, Gomez F: The nature of senile changes of the human olfactory bulb and tract, *Arch Otolaryngol* 67:167, 1958.

50. Logemann J: *Manual for the videofluorographic study of swallowing, ed. 2,* Austin, Pro-Ed, 1993.

51. Makila E: Oral health among the inmates of old people's homes: salivary secretions, *Proc Finn Dent Soc* 73:64, 1977.

52. McGuirt WF, Davis SP: Demographic portrayal and outcome analysis of head and neck cancer surgery in the elderly, *Arch Otolaryngol Head Neck Surg* 121:150, 1995.

53. Mellert TK and others: Characterization of the immune barrier in human olfactory mucosa, *Otolaryngol Head Neck Surg* 106:181, 1992.

54. Morgan RF and others: Head and neck surgery in the aged, *Am J Surg* 144:449, 1982.

55. Mueller PB, Sweeney RJ, Baribeau LJ: Acoustic and morphologic study of the senescent voice, *Ear Nose Throat J* 63:292, 1984.

56. Murty GE, Carding PN, Kelly PJ: Combined glottographic changes in the elderly, *Clin Otolaryngol* 16:532, 1991.

57. Nadol JB, Schuknecht HF: The pathology of peripheral vestibular disorders in the elderly, *Ear Nose Throat J* 68:930, 1989.

58. Naessen R: An enquiry on the morphological characteristics and possible changes with age in the olfactory region of man, *Acta Otolaryngol (Stockh)* 71:49, 1971.

59. Nakashima T, Kimmelman CP, Snow JB Jr: Immunohistopathologic analysis of olfactory degeneration caused by ischemia, *Otolaryngol Read Neck Surg* 93:40, 1985.

60. Nedelman CI, Bernick S: The significance of age changes in human alveolar mucosa and gum, *J Prosthet Dent* 39:495, 1978.

61. Nixon JC, Glorig A: Changes in air and bone conduction thresholds, *J Laryngol* 76:288, 1962.

62. Orma EJ, Koskenoja M: Postural dizziness in the aged, *Geriatrics* 12:49, 1957.

63. Paik SI and others: Human olfactory biopsy: the influence of age and receptor distribution, *Arch Otolaryngol Head Neck Surg* 118:731, 1982.

64. Parker DR and others: The relationship of nonspecific airway responsiveness and atopy to the rate of decline in lung function, *Am Rev Respir Dis* 141:589, 1990.

65. Patterson CN: The aging nose: characteristics and correction, *Otolaryngol Clin North Am* 13:275, 1980.

66. Pressman JJ, Keleman G: Physiology of the larynx, *Physiol Rev* 35:513, 1955.

67. Ramig LA: Effects of physiologic aging on vowel spectral noise, *J Gerontology* 38:223, 1983.

68. Ramig LA, Ringel RL: Effects of physiologic aging on selected acoustic characteristics of voice, *J Speech Hearing* 26:22, 1983.

69. Ramig LA and others: Acoustic analysis of voice in amyotrophic lateral sclerosis: a longitudinal case study, *J Speech Hear Res* 55:2, 1990.

70. Robbins J and others: Oropharyngeal swallowing in normal adults of different ages, *Gastroenterology* 103:823, 1992.

71. Rosen S, Olin K: Hearing loss in coronary heart disease, *Arch Otolaryngol* 82:836, 1965.

72. Sakakura Y and others: Nasal mucociliary clearance under various conditions, *Acta Otolaryngol (Stockh)* 96:167, 1983.

73. Santos AL, Gelperin A: Surgical mortality in the elderly, *J Am Geriatr Soc* 23:42, 1975.

74. Schiffman SS: Taste and smell in disease (first of two parts), *N Engl J Med* 308:1275, 1983.

75. Scott J: Quantitative age changes in the histological structure of human submandibular salivary glands, *Arch Oral Biol* 22:221, 1977.

76. Settipane GA, Chafee FH: Nasal polyps in asthma and rhinitis, a review of 6,037 patients, *J Allergy Clin Immunol* 59:17, 1997.

77. Seymour DG, Pringle R: Post-operative complications in the elderly surgical patient, *Gerontology* 29:262, 1983.

78. Shaker R, Lang I: Effects of aging on the deglutitive oral, pharyngeal, and esophageal motor function, *Dysphagia* 9:221, 1994.

79. Shapiro DP: Geriatric demographics and the practice of otolaryngology, *Ear Nose Throat J* 78:6, 1999.

80. Shipp T and others: Acoustic and temporal correlates of perceived age, *J Voice* 6:211, 1992.

81. Simpson WJ: Thyroid malignancy in the elderly, *Geriatrics* 37:119, 1982.

82. Sinha UK and others: Temporal bone findings in Alzheimer's disease, *Laryngoscope* 106:1, 1996.

83. Smith CG: Age incidence of atrophy of olfactory nerves in man, *J Comp Neurol* 77:589, 1942.
84. Snow JB Jr.: *Clinical disorders of olfaction and gustation in the aged.* In Goldstein JC and others, editors: *Geriatric otolaryngology,* Toronto, 1989, Decker, pp 92–96.
85. Sonies BC and others: Durational aspects of the oral phase of swallow in normal aging adults, *Dysphagia* 3:1, 1988.
86. Sorbinni CA and others: Arterial oxygen tension in relation to age in healthy subjects, *Respiration* 25:3, 1986.
87. Strehler BL: *Aging in cellular level.* In Rossman I, editor: *Clinical geriatrics,* Philadelphia, 1971, Lippincott.
88. Sunberg J: *The science of the singing voice,* De Kalb, Illinois, Northern Illinois University Press, 1987.
89. Tanaka S, Hirano M, Chijiwa K: Some aspects of vocal fold bowing, *Ann Otolaryngol Rhinol Laryngol* 103(5 pt 1):357, 1994.
90. Tracy JF and others: Preliminary observations on the effects of age on oropharyngeal deglutition, *Dysphagia* 4:90, 1989.
91. Trupe EH, Siebens H, Siebens A: Prevalence of feeding and swallowing disorders in a nursing home, *Arch Phys Med Rehabil* 65:651, 1984.
92. Tucker HM: Laryngeal framework surgery in the management of the aged larynx, *J Otol Rhinol Laryngol* 97:534, 1988.
93. Van der Veken PJ and others: Age related CT-scan study of the incidence of sinusitis in children, *Am J Rhinol* 6:45, 1992.
94. Wolf GT: *Aging, the immune system and head and neck cancer.* In Goldstein JC, Kashima HK, Koopmann CF, editors: *Geriatric otolaryngology,* Burlington, Vermont, 1989, BC Decker.
95. Woo P and others: Dysphonia in the aging: physiology versus disease, *Laryngoscope* 102:139, 1992.

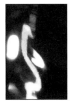

CHAPTER TWELVE

GENETICS AND OTOLARYNGOLOGY

‖ William J. Kimberling

INTRODUCTION

Genetics plays a role in just about everything, although the magnitude of that role may be, in a few cases, barely detectable. It is important—and quickly becoming even more so—for the otolaryngologist to understand genetics to carry out his or her medical obligations effectively. There are hundreds of syndromes that affect the head and neck,[25] and people with most of these syndromes come under the care of an ear, nose, and throat (ENT) surgeon at one time or another during their lives. Furthermore, hearing is an important aspect of the otolaryngologist's practice, and more than 50 different genes have been identified that cause nonsyndromic hearing loss (see the Hereditary hearing loss home page at *http://dnalab-www.uia.ac.be/dnalab/hhh/*). The identification of the basic dysfunction underlying all of these single-gene disorders is the first step to effective prevention and treatment, whether surgical or pharmacologic. An understanding of complex (presumably polygenic) disorders has become an extremely important objective for medical research. Liability for a variety of diseases (e.g., head and neck cancer, otosclerosis, otitis media, dyslexia) is controlled by several genes.[2,18,28,46] It is felt that the day is near when knowledge about an individual's genotype will identify those who are at high risk for developing these and other disorders.[8]

The genome revolution has placed mankind at the brink of the development of new and exciting therapies for both rare and common genetic disorders. It has thus become increasingly important for the ENT practitioner to recognize those disorders that have a strong genetic component and to be aware of the new and developing approaches to their treatment.

THE GENOME

The term *genome* refers to the collection of all of the genes that an organism possesses. It has been estimated that there are between 40,000 and 140,000 genes in the human genome. The genes are assembled into lengthy strands of deoxyribonucleic acid (DNA), which are organized linearly into chromosomes. The chromosomes are made up of the DNA that forms the genes and the intervening DNA as well as chromatin, which is a protein that assists in the maintenance of the structure and regulation of chromosomal expression. The nuclei of most human cells contain 46 chromosomes that are organized as 23 pairs. Except for the mitochondria, all genes that are contained within the human genome lie on one or the other of these chromosomes. The linear order of the genes on the chromosomes allows one to create maps of the human gene order; these maps are generally invariant throughout any given species. It is these maps that allow us to associate specific genes with specific traits through *gene mapping*.[48,64] Genes are transmitted in groups that correspond with the chromosomes. Aside from cases of the exception known as "crossing over," all of the genes of one chromosome (e.g., the paternal one) are transmitted together to the exclusion of the other one. *Crossing over* allows one chromosome to become a mosaic of both paternal and maternal genes; the frequency with which crossing over occurs has been studied and forms the basis for one of the two ways of measuring distances between genes. The physical distance between two genes is the number of bases between genes and is measured in megabases or kilobases. The genetic distance between two genes, however, is based on the frequency of observed recombination between them and can only be estimated by the study of informative matings and offspring. Genetic distance is the result of a biologic phenomenon and is imperfectly correlated with physical distance. The order of genes on a chromosome is constant.

The amount of information stored in the genome is tremendous. In the human genome there are approximately 3×10^9 base pairs of DNA that make up the haploid genome. The largest chromosome, 1, contains about 10% of the total, whereas the smallest autosome, 21, contains about 2.5%. Given that the estimated number of genes is between 40,000 and 140,000, the expected number of genes per megabase is between 12 and 46. The average high resolution band is about three megabases in size and would be expected to contain between 36 and 138 genes.

Another way of appreciating the size of the genome is to compare the amount of information in it with that in the typical encyclopedia. The encyclopedia would need to have 200 volumes of 1000 pages each to contain the information found in the human genome. In this analogy, gene size would vary from about a third of a page up to several pages. In actuality, the human genetic encyclopedia is packaged into 23 volumes, and the genes are not as easily demarcated as are chapters in a real encyclopedia. However, the analogy serves us well when we are trying to understand the importance of deciphering the genome. This biologic encyclopedia is in truth a manual for the construction and maintenance of a human being. By understanding the information contained within the genes, we will come to understand the basics of our own biology.

Unfortunately, the information in the genome is simply not organized into rational groupings. Part of the purpose of the genome project has been to develop an index of the genome that will allow researchers who are trying to connect specific genes with specific disorders to do so efficiently.[13,14] From the perspective of the otolaryngologist, this means first that better diagnoses will become available and ultimately that better therapies will emerge as more is learned about the basic nature of hereditary disorders that affect hearing, speech, and the structures of the head and neck.

The genome revolution has placed mankind at the brink of the development of new and exciting therapies for both rare and common genetic disorders.[15] It will thus become increasingly important for the ENT practitioner to recognize those disorders that have a strong genetic component.

DNA STRUCTURE AND THE GENETIC CODE

Humans store genetic information in DNA, which is a linear polymer made up of four different nucleotides: adenine (A), guanine (G), thymidine (T), and cytosine (C). Nucleotides (also called bases) are linked together by phosphodiester bonds into a single strand. Nucleotides also have the capability of pairing with each other (A with T and G with C) through hydrogen bonds. Two strands of DNA can pair with each other in a complementary fashion (again, A with T and G with C) to form a double helix. The two strands are perfectly complementary; for example, if one strand has an order of ATGGGCCATA, its complement would

be TACCCGGTAT. During replication, the two strands separate, and the base sequence of each strand would dictate the construction of a new, complementary strand. In this way, the sequence of the double strands is preserved in the two new identical double strands that are produced.

A single strand has an orientation that reflects the direction of the phosphodiester bond, which is usually referred to as going from the 5' to the 3' end; genes are transcribed in this direction. Because there is a double helix, the actual transcription occurs from only one strand, called the *template strand.* The antiparallel strand is referred to as the *coding strand,* because its base sequence corresponds with the sequence of the message; however, uracil is substituted for thymidine.

The sequence of bases is what determines all parts of the gene, and it specifically determines the sequence of amino acids in the protein that results for the process of translation. The nucleotides within the coding region are arranged in groups of three, called *codons,* which determine the precise amino acid sequence. Because there are four bases, there are 64 possible combinations of nucleotides, but only 20 amino acids. The code is said to be degenerate, because most amino acids are specified by more than one codon. For example, the code for valine can be GTT, GTC, GTA, or GTG. The third nucleotide can vary for most amino acids and is often call the *wobble nucleotide.* A specific codon, ATG, codes for methionine and also indicates the beginning of a coding sequence. There are three stop codons: TAA, TAG, and TGA. An example of a sequence obtained for three individuals in provided in Figure 12-1.

GENE STRUCTURE AND EXPRESSION

The definition of a gene has gone through several stages and is now neither simple nor straightforward. The gene is the basic unit of biologic information that can be transmitted from parents to offspring, and it typically provides information about structural or functional components of the cell. The information transfer occurs not only between parent and daughter cells but between the nucleus and cytoplasmic machinery. It is the transfer of this information that we call *inheritance* when it occurs between parent and child and *expression* when between the nucleus and the cell proper. Gene structure has presumably evolved in a way that facilitates the transfer of genetic information, but the true molecular boundaries that define any specific gene are often poorly recognized.

The basic eukaryotic gene is made up of exons and introns. Exons make up the coding part of the gene; the intron is DNA that is interspersed between the exons. During the process of creating a message,

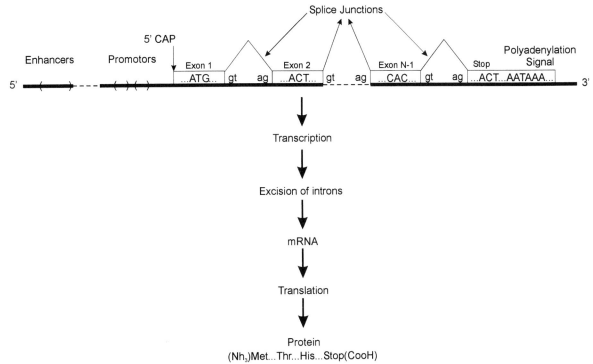

Figure 12-1. Gene structure and transcription. The ultimate primary function of most genes is to produce a protein in a cell at a time at which it is needed. Genes have structures that are adapted to this function. Not only does a gene have syntax that establishes the amino acid sequence of the protein, but it also has punctuation that controls its expression. The exons make up the coding or information content of the gene; these are interspersed with introns, which are DNA sequences with a function that is only poorly understood. There is poorer evolutionary conservation of introns, which suggests that that the code they represent is more tolerant of change. Although the primary regulatory regions occur as 5′ enhancers and promotors, regulation can occur at any place along the genes, in the introns, in the 3′ tail end of the gene, or even on the other chromosome, which demonstrates the so-called "trans elements." The first step of expression is transcription. The gene is transcribed from the 5′ cap to the end of the polyadenylation signal. This transcript contains both introns and exons, and so the next step is for the introns to be excised. Recognizable splice-site junctions are needed for this to occur normally, and so are other sites that assist in the recognition of the appropriate splice sites. The final mRNA product contains the code that is necessary for the final step of translation, after which a protein is made.

introns are spliced out of the message, thus leaving only the exons to be translated into protein. The gene is thus an interrupted sequence of code that must be further processed into a useable message. Figure 12-1 illustrates how the structure of the gene is related to the process of transcription. During transcription, the whole gene is copied—exons and introns together—into a pre-message. The pre-message is then processed by excising the introns and joining the exons together to make a series of bases that code for a protein. The sites at which the excisions and rejoining take place are called *splice sites,* and specific sequences of bases are used to signal the cellular machinery to recognize these places. There are specific start and end points

for the transcription of the gene as well; within the genes, there are specific signals in the form of three-base sequences (the start and stop codons) that indicate where translation into protein is to begin and end. The gene is thus made up of a coding sequence and punctuation.

In addition to the basic structure of a gene, there are elements that are both 5′ and 3′ of the gene that regulate its expression. These are called *cis-acting elements,* because they are on the same strand of DNA as the gene they regulate. Some of the regulatory elements may be inside of one or more introns. In fact, the first few introns of a gene frequently contain such regulatory elements. Although some of the

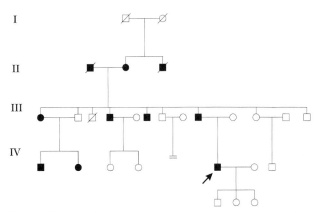

Figure 12-2. Pedigree typical of a dominantly inherited trait; in this case, autosomal dominant congenital deafness. The arrow points to the proband of the family (a proband is the person though whom the family came to your attention). Note that the pattern of transmission in the family covers multiple generations and that both sexes are affected equally. A slash though a circle or square indicates that the person is deceased.

cis-acting elements are close to the actual start of the gene, others may be as much as 50 kilobases in front of (upstream) or in back of (downstream) the genes. Regulatory elements act predominantly by controlling the rate of transcription, and they respond to signals in the nucleoplasm to control the cellular specificity of gene action.

A basic understanding of gene structure is critical to an understanding of how mutations can disrupt gene function. Mutations can change the code, the punctuation, or the elements that regulate the expression of the gene; their detection and analysis are discussed in more detail below.

THE MOLECULAR BASIS OF PATTERNS OF INHERITANCE

There are three broad categories of genetic disease: chromosomal, monogenic, and complex. Chromosomal disorders are those in which relatively large segments of one or more chromosomes occur in only one copy or in more than the expected two copies. Examples would be Down's syndrome (trisomy 21) and Turner syndrome (missing an X or a Y, depending on your perspective). The term *single-gene disorder* refers to the large group of disorders that are due to mutations in only one gene. Many hearing loss disorders are known to be to the result of mutations in specific genes; almost all single-gene disorders show a specific pattern of inheritance (e.g., dominant, recessive, X-linked). Complex traits are those in which the genetics are not clear. The commonly accepted idea is that complex disorders—like cleft lip or palate, a reading

disability, cancer, and hypertension, to name a few—are the result of the interaction between several genes, the environment, and random factors. The otolaryngologist will encounter each category. Chromosomal disorders are generally quite severe but will frequently present with hearing and head and neck problems. Single-gene disorders are also severe, but many are not associated with multiple anomalies and/or mental retardation. The bulk of an ENT physician's practice will involve individuals with complex disorders, because these are typically more frequent.

Chromosomal Disorders

With some exceptions, chromosomal disorders are generally not heritable. Physical abnormalities associated with chromosomal imbalance are the result of rather extensive duplications or deletions of genetic material involving multiple genes. The most common chromosomal disorder that involves the autosomes is trisomy 21.[1] Chromosomal disorders can be classified into one of four groups:

1) Aneuploidy: the excess or loss of an intact chromosome.
2) Deletion: the breakage or loss of a piece of a chromosome.
3) Duplication: the insertion of an extra partial copy of a chromosome onto an existing chromosome. This sometimes involves a different chromosome, and it is often a tandem duplication that yields a second copy of the same set of genes just adjacent to the duplicated segment.
4) Rearrangement: two breaks of a chromosome or chromosomes and the subsequent refusion of the ends of the chromosome into a different order. When this involves two different chromosomes, it is called a *translocation*; when the same chromosome is involved and the order is reversed, it is called an *inversion*.

A chromosomal abnormality can occur in all or just some of the cells; the latter instance is called *mosaicism.* For example, most malignant cell lines show extensive chromosomal mosaicism, with multiple cell lines present in the tumor. Many females with only one X chromosome (designated as 45,X) are mosaic with a minor cell line that has a normal female constitution, 46,XX. The degree of mosaicism and the distribution in different tissues is believed to determine the severity of some cytogenetic disorders.

Aneuploidies

A *trisomy* is demonstrated when three copies of a whole chromosome occur in an offspring. This happens because of nondisjunction, which is the movement of a pair of chromosomes to one pole during cell division; this results in one daughter cell lacking that chromosome and the other daughter cell possessing an extra copy of that chromosome.[45] The three major autosomal trisomies are 21, 18, and 13.

Trisomies 13 and 18 are not compatible with long life, and the average life span individuals with either of these conditions is less than 1 year. The majority of infants with trisomy 13 are profoundly deaf and have a cleft lip and palate in addition to multiple other congenital anomalies.[16,36] Hearing loss is frequent in trisomy 18 as well.[21] However, hearing and head and neck anomalies are unlikely to be a serious concern because of the limited survival.

Patients with trisomy 21 have ears that are smaller than normal. About 75% have hearing loss, which can be sensory-neural, conductive, or mixed.[74] The prognosis of a child with trisomy 21 is generally good, and correction to normal hearing is important for helping such a child achieve maximal abilities.[11]

The common aneuploidies that involve the sex chromosomes include 45,X (Turner's syndrome, phenotypic female) and 47,XXY (Klinefelter's syndrome, phenotypic male). Although profound hearing loss is infrequent, mild to moderate hearing loss is common in 45,X individuals.[27,29,50] Females with Turner's syndrome are highly susceptible to otitis media, but whether this changes with hormone replacement therapy remains to be investigated.[3,29,59] About 25% of children with Klinefelter's syndrome have a mild sensory-neural hearing loss.[5,26] Hearing losses in both Turner's and Klinefelter's syndromes too often remain undetected.

Chromosomal Rearrangements

Usually aneuploidies are not heritable; however, rearrangements, translocation, and inversions can be. There is a heritable form of trisomy 21 that involves a translocation between chromosome 21 and another chromosome, usually chromosome 14. This is a so-called "centric fusion" translocation that results in the loss of both short arms and the fusion of the two long arms of chromosomes 21 and 14. A balanced chromosome complement would be 45 chromosomes. Because of the abnormal way in which the chromosomes need to be paired, this translocation sets the stage for an abnormal separation of chromosomes during meiosis. The result can be a balanced carrier, like the parent (a normal), or a carrier who has three copies of chromosome 21 material. Both translocations and inversions can be heritable and could result in a family that has multiple instances of children with multiple anomalies. The heritable forms can be distinguished by a straightforward cytogenetic evaluation.

Single-Gene Disorders

The terms *dominant* and *recessive* usually refer to the pattern of inheritance of a particular disorder, but, more importantly, they communicate the way in which combinations of two alleles produce a specific (usually abnormal) phenotype. With a dominant inheritance pattern, individuals who carry one copy of the mutant allele (heterozygote) or two copies of the mutant allele (homozygote) are equally affected. With recessive inheritance, a person must be homozygous for the mutant alleles; individuals who are heterozygous are normal. When using these terms to describe a disease, if we call a disease dominant, then normal is recessive, and vice versa. True dominance and recessivity are probably uncommon. Branchiootorenal syndrome is described as dominant,[19] but it is uncommon, and a true mutant homozygous individual has probably never been born. Most geneticists would expect that patients with the homozygous mutant form would have a more severe phenotype, one that is possibly even lethal. Similarly, one might expect that patients with many of the recessive nonsyndromic deafness disorders could have a mild manifestation in the heterozygote possibly contributing to the liability of the development of age-related hearing loss. An example of true dominance occurs with Huntington's disease, in which a homozygous patient that is affected has the same phenotype as heterozygous individuals.[43,78]

Dominant Disorders

Figure 12-2 shows a typical family pedigree of an autosomal dominant disorder. Under full penetrance, each affected individual will have an affected parent. Because they are heterozygous, each affected individual has a 50% chance of transmitting the abnormal gene to offspring, each of whom would be similarly affected. The only reasonable instance in which a person could be homozygous and affected would be if both parents were affected. Dominant mutations are recognized through their pattern of inheritance, which typically shows vertical transmission and the involvement of several generations and several sibships.

Affected patients are typically equally distributed between the sexes. However, a few sex-limited and sex-modified dominant disorders do exist.[47]

Dominance occurs with X-linked genes as well. The biochemical basis of the action of dominance is the same, but the pattern of inheritance is distinctly different. Twice as many females as males are expected to be affected. X-linked dominant pedigrees can mimic the characteristics of an autosomal dominant one, but they would not be expected to show male-to-male transmission. When the distinction between autosomal and X-linked dominant is in question, the

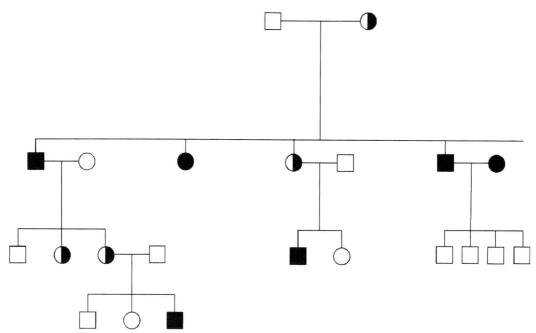

Figure 12-3. X-linked recessive disorders show a very characteristic pattern of inheritance. Females are carriers, and they are usually asymptomatic. They are indicated here by the half-colored circle; the diagnosis of carrier status was done here by inference from the parents having an affected son; however, for many disorders, carrier tests are available.

observation of male-to-male transmission establishes an autosomal position of the gene.

There are three major mechanisms by which dominant genes generally influence phenotype: haploinsufficiency, the dominant-negative effect, and the two-hit effect.[71,80] *Haploinsufficiency* refers to the situation in which the inactivation of one gene reduces the gene product to a point where it is insufficient to maintain some cellular function at its normal level. Genes that contain proteins that regulate metabolic activity or transport are likely candidates for this mechanism. A *dominant-negative effect* occurs when the gene product actively interferes with normal cellular processes; the gene is producing a protein that either has acquired a new function or that competes with the action of the normal protein. The *two-hit effect* refers to the situation (e.g., retinoblastoma) in which one allele is inactive, and the disease results from its homologue being inactivated by mutation. At the organism level, the inheritance appears to be dominant, but the mechanism of action at the cellular level is recessive. This is an important mechanism for the development of tumors in dominantly inherited cancer syndromes, and it is probably the mechanism of the carotid body tumor. The mechanism by which a dominant gene causes pathology is an important consideration in the search for treatments. For those disorders that are caused by insufficient gene

products, the addition of a gene (or accompanying products) may be considered a reasonable approach to treatment and is likely to be easier to achieve. A dominant-negative effect, however, requires that the action of the gene and/or its product be stopped; this is a far more difficult task conceptually than is that of product replacement.

Examples of dominantly inherited disorders that are important in otolaryngology include all of the dominantly inherited nonsyndromic hearing losses, Waardenburg syndrome,[54,80] branchiootorenal syndrome,[41,63] Treacher-Collins syndrome,[40,52] and many others.[25]

Recessive Disorders

Autosomal recessive disorders result only when a person has two abnormal copies of the same gene. Because the affected person must be homozygous, both unaffected parents are heterozygous and thus carriers. In many families, the heritability of a recessive trait is not obvious. Given today's small family sizes, most individuals with recessive disorders present to the clinician as singleton cases lacking any family history of the same disorder. More than 50% of all cases of Usher's syndrome in the United Sates represent the only affected individuals in their respective families; most of the rest have a few affected siblings. When normal parents have a child with a recessive disorder, the chance of it occurring in any other children they may have is 25%. Although many of the unaffected relatives may also be normal heterozygotes (e.g., aunts and uncles have a 50% chance of being a carrier; first cousins have a 25% chance), one only infrequently observes recurrence outside of the initial sibship involved. One important clue to recessive inheritance is the presence of consanguinity. Important disorders that are inherited via autosomal recessive routes include nonsyndromic deafness,[6] Pendred's syndrome,[55,79] Usher's syndrome,[35,51] Alstrom's syndrome,[58] and many others.[25]

It is the nature of recessive disorders that the abnormal gene is in a much higher frequency than would be appreciated on the basis of the relative rarity of the disorder. For example, Usher's syndrome type Ib, which is due to a defect of *MYO7A*,[76] is present in about one out of 25,000 births; heterozygote frequency is estimated at about one of every 80 persons. For every affected person, there are more than 300 heterozygotes; if there are 10,000 patients with type Ib Usher's syndrome in the United States, there should be 3,000,000 carriers. For all rare recessive conditions, most of the gene pool resides with the asymptomatic carriers. In some disorders, the carrier rate is quite high; connexin 26 deafness (caused by a

defect of *DFNB1*) is the most common form of deafness in the United States,[23] and carrier rates may be as high as one in every 25 persons. Some recessive disorders appear to have a high frequency in certain populations. For example, cystic fibrosis is common among people of European extraction,[7] Tay-Sachs among Ashkenazi Jews,[39] and sickle cell anemia (hemoglobin beta S disease) in individuals of African ancestry.[4,56]

Sometimes the increase in frequency of certain conditions in certain populations is a result of what is referred to as the *founder effect,* which is usually believed to be caused by certain patterns of selection, such as those that are seen when the heterozygote has a selective advantage over both homozygotes (e.g., sickle cell anemia). A good example of the founder effect is the very high frequency of Usher's syndrome type IC (due to a defect in the harmonin gene) among the French Acadians of Louisiana.[9] This gene is presumed to have been present in a few individuals who represented a significant part of the small number of immigrants to that region. The French Acadians stayed genetically isolated, and their numbers increased. Because of the chance occurrence of the gene in the founder population, the high frequency was maintained to this day. Selection was important

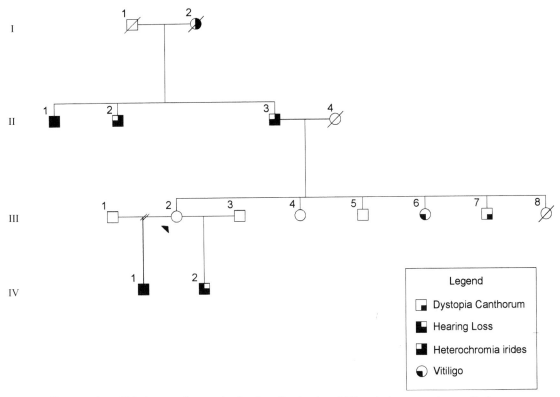

Figure 12-4. This is a pedigree of a family with dominant Waardenburg syndrome. It shows variable expression and non-penetrance. Such variability is usual for many dominant hearing related disorders.

when establishing the high frequency of the hemoglobin beta s allele in Africans. One of the most interesting genetic puzzles now surrounds the reason for the high frequency of connexin 26 deafness alleles. If this is due to a founder effect, then why is there a high frequency of different mutations in Jews, Europeans, and Asians? The high frequency across ethnic lines suggests that the heterozygotes may have (or may have had) a selective advantage over the homozygous normal.

X-linked genes may also harbor recessive mutations. The molecular mechanisms are the same, but the pattern of inheritance is unique and remarkable. Females, who have two X chromosomes, are heterozygotes/carriers. Males, with only one X, are affected; they have only one copy of the abnormal gene, because the Y chromosome carries little in the way of genetic information. The pattern of inheritance is shown in Figure 12-3. Carrier females have a 50% chance of transmitting the abnormal gene, which means that half of a carrier female's sons will be affected and that half of her daughters will be carriers as well. An affected male cannot transmit the gene to his sons, because he would need to transmit a Y to have a son; however, all of his daughters would be carriers, which would mean that 25% of his grandsons could be affected. The two best known X-linked traits are hemophilia[10] and Duchenne's muscular dystrophy.[66] X linkage plays only a minor role in nonsyndromic hearing loss. To otolaryngologists, perhaps the most notable disorders are X-linked deafness with perilymphatic gusher,[13,31] Alport's syndrome,[33,68] and Mohr-Tranebjaerg's syndrome.[72]

Biochemical defects underlying recessive disorders were among the first for human geneticists to understand. Early work in human genetics focused on metabolic defects. Many recessive disorders were found to be due to enzyme deficiencies that interrupted a specific metabolic pathway. Heterozygotes had sufficient enzymes for a typically dosage-tolerant pathway to operate and maintain a normal phenotype. Pathology results either because some product is lacking or because the interruption of the pathway diverts the metabolism to the excessive production of a toxic substance. Some metabolic disorders are treatable by either supplying the missing product(s) or enzyme or by removing or reducing toxins. Refsum's disease is a metabolic disorder that involves the inability to metabolize phytanic acid, thereby causing a lysosomal storage disorder.[77] The symptoms of Refsum's syndrome can be minimized by consuming a diet that is low in phytanic acid. From the perspective of potential gene therapy, recessive disorders seem ideal, because replacement of the gene—if active—should replace the missing protein. Most recessive disorders are the result of almost total ablation of the gene function, and a reasonably normal phenotype would be expected with only minor restoration of gene function and protein levels.

Penetrance and Expressivity

Penetrance is a frequently misused word; it should refer to a simple "yes" or "no" with regard to the presence of *any* aspect of the phenotype. A genetic disorder is said to show reduced penetrance if some cases fail to show the phenotype (i.e., if the geneticist is

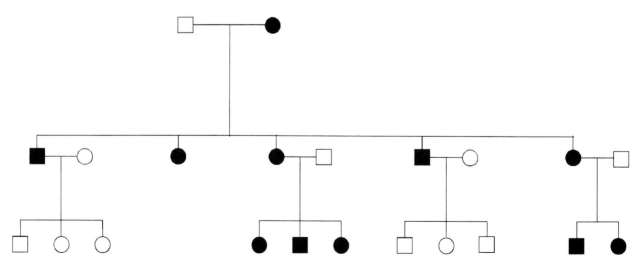

Figure 12-5. Mitochondrial disorders show several generations involved. Transmission is from a mother to all of her children. Males do not transmit the disease to their children. There can be variable expression, which is sometimes due to variable proportions of the mutant-and wild-type Mitochondria.

unable to make a clinical diagnosis). For example, Figure 12-6 shows a pedigree of a family with Waardenburg's syndrome type I (MIM #193500). Waardenburg's syndrome is an autosomal dominant disorder that is characterized by variable hearing loss, pigmentary anomalies (i.e., white forelock, heterochromia irides, vitiligo) and a characteristic broad face with widely spaced inner canthi.[44] Mutations of the *PAX3* gene on chromosome 2 are responsible for the majority of cases of this type of Waardenburg's syndrome.[1,70] There is considerable variability in the extent to which the different symptoms appear in different family members. Individual 3-7 described in Figure 12-6 has dystopia canthorum but no pigmentary anomaly or hearing loss. Still, the gene would be considered to be penetrant, because the diagnosis can be made as a result of the presence of dystopia. On the other hand, individual 3-2 shows none of the characteristics of the mutant *PAX3* gene, and her genotype can only be inferred by the presence of her two affected children.

The term *expressivity* is used to describe the continuum of the severity of the phenotype. *Zero expression* is equivalent to nonpenetrance. The expressivity of dominant genes is often quite variable, whereas that of recessive disorder is more consistent, especially within families. *Variable expression* implies that there is some mechanism by which the severity of the disorder can be modified; these mechanisms may include background genes and/or environmental effects. The investigation of the causes of variable expression may lead to new approaches to therapy.

Pleiotropism is a term used to describe a gene that affects multiple organ systems in an apparently unconnected manner. For example, branchiootorenal syndrome can influence renal development as well as hearing.

Oligogenic Disorders

Some disorders are believed to be caused by the interactions among a few genes. Deafness as a result of connexins 26 and 30 is one possible example. The two genes, *GJB2* and *GJB6*, are adjacent each other on chromosome 13, and deafness has been observed in children with mutations in each of the two genes, each on separate homologues.[15,37,49] This is a digenic effect, and it has also been proposed to occur in certain cases of retinitis pigmentosa.[32,57] In the case of deafness, it is not yet clear whether the effect is truly digenic or whether the deletion in *GJB6* interferes with the control of expression of *GJB2*. It would be expected that many human disorders may have their severity and/or their pleiotropic effects modified by other major genes.

X Linkage

Pedigrees of dominant and recessive X-linked disorders are discussed above and are presented in Figures 12-3 and 12-5. X-linked dominant and recessive traits show more variable expression in females than in males. One reason for this has to do with inactivation of one X chromosome in females, a phenomenon that is also referred to as *Lyon's hypothesis*. One X from each chromosome is randomly selected to be inactivated early during development, and all of the daughter cells will have the same X inactivated; this occurs in all cells except germinal line cells. When a female is heterozygous for an X-linked gene, the fraction of cells that have the normal gene inactivated would be expected to vary but to be around 50%. If, by chance, a significant proportion of normal genes are inactivated, a mild phenotype may result; this has been observed in patients with hemophilia and muscular dystrophy. The impact of X inactivation on the few X-linked hearing loss disorders has not been extensively studied. Occasionally, a fully affected female will be observed; many such patients have one or another form of Turner's syndrome, others may have nonrandom X inactivation, and few may be true homozygotes.

Sporadic Cases

When only one case of a particular disorder occurs in a family, its heritability is not evident; this is an especially frequent event with childhood deafness. The

USH2A Exon 4 653 T>A mutation

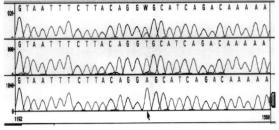

Figure 12-6. Sequencing is currently the best way of determining the genetic constitution of a gene or of part of a gene. This figure shows sequencing that was done to identify the mutation found in a patient with Usher's syndrome type IIa. Each row corresponds to a separate person. The arrow indicates the precise base position at which the mutation was found. The peaks and their colors correspond with each of the four bases in DNA. The control/normal sequence is shown in the middle frame. At position 653 in exon 4, there has been a change in the T (thymine) to an A (adenine). The affected patient in the bottom frame shows only an A at that position, which indicates that he is most likely homozygous for the mutation. His parent is shown in the first frame, and it is evident at that position that both the adenine and thymine bases are being detected by the sequencing reaction; this is typical of a heterozygote. To view this image in color, please go to *www.ototext.com* or the Electronic Image Collection CD, bound into your copy of Cummings Otolaryngology—Head and Neck Surgery, 4th edition.

etiology of the sporadic case can be dominant as a result of a new mutation that has not yet had an opportunity to be transmitted and show the typical inheritance pattern. A sporadic case could also be recessive, because most recessive disorders present as sporadic cases. X linkage, if the patient is male, is also a possibility, and so are more complex patterns of inheritance. In the case of childhood hearing loss, obviously there are many nongenetic factors that may be responsible as well. The pattern of inheritance can help with the diagnosis of many ENT-related disorders, but close examination of the clinical phenotype is critical, especially for sporadic cases.

Mitochondrial Disorders

The mitochondria represent the only nonchromosomal DNA that is inherited. Each cell has several hundred copies of usually identical mitochondria. Mitochondria are inherited solely through the maternal line, with the father giving few if any mitochondria to his offspring. This makes for a curious pattern of inheritance; all of the children of an affected mother are affected, but there is never transmission through the father (see Figure 12-6). Susceptibility to aminoglycoside-induced hearing loss is the result of a mutation *(A1555G)* in the *12S* rRNA gene of the mitochondrion.[30,73,75] There are other, more severe disorders that result from mitochondria mutations. One is the Kearns-Sayre's syndrome, in which the hearing loss is extremely variable[67]; this is presumably because not all of the mitochondria carry the causative mutations. A mixed population is called *heteroplasmy;* this is a frequent occurrence in those disorders that may well be lethal if all the mitochondria carried the mutant gene (homoplasmy).

Complex Traits

Common disorders are believed to involve some mix of genetic and environmental causes. The genetics that underlie such traits have been labeled *multifactorial* or *polygenic.* Data indicate that several genes interact to produce a liability for a particular abnormal phenotype; each gene is presumed to have a small effect. Actually, the number of genes involved remains unknown, and it is possible that some complex disorders could be due to a few major genes that have very reduced penetrances. The idea of using linkage and gene mapping to identify liable genes has become appealing during the last decade, primarily because of the great interest in such common disorders and because molecular- and gene-mapping tools have only recently become available. Some types of neurosensory hearing loss are thought to be inherited in a complex manner. Naturally, age-related hearing loss (presbycusis) is a likely possibility.[17,60] Liability for

otitis media has also been hypothesized to be under some genetic control.[24] In the previous section, it was mentioned that liability for aminoglycoside-induced hearing loss is associated with a change in a mitochondrial gene. It would be reasonable to expect that other liabilities for infection (e.g., rubella) may be under genetic control.[61] The discovery of liability genes promises to have a great payoff in terms of the diagnosis of high-risk groups, as well as new possibilities for treatments that might mimic whatever mechanisms the genes use to confer resistance.

Genetic Heterogeneity

Genetic heterogeneity refers to the existence of cases with similar phenotypes but with differing causes. Childhood deafness, Usher's syndrome, and retinitis pigmentosa are good examples of this phenomenon. With Usher's syndrome, there are at least seven different genes that all cause the severe form of Usher's syndrome.[34] The phenotypes appear to be indistinguishable, and a differential diagnosis can be made only with molecular testing. However, if a man with Usher's syndrome type Ib produces offspring with a woman with Usher's syndrome type Id, all of the children would be expected to be have hearing and normal vision, but they would be carriers of both Usher's syndrome types Ib and Id.

TESTING HUMAN DNA

DNA and ribonucleic acid (RNA) have two useful properties. One is that of easy replication; DNA likes to make copies of itself. The second is their ability to hybridize; they are sticky. If you start with a double strand of DNA and heat it sufficiently, the two strands will dissociate (melt) into a mixture of single-stranded nucleic acid chains. If you then cool this mixture, complementary strands will reassociate (hybridize). The replication property is what makes the polymerase chain reaction (PCR) work, and the hybridization property has allowed a variety of DNA and RNA detection systems to be developed.

Polymerase Chain Reaction

PCR is a method of amplifying targeted sequences of DNA.[42] Oligonucleotide primers are constructed that are complementary to the 5' and 3' ends of the DNA fragment to be amplified. The size of the fragment is typically only a few hundred bases, but techniques like long PCR may involve several thousand bases. A specific thermostabile DNA polymerase is used. The DNA is heated until it melts, and the temperature is then slowly lowered; at the time at which the primers anneal to the test DNA, the PCR is run and the fragment is duplicated. The heating-cooling cycle is then repeated 20 to 30 times; each time, the DNA fragment between the two primers is duplicated, and we eventually end up with several thousand fragments that each have the same length and DNA sequence. PCR is easy to carry out and can be used on minimal samples of DNA; these large quantities of manufactured DNA can then be subjected to a variety of experimental investigations. For example, the DNA can be electrophoresed, stained with ethidium bromide or silver stain, and visualized on a simple agarose or acrylamide gel. The size of the fragment and—more importantly—slight changes in its size can be easily noted. The DNA can be directly used in a sequencing reaction to verify that the sequence of the fragment is as expected. Almost all modern molecular diagnostics start with PCR.

Nucleic Acid Hybridization and Southern Blotting

The early 1980s analysis of genes involved a blotting procedure developed by E. M. Southern that involved hybridizing DNA in a solution (the probe), with the DNA on a stable membrane support, usually filter paper.[65] The probe is labeled with radiolabeled bases (fluorescent tags can be used as well), and the migration of the target DNA can be visualized by autoradiography. Southern hybridization of genomic DNA has limited use in today's molecular genetics laboratories; however, it is still useful for detecting and analyzing large fragments of DNA.

DNA Chips

DNA chips are referred to in two contexts: one when they are used for the analysis of patterns of gene expression,[38] and the other when they are used for the detection of single-base variation in individuals.[14,53] There are several different chip systems, but the basis of the functionality of the chip lies in the ability of antiparallel nucleic acid strands to hybridize.

Oligonucleotides that are typically 8 to 20 bases long and that are each of known sequence are arrayed onto a surface by a photolithographic method. These oligonucleotides can be linked, for example, to a fluorescent detection system. When bathed in a sample, RNA or DNA with homology to the oligonucleotides on the chip can be detected. One use of chips is to analyze changes in the pattern of expression of cells as they change; for example, they have been used to determine which genes are up- and down-regulated during the process of repair after cochlear cells have be damaged by high levels of noise.[69] Chips can help determine which (if any) genes change their pattern of expression in response to different disease processes.

Chips can also be used to detect single-base differences. Many single-base changes are polymorphic (i.e., they have a frequency of heterozygosity of more than 2%); these are called single-nucleotide polymorphisms. There are thousands of these polymorphisms, and they can be employed effectively for the mapping of complex disorders. Not all single-base changes are clinically neutral; some inactivate or change the gene in which they occur. Chips are an inexpensive and rapid way of detecting single-gene pathologic mutations, and they are likely to become the principle means of diagnosis of many genetic disorders. Unfortunately, chips cannot be used to detect novel mutation, so the lack of a positive hit does not disprove a diagnosis.

Mutation Testing

The detection of pathologic mutations is the essential step toward making a definite molecular diagnosis. Although there are several different strategies to use, the initial evaluation will depend on whether you are looking for a known mutation or whether the patient has a novel mutation that has never been seen before. When the mutation is known, molecular techniques that focus on specific base changes can be employed. One method relies on changes in restriction sites. A *restriction enzyme* is one that recognizes a specific short sequence of bases (usually four to eight bases long) and that cleaves the DNA at that site or nearby. The DNA site that is recognized by a restriction enzyme is usually palindromic, which means that the sequence reads the same in both directions. For example, the restriction enzyme *Taq I* recognizes the palindromic sequence TCGA and the complementary AGCT, and it cuts the DNA between the T and the C. If there is a change in DNA, it can either disrupt an existing restriction site or create a new one; this can be detected by amplifying the appropriate DNA fragment, cutting it with the restriction enzyme, and running the product on an electrophoresis gel. Fragments with one or more restriction sites will show multiple bands; if a restriction site is added or lost, it can be easily detected by noting the position and number of DNA bands. However, not all DNA changes involve a restriction site. Methods based on the innate annealing capacity of DNA can also be employed. The use of DNA chips in this regard was discussed above.

It is generally thought that screening for known mutations in a gene is a reasonable and less expensive strategy for making a molecular diagnosis. However, if a patient does not show one of the known mutations, this does not rule the patient out as having a pathologic mutation; it could be that the mutation has not yet been observed. In fact, many mutations are extremely rare and occur in only one case or family. Many mutations are limited to a specific family because they have not had time to spread throughout the population. As a result, molecular diagnosis must rely on techniques that can pick up novel mutations. Direct sequencing of a gene is one approach, and it is illustrated in Figure 12-7. However, if the gene is large, the sequencing effort can be time consuming and expensive. There are two popular methods that help with screening DNA for mutations: heteroduplex testing and single strand conformation polymorphism (SSCP). In heteroduplex testing, a fragment is amplified, heated, and allowed to anneal with itself.[20,22] If the patient is heterozygous, then the fragment will contain two populations of DNA: one with each of the two DNA variants. When the DNA is heated, it melts. Then, when it cools, it anneals back onto itself. However, three different forms of double-stranded DNA will be formed. Two forms will be like the original mother strands; the third, however, will contain two strands that have mismatched bases—a so-called *heteroduplex*. This produces a double strand that will migrate slightly differently under certain conditions. This can be easily visualized using a dematuring high performance liquid chromatography (DHPLC) (Figure 12-7). After a potential mutation is recognized, the

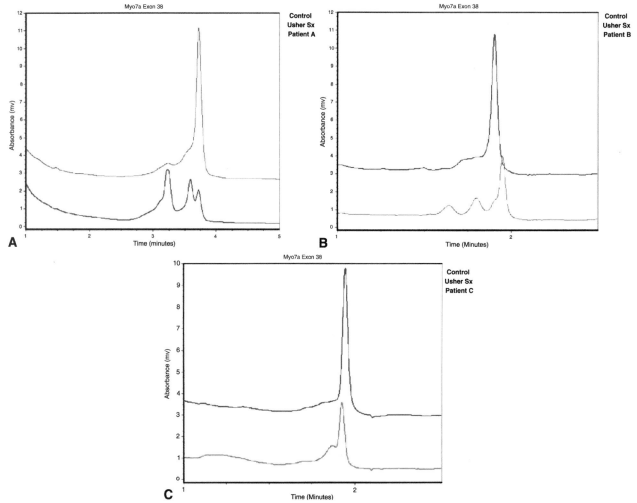

Figure 12-7. DHPLC using a WAVE apparatus is a common method of screening for mutations. This figure shows the results of DHPLC for three different mutations of exon 38 of the *MYO7A* gene, which causes Usher's syndrome type Ib. A fragment of DNA is amplified by polymerase chain reaction, heated to disassociation, and then cooled. Upon reannealing, four different double-stranded molecules are possible, two of which represent the original fragments. The other two will have double strands that differ slightly (e.g., at only one base) and that cause a slight conformational change that alters their mobility; this is observed as an additional peak or peaks when run out on a column. When a peak is observed, the exact nature of the change must be determined by sequencing. To view this image in color, please go to *www.ototext.com* or the Electronic Image Collection CD, bound into your copy of Cummings Otolaryngology—Head and Neck Surgery, 4th edition.

fragment can then be sequenced, and the specific base change can be precisely identified. Other methods of mutation detection include allele-specific oligonucleotide hybridization, reverse dot blots, and amplification refractory mutations systems.[12]

ETHICAL ISSUES

Genetics has raised a host of ethical issues that had not been of much concern before the 1990s. From the physician's perspective, one issue relates to his or her "duty" to inform patients who are at risk for genetic disorders. If a woman is found to carry breast cancer liability alleles on the *BRCA1* gene, is it the physician's responsibility to make sure that this patient communicates the possibility of risk to her female relatives? There is clearly a conflict here between the patient's right to privacy and the responsibility to "do good" by informing women for whom this extra diligence just might be life saving. Any genetic diagnosis carries with it the potential that a person other than the primary patient could be involved. The diagnosis of *GJB2* hearing loss identifies siblings, cousins, and other relatives as potential heterozygotes who have an increased risk of having a child with profound deafness. It is not always the case that family members want the information, either. Although the issue is still argued, the general consensus is that the flow of information must come from the patient or an immediate family member, in the case of a minor.

THE UTILITY OF MOLECULAR GENETICS IN OTOLARYNGOLOGY

The main role of molecular genetics in medical science is as a diagnostic tool. At the present time, the emphasis is on disorders that are caused by major genes. DNA testing can be used to definitively establish a diagnosis. This aids in the establishment of a prognosis, the elimination of the need for further expensive (and perhaps invasive) clinical testing, and the provision of information to the family about the likelihood of the disorder in other family members.

REFERENCES

1. Antonarakis SE, Lyle R, Deutsch S and others: Chromosome 21: a small land of fascinating disorders with unknown pathophysiology, *Int J Dev Biol* 46: 89, 2002.
2. Baldwin CT and others: Mutations in PAX3 that cause Waardenburg syndrome type I: ten new mutations and review of the literature, *Am J Med Genet* 58:115, 1995.
3. Balmain A, Gray J, Ponder B: The genetics and genomics of cancer, *Nat Genet* 33(suppl):238, 2003.
4. Barrenasa M, Landin-Wilhelmsenb K, Hansonc C: Ear and hearing in relation to genotype and growth in Turner syndrome, *Hear Res* 144:21, 2000.
5. Beighton P, Botha MC: Inherited disorders in the black population of southern Africa. Part I. Historical and demographic background; genetic haematological conditions, *S Afr Med J* 69:247, 1986.
6. Bender B and others: Speech and language development in 41 children with sex chromosome anomalies, *Pediatrics* 71:262, 1983.
7. Bitner-Glindzicz M: Hereditary deafness and phenotyping in humans, *Br Med Bull* 63:73, 2002.
8. Bobadilla JL and others: Cystic fibrosis: a worldwide analysis of CFTR mutations—correlation with incidence data and application to screening, *Hum Mutat* 19:575, 2002.
9. Botstein D, Risch N: Discovering genotypes underlying human phenotypes: past successes for Mendelian disease, future approaches for complex disease, *Nat Genet* 33(suppl):228, 2003.
10. Boughman JA, Vernon M, Shaver KA: Usher syndrome: definition and estimate of prevalence from two high risk populations, *J Chron Dis* 36:595, 1983.
11. Cahill MR, Colvin BT: Haemophilia, *Postgrad Med J* 73:201, 1997.
12. Chapman RS and others: Predicting language production in children and adolescents with Down syndrome: the role of comprehension, *J Speech Lang Hear Res* 43:340, 2000.
13. Collins FS: The Genome Project and human health, *FASEB J* 5:77, 1991.
14. Collins FS and Guttmacher AE: Genetics moves into the medical mainstream, *JAMA* 286:2322, 2001.
15. Collins FS, Green ED, Guttmacher AE and others: A vision for the future of genomics research, *Nature* 422:835, 2003.
16. Cotton RG: Current methods of mutation detection, *Mutat Res* 285:125, 1993.
17. Cremers CW and others: X-linked mixed deafness syndrome with congenital fixation of the stapedial footplate and perilymphatic gusher (DFN3), *Adv Otorhinolaryngol* 61:161, 2002.
18. De Benedetti VM and others: DNA chips: the future of biomarkers, *Int J Biol Markers* 15:1, 2000.
19. del Castillo I and others: A deletion involving the connexin 30 gene in nonsyndromic hearing impairment, *N Engl J Med* 346:243, 2002.
20. Delatycki M, Gardner RJ: Three cases of trisomy 13 mosaicism and a review of the literature, *Clin Genet* 51:403, 1997.
21. DeStefano AL and others: Genomewide linkage analysis to presbycusis in the Framingham Heart Study, *Arch Otolaryngol Head Neck Surg* 129:285, 2003.
22. Fisher SE, DeFries JC: Developmental dyslexia: genetic dissection of a complex cognitive trait, *Nat Rev Neurosci* 3:767, 2002.
23. Fraser FC and others: Genetic aspects of the BOR syndrome—branchial fistulas, ear pits, hearing loss, and renal anomalies, *Am J Med Genet* 2:241, 1978.
24. Frueh FW, Noyer-Weidner M: The use of denaturing high-performance liquid chromatography (DHPLC) for the analysis of genetic variations: impact for diagnostics and pharmacogenetics, *Clin Chem Lab Med* 41:452, 2003.
25. Gandolfi A, Horoupian DS, De Teresa RM: Pathology of the auditory system in autosomal trisomies with morphometric and quantitative study of the ventral cochlear nucleus, *J Neurol Sci* 51:43, 1981.
26. Ganguly A: An update on conformation sensitive gel electrophoresis, *Hum Mutat* 19:334, 2002.
27. Gasparini P and others: High carrier frequency of the 35delG deafness mutation in European populations. Genetic Analysis Consortium of GJB2 35delG, *Eur J Hum Genet* 8:19, 2000.
28. Goodwin JH, Post JC: The genetics of otitis media, *Curr Allergy Asthma Rep* 2:304, 2002.

29. Gorlin RJ, Toriello HV, Cohen MM: *Hereditary hearing loss and its syndromes.* Oxford, England, Oxford University Press, 1995

30. Grand RJ and others: Unusual case of XXY Klinefelter's syndrome with pancreatic insufficiency, hypothyroidism, deafness, chronic lung disease, dwarfism and microcephaly, *Am J Med* 41:478, 1966.

31. Gungor N and others: High frequency hearing loss in Ullrich-Turner syndrome, *Eur J Pediatr* 159:740, 2000.

32. Ha PK, Califano JA: The molecular biology of laryngeal cancer, *Otolaryngol Clin North Am* 35:993, 2002.

33. Hultcrantz M: Ear and hearing problems in Turner's syndrome, *Acta Otolaryngol* 123:253, 2003.

34. Hutchin TP, Cortopassi GA: Mitochondrial defects and hearing loss, *Cell Mol Life Sci* 57:1927, 2000.

35. Johnson J, Lalwani AK: Sensorineural and conductive hearing loss associated with lateral semicircular canal malformation, *Laryngoscope* 110(10 Pt 1):1673, 2000.

36. Kajiwara K, Berson EL, Dryja TP: Digenic retinitis pigmentosa due to mutations at the unlinked peripherin/RDS and ROM1 loci, *Science* 264:1604, 1994.

37. Kashtan CE: Alport syndrome. An inherited disorder of renal, ocular, and cochlear basement membranes, *Medicine (Baltimore)* 78:338, 1999.

38. Kimberling WJ, Moller C: Clinical and molecular genetics of Usher syndrome, *J Am Acad Audiol* 6:63, 1995.

39. Kimberling WJ, Orten D, Pieke-Dahl S: Genetic heterogeneity of Usher syndrome, *Adv Otorhinolaryngol* 56:11-18, 2000.

40. Lehman CD and others: Trisomy 13 syndrome: prenatal US findings in a review of 33 cases, *Radiology* 194:217, 1995.

41. Lerer I and others: A deletion mutation in GJB6 cooperating with a GJB2 mutation in trans in non-syndromic deafness: a novel founder mutation in Ashkenazi Jews, *Hum Mutat* 18:460, 2001.

42. Luo Z, Geschwind DH: Microarray applications in neuroscience, *Neurobiol Dis* 8:183, 2001.

43. Mahuran DJ and others: The molecular basis of Tay-Sachs disease: mutation identification and diagnosis, *Clin Biochem* 23:409, 1990.

44. Marsh KL, Dixon MJ: Treacher Collins syndrome, *Adv Otorhinolaryngol* 56:53, 2000.

45. Misra M, Nolph KD: Renal failure and deafness: branchio-oto-renal syndrome, *Am J Kidney Dis* 32:334, 1998.

46. Mullis KB: Target amplification for DNA analysis by the polymerase chain reaction, *Ann Biol Clin (Paris)* 48:579, 1990.

47. Myers RH and others: Homozygote for Huntington disease, *Am J Hum Genet* 45:615, 1989.

48. Newton VE: Clinical features of the Waardenburg syndromes, *Adv Otorhinolaryngol* 61:201, 2002.

49. Nicolaidis P, Petersen MB: Origin and mechanisms of non-disjunction in human autosomal trisomies, *Hum Reprod* 13:313, 1998.

50. Niedermeyer HP, Arnold W: Etiopathogenesis of otosclerosis, *ORL J Otorhinolaryngol Relat Spec* 64:114, 2002.

51. Ostrer H: Invited review: sex-based differences in gene expression, *J Appl Physiol* 91:2384, 2001.

52. Ott J: *Analysis of human genetic linkage,* ed 3. Baltimore: Johns Hopkins University Press, 1999.

53. Pallares-Ruiz N and others: A large deletion including most of GJB6 in recessive non syndromic deafness: a digenic effect? *Eur J Hum Genet* 10:72, 2002.

54. Parker KL and others: Screening girls with Turner syndrome: the National Cooperative Growth Study experience, *J Pediatr* 143:133, 2003.

55. Petit C: Usher syndrome: from genetics to pathogenesis, *Annu Rev Genomics Hum Genet* 2:271, 2001.

56. Posnick JC, Ruiz RL: Treacher Collins syndrome: current evaluation, treatment, and future directions, *Cleft Palate Craniofac J* 37:434, 2000.

57. Ravine D: Automated mutation analysis, *J Inherit Metab Dis* 22:503, 1999.

58. Read AP: Waardenburg syndrome, *Adv Otorhinolaryngol* 56:32, 2000.

59. Reardon W, Trembath RC: Pendred syndrome, *J Med Genet* 33:1037, 1996.

60. Reed W, Vichinsky EP: New considerations in the treatment of sickle cell disease, *Annu Rev Med* 49:461, 1998.

61. Runte M, Dekomien G, Epplen JT: Evaluation of RDS/Peripherin and ROM1 as candidate genes in generalised progressive retinal atrophy and exclusion of digenic inheritance, *Anim Genet* 31:223, 2000.

62. Russell-Eggitt IM and others: Alstrom syndrome. Report of 22 cases and literature review, *Ophthalmology* 105:1274, 1998.

63. Sculerati N and others: Otitis media and hearing loss in Turner syndrome, *Arch Otolaryngol Head Neck Surg* 116:704, 1990.

64. Seidman MD, Ahmad N, Bai U: Molecular mechanisms of age-related hearing loss, *Ageing Res Rev* 1:331, 2002.

65. Shaver KA, Boughman JA, Nance WE: Congenital rubella syndrome and diabetes: a review of epidemiologic, genetic, and immunologic factors, *Am Ann Deaf* 130:526, 1985.

66. Shore EM, Kaplan FS: Tutorial. Molecular biology for the clinician. Part II. Tools of molecular biology, *Clin Orthop* 320:247, 1995.

67. Smith RJ, Schwartz C: Branchio-oto-renal syndrome, *J Commun Disord* 31:411, 1998.

68. Smith SD: Overview of genetic auditory syndromes, *J Am Acad Audiol* 6:1, 1995.

69. Southern EM: Detection of specific sequences among DNA fragments separated by gel electrophoresis, *J Mol Biol* 98:503, 1975.

70. Sussman M: Duchenne muscular dystrophy, *J Am Acad Orthop Surg* 10:138, 2002.

71. Swift AC, Singh SD: Hearing impairment and the Kearns-Sayre syndrome, *J Laryngol Otol* 102:626, 1988.

72. Tachibana M: Alport syndrome, *Adv Otorhinolaryngol* 56:19, 2000.

73. Taggart RT and others: Gene expression changes in chinchilla cochlea from noise-induced temporary threshold shift, *Noise Health* 3:1, 2001.

74. Tassabehji M and others: Mutations in the PAX3 gene causing Waardenburg syndrome type 1 and type 2, *Nat Genet* 3:26, 1993.

75. Tomlinson IP, Roylance R, Houlston RS: Two hits revisited again, *J Med Genet* 38:81, 2001.

76. Tranebjaerg L, Jensen PK, van Ghelue M: X-linked recessive deafness-dystonia syndrome (Mohr-Tranebjaerg syndrome), *Adv Otorhinolaryngol* 56:176, 2000.

77. Usami S and others: Sensorineural hearing loss caused by mitochondrial DNA mutations: special reference to the A1555G mutation, *J Commun Disord* 31:423, 1998.

78. Van Buggenhout GJ and others: Down syndrome in a population of elderly mentally retarded patients: genetic-diagnostic survey and implications for medical care, *Am J Med Genet* 85:376, 1999.

79. Van Camp G, Smith RJ: Maternally inherited hearing impairment, *Clin Genet* 57:409, 2000.

80. Weil D and others: Defective myosin VIIa gene responsible for Usher syndrome type 1B, *Nature* 374:60, 1995.

81. Weinstein R: Phytanic acid storage disease (Refsum's disease): clinical characteristics, pathophysiology and the role of therapeutic apheresis in its management, *J Clin Apheresis* 14:181, 1999.

82. Wexler NS and others: Homozygotes for Huntington's disease, *Nature* 326:194, 1987.

83. Wilcox ER and others: The PDS gene, Pendred syndrome and non-syndromic deafness DFNB4, *Adv Otorhinolaryngol* 56:145, 2000.

84. Wilkie AO: The molecular basis of genetic dominance, *J Med Genet* 31:89, 1994.

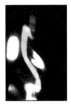

CHAPTER THIRTEEN

FUNDAMENTALS OF MOLECULAR BIOLOGY AND GENE THERAPY

Bert W. O'Malley, Jr.
Daqing Li
Hinrich Staecker

INTRODUCTION

Molecular biology is a relatively young scientific field, with its major thrust arising from the discovery of methods to study and manipulate DNA in the 1970s. The rapid advances in this arena, however, enabled actual clinical application by the 1980s and 1990s. No longer does molecular biology reside solely within the research laboratory. Many diagnostic laboratory tests routinely used in clinical medicine as well as the development and mass production of pharmaceuticals make use of molecular biology techniques. The surge of molecular biology and the new understanding of genes and the products of their expression have allowed the emergence of a rising field heralded as "gene therapy." This rapidly expanding field is founded on the ability to introduce genetic material into the body to treat disease or alter an ongoing pathologic process.

The purpose of this chapter is not to discuss molecular biology in detail. Rather, the purpose is to review basic molecular terminology and to introduce the concept of gene and molecular therapy. Emphasis will be placed on the rationale, methods, and progress to date for clinical application of this exciting and even controversial therapy.

MOLECULAR BIOLOGY: FUNDAMENTALS

The basic premise of molecular biology is to study cell function and regulation at the level of the genome. With this understanding comes insight into human disease because aberrances in cell function or regulation are the basis for most diseases. The following section reviews fundamental terminology and concepts on how information travels from the genetic code to the functional protein level. Included is a brief discussion on cell cycling, which is an important concept in tumor molecular biology.

Gene Expression

The information for conducting all aspects of cellular function is contained within molecules of DNA located in the nucleus. The actual length of a human DNA strand is 1.8 M, however, it is coiled around nuclear proteins called *histones* that structure the folds and loops of DNA to allow compression into the microscopic size of the cell's nucleus. Each strand of DNA contains thousands of genes, which are specific subunit sequences that are coded for the information required to synthesize a protein. One molecule of double-stranded DNA and its genes make up each of a cell's 46 total chromosomes. Although every cell in the human body contains the same DNA, the expression of individual genes are not the same. Gene expression will vary depending on the cells function. These differences in gene expression result in the multiple cell and tissue phenotypes that constitute the human body as a whole.

The process by which a gene codes for a specific protein begins with *transcription*, which is the formation of a single-stranded RNA molecule, which compliments a single strand of the DNA subunit (Figure 13-1). This RNA molecule is subsequently modified to become the messenger, which brings the genetic information or directions from the nucleus to the cell's cytoplasm where the actual synthesis of the functional protein occurs. After reaching the cytoplasm, the process of translation begins (Figure 13-1). During translation, the message from the RNA molecule directs the construction of a protein from its basic subunit, the amino acid. Once a protein is formed, it may require further modification or control steps to enable its designated function. These modifications include the addition of sugars, lipids, or phosphates to the protein backbone. These internal control steps are mediated by existing cytoplasmic enzymes, which, if defective, can also lead to defined diseases. Once a protein is formed within the cell cytoplasm, it can reside in the cell or be released to affect other tissues within the body. Depending on the original genetic program for the protein, it may serve its purpose and be rapidly degraded, or it may enter the circulation or reside in local or distant tissues for an extended period. Although stated simply above, both transcription and translation are complex processes that have many more modification and regulatory steps governed by regulatory genes and their protein products. When these delicate control mechanisms are lost, a disease state or a state of abnormal cell proliferation can ensue, as is exemplified in the development of cancer.

Cell Division

Disorders in cell function can lead either to cell death or proliferation. Abnormal stimulation of cell proliferation is the basis for the development of cancer. For a cell to divide, it must progress through the various phases of growth and reproduction that constitute what is called the *cell cycle* (Figure 13-2). The principal components of the cell cycle are the replication nuclear DNA and its distribution among the progeny cells (i.e., daughter cells). The first phase of the cell cycle is called *G1*, and it is here that all the enzymes, nucleic acids, and other factors are produced that will enable DNA replication or "synthesis," which occurs in the *S phase*. Once the DNA is replicated, a period of cell growth and duplication of cellular proteins and

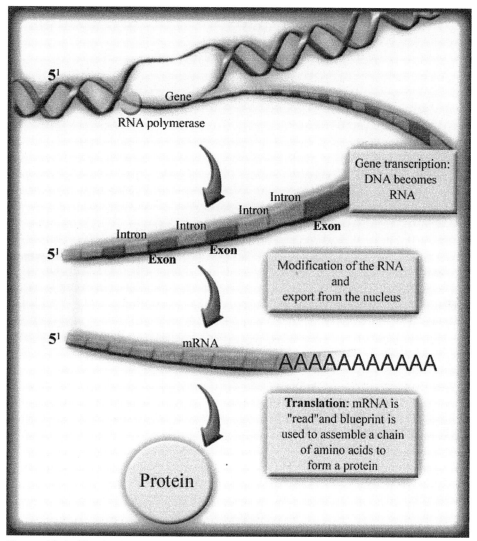

Figure 13-1. The basic steps involved in gene expression. Genes are copied within the nucleus by RNA polymerase resulting in production of a complementary RNA strand. This is processed to produce mRNA. The mRNA exits the nucleus and undergoes "translation" by ribosomes to form a protein product.

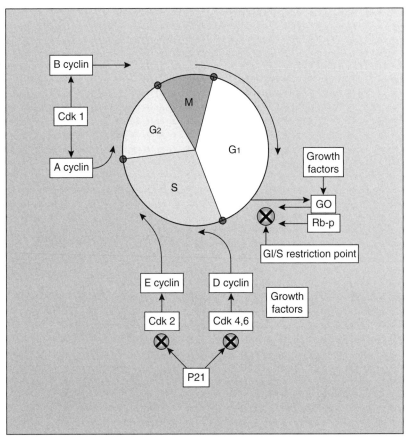

Figure 13-2. Cell cycle. The various phases of the entire cell cycle are depicted, which typically last 10 to 25 hours in animals. Only 1 hour is spent in the M phase. The longest and most variable phase is G1, which can range from 4 to 24 hours. Also depicted are regulation of the cell cycle, many elements of which are targets of gene and molecular therapy.

structures occurs in a period called *G2*. After this cell growth, the actual distribution of the replicated DNA and the physical division of the parent cell into two daughter cells occur in the *M phase,* which takes approximately 1 hour. After cell division, the cell cycle process can begin again, or the cell may enter a state of rest called *G0*. The signal to divide can either come from internal factors or exogenous growth factors, which bind to cell surface receptors and stimulate a cascade of events, which lead to division. Important internal control mechanisms exist at the genetic level, which help regulate cell cycling. The "negative regulatory" genes that code for proteins inhibiting abnormal cell proliferation are called *tumor suppressor genes*. A mutation or loss of a tumor suppressor gene is a basic step in the development of many human cancers. Cell cycling can also be abnormally induced by cellular *oncogenes*, which naturally exist within cells but are typically kept dormant either by tumor suppressor genes or other regulatory mechanisms. Loss of negative regulation from tumor suppressor genes or amplification or mutation of the actual oncogene has also been associated with cancer formation. Continued molecular research will provide further understanding of cell cycle regulation and may lead to novel therapies for treating human cancer.

A discussion of basic molecular biology techniques, which have provided the means to understand gene expression, regulation, and cell cycling, can be found in Chapter 16.

GENE THERAPY

Arising from the dramatic progress in molecular and cellular biology is an exciting and even controversial new field of clinical research and human investigation. This new field of translational research, known as *gene therapy*, focuses on the transfer of therapeutic genes to normal or abnormal target cells. During the advent of gene therapy, the initial clinical targets were rare inherited diseases such as adenosine deaminase deficiency, which results in a deadly systemic immune deficiency, enzymatic deficiencies resulting in liver failure, or coagulation pathway deficiencies resulting in various types of hemophilia. In the past

5 years, however, it has become clear that gene therapy may have its most immediate and effective role in treating more common diseases such as cancer, cystic fibrosis, arthritis, and atherosclerosis.[51] As the field of gene therapy continues its rapid advancement, the techniques and therapies will not be restricted to the practices of geneticists and specialists in rare inherited diseases. It is likely that gene therapy will be a standard regimen available to both internists and surgeons in the course of routine clinical care.

Principles and Concepts
Basic Principle

The basic principle of gene therapy is that normal or therapeutic genes can be introduced into body tissues to treat a disease. In many genetic diseases, this may involve introducing a normal gene into the body to carry out the function that is defective because of the inheritance of a mutant gene. An example of this is hemophilia, in which individuals at the time of birth lack a normal gene for clotting factor VIII and can experience prolonged bleeding. The transfer of a normal factor VIII gene into the patient's endothelial cells or hepatocytes could restore the ability of these cells to secrete factor VIII and could therefore restore the bleeding time to normal. Acquired diseases such as cancer can also be treated with gene therapy. For example, one of the first clinical trials focused on the treatment of melanoma.[61] In this clinical trial, lymphocytes that had infiltrated the tumors (tumor-infiltrating lymphocytes; TIL) were purified from a tumor at the time of surgical resection. The TIL cells were then grown in the laboratory, and the gene for tumor necrosis factor (TNF) was introduced into the cells. The genetically engineered cells were subsequently transfused into the patient with the expectation that they would preferentially migrate to the site of residual tumor, delivering a therapeutic dose of TNF.

The potential for gene therapy of diseases such as hemophilia or cancer illustrate several essential points about somatic gene therapy in general.

Somatic vs Germ Cell Gene Therapy

Gene therapy has two possible target cell types. The first and presently used targets are the somatic cells, or those cells that constitute the organs and postnatal tissues of the body. The second potential target is the germ cells, or those cells that produce the sperm or ovum and are passed on to a person's offspring. Many different organs and cell types are targets for somatic gene therapy, including bone marrow, liver, tumor cells, muscle, skin, endothelium, thyroid, and others (Figure 13-3). Genetic manipulation and therapy at these sites does not alter the inherited genetic material and raises few novel ethical or social issues.[49]

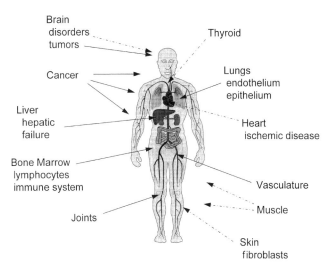

Figure 13-3. Somatic targets for gene therapy. Many different cell types are potential targets for gene therapy. Solid arrows represent tissue targets presently under human clinical trial investigation, and dotted arrows represent targets under investigation in animal models. Current gene therapy laboratory and clinical investigation explicitly excludes manipulation of germ cells (sperm and ovum) which may pass genes to future generations.

Genetic manipulation of the sperm or ovum, however, could prevent inherited diseases by altering the genetic constitution of offspring. Although this is an appealing idea on the surface, there are serious technical and safety issues as well as profound ethical concerns involved. Currently, gene therapy is restricted to somatic cells, and genetic manipulation of human germ cells would be prohibited under existing recombinant DNA guidelines.[58]

Homologous Recombination

It is possible to introduce a gene into a targeted cell in such a way that the defective region of the existing genetic material will be excised and replaced with a new gene sequence. This process known as *homologous recombination* and has been used to restore mutant genes to normal embryonic mouse cells. Homologous recombination methods, however, are presently ineffective for human gene therapy because of the very low efficiency of actual gene transfer (1 in 10^5–10^7 targeted cells).[74] Current gene therapy strategies are much more efficient than attempts at homologous recombination and involve the introduction of new genetic material into cells to express a therapeutic gene product. Gene therapy, therefore, is not only applicable for treating single gene disorders but can be used for any disorder in which the expression of a gene product has a therapeutic effect.

Therapeutic Mechanism

The gene that is delivered to a target cell is not itself therapeutic. Rather, it is the product encoded by the gene, which is responsible for the resulting therapeutic effect. The gene product is typically a protein, which has a specific function such as a hormone or cytokine, but could also be a bioactive RNA molecule or a regulatory molecule (RNA or protein) that alters the regulation of pathologic processes. Thus, although gene therapy commonly focuses on methods for delivering genes to cells, it is the ability to achieve expression of the gene product at therapeutic levels that ultimately determines the effectiveness and efficacy of therapy.

Permanent vs Temporary Gene Therapy

A common perception is that the goal of gene therapy is to "permanently" introduce a therapeutic gene into a patient. Permanent gene therapy, however, may not be necessary or optimal in a clinical setting. As a general principal, permanent gene therapy could prove more desirable when the methods required for introducing the gene into the patient involve significant surgical procedures or substantial risk to the patients such as in the case of organ resection, cellular transplantation, or stereotactic injection under anesthesia. To achieve permanent gene therapy, the gene that is introduced into the patient should be expressed indefinitely. The gene must also demonstrate appropriate regulation in response to both normal and pathologic situations, and there should be no detrimental consequences of this gene expression in later life. In considering diseases such as growth hormone deficiency or juvenile diabetes, correction by permanent gene transfer would require precise regulation of the gene products to ensure both short-term efficacy and long-term safety. This tight control and regulation of transferred genetic material is not feasible with present techniques.

For many diseases such as cancer, cystic fibrosis, arthritis, and disorders requiring surgery, insertion of a "temporary" gene into a patient's tumor, residual tumor, or other target cells could produce a selected beneficial therapy over a limited period of time. For example, the treatment of a tumor or area of residual tumor after surgery may only require a one-time, limited expression of a gene that either produces a substance directly toxic to the cancer cell or a cytokine or other factor that can initiate an antitumor immune response. Instead of permanent gene therapy, repeat gene transfer over a period of time could also prove effective, as in the case of radiation therapy or possible chemotherapy regimens. Repeat gene transfer may also find a role in the treatment of arthritis and other chronic diseases. With respect to surgical procedures, the use of gene therapy to enhance wound healing or tissue regeneration after an injury might only require gene expression for a period of days or weeks. Another new frontier on the near horizon is gene therapy, which can be administered repetitively by minimally invasive or noninvasive routes such as intramuscular, intravenous, or even oral administration. This novel future application could allow the establishment of steady-state gene product levels, which parallels present medical regimens and enables the physician to adjust the dose and schedule of administration to the patient's needs.

Therapeutic Levels of Gene Expression

Effective gene therapy requires not only the delivery of genes to the appropriate target cell within the body but the expression of the therapeutic gene product at appropriate levels. It is the ability to achieve adequate gene expression that will determine the efficacy and therapeutic index of gene therapy. There are several ways to achieve appropriate expression of a therapeutic gene product.

Specific genetic elements called *promoters* and *enhancers* that normally control the rate of therapeutic product expression can be incorporated into the gene transfer vehicles. These elements can also control the level of gene expression, restrict it to specific cell types, and provide regulated gene expression in response to endocrine or pharmacologic factors. For example, gene therapy for diabetes will certainly require the incorporation of genetic elements that provide normal regulation of insulin levels by glucose.

Promoter and enhancer elements derived from different genes can be combined to provide an improved effect. In this way, vectors can be designed to produce gene products at high levels from a cell that normally produces only low levels or to constitute expression of a gene product from a cell that does not normally produce that particular gene product. For example, clotting factors or peptide hormones can be expressed from muscle cells after gene transfer using vehicles that incorporate the promoter and enhancer elements from muscle-specific genes such as skeletal actin or myosin. In considering cancer gene therapy, highly efficient viral promoters can be mixed and matched with a variety of gene-delivery vehicles that will result in high levels of expression of therapeutic antitumor genes directly from the targeted cancer cells.

Another important regulatory mechanism resides in the natural actions of a cell, tissue, or organ. As is the case with conventional pharmaceuticals, the basic principles of drug distribution, metabolism, and elimination within the cells and tissues of the body will provide additional means for regulating the level of the gene product.

Why Gene Therapy?

An important universal question asks what advantages gene therapy has over the present accepted medical and surgical treatments that would warrant clinical investigation and application in routine patient care. In response to this basic question are several reasons why gene therapy might become a first-line treatment in clinical practice.

New Therapeutic Approach

With the rapid evolution of molecular biology over the past decade, an increasing number of basic biologic phenomena and pathologic conditions are now understood in terms of the events that take place on a molecular level between genes and their gene products. According to both experimental animal models and early human clinical trials, it is now possible to alter processes such as immunity, growth, development, regeneration, and malignancy on a molecular level using gene transfer. Therapeutic gene transfer provides a novel approach to diseases that are not satisfactorily managed using conventional pharmacologic or surgical intervention. As a general example, using gene therapy to reconstitute deficient functions resulting from failing organs or tissues may provide an alternative to allogenic transplantation of bone marrow, solid organs, or individual cells.

Site-Specific Gene Expression

Using the techniques and principles of gene transfer, therapeutic products can be released from specific cell types in precise locations within the body. This concept of site-specific gene expression provides a valuable advantage for gene therapy. Therapeutic proteins such as cytokines or growth factors can be expressed in precise locations, rather than administering similar products via a systemic route. The highest concentration of the therapeutic product will therefore be focused at the desired site of action. For example, gene transfer can be used to express products specifically in the epidermal or dermal layers of the skin without affecting underlying connective tissue, nerves, muscles, or vessels. Such spatial specificity will minimize untoward consequences or toxicity in organs or other vital structures outside of the site being treated.

Improved Efficacy and Safety

Gene therapy establishes the expression of normal, human proteins acting in a directed therapeutic fashion within the body. Based on this concept, gene therapy may prove to be more efficacious and safer than the application of proteins purified from microorganisms, animals, or human populations, which carry the attendant risk of transmitting pathogens or inciting allergic reactions. Moreover, gene therapy can be used to achieve regulated, physiologic expression of gene products, which may further improve efficacy. By altering the dose or schedule of gene administration to a patient, it will be possible to optimize the level, effect, and safety of the gene product.

Improved Routes of Administration and Compliance

Most standard medications have short half-lives and need to be administered by frequent oral dosing, injections, or even constant infusions to achieve an optimal therapeutic effect. Gene therapy, however, provides continuous endogenous expression of natural protein products and requires less frequent administration (of the gene) ranging from one time to weekly or monthly treatments, depending on the disease target and gene transfer strategy. As is known to all clinicians, decreasing the frequency of administration improves acceptance and compliance with therapeutic regimens.

Preventative Medicine and a Reduction in Health Care Costs

As molecular and genetic research continues to identify factors that predispose individuals to diseases such as atherosclerosis, cancer, diabetes, infections, or degenerative disorders, the application of gene therapy may allow a physician to alter the expression of these factors in a preventative manner. Of particular importance is the ability to deliver therapy over a long period in clinically asymptomatic or minimally symptomatic patients who have inherited or acquired progressive diseases—a combination of circumstances that is traditionally associated with poor compliance. For example, treating a diabetic patient with gene therapy early in the stages of the disease may prevent morbidity later in life that occurs even with conventional exogenous insulin therapy. Also, combining the advances in molecular diagnostics of cancer may allow replacement of lost or defective critical tumor-suppressor genes in normal or premalignant tissues, thereby preventing the progression of the defective tissue into cancer.

Because gene therapy can establish continuous release of a therapeutic product with one-time treatment or infrequent dosing, its use for prevention is more practical and affordable than conventional therapies. The practice of preventative gene therapy to diminish morbidity and early mortality and the use of more affordable treatment regimens will ultimately reduce the rapidly growing cost of health care.

Methods for Gene Transfer

A major focus in the field of gene therapy is the development of vehicles for introducing genetic material into selected target cells. Two general classes of gene vehicles and transfer methods can be distinguished: (1) DNA-mediated gene transfer involves the administration of DNA alone to the patient in various formulations such as in saline or lipid complex mediums. (2) Viral-mediated gene transfer involves packaging a therapeutic gene into a defective virus particle and using the natural process of viral infection to introduce the gene. The purpose of viral-mediated gene transfer is to exploit the efficient and often complex mechanisms that viruses have evolved to introduce their viral genes into human cells during infections.

DNA-Mediated Gene Transfer

The process of DNA-mediated gene transfer is called *transfection*, and the vehicle through which a therapeutic gene is transferred into a cell is called a *vector*. Functional DNA vectors are circular molecules of DNA that contain various additional genetic elements required to achieve expression of the gene product at therapeutic levels (Figure 13-4). Included in these are the special elements (promoter and enhancer) that direct gene expression and elements that determine the processing and persistence of genetic material within the cell.

The delivery of DNA vectors into cells is possible via a variety of techniques. One classic method is to simply microinject DNA directly into the cell nucleus.[5] This method is both time consuming and inefficient for achieving large numbers of transfected cells. Although this method is common in the laboratory with in vitro studies, its technical limitations prohibit effective application to living animal models or human subjects. A more efficient process, which is also is limited to in vitro application, is the process of electroporation, in which cultured cells are exposed to DNA in the presence of a strong electrical pulse.[7] The electrical pulse creates pores in the cell membrane, which allows electrophoresis of DNA into the cell.

It is possible to effectively introduce genes into muscle[79] or thyroid[68] simply by injecting DNA into these tissues in vivo, where the process of endocytosis enables cellular uptake. This is not true of other tissues examined to date. Gene transfer into other organs requires special methods to enhance the uptake of DNA into the specific target cells. A common alternative method is the use of cationic lipids, which encase DNA vectors and fuse with the target cell membrane[19] to enhance intracellular gene uptake. This process has been termed *lipofection*. Another method is to couple the DNA vector to proteins that bind to specific receptors on the target cell leading to uptake of the DNA by receptor-mediated endocytosis.[75,80] A recent technical advance is the development of the "gene gun," which uses electrical currents and magnetic properties to project DNA vectors that are coated with microscopic gold particles into the target cells.[82] Another less common technique still under early investigation involves using select viral components to enhance vector movement across the cell membrane and into the cell.[14,76]

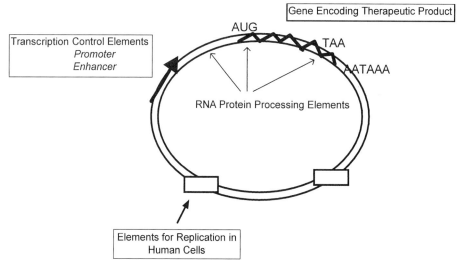

Figure 13-4. Schematic structure of a plasmid DNA vector. Plasmid DNA vectors are circular molecules of DNA encoding a therapeutic gene product. DNA vectors contain special elements required to achieve expression of the gene product at therapeutic levels. Promoter and enhancer regions regulate the transcription of plasmid DNA into RNA, and specific processing elements regulate the translation of RNA into protein. A DNA vector may be complexed with protein, lipids, or synthetic organic compounds that enhance vector uptake or provide cell uptake specificity.

An important point to understand is that DNA-mediated gene transfer typically results in only transient residence of the therapeutic genes in the targeted cell. DNA vectors, which are introduced into cells, are degraded and eliminated from the cell over time. Different cell types eliminate the introduced genetic material at different rates. In muscle, for example, DNA vectors may persist in cells for many months and continue to express gene products.[79] In contrast, DNA vectors injected into the thyroid have a shorter half-life and the gene product is eliminated after 2 days.[68] Vectors introduced into the liver are eliminated with a half-life of approximately 1 to 2 hours and expression is significantly reduced after 6 to 24 hours.[70]

Although permanent incorporation of genes into cells occurs rarely after DNA-mediated gene transfer in cultured cells ($<1:10^5$ cells), this phenomenon has not been observed in vivo. DNA vectors are therefore considered "safe" because they do not incorporate into the recipient cells chromosome in vivo and thus should not present a theoretic risk inherent to altering a cells genome. Moreover, they have not demonstrated significant toxicity to recipient tissues or any anti-DNA immune response.

DNA vectors can thus be delivered repeatedly, which overcomes the potential limitation of transient therapeutic gene expression. The transient nature of gene expression does have an advantage in certain clinical scenarios because the therapeutic gene can be administered by conventional oral, intramuscular, or intravenous routes to provide its beneficial effect over a predictable and extended period. In contrast to conventional medications with short half-lives, DNA-mediated gene therapy could lead to prolonged expression of a gene product at continuous levels, eliminating the need for continuous infusions or enhancing compliance by minimizing the frequency of injections.

Viral-Mediated Gene Transfer

The majority of research to date has focused on developing methods for using viruses as vectors. Viral-mediated gene transfer involves the construction of synthetic virus particles that lack pathogenic functions, are incapable of replication, contain a therapeutic gene within the viral genome, and can deliver this gene to cells by the process of infection. Certain viruses have the property of permanently integrating their genes into the chromosomes of the infected cell; therefore, select forms of viral-mediated gene transfer can lead to permanent gene therapy.

Retroviruses as Gene Transfer Vehicles

The original prototypes for viral-mediated gene transfer are retroviral vectors derived from the Moloney murine leukemia virus.[35,43] Retroviral vectors were chosen as vehicles because of several useful properties. First, "defective" virus particles can be constructed that contain therapeutic genes and are capable of infecting cells, but which contain no viral genes and express no pathogenic viral gene products. A general scheme for constructing a defective retroviral particle is illustrated in Figure 13-4. Second, retroviral vectors are capable of permanently integrating the therapeutic genes they carry into the chromosomes of the target cell. Because of this property, retroviral vectors are well suited for treating diseases that require permanent gene expression. Third, modifications can be made in retroviral vectors and in the cell lines producing vectors that result in enhanced safety features. Previous experience in animal models[10,11] and initial experiences in clinical trials suggests that these vectors have a high margin of safety.

A major limitation for this strategy is that retroviruses will only integrate into actively dividing cells and the efficiency of retroviral infection is relatively low. It is therefore difficult to generate the large numbers of transduced cells that are required for effective gene expression. Perhaps the most serious problem, however, has been the difficulty in achieving stable, regulated expression from retroviral vectors in cells that permanently carry these genes despite the known permanent integration. Cells are apparently able to shut off expression from retroviral vectors under certain conditions that have not been clearly defined.

Adenoviruses as Gene Transfer Vehicles

A recent focus of gene therapy has been the development of adenovirus vectors as powerful and effective vehicles for gene transfer.[3] An overview for the construction of a replication-defective adenoviral vector is shown in Figure 13-5. Adenoviral vectors differ from retroviral vectors in that they remain episomal; that is, they do not integrate their genes into the target cell's chromosome. Compared with retroviral vectors, adenoviral vectors demonstrate the significant advantage of infecting a wide variety of both dividing and nondividing cells in vitro and in vivo with a high level of efficiency.[4,6,52] Using adenoviral gene transfer, expression of the therapeutic gene is possible for a period of several weeks to months. Although current technologies enable the construction of adenoviral vectors, which cannot proliferate, they are not completely defective and will express a series of viral gene products. Under certain conditions, adenoviral vectors remain capable of inducing an inflammatory response and subsequent cell lysis. The potential disadvantages of impermanent gene expression and possible limiting inflammatory responses has been addressed with further manipulation of the adenovirus

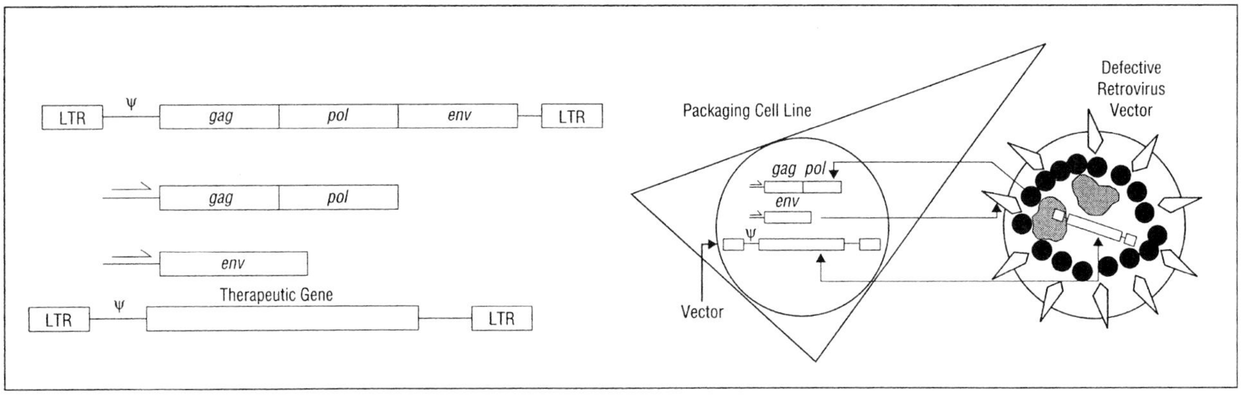

Figure 13-5. Construction of a replication-defective retroviral vector. **A,** The Moloney leukemia virus genome encodes three polyproteins gag, pol, and env, which together consti-tute a retroviral particle. The *gag* and *pol* genes encode the inner core of the retrovirus as well as enzymes required for processing the retroviral gene after infection of the target cell. The *env* gene forms the outer envelope of the virus and recognizes a specific receptor on target cells. Defective retroviral vectors are made using several recombinant genes: one that expresses the gag-pol polyprotein, one that encodes the env protein, and one that contains the therapeutic gene in conjunction with two LTR (promoter and enhancer) sequences and the psi (packag-ing) sequence. **B,** A packaging cell line expresses *gag, pol,* and *env* from the constructs shown in **A.** When a vector containing the therapeutic gene with the LTR and psi sequences is introduced into this cell, a nonpathogenic viral particle will be assembled from the gag, pol, and env proteins that is capable of carrying the therapeutic sequence into cells by the process of infection. (Reprinted from O'Malley BW Jr., Ledley FD: *Arch Otolaryngol Head Neck Surg* 119:1100, 1993, Copyright 1993, American Medical Association. Used with permission.)

genetic backbone to create new vectors that remain for months in the target cell, express fewer viral pro-teins, and have greatly reduced inflammatory responses.[17] Although the safety of adenoviral vectors for gene therapy has not been studied as extensively as retroviral vectors, there is considerable experience with the use of attenuated adenovirus in animal mod-els and in human subjects, which suggests that there is a high margin of safety.[4,6,13,52]

Other Viral Vectors

There exist other viruses that exhibit properties that may be useful for gene transfer, but experimentation with these vectors is still in the early stages. Herpesvirus is capable of infecting cells and persisting indefinitely in a latent state. Vectors using herpesvirus have been constructed that are replication defective and capable of expressing recombinant genes for pro-longed periods of time in animal models.[23] These viruses are not completely defective, and they con-tinue to express many viral proteins that can be cyto-pathic, a property that severely limits herpesvirus for present gene therapy applications.

The human papillomavirus has the ability to persist indefinitely in the host cell as an independent, extra-chromosomal element. This papillomavirus, however, has detrimental transforming potential that must be eliminated before it can be used as a vector for gene

therapy. Another viral vector on the horizon is based on the adeno-associated virus, which, like the retro-virus, can provide a completely defective vector that permanently integrates in the chromosomes of the target cell.[65] Unlike retrovirus, adeno-associated virus integrates in a predictable location within the infected cell, which could make these vectors safer than those that integrate randomly in the genome. A disadvan-tage of the adeno-associated virus us that a wild-type "helper virus" is required to help produce the thera-peutic recombinant vector. The "safe" recombinant vector must then be purified from the potentially cytotoxic helper virus before amplification. Further investigation is required to define the role and safety of adeno-associated virus in clinical application. A summary of viral vector characteristics and gene transfer principles is shown in Table 13-1 and Figures 13-6 and 13-7.

Strategies

Two general strategies exist for administering gene therapy (Figure 13-8). The first and earliest conceived strategy is ex vivo gene therapy, in which tissue from a patient is removed by a surgical biopsy, cells are iso-lated and grown in culture, genes are inserted into these cells (typically using retroviral vectors), and the cells are then reimplanted in the body by autologous transplantation. The second is in vivo gene therapy, in

TABLE 13-1

Viral Vectors Currently Used for Gene Therapy

	Adenovirus	Retrovirus/Lentivirus	Adeno-Associated	Herpes Simplex
Infectivity	Broad	Dividing cells/non-dividing cells	Broad	Broad/neurons
Integration	Episomal	Random chromosomal	Specific chromosomal integration	Episomal integration
Viral titer	High	Low	Low	Low
Max. insert size	Intermediate (approx. 8 kb)	Intermediate (approx. 10 kb)	Small (approx. 5 kb)	Large (approx. 36 kb)
Risks	Immune response	Mutagenesis tumorigenesis	Wild-type virus contamination	Cytopathogenicity
Viral production	Helper-free	Helper-free	Helper virus	Helper virus and helper-free vector

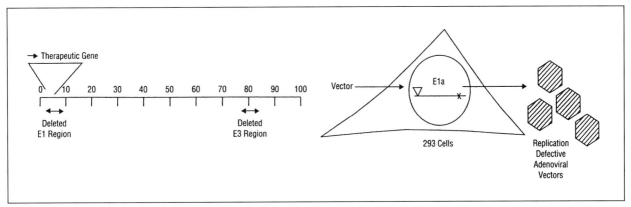

Figure 13-6. Construction of a replication-defective adenoviral vector. **A,** Adenoviral vectors are constructed using a deleted adenoviral genome that lacks the *E3* gene as well as the *E1* gene that is required for producing a proliferating adenovirus particle. Recombinant genes are inserted into the site of the *E1* gene. **B,** Adenoviral particles are produced in the 293 cell line that is able to express *E1* and is thus capable of assembling a viral particle containing only the recombinant viral genome with the therapeutic gene. (Reprinted from O'Malley BW Jr., Ledley FD: *Arch Otolaryngol Head Neck Surg* 119:1100, 1993, Copyright 1993, American Medical Association. Used with permission.)

which DNA or viral vectors (predominantly adenoviral vectors to date) are administered directly to patients.

Ex Vivo Gene Therapy

The initial clinical trials of gene transfer and gene therapy used the ex vivo strategy to deliver genes to lymphocytes, hepatocytes, tumor cells, fibroblasts, or bone marrow stem cells.[1,42] The intent of ex vivo gene therapy is to create a population of cells within the body, which permanently express a therapeutic function. Thus, ex vivo strategies for gene therapy commonly make use of retroviral vectors because they integrate into the target cells and theoretically result in permanent therapeutic gene expression.

The initial attraction of ex vivo gene therapy stemmed from the concept that gene transfer could be performed in the laboratory under controlled conditions without exposing the patient directly to a viral or DNA vector. Ex vivo strategies, however, require methods for cellular transplantation to return the genetically manipulated cells back into the patient. Whereas bone marrow transplantation, lymphocyte transfusion, and skin grafting are accepted clinical procedures, there is little precedent for the transplantation of cells into solid organs. At present, this approach continues to be a difficult field of surgical research. Methods have been described for transplanting hepatocytes,[37] thyroid follicular cells,[50]

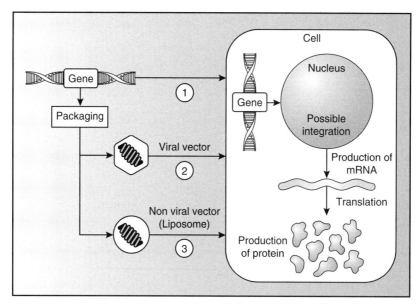

Figure 13-7. Transfer of genes can be achieved through several different delivery mechanisms. Gene transfer was originally described in muscle using naked DNA injected directly into muscle (1). This generally is considered a low-efficiency method of gene transfer but may be very useful for the development of DNA vaccination strategies. Packaging into viral vectors (2) allows for the most efficient gene transfer but is associated with safety concerns. Nonviral vector technology (3) involves coated or condensing the gene construct to allow easy passage into the cell. It is less efficient than viral vector-mediated gene transfer but is considered safer. The final common pathway for all gene delivery is production of a protein resulting in a change in cell phenotype. Alternate gene therapy strategies being developed use inhibitory RNA to decrease the expression of certain genes.

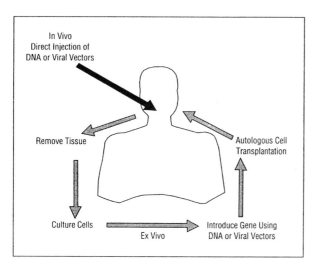

Figure 13-8. Strategies for ex vivo and in vivo gene therapy. In vivo strategies for gene therapy involve the direct administration of DNA or viral vectors to the patients by conventional routes of injection (*black arrows*). Ex vivo strategies involve removing tissue from patients, growing cells in culture, introducing genes into these cells in the laboratory, and then returning the genetically modified cells to the patient by autologous transplantation (*shaded arrows*). (Reprinted from O'Malley BW Jr., Ledley FD: *Arch Otolaryngol Head Neck Surg* 119:1100, 1993, Copyright 1993, American Medical Association. Used with permission.)

myoblasts,[2] or fibroblasts,[66] although the effectiveness of these methods has not yet been established in clinical practice. In the above models, the number of cells that can be transplanted into the body may limit the amount of the therapeutic gene product that can be expressed by ex vivo methods.[37]

In Vivo Gene Therapy

A major recent focus in gene therapy is the application of in vivo strategies for gene therapy in which genes are administered directly to patients using viral or DNA vectors. Investigations in animal models with retroviral vectors have demonstrated that it is possible to infect dividing cells in the liver, endothelium, lung, or tumors in vivo.[1,42] Studies using adenoviral vectors have demonstrated infection of both dividing and nondividing cells in the pulmonary epithelium,[40] liver,[71] muscle,[72] a variety of tumors,[6,52] and other tissues in vivo. Other studies have demonstrated the feasibility of delivering DNA vectors to organs including muscle,[79] thyroid,[68] liver,[80] and joints[83] in vivo.

Whereas the goal of ex vivo gene therapy is to permanently introduce a recombinant gene into a patient's cells, the primary goal of in vivo strategies can vary depending on the tissue and disease for which the treatment has been designed. In vivo gene therapy can be performed with single treatments for certain tumors[6,52] or administered intermittently in response to acute disease or chronically to establish steady-state levels of the therapeutic gene product. The in vivo strategy correlates with conventional regimens of medical therapy, however the gene therapy could provide prolonged or improved effects. Furthermore, the in vivo strategy facilitates the combination of conventional medical treatments or surgical procedures with gene therapy to potentially provide synergistic effects. It is the development of in vivo and relatively noninvasive methods for gene delivery that may allow the widespread application of gene therapy to the routine problems of medicine and surgery.

Applications of Somatic Gene Therapy in Otolaryngology

Gene therapy is relatively new to the field of otolaryngology—head and neck surgery. Its applications are broad and important, and advances in overlapping medical and surgical fields can be applied to the diseases and clinical scenarios common to otolaryngologists. The remainder of this chapter will review the various applications arising from ongoing basic research and proposed clinical trials.

Inherited Disease

A variety of inherited diseases are associated with head and neck pathology such as sinus disease in cystic fibrosis; hearing loss in Usher's, Alport's, or Pendred's syndrome; and goiter in certain forms of congenital hypothyroidism. In some of these diseases it might be possible to place a normal gene in appropriate cells to carry out the function of the inherited, mutant gene. For example, the first clinical trial of gene therapy for cystic fibrosis involved the introduction of a normal cystic fibrosis transmembrane conductance regulator (CFTR) gene into the nasal mucosa using adenoviral vectors.[84] The intention of this study was to assess expression of the CFTR gene in the respiratory epithelium and determine any toxic or inflammatory adverse effects. This trial provided a foundation for future studies in which the CFTR gene would be replaced throughout the respiratory tract using viral or DNA vectors.[12]

Head and Neck Oncology

Many of the initial clinical trials of somatic gene therapy are focused on the treatment of cancer. Gene therapy for the head and neck oncology patients remains a focal point for this emerging strategy. The original head and neck tumor target was melanoma, but squamous cell carcinoma quickly became the target of choice for human clinical trials. Various

approaches for treating cancer by gene therapy have been proposed (Figure 13-9) and are applicable to common head and neck tumors.

New investigations and advances in both viral and nonviral gene therapy technologies should also prove valuable in overcoming many of the obstacles in the application of gene therapy to cancer. One such recent advance is the application of replication-selective oncolytic viruses, which will be discussed later in the chapter. Another advance and rapidly growing field is that of "tumor targeting," whereby the viral or nonviral vehicle carrying the therapeutic gene is either engineered or formulated to avoid classic receptor or vehicle-binding mechanisms and is retargeted to tumor-specific surface receptors or proteins. The preclinical studies and progress to date with vector targeting is beyond the scope of this chapter.

Genetic Modification of Tumor-Infiltrating Lymphocytes

Although the first clinical trial of gene therapy involved only the introduction of marker genes into TIL cells, which infiltrate solid tumors such as melanoma, this trial founded the principle, feasibility, and safety of gene transfer into human patients. The original interest in TIL cells stems from prior studies demonstrating that adoptive transfer of TIL cells

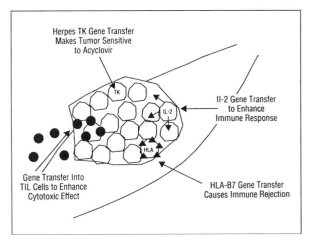

Figure 13-9. Strategies for gene therapy of cancer. Several different strategies have been described for treating cancers by gene therapy. These include expression of cytokines such as interleukin-2 within tumor cells to enhance the immune response against tumor-specific antigens; introduction of a foreign transplantation antigen such as HLA-B7 to induce immune rejection; introduction of cytokines into tumor-infiltrating lymphocytes (TIL cells) to enhance their cytopathic effect; and introducing genes such as herpes TK to make tumor cells sensitive to drugs such as acyclovir or ganciclovir. (Reprinted from O'Malley BW Jr., Ledley FD: *Arch Otolaryngol Head Neck Surg* 119:1191, 1993, Copyright 1993, American Medical Association. Used with permission.)

coupled with the administration of interleukin-2 (IL-2) could cause significant tumor regression in some patients with malignant melanoma.[64] TIL cells, however, are relatively inefficient in destroying tumors despite their ability to selectively infiltrate tumor sites.

Gene therapy is therefore an ideal strategy to increase the antitumor potential of TIL cells by providing concurrent expression of stimulatory proteins such as cytokines. In an early melanoma trial, TIL cells are harvested from the tumors of patients, and a gene for TNF is introduced into these cells.[63] When these genetically engineered cells are transfused into the patient, they are expected to hone in on the tumor and express the antitumor TNF. The expression of high levels of TNF is expected to cause tumor cell lysis with minimal systemic exposure to this toxic protein.[15]

Another clinical trial for cancer patients uses autologous cancer cells modified with a gene that produces IL-2, a cytokine that increases the immunogenicity of cancer cells and suppresses tumor growth.[62] This strategy involves transfer of the gene for IL-2 directly into a patient's tumor, which results in the local formation of tumor-specific cytolytic TIL cells. An excisional biopsy of a draining lymph node allows harvesting of sensitized TIL cells that are multiplied in culture and then transfused back into the patient. The TIL cells are now sensitized to the specific tumor, and when infused into the patient, will hone in on any cancer tissue or cells and enact a cytolytic response. This protocol focuses on patients with primary or metastatic cancer for which standard therapy has proved ineffective.

Direct In Vivo Stimulation of an Antitumor Immune Response

This method of cancer therapy involves introducing genes for various cytokines directly into tumor cells to increase the natural immune response to tumor-specific antigens. The human body has natural cellular and humoral immune effectors that inhibit or prevent tumor cell growth. Examples of such effectors include major histocompatibility complex (MHC)-restricted cytotoxic T cells, natural killer cells, and lymphokine-activated killer cells. The majority of human malignancies, however, arise in immunocompetent individuals, which implies that tumor cells escape the body's natural immune defenses. Tumors are also known to lack or demonstrate deficiencies in the expression of class I MHC antigens, which prevents recognition and attack by cytotoxic T cells.[29]

In animal models, the transfer of the gene for foreign class I MHC histocompatibility leukocyte antigen (HLA)-B7 into colon carcinoma, melanoma, and sar-

coma cell lines has resulted in cytolytic activity from splenic lymphocytes.[47] In this immunologic gene therapy strategy, the gene for HLA-B7 expression is transferred into a cutaneous melanoma lesion of patients who have primary or recurrent tumors or distant metastases that have not responded to conventional therapy.[47] Expression of the HLA-B7 antigen on the melanoma cells is expected to lead to rejection of the primary tumor and metastases by the immune system. B7 gene therapy using nonviral vectors has been approved for a multitumor phase I clinical trial that includes head and neck squamous cell carcinoma.

In a head and neck cancer animal model, the use of adenoviral-mediated delivery of the cytokine IL-2 in combination with a cytotoxic gene has demonstrated synergistic effects on tumor regression.[53] The proposed mechanism is the stimulation of a cytotoxic T-cell immune response magnified by released tumor antigens and cellular debris created by the cytotoxic gene. This work will provide the foundation for future human clinical trials using combination therapy in head and neck patients.

Cytotoxic or Suicide Gene Therapy Strategies

Methods have been described for altering the response of tumor cells to chemotherapeutic agents. One experimental approach involves infecting tumor cells by direct injection with a retrovirus that encodes the thymidine kinase gene from herpesvirus.[56] Since retroviruses infect dividing cells, this virus will selectively enter growing tumor cells, causing them to express the herpes thymidine kinase gene and making them susceptible to chemotherapy with ganciclovir or acyclovir. Because these drugs are relatively nontoxic to the immune system, this treatment not only eliminates the fraction of cells, which are infected with the virus, but also allows for a more general immune response against tumor-specific antigens.

Based on the low efficiency of retrovirus application in animal model and human application, highly efficient adenovirus vectors have been created, which are capable of transferring the thymidine kinase gene directly to tumor cells.[52] This system has been effective in animal models and received approval from the U.S. Food and Drug Administration for a phase I clinical trial in 1996 but was not completed because of insufficient funding.

Modifying Oncogenes and Tumor Suppressor Genes

The discovery of oncogenes and tumor suppressor genes that are involved in the transformation of normal cells into tumor cells has stimulated new approaches for molecular therapy. Oncogenes are naturally present in cells and have proposed functions involving growth and differentiation until a mutation or overexpression activates them to oncogenic potential. Tumor suppressor genes are also naturally occurring, and their expression prevents unrestrained cell proliferation. A deletion or mutation that results in loss of tumor suppressor gene function will therefore allow uncontrolled cell growth. Mutations in the tumor suppressor genes *p53* and *p16* have been detected in a variety of human tumors and a majority of head and neck cancers.[59] (Refer to Chapter 14 for a thorough discussion of tumor suppressor genes and their relation to head and neck cancer.)

Ongoing research in these areas will provide the foundational understanding needed to develop schemes for screening patients for specific oncogenes and tumor suppressor genes and will allow for correction by gene transfer mechanisms. With respect to activated oncogenes, gene therapy may prove effective in blocking the production of oncogenic proteins. In lung cancer experiments, for example, cell lines containing the activated oncogene *K-ras* were transfected with a *K-ras* segment oriented in an antisense direction.[45] Transcription of the anitsense DNA produced messenger RNA (mRNA) that hybridized with the activated mutant mRNA and blocked its translation into the oncogenic protein. This resulted in significant inhibition of tumor cell growth. Although encouraging, this strategy does not reverse the activated oncogene; therefore, strategies must be designed to enable permanent antisense mRNA production before any clinical benefit can be achieved.

Gene transfer of tumor suppressor genes for the treatment of head and neck cancer is another strategy under current investigation. Using nude mouse models, adenovirus-mediated delivery of *p53* has resulted in stimulation of apoptosis and subsequent squamous cell cancer regression.[9] This approach to gene therapy of cancer, however, could prove difficult because it requires the transfer of tumor suppressor genes into a majority of tumor cells. Furthermore, the expression of the suppressor gene is transient, and the tumor regression in these studies has not been permanent. Adenovirus-mediated *p53* gene therapy has moved from phase I to early phase III clinical trials for squamous cell carcinoma of the head and neck.

Conditionally Replicating Adenovirus Therapy

Until very recently, all viral vectors used in gene therapy strategies were replication incompetent. Although the use of replication incompetent or "nonpathogenic" viruses was based on safety precautions, the strategy does not take advantage of the powerful ability of viruses. That is, viruses have the ability to easily infect target cells, replicate, and release viral particles, thereby killing target cells and spreading to

surrounding target cells to continue this process. Continued research and investigation in the fields of molecular biology and the genetics of cancer have led to a greater understanding of the principles of viral replication and the genetics of carcinogenesis. This greater understanding has allowed the development of replication-selective oncolytic viruses for use as novel anticancer therapies.

Conditionally replicating viruses have been engineered to selectively infect and replicate in targeted tumor cells that have inherent genetic defects such as loss of *p53* gene expression. Tumor cells that lack *p53* expression allow select viral replication that kills the host tumor cell, and then subsequent spread and infection of surrounding tumor cells results in further tumor kill. This modification of classic suicide gene therapy into suicide viral therapy may prove to be a key advance in overcoming limitations of gene transfer efficiency in the presently available replication-incompetent adenoviral vectors.

The first replication-selective viral vector to move from preclinical studies to human cancer clinical trials was the Onyx-015 adenovirus, also known as dl1520.[32,41] The key alteration that made this adenovirus replication selective was the deletion of the gene that codes for the *p53*-binding protein, E1B-55kDa. Typically, the adenovirus achieves replication in part through a process by which the E1B-55kDa protein binds a host cell's *p53*, thereby allowing the cell to enter the S phase of cell cycle activity. The dl1520 adenovirus with its deletion of the *E1B* gene will not express the E1B-55kDa *p53*-binding protein on infection of a target cell. The lack of E1B-55kDa expression will inhibit viral replication. However, in target cells that lack normal *p53* expression, the dl1520 virus will maintain its ability to replicate, lyse a target cell, and spread to nearby cells. Because the majority of cancers have a loss of normal *p53* function, cancer cells are the ideal target for an *E1B*-deleted replication-selective adenovirus therapy. There are many other evolving strategies for oncolytic viral vector therapy, and it is not the purpose of this chapter to discuss the present state of this novel therapy in detail. However, it is important to mention replication-selective oncolytic viral therapy because it may be thought of as a type of gene-dependent suicide therapy.

Antiangiogenesis

An approach with future potential in cancer gene therapy involves introducing genes that inhibit angiogenesis in the vicinity of a tumor.[21] A decrease or regression of important vascular supply by the action of antiangiogenesis factors has been shown to cause significant tumor regression in mouse melanoma models. Continued development and investigation of inhibitors of growth and angiogenesis coupled with the packaging of these factors into vectors for gene transfer in vivo may provide alternative or adjuvant therapies for both benign vascular and malignant tumors of the head and neck.

Plastic and Reconstructive Surgery

Great potential for gene therapy exists in the area of plastic and reconstructive surgery. The principle concept of gene therapy as applied to this field will be the expression of growth-regulating factors to enhance repair or regeneration of damaged tissues and to induce local proliferation to fill surgical defects. By introducing genes into cells within a surgical site, local expression of growth factors can be constituted at levels that maximize the therapeutic response. The use of gene transfer to release growth factors, as opposed to simply injecting suspensions of purified factors, will enable regulated expression of the product over a programmed period with restriction of the product to specific targeted layers of tissue. The combination of this property with the incorporation of proper regulatory elements could minimize associated toxicities or unwanted proliferation of nearby tissues.

Reconstructive Tissue Flaps and Wound Healing

A common problem encountered in the use of local or regional flaps is distal flap necrosis with atrophy or even partial loss.[46] Timely angiogenesis and neovascularization is essential for the survival of these tissues as well as healing of the surgical wound. This process of angiogenesis is stimulated by various growth factors such as basic fibroblast growth factor (bFGF) and heparin binding growth factor.[22] Using gene transfer techniques, a gene encoding an angiogenesis factor could be introduced into cells within a reconstructed tissue, recipient site, or primary wound defect. Subsequent to this gene therapy, an accelerated and magnified vascular response resulting from local expression of angiogenic factors could promote healing with improved tissue survival. The use of gene therapy may prove to be very important in free tissue flaps where failure often occurs because of inadequate venous efflux leading to vascular engorgement and tissue destruction.

There are multiple other growth factors that influence the process of tissue repair and regeneration. Examples include transforming growth factors (e.g., TGFα, TGFa), insulin-like growth factors (e.g., IGF-I, IGF-II), platelet-derived growth factors (PDGF), nerve growth factors, and others. Different combinations of these factors can be used to enhance regeneration of vascular tissue, muscle, epithelium, and even nerves.[26] IGF-1 is especially important in maintaining mus-

cle mass and differentiation and may even be able to promote reinnervation of damaged muscle.

bFGF, epidermal growth factor, and TGF-a are potent growth stimulators in dermal layers and may prove advantageous in the management of soft tissue defects caused by trauma or resulting from surgery, a particularly difficult problem for the reconstructive surgeon. For example, the gene for a therapeutic growth factor could be transferred into the surgical defect created by a tongue-jaw-neck resection for oral squamous cell cancer. The local programmed production of healing and growth factors resulting from the direct gene therapy would then stimulate the growth of muscle, fascia, blood vessels, or dermal structures. This growth response would decrease the size of the defect while providing added strength and vascularized tissue to prevent wound dehiscence or extrusion or infection of reconstruction plates. Because of the ability to increase muscle and connective tissue mass and retard atrophy, much smaller flaps could be taken that reduce the overall morbidity and cosmetic defect at the donor site.

Skin Grafting

Skin Grafts are an Attractive Target for Somatic Gene therapy because of the proven feasibility of cultivating epidermal cells ex vivo and subsequently engrafting these cells successfully in patients. Furthermore, previous studies have established the feasibility of effective gene transfer into skin grafts in animal models.[44]

The survival of skin grafts is dependent on adequate nutrition and oxygenation of the graft as well as removal of waste products. Until the blood supply is established, the recipient bed is responsible for the fibrous and plasma exudate through which nutrition is supplied and metabolic wastes are transferred.[54] Gene therapy to increase vascularization or provide local growth factors for the dermal or epidermal layers (depending on the thickness of the graft) could promote early graft take and overall improved strength survival. As a protective mechanism, gene transfer of various cytokines, complements, or antimicrobial factors may prove effective in preventing infection. This particular application could prove invaluable in burn patients who require extensive skin grafting and in cases in which grafting is performed over irradiated tissues, ulcers, or prostheses, where survival is typically poor.

Repair and Regeneration of Irradiated Tissue

Morbidity associated with primary or postoperative radiation therapy is common in patients with head and neck cancer. Inflammation, fibrosis, pain, and even wound breakdown with infection are problems encountered in our patients receiving radiation therapy.[55]

Despite efforts to narrow the x-ray field and block surrounding structures, there is still substantial damage to superficial and nearby tissues. Growth factors such as ECGF[28] have been shown to enhance viability and vascularity in irradiated soft tissue in animal models. Gene transfer of reparative factors such as ECGF may provide spatially precise and regulated expression of reparative factors within the field of radiation and may result in reduced toxicity and overall morbidity.

Applications in Otology/Neurotology

At present, progress with inner ear gene therapy is purely at the experimental stage.[73] Within the auditory system, several vectors have been studied and shown to successfully transfer functional ectopic genes into the mammalian auditory system. Adenoviruses have been shown to transfer functional marker genes such as β-galactosidase (β gal) and green fluorescent protein (gfp) as well as genes that alter the biology of the inner ear such as glial-derived neurotrophic factor (GDNF) to the auditory system.[57,78,81] Alternate vectors include herpesvirus-derived vectors[16,69] that have the advantage of being strongly neurotropic and expressing the transgene for prolonged periods.[69] Adeno-associated virus and liposome packaged plasmids have also been effectively transferred into the cochlea.[33,77] The preservation of hearing in animals treated with infusion of adenoviral vectors into the cochlea and vestibule has recently been demonstrated.[38]

For long-term application of gene therapy for auditory disease, several criteria need to be met. Otologic disease generally is not associated with mortality, therefore unlike gene therapy for cancer, vectors need to have low immunogenicity and cytotoxicity. Vectors have to be replication deficient and nononcogenic and must express their transgene for prolonged periods. Advances in vector design will make it possible to apply the rapidly growing knowledge of inner ear biology to human disease.

Human Gene Therapy and Clinical Trials
Ethical and Social Considerations

Over the past decade, there has been extensive debate about the proprietary and social implications of gene therapy.[20] It is now generally accepted that the implantation of therapeutic genes into somatic cells is conceptually similar to the implantation of cells, organs, or artificial devises for therapeutic purposes, and it raises few novel ethical or social issues.[34] No governmental or religious sector in this country has raised objections to gene therapy research in somatic cells, and the pubic seems to understand the intent to develop novel therapies. In designing gene therapy

clinical trials, careful attention has been directed to ensuring no risk to nonsubjects, to observing the conventional principles of balancing risk vs benefit, and to ensuring fairness, privacy, and confidentiality. Clinical trials of gene therapy are, in fact, not significantly different than trials of nongenetic technologies.

Regulatory Agencies and Approval for Clinical Trials

Because of the unusual public and professional concern about gene therapy, a special review process has been established in which clinical trials are reviewed by both local and federal agencies. Within each medical institution or hospital, an internal review board and biosafety committee have been established to review and monitor human clinical trial proposals and progress. On a federal level, the Recombinant DNA Advisory Committee of the U.S. National Institutes of Health (NIH) and the U.S. Food and Drug Administration have also established a strict review process as outlined in *Points to Consider in the Design and Submission of Human Somatic Cell Gene Therapy Protocols*.[58] These guidelines sanction the application of gene therapy for medical purposes only and explicitly proscribe genetic manipulation of germ cells.

As concerns about the social implications of genetic engineering have abated, increasing attention has been focused on developing models for clinical trials and the clinical issues involved in performing such clinical trials. These issues include establishing procedures for patient selection, documents for informed consent, standards for clinical care, sources of funding, and mechanisms for long-term follow-up.[36]

Status of Clinical Trials Overall

The first gene therapy clinical trial began at the NIH in 1989 and demonstrated that gene transfer could be performed safely and with public acceptance.[30] This original trial involved "gene marking" studies in which a gene with no therapeutic potential was introduced into various cells before they were transplanted into the body to assist in the quantitative study of these cells in vivo. The initial clinical trial at the NIH in 1989 used a retrovirus to introduce a "marker gene" into TILs and demonstrated that these cells would preferentially infiltrate tumors when reimplanted in the body.[64]

The first true therapeutic trial of gene therapy involved retroviral transfer of a gene for adenosine deaminase into the peripheral blood lymphocytes of patients with severe combined immunodeficiency due to mutations in this enzyme.[42] In this temporary therapy, the gene persisted for several weeks, correlating to the survival time of lymphocytes after transfusion and resulting in a significant improvement of the immune status of these patients.

The clinical targets in active gene therapy trials have broadened to include familiar hypercholesterolemia, cystic fibrosis, arthritis, AIDS, Gaucher's disease, leukemia, and solid tumors.[25] The majority of clinical trials focus on novel treatments for cancer or marking trials of hematopoietic cells. The marking of hematopoietic cells has been applied to understand important questions regarding the tumor selectivity of TILs and issues in bone marrow transplantation. For the direct treatment of cancer, targets include melanoma, neuroblastoma, mesothelioma, and brain, colon, breast, prostate, lung, renal, and head and neck cancer. The gene therapy strategies include gene transfer of specific cytokines, cytotoxic genes, and tumor suppressor genes into established, advanced, or recurrent tumors.

As of July of 2002, there have been 636 human gene therapy clinical trials that have been either initiated or completed worldwide, with an estimated patient enrollment of 5000.[24,27,39,60] A summary of the progression of patient enrollment is depicted in Figure

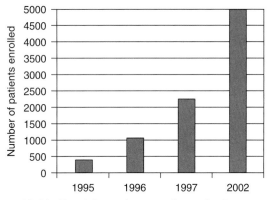

Figure 13-10. Trend for patient enrollment for human gene therapy trials from July 1995 through July 2002.

13-10, and a breakdown of the trials by diseases appears in Figure 13-11. Of these human clinical trials, approximately 505 have been or are being conducted in the United States, with the next highest number of trials at 43 for the United Kingdom. Of these total human clinical trials, 403 are directed at cancer and 55 of these cancer trials are evaluating suicide gene therapy.

With respect to the vectors being used, Figure 13-12 shows the distribution to date. The retrovirus remains the most commonly studied vector, present in approximately 34% of all trials. The adenovirus has advanced to a close second at 27% of all trials. The largest increase over the past 5 years has been in the strategy of nonviral gene delivery, with approximately 23% of all trials focusing on this method. The distribution within nonviral trials is evenly split between lipid-mediated and naked plasmid–mediated gene transfer.

The ongoing or completed clinical trials for suicide gene therapy and cancer overall have provided a few important points for human gene therapy investigation. The first point is that retroviral, adenoviral, and DNA-mediated vectors are at present overall safe vehicles for gene transfer. Except for the unfortunate death of a young man in 1999 who was enrolled in a gene therapy trial for congenital liver disease, there have been rare and limited occurrences of adverse effects with the collection of vectors and genes under investigation.[27,60] There have been no significant adverse events with nonviral or DNA-mediated gene transfer in human trials to date. The second important point is that gene transfer and expression in human cancer cells in vivo is possible with both viral and nonviral strategies. The last point is that tumor responses or reports of regression must be interpreted cautiously because the majority of trials remain in phase I or phase I/II and have limited controls for measuring outcomes.

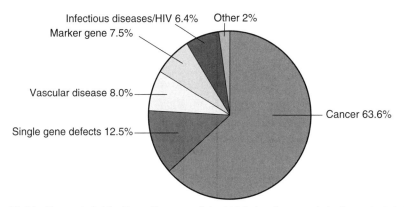

Figure 13-11. Percent distribution of human clinical trials by disease state through July 2002.

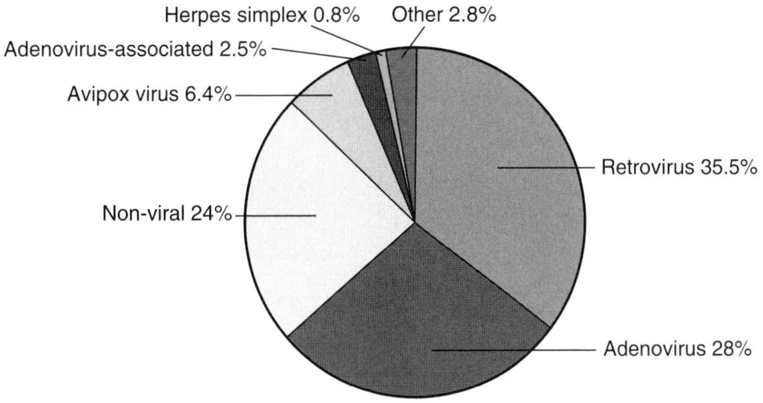

Figure 13-12. Percent distribution of vectors used in human clinical trials through July 2002.

At this early stage of human clinical trial investigation, the studies have focused on patients with advanced or incurable cancer. Although this patient population is a standard choice for establishing the safety of novel therapies, the greatest chance of eventual success with presently available suicide gene therapy strategies can be found among patients with less advanced disease. Another important potential for suicide gene therapy is in combination with immune therapies or standard therapy, such as with surgery or radiation. As advancements in both preclinical development and clinical application continue, suicide gene therapy should achieve a role in the treatment of cancer.

Safety Update for Adenovirus Gene Therapy in Patients with Head and Neck Cancer

Safety with adenovirus vectors in humans with head and neck squamous cell carcinoma (HNSCC) has been widely studied with both Adp53 and Onyx15 conditionally replicating virus for intratumor injection.[8,18,31,48,67] In these human studies, adenovirus injections have been given six or more times to patients with head and neck cancer. Despite the generation of serum antibodies to adenovirus, there have been no significant toxicities identified. Also, investigators claim that these antibodies do not appear to be a limiting factor for effective gene transfer and expression in their human HNSCC trials. The strategy of intratumor injection has been hypothesized as a key issue in limiting the presence of circulating adenovirus vector and thus liver exposure, infection, and subsequent transaminase elevation and toxicity. Collectively, these studies of over 200 HNSCC patients receiving intratumor injections have shown only two transient elevations in liver AST, and otherwise no serious adverse events directly related to the adenovirus gene therapy have been seen.[18] We have also performed preclinical safety experiments in our murine animal model that support the findings in the human trials.[67]

CONCLUSION

The founding work in molecular biology over the past 30 years has enabled clinical application in the realm of gene therapy. Now there are over 600 completed or ongoing clinical trials, and the pace continues. No longer is gene therapy simply a speculative approach for treating disease in the distant future. While the methods of gene therapy are still evolving, current methods are already sufficiently advanced so as to be used in trials of gene therapy for select diseases and to be incorporated into clinically efficacious pharmaceutical products. Gene therapy has great potential not only for the treatment of inherited diseases, but also for providing new treatments for complex diseases such as cancer and for the development of novel adjuvants to standard medical or surgical interventions. Gene therapy technologies should have a significant impact on the quality of medicine, while at the same time providing the additional benefit of cost reduction. As the field rapidly advances, increasing opportunities should arise for physicians to apply these technologies in clinical trials and, eventually, clinical practice.

REFERENCES

1. Anderson WF: Human gene therapy, *Science* 256:808–813, 1992.
2. Ban E, Leiden JM: Systemic delivery of recombinant proteins by genetically modified myoblasts, *Science* 254:1507–1509, 1991.
3. Berkner KL: Development of adenovirus vectors for the expression of heterologous genes, *BioTechniques* 6:616–629, 1988.
4. Brody SL, Crystal RG: Adenovirus-mediated in vivo gene transfer, *Ann NY Acad Sci* 716:90–101, 1994.
5. Capecchi MR: High efficiency transformation by direct microinjection of DNA into cultured mammalian cells, *Cell* 22:479–488, 1980.

6. Chen S-H and others: Gene therapy for brain tumors: regression of experimental gliomas by adenovirus-mediated gene transfer in vitro, *Proc Natl Acad Sci USA* 91:3054–3057, 1994.

7. Chu G, Hayakawa H, Berg P: Electroporation for the efficient transfection of mammalian cells with DNA, *Nucleic Acids Res* 15:1311–1326, 1987.

8. Clayman GL and others: Adenovirus-mediated p53 gene transfer in patients with advanced recurrent head and neck squamous cell carcinoma, *J Clin Oncol* 16:2221–2232, 1998.

9. Clayman GL and others: In vivo molecular therapy with p53 adenovirus for microscopic residual head and neck squamous carcinoma, *Cancer Res* 55:1–6, 1995.

10. Cornetta K, Morgan RA, Anderson WF: Safety issues related to retroviral mediated gene transfer in humans, *Hum Gene Ther* 2:5–14, 1991.

11. Cornetta K and others: Amphotropic murine leukemia retrovirus is not an acute pathogen for primates, *Hum Gene Ther* 1:15–30, 1990.

12. Crystal RG: Gene therapy strategies for pulmonary disease, *Am J Med* 92:44–52, 1992.

13. Crystal RG and others: Administration of an adenovirus containing the human CFTR cDNA to the respiratory tract of individuals with cystic fibrosis, *Nat Genet* 8:42–51, 1994.

14. Curiel DT and others: Adenovirus enhancement of transferrin polylysine mediated gene delivery, *Proc Natl Acad Sci USA* 88:8850–8854, 1991.

15. Debs RJ and others: Immunomodulatory and toxic effects of free and liposome-encapsulated tumor necrosis factor alpha in rats, *Cancer Res* 50:375–380, 1990.

16. Derby ML and others: Gene transfer into the mammalian inner ear using HSV-1 and vaccinia virus vectors, *Hear Res* 134:1–8, 1999.

17. Engelhardt JF and others: Ablation of E2A in recombinant adenoviruses improves transgene persistence and decreases inflammatory response in mouse liver, *Proc Natl Acad Sci USA* 91:6196–6200, 1994.

18. *FDA Safety Alert Reports, 2000, Aventis Studies T-202 and T-207 with RPR/INGN Adp53 in patients with squamous cell cancer of the head and neck.* Washington DC, U.S. Food and Drug Administration, 2000.

19. Felgner PL and others: Lipofection: a highly efficient, lipid mediated DNA transfection procedure, *Proc Natl Acad Sci USA* 84:7413–7417, 1987.

20. Fletcher JC: Evolution of ethical debate about human gene therapy, *Hum Gene Ther* 1:55–68, 1990.

21. Folkman J: Angiogenesis and its inhibitors, *Important Adv Oncol* 42–62, 1985.

22. Folkman J, Klagsbrun M: Angiogenic factors, *Science* 235:442–447, 1987.

23. Geller AI and others: An efficient deletion mutant packaging system for defective herpes simplex virus vectors: potential applications to human gene therapy and neuronal physiology, *Proc Natl Acad Sci USA* 87:8950–8954, 1990.

24. Gene Therapy Clinical Trials, Charts and Statistics *J Gen Med* @ John Wiley & Sons Website.

25. Hanania EG and others: Recent advances in the applicatio of gene therapy to human disease, *Am J Med* 99:537–552, 1995.

26. Hansson HA and others: Regenerating human nasal mucosa cells express peptide growth factors, *Arch Otolaryngol Head Neck Surg* 117:1368–1378, 1991.

27. Hollon T: Gene therapy-a loss of innocence, *Nat Med* 6:1–2, 2000.

28. Hom DB, Girma A, Chang WS: Endothelial cell growth factor (ECGF) application to irradiated soft tissue, *Laryngoscope* 103:165–170, 1993.

29. Isakov N and others: Loss of expression of transplantation antigens encoded by H-2K locus on Lewis lung carcinoma cells and its relevance to the tumor's metastatic properties, *J Cancer Inst* 71:139–145, 1983.

30. Kanzaki S and others: From gene identification to gene therapy, *Audiol Neurootol* 7:161–164, 2002.

31. Kirn D: Oncolytic virotherapy for cancer with the adenovirus dl1520 (Onyx-015): results of phase I and II trials, *Expert Opin Biol Ther* 1:525–38, 2001.

32. Kirn D and others: The emerging fields of suicide gene therapy and virotherapy, *Trends Mol Med* 8:S68–S73, 2002.

33. Lalwani AK and others: Green fluorescent protein as a reporter for gene transfer studies in the cochlea, *Hear Res* 114:139–147, 1997.

34. Ledley FD: Clinical considerations in the design of protocols for somatic gene therapy, *Hum Gene Ther* 2:77–84, 1991.

35. Ledley FD: *Human gene therapy.* In Jacobson GK, Jolly SO, editors: *Biotechnology, a comprehensive treatise,* vol 7b. Weinheim, 1989, VCH Verlagsgesellschaft, pp 399–461.

36. Ledley FD and others: The challenge of follow-up for clinical trials of somatic gene therapy, *Hum Gene Ther* 3:657–664, 1991.

37. Ledley FD and others: Development of a clinical protocol for hepatic gene transfer: lessons learned in pre-clinical studies, *Pediatr Res* 33:313–320, 1993.

38. Luebke AE and others: A modified adenovirus can transfect cochlear hair cells in vivo without compromising cochlear function, *Gene Ther* 8:789–794, 2001.

39. Marcel T, Grausz JD: The TMC worldwide gene therapy enrollment report, end 1996, *Hum Gene Ther* 8:775–880, 1997.

40. Mastrogeli A and others: Diversity or airway epithelial cell targets for in vivo recombinant adenovirus-mediated gene therapy, *J Clin Invest* 91:225–234, 1993.

41. McCormick F: Interactions between adenovirus proteins and the p53 pathway: the development of ONYX-015, *Semin Cancer Biol* 10:453–459, 2000.

42. Miller AD: Human gene therapy comes of age, *Nature* 357:455–460, 1992.

43. Miller AD: Retrovirus packaging cells, *Hum Gene Ther* 61:5–14, 1990.

44. Morgan JR and others: Expression of an exogenous growth hormone gene by transplantable human epidermal cells, *Science* 237:1476–1479, 1987.

45. Mukhopadhyay T and others: Specific inhibition of K-ras expression and tumorigenicity of lung cancer cells by antisense RNA, *Cancer Res* 51:1744, 1991.

46. Myers MB, Cherry G: Causes of necrosis in pedicle flaps, *Plast Reconstr Surg* 42:43–50, 1983.

47. Nabel GJ and others: Clinical protocol: immunotherapy of malignancy by in vivo gene transfer into tumors, *Hum Gene Ther* 3:399–410, 1992.

48. Nemunaitis J and others: Phase II trial of intratumoral administration of ONYX-015, a replication-selective adenovirus, in patients with refractory head and neck cancer, *J Clin Oncol* 19:289–298, 2001.

49. Office of Technology Assessment: Human gene therapy [background paper]. Washington, DC, U.S. Government Printing Office, 1984.

50. O'Malley BW Jr, Finegold MJ, Ledley FD: Autologous, orthotopic thyroid follicular cell transplantation: a surgical component of ex vivo somatic gene therapy, *Otolaryngol Head Neck Surg* 108:51–62, 1993.

51. O'Malley BW Jr, Ledley FD: Somatic gene therapy: methods for the present and future, *Arch Otolaryngol Head Neck Surg* 119:1100–1107, 1993.

52. O'Malley BW Jr and others: Adenovirus-mediated gene therapy for head and neck cancer in a nude mouse model, *Cancer Res* 55:1080–1085, 1995.
53. O'Malley BW Jr and others: Combination gene therapy for oral cancer in a murine model, *Cancer Res* 56:1737–1741, 1996.
54. Paparella MM and others: *Otolaryngology,* vol IV. *Plastic and reconstructive surgery.* Philadelphia, 1991, W.B. Saunders, p 2639.
55. Parson JT: *The effects of radiation on normal tissues of the head and neck.* In Million RR, Cassissi NJ, editors: *Management of head and neck cancer: a multidisciplinary approach.* Philadelphia, 1984, JB Lippincott, p 173.
56. Ram Z and others: In situ retroviral-mediated gene transfer for the treatment of brain tumors in rats, *Cancer Res* 53;83–88, 1993.
57. Raphael Y, Frisancho JC, Roessler BJ: Adenoviral-mediated gene transfer into guinea pig cochlear cells in vivo, *Neurosci Lett* 207:137–141, 2000.
58. Recombinant DNA Advisory Committee: Points to consider in the design and submission of human somatic cell gene therapy protocols. *Federal register,* vol 54, no 169, pp 36698-36703. (Reprinted in *Hum Gene Ther* 1:93–103, 1990.)
59. Reed A and others: High frequency of P16 (CDKN2/MTS-1/INK4A) inactivation in head and neck squamous cell carcinoma, *Cancer Res* (in press).
60. Rochlitz CF: Gene therapy of cancer, *Swiss Med Wkly* 131 (1-2):4–9, 2001.
61. Rosenberg SA: Gene therapy for cancer, *JAMA* 268:2416–2419, 1992.
62. Rosenberg SA and others: Clinical research project: immunization of cancer patients using autologous cancer cells modified by insertion of the gene for interleukin-2, *Hum Gene Ther* 3:75–90, 1992.
63. Rosenberg SA and others: Clinical research project: Immunization of cancer patients using autologous cancer cells modified by insertion of the gene for tumor necrosis factor, *Hum Gene Ther* 3:57–73, 1992.
64. Rosenberg SA and others: Gene transfer into humans: immunotherapy of patients with advanced melanoma, using tumor-infiltrating lymphocytes modified by retroviral gene transduction, *N Engl J Med* 323:570–578, 1990.
65. Samulski RJ, Chang LS, Shenk T: Helper free stocks of recombinant adeno associated viruses: normal integration does not require viral gene expression, *J Virol* 63:3822–3828, 1989.
66. Scharfmann R, Axelrod JH, Verman IM: Long-term in vivo expression of retrovirus-mediated gene transfer in mouse fibroblast implants, *Proc Natl Acad Sci USA* 88:4676–4630, 1991.
67. Sewell DA and others: Safety of in vivo adenovirus-mediated thymidine kinase treatment of oral cancer, *Arch Otolaryngol* 123:1298–1302, 1997.
68. Sikes ML and others: In vivo gene transfer into rabbit thyroid follicular cells by direct DNA injection, *Hum Gene Ther* 5:837–884, 1994.
69. Staecker H and others: Gene expression in the mammalian cochlea: a study of multiple vector systems, *Acta Otolaryngol* 121:157–63, 2001.
70. Stankovics J and others: Overexpression of human methylmalonyl CoA mutase in mice after in vivo gene transfer with asialoglycoprotein/polylsine/DNA complexes, *Hum Gene Ther* 5:1095–1104, 1994.
71. Stratford-Perricaudet LD and others: Evaluation of the transfer and expression in mice of an enzyme encoding gene using a human adenovirus vector, *Hum Gene Ther* 3:241–256, 1990.
72. Stratford Perricaudet LD and others: Widespread long term gene transfer to mouse skeletal muscles and heart, *J Clin Invest* 90(2):626–630, 1992.
73. Van De Water TR and others: Gene therapy in the inner ear, *Ann NY Acad Sci* 884: 345–360, 1999.
74. Vega MA: Prospects for "homologous recombination" in human gene therapy, *Hum Genet* 87:245–253, 1991.
75. Wagner E and others: Influenza virus hemagglutinin HA 2 N terminal fusogenic peptides augment gene transfer by transferrin polylysine DNA complexes: toward a synthetic virus like gene transfer vehicle, *Proc Natl Acad Sci USA* 89:7934–7938, 1992.
76. Wagner E and others: Transferrin polycation conjugates as carriers for DNA uptake into cells, *Proc Natl Acad Sci USA* 87:3410–3414, 1990.
77. Wareing M and others: Cationic liposome mediated transgene expression in the guinea pig cochlea, *Hear Res* 128:61–69, 1999.
78. Weiss MA and others: Viral-mediated gene transfer in the cochlea, *Int J Dev Neurosci* 15(4/5):577–583, 1997.
79. Wolff JA and others: Direct gene transfer into mouse muscle in vivo, *Science* 247:1465–1468, 1990.
80. Wu GY, Wu CH: Receptor mediated in vitro gene transformation by a soluble DNA carrier system, *J Biol Chem* 262:4429–4432, 1987.
81. Yagi M and others: Hair cell protection from aminoglycoside ototoxicity by adeno-virus-mediated overexpression of glial cell lined-derived neurotrophic factor, *Hum Gene Ther* 10:813–23, 1999.
82. Yang NS and others: In vivo and in vitro gene transfer to mammalian somatic cells by particle bombardment, *Proc Natl Acad Sci USA* 87:9568–9572, 1990.
83. Yovandich J and others: Gene transfer to synovial cells by intra-articular administration of plasmid DNA, *Hum Gene Ther* 6:603–610, 1995.
84. Zabner J and others: Adenovirus-mediated gene transfer transiently corrects the chloride transport defect in nasal epithelium of patients with cystic fibrosis, *Cell* 75:207–216, 1993.

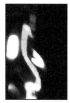

CHAPTER FOURTEEN

MOLECULAR BIOLOGY OF HEAD AND NECK CANCER

Patrick K. Ha
David Goldenberg
Matthew Walpoe
Joseph A. Califano, III

INTRODUCTION

The understanding of the molecular basis of head and neck cancer has continued to increase at a more accelerated pace over the past 5 years. This is a result of technologic advances in molecular biology, as well as an increase in the breadth and depth of molecular biologic research in head and neck cancer in general. As a result, a comprehensive and detailed review of all of the recent advances in head and neck molecular biologic research is beyond the scope of this chapter. The aim of this chapter, therefore, is to provide an overview of recent advances in the field for the general otolaryngologist, as well as to highlight specific areas of inquiry that may spur further interest by a more specialized reader. This chapter details many of the recent advances in the understanding of the molecular genetic pathway of cancer development in head and neck, with a focus on head and neck squamous cell carcinoma (HNSC).

Tumor-specific genetic alterations, as well as other molecular alterations, will be discussed and related to a molecular genetic progression model for HNSC. The impact of molecular genetics on the understanding of field cancerization will also be explored, as well as the molecular basis of environmental factors related to HNSC. Advances in molecular detection and surveillance of HNSC will be discussed, in addition to the molecular basis for novel, targeted therapies based on molecular alterations in HNSC.

BACKGROUND

There are over 40,000 new cases of head and neck cancer every year in the United States, predominantly consisting of squamous cell carcinoma of the upper aerodigestive tract.[74] Advances in surgery, chemotherapy, and radiation therapy have improved the resultant morbidity of treatment, although overall survival rates remain largely unchanged. Clearly, further insight into the molecular basis of head and neck cancer in general could lead to advances in screening, diagnosis, and treatment with improved clinical outcome. The understanding of cancer and its molecular genetic underpinnings has grown rapidly within the past decade. Significant progress has been made in the fields of tumor genetics, protein function, environmental influences, premalignant disease, and molecular diagnostics.

The mechanisms underlying carcinogenesis in the head and neck are similar to those mechanisms and principles found in other solid tumors. Currently, it is generally accepted that cancer arises from the progressive accumulation of genetic alterations that lead to a selection of a clonal population of transformed cells.[43] In an attempt to classify and understand the biology of sporadic and hereditary retinoblastoma, Knudson[87] first put forth his model of the "two-hit" hypothesis in 1971. He described a model in which two copies of the parentally inherited *Rb* gene were inactivated either by mutation or by loss of chromosomal material, leading to development of hereditary or sporadic retinoblastoma. A model of tumor progression was synthesized by Vogelstein into three basic tenets: (1) cancer arises as the result of inactivation of tumor suppressor genes (TSGs) or activation of protooncogenes; (2) there is a defined order of genetic events that lead to development of a malignant phenotype; however, (3) variations in the order of events can occur, and it is ultimately the net accumulation of genetic events that determines the phenotypic expression of malignancy.[43]

The breadth of possible genetic alterations leading to a phenotypic expression of malignancy has grown, although the end targets of genetic alterations almost always involve inactivation of TSGs, activation of protooncogenes, or both. TSGs are those that are normally present in cells and whose function is to regulate and repress cellular functions that, when left unchecked, would lead to expression of a cancer phenotype. Protooncogenes are those genes that, when altered either by aberrant, constitutive activation or amplification, result in inappropriate overexpression or increased activity that results in expression of a malignant phenotype. Alterations of both TSGs and protooncogenes can be caused by several mechanisms, including endogenous mutation, environmental carcinogens, or as a result of the disruption of normal cellular functions by viral, chemical, or other factors. These alterations in the DNA level lead to changes in sequence or quantity of messenger ribonucleic acid (mRNA) intermediates, with subsequent translation into aberrant protein products or an altered level of normal proteins. Ultimately, these genetic alterations lead to a malignant phenotype that can include altered cell proliferation, invasion, metastasis, altered immunogenicity, resistance to therapy, and genetic instability, as well as other phenotypic characteristics common to malignancy.

In 1993, Renan[143] put forth a statistical model suggesting that between 6 and 10 independent genetic alterations need to accumulate before the development of HNSC. The precise number of necessary events required for carcinogenesis is unlikely to be defined. Rather, the conclusion from this analysis is that HNSC likely requires many genetic alterations in its development compared with other solid tumors. This series of genetic changes that must occur for frank malignancy to arise is a result of the 20- to 25-year latency period seen in head and neck cancer. During this time, a cumulative exposure to carcinogens—particularly tobacco, perhaps augmented by alcohol—is believed to be the predominant cause of specific genetic alterations acquired during HNSC progression.

Through the examination of premalignant and invasive lesions, many of these initial genetic alterations have been well described in head and neck cancer, and a genetic progression model has been created to detail the evolution of genetic alterations.[19] In addition, a recent transcriptional progression model has also been described.[58] These genetic and transcriptional alterations have been correlated with the histopathologic stage of premalignant and malignant mucosal lesions to define the order and time course of molecular alterations in the development of HNSC. Early events in the development of malignancy offer an opportunity for molecular prognostic characterization and early detection.

The broad range of DNA, RNA, and protein-based molecular alterations are set within the context of tumor development defined by genomic alteration in the tumor cell. In addition to specific gene products, many of these alterations are characterized within different sets of molecular pathways, defined as a set of genes and resulting protein products that participate in a highly coordinated and linked fashion to provide for a specific function for the cell. These pathways include those functions mentioned above, such as cellular division, differentiation, motility, cell signaling, immune recognition, angiogenesis, and apoptosis or cell death. As knowledge about the multiple, specific alterations present in solid tumors increases, it has become more apparent that multiple, diverse alterations in tumor cells allow for a coordinated inactivation or activation of a specific, single molecular pathway. The implication of these observations is that solid tumors do not require obligatory inactivation of a particular gene, but require alteration of critical pathways of cellular functions through a variety of mechanisms that are often complementary in their focus on a single pathway. Alterations that include the epidermal growth factor (EGF) cascade and the nuclear factor kappa B (NFκB) pathway are examples of systems that are profoundly altered in HNSC via multiple mechanisms, although genetic alterations responsible for these changes continue to be under active investigation. This underscores the fact that significant perturbations in cellular homeostasis can be detected initially on a DNA, RNA, protein, or phenotypic level, and that further study is still required to connect genetic alteration with alterations in transcription, translation, expression, and ultimate biologic behavior.

ENVIRONMENTAL EXPOSURE

Head and neck cancer is associated with environmental toxins, such as tobacco and alcohol. These two exposures in combination have been shown to synergistically increase the risk of development of HNSC, and the molecular mechanisms behind these alterations involving DNA damage and mutations, DNA adduct formation, and detoxifying enzymes are being examined. Indeed, such intense carcinogen exposure and a relative inability to up-regulate detoxification mechanisms may contribute to the molecular alterations seen in head and neck cancer.

Tobacco smoke is known to contain over 55 mutagenic compounds, including aromatic heterocyclic radicals and epoxides.[51] One of the family of enzymes responsible for the detoxification and processing of such harmful chemicals is known as *glutathione S-transferase* (GST). There are five separate loci for the production of different GST subtypes that are responsible for detoxifying many different compounds. There also exist several polymorphisms within these subtypes—these subtypes may delineate those people more at risk of developing cancer in the face of tobacco smoke exposure. One large case-controlled study looked at the effects of two specific polymorphisms, GSTM3 and GSTP1.[78] The investigators reported that those people with a GSTM3 polymorphism had a two-fold higher risk of developing laryngeal cancer. However, in a large meta-analysis, Geisler and Olshan[51] reported inconsistent results across 24 studies looking at the role of GSTM1 and GSTT1. They concluded that there are likely subtle effects of polymorphisms on detoxifying enzyme function and the complexity of detoxification processes in general, and that large population-based studies need to be performed before the effects of tobacco smoke in subjects with these alterations can be correctly ascertained. Variations in other detoxifying enzymes such as UDP-glucuronosyltransferase (UGT) have been implicated in an increased risk of head and neck cancer as well.[196] A low-activity UGT genotype was associated with 3.7-fold greater odds of developing laryngeal cancer in smokers; the odds ratio increased to 6.1 in heavy smokers and was not increased in those who never smoked, suggesting that this enzyme is involved in tobacco smoke detoxification and that the genotype can predict the phenotype in this situation. In summary, the molecular mechanisms behind tobacco smoke detoxification are beginning to be elucidated, but further work needs to be performed to be able to accurately predict those people more susceptible to the development of cancer when subjected to this environmental exposure.

Although these detoxifying enzymes play a role in clearing carcinogens, they may also inactivate chemotherapeutic agents delivered in an attempt to kill offending tumor cells. One study examining a different subtype of glutathione-S-transferase, *GST* π, found that those patients with high levels of this enzyme had a worsened overall survival when treated with neoadjuvant chemotherapy, likely due to the clearance of the drug by the *GST* π.[154] These studies indicate that profiling the level of individual patients' responses to carcinogens or chemotherapeutic agents may be possible by characterizing their ability to detoxify these agents.

Another environmental risk thought to be important in the development of certain forms of head and neck cancer is the human papillomavirus (HPV). HPV is a double-stranded papovavirus that encodes for several proteins necessary for its propagation; these proteins have the ability to disrupt normal cellular functions to allow for viral replication. There are over 70 subtypes found in nature known to infect humans, although the majority of these have no appreciable effect. HPV types 16 and 18 have been implicated in

the cervix as being a major etiologic risk for the development of cancer. This is thought to be due to the E6 and E7 viral protein-mediated degradation of *p53* (a major TSG involved in genomic integrity, proliferation, apoptotic, DNA repair, and other pathways) and disruption of *Rb* (involved in the regulation of the G_1S cell cycle transition).[82,83,185] Because of HPV's affinity for epithelial cells and the potential common exposure risks, many researchers have drawn a parallel to a head and neck carcinoma model. Several conflicting studies have been performed, detailing a wide range of prevalence of HPV in head and neck tumors, perhaps due to the different methods of detection that have inherent sensitivity and specificity shortcomings.[106]

The prevalence of HPV in oral cavity premalignant and malignant lesions ranges from 0% to 100%, depending on the study one examines.* Likewise, there has been confusion as to the prevalence of HPV found in the oral cavity of normal individuals without any lesions; ranges between 0% and 60% have been reported.[12,40,90] These studies point to the fact that there are many different molecular techniques with differing sensitivities that can overrepresent or underrepresent the true contribution of HPV to oral cancer.[106]

In contrast, the presence of HPV in a high proportion of oropharyngeal tumors has been confirmed by a variety of standard molecular techniques. An inverse relationship between *p53* alteration and HPV positivity was also noted, implying that HPV gene product may inactivate portions of the *p53* pathway.[54,60,128] In addition, these studies have demonstrated improved survival for patients with HPV-positive tumors. The inverse relationship between *p53* alteration and HPV positivity in tumors is an example of complementary alterations needed, *p53* gene point mutation or HPV E6 protein production, to deregulate a single pathway (i.e., *p53*). One of the largest population-based studies looked at 900,000 individuals, their antibody status to HPV-16, smoking status, and the development of head and neck cancer.[109] The results suggested that there was indeed an increased risk (odds ratio, 2.2) independent of smoking status for head and neck cancer in those people infected with HPV-16, with a mean interval of 8 years between HPV immunoreactivity and cancer development. Furthermore, most of this risk involved oropharynx tumors; there was a 14-fold risk for developing oropharyngeal cancer in HPV-positive persons. The results of this population-based study are corroborated by much of the molecular literature, suggesting that oropharyngeal tumors are much more likely to have HPV DNA incorporated into their genome than other subsites of head and neck cancer.[45,54,128]

---

*References 12, 23, 46, 47, 68, 149, 170, 171.

Many of these studies looking for the prevalence of HPV in head and neck cancer included samples taken from the larynx, but again, the wide range of reported estimates calls into question the contribution of HPV to malignancy in the larynx. Indeed, some reports focused solely on the larynx indicate that the prevalence of HPV is low, such that it is likely to not play a major role in carcinogenesis.[96,104] However, one recently published study demonstrated that roughly one third of laryngeal tumors had evidence of HPV DNA.[1] Evidence in oral cavity squamous cell carcinoma has also been debated. Prior reports have shown rates of HPV-16 positivity to range from 0% to 100%, but a recent study attempted to use quantitative polymerase chain reaction techniques to eliminate these technical biases.[59] Researchers found that the incidence of HPV-16 in oral cavity premalignant or malignant lesions was quite low, on the order of 1% to 3%, suggesting that many studies likely overestimate the true prevalence caused by inherent errors in technique. Overall, it is clear that HPV plays a significant role in the development of cancer in a subset of head and neck malignancies, namely those involving the oropharynx. When examined with rigorous molecular techniques, its contribution to other anatomic subsites within the head and neck appears to be less clear. Further studies will reveal why HPV tends to cluster in tonsillar tissue, as well as the mechanism behind its ability to transform cells into a malignant phenotype.

TUMOR SUPPRESSOR GENE INACTIVATION AND ALLELIC LOSS

Knudson's hypothesis, as alluded to earlier,[87] demonstrated the inactivation of both parental alleles of a TSG leading to a malignant phenotype. In sporadic and inherited tumors, the loss of TSGs can occur with a mutation of one allele and a loss of the other allele through other mechanisms—in effect, this would equal a loss of expression of both alleles, leading to a functional deficit of the TSG product. Therefore, deletions of one or both alleles can serve as an identifier for potential areas where putative TSGs may reside. The identification of *p53* as a target of inactivation in sporadic colon cancer serves as one of the first successes of this positional cloning approach. Investigators determined that chromosome 17p was frequently deleted in colon cancer. As the locus was further mapped, *p53* was characterized as the target of 17p13 loss[43] and was subsequently characterized as one of the most commonly mutated genes in human malignancy.[69]

Whereas the assays describing gross chromosomal alteration discussed above identify large regions of loss or gain, more specific assays looking for allelic loss involve the use of the polymerase chain reaction to amplify microsatellite markers. Microsatellites are tandem repeat sequences, often in noncoding regions, scattered throughout the human genome. After amplification, the balance of maternal and paternal alleles found in matched normal tissue is compared with those of the tumor or lesion; in this fashion, alleles that are relatively lost or gained can be identified in the samples of interest. This allelic loss is also known as *loss of heterozygosity* (LOH).

Because these microsatellite repeats are located throughout the genome, one can finely map the region containing the gene of interest by looking at the pattern of loss surrounding the area with microsatellite markers known to be flanking that region. Furthermore, tumors can be characterized and identified by patterns of common microsatellite loss.

Using 58 such microsatellite markers on 29 primary tumor samples, an initial comprehensive allelotype of head and neck cancer was performed detailing the proportion of allelic imbalance found on each chromosomal arm.[115] Many hot spots were identified such as 3p (67%), 11q (61%), 17p (52%), and 13q (54%). However, the most frequent loss occurred at chromosome 9p21 (70%).[182] Two of the putative TSGs in this location are known as *p16* (CDKN2/MTS1) and *p14/ARF,* which are produced by alternately spliced transcripts that share the same genomic locus. *p16* works to prohibit cells from entering the cell cycle by inhibiting cyclins CDK4 and CDK6, which then block the phosphorylation of *Rb,* leading to the downstream prevention of the cell traversing the G1 growth phase into the S phase.[62] Inhibition of this cell cycle progression leads to growth arrest of the cell; if this regulatory pathway is disrupted, the cell loses one of the mechanisms by which division and propagation cease. *p14/ARF* is involved in the activation of the *p53* response pathway by inhibiting the association of *p53* with *MDM2,* a *p53* inhibitor. However, very few sequence mutations in the *p16-p14* locus were identified in head and neck tumors,[17] suggesting that there were alternative means of gene silencing occurring.

To explain this apparent paradox, researchers discovered that homozygous deletions of the *p16* locus occurred in approximately 50% of head and neck cancers.[16] Furthermore, promoter hypermethylation has emerged as one of the mechanisms behind gene silencing that does not involve sequence mutations. Methyl groups on cytosine followed by guanine (CpG)-rich regions of gene promoter sequences have the ability to inhibit transcription of that gene, thereby leading to a functional loss of that allele. Both of these phenomena were noted with *p16* and helped to explain the relatively small prevalence of point mutations found in the gene. These findings corresponded with the immunohistochemical studies that determined there was an absence of *p16* product detection in tumors.[139] Additionally, the investigators determined that 66% of their tumor samples demonstrated homozygous deletions, and 21% had promoter hypermethylation, confirming the mechanisms of loss of *p16*.

Another region of interest identified by allelic loss is chromosome 17p; this is the site of *p53*. *p53* has been implicated in several cellular regulatory pathways including DNA repair, control of the cell cycle, and apoptosis.[156] Boyle and colleagues[13] reported a rising prevalence of *p53* mutations concurrent with increasing histologic severity up to 45% of invasive cancers of the head and neck. Indeed, the importance of this TSG in head and neck cancer is pervasive—many of the therapies discussed later attempt to use this gene in the prevention of malignant progression.

Although chromosome 3p demonstrates allelic imbalance in over about two thirds of head and neck cancers, the gene(s) at this locus has (have) not yet been well characterized. Investigators have mapped three distinct regions of loss, raising the possibility that there are in fact three different tumor suppressor loci.[98,190] The FHIT gene was recently cloned from the 3p locus, and it has been shown to have altered transcripts in aerodigestive tract malignancies.[121] However, a genetic correlation of specific gene inactivation in primary tumors with 3p loss has not yet been demonstrated. Future studies will likely identify the genes on this chromosomal arm responsible for cancer progression.

Similarly, chromosome 13q demonstrates LOH in approximately 60% of head and neck tumors, although only a few candidate genes have been identified with limited success. The *Rb* gene locus resides at this site, as well as *BRCA2,* although these genes do not appear to be consistently affected in those tumors with loss of 13q.[116,193] With time, these and other regions demonstrating loss may yield more TSGs involved in head and neck cancer.

PROTOONCOGENE AMPLIFICATION

Although allelic loss is certainly more common than gain, there are some genes that, on amplification of a normal gene product or a mutated gene product, provide an increased stimulus for the cell to grow and divide. Amplification of 11q13 occurs in approximately one third of head and neck cancers; the cyclin D1 (also known as *PRAD1* or *CCND1*) gene resides at this locus and is amplified in a significant proportion of HNSC. Cyclin D1 phosphorylates *Rb*, thereby activating it and leading to progression through the cell cycle, from the G1 (growth) phase to the S (synthesis) phase. Recall that *p16*'s normal function is to downregulate the phosphorylation of *Rb* by inhibiting

cyclin D1. Despite these related and opposing functions, it has been demonstrated that the loss of *p16* and the gain of cyclin D1 are independent mechanisms leading to cell cycle dysregulation.[122]

Amplification of chromosome 3q has also been demonstrated, and a *p53* homologue with several splice variants has been identified,[179] although its function is still under investigation. The proteins *p40/p51/p63* were identified and mapped to the distal region of 3q by using microsatellite markers. However, rather than the allelic loss at this locus that one would expect given its homology to *p53*, an amplification of these genes was detected. Fifty-four percent of primary head and neck tumors showed allelic imbalance at this site, and by fluorescence in situ hybridization (FISH) techniques, the majority of cancer cells were found to have an increased copy number of this locus, suggesting that this region plays a role in head and neck cancer.[192] In subsequent experiments,[66] the overexpression of one of the splice variants, *p40,* was noted to lead to larger colonies in rat tumor cells in vitro, as well as larger squamous cell tumors in nude mice. Therefore, while the function of these *p53* homologues is not entire clear, it is apparent that they are amplified in squamous cell carcinomas and may have an oncogenic role rather than a tumor-suppressive role.

Recently, a large series of 609 HNSCs were analyzed using FISH to determine amplification rates of candidate protooncogenes. These data showed an overall prevalence of amplification of 34.5% for cyclin D1, 12.7% for the EGF receptor, 8.8% for *myc* (a well-described oncogene), 6.2% for ZNF217, and 3.6% for ERBB2 (a protooncogene implicated in multiple pathways involved in cell growth and proliferation). In addition, cyclin D1 amplifications were highly associated with the pharyngeal site in primary carcinomas, implying that this is an alternate mechanism to dysregulate[Au5] the cell cycle in oropharynx cancers that is not required in other subsites.[48] This may indicate that cyclin D1 amplification and oncogenic HPV integration provide for a complementary mechanism of *p53* inactivation in oropharyngeal tumors.

CYTOGENETIC ALTERATIONS

Molecular alterations leading to cancer may be due to large chromosomal translocations, deletions, and amplifications such as those found in many leukemias and lymphomas. In head and neck cancer, it has been well documented that the progression to cancer is accompanied by increasing aneuploidy.[195] These studies have been performed in laryngeal premalignancies and demonstrate tetraploidy in the dysplastic and carcinoma in situ lesions, but not in normal epithelium and rarely in hyperplastic lesions.[184]

Certain regions of the genome prone to loss or gain have been identified in head and neck and laryngeal cell lines and tumor specimens. Specifically, studies have identified large chromosomal deletions on 3p, 5q, 8p, 9p, 18q, and 21q and areas of loss on 3q, 5p, 7p, 8q, and 11q.[21,32,65,77,183] One study demonstrated that metastatic tumors of the larynx have a higher average number of chromosomal alterations and the metastases showed more loss at chromosomes 13, 8p, and 9q compared with primary tumors.[88] The accumulation of gross chromosomal abnormalities with increasing histopathologic severity and the apparent increase in chromosomal change with a metastatic phenotype suggest that there may be defective chromosomal integrity mechanisms that cannot stably maintain the genome in premalignant lesions of the head and neck.

The technique of comparative genomic hybridization (CGH) was first described by Kallioniemi and others in 1992.[80] This method was designed to screen a cell's entire genome for gross alterations in the gain or loss of copy number, also known as *allelic imbalance.* The technique is based on hybridizing normal and tumor DNA that has been differentially labeled with either green or red fluorophores onto a reference metaphase spread. The labels are then read, and a difference in intensity at any one locus is interpreted as allelic imbalance. CGH is well suited for determining these types of alterations throughout the entire genome, up to a resolution of 5 to 10 mega base pairs. The limitations of CGH are that it is still somewhat coarse in resolution and it is unable to detect rearrangements that do not result in loss of DNA (i.e., translocations or inversions).

Many studies have used CGH to examine head and neck tumors and their areas of frequent loss or gain.[11,15,164] One study suggested that certain patterns of chromosomal loss and gain were significantly associated with survival and disease-free interval.[10] There has been remarkable consistency in the areas most frequently affected. For example, all of these studies identified the 3q region as being a hot spot area for amplification and 3p as being an area for loss of chromosomal material. This information helped lead to the discovery of a novel *p53* homologue known as *p40,* mapped to the distal region of chromosome 3q, which has been shown to be amplified in a majority of head and neck cancer samples.[192]

The technique of karyotyping, or looking at the chromosomal banding pattern of DNA in metaphase preparations from head and neck cancer cell lines, was used both in primary tumors[134] and in cell lines.[21,32,77,183] The gross banding pattern alterations could be suggestive of large regions of chromosomal loss, as well as indicating ploidy. It was clear that there

are many gross chromosomal abnormalities that could be detected through this means, although the complexity of alterations could not fully be appreciated with these limited techniques. The addition of fluorescent dyes hybridized to the genome, known as *spectral karyotyping* (SKY), provided an even greater ability to determine break points and translocations.[152] This technique involves hybridizing probes with various labeled antibodies onto a metaphase spread, such that each chromosome is indicated by a different color. Therefore, the entire genome can be examined simultaneously, and complex rearrangements or translocations can be easily detected. However, because each chromosome is painted uniformly, this modality cannot detect structural changes within a chromosome.

For hematologic malignancies that are often a result of translocation events, SKY has proved to be very powerful.[135] Other more genetically complex tumors have been shown to possess many of the same regions of chromosomal loss and translocation. Head and neck malignancies have also been studied in search of patterns of chromosome break points and rearrangements.[10,76] Studies using a combination of SKY and CGH have shown that the two techniques are largely complementary, each providing different information, but overall providing consistent findings in head and neck tumors.[158,166]

PROTEIN-BASED ALTERATIONS

Although genetic amplification is the basis for RNA and protein overexpression, it is not the only significant mechanism by which this can occur. Upregulation of DNA transcription and translation can occur in the absence of an increased number of gene copies. Several gene products have been implicated in cancer progression in this fashion and can still provide meaningful targets for cancer detection and possible therapeutic interventions.

EGF, through a tyrosine kinase pathway, is known to influence cell division, migration, adhesion, differentiation, and apoptosis.[188] The level of expression of EGF has been shown to be a predictor of recurrence and poor prognosis in head and neck cancer.[34,167] It has also been shown that EGF receptor (EGFR) protein overexpression is an early event, as it rises with increasing severity of dysplasia in premalignant lesions.[56] In laryngeal cancer specifically, researchers discovered that EGFR levels were significant independent predictors of metastasis-free survival,[2] as well as overall survival,[105] although these series contained a limited number of patients, and the results have not been replicated in large trials.

One family of downstream targets of EGFR has been identified: signal transducers and activators of transcription (STATs) are phosphorylated and activated by the tyrosine kinase region of EGFR. These STATs can then bind to DNA promoters and regulate gene expression.[63] STAT3 expression has been shown to be an early event in head and neck carcinogenesis and to have an antiapoptotic role in a head and neck xenograft model, suggesting that it plays an important role in cancer progression.[57]

The matrix metalloproteinase (MMP) family of genes and gene products has been studied as potential markers for metastasis because of their ability to degrade collagen, giving those cells the theoretic ability to invade the basement membrane and metastasize. Studies performed on head and neck cell lines[178] and tumor tissue[119] suggest that MMP protein levels are indeed elevated and can help explain one of the mechanisms for tumor spread. In a small study,[99] investigators examined eight primary laryngeal tumors and found a widespread increase in MMP expression levels. One study[120] in head and neck cancer cell lines suggests that EGF levels led to an increase in MMP-9 expression, implying that the EGFR signaling pathway may be involved in tumor invasion and spread via MMP pathways, as well as the known tyrosine kinase pathways.

Another protein overexpresesd in larynx cancer, known as *eIF4e,* has been examined. It has been implicated in increasing the translation of growth promoting, angiogenic, and metastatic factors. Researchers found that 100% of their laryngeal cancer samples demonstrated increased levels of this protein, and using this marker they were able to significantly predict recurrence based on analysis of tumor margins.[113]

NFκB describes a specific heterodimer within a family of transcription factors that serve many functions, including the activation of inflammatory cytokines and angiogenic factors. There are five known subtypes in mammalian cells: *p50, p52, c-rel, RelA,* and *RelB.* These proteins all share a common N-terminus region, known as the *Rel* homology domain. The *Rel* homology domain serves to bind nuclear DNA, dimerize, and bind inhibitor (*IkB*). It is through this *Rel* domain that different combinations of dimers exist, either as homodimers or heterodimers. The C-terminal domains of the different proteins have different functions and can be either inhibitory or activating in nature. *NFκB* refers to a specific heterodimer form, *p50-RelA.*

The *Rel/NFκB* protein normally lies dormant in the cytoplasm, bound by inhibitors (*IkB*). Binding of *IkB* in the cytoplasm hides the nuclear localization site, thereby keeping these complexes inactive. Degradation of the *IkB* proteins can be induced by inflammatory cytokines, leading to translocation of active *Rel/NF-κB* proteins to the nucleus where it can have a variety of functions, either inhibitory or activating.[24] These transcription factors have been shown to control many different cellular functions, including immune and inflammatory responses, as well as regulation of apoptosis and cell proliferation.[138]

NFκB has been examined within head and neck cancer models for its potential role in carcinogenesis. Murine tumor models first suggested that the activation of *NFκB* led to malignant transformation.[36,93] Since then, further work has been performed establishing the mechanism behind this association. It is well known that head and neck cancers produce inflammatory cytokines.[25,29,100,189] Binding sites between inflammatory cytokines such as interleukin (IL)-1, IL-6, granulocyte-macrophage colony-stimulating factor (GM-CSF), and *NFκB/RelA* transcription factors have been identified,[3,35,111,175] suggesting that *NFκB* and its family may play a role in the inflammatory cascade, specifically in tumor models. In head and neck cancer cell lines, the activation of *NFκB* led to further production of IL-8, a modulator of angiogenesis and the inflammatory response.[124] Another study using head and neck cancer cell lines demonstrated that inhibition of *NFκB* led to decreased cell proliferation, suggesting that *NFκB* plays an important role in the regulation of growth, although the exact mechanism remains unknown.[38] Expression microarray technology was used to examine a metastatic murine squamous carcinoma model, revealing a cluster of altered genes related to the *NFκB* signaling pathway.[37]

In summary, *NFκB* has been shown to be involved in the inflammatory pathway known to be active in head and neck cancer and other tumor models. It appears to have a role in the regulation of cellular proliferation, angiogenesis, and modulation of cytokine production, but its exact mechanism behind carcinogenesis remains somewhat unclear. Further studies are underway to determine the pathways behind its action and the possible uses for therapeutic interventions.

GENETIC PROGRESSION MODEL

The correlation of loci that display allelic imbalance due to chromosomal loss and gain with varying grades of dysplasia in premalignant lesions has led to the creation of a progression model involving TSGs and protooncogenes, respectively. The histologic progression of hyperplasia, dysplasia (mild, moderate, and severe), carcinoma in situ, and finally invasive carcinoma provided the structure in which genetic alterations were framed. A genetic progression model was created to examine lesions in each of these categories for similar patterns of allelic imbalance.[19] Even in the earliest of lesions, there were clonal, genetic changes; 30% of benign hyperplastic lesions had loss at 9p21 or

3p, indicating that these losses and the corresponding inactivation of *p16* and *p14/aRF* and putative 3p TSGs are among the first genetic alterations to occur in the progression to cancer. Because of these early genetic alterations, the model offers the hope that there are possible molecular interventions that could be developed to prevent these early lesions from progressing, even before frank malignancy occurs. Further description of the precise genetic alterations is a continuing area of investigation.

PROGNOSTIC FACTORS

A plethora of molecular prognostic factors have been reported by scores of investigators over the past decade. Generally, it is observed that an increasing burden of molecular alterations correlates with poor prognosis, therapeutic resistance, and recurrence, in keeping with the concept that aggressive tumors possess more profound and extensive genetic alterations. It is beyond the scope of this chapter to detail all of the prognostic factors reported in the literature, and the reader is referred to review articles for an overview of this area.[73] In short, a clear consensus from multiple investigators regarding molecular alterations that provide prognostic information independent of conventional clinical prognostic factors for invasive HNSC has been lacking.

However, it has been shown that the pattern of genetic alteration has prognostic significance for premalignant lesions. The loss of chromosomes 9p21 and 3p14 was determined to be a more frequent event in those patients with premalignant disease who progressed to develop HNSC, compared with those patients without LOH at these loci.[101] In another study, patients with loss of only 3p and 9p had a significant risk for progression to cancer (3.8-fold increase), whereas those patients with additional losses (4q, 8p, 11q, or 17p) had an even larger (33-fold) increase in the risk of progression to cancer.[145] In a large study of 150 prospectively accrued patients with oral leukoplakia, aneuploidy was seen to be highly predictive of subsequent development of oral cancer with a mean follow-up of over 8 years.[168] These studies indicate that gross chromosomal alteration is an early predictor of development into invasive cancer.

FIELD CANCERIZATION

Slaughter and others[161] first coined the term *field cancerization* in a study examining the epithelium surrounding invasive cancers, the same year that Watson and Crick aneuploidy described the double-helix structure of DNA. Slaughter and colleagues recognized there were histopathologic changes in the epithelia surrounding invasive oral tumors and reported an increased incidence of second primary tumors, usually close to the initial tumor. Other investigators subsequently confirmed an increased incidence of second primary tumors in the upper aerodigestive tract in those patients with initial head and neck primary tumors.[26,94,173]

Thus, field cancerization originally was a clinical concept describing a mucosal surface in the region near an invasive tumor with premalignant changes and the propensity for second primary tumor development in adjacent mucosa. With the advent of contemporary molecular genetic understanding of malignancy, two theories provide possible explanations for this finding: (1) the areas of abnormality represent independent clones, with a unique pattern of genetic alterations; or (2) these areas of abnormality are genetically related and originate from a common cellular clone. Although these theories are not exclusive, genetic studies performed seem to increasingly suggest that the latter is true, and that lateral spread of progenitor clones throughout squamous mucosal surfaces is a fairly common phenomenon.

Using microsatellite analysis and X-chromosome inactivation, studies have been performed looking at metachronous and synchronous lesions from distinct anatomic sites to examine whether they are clonally related. One such study[6] looked at second primary head and neck tumors, and the findings suggested that the second lesions originated from a common clone.

In a study examining serial biopsies of head and neck premalignant lesions that ultimately progressed to invasive cancer, an accumulated pattern of microsatellite loss was found, with the cancer demonstrating all of the identical losses as the previous premalignant lesions.[18] This study, along with others,[127] builds a case that lesions separated by time or distance share a common clonal origin.

Many studies supporting the theory of malignancy originating from a common clone have also been performed in esophageal cancer. Dysplasias adjacent to adenocarcinomas often share genetic alterations,[144] and a small study of metachronous esophageal mucosa progressing from metaplasia to dysplasia and then to adenocarcinoma share common cytogenetic alterations.[136,137] These concepts have also been shown in a cohort of patients without a history of carcinogen exposure, defining a phenotypic subtype that displays clonal field cancerization.[127] In addition, evidence has demonstrated that expansion of clonal alterations may be more extensive than initially thought in the oral cavity in a conventional presentation of oral cancer.[125] The precursor clones have even been found to migrate or expand up to 9 cm in the esophagus.[131]

A further refinement on this model is that the early genetic alterations may be clonal, with subsequent alterations demonstrating discordance, so the final pattern may be different. For example, the early genetic events such as 3p and 9p21 loss may precede *p53* mutation,[27] so common clones need to be identified by their shared early events. Therefore, the concept of field cancerization is likely a reflection that at least a proportion of lesions derived from lateral migration and subsequent expansion of clonally related cells develop histologic alterations surrounding the primary lesion, and ultimately lead to an increased incidence of subsequent primary tumors.

MOLECULAR DIAGNOSTICS

The discovery of genetic alterations and mutations serves to elucidate the pathways important in carcinogenesis. Furthermore, they open the door to the development of novel assays for early detection, or detection of minimal presence of malignant cells, including the molecular analysis of surgical margins for microscopic tumor foci. Due to the multistep accumulation of genetic events in head and neck cancer, as well as the accessibility on physical examination, lesions in this region offer ideal conditions for molecular testing.

However, because individual tumors often exhibit different molecular alterations, it has been difficult to identify a single assay that is useful in all cancer types. In addition, the assays must be extremely sensitive, able to pick up single tumor cells in a vast sea of normal cells. It has been noted that circulating DNA is often shed by different organs and can be detected by molecular means.[75] Many studies have taken advantage of this and have attempted to search for molecular mutations in blood, serum, plasma, saliva, sputum, bile, feces, and other fluids. Initial strategies involved the identification of genetic alterations in a tumor sample with subsequent analysis of matched bodily fluids such as saliva or serum for identical alterations.[44,157] The disadvantage is that these assays are dependent on an initial lesion sample that possesses an identifiable genetic alteration and may not apply universally to a high-risk population for which molecular lesions have not yet been characterized.

Promoter hypermethylation (a means of gene silencing) has also been used as a marker for uniquely identifying tumor cells. This strategy was used in detecting abnormalities in the serum of patients with lung cancer[42] and in urine samples of patients with bladder cancer.[41] Adenomatous polyposis coli gene hypermethylation in lung cancer was examined in primary tissue, serum, and plasma, and approximately half of the samples demonstrated appreciable amounts of this methylated gene. Detection of high levels of methylation in the primary lung tissue was an independent predictor of poor survival in this study.[181] In HNSC patients, a study examined a panel of four genes known to have promoter hypermethylation (*p16*, O6-methylguanine-DNA methyltransferase, *GST-pi*, and death associated protein-kinase) in primary tumors, and a similar pattern of DNA methylation was also detected in serum DNA in 42% of the cases.[148] Because not all tumors have identifiable methylated genes in HNSC, it has been difficult to create an assay that is sensitive enough for clinical use.

Allelic loss within tumor cells has proved to be difficult to exploit due to the inability of assays to selectively detect those altered cells. To circumvent this problem, large microsatellite panels have been selected to enrich areas of allelic alteration, including instability or shift. This includes microsatellite repeat sequences that have undergone unique alterations in repeat length in candidate tumors, which have also been examined in the population of patients with HNSC.[163] Using oral rinses, 92% of oral lesions with allelic loss or allelic length alteration could be detected, with a threshold of detection of 1 tumor cell in 100 normal cells. However, the mechanism behind microsatellite instability/allelic alteration is not well understood, and it requires many markers for detection because a minority of tumor samples will exhibit alteration at any given microsatellite locus.

The analysis of surgical margins for microscopic residual tumor cells has been performed taking advantage of *p53* mutations.[14] Using unique single-stranded DNA probes complementary to each type of mutation, the investigators were able to identify histologically clear margins that were positive for *p53* mutations. Those patients with molecularly negative margins had a statistically significant decrease in local recurrence. One recent study looked at histologically negative surgical margins and lymph nodes from HNSC resections for microsatellite alterations; in a small sample, they found that molecularly positive margins were an independent predictor of local recurrence.[150] In a different study, researchers were able to detect HPV in the serum of patients with HNSC, and the metastatic tumors were more likely to possess HPV DNA.[20] Other investigators have used immunohistochemical means to detect altered cells in surgical margins, with an ability to predict a shorter disease-free interval for those patients with immunohistochemically positive margins.[114] Currently, a multiinstitutional trial using this margin analysis strategy for *p53* mutations in a prospective fashion is underway under the supervision of the Eastern Cooperative Oncology Group (ECOG). Such detection schemes provide the hope that, in the future, more simple and feasible assays can be created to assist with clinical judgments and patient care.

A myriad of studies attempting to take advantage of other known molecular alterations in head and neck and laryngeal primary tumors have been performed to predict prognosis, lymph node metastasis, and local recurrence. Although these and other reports often provide suggestions that these molecular analyses can be predictive of outcomes, the studies are often hampered by small sample sizes and an inability to adequately control for factors such as tumor stage, smoking status, and age. Thus, these studies suggest that molecular markers are feasible to use in clinical settings, but they have not been rigorously tested. To date, large, prospective studies have not been performed to adequately assess any of the possible molecular prognostic markers in primary tumors for their potential clinical relevance.

MOLECULAR-DIRECTED THERAPY

The accessibility of the mucosa of the head and neck regions provides easy access for the direct delivery of therapeutic agents. The genetic and protein alterations described above provide many possible targets for therapeutic intervention. The purpose of a molecular understanding of cancer is that knowledge of the etiology and pathway of disease will allow for more effective treatment with enhanced safety. However, defining the appropriate molecular target has proved difficult, and devising an appropriate means to deliver therapy to abnormal cells without affecting normal tissue has been challenging as well. Nonetheless, there are currently several promising avenues of investigation.

As described previously, the EGF family of receptors has been known to be up-regulated in head and neck cancers. This finding was first reported in breast cancer with the discovery that 30% of breast cancers overexpressed the *HER2/neu* oncogene,[159] which is homologous to the EGF receptor. These patients fared worse than those who did not overexpress the EGFR homologue. This finding has led to the creation of trastuzumab (Herceptin), a monoclonal antibody that binds and blocks the growth factor receptor on *HER2*.[108] Herceptin has been used in phase III trials as adjuvant treatment for node-positive tumors in nonmetastatic breast cancer. Currently, trials are underway in head and neck cancer to try to capitalize on the success of this agent in breast cancer treatment. (This is described in greater detail in the subsequent "Immunotherapy" section.)

Another approach to altering the EGF pathway is by inhibiting tyrosine kinase activity, which is the active portion of the EGF receptor/ligand complex. Specific compounds have been specifically designed to target the tyrosine kinase domain of this receptor (for example, ZD1839, or Iressa), which can be delivered orally with good pharmacokinetic properties.[4] It has been found that not only is this drug effective in blocking the EGF receptor, it is also effective in suppressing the growth of cell lines overexpressing HER.[107] Clinical trials of these compounds are beginning in patients with breast cancer and head and neck cancer as well.

Gene therapy involves the alteration or introduction of DNA into tumor cells that will either lead to cell killing or correction of the molecular defect in a specific population of affected cells. The overwhelming challenge is to provide a selective ability for the introduced DNA to target or kill nearly all tumor cells, while sparing normal tissue. Many different methods of gene transfer systems have been attempted, including adenovirus, retrovirus, liposomal mediated delivery, electroporation, and direct injection, each with limited success.

One of the first attempts at gene therapy in the head and neck involved replacement of the *p53* gene. The hope was that by restoring the gene, cells that were defective in the apoptosis pathway could then proceed to lysis. Wild-type *p53* was replaced using an adenovirus vector as a surgical adjuvant therapy in patients with locoregionally advanced head and neck cancer with some success.[28] Other studies have been performed using different tumor sites, although the results were somewhat equivocal. The delivery of the corrected gene must be made to all of the tumor cells for the wild type *p53* to be inserted—studies have shown that the tumors may have lost receptors necessary for adenoviral binding and gene delivery.[172] Rather than relying solely on replacement of this gene, other investigators are trying combination therapy with radiation[130] or chemotherapy[118] to further sensitize those cells to go into the apoptotic pathway.

The ONYX O-15 adenovirus was created in an attempt to select those cells with *p53* mutations.[9] The ONYX virus is unable to replicate when wild type *p53* is present; only when exposed to proteins that inactivate *p53* is the virus able to replicate, lyse the cell, and spread to neighboring cells. A phase II trial in patients with recurrent head and neck cancer was performed: one group received ONYX-O15 injections in combination with intravenous cisplatin and 5-fluorouracil, and one group received chemotherapy alone.[84] After 6 months, the investigators noted that the tumors treated with ONYX and chemotherapy did not progress, whereas those treated with chemotherapy alone all progressed. Phase II trials of the direct tumor injection of ONYX-015 alone have also been performed in patients with refractory head and neck cancer demonstrating modest success; 10% to 14% of patients had partial to complete responses, although overall survival was not significantly affected.[117]

Despite early success, future trials with the ONYX virus are currently on hold.

Phase I trials have been performed with a lipid-mediated transfer through direct tumor injection of *E1A*[184] (an adenovirus gene that induces apoptosis of cancer cells and sensitizes cancer cells to chemotherapeutic agents). *HER2/neu* levels were assayed as a surrogate biomarker end point, and two of five patients who demonstrated overexpression of the receptor at baseline had a down-regulation of receptor levels. Further studies looking at the use of this drug in combination therapies are likely to be pursued.

IMMUNOTHERAPY

Immunotherapy, defined broadly as any manipulation of the immune system to achieve a desired treatment effect, is a relatively new but promising therapeutic strategy for the treatment of cancer. The increasing popularity of this therapeutic technique stems in large part from the fact that immune cells can theoretically be specifically targeted without the need for potentially toxic foreign chemicals or agents. In addition, immunotherapy can be integrated and even enhanced by existing therapies such as surgery, chemotherapy, and radiation. Like vaccination against infectious diseases, tumor vaccines rely on the concept of exploiting antigenic components of target cells. This therapeutic modality is based on the assumptions that: (1) the tumors express antigens or neoepitopes that are either not found or present in low levels on normal cells; and (2) the immune system can be appropriately activated to exterminate such cells. However, unlike many microbial organisms, neoplastic cells derived from a patient's own tissues vary only slightly from normal cells. In addition, many potential antigens expressed by these cells have been constitutively present throughout development and therefore are not recognized as foreign. This is because the immune system has evolved a network of sophisticated checkpoints to prevent autoimmunity collectively known as "tolerance." This includes mechanisms such as positive and negative thymic selection, as well as peripheral means such as anergy, suppression, and ignorance, all designed to prevent recognition of "self" antigens as "other."

Unfortunately, in HNSC, the presence of tolerance is further confounded by the fact that in these patients' T cells, lymphocytes that coordinate recognition of foreign antigens in normal cells are often dysfunctional. A high proportion of both tumor-infiltrating lymphocytes (TILs) and peripheral blood lymphocytes (PBLs) in patients with HNSC have fragmented DNA and express markers such as annexin V that indicate the occurrence of apoptosis (programmed cell death).[39,67,89,141,186] In addition, both TILs and PBLs have an impaired ability to proliferate and transduce integral signaling pathways.[89,140-142,186] This functional inactivation may be related to a lack of expression of the z portion of the CD3 T-cell receptor complex that is essential for signaling transduction, as well as increased expression of FAS ligand.[141] It is predominantly CD8+ T cells that display these dysfunctional attributes, whereas CD4+ T cells remain comparatively unaffected.[146,186]

The deficits seen in both TIL and PBL appear to have significant clinical significance in patients with HNSC. HNSC patients with a high percentage of apoptotic TIL have a significantly lower 5-year survival rate than those that do not.[140] Patients with HNSC have significantly lower levels of thymic output of naïve T cells than healthy control subjects.[186] This indicates that patients with such deficits do not compensate well for frequent T-cell apoptosis.

Despite the fact that patients with HNSC display this degree of relative immunosuppression, there has been a recent increase in the number of translational and clinical immunotherapeutic trials in HNSC. Early attempts at immunotherapy in patients with HNSC mainly focused on the administration of nonspecific agents such as the cytokine IL-2.[112,187] However, it was found that only a small minority of patients responded to IL-2 and similar agents, and these responses were usually of short duration. More recent studies have focused on ways to improve response rates and extend remissions with cytokines through a variety of strategies. Treating peripheral blood mononuclear cells from HNSC patients with the combination of IL-2 and IL-12 improved cytolytic activity compared with treatment using either alone.[136] In addition, the lack of response to IL-2 may be due to inadequate expression of this cytokine at the tumor site.[123] This hypothesis was reinforced by the demonstration of regression of a significant proportion of implanted murine floor of mouth tumors after peritumoral injection of vaccinia virus that had been transduced with IL-2.[132] Other investigators have hypothesized that the potential reason for lack of efficacy with IL-2 and other cytokines in HNSC may be a lack of sufficient costimulation, an essential element for T-cell activation.[174]

Recently, in a phase II clinical trial, there was an attempt to improve the response of HNSC patients to cytokine-based therapy by using the natural cytokine mixture (IRX-2), in 15 patients with stage II–IV HNSC.[5] Patients were given a 21-day cycle of perilymphatic IRX-2 in combination with cyclophosphamide, indomethacin, and zinc with surgery, radiation, or both. Although it is difficult to draw substantial conclusions from this study based on the low number of patients enrolled with a variety of clinical presentations, a complete response was seen in one patient and a partial response was seen in several others. The treatment regimen was well tolerated, and all patients enrolled in the trial had evidence of a histologic response. Based on these encouraging results, a phase III trial including a larger number of patients is planned for the near future.

In addition to cytokine therapy, antibody targeting of oncogenic proteins in HNSC has shown some therapeutic promise. IMC-225, a human-mouse chimerized monoclonal antibody directed against the EGFrR, originally developed for colon carcinoma, has been used in clinical trials in HNSC. The mechanism of action of IMC-225 appears to be that it binds to the extracellular domain of the EGFR in a manner that prevents binding by natural ligands, such as EGF and tumor necrosis factor α. Via this binding blockade, IMC-225 inhibits up-regulation of several signaling pathways including those that promote tumor cell cycle progression, angiogenesis, and metastasis.[64] In a phase Ib clinical trial, IMC-22 was combined with cisplatin.[155] Patients in this trial demonstrated high levels of EGFR saturation, and 67% of subjects showed a partial response, whereas 22% demonstrated complete responses to this regimen.

HER-2/neu (*erB2-2*), a second member of the EGFR family, is overexpressed in approximately 40% of oral squamous cell carcinomas[191] and also has been targeted for antibody therapy. Imajo and colleagues showed the *HER-2/neu* monoclonal antibody rhumAbHER2 was effective at inhibiting growth of oral squamous cell carcinoma lines in culture.[180] This effect was augmented by the combining rhumAbHER2 with radiation therapy. In addition to rhumAbHER2, trastuzumab (Herceptin) has induced response rates in 10% to 20% of women with refractory *HER-2/neu* overexpressing breast carcinomas.[153] The number of responders to this agent increases to nearly 50% when combined with chemotherapy.[160]

Although monoclonal antibodies hold much therapeutic promise, much effort is being spent to develop immunotherapeutic strategies that induce adaptive immune responses that are sufficient to eradicate tumor, while not affecting normal host tissues. One of the most attractive ways to achieve this is via whole-cell, dendritic (antigen-presenting) cell– and peptide-based vaccinations. One study examined the efficacy of an autologous whole-cell vaccine and adoptive T-cell immunotherapy in 17 patients with unresectable HNSC.[177] Patients were first given an injection of irradiated autologous T cells at a single site, followed by three injections of GM-CSF at that site. Approximately 10 days later, the draining lymph nodes were excised and the T cells isolated. These were then expanded in culture in the presence of IL-2 and enterotoxin A, and then reinjected into these patients. Overall, the vaccines were well tolerated with minimal adverse effects. Three patients experienced stabilization of disease, and one patient was disease free 4 years after the implementation of therapy. Although these results are promising, it should be noted that autologous tumor vaccines are expensive and labor intensive.

In addition to whole-cell vaccines, dendritic cell–based vaccines are being developed for HNSC. Dendritic cells are powerful professional antigen-presenting cells that have the ability to phagocytose apoptotic cells and then present peptides to T cells, a process called *cross-priming*.[72] Dendritic cells exposed to the proper antigenic proteins can serve as a vehicle for antigen presentation and T cell priming. This concept was recently illustrated in a DBA2/J mouse model of HNSC.[162] Mice that were treated with this vaccine regimen demonstrated a significant decrease in tumor burden verses than control mice, with little evidence of toxicity.

Despite the fact that using irradiated tumor cells is an efficacious therapeutic technique, targeting antigens known to activate T cells has the potential to lead to a more specific and robust immune response. Although there are no HNSC-specific antigens as of yet, there are a variety of immunogenic proteins present in these tumors that have been shown in other tissue types to be effective targets of vaccination. For example, carcinoembryonic antigen (CEA) has been shown to be a safe and efficacious target in patients with tumors of the digestive tract.[103] In addition, patients can mount CEA-specific T-cell responses that are capable of lysing colorectal carcinoma cells.[30] Recently, Van Waes and colleagues[81] evaluated the feasibility of targeting CEA with a vaccine in head and neck cancer. This group demonstrated that CEA was expressed in between 50% and 100% of HNSC tumors, depending on the site. In a slightly different vein, Ishikawa and colleagues[92] found that a high percentage of patients with various head and neck cancers expressed several isoforms of the melanoma antigen E (MAGE) tumor-associated antigen. This protein is an attractive target for immunotherapy because it is expressed in a variety of tumors and is comparatively absent in noncancerous tissues. MAGE proteins have been shown to be effective targets in melanoma[147] and therefore offer a potential target for immunotherapy in HNSC. Lastly, as alluded to above, HPV is a factor in the development of a subset of head and neck cancers.[53] As HPV vaccines have shown efficacy in trials of women with cervical carcinoma[110] and patients with HPV-expressing tumors infected with the same isotype (type 16),[53] a vaccine trial targeting this strain of HPV in patients at high risk for oral squamous cell carcinoma holds great therapeutic promise, in particular as a prophylactic vaccine given before tumor development, in a manner analogous to strategies described for cervical cancer.[86]

Immunotherapy for HNSC is a relatively new but promising therapeutic strategy. Difficulties with achieving efficacy with this approach are due mainly to problems with host tolerance and the relative immunosuppression of patients with HNSC. Despite this fact, both clinical and translational trials with cytokines, monoclonal antibodies, and a variety of other strategies have yielded promising results with little evidence of host toxicity. In HNSC and other tumor types, immunotherapy has been implemented successfully in patients undergoing a variety of other therapeutic modalities, often in patients with end-stage disease. Future efforts will hopefully find ways to circumvent immune tolerance and overcome malignancy-related immune dysfunction to produce regimens with better efficacy.

CHEMOPREVENTION

Much of the therapy of head and neck cancer is focused on treating the disease after it has already progressed to malignancy. However, since head and neck cancer often presents initially with premalignant disease, and there is a defined set of high-risk individuals, many researchers have begun the search for agents that can either prevent disease from occurring, prevent recurrent disease, or prevent disease progression.

The concept of chemoprevention was first proposed by Sporn and colleagues,[165] who looked at the protective effects of vitamin A and its derivatives on carcinogenesis. The mechanism of action is thought to be via binding of retinoic acid receptor molecules,[85,91] which then function as angiogenic and growth-regulating factors.[97,169] In a landmark study, the utilization of high-dose 13-cis retinoic acid in patients with known head and neck cancers proved helpful in preventing the development of second primary tumors[71] and in the treatment of oral leukoplakias,[70] although there was significant toxicity associated with this therapy, including skin lesions, conjunctivitis, and cheilitis. Furthermore, when therapy was discontinued, the risk of disease development returned to baseline after about 2 years.[7] Therefore, the investigation of a low-dose, prospective treatment regimen that has shown promise is underway, as well as many other studies looking at different formulations involving the retinoic acid receptor pathway.

Cyclooxygenase (COX)-1 and -2 inhibitors have also been studied as possible mediators of prostaglandins and inflammation that often accompanies many different tumors. Prostaglandins have long been known to be elevated in head and neck cancers as well, presumably due to the up-regulation of COX-1 and -2.[8,79] Animal models suggested that aspirin or ibuprofen

could inhibit the formation of buccal tumors.[31,129] Colon cancer was among the first tumors studied widely in humans, beginning with epidemiologic evidence that aspirin reduced the risk of colon cancer development.[176] Sulindac was shown prospectively to reduce the number and size of colonic polyps in patients afflicted with this disease.[52] Studies also followed in colorectal, breast, lung, and esophageal carcinomas.* The mechanism behind the effect of COX-2 inhibitors appears to be multifactorial.[33,95] The overexpression of COX-2 leads to decreased apoptosis, thereby prolonging the life span of abnormal cells. Furthermore, inflammation may be a risk factor for epithelial carcinogenesis because it is often found in these malignancies. Angiogenesis may also be tied in to the COX-2 pathway because vascular endothelial growth factor (VEGF) expression is elevated by high COX-2 levels.[50] Thus, there are several mechanistic reasons why COX-2 inhibitors would be beneficial in preventing recurrence, development, or progression of head and neck lesions, especially in high-risk patients. These prospective studies are currently underway in human subjects.

Newer perspectives are also gained in the area of chemoprevention. Retinoids have been shown to regulate cell growth by activating retinoic acid receptor and retinoid X receptor genes, and they have shown a chemopreventive effect in premalignant head and neck lesions. The treatment of head and neck cell lines has been shown to inhibit growth[169] and may have some antiangiogenic effects as well.[97] The effects of 13-cis retinoic acid, interferon α, and α-tocopherol were studied in 22 patients with high-grade premalignant lesions of the head and neck and were examined for subsequent molecular and histologic alterations.[102] The histologic responses were often more pronounced than the molecular alterations, but further studies need to be performed in large populations to determine their efficacy.

CONCLUSIONS

Novel techniques have led to the discovery of many genes and gene products important in the development of HNSC and laryngeal cancer. TSGs and oncogenes have been identified, and many of their roles have been elucidated in a genetic progression model. As these molecular pathways are better understood, the information obtained will increasingly be used to guide patient therapy. Specifically, advances will likely be made in: (1) molecular characterization of steps leading to HNSC; (2) molecular screening, staging, and surveillance; (3) molecularly based therapy including gene transfer and small molecule therapy

---

*References 22, 49, 55, 61, 133, 151.

directed at specific molecular pathways involved in neoplasia; and (4) chemopreventive therapy for high-risk patients after molecular characterization of those patients who are at high risk for development of HNSC.

REFERENCES

1. Almadori G and others: Human papillomavirus infection and epidermal growth factor receptor expression in primary laryngeal squamous cell carcinoma, *Clin Cancer Res* 7:3988–3993, 2001.
2. Almadori G and others: Epidermal growth factor receptor expression in primary laryngeal cancer: an independent prognostic factor of neck node relapse, *Int J Cancer* 84:188–191, 1999.
3. Bailly S and others: The transcription factor AP-1 binds to the human interleukin 1 alpha promoter, *Eur Cytokine Netw* 7:125–128, 1998.
4. Barker AJ and others: Studies leading to the identification of ZD1839 (IRESSA): an orally active, selective epidermal growth factor receptor tyrosine kinase inhibitor targeted to the treatment of cancer, *Bioorg Med Chem Lett* 11:1911–1914, 2001.
5. Barrera JL and others: Combination immunotherapy of squamous cell carcinoma of the head and neck: a phase 2 trial, *Arch Otolaryngol Head Neck Surg* 126:345–351, 2000.
6. Bedi GC and others: Multiple head and neck tumors: evidence for a common clonal origin, *Cancer Res* 56:2484–2487, 1996.
7. Benner SE and others: Prevention of second primary tumors with isotretinoin in patients with squamous cell carcinoma of the head and neck: long-term follow-up, *J Natl Cancer Inst* 86:140–141, 1994.
8. Bennett A and others: Prostaglandin-like material extracted from squamous carcinomas of the head and neck, *Br J Cancer* 41:204–208, 1990.
9. Bischoff JR and others: An adenovirus mutant that replicates selectively in p53-deficient human tumor cells, *Science* 274:373–376, 1996.
10. Bockmuhl U and others: Genetic imbalances with impact on survival in head and neck cancer patients, *Am J Pathol* 157:369–375, 2000.
11. Bockmuhl U and others: Genomic alterations associated with malignancy in head and neck cancer, *Head Neck* 20:145–151, 1998.
12. Bouda M and others: "High risk" HPV types are frequently detected in potentially malignant and malignant oral lesions, but not in normal oral mucosa, *Mod Pathol* 13:644–653, 2000.
13. Boyle JO and others: Gene mutations in saliva as molecular markers for head and neck squamous cell carcinomas, *Am J Surg* 168:429–432, 1994.
14. Brennan JA and others: Molecular assessment of histopathological staging in squamous-cell carcinoma of the head and neck, *N Engl J Med* 332:429–435, 1995.
15. Brzoska PM and others: Frequent novel DNA copy number increase in squamous cell head and neck tumors, *Cancer Res* 55:3055–3059, 1995.
16. Cairns P and others: Frequency of homozygous deletion at p16/CDKN2 in primary human tumours, *Nat Genet* 11:210–212, 1995.
17. Cairns P and others: Rates of p16 (MTS1) mutations in primary tumors with 9p loss, *Science* 265:415–417, 1994.
18. Califano J and others: Genetic progression and clonal relationship of recurrent premalignant head and neck lesions, *Clin Cancer Res* 6:347–352, 2000.
19. Califano J and others: Genetic progression model for head and neck cancer: implications for field cancerization, *Cancer Res* 56:2488–2492, 1996.
20. Capone RB and others: Detection and quantitation of human papillomavirus (HPV) DNA in the sera of patients with HPV-associated head and neck squamous cell carcinoma, *Clin Cancer Res* 6:4171–4175, 2000.
21. Carey TE, Van Dyke DL, Worsham MJ: Nonrandom chromosome aberrations and clonal populations in head and neck cancer, *Anticancer Res* 13:2561–2567, 1993.
22. Castonguay A, Rioux N: Inhibition of lung tumourigenesis by sulindac: comparison of two experimental protocols, *Carcinogenesis* 18:491–496, 1997.
23. Chang F and others: Human papillomavirus (HPV) infections and their associations with oral disease, *J Oral Pathol Med* 20:305–317, 1991.
24. Chen FE, Ghosh G: Regulation of DNA binding by Rel/NF-kappaB transcription factors: structural views, *Oncogene* 18:6845–6852, 1999.
25. Chen Z and others: Expression of proinflammatory and proangiogenic cytokines in patients with head and neck cancer, *Clin Cancer Res,* 5:1369–1379, 1999.
26. Christensen PH and others: Hyperfrequency of pulmonary cancer in a population of 415 patients treated for laryngeal cancer, *Laryngoscope* 97:612–614, 1987.
27. Chung KY and others: Discordant p53 gene mutations in primary head and neck cancers and corresponding second primary cancers of the upper aerodigestive tract, *Cancer Res* 53:1676–1683, 1993.
28. Clayman GL and others: Adenovirus-mediated p53 gene transfer in patients with advanced recurrent head and neck squamous cell carcinoma, *J Clin Oncol* 16:2221–2232, 1998.
29. Cohen RF and others: Interleukin-8 expression by head and neck squamous cell carcinoma, *Arch Otolaryngol Head Neck Surg* 121:202–209, 1995.
30. Conry RM and others: Safety and immunogenicity of a DNA vaccine encoding carcinoembryonic antigen and hepatitis B surface antigen in colorectal carcinoma patients, *Clin Cancer Res* 8:2782–2787, 2002.
31. Cornwall H, Odukoya O, Shklar G: Oral mucosal tumor inhibition by ibuprofen, *J Oral Maxillofac Surg* 41:795–800, 1983.
32. Cowan JM, Beckett MA, Weichselbaum RR: Chromosome changes characterizing in vitro response to radiation in human squamous cell carcinoma lines, *Cancer Res* 53:5542–5547, 1993.
33. Dannenberg AJ and others: Cyclo-oxygenase 2: a pharmacological target for the prevention of cancer, *Lancet Oncol* 2:544–551, 2001.
34. Dassonville O and others: Expression of epidermal growth factor receptor and survival in upper aerodigestive tract cancer, *J Clin Oncol* 11:1873–1878, 1993.
35. Dendorfer U, Oettgen P, Libermann TA: Multiple regulatory elements in the interleukin-6 gene mediate induction by prostaglandins, cyclic AMP, and lipopolysaccharide, *Mol Cell Biol* 14:4443–4454, 1994.
36. Dong G and others: The host environment promotes the constitutive activation of nuclear factor-kappaB and proinflammatory cytokine expression during metastatic tumor progression of murine squamous cell carcinoma, *Cancer Res* 59:3495–3504, 1999.

37. Dong G and others: Molecular profiling of transformed and metastatic murine squamous carcinoma cells by differential display and cDNA microarray reveals altered expression of multiple genes related to growth, apoptosis, angiogenesis, and the NF-kappaB signal pathway, *Cancer Res* 61:4797–4808, 2001.

38. Duffey DC and others: Expression of a dominant-negative mutant inhibitor-kappaBalpha of nuclear factor-kappaB in human head and neck squamous cell carcinoma inhibits survival, proinflammatory cytokine expression, and tumor growth in vivo, *Cancer Res* 59:3468–3474, 1999.

39. Dworacki G and others: Decreased zeta chain expression and apoptosis in CD3+ peripheral blood T lymphocytes of patients with melanoma, *Clin Cancer Res* 7:947S–957S, 2001.

40. Eike A and others: Human papillomavirus (HPV) is rarely present in normal oral and nasal mucosa, *Clin Otolaryngol* 20:171–173, 1995.

41. Eisenberger CF and others: Diagnosis of renal cancer by molecular urinalysis, *J Natl Cancer Inst* 91:2028–2032, 1999.

42. Esteller M and others: Detection of aberrant promoter hypermethylation of tumor suppressor genes in serum DNA from non-small cell lung cancer patients, *Cancer Res* 59:67–70, 1999.

43. Fearon ER, Vogelstein B: A genetic model for colorectal tumorigenesis, *Cell* 61:759–767, 1990.

44. Fliss MS and others: Facile detection of mitochondrial DNA mutations in tumors and bodily fluids, *Science* 287:2017–2019, 2000.

45. Fouret P and others: Human papillomavirus in head and neck squamous cell carcinomas in nonsmokers, *Arch Otolaryngol Head Neck Surg* 123:513–516, 1997.

46. Fouret P and others: Human papillomavirus infection in the malignant and premalignant head and neck epithelium, *Diagn Mol Pathol* 4:122–127, 1995.

47. Franceschi S and others: Human papillomavirus and cancers of the upper aerodigestive tract: a review of epidemiological and experimental evidence, *Cancer Epidemiol Biomarkers Prev* 5:567–575, 1996.

48. Freier K and others: Tissue microarray analysis reveals site-specific prevalence of oncogene amplifications in head and neck squamous cell carcinoma, *Cancer Res* 63:1179–1182, 2003.

49. Funkhouser EM, Sharp GB: Aspirin and reduced risk of esophageal carcinoma, *Cancer* 76:1116–1119, 1995.

50. Gallo O and others: Cyclooxygenase-2 pathway correlates with VEGF expression in head and neck cancer: implications for tumor angiogenesis and metastasis, *Neoplasia* 3:53–61, 2001.

51. Geisler SA, Olshan AF: GSTM1, GSTT1, and the risk of squamous cell carcinoma of the head and neck: a mini-HuGE review, *Am J Epidemiol* 154:95–105, 2001.

52. Giardiello FM and others: Treatment of colonic and rectal adenomas with sulindac in familial adenomatous polyposis, *N Engl J Med* 328:1313–1316, 1993.

53. Gillison ML, Shah KV: Human papillomavirus-associated head and neck squamous cell carcinoma: mounting evidence for an etiologic role for human papillomavirus in a subset of head and neck cancers, *Curr Opin Oncol* 13: 183–188, 2001.

54. Gillison ML and others: Evidence for a causal association between human papillomavirus and a subset of head and neck cancers, *J Natl Cancer Inst* 92:709–720, 2000.

55. Giovannucci E and others: Aspirin and the risk of colorectal cancer in women, *N Engl J Med* 333:609–614, 1995.

56. Grandis JR, Tweardy DJ, Melhem MF: Asynchronous modulation of transforming growth factor alpha and epidermal growth factor receptor protein expression in progression of premalignant lesions to head and neck squamous cell carcinoma, *Clin Cancer Res* 4:13–20, 1998.

57. Grandis JR and others: Constitutive activation of Stat3 signaling abrogates apoptosis in squamous cell carcinogenesis in vivo, *Proc Natl Acad Sci USA* 97:4227–4232, 2000.

58. Ha PK and others: A transcriptional progression model for head and neck cancer, *Clin Cancer Res* 9:3058–3064, 2003.

59. Ha PK and others: Real-time quantitative PCR demonstrates low prevalence of human papillomavirus type 16 in premalignant and malignant lesions of the oral cavity, *Clin Cancer Res* 8:1203–1209, 2002.

60. Haraf DJ and others: Human papilloma virus and p53 in head and neck cancer: clinical correlates and survival, *Clin Cancer Res* 2:755–762, 1996.

61. Harris RE, Namboodiri KK, Farrar WB: Nonsteroidal antiinflammatory drugs and breast cancer, *Epidemiology* 7:203–205, 1996.

62. Hartwell LH, Kastan MB: Cell cycle control and cancer, *Science* 266:1821–1828, 1994.

63. Heim MH and others: Contribution of STAT SH2 groups to specific interferon signaling by the Jak-STAT pathway, *Science* 267:1347–1349, 1995.

64. Herbst RS, Kim ES, Harari PM: IMC-C225, an anti-epidermal growth factor receptor monoclonal antibody, for treatment of head and neck cancer, *Expert Opin Biol Ther* 1:719–732, 2001.

65. Hermsen M and others: New chromosomal regions with high-level amplifications in squamous cell carcinomas of the larynx and pharynx, identified by comparative genomic hybridization, *J Pathol* 194:177–182, 2001.

66. Hibi K and others: AIS is an oncogene amplified in squamous cell carcinoma, *Proc Natl Acad Sci U S A* 97:5462–5467, 2000.

67. Hoffmann TK and others: Spontaneous apoptosis of circulating T lymphocytes in patients with head and neck cancer and its clinical importance, *Clin Cancer Res* 8:2553–2562, 2002.

68. Holladay EB, Gerald WL: Viral gene detection in oral neoplasms using the polymerase chain reaction, *Am J Clin Pathol* 100:36–40, 1993.

69. Hollstein M and others: p53 mutations in human cancers, *Science* 253:49–53, 1991.

70. Hong WK and others: 13-cis-retinoic acid in the treatment of oral leukoplakia, *N Engl J Med* 315:1501–1505, 1986.

71. Hong WK and others: Prevention of second primary tumors with isotretinoin in squamous-cell carcinoma of the head and neck, *N Engl J Med* 323:795–801, 1990.

72. Huang AY and others: Role of bone marrow-derived cells in presenting MHC class I-restricted tumor antigens, *Science* 264:961–965, 1994.

73. Hussein MR, Cullen K: Molecular biomarkers in HNSCC: prognostic and therapeutic implications, *Expert Rev Anticancer Ther* 1:116–124, 2001.

74. Jemal A and others: Cancer statistics, 2002, *CA Cancer J Clin* 52:23–47, 2002.

75. Jen J, Wu L, Sidransky D: An overview on the isolation and analysis of circulating tumor DNA in plasma and serum, *Ann N Y Acad Sci* 906:8–12, 2000.

76. Jin C and others: Nonrandom pattern of cytogenetic abnormalities in squamous cell carcinoma of the larynx, *Genes Chromosomes Cancer* 28:66–76, 2000.

77. Jin Y and others: Chromosome abnormalities in eighty-three head and neck squamous cell carcinomas: influence of culture conditions on karyotypic pattern, *Cancer Res* 53:2140–2146, 1993.

78. Jourenkova-Mironova N and others: High-activity microsomal epoxide hydrolase genotypes and the risk of oral, pharynx, and larynx cancers, *Cancer Res* 60:534–536, 2000.

79. Jung TT, Berlinger NT, Juhn SK: Prostaglandins in squamous cell carcinoma of the head and neck: a preliminary study, *Laryngoscope* 95:307–312, 1985.

80. Kallioniemi A and others: Comparative genomic hybridization for molecular cytogenetic analysis of solid tumors, *Science* 258:818–821, 1992.

81. Kass ES and others: Carcinoembryonic antigen as a target for specific antitumor immunotherapy of head and neck cancer, *Cancer Res* 62:5049–5057, 2002.

82. Kessis TD and others: p53 gene mutations and MDM2 amplification are uncommon in primary carcinomas of the uterine cervix, *Am J Pathol* 143:1398–1405, 1993.

83. Kessis TD and others: Human papillomavirus 16 E6 expression disrupts the p53-mediated cellular response to DNA damage, *Proc Natl Acad Sci USA* 90:3988–3992, 1993.

84. Khuri FR and others: A controlled trial of intratumoral ONYX-015, a selectively-replicating adenovirus, in combination with cisplatin and 5-fluorouracil in patients with recurrent head and neck cancer, *Nat Med* 6:879–885, 2000.

85. Klaassen I and others: Expression of retinoic acid receptor gamma correlates with retinoic acid sensitivity and metabolism in head and neck squamous cell carcinoma cell lines, *Int J Cancer* 92:661–665, 2001.

86. Koutsky LA and others: A controlled trial of a human papillomavirus type 16 vaccine, *N Engl J Med* 347:1645–1651, 2002.

87. Knudson AG, Jr: Mutation and cancer: statistical study of retinoblastoma, *Proc Natl Acad Sci USA* 68:820–823, 1971.

88. Kujawski M and others: Recurrent DNA copy number losses associated with metastasis of larynx carcinoma, *Genes Chromosomes Cancer* 26:253–257, 1999.

89. Kuss I and others: Clinical significance of decreased zeta chain expression in peripheral blood lymphocytes of patients with head and neck cancer, *Clin Cancer Res* 5:329–334, 1999.

90. Lawton G and others: Human papillomaviruses in normal oral mucosa: a comparison of methods for sample collection, *J Oral Pathol Med* 21:265–269, 1992.

91. Le Q and others: Modulation of retinoic acid receptor function alters the growth inhibitory response of oral SCC cells to retinoids, *Oncogene* 19:1457–1465, 2000.

92. Lee KD and others: Expression of the MAGE–1, -2, -3, -4, and -6 genes in non-squamous cell carcinoma lesions of the head and neck, *Acta Otolaryngol* 116:633–639, 1996.

93. Li JJ and others: Inhibitors of both nuclear factor-kappaB and activator protein-1 activation block the neoplastic transformation response, *Cancer Res* 57:3569–3576, 1997.

94. Licciardello JT, Spitz MR, Hong WK: Multiple primary cancer in patients with cancer of the head and neck: second cancer of the head and neck, esophagus, and lung, *Int J Radiat Oncol Biol Phys* 17:467–476, 1989.

95. Lin DT and others: Cyclooxygenase-2: a novel molecular target for the prevention and treatment of head and neck cancer, *Head Neck* 24:792–799, 2002.

96. Lindeberg H, Krogdahl A: Laryngeal cancer and human papillomavirus: HPV is absent in the majority of laryngeal carcinomas, *Cancer Lett* 146:9–13, 1999.

97. Lingen MW, Polverini PJ, Bouck NP: Retinoic acid and interferon alpha act synergistically as antiangiogenic and antitumor agents against human head and neck squamous cell carcinoma, *Cancer Res* 58:5551–5558, 1998.

98. Maestro R and others: Three discrete regions of deletion at 3p in head and neck cancers, *Cancer Res* 53:5775–5779, 1993.

99. Magary SP and others: Expression of matrix metalloproteinases and tissue inhibitor of metalloproteinases in laryngeal and pharyngeal squamous cell carcinoma: a quantitative analysis, *Otolaryngol Head Neck Surg* 122:712–716, 2000.

100. Mann EA and others: Cytokine expression by head and neck squamous cell carcinomas, *Am J Surg* 164:567–573, 1992.

101. Mao L and others: Frequent microsatellite alterations at chromosomes 9p21 and 3p14 in oral premalignant lesions and their value in cancer risk assessment, *Nat Med* 2:682–685, 1996.

102. Mao L and others: Phenotype and genotype of advanced premalignant head and neck lesions after chemopreventive therapy, *J Natl Cancer Inst* 90:1545–1551, 1998.

103. Marshall JL and others: Phase I study in cancer patients of a replication-defective avipox recombinant vaccine that expresses human carcinoembryonic antigen, *J Clin Oncol* 17:332–337, 1999.

104. Matzow T and others: Low detection rate of HPV in oral and laryngeal carcinomas, *Acta Oncol* 37:73–76, 1998.

105. Maurizi M and others: Prognostic significance of epidermal growth factor receptor in laryngeal squamous cell carcinoma, *Br J Cancer* 74:1253–1257, 1996.

106. Miller CS, White DK: Human papillomavirus expression in oral mucosa, premalignant conditions, and squamous cell carcinoma: a retrospective review of the literature, *Oral Surg Oral Med Oral Pathol Oral Radiol Endod* 82:57–68, 1996.

107. Moasser MM and others: The tyrosine kinase inhibitor ZD1839 ("Iressa") inhibits HER2-driven signaling and suppresses the growth of HER2-overexpressing tumor cells, *Cancer Res* 61:7184–7188, 2001.

108. Mokbel K, Hassanally D: From HER2 to herceptin, *Curr Med Res Opin* 17:51–59, 2001.

109. Mork J and others: Human papillomavirus infection as a risk factor for squamous-cell carcinoma of the head and neck, *N Engl J Med* 344:1125–1131, 2001.

110. Muderspach L and others: A phase I trial of a human papillomavirus (HPV) peptide vaccine for women with high-grade cervical and vulvar intraepithelial neoplasia who are HPV 16 positive, *Clin Cancer Res* 6:3406–3416, 2000.

111. Mukaida N and others: Molecular mechanism of interleukin-8 gene expression, *J Leukoc Biol* 56:554–558, 1994.

112. Musiani P and others: Effect of low doses of interleukin-2 injected perilymphatically and peritumorally in patients with advanced primary head and neck squamous cell carcinoma, *J Biol Response Mod* 8:571–578, 1989.

113. Nathan CA and others: Correlation of p53 and the proto-oncogene eIF4E in larynx cancers: prognostic implications, *Cancer Res;* 60:3599–3604, 2000.

114. Nathan CA and others: Molecular analysis of surgical margins in head and neck squamous cell carcinoma patients, *Laryngoscope* 112:2129–2140, 2002.

115. Nawroz H and others: Allelotype of head and neck squamous cell carcinoma, *Cancer Res* 54:1152–1155, 1994.

116. Nawroz-Danish HM and others: Lack of BRCA2 alterations in primary head and neck squamous cell carcinoma, *Otolaryngol Head Neck Surg* 119:21–25, 1998.

117. Nemunaitis J and others: Adenovirus-mediated p53 gene transfer in sequence with cisplatin to tumors of patients with non-small-cell lung cancer, *J Clin Oncol* 18:609–622, 2000.

118. Nielsen LL and others: Adenovirus-mediated p53 gene therapy and paclitaxel have synergistic efficacy in models of human head and neck, ovarian, prostate, and breast cancer, *Clin Cancer Res* 4:835–846, 1998.

119. O-Charoenrat P, Rhys-Evans PH, Eccles SA: Expression of matrix metalloproteinases and their inhibitors correlates with invasion and metastasis in squamous cell carcinoma of the head and neck, *Arch Otolaryngol Head Neck Surg* 127:813–820, 2001.

120. O-Charoenrat P and others: Overexpression of epidermal growth factor receptor in human head and neck squamous carcinoma cell lines correlates with matrix metalloproteinase-9 expression and in vitro invasion, *Int J Cancer* 86:307–317, 2000.

121. Ohta M and others: The FHIT gene, spanning the chromosome 3p14.2 fragile site and renal carcinoma-associated t(3;8) breakpoint, is abnormal in digestive tract cancers, *Cell* 84:587–597, 1996.

122. Okami K and others: Cyclin D1 amplification is independent of p16 inactivation in head and neck squamous cell carcinoma, *Oncogene* 18:3541–3545, 1999.

123. O'Malley BW Jr and others: Limitations of adenovirus-mediated interleukin-2 gene therapy for oral cancer, *Laryngoscope* 109:389–395, 1999.

124. Ondrey FG and others: Constitutive activation of transcription factors NF-(kappa)B, AP-1, and NF-IL6 in human head and neck squamous cell carcinoma cell lines that express pro-inflammatory and pro-angiogenic cytokines, *Mol Carcinog* 26:119–129, 1999.

125. Partridge M and others: A case-control study confirms that microsatellite assay can identify patients at risk of developing oral squamous cell carcinoma within a field of cancerization, *Cancer Res* 60:3893–3898, 2000.

126. Partridge M and others: Field cancerisation of the oral cavity: comparison of the spectrum of molecular alterations in cases presenting with both dysplastic and malignant lesions, *Oral Oncol* 33:332–337, 1997.

127. Partridge M and others: Profiling clonality and progression in multiple premalignant and malignant oral lesions identifies a subgroup of cases with a distinct presentation of squamous cell carcinoma, *Clin Cancer Res* 7:1860–1866, 2001.

128. Paz IB and others: Human papillomavirus (HPV) in head and neck cancer: an association of HPV 16 with squamous cell carcinoma of Waldeyer's tonsillar ring, *Cancer* 79:595–604, 1997.

129. Perkins TM, Shklar G: Delay in hamster buccal pouch carcinogenesis by aspirin and indomethacin, *Oral Surg Oral Med Oral Pathol* 53:170–178, 1982.

130. Pirollo KF and others: p53 mediated sensitization of squamous cell carcinoma of the head and neck to radiotherapy, *Oncogene* 14:1735–1746, 1997.

131. Prevo LJ and others: p53-mutant clones and field effects in Barrett's esophagus, *Cancer Res* 59:4784–4787, 1999.

132. Qin H and others: Gene therapy for head and neck cancer using vaccinia virus expressing IL-2 in a murine model, with evidence of immune suppression, *Mol Ther* 4:551–558, 2001.

133. Rao CV and others: Chemoprevention of colon carcinogenesis by sulindac, a nonsteroidal anti-inflammatory agent, *Cancer Res* 55:1464–1472, 1995.

134. Rao PH and others: Cytogenetic analysis of 11 squamous cell carcinomas of the head and neck, *Cancer Genet Cytogenet* 77:60–64, 1994.

135. Rao PH and others: Multicolor spectral karyotyping identifies new recurring breakpoints and translocations in multiple myeloma, *Blood* 92:1743–1748, 1998.

136. Rashleigh SP and others: Interleukins 2 and 12 activate natural killer cytolytic responses of peripheral blood mononuclear cells from patients with head and neck squamous cell carcinoma, *Arch Otolaryngol Head Neck Surg* 122:541–547, 1996.

137. Raskind WH and others: Persistent clonal areas and clonal expansion in Barrett's esophagus, *Cancer Res* 52:2946–2950, 1992.

138. Rayet B, Gelinas C: Aberrant rel/nfkb genes and activity in human cancer, *Oncogene* 18:6938–6947, 1999.

139. Reed AL and others: High frequency of p16 (CDKN2/MTS-1/ INK4A) inactivation in head and neck squamous cell carcinoma, *Cancer Res* 56:3630–3633, 1996.

140. Reichert TE and others: Absent or low expression of the zeta chain in T cells at the tumor site correlates with poor survival in patients with oral carcinoma, *Cancer Res* 58:5344–5347, 1998.

141. Reichert TE and others: Mechanisms responsible for signaling and functional defects, *J Immunother* 21:295–306, 1998.

142. Reichert TE and others: Signaling abnormalities, apoptosis, and reduced proliferation of circulating and tumor-infiltrating lymphocytes in patients with oral carcinoma, *Clin Cancer Res* 8:3137–3145, 2002.

143. Renan MJ: How many mutations are required for tumorigenesis? Implications from human cancer data, *Mol Carcinog* 7:139–146, 1993.

144. Riegman PH and others: Genomic alterations in malignant transformation of Barrett's esophagus, *Cancer Res* 61:3164–3170, 2001.

145. Rosin MP and others: Use of allelic loss to predict malignant risk for low-grade oral epithelial dysplasia, *Clin Cancer Res* 6:357–362, 2000.

146. Saito T and others: Spontaneous apoptosis of CD8+ T lymphocytes in peripheral blood of patients with advanced melanoma, *Clin Cancer Res* 6:1351–1364, 2000.

147. Salgaller ML and others: Generation of specific anti-melanoma reactivity by stimulation of human tumor-infiltrating lymphocytes with MAGE-1 synthetic peptide, *Cancer Immunol Immunother* 39:105–116, 1994.

148. Sanchez-Cespedes M and others: Gene promoter hypermethylation in tumors and serum of head and neck cancer patients, *Cancer Res* 60:892–895, 2000.

149. Sand L and others: Human papilloma viruses in oral lesions, *Anticancer Res* 20:1183–1188, 2000.

150. Sardi I and others: Prediction of recurrence by microsatellite analysis in head and neck cancer, *Genes Chromosomes Cancer* 29:201–206, 2000.

151. Schreinemachers DM, Everson RB: Aspirin use and lung, colon, and breast cancer incidence in a prospective study, *Epidemiology* 5:138–146, 1994.

152. Schrock E and others: Multicolor spectral karyotyping of human chromosomes, *Science* 273:494–497, 1996.

153. Shak S: Overview of the trastuzumab (Herceptin) anti-HER2 monoclonal antibody clinical program in HER2-overexpressing metastatic breast cancer: Herceptin Multinational Investigator Study Group, *Semin Oncol* 26:71–77, 1999.

154. Shiga H and others: Prognostic value of p53, glutathione S-transferase pi, and thymidylate synthase for neoadjuvant cisplatin-based chemotherapy in head and neck cancer, *Clin Cancer Res* 5:4097–4104, 1999.

155. Shin DM and others: Epidermal growth factor receptor-targeted therapy with C225 and cisplatin in patients

with head and neck cancer, *Clin Cancer Res* 7:1204–1213, 2001.

156. Sidransky D, Hollstein M: Clinical implications of the p53 gene, *Annu Rev Med* 47:285–301, 1996.

157. Sidransky D and others: Identification of p53 gene mutations in bladder cancers and urine samples, *Science* 252:706–709, 1991.

158. Singh B and others: Molecular cytogenetic characterization of head and neck squamous cell carcinoma and refinement of 3q amplification, *Cancer Res* 61:4506–4513, 2001.

159. Slamon DJ and others: Human breast cancer: correlation of relapse and survival with amplification of the HER-2/neu oncogene, *Science* 235:177–182, 1987.

160. Slamon DJ and others: Use of chemotherapy plus a monoclonal antibody against HER2 for metastatic breast cancer that overexpresses HER2, *N Engl J Med* 344:783–792, 2001.

161. Slaughter DP, Southwick HA, Wmejkal W: "Field cancerization" in oral stratified squamous epithelium: clinical implications of multicentric origin, *Cancer* 6: 963–968, 1953.

162. Son YI and others: Dendritic cells pulsed with apoptotic squamous cell carcinoma have anti-tumor effects when combined with interleukin-2, *Laryngoscope* 111:1472–1478, 2001.

163. Spafford MF and others: Detection of head and neck squamous cell carcinoma among exfoliated oral mucosal cells by microsatellite analysis, *Clin Cancer Res* 7:607–612, 2001.

164. Speicher MR and others: Comparative genomic hybridization detects novel deletions and amplifications in head and neck squamous cell carcinomas, *Cancer Res* 55:1010–1013, 1995.

165. Sporn MB and others: Prevention of chemical carcinogenesis by vitamin A and its synthetic analogs (retinoids), *Fed Proc* 35:1332–1338, 1976.

166. Squire JA and others: Molecular cytogenetic analysis of head and neck squamous cell carcinoma: by comparative genomic hybridization, spectral karyotyping, and expression array analysis, *Head Neck* 24:874–887, 2002.

167. Stanton P and others: Epidermal growth factor receptor expression by human squamous cell carcinomas of the head and neck, cell lines and xenografts, *Br J Cancer* 70:427–433, 1994.

168. Sudbo J and others: DNA content as a prognostic marker in patients with oral leukoplakia, *N Engl J Med* 344:1270–1278, 2001.

169. Sun SY and others: Identification of receptor-selective retinoids that are potent inhibitors of the growth of human head and neck squamous cell carcinoma cells, *Clin Cancer Res* 6:1563–1573, 2000.

170. Syrjanen SM, Syrjanen KJ, Happonen RP: Human papillomavirus (HPV) DNA sequences in oral precancerous lesions and squamous cell carcinoma demonstrated by in situ hybridization, *J Oral Pathol* 17:273–278, 1988.

171. Syrjanen SM, Syrjanen KJ, Lamberg MA: Detection of human papillomavirus DNA in oral mucosal lesions using in situ DNA-hybridization applied on paraffin sections, *Oral Surg Oral Med Oral Pathol* 62:660–667, 1986.

172. Takayama K and others: The levels of integrin alpha v beta 5 may predict the susceptibility to adenovirus-mediated gene transfer in human lung cancer cells, *Gene Ther* 5:361–368 1998.

173. Tepperman BS, Fitzpatrick PJ: Second respiratory and upper digestive tract cancers after oral cancer, *Lancet* 2:547–549, 1981.

174. Thomas GR and others: IL-12- and IL-2-induced tumor regression in a new murine model of oral squamous-cell carcinoma is promoted by expression of the CD80

175. Thomas RS and others: ETS1, NFkappaB and AP1 synergistically transactivate the human GM-CSF promoter, *Oncogene* 14:2845–2855, 1997.

176. Thun MJ, Namboodiri MM, Heath CW Jr: Aspirin use and reduced risk of fatal colon cancer, *N Engl J Med* 325: 1593–1596, 1991.

177. To WC and others: Systemic adoptive T-cell immunotherapy in recurrent and metastatic carcinoma of the head and neck: a phase 1 study, *Arch Otolaryngol Head Neck Surg* 126:1225–1231, 2000.

178. Tokumaru Y and others: Activation of matrix metalloproteinase-2 in head and neck squamous cell carcinoma: studies of clinical samples and in vitro cell lines co-cultured with fibroblasts, *Cancer Lett* 150:15–21, 2000.

179. Trink B and others: A new human p53 homologue *Nature* 4:747–748, 1998.

180. Uno M and others: Anti-HER2-antibody enhances irradiation-induced growth inhibition in head and neck carcinoma, *Int J Cancer* 94:474–479, 2001.

181. Usadel H and others: Quantitative adenomatous polyposis coli promoter methylation analysis in tumor tissue, serum, and plasma DNA of patients with lung cancer, *Cancer Res* 62:371–375, 2002.

182. van der Riet P and others: Frequent loss of chromosome 9p21–22 early in head and neck cancer progression, *Cancer Res* 54:1156–1158, 1994.

183. Van Dyke DL and others: Recurrent cytogenetic abnormalities in squamous cell carcinomas of the head and neck region, *Genes Chromosomes Cancer* 9:192–206, 1994.

184. Veltman JA and others: Chromosome instability as an indicator of malignant progression in laryngeal mucosa, *J Clin Oncol* 18:1644–1651, 2000.

185. Werness BA, Levine AJ, Howley PM: Association of human papillomavirus types 16 and 18 E6 proteins with p53, *Science* 248:76–79, 1990.

186. Whiteside TL: Apoptosis of immune cells in the tumor microenvironment and peripheral circulation of patients with cancer: implications for immunotherapy, *Vaccine* 20 (Suppl 4):A46–A51, 2002.

187. Whiteside TL and others: Evidence for local and systemic activation of immune cells by peritumoral injections of interleukin 2 in patients with advanced squamous cell carcinoma of the head and neck, *Cancer Res* 53:5654–5662, 1993.

188. Woodburn JR: The epidermal growth factor receptor and its inhibition in cancer therapy. *Pharmacol Ther* 82:241–250, 1999.

189. Woods KV and others: Variable expression of cytokines in human head and neck squamous cell carcinoma cell lines and consistent expression in surgical specimens, *Cancer Res* 58:3132–3141, 1998.

190. Wu CL and others: Deletion mapping on the short arm of chromosome 3 in squamous cell carcinoma of the oral cavity, *Cancer Res* 54:6484–6488, 1994.

191. Xia W and others: Strong correlation between c-erbB-2 overexpression and overall survival of patients with oral squamous cell carcinoma, *Clin Cancer Res* 3:3–9, 1997.

192. Yamaguchi K and others: Frequent gain of the p40/p51/p63 gene locus in primary head and neck squamous cell carcinoma, *Int J Cancer* 86:684–689, 2000.

193. Yoo GH and others: Infrequent inactivation of the retinoblastoma gene despite frequent loss of chromosome

13q in head and neck squamous cell carcinoma, *Cancer Res* 54:4603–4606, 1994.

194. Yoo GH and others: Phase I trial of intratumoral liposome E1A gene therapy in patients with recurrent breast and head and neck cancer, *Clin Cancer Res* 7:1237–1245, 2001.

195. Zatterstrom UK and others: Prognostic factors in head and neck cancer: histologic grading, DNA ploidy, and nodal status, *Head Neck* 13:477–487, 1991.

196. Zheng Z and others: Tobacco carcinogen-detoxifying enzyme UGT1A7 and its association with orolaryngeal cancer risk, *J Natl Cancer Inst* 93:1411–1418, 2001.

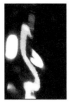

CHAPTER FIFTEEN

OUTCOMES RESEARCH

‖ Bevan Yueh

INTRODUCTION

The time is past when physicians chose treatment based solely on their personal notions of what was best. This era, although chronologically recent, is now conceptually distant. In a health care environment altered by abundant information on the Internet and continual oversight by managed care organizations, patients and insurers are now active participants in selecting treatment. Personal notions ("expert opinions") are replaced by objective evidence. And the physician's sense of what is best is being supplemented by patients' perspectives on outcomes after treatment.

Outcomes research (clinical epidemiology) is the scientific study of treatment effectiveness. The word "effectiveness" is a critical one, because it pertains to the success of treatment in populations found in actual practice in the real world, as opposed to treatment success in the controlled populations of randomized clinical trials in academic settings ("efficacy").[6,33] Success of treatment can be measured using patient survival, costs, and physiologic measures, but frequently health-related quality of life is a primary consideration.

Therefore, to gain scientific insight into these types of outcomes in the observational (nonrandomized) setting, outcomes researchers need to be fluent with methodological techniques that are borrowed from a variety of disciplines, including epidemiology, biostatistics, economics, management science, and psychometrics. A full description of the techniques in clinical epidemiology[28] is clearly beyond the scope of this chapter. The goal of this chapter is to provide a primer on the basic concepts in effectiveness research, and to provide a sense of the breadth and capacity of outcomes research and clinical epidemiology.

History

In 1900, Dr. Ernest Codman proposed to study what he termed the "end-results" of therapy at the Massachusetts General Hospital.[14] He asked his fellow surgeons to report the success and failure of *each* operation and developed a classification scheme by which failures could be further detailed. During the next two decades, his attempts to introduce systematic study of surgical end-results were scorned by the medical establishment, and his prescient efforts to study surgical outcomes gradually faded.

During the next 50 years, the medical community accepted the randomized clinical trial (RCT) as the dominant method for evaluating treatment.[46] By the 1960s, the authority of the RCT was rarely questioned.[106] However, a landmark 1973 publication by Wennberg and Gittelsohn spurred a sudden reevaluation of the value of observational (nonrandomized) data. These authors documented significant geographic variation in rates of surgery.[107] Tonsillectomy rates in 13 Vermont regions varied from 13 to 151 per 10,000 persons, even though there was no variation in the prevalence of tonsillitis. Even in cities with similar demographics and similar access to health care (Boston and New Haven), rates of surgical procedures varied tenfold. These findings raised the question of whether the higher rates of surgery represented better care or unnecessary surgery.

Researchers at the Rand Corporation sought to evaluate the appropriateness of surgical procedures. Supplementing relatively sparse data in the literature about treatment effectiveness by presenting statistics at expert opinion conferences, these investigators argued that rates of inappropriate surgery were high.[108] However, utilization rates did not correlate with rates of inappropriateness, and therefore did not explain all the variation in surgical rates.[12,62] To some, this suggested that the practice of medicine was anecdotal and inadequately scientific.[44] In 1988, a seminal editorial by physicians from the Health Care Financing Administration argued that a fundamental change towards study of treatment effectiveness was necessary.[82] These events subsequently led Congress to establish the Agency for Health Care Policy and

Research in 1989. The agency has since been renamed the Agency for Healthcare Research and Quality (AHRQ), which was charged with "systematically studying the relationships between health care and its outcomes."

In the past decade, outcomes research and the AHRQ have become integral to understanding treatment effectiveness and establishing health policy. Randomized trials cannot be used to answer all clinical questions, and outcomes research techniques can be used to gain considerable insights from observational data (including data from large administrative data bases). With current attention on evidence-based medicine and quality of care, a basic familiarity with outcomes research is more important than ever.

KEY TERMS AND CONCEPTS

The fundamentals of clinical epidemiology are best understood by thinking about an episode of treatment: a patient presents at baseline with an index condition, receives treatment for that condition, and then experiences a response to treatment. Assessment of baseline state, treatment, and outcomes are all subject to bias. We will begin with a brief review of bias and confounding.

Bias and Confounding

Bias occurs when "compared components are not sufficiently similar."[28] The compared components may involve any aspect of the study. For example, *selection* bias exists if, when comparing patients who have surgical resection to patients who undergo chemoradiation, researchers determine that oncologists avoid treating patients with renal or liver failure. This makes the comparison unfair because, on average, the surgical cohort will accrue patients who are more ill. *Treatment* bias occurs if we attempt to compare standard stapedotomy with laser stapedotomy, but one procedure is performed by an experienced surgeon and the other is performed by resident staff.

Similar to bias, confounding also has the potential to distort the results. However, confounding refers to specific variables. Confounding occurs when a variable thought to cause an outcome is actually not responsible, because of the unseen effects of another variable. Consider the hypothetical (and obviously faulty) case where an investigator postulates that nicotine-stained teeth cause laryngeal cancer. Despite a strong statistical association, this relationship is not causal, because another variable—cigarette smoking—is responsible. Cigarette smoking is confounding because it is associated with both the outcome (laryngeal cancer) and the supposed baseline state (stained teeth).

Assessment of Baseline

Most physicians are aware of the confounding influences of age, gender, ethnicity, and race. However, accurate baseline assessment also means that investigators should carefully define the disease under study, account for disease severity, and consider other important variables such as comorbidity.

Definition of Disease

It would seem obvious that the first step is to establish diagnostic criteria for the disease under study. Yet this is often incomplete. Inclusion criteria should include all relevant portions of the history, the physical examination, and laboratory and radiographic data. For example, the definition of chronic sinusitis may vary by pattern of disease (e.g., persistent vs recurrent acute infections), duration of symptoms (3 months vs 6 months), and diagnostic criteria for sinusitis (clinical exam vs ultrasound vs CT vs sinus taps and cultures). All of these aspects must be delineated to place studies into proper context.

In addition, advances in diagnostic technology may introduce a bias called stage migration.[26] In cancer treatment, stage migration occurs when more sensitive technologies (such as CT scans in the past and PET scans now) may "migrate" patients with previously undetectable metastatic disease out of an early stage (improving the survival of that group), and place them into a stage with otherwise advanced disease (improving this group's survival as well).[10,88] The net effect is that there is improvement in stage-specific survival, but no change in overall survival.

Disease Severity

The severity of disease strongly influences response to treatment. This reality is second nature for oncologists, who use TNM stage to select treatment and interpret survival outcomes. It is intuitively clear that the more severe the disease, the more difficult it will be (on average) to restore function. Yet, this concept has not been fully integrated into the study and practice of common otolaryngologic diseases such as sinusitis and hearing loss.

Recent progress has been made in sinusitis. Kennedy identified prognostic factors for successful outcomes in patients with sinusitis and has encouraged the development of staging systems.[58] Several staging systems have now been proposed, but most systems rely primarily on radiographic appearance.[41,65,66] Clinical measures of disease severity (symptoms and findings) are not typically included in staging systems. Although the Lund-Mackay staging system is reproducible,[69] this radiographic staging systems has correlated poorly with clinical disease.[4,48,94] However, the Harvard staging system has been reproducible[69] and may predict response to treatment.[91] The development and validation of reliable staging systems for other common disorders and the integration of these systems into patient care are pressing challenges in otolaryngology.

Comorbidity

Comorbidity refers to the presence of concomitant disease unrelated to the "index disease" (the disease under consideration), which may affect the diagnosis, treatment, and prognosis for the patient.[11,32,79] Documentation of comorbidity is important, because the failure to identify comorbid conditions such as liver failure may result in inaccurately attributing poor outcomes to the index disease being studied.[80] This baseline variable is most commonly considered in oncology, because most models of comorbidity have been developed to predict survival.[11,77] Given its impact on costs, utilization, and quality of life, comorbidity should be incorporated in studies of non-oncologic diseases as well.

Assessment of Treatment
Control Groups

Reliance on case series to report results of surgical treatment is time-honored. It is also inadequate for establishing cause and effect relationships. An evaluation of endoscopic sinus surgery reports revealed that only 4 of 35 studies used a control group.[63] Without a control group, the investigator cannot establish that the observed effects of treatment were directly related to the treatment itself.[28]

It is also particularly crucial to recognize that the scientific rigor of the study will vary with the suitability of the control group. The more fair the comparison, the more rigorous the results. Therefore, a randomized cohort study, where subjects are randomly allocated to different treatments, is more likely to be free of biased comparisons than observational cohort studies, where treatment decisions are made by an individual, a group of individuals, or a health care system. Within observational cohorts, there are also different levels of rigor. In a recent evaluation of critical pathways in head and neck cancer, a "positive" finding in comparison with a historical control group (a comparison group assembled in the past) was not significant when compared with a concurrent control group.[109]

Assessment of Outcomes
Efficacy

The distinction between efficacy and effectiveness, briefly discussed earlier in this chapter, illustrates one of the fundamental differences between randomized trials and outcomes research. Efficacy refers

to whether a health intervention, in a controlled environment, achieves better outcomes than does placebo. Two aspects of this definition need emphasis. First, efficacy is a comparison to placebo. As long as the intervention is better, it is efficacious. Second, controlled environments shelter patients and physicians from problems in actual clinical settings. For example, randomized efficacy trials of medications provide continuing reminders for patients to use their medications, and patients who do not adhere to the regimen are dropped from further study.

Effectiveness

An efficacious treatment that retains its value under usual clinical circumstances is effective. Effective treatment must overcome a number of barriers not encountered in the typical trial setting. For example, disease severity and comorbidity may be worse in the community, since healthy patients tend to be enrolled in (non-oncologic) trials. Patient adherence to treatment may also be imperfect. Consider CPAP treatment for patients with obstructive sleep apnea. Although the CPAP is efficacious in the sleep laboratory, the positive pressure is ineffective if the patients don't wear the masks when they return home.[102] A different challenge is present for surgical treatments, since community physicians learning a new procedure cannot be expected to perform it as effectively as the surgeon investigator who pioneered its development.

FUNDAMENTALS OF STUDY DESIGN

A variety of study designs are used to gain insight into treatment effectiveness. Each has advantages and disadvantages. The principle trade-off is complexity vs rigor, because rigorous evidence demands greater effort. An understanding of the fundamental differences in study design can help to interpret the quality of evidence, which has been formalized by the evidence-based medicine (EBM) movement. EBM is the "conscientious, explicit, and judicious use of current best evidence in making decisions about the care of individual patients."[86] EBM is discussed in detail elsewhere in this book, but is mentioned here because of its overlap with clinical epidemiology. We will summarize the major categories of study designs, with reference to the EBM hierarchy of levels of evidence (Table 15-1).[15,86]

Randomized Clinical Trial

Randomized clinical trials (RCT) represent the highest level of evidence, because the controlled, experimental nature of the RCT allows the investigator to establish a causal relationship between treatment and subsequent outcome. The random distribution of

TABLE 15-1

SUMMARY OF STUDY DESIGNS

Design	Advantages	Disadvantages	Level of Evidence
Randomized clinical trial	• Only design to prove causation • Unbiased distribution of confounding	• Expensive and complex • Typically targets efficacy	1, if high quality RCT 2, if low quality RCT
Observational (cohort) study	• Cheaper than RCT • Clear temporal directionality from treatment to outcome	• Difficult to find suitable controls • Confounding	2, with control group 4, if no control group
Case-control study	• Cheaper than cohort study • Efficient study of rare diseases or delayed outcomes	• Must rely on retrospective data • Directionality between exposure and outcome unclear	3
Case series	• Cheap and simple	• No control group • No causal link between treatment and outcome	4
Expert opinion	N/A	N/A	5

patients also allows unbiased distribution of baseline variables and minimizes the influence of confounding. Although randomized trials have generally been used to address efficacy, modifications can facilitate insight into effectiveness as well. RCTs with well-defined inclusion criteria, double-blinded treatment and assessment, low losses to follow-up, and high statistical power are considered high-quality RCTs and represent level 1 evidence. Lower quality RCTs are rated level 2 evidence.

Observational Study

In observational studies, sometimes called cohort studies, patients are identified at baseline before treatment (or "exposure," in standard epidemiology cohort studies investigating risk factors for disease). This is similar to randomized trials. However, these studies assemble patients who receive routine clinical care. Inclusion criteria are substantially less stringent, and treatment is assigned by the provider in the course of clinical care. Maintenance of the cohort is also straightforward, since there is no need to keep patients and providers doubly-blinded.

The challenge in cohort studies is to find an appropriate control group. Rigorous prospective and retrospective cohort studies with a suitable control group represent high-quality studies, and can represent level 2 evidence. To obtain insight into comparisons of treatment effectiveness, these studies need to use sophisticated statistical and epidemiological methods to overcome the biases discussed earlier in this chapter. Even with these techniques, there is the risk that

unmeasured confounding variables will distort the comparison of interest. Poor-quality cohorts without control groups or inadequate adjustment for confounding variables are considered level 4 evidence, since they are essentially equivalent to a case series, as discussed later.

Case-Control Study

Case-control studies are typically used by traditional epidemiologists to identify risk factors for the development of disease. In such cases, the disease becomes the "outcome." Randomized and observational studies identify patients before "exposure" to a treatment (or a pathogen) and then follow patients forward in time to observe the outcome. In contrast, case-control studies use the opposite temporal direction. This design is particularly valuable when prospective studies are not feasible, either because the disease is too rare or because the time interval between baseline and outcome is prohibitively long.

For example, a prospective study of an association between a proposed carcinogen (e.g., gastroesophageal reflux) and laryngeal cancer would require a tremendous number of patients and decades of observation. However, by identifying patients with and without laryngeal cancer, and comparing relative rates of carcinogen exposure, a case-control study can obtain a relatively quick answer.[24] It should be noted that because the temporal relationship between exposure and outcome is not directly observed, no causal judgments are possible. These studies are considered level 3 evidence.

Case Series and Expert Opinion

Case series are the least sophisticated format. As discussed earlier, no conclusions about causal relationships between treatment and outcome can be made because of uncontrolled bias and the absence of any control group. These studies are considered level 4 evidence. If case studies are unavailable, then expert opinion is used to provide level 5 evidence.

Other Study Designs

Numerous other important study designs in outcomes research exist, but a detailed discussion of these techniques is beyond the scope of this chapter. The most common approaches include decision analyses,[57,74] cost-identification and cost-effectiveness studies,[43,59,85] secondary analyses of administrative databases,[31,47,70] and meta-analyses.[30,84] Critiques of these techniques are referenced for completeness.

Grading of EBM Recommendations

EBM uses the levels of evidence described earlier to grade treatment recommendations (Table 15-2).[9] The presence of high-quality RCTs allows treatment recommendations for a particular intervention to be ranked as grade A. If no RCTs are available, but level 2 (observational study with a control group) or 3 (case-control study) evidence exists, the treatment recommendations are ranked as grade B. The presence of only a case series would result in a grade C recommendation. If even case series are unavailable and only expert opinion is available, the recommendation for the index treatment is considered grade D.

MEASUREMENT OF CLINICAL OUTCOMES

Clinical studies have traditionally used outcomes such as mortality and morbidity, or other "hard" laboratory or physiologic endpoints,[27] such as blood pressure, white cell counts, or radiographs. This practice has persisted despite evidence that interobserver variability of accepted "hard" outcomes such as chest x-ray findings and histological reports are distressingly high.[23] In addition, clinicians rely on "soft" data, such as pain relief or symptomatic improvement to determine whether patients are responding to treatment. But because it has been difficult to quantify these variables, these outcomes were largely ignored until the millennium.

Psychometric Validation

An important contribution of outcomes research has been the development of questionnaires to quantify these "soft" constructs, such as symptoms, satisfaction, and quality of life. A rigorous psychometric validation process is typically followed to create these questionnaires (more often referred to as *scales* or *instruments*). These scales can then be administered to patients to produce a numerical score. I will briefly introduce the validation process. A more complete description can be found elsewhere.[73,90,96] The three major steps in the process are the establishment of reliability, validity, and responsiveness.

- Reliability. A reliable scale reproduces the same result in precise fashion. For example, assuming there is no clinical change, a scale administered today and next week should produce the same result. This is called *test-retest reliability*. Other forms of reliability include internal consistency and inter-observer reliability.[67,96]
- Validity. A valid scale measures what it is purported to measure. This concept is initially difficult to appreciate. Since these scales are designed to measure constructs that have not previously been measured, and since the constructs are difficult to define in the first place (e.g., quality of life), how does one determine what the scales are supposed to measure? The abbreviated answer is that the scales should behave in the hypothesized way. A simple example of an appropriate hypothesis is that a proposed cancer-specific quality-of-life scale should correlate strongly with pain, tumor stage, and disfigurement, but less strongly with age and gender. For more complete discussion, several excellent references are listed.[29,67,73,90,96]
- Responsiveness. A responsive scale is able to detect clinically important change.[21] For instance, a scale may distinguish a moderately hearing impaired individual from a deaf individual. Such a scale is "valid." But can it detect a different score if the individual's hearing improves mildly after surgery? Alternatively, the minimum improvement in score that represents a clinically important change might be provided.[51,53]

Categories of Outcomes

In informal use, the terms *health status*, *function*, and *quality of life* are frequently used interchangeably.

TABLE 15-2

RELATIONSHIPS BETWEEN GRADE OF RECOMMENDATION AND LEVEL OF EVIDENCE

Grade of Recommendation	Level of Evidence
A	1
B	2 or 3
C	4
D	5

However, these terms have important distinctions in the health services literature. Health status describes an individual's physical, emotional, and social capabilities and limitations. Function refers to how well an individual is able to perform important roles, tasks, or activities.[73] Quality of life (QOL) differs because the central focus is on the value that individuals place on their health status and function.[73]

Because many aspects of QOL are unrelated to a patient's health status (e.g., income level, marital and family happiness), outcomes researchers typically focus on scales that measure only health-related quality of life (HRQOL). HRQOL scales may be categorized as either generic or disease-specific. Generic (or general) scales are used for QOL assessment in a broad range of patients. The principal advantage of generic measures is that they facilitate comparison of results across different diseases. For example, how does the QOL of a heart transplant patient compare to that of a cancer patient? Disease-specific scales, on the other hand, are designed to assess specific patient populations. Because these scales can focus on a narrower range of topics, they tend to be more responsive to clinical change in the population under study. To benefit from the advantages of each type of scale, rigorous studies often use both a generic and a disease-specific scale to assess outcomes.

In addition to these measures, a number of other outcomes are increasingly popular. These include patient satisfaction, costs and charges,[74,109] health care utilization, and patient preferences (utilities, willingness to pay).[16,37,109] Descriptions of these methods are referenced for completeness.

EXAMPLES OF OUTCOMES MEASURES

As mentioned earlier in this chapter, one of the principal contributions of outcomes research has been the development of scales to measure HRQOL and related outcomes. I will briefly discuss several validated scales that are relevant to otolaryngology. Unless otherwise indicated, these scales are completed by the patient. The references contain details about validation data, and most also include a listing of sample questions and scoring instructions. The most widely used scales in each category are listed in Table 15-3.

Generic Scales

The best known and most widely used outcomes instrument is the Medical Outcomes Study Short Form-36, commonly called the SF-36.[101] This 36-item scale is designed for adults and surveys general health status. It produces scores in eight health categories (e.g., vitality, bodily pain, limitations in physical activities). The SF-36 also generates two summary scores on overall physical and mental health status. Normative population scores are available, and the scale has been translated into numerous languages.

TABLE 15-3

Outcomes Measures Relevant to Otolaryngology*

Disease Category Examples

Generic	Health status	SF-36[101]
	Quality of life	WHOQOL[98]
	utility	QWB[55]
Head and neck cancer	General	UWQOL,[81] FACT,[8] EORTC[5]
	Radiation-specific	QOL-RTI/H&N[99]
	Clinician-rated	PSS[64]
Otologic	General	HHIE[100]
	Conductive loss	HSS[93]
	Amplification	APHAB,[16] EAR[89]
	Dizziness	DHI[50]
	Tinnitus	THI[60]
Rhinologic	Nasal obstruction	NOSE[95]
	Chronic sinusitis	SNOT-20,[78] CSS[42]
Pediatric	Tonsillectomy	TAHSI[92]
	Otitis media	OM-6[83]
	Sleep apnea	OSD-6,[18] OSA-18[36]
Other	Adult sleep apnea	FOSQ,[103] SAQLI[34]
	Swallowing	MDADI,[13] SWAL-QOL[68]
	Voice	VHI,[49] VOS[39]
	Cosmetic	ROE, BOE[1]

*Refer to text for additional scales.

Instructions, numerous reference publications, and other related information can be found at the SF-36 Web site (www.sf36.com).

A variety of other popular generic scales are available as well and are referenced at the site. Another health status measure is the Sickness Impact Profile.[3] The Quality of Well Being (QWB[55,56]) and the Health Utilities Index (HUI[25,37]) measure patient preferences, or utilities, and the World Health Organization's QOL scale (WHOQOL[98]) is a measure of generic quality of life.

Head and Neck Cancer

In 2002, the National Institutes of Health (NIH) sponsored a conference to achieve consensus on the methods used to measure and report QOL assessment in head and neck cancer.[110] There was agreement that an adequate number of scales already exist to measure general QOL in head and neck cancer patients. The three most popular scales at that time were the European Organization for Research and Treatment of Cancer Quality of Life Questionnaire (EORTC-HN35[5]), the University of Washington Quality of Life scale (UW-QOL[19,45,81]), and the Functional Assessment of Cancer Therapy Head and Neck module (FACT-HN[8]). Both the EORTC-HN35 and FACT-HN instruments offer additional modules that measure general cancer QOL in addition to the head-and-neck cancer-specific modules, but are longer than the 12-item UW-QOL scale.

A clinician-rated scale—in which the clinician completes the scale, rather than the patient—that has achieved widespread use is the Performance Status Scale, a 3-item instrument that correlates well with many of the already-mentioned cancer scales.[64] A number of other excellent, validated patient-completed scales are also available, including the Head and Neck Quality of Life (HNQOL[97]) and the Head & Neck Survey (H&NS[40]), although these scales have not been used as widely. Several validated scales that focus on QOL of patients undergoing radiation are also in use.[7,99]

Otologic Disease

The most widely used validated measure to quantify hearing-related QOL is the Hearing Handicap Inventory in the Elderly (HHIE), a 25-item scale with two subscales that measure the emotional and social impact of hearing loss.[100,104] The minimum change in score that corresponds to a clinically important difference has been established.[72] However, the scale does not distinguish between conductive or sensorineural hearing loss. The Hearing Satisfaction Scale (HHS) is specifically designed to measure outcomes after treatment for conductive hearing loss. It therefore

addresses side effects or complications of treatment and is brief (15 items).[93]

Numerous validated measures exist to assess outcomes after hearing amplification. One popular scale is the Abbreviated Profile of Hearing Aid Benefit (APHAB).[16] This 24-item scale measures four aspects of communication ability. Values corresponding to minimally clinically important clinical change have also been established.[17] The Effectiveness of Auditory Rehabilitation (EAR) scale addresses comfort and cosmesis issues associated with hearing aids that are overlooked in many hearing aid scales.[89] There are two brief 10-item modules. The Inner EAR addresses intrinsic issues of hearing loss such as functional, physical, emotional, and social impairment. The Outer EAR covers extrinsic factors such as the comfort, convenience, and cosmetic appearance of hearing aids.

Individuals interested in pursuing research on hearing amplification should also be aware of a number of other validated scales. Only a partial listing is referenced here.[20,22,38,87] In addition to these scales, there are several excellent, validated scales that assess other aspects of otologic disease including dizziness[50] and tinnitus.[60]

Rhinologic Disease

The ability to assess outcomes in chronic rhinosinusitis has dramatically improved with the development of disease-specific scales. The two most widely used scales are the Sinonasal Outcome Test (SNOT-20[78]) and the Chronic Sinusitis Survey (CSS[42]). The SNOT-20 has 20 items, has been extensively validated, and is a shortened version of the 31-item Rhinosinusitis Outcome Measure.[75] It is responsive to clinical change and has established scores that reflect minimally clinically important differences. The CSS is a shorter scale that consists of two components. The severity-based component has four items, and the duration-based component asks about duration of both symptoms and medication use. In addition to the SNOT-20 and CSS, there are a number of other excellent validated sinusitis scales.[2,54]

In 2003, the American Academy of Otolaryngology-Head and Neck Surgery Foundation commissioned the National Center for the Promotion of Research in Otolaryngology (NC-PRO) to develop and validate a disease-specific instrument for patients with nasal obstruction for a national outcomes study. The Nasal Obstruction Symptom Evaluation (NOSE) scale is a five-item instrument that is valid, reliable, and responsive.[95]

Pediatric Diseases

An important difference between measuring outcomes in adults and children is that younger children may be unable to complete the scales by themselves. In these cases, the instruments need to be completed by proxy, typically a parent or other care giver. This difference in perspective should be kept in mind when interpreting the results of pediatric studies. A good generic scale, similar to the SF-36 for adults, is the Child Health Questionnaire (CHQ[61]). This is also a widely used instrument that has been extensively validated and translated into numerous languages. The CHQ is a health status measure designed for children 5 years of age and older, and can be completed directly by children 10 years of age and older.

A number of excellent, validated disease-specific scales exist for children. The Otitis Media scale (OM-6) is a brief, 6-item scale useful for the evaluation of otitis media-related QOL in children.[83] The OM-6 has been shown to be reliable, valid, and responsive, and has been widely adopted. Two scales are pertinent to children with obstructive sleep disorders, the OSA-18[36] and the OSD-6.[18] A scale has also been developed for studying tonsil and adenoid health in children.[92]

Other Disorders

Several validated scales are in use to assess HRQOL in adults with obstructive sleep apnea. The most widely used are the 30-item Functional Outcomes of Sleep Questionnaire (FOSQ[103]) and the 50-item Calgary Sleep Apnea Quality of Life Index (SAQLI[34,35]). Clinicians interested in a more brief instrument may wish to consider the Symptoms of Nocturnal Obstruction and Respiratory Events (SNORE-25[76]). The eight-item Epworth Sleepiness Scale is commonly used to assess the degree of daytime sleepiness.[52]

Two scales specific to swallowing are available. The MD Anderson Dysphagia Inventory (MDADI[13]) is a brief, 20-item scale intended to measure dysphagia in head and neck cancer patients. The SWAL-QOL is longer (44 items), but validated for use in a more general population.[63] Finally, several instruments have been developed to assess outcomes in voice[39,49] and facial plastic surgery.[1]

SUMMARY AND FUTURE DIRECTIONS

Outcomes research is the scientific analysis of treatment effectiveness. From the early 1990s into the early twenty-first century, outcomes research has contributed substantially to the national debate on health resource allocation. Outcomes research provides insight into the value of otolaryngology treatments and methods for quantifying important outcomes that were previously too "soft" to measure. Better appreciation of outcomes research will improve the level of evidence about important treatments and operations. The impact of outcomes research is now beginning to extend into deliberations about quality of care, as the

health care system moves to establish standards for patient safety. The Leapfrog Group, a coalition of the largest public and private organizations that provide health care benefits for its employees, uses its collective purchasing power to ensure that its employees have access to and more informed choices about high-quality health care. Policymakers will increasingly look to outcomes research for insight into how to measure quality and safety, in addition to effectiveness.

It is imperative that clinicians be familiar with these basic principles. Otolaryngologists should participate in local and national outcomes research efforts to improve the evidence supporting successful otolaryngology interventions and to provide informed physician perspective in a health care environment that is increasingly driven by third-party participants.

REFERENCES

1. Alsarraf R: Outcomes instruments in facial plastic surgery, *Facial Plast Surg Clin North Am* 18:77–86, 2002.
2. Benninger MS, Senior BA: The development of the rhinosinusitis disability index, *Arch Otolaryngol Head Neck Surg* 123:1175–1179, 1997.
3. Bergner M and others: The sickness impact profile: development and final revision of a health status measure, *Med Care* 19:787–805, 1981.
4. Bhattacharyya T, Piccirillo J, Wippold FJ, II: Relationship between patient-based descriptions of sinusitis and paranasal sinus computed tomographic findings, *Arch Otolaryngol Head Neck Surg* 123:1189–1192, 1997.
5. Bjordal K and others: Quality of life in head and neck cancer patients: validation of the European Organization for Research and Treatment of Cancer Quality of Life Questionnaire-H&N35, *J Clin Oncol* 17:1008–1019, 1999.
6. Brook RH, Lohr KN: Efficacy, effectiveness, variations, and quality. Boundary-crossing research, *Med Care* 23:710–722, 1985.
7. Browman GP and others: The head and neck radiotherapy questionnaire: a morbidity/quality-of-life instrument for clinical trials of radiation therapy in locally advanced head and neck cancer, *J Clin Oncol* 11:863–872, 1993.
8. Cella DF and others: The Functional Assessment of Cancer Therapy scale: development and validation of the general measure, *J Clin Oncol* 11:570–579, 1993.
9. Centre for Evidence-Based Medicine: *http://www.cebm.net/*. Accessed May 6, 2003.
10. Champion GA, Piccirillo JF: The impact of computer tomography on pretherapeutic staging of patients with laryngeal cancer: demonstration of the Will Rogers' phenomenon. *Head Neck,* in press.
11. Charlson ME and others: A new method of classifying prognostic comorbidity in longitudinal studies: development and validation, *J Chronic Dis* 40:373–383, 1987.
12. Chassin MR and others: Does inappropriate use explain geographic variations in the use of health care services? A study of three procedures *JAMA* 258:2533–2537, 1987.
13. Chen AY and others: The development and validation of a dysphagia-specific quality-of-life questionnaire for patients with head and neck cancer: the MD Anderson dysphagia inventory, *Arch Otolaryngol Head Neck Surg* 127:870–876, 2001.

14. Codman EA: The product of a hospital, *Surg Gyn Obst* 18:491–496, 1914.

15. Cook DJ and others: Rules of evidence and clinical recommendations on the use of antithrombotic agents, *Chest* (Suppl) 102(4):305S–311S, 1992.

16. Cox RM, Alexander GC: The abbreviated profile of hearing aid benefit, *Ear Hear* 16:176–186, 1995.

17. Cox RM: Administration and Application of the APHAB, *www.ausp.memphis.edu/harl*, 1996.

18. de Serres LM and others: Measuring quality of life in children with obstructive sleep disorders, *Arch Otolaryngol Head Neck Surg* 126:1423–1429, 2000.

19. Deleyiannis FW, Weymuller EA, Jr., Coltrera MD: Quality of life of disease-free survivors of advanced (stage III or IV) oropharyngeal cancer, *Head Neck* 19:466–473, 1997.

20. Demorest ME, Erdman SA: Scale composition and item analysis of the Communication Profile for the Hearing Impaired, *J Speech Hear Res* 29:515–535, 1986.

21. Deyo RA, Diehr P, Patrick DL: Reproducibility and responsiveness of health status measures. Statistics and strategies for evaluation, *Control Clin Trials* (Suppl) 12(4 suppl):142S–158S,1991.

22. Dillon H, James A, Ginis J: Client Oriented Scale of Improvement (COSI) and its relationship to several other measures of benefit and satisfaction provided by hearing aids, *J Am Acad Audiol* 8:27–43, 1997.

23. Elmore JG and others: Variability in radiologists' interpretations of mammograms, *N Engl J Med* 331: 1493–1499, 1994.

24. El-Serag HB and others: Gastroesophageal reflux disease is a risk factor for laryngeal and pharyngeal cancer, *Am J Gastroenterol* 96:2013–2018, 2001.

25. Feeny D and others: Multi-attribute health status classification systems. Health Utilities Index, *Pharmacoeconomics* 7:490–502, 1995.

26. Feinstein AR, Sosin DM, Wells CK: The Will Rogers phenomenon. Stage migration and new diagnostic techniques as a source of misleading statistics for survival in cancer, *N Engl J Med* 312:1604–1608, 1985.

27. Feinstein AR: Clinical biostatistics. XLI. Hard science, soft data, and the challenges of choosing clinical variables in research, *Clin Pharmacol Ther* 22:485–498, 1977.

28. Feinstein AR: *Clinical epidemiology: the architecture of clinical research*. Philadelphia, W. B. Saunders Company, 1985.

29. Feinstein AR: *Clinimetrics*. New Haven, CT, Yale University Press, 1987.

30. Feinstein AR: Meta-analysis: statistical alchemy for the 21st century, *J Clin Epidemiol,* 48:71–79, 1995.

31. Feinstein AR: Para-analysis, faute de mieux, and the perils of riding on a data barge, *J Clin Epidemiol* 42:929–935, 1989.

32. Feinstein AR: The pre-therapeutic classification of comorbidity in chronic disease, *J Chronic Dis* 23:455–469, 1970.

33. Flay BR: Efficacy and effectiveness trials (and other phases of research) in the development of health promotion programs, *Prev Med* 15:451–474, 1986.

34. Flemons WW, Reimer MA: Development of a disease-specific health-related quality of life questionnaire for sleep apnea, *Am J Respir Crit Care Med* 158:494–503, 1998.

35. Flemons WW, Reimer MA: Measurement properties of the Calgary sleep apnea quality of life index, *Am J Respir Crit Care Med* 165:159–164, 2002.

36. Franco RA, Jr., Rosenfeld RM, Rao M: First place—resident clinical science award 1999. Quality of life for children with obstructive sleep apnea, *Otolaryngol Head Neck Surg* 123:9–16, 2000.

37. Furlong WJ and others: The Health Utilities Index (HUI) system for assessing health-related quality of life in clinical studies, *Ann Med* 33:375–384, 2001.

38. Giolas TG: The measurement of hearing handicap revisited: a 20-year perspective, *Ear Hear* 11(5 Suppl): 2S–5S,1990.

39. Gliklich RE, Glovsky RM, Montgomery WW: Validation of a voice outcome survey for unilateral vocal cord paralysis, *Otolaryngol Head Neck Surg* 120:153–158, 1999.

40. Gliklich RE, Goldsmith TA, Funk GF: Are head and neck specific quality of life measures necessary? *Head Neck* 19:474–480, 1997.

41. Gliklich RE, Metson R: A comparison of sinus computed tomography (CT) staging systems for outcomes research, *Am J Rhinol* 8:291–297, 1994.

42. Gliklich RE, Metson R: Techniques for outcomes research in chronic sinusitis, *Laryngoscope* 105:387–390, 1995.

43. Gold MR and others: Cost-effectiveness in health and medicine. New York, Oxford University Press, 1996.

44. Gray BH: The legislative battle over health services research, *Health Affairs* 11:38–66, 1992.

45. Hassan SJ, Weymuller E, Jr.: Assessment of quality of life in head and neck cancer patients, *Head Neck* 15:485–496, 1993.

46. Hill AB: The clinical trial, *Brit Med Bull* 7:278–282, 1951.

47. Hoffman HT and others: The National Cancer Data Base report on cancer of the head and neck, *Arch Otolaryngol Head Neck Surg* 124:951–962, 1998.

48. Hwang PH and others: Radiologic correlates of symptom-based diagnostic criteria for chronic rhinosinusitis, *Otolaryngol Head Neck Surg* 128:489–496, 2003.

49. Jacobson BH and others: The voice handicap index (VHI): development and validation, *Am J Speech Lang Pathol* 6:66–70, 1997.

50. Jacobson GP, Newman CW: The development of the Dizziness Handicap Inventory, *Arch Otolaryngol Head Neck Surg* 116:424–427, 1990.

51. Jaeschke R, Singer J, Guyatt GH: Measurement of health status. Ascertaining the minimal clinically important difference, *Control Clin Trials* 10:407–415, 1989.

52. Johns MW: Reliability and factor analysis of the Epworth Sleepiness Scale, *Sleep* 15:376–381,1992.

53. Juniper EF and others: Determining a minimal important change in a disease-specific Quality of Life Questionnaire, *J Clin Epidemiol* 47:81–87, 1994.

54. Juniper EF, Guyatt GH: Development and testing of a new measure of health status for clinical trials in rhinoconjunctivitis, *Clin Exp Allergy* 21:77–83, 1991.

55. Kaplan RM, Atkins CJ, Timms R: Validity of a quality of well-being scale as an outcome measure in chronic obstructive pulmonary disease, *J Chronic Dis* 37:85–95, 1984.

56. Kaplan RM and others: The Quality of Well-Being Scale: critical similarities and differences with SF-36, *Int J Qual Health Care* 10:509–520, 1998.

57. Kassirer JP and others: Decision analysis: a progress report, *Ann Intern Med* 106:275–291, 1987.

58. Kennedy DW: Prognostic factors, outcomes and staging in ethmoid sinus surgery. *Laryngoscope* (Suppl) 102:1–18 1992.

59. Kezirian EJ, Yueh B: Accuracy of terminology and methodology in economic analyses in otolaryngology, *Otolaryngol Head Neck Surg* 124:496–502, 2001.

60. Kuk FK and others: The pyschometric properties of a tinnitus handicap questionnaire, *Ear Hear* 11:434–445, 1990.

61. Landgraf JM and others: Canadian-French, German and UK versions of the Child Health Questionnaire: methodology and preliminary item scaling results, *Qual Life Res* 7:433–445, 1998.

62. Leape LL and others: Does inappropriate use explain small-area variations in the use of health care services? *JAMA* 263:669–672, 1990.

63. Lieu J, Piccirillo JF: Methodologic assessment of studies on endoscopic sinus surgery, *Arch Otolaryngol Head Neck Surg* 129(11):1230–1235, 2003.

64. List MA and others: The Performance Status Scale for Head and Neck Cancer Patients and the Functional Assessment of Cancer Therapy-Head and Neck Scale. A study of utility and validity, *Cancer* 77:2294–2301, 1996.

65. Lund VJ, Kennedy DW: Staging for rhinosinusitis, *Otolaryngol Head Neck Surg* 117:S35–40, 1997.

66. Lund VJ, Mackay IS: Staging in rhinosinusitis, *Rhinology* 31:183–184, 1993.

67. McDowell I, Jenkinson C: Development standards for health measures, *J Health Serv Res Policy* 1:238–246, 1996.

68. McHorney CA and others: The SWAL-QOL and SWAL-CARE outcomes tool for oropharyngeal dysphagia in adults: III. Documentation of reliability and validity, *Dysphagia* Spring 17:97–114, 2002.

69. Metson R and others: Comparison of sinus computed tomography staging systems, *Otolaryngol Head Neck Surg* 117:372–379, 1997.

70. Mitchell JB and others: Using Medicare claims for outcomes research, *Med Care* (Suppl) 32:JS38–51, 1994.

71. Nease RF, Jr., and others: Variation in patient utilities for outcomes of the management of chronic stable angina. Implications for clinical practice guidelines, *JAMA* 273:1185–1190, 1995.

72. Newman CW and others: Practical method for quantifying hearing aid benefit in older adults, *J Am Acad Audiol* 2:70–75, 1991.

73. Patrick DL, Erickson P: Health status and health policy: quality of life in health care evaluation and resource allocation. New York, Oxford University Press, 1993.

74. Pauker SG, Kassirer JP: Decision analysis, *N Engl J Med* 316:250–258, 1987.

75. Piccirillo JF and others: Psychometric and clinimetric validity of the 31-item rhinosinusitis outcome measure, *Am J Rhin* 9:297–306, 1995.

76. Piccirillo JF and others: Obstructive sleep apnea treatment outcomes pilot study, *Otolaryngol Head Neck Surg* 118:833–844, 1998.

77. Piccirillo JF and others: Development of a new head and neck cancer-specific comorbidity index, *Arch Otolaryngol Head Neck Surg* 128:1172–1179, 2002.

78. Piccirillo JF, Merritt MG, Jr., Richards ML. Psychometric and clinimetric validity of the 20-Item Sino-Nasal Outcome Test (SNOT-20), *Otolaryngol Head Neck Surg* 126:41–47, 2002.

79. Piccirillo JF: Importance of comorbidity in head and neck cancer, *Laryngoscope* 110:593–602, 2000.

80. Pugliano FA, Piccirillo JF: The importance of comorbidity in staging upper aerodigestive tract cancer, *Curr Opin Otolaryngol Head Neck Surg* 4:88–93, 1996.

81. Rogers SN and others: The addition of mood and anxiety domains to the University of Washington quality of life scale, *Head Neck* 24:521–529, 2002.

82. Roper WL and others: Effectiveness in health care. An initiative to evaluate and improve medical practice, *N Engl J Med* 319:1197–1202, 1988.

83. Rosenfeld RM and others: Quality of life for children with otitis media, *Arch Otolaryngol Head Neck Surg* 123:1049–1054, 1997.

84. Rosenfeld RM: How to systematically review the medical literature, *Otolaryngol Head Neck Surg* 115:53–63, 1996.

85. Russell LB and others: The role of cost-effectiveness analysis in health and medicine. Panel on Cost-Effectiveness in Health and Medicine, *JAMA* 276:1172–1177, 1996.

86. Sackett DL and others: Evidence based medicine: what it is and what it isn't, *BMJ* 312:71–72, 1996.

87. Schum DJ: Test-retest reliability of a shortened version of the hearing aid performance inventory, *J Am Acad Audiol* 4:18–21, 1993.

88. Schwartz DL and others: Staging of head and neck squamous cell cancer with extended-field FDG-PET, *Arch Otolaryngol Head Neck Surg* 129(11) 1173–1178, 2003.

89. Souza P and others: Sensitivity of self-assessment questionnaires to differences in hearing aid technology. Paper presented at: International Hearing Aid Research Conference; August 2002; Lake Tahoe, NV.

90. Stewart AL, Ware JE: Measuring functioning and well-being: the medical outcomes study approach. Durham, North Carolina, Duke University Press, 1992.

91. Stewart MG and others: Does the severity of sinus computed tomography findings predict outcome in chronic sinusitis? *Otolaryngol Head Neck Surg* 123:81–84, 2000.

92. Stewart MG and others: Validation of an outcomes instrument for tonsil and adenoid disease, *Arch Otolaryngol Head Neck Surg* 127:29–35, 2001.

93. Stewart MG and others: Development of a new outcomes instrument for conductive hearing loss, *Am J Otology* 18:413–420, 1997.

94. Stewart MG and others: Severity staging in chronic sinusitis: are CT scan findings related to patient symptoms? *Am J Rhinol* 13:161–167, 1999.

95. Stewart MG and others: Development and Validation of the Nasal Obstruction Symptom Evaluation Scale. *Otolaryngol Head Neck Surg,* in press.

96. Streiner DL, Norman GR: *Health measurement scales: a practical guide to their development and use,* ed 2, Oxford, England, Oxford University Press, 1995.

97. Terrell JE and others: Head and neck cancer-specific quality of life: instrument validation, *Arch Otolaryngol Head Neck Surg* 123:1125–1132, 1997.

98. The WHOQOL Group: Development of the World Health Organization WHOQOL-BREF quality of life assessment, *Psychol Med* May 28:551–558, 1998.

99. Trotti A and others: Development of a head and neck companion module for the quality of life-radiation therapy instrument (QOL-RTI), *Int J Radiat Oncol Biol Phys* 42:257–261, 1998.

100. Ventry IM, Weinstein BE: The Hearing Handicap Inventory for the Elderly: a new tool, *Ear Hear* 3:128–134, 1982.

101. Ware JE: *SF-36 health survey manual and interpretation guide.* Boston, MA, The Health Institute, 1993.

102. Weaver EM: Sleep apnea devices and sleep apnea surgery should be compared on effectiveness, not efficacy, *Chest* 123:961–962, 2003.

103. Weaver TE and others: An instrument to measure functional status outcomes for disorders of excessive sleepiness, *Sleep* 20:835–843, 1997.

104. Weinstein BE, Ventry IM: Audiometric correlates of the Hearing Handicap Inventory for the Elderly, *J Speech Hear Disord* 48:379–384, 1983.

105. Weinstein MC and others: Recommendations of the Panel on Cost-effectiveness in Health and Medicine, *JAMA* 276: 1253–1258, 1996.

106. Weinstein MC: Allocation of subjects in medical experiments, *New Engl J Med* 291:1278–1285, 1974.

107. Wennberg J, Gittelsohn: Small area variations in health care delivery, *Science* 182:1102–1108, 1973.

108. Winslow CM and others: The appropriateness of carotid endarterectomy, *N Engl J Med* 318:721–727, 1988.

109. Yueh B and others: A critical evaluation of critical pathways in head and neck cancer, *Arch Otolaryngol Head Neck Surg* 129:89–95, 2003.

110. Yueh B: Measuring and Reporting Quality of Life in Head and Neck Cancer, 2002; McLean, Virginia.

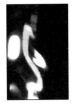

CHAPTER SIXTEEN

INTERPRETING MEDICAL DATA

‖ Richard M. Rosenfeld

INTRODUCTION

In every chapter of this book, whether it relates to clinical medicine or basic science, the authors draw on their own experience and the experience of others to form systematic conclusions. Experience yields data, and interpreting data is the heart and soul of the cumulative process called science. Data interpretation is also a centerpiece of evidence-based medicine, defined as the "... conscientious, explicit and judicious use of current best evidence in making decisions about the care of individual patients."[44] Learning how to interpret medical data will make you a better clinician, researcher, and teacher.

Effective data interpretation is a habit: a combination of knowledge, skill, and desire.[13] My goal is primarily to light the fires of desire, because I cannot possibly convey all the knowledge and skill in the space of this chapter. Instead, I will focus on the fundamental principles that underlie *all* data interpretation, regardless of the specific situation or statistical test to which they are applied. If you understand and apply these principles, you will be able to tackle the most complex data set or analytical problem.

By applying the seven habits (Table 16-1) outlined in this chapter, all otolaryngologists—regardless of their level of statistical knowledge or lack thereof—can interpret data. The numerous tables that accompany the text are designed as stand-alone reminders, and often contain keywords with definitions endorsed by the International Epidemiological Association.[31] I will also discuss the practice of data interpretation, including specific hypothesis tests, sample size determination, and common statistical deceptions encountered in the otolaryngology literature. You do not have to be a numerical wizard to understand data; all you need are patience, persistence, and a few good habits that will help settle the dust following the clash of statistics with the human mind.

The Seven Habits of Highly Effective Data Users

The seven habits that follow are the key to understanding data.[42] They embody fundamental principles of epidemiology and biostatistics that are developed in a logical and sequential fashion. Table 16-1 gives an overview of the seven habits and their corresponding principles and keywords.

Habit 1: Check Quality Before Quantity

Bias is a four-letter word that is easy to ignore, but difficult to avoid.[46] Data collected specifically for research (Table 16-2) are likely to be unbiased—they reflect the true value of the attribute being measured. In contrast, data collected during routine clinical care will vary in quality depending on the specific methodology applied.[46]

Experimental studies, such as randomized trials, often yield high-quality data because they are performed under carefully controlled conditions. In observational studies, however, the investigator is simply a bystander who records the natural course of health events during clinical care. Although more reflective of "real life" than a contrived experiment, observational studies are more prone to bias. Comparing randomized trials with outcomes studies highlights the difference between experimental and observational research (Table 16-3).

The presence or absence of a control group has a profound influence on data interpretation. An uncontrolled study—no matter how elegant—is purely descriptive.[36] Nonetheless, authors of case series often delight in unjustified musings on efficacy, effectiveness, association, and causality. Without a control or comparison group, treatment effects cannot be distinguished from other causes of clinical change (Table 16-4). Some of these causes are found in Figure 16-1, which depicts change in health status after a healing encounter as a complex interaction of three primary factors [8,37]:

TABLE 16-1

THE SEVEN HABITS OF HIGHLY EFFECTIVE DATA USERS

Habit	Underlying Principles	Keywords
1. Check quality before quantity	All data are not created equal; fancy statistics cannot salvage biased data from a poorly designed and executed study	Bias, accuracy, research design, confounding, causality
2. Describe before you analyze	Special data require special tests; improper analysis of small samples or data with an asymmetric distribution gives deceptive results	Measurement scale, frequency distribution, descriptive statistics
3. Accept the uncertainty of all data	All observations have some degree of random error; interpretation requires estimating the associated level of precision or confidence	Precision, random error, confidence intervals
4. Measure error with the right statistical test	Uncertainty in observation implies certainty of error; positive results must be qualified by the chance of being wrong; negative results by the chance of having missed a true difference	Statistical test, type I error, P value, type II error, power
5. Put clinical importance before statistical significance	Statistical tests measure error, not importance; an appropriate measure of clinical importance must be checked	Effect size, statistical significance, clinical importance
6. Seek the sample source	Results from one data set do not necessarily apply to another; findings can be generalized only for a random and representative sample	Population, sample, selection criteria, external validity
7. View science as a cumulative process	A single study is rarely definitive; data must be interpreted relative to past efforts and by their implications for future efforts	Research integration, level of evidence, meta-analysis

1. What was actually done? Specific effect(s) of therapy, including medications, surgery, physical manipulations, and alternative or integrative approaches.
2. What would have happened anyway? Spontaneous resolution, including natural history, random fluctuations in disease status, and regression to a mean symptom state.
3. What was imagined to have been done? Placebo response, defined as a change in health status resulting from the symbolic significance attributed by the patient (or proxy) to the encounter itself. A placebo response is most likely to occur when the patient receives a meaningful and personalized explanation, feels care and concern expressed by the healer, and achieves control and mastery over illness (or believes that the healer can control the illness).

The placebo response differs from the traditional definition of placebo as an inactive medical substance. Whereas a placebo can elicit a placebo response, the latter can occur without the former. A placebo response results from the psychological or symbolic importance attributed by the patient to any nonspecific event in a healing environment. These events include touch, words, gestures, locale ambiance, and social interactions.[15] Many of these factors are encompassed in the term *caring effects*,[26] which have been central to medical practice in all cultures throughout history.

When data from a comparison or control group are available, inferential statistics may be used to test hypotheses and measure associations. Causality may also be assessed when the study has a time-span component, either retrospective or prospective (see Table 16-2). Prospective studies measure incidence (new events), whereas retrospective studies measure prevalence (existing events). Unlike time-span studies, cross-sectional inquiries measure association not causality. Examples include surveys, screening programs, and evaluation of diagnostic tests. Experimentally planned interventions are ideal for assessing cause-effect relationships, because observational studies are prone to innate distortions or biases caused by individual judgments and other selective decisions.[17]

Another clue to data quality is study type,[40] but this cannot replace the four questions in Table 16-2. Note the variability in data quality for the study types listed

TABLE 16-2

EFFECT OF STUDY DESIGN ON DATA INTERPRETATION

Aspect of Study Design	Effect on Data Interpretation
How were the data originally collected?	
Specifically for research	Interpretation is facilitated by quality data collected according to an a priori protocol
During routine clinical care	Interpretation is limited by the consistency, accuracy, availability, and completeness of the source records
Is the study experimental or observational?	
Experimental study with conditions under direct control of the investigator	Low potential for systematic error (bias); bias can be reduced further by randomization and masking (blinding)
Observational study without intervention other than to record, classify, analyze	High potential for bias in sample selection, treatment assignment, measurement of exposures and outcomes
Is there a comparison or control group?	
Comparative or controlled study with two or more groups	Permits analytic statements concerning efficacy, effectiveness, and association
No comparison group present	Permits descriptive statements only, because of improvements from natural history and placebo effect
What is the direction of study inquiry?	
Subjects identified prior to an outcome or disease; future events recorded	Prospective design measures incidence (new events) and causality (if comparison group included)
Subjects identified after an outcome or disease; past histories are examined	Retrospective design measures prevalence (existing events) and causality (if comparison group included)
Subjects are identified at a single time point, regardless of outcome or disease	Cross-sectional design measures prevalence (exiting events) and association (if comparison group included)

in Table 16-5, particularly the observational designs. Randomization balances baseline prognostic factors (known and unknown) among groups, including severity of illness and the presence of comorbid conditions. Because these factors also influence a clinician's decision to offer treatment, nonrandomized studies are prone to allocation (susceptibility) bias (see Table 16-3) and false-positive results.[16] A typical example occurs when the survival of surgically treated cancer patients is compared with nonsurgical controls (e.g., radiation or chemotherapy). Without randomization, the surgical group will generally have a more favorable prognosis—independent of therapy—because the customary criteria for operability (special

TABLE 16-3

COMPARISON OF RANDOMIZED CLINICAL TRIALS AND OUTCOMES STUDIES

Characteristic	Randomized Clinical Trial	Outcomes Study
Level of investigator control	Experimental	Observational
Treatment allocation	Random assignment	Routine clinical care
Patient selection criteria	Restrictive	Broad
Typical setting	Hospital or university based	Community based
Endpoint definitions	Objective health status	Subjective quality of life
Endpoint assessment	Masked (blinded)	Unmasked
Statistical analysis	Comparison of groups	Multivariate regression
Potential for bias	Low	Very high
Ability to be generalized	Potentially low	Potentially high

TABLE 16-4

Explanations for Favorable Outcomes in Treatment Studies

Explanation	Definition	Solution
Bias	Systematic variation of measurements from their true values; may be intentional or unintentional	Accurate, protocol-driven data collection
Chance	Random variation without apparent relation to other measurements or variables (e.g., getting lucky)	Control or comparison group
Natural history	Course of a disease from onset to resolution; may include relapse, remission, and spontaneous recovery	Control or comparison group
Regression to the mean	Symptom improvement independent of therapy, as sick patients return to a mean level after seeking care	Control or comparison group
Placebo effect	Beneficial effect caused by the expectation that the regimen will have an effect (e.g., power of suggestion)	Control or comparison group with placebo
Halo effect	Beneficial effect caused by the manner, attention, and caring of a provider during a medical encounter	Control or comparison group treated similarly
Confounding	Distortion of an effect by other prognostic factors or variables for which adjustments have not been made	Randomization or multivariate analysis
Allocation (susceptibility) bias	Beneficial effect caused by allocating subjects with less severe disease or better prognosis to treatment group	Randomization or comorbidity analysis
Ascertainment (detection) bias	Favoring the treatment group during outcome analysis (e.g., statistical rounding up for treated subjects, statistical rounding down for controls)	Masked (blinded) outcome assessment

anatomic conditions and no major comorbidity) also predispose to favorable results.

The relationship between data quality and interpretation is illustrated in Table 16-6 using hypothetical studies to determine whether tonsillectomy causes baldness. Note how a case series (examples 1 and 2) can have either a prospective or retrospective direction of inquiry depending on how subjects are identified. Contrary to common usage, all case series are not "retrospective reviews." Only the controlled studies (examples 3–7) can measure associations, and only the controlled studies with a time-span component (examples 4–7) can assess causality. The nonrandomized studies (examples 3–6), however, require adjustment for potential confounding variables—baseline prognostic factors that may be associated with both tonsillectomy and baldness and therefore influence results. As noted previously, adequate randomization ensures balanced allocation of prognostic factors among groups, thereby avoiding the issue of confounding.

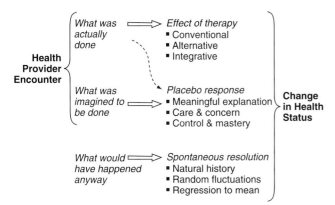

Figure 16-1. Model depicting change in health status after a healing encounter. Dashed arrow shows that a placebo response may occur from symbolic significance of the specific therapy given or from interpersonal aspects of the encounter.

Habit 2: Describe Before You Analyze

Statistical tests often make assumptions about the underlying data. Unless these assumptions are met, the test will be invalid. If you describe before you analyze, you avoid trying to unlock the mysteries of square data by using a round key.

TABLE 16-5

RELATIONSHIP OF STUDY TYPE TO STUDY METHODOLOGY

Study Type	How were the Data Originally Collected?	Is there a Control or Comparison Group?	What is the Direction of Study Inquiry?
Experimental studies			
Basic science	Research	Yes or no	Prospective or cross-sectional
Clinical	Research	Yes or no	Prospective or cross-sectional
Randomized	Research	Yes	Prospective
Observational studies			
Cohort	Clinical care or research	Yes or no	Prospective
Historical cohort	Clinical care	Yes	Prospective
Outcomes research	Clinical care or research	Yes or no	Prospective
Case-control	Clinical care	Yes	Retrospective
Case series	Clinical care	Yes or no	Retrospective or prospective
Survey	Clinical care or research	Yes or no	Cross-sectional
Diagnostic test	Clinical care or research	Yes or no	Cross-sectional

Data description begins by defining the measurement scale that best suits the observations. Categorical (qualitative) observations fall into one or more categories and include dichotomous, nominal, and ordinal scales (Table 16-7). Numerical (quantitative) observations are measured on a continuous scale and are further classified by the underlying frequency distribution (i.e., the plot of observed values vs the frequency of each value). Numerical data with a symmetric (normal) distribution are symmetrically placed around a central crest or trough (i.e., bell-shaped curve). Numerical data with an asymmetric distribution are skewed (shifted) to one side of the center, have a sloping "exponential" shape that resembles a forward or backward J, or contain some unusually high or low outlier values.

Depending on the measurement scale, data may be summarized using one or more of the descriptive statistics in Table 16-8. Note that when summarizing numerical data, the descriptive method varies according to the underlying distribution. Numerical data with a symmetric distribution are best summarized with the mean and standard deviation (SD), because 68% of the observations fall within the mean ± 1 SD and 95% fall within the mean ± 2 SD. In contrast, asymmetric numerical data are best summarized with the median, because even a single outlier can strongly influence the mean. If a series of 5 patients are followed after sinus surgery for 10, 12, 15, 16, and 48 months, the mean duration of follow-up is 20 months, but the median is only 15 months. In this case a single outlier—48 months—distorts the mean.

Although the mean is appropriate only for numerical data with a symmetric distribution, it is often applied regardless of the underlying symmetry. An easy way to

determine whether the mean or median is appropriate for numerical data is to calculate both; if they differ significantly, the median should be used. Another way is to examine the SD. When the SD is very large (e.g., larger than the mean value with which it is associated), the data often have an asymmetric distribution and should be described by the median and interquartile range. When in doubt, the median should always be used over the mean.[18]

A special form of numerical data is called censored (Table 16-7). Data are censored when three conditions apply: (1) the direction of study inquiry is prospective; (2) the outcome of interest is time-related; and (3) some subjects die, are lost, or have not yet had the outcome of interest when the study ends. Interpreting censored data is called survival analysis, because of its use in cancer studies where survival is the outcome of interest. Survival analysis permits full utilization of censored observations by including them in the analysis up to the time the censoring occurred. If censored observations are instead excluded from analysis (e.g., exclude all patients with less than 3 years follow-up in a cancer study), the resulting survival rates will be biased and sample size will be unnecessarily reduced.

A survival curve starts with 100% of the study sample alive and shows the percentage still surviving at successive times for as long as information is available. The curve may be applied not only to survival as such, but also to the persistence of freedom from a disease or complication or some other endpoint. For example, one could estimate the 3-year, 5-year, or 10-year rates for cholesteatoma recurrence, or the future "survival" of tonsils (e.g., no need for tonsillectomy) in a cohort of children after adenoidectomy alone. Several statistical methods are available for

TABLE 16-6

DETERMINING WHETHER TONSILLECTOMY CAUSES BALDNESS: STUDY DESIGN VS INTERPRETATION*

Study Design	Study Execution	Interpretation
1. Case series, retrospective	A group of bald subjects are questioned as to whether or not they ever had tonsillectomy	Measures prevalence of tonsillectomy in bald subjects; cannot assess association or causality
2. Case series, prospective	A group of subjects who had, or who are about to have, tonsillectomy are examined later for baldness	Measures incidence of baldness after tonsillectomy; cannot assess association or causality
3. Cross-sectional study	A group of subjects are examined for baldness and for presence or absence of tonsils at the same time	Measures prevalence of baldness and tonsillectomy and their association; cannot assess causality
4. Case-control study	A group of bald subjects and a group of non-bald subjects are questioned about prior tonsillectomy	Measures prevalence of baldness and association with tonsillectomy; limited ability to assess causality
5. Historical cohort study	A group of subjects who had prior tonsillectomy and a comparison group with intact tonsils are examined later for baldness	Measures incidence of baldness and association with tonsillectomy; can assess causality when adjusted for confounding variables
6. Cohort study (longitudinal)	A group of non-bald subjects about to have tonsillectomy and a non-bald comparison group with intact tonsils are examined later for baldness	Measures incidence of baldness and association with tonsillectomy; can assess causality when adjusted for confounding variables
7. Randomized controlled trial	A group of non-bald subjects with intact tonsils are randomly assigned to tonsillectomy or observation and examined later for baldness	Measures incidence of baldness and association with tonsillectomy; can assess causality despite baseline confounding variables

*Studies are listed in order of increasing ability to establish a causal relationship.

analyzing survival data. The Kaplan-Meier (product-limit) method records events by exact dates and is suitable for small and large samples. Conversely, the life table (actuarial) method records events by time interval (e.g., every month, every year) and is most commonly used for large samples in epidemiological studies.

The odds ratio, relative risk, and rate difference (see Table 16-8) are useful ways of comparing two groups of dichotomous data.[9] A retrospective (case-control)

TABLE 16-7

MEASUREMENT SCALES FOR DESCRIBING AND ANALYZING DATA

Scale	Definition	Examples
Dichotomous	Classification into either of two mutually exclusive categories	Breast feeding (yes/no), sex (male/female)
Nominal	Classification into unordered qualitative categories	Race, religion, country of origin
Ordinal	Classification into ordered qualitative categories, but with no natural (numerical) distance between their possible values	Hearing loss (none, mild, moderate), patient satisfaction (low, medium, high), age group
Numerical	Measurements with a continuous scale, or a large number of discrete ordered values	Temperature, age in years, hearing level in decibels
Numerical (censored)	Measurements on subjects lost to follow-up or in whom a specified event has not yet occurred at the end of a study	Survival rate, recurrence rate, or any time-to-event outcome in a prospective study

study of tonsillectomy and baldness might report an odds ratio of 1.6, indicating that bald subjects were 1.6 times more likely to have had tonsillectomy than were non-bald controls. In contrast, a prospective study would report results using relative risk. A relative risk of 1.6 means that baldness was 1.6 times more likely to develop in tonsillectomy subjects than in nonsurgical controls. Finally, a rate difference of 30% in a prospective trial or experiment reflects the increase in baldness caused by tonsillectomy, above and beyond what occurred in controls. No association exists between groups when the rate difference equals 0, or the odds ratio or relative risk equals one (unity).

Two groups of ordinal or numerical data are compared with a correlation coefficient (Table 16-8). A coefficient (r) of 0 to .25 indicates little or no relationship, .25 to .49 a fair relationship, .50 to .74 a moderate to good relationship, and greater than .75 a good to excellent relationship. A perfect linear relationship would yield a coefficient of 1.00. When one variable varies directly with the other, the coefficient is positive. A negative coefficient implies an inverse association. Sometimes the correlation coefficient is squared (R^2) to form the coefficient of determination, which estimates the percentage of variability in one measure that is predicted by the other.

Habit 3: Accept the Uncertainty of all Data

Uncertainty is present in all data because of the inherent variability in biologic systems and in our ability to assess such systems.[43] It is impossible to reproduce the exact same results time after time. If you measure hearing in 20 healthy volunteers on 5 different days, how likely would it be to get the same mean result each time? Very unlikely, because audiometry has a variable behavioral component that depends on the subject's response to a stimulus and the examiner's perception of that response. Similarly, if you measured hearing in 5 groups of 20 healthy volunteers each, how likely would it be to get the same mean hearing level in each group? Again unlikely, because of variations between individuals. We would get a range of similar results, but rarely the exact same result on repetitive trials.

Uncertainty must be dealt with when interpreting data, unless the results are meant to apply only to the particular group of patients, animals, cell cultures,

TABLE 16-8

DESCRIPTIVE STATISTICS

Descriptive Measure	Definition	When to Use it
Central tendency		
Mean	Arithmetic average	Numerical data that are symmetric
Median	Middle observation; half the values are smaller and half are larger	Ordinal data; numerical data with an asymmetric distribution
Mode	Most frequent value	Nominal data; bimodal distribution
Dispersion		
Range	Largest value minus smallest value	Emphasizes extreme values
Standard deviation	Spread of data about their mean	Numerical data that are symmetric
Percentile	Percentage of values that are equal to or below that number	Ordinal data; numerical data with an asymmetric distribution
Interquartile range	Difference between the 25th percentile and 75th percentile	Ordinal data; numerical data with an asymmetric distribution
Outcome		
Survival rate	Proportion of subjects surviving, or with some other outcome, after a time interval (e.g., 1 year, 5 years, etc.)	Numerical (censored) data in a prospective study
Odds ratio	Odds of a disease or outcome in subjects with a risk factor divided by odds in controls	Dichotomous data in a retrospective or prospective controlled study
Relative risk	Incidence of a disease or outcome in subjects with a risk factor divided by incidence in controls	Dichotomous data in a prospective controlled study
Rate difference*	Event rate in treatment group minus event rate in control group	Compares success or failure rates in clinical trial groups
Correlation coefficient	Degree to which two variables have a linear relationship	Numerical or ordinal data

*Also called the absolute risk reduction.

DNA strands, etc., in which the observations were initially made. Recognizing this uncertainty, we call each of the descriptive measures in Table 16-8 a point estimate, specific to the data that generated it. In medicine, however, we seek to pass from observations to generalizations, from point estimates to estimates about other populations. When this process occurs with calculated degrees of uncertainty, we call it inference.

Here's a brief example of clinical inference. After treating five vertiginous patients with vitamin C, you remark to a colleague that four had excellent relief of their vertigo. She asks, "How confident are you of your results?" "Quite confident," you reply, "there were five patients, four got better, and that's 80%." "Maybe I wasn't clear," she interjects, "how confident are you that 80% of vertiginous patients you see in the next few weeks will respond favorably, or that 80% of similar patients in my practice will do well with vitamin C?" "In other words," she continues, can you *infer* anything about the real effect of vitamin C on vertigo from only five patients?" Hesitatingly you retort "I'm pretty confident about that number 80%, but maybe I'll have to see a few more patients to be sure."

The real issue, of course, is that a sample of only five patients offers low precision (repeatability). How likely is it that the same results would be found if five new patients were studied? Actually, we can state with 95% confidence that 4 out of 5 successes in a single trial is consistent with a range of results from 28% to 99% in future trials. This 95% confidence interval may be calculated manually or with a statistical program, [5,23] and tells us the range of results consistent with the observed data. Thus, if this trial were repeated, we could obtain a success rate as low as 28%, not very encouraging compared with the original point estimate of 80%. To make an analogy to a mutual fund prospectus, past performance is no guarantee of future results. Statistics, however, allow us to estimate future performance with a calculated degree of uncertainty.

Precision may be increased (uncertainty may be decreased) by using a more reproducible measure, by increasing the number of observations (sample size), or by decreasing the variability among the observations. The most common method is to increase the sample size, because we can rarely reduce the variability inherent in the subjects we study. Even a huge sample of perhaps 50,000 subjects still has some degree of uncertainty, but the 95% confidence interval will be quite small. Realizing that uncertainty can never completely be avoided, we use statistics to estimate precision. Thus, when data are described using the summary measures listed in Table 16-8, a corre-sponding 95% confidence interval should accompany each point estimate.

Precision differs from accuracy. *Precision* relates to random error and measures repeatability. *Accuracy* relates to systematic error (bias) and measures nearness to the truth. A precise otologist may always perform a superb mastoidectomy, but an accurate otologist performs it on the right patient. A precise surgeon cuts on the exact center of the line, but an accurate surgeon first checks the line to be sure it is in the right place. Succinctly put, precision is doing things right and accuracy is doing the right thing. Precise data include a large enough sample of carefully measured observations to yield repeatable estimates. Accurate data are measured in an unbiased manner so that the reflect what is truly purported to be measured. When we interpret data, we must estimate both precision and accuracy.

Before moving on to Habit 4, let me briefly summarize Habits 1, 2, and 3. Habit 1, "Check quality before quantity," determines whether the data are worth interpreting. Assuming they are, we move to Habit 2, "Describe before you analyze," and summarize the data using appropriate measures of central tendency, dispersion, and outcome for the particular measurement scale(s) involved. Next, we "Accept the uncertainty of all data" as noted in Habit 3, and qualify the point estimates in Habit 2 with 95% confidence intervals to measure precision. When precision is low (e.g., the confidence interval is wide), we proceed with caution. Otherwise, we proceed to Habits 4, 5, and 6, which deal with errors and inference.

Habit 4: Measure Error with the Right Statistical Test

To err is human—and statistical. When comparing two or more groups of uncertain data, errors in inference are inevitable. If we conclude the groups are different, they may actually be equivalent. If we conclude they are the same, we may have missed a true difference. Data interpretation is an exercise in modesty, not pretense—any conclusion we reach may be wrong. The ignorant data analyst ignores the possibility of error; the savvy analyst estimates this possibility by using the right statistical test.[10]

Now that we've stated the problem in English, let's restate it in thoroughly confusing statistical jargon (Table 16-9). We begin with some testable hypothesis about the groups we are studying, such as "Gibberish levels in Group A differ from those in Group B." Rather than keep it simple, we now invert this to form a null hypothesis: "Gibberish levels in Group A are equal to those in Group B." Next we fire up our personal computer, enter the gibberish levels for the subjects in both groups, choose an appropriate statistical test, and wait for the omnipotent P value to emerge.

The P value tells us the probability making a type I error: rejecting a true null hypothesis In other words, if $P = .10$ we have a 10% chance of being wrong when we declare Group A differs from Group B, based on the observed data. Alternatively, there is a 10% probability that the difference in gibberish levels is explainable by random error—we can't be certain that uncertainty isn't the cause. In medicine, $P < .05$ is generally considered low enough to safely reject the null hypothesis. Conversely, when $P > .05$ we accept the null hypothesis of equivalent gibberish levels. Nonetheless, we may be making a type II error by accepting a false null hypothesis. Rather than state the probability of a type II error directly (which would make too much sense), we state it indirectly by specifying power (Table 16-9). Clear as mud, right?

TABLE 16-9

GLOSSARY OF STATISTICAL TERMS ENCOUNTERED WHEN TESTING HYPOTHESES

Term	Definition
Hypothesis	A supposition, arrived at from observation or reflection, that leads to predictions that can be tested and refuted
Null hypothesis	Results observed in a study, experiment, or test are no different from what might have occurred because of chance alone
Statistical test	Procedure used to reject or accept a null hypothesis; statistical tests may be parametric, nonparametric (distribution-free), or exact
Type I (alpha) error	Rejecting a true null hypothesis (false positive error); declaring that a difference exists when in fact it does not
P value	Probability of making a type I error; $P < .05$ indicates a statistically significant result that is unlikely to be caused by chance
Type II (beta) error	Accepting a false null hypothesis (false negative error); declaring that a difference does not exist when in fact it does
Power	Probability that the null hypothesis will be rejected if it is indeed false; mathematically, power is 1.00 minus type II error

Now let's digress from principles to practice. We'll use two hypothetical studies for this purpose. The first is an observational, prospective study to determine whether tonsillectomy causes baldness: 20 patients undergoing tonsillectomy and 20 controls are examined 40 years after tonsillectomy and the incidence of baldness is compared. The second study will use the same groups, but will determine whether tonsillectomy causes hearing loss. This will allow us to explore statistical error from the perspective of a dichotomous outcome (bald vs non-bald) and a numerical outcome (hearing level in decibels).

Suppose that baldness develops in 80% of tonsillectomy patients (16/20) but in only 50% of controls (10/20). If we infer that, based on these results in 40 specific patients, tonsillectomy predisposes to baldness in general, what is our probability of being wrong (type I error)? Because $P = .10$ (Fisher exact test) there is a 10% chance of type I error, so we are reluctant to associate tonsillectomy with baldness based on this single study. Intuitively, however, a rate difference of 30% seems like a big difference. So what is our chance of being wrong when we conclude it is *not* significant (type II error)? The probability of a type II error (false-negative result) is actually 48% (same as saying 52% power), which means we may indeed be wrong in accepting the null hypothesis. Therefore, we need a larger study before any definitive conclusions can be drawn.

Intrigued by our initial findings, we repeat the tonsillectomy study with twice as many patients in each group. Suppose that baldness again develops in 80% of tonsillectomy patients (32/40), but only 50% of controls (20/40). The rate difference is still 30%, but now $P = .01$ (Fisher exact test). We therefore conclude that tonsillectomy is associated with baldness, with only a 1% chance of making a type I error (false-positive result). By increasing the number of subjects studied, we increased precision to a level where we could move from observation to generalization with a tolerable level of uncertainty.

Returning to our earlier study of 20 tonsillectomy patients and 20 controls, we find that the hearing levels for the groups are 25 ± 9 decibels (dB) and 20 ± 9 dB, respectively (mean value $\pm$ SD). What is our chance of being wrong if we infer that post-tonsillectomy patients have hearing levels 5 dB lower than controls? Because $P = .09$ (t test), there is a 9% probability of a type I error. If, however, we conclude there is no true difference between the groups, we have a 58% chance of making a type II error. Thus, we can say little about the impact of tonsillectomy on hearing based on this study, because power is only 42%. In general, studies with "negative" findings should be interpreted by power not P values.

When making inferences about numerical data, precision may be increased by studying more subjects, or subjects with less variability in their responses. For example, suppose that we again study 20 tonsillectomy patients and 20 controls, but this time the hearing levels are 25 ± 3 dB and 20 ± 3 dB. Although the difference remains 5 dB, the standard deviation is only 3 for this study, compared with 9 for the preceding study. For whatever reason, the second subjects had more consistent (less variable) responses. What effect does this reduced variability have on our ability to make inferences? We now obtain $P < .001$ (t test), indicating less than a 1:1000 probability of a type I error if we conclude that the hearing levels truly differ.

All statistical tests measure error. Choosing the right test for a particular situation is determined by (1) whether the observations come from independent or related samples; (2) whether the purpose is to compare groups or to associate an outcome with one or more predictor variables; and (3) the measurement scale of the variables (see Tables 16-10 and 16-11).[14] Despite the myriad tests available, the principles underlying each remain constant.

Two events are independent if the occurrence of one is in no way predictable from the occurrence of the other. A common example of independent samples is two or more parallel (concurrent) groups in a clinical trial or observational study. Conversely, related samples include paired organ studies, subjects matched by age and sex, and repeated measures on the same subjects (e.g., before and after treatment). Measurement scales have been previously discussed, but the issue of frequency distribution deserves emphasis. The parametric tests discussed in Tables 16-10 and 16-11 assume an underlying symmetric distribution for data. If the data are sparse, asymmetric, or plagued with outliers, then a "nonparametric" test must be used.

Using the wrong statistical test to estimate error invalidates results. For example, suppose we measure intelligence quotient (IQ) in 20 subjects before and after tonsillectomy, and find that the mean IQ increases from 125 to 128. This 3-point increase $P = .29$ (t test, independent samples), suggests a high probability (29%) of reaching a false-positive conclusion. However, the observations in this example are related—before and after IQ tests in the same subjects. What is really of interest is the mean change in IQ for each subject (related samples), not how the mean IQ of all subjects before surgery compares with the mean IQ of all subjects postoperatively (independent samples). When the proper statistical test is used (t test, paired samples), $P = .05$ suggests a true association. Related (matched) samples are common

in biomedical studies and should never be analyzed as though they were independent.

Habit 5: Put Clinical Importance Before Statistical Significance

Results are statistically significant when the probability of a type I error is low enough ($P < .05$) to safely reject the null hypothesis. If the statistical test compared two groups, we conclude that the groups differ. If the statistical test compared three or more groups, we conclude that global differences exist among them. If the statistical test related predictor and outcome variables (regression analysis), we conclude that the predictor variables explain more variation in the outcome than would be expected by chance alone. These generalizations apply to all the statistical tests in Tables 16-10 and 16-11.

The next logical question after "Is there a difference?" (indicating statistical significance) is "How big a difference is there?" (indicating clinical importance). Unfortunately, most data interpretation stops with the P value, and the second question is never asked. For example, a clinical trial of nonsevere acute otitis media found amoxicillin superior to placebo as initial treatment ($P = .009$).[29] Before we agree with the author's recommendation for routine amoxicillin therapy, let's look more closely at the magnitude of clinical effect. Initial treatment success occurred in 96% of amoxicillin-treated children vs 92% of controls, yielding a 4% rate difference favoring drug therapy. Alternatively, we must treat 25 subjects (100/4) with amoxicillin to increase the success rate by one subject over what would occur from placebo alone. Is this clinically important? Maybe, or maybe not.

Statistically significant results must be accompanied by a measure of effect size, which reflects the magnitude of difference between groups.[32] Otherwise, findings with minimal clinical importance may become statistically significant when a large number of subjects are studied. In the preceding example, the 4% difference in success rates was highly statistically significant because more than 1000 episodes of otitis media contributed to this finding. Large numbers provide high precision (repeatability), which in turn reduces the likelihood of error. The final result is a hypnotically tiny P value, which may reflect a clinical difference of trivial importance.

Common measures of effect size when comparing groups include the odds ratio, relative risk, and rate difference (see Table 16-8). For example, in the hypothetical study of tonsillectomy and baldness discussed earlier in this chapter the rate difference was 30% ($P = .01$), with a 95% confidence interval of 10% to 50%. Therefore, we are 95% confident that tonsillectomy increases the rate of baldness between 10% and

TABLE 16-10

STATISTICAL TESTS FOR INDEPENDENT SAMPLES

Situation	Parametric Test	Nonparametric Test
Comparing two groups of data		
Numerical scale	*t* test	Mann-Whitney U,* median test
Numerical (censored) scale	Mantel-Haenszel life table	Wilcoxon, log-rank, Mantel-Cox
Ordinal scale	—	Mann-Whitney U, median test, chi-square test for trend
Nominal scale	—	Chi-square, log-likelihood ratio
Dichotomous scale	—	Chi-square, Fisher exact test, odds ratio, relative risk
Comparing three or more groups of data		
Numerical scale	One-way ANOVA†	Kruskal-Wallis ANOVA
Ordinal scale	—	Kruskal-Wallis ANOVA, chi-square test for trend
Dichotomous or nominal scale	—	Chi-square, log-likelihood ratio
Associating an outcome with predictor variables		
Numerical outcome, one predictor	Pearson correlation	Spearman rank correlation
Numerical outcome, two or more predictor variables	Multiple linear regression, two-way ANOVA	—
Numerical (censored) outcome	Proportional hazards (Cox) regression	—
Dichotomous outcome	Discriminant analysis	Multiple logistic regression
Nominal or ordinal outcome	Discriminant analysis	Log-linear model

*The Mann-Whitney U test is equivalent to the Wilcoxon rank-sum test.
†ANOVA=analysis of variance.

50%, with only a 1% chance of a type I error (false-positive). Alternatively, results could be expressed in terms of relative risk. For the tonsillectomy study, relative risk is 1.6 (the incidence of baldness was 1.6 times higher after surgery), with a 95% confidence interval of 1.1 to 2.3. Effect size and 95% confidence limits may be calculated manually[14,29,32,52] or with a computer program.[5]

Effect size is measured by the correlation coefficient (r) when an outcome variable is associated with one or more predictor variables in a regression analysis (see Table 16-10). Suppose that a study of thyroid surgery reports that shoe size had a statistically significant association with intraoperative blood loss (multiple linear regression, $P = .04$, $r = .10$). A correlation of only .10 implies little or no relationship (see

TABLE 16-11

STATISTICAL TESTS FOR RELATED (MATCHED, PAIRED, OR REPEATED) SAMPLES

Situation	Parametric Test	Nonparametric Test
Comparing two groups of data		
Dichotomous scale	—	McNemar test,
Ordinal scale	—	Sign test, Wilcoxon signed rank test
Numerical scale	Paired *t* test	Sign test, Wilcoxon signed rank test
Comparing three or more groups of data		
Dichotomous scale	—	Cochran *Q* test, Mantel-Haenszel Chi-square
Ordinal scale	—	Friedman ANOVA*
Numerical scale	Repeated measures ANOVA	Friedman ANOVA

*ANOVA=analysis of variance.

my discussion of "Describe before you analyze" earlier in this chapter), and an R^2 of .01 means that only 1% of the variance in survival is explainable by shoe size. Who cares whether the results are "significant" when the effect size is clinically irrelevant, not to mention nonsensical. Besides, when $P = .04$ we have a 4% chance of being wrong when we reject the null hypothesis, which may in fact be the case here. A nonsensical result should prompt a search for confounding factors that may not have been included in the regression, such as the tumor, node, metastasis (TNM) stage; comorbid conditions; duration of surgery; etc.

Confidence intervals (CI) are more appropriate measures of clinical importance than P values, because they reflect *both* magnitude and precision.[7,23] When a study reports "significant" results, the lower limit of the 95% CI should be scrutinized. A value of minimal clinical importance suggests low precision (inadequate sample size). When a study reports "nonsignificant" results, the upper limit of the 95% CI should be scrutinized. A value indicating a potentially important clinical effect suggests low statistical power (false negative finding). Confidence intervals are essential for interpreting effect size, which is a critical concept in evidence-based medicine.[25]

Habit 6: Seek the Sample Source

When we interpret medical data, we ultimately seek to make inferences about some target population based on results in a smaller sample (Table 16-12). Rarely is it possible to study every patient, medical record, DNA strand, or fruit fly with the condition of interest. Nor is it necessary—inferential statistics allow us to generalize from the few to the many, provided that the few we study are a random and representative sample of the many. However, random and representative samples rarely arise from divine providence. Therefore, you must always seek the sample source before generalizing your interpretation of the data beyond the confines of the study that produced it.

As an example of sampling, consider a new antibiotic that is touted as superior to an established standard for treating acute otitis media. When you review that data on which this statement is based, you learn that the study endpoint was bacteriologic efficacy—the ability to sterilize the middle ear after treatment. Further, the only patients included in the study were those whose initial tympanocentesis revealed an organism with in vitro sensitivity to the new antibiotic. Patients with no growth or resistant bacteria were excluded. Can you apply these results to your clinical practice? Most likely not, because you probably don't limit your practice to patients with sensitive bacteria. In other words, the sample of patients included in the study is not representative of the target population in your practice.

A statistical test is valid only when the study sample is random and representative. Unfortunately, these assumptions are frequently violated or overlooked.

TABLE 16-12

GLOSSARY OF STATISTICAL TERMS RELATED TO SAMPLING AND VALIDITY

Term	Definition
Target population	Entire collection of items, subjects, patients, observations, etc., about which we want to make inferences; defined by the selection criteria (inclusion and exclusion criteria) for the study
Accessible population	Subset of the target population that is accessible for study, generally because of geographic or temporal considerations
Study sample	Subset of the accessible population that is chosen for study
Sampling method	Process of choosing a sample from a larger population; the method may be random or nonrandom, representative or nonrepresentative
Selection bias	Error caused by systematic differences between a study sample and target population; examples include studies on volunteers, and those conducted in clinics or tertiary care settings
Sample size determination	Process of deciding, before a study begins, how many subjects should be studied; based on the incidence or prevalence of the condition under study, anticipated differences between groups, the power that is desired, and the allowable level of type I error
Internal study validity	Degree to which conclusions drawn from a study are valid for the study sample; results from proper study design, unbiased measurements, and sound statistical analysis
External study validity (ability to be generalized)	Degree to which conclusions drawn from a study are valid for a target population (beyond the subjects in the study); results from representative sampling and appropriate selection criteria

A random sample is necessary because most statistical tests are based on probability theory—playing the odds. The odds apply only if the deck is not stacked and the dice are not rigged (i.e., all members of the target population have an equal chance of being sampled for study). Investigators, however, typically have access to only a small subset of the target population because of geographic or temporal constraints. When they choose an even smaller subset of this accessible population to study, the method of choosing (sampling method) affects our ability to make inferences about the original target population.

Of the sampling methods listed in Table 16-13, only a random sample is theoretically suitable for statistical analysis. Nonetheless, a consecutive or systematic sample offers a relatively good approximation, and provides data of sufficient quality for most statistical tests. The worst sampling method occurs when subjects are chosen based on convenience or subjective judgments about eligibility. Applying statistical tests to the resulting convenience (grab) sample is the equivalent of asking a professional card counter to help you win a blackjack game when the deck is stacked and cards are missing—all bets are off because probability theory will not apply. A brute force sample of the entire population is also unsatisfactory, because lost, missing, or incomplete units tend to differ systematically from those that are readily accessible.

To "seek the sample source" is to identify the sampling method and selection criteria (inclusion and exclusion criteria) that were applied to the target population to obtain the study sample. When the process appears sound, we conclude that the results can be generalized and are externally valid (see Table 16-12).

If the process appears flawed, we cannot interpret or extrapolate the results beyond the confines of the study sample. For example, a nasal spray that is effective for tree pollen allergy in patients referred to a tertiary rhinology center would offer uncertain benefit for patients with dust mite allergy treated by a family practitioner. Similarly, patients studied by otolaryngologists generally have more severe and chronic disease than the population at large or the population seen by primary care physicians. Volunteers and hospital-based patients are further examples of biased samples with little potential for generalization.

The impact of sampling on the ability to generalize is particularly important when interpreting a diagnostic test.[45] For instance, suppose an audiologist develops a new test for diagnosing middle ear effusion (MEE). After testing 1000 children, she reports that 90% of children with a positive result did in fact have MEE. This is a positive predictive value of 90%. Yet when you screen random kindergarten children for MEE, the positive predictive value of the test is only 50%. Why does this occur? Because the baseline prevalence of MEE is lower in the kindergarten class (10% have MEE) than in the referral-based audiology population in which the test was developed (50% have MEE). Whereas the sensitivity and specificity of the test are unchanged in both situations, the predictive value is related to baseline prevalence (Bayes, theorem). Therefore, the ultimate utility of the test depends on the sample to which it will be applied.

Habit 7: View Science as a Cumulative Process

A single study—no matter how elegant or seductive—is rarely definitive. Science is a cumulative process

---

TABLE 16-13

METHODS FOR SAMPLING A POPULATION

Method	How it is Performed	Comments
Brute force sample	Includes all units of study (charts, patients, laboratory animals, or journal articles) accessible to the researchers	Time-consuming and unsophisticated; bias-prone because missing units are seldom randomly distributed
Convenience (grab) sample	Units are selected on the basis of accessibility, convenience, or subjective judgments about eligibility	Assume this method when none is specified; study results cannot be generalized because of selection bias
Consecutive sample	Every unit is included over a specified time interval, or until a specified number is reached	Excellent method when intake period is long enough to adequately represent seasonal and other temporal factors
Systematic sample	Units are selected using some simple, systematic rule, such as first letter of last name, date of birth, or day of week	Less biased than a grab sample, but problems may still occur because of unequal selection probabilities
Random sample	Units are assigned numbers then selected at random until a desired sample size is attained	Best method; bias is minimized because all units have a known (and equal) probability of selection

that requires a large body of consistent and reproducible evidence before conclusions can be formed.[33] When interpreting an exciting set of data, the cumulative basis of science is often overshadowed by the seemingly irrefutable evidence at hand. At least until a new study, by different investigators in a different environment, adds a new twist.

Habit 7 is the process of integration: reconciling our findings with the existing corpus of known similar research. It is the natural consequence—Habits 1 through 3 deal with description and Habits 4 through 6 deal with analysis. Thus, we can summarize data interpretation with three words: describe, analyze, and integrate. This is a sequential process in which each step lays the foundation for subsequent ones, just as occurs for the six habits that underlie them.

Research integration begins by asking "Do the results make sense?" Statistically significant findings that are biologically implausible, or that are inconsistent with other known studies, can often be explained by hidden biases or design flaws that were initially unsuspected (Habit 1). Improbable results can become statistically significant through biased data collection, natural history, placebo effects, unidenti-

fied confounding variables, or improper statistical analysis. A study with design flaws or improper statistical analysis is said to have low internal validity (see Table 16-12) and should be reanalyzed or discarded.

At the next level of integration, we compare the study design that produced the current data with the design of other published studies. The level of evidence generally increases as we progress from uncontrolled observational studies (e.g., case reports, case series), to controlled observational studies (e.g., cross-sectional, retrospective, prospective) to controlled experiments (e.g., randomized trials).[25] Levels of research evidence are most often applied to studies of therapy or prevention (Table 16-14), but can also be defined for diagnosis and prognosis.[38] Grades of recommendation (Table 16-15) are assigned based on the quality and consistency of supporting research evidence. Note that "expert opinion" or consensus, a commonly used method in otolaryngology, qualifies only as a grade D recommendation.

Bentsianov and colleagues[3] assessed the levels of supporting evidence for therapeutic recommendations in leading otolaryngology journals. Of 1019 articles published in 1999, 72% were clinical research and

TABLE 16-14

LEVELS OF RESEARCH EVIDENCE FOR CLINICAL RECOMMENDATIONS*

Level	Therapy or Prevention	Diagnosis	Prognosis
1	Randomized controlled trial; systematic review of randomized trials; "all or none" case series	Validating cohort study with good reference standard; CDR[†] tested at one clinical center; SpPins[‡] and SpNouts[#]	CDR validated in a single population or in cohort study with >80% follow-up; "all or none" case series
2	Prospective controlled study: cohort study, outcomes research, ecological study	Exploratory cohort study with good reference standard; derivation of CDR; or CDR tested on split-sample or data base	Retrospective cohort study or follow-up of untreated controls; derivation or CDR; or CDR tested on split-sample; outcomes research
3	Retrospective controlled study: case-control study	Nonconsecutive study, or without consistently applied reference standards	—
4	Case series and poor quality cohort and case-control studies	Case-control study, or poor or nonindependent reference standard	Case-series and poor quality prognostic cohort studies
5	Expert opinion without explicit critical appraisal; or based on physiology, bench research, or "first principles"	Expert opinion without explicit critical appraisal; or based on physiology, bench research, or "first principles"	Expert opinion without explicit critical appraisal; or based on physiology, bench research, or "first principles"

*Adapted from Phillips and others: Levels of evidence and grades of recommendation. Oxford Centre for Evidence-based Medicine, *http://www.cebm.net/levels_of_evidence.asp* (cited 3/25/03).
[†]CDR = clinical decision rule (algorithm or scoring system that leads to a prognostic estimation).
[‡]SpPn = specificity is so high that positive result rules-in the diagnosis.
[#]SpNout = sensitivity is so high that a negative result rules-out the diagnosis.

TABLE 16-15

GRADES OF RECOMMENDATION BASED ON LEVEL OF SUPPORTING EVIDENCE*

Grade	Level of Supporting Evidence as Defined in Table 16-14
A	Consistent level 1 studies
B	Consistent level 2 or 3 studies or extrapolations† from level 1 studies
C	Level 4 studies or extrapolations from level 2 or 3 studies
D	Level 5 evidence or troublingly inconsistent or inconclusive studies of any level

*Adapted from Phillips and others: Levels of evidence and grades of recommendation. Oxford Centre for Evidence-based Medicine, *http://www.cebm.net/levels_of_evidence.asp* (cited 3/25/03).
†Extrapolations are where data is used in a situation that has potentially clinically important differences than the original study situation.

36% made therapeutic recommendations. The level of evidence for positive studies was lower than for negative studies, with twice as many negative recommendations supported by randomized trials or controlled studies (analytic research). Similarly, the level of evidence for surgery was lower than for medical therapy, with 3 times as many medical recommendations supported by analytic research. The authors concluded that a dual evidence standard appears to exist for negative vs positive studies and for medical vs surgical recommendations in the otolaryngology literature.

Quantitative data integration ranges from simple tabular listings to sophisticated health services, including systematic reviews, practice guidelines, decision analyses, and economic analyses.[25] Systematic reviews or meta-analyses are an ideal way to synthesize results from a group of logically related randomized trials or, less commonly, observational studies.[41] The "bottom line" in a systematic review typically includes a summary measure of effect size (e.g., rate difference), a 95% confidence interval, and a statistical test for heterogeneity among source articles. Graphical comparison of studies using forest and funnel plots helps assess publication trends, small-study bias, overall ability to be combined, and consistency of included studies.[51] Excellent statistical software is available for quantitative and graphical data synthesis.[6]

At this point, I urge you to review the seven habits outlined in Table 16-1. The same fundamental principles may be applied to interpreting your own data, interpreting someone else's data (e.g., a journal article), reviewing an unpublished manuscript for a jour-

nal, and reviewing a grant application for a funding agency. I have purposely avoided listing specific formulae and calculations throughout this presentation to keep you focused on the forest, not the trees. For the tree lovers among you, I recommend the basic book by Dawson-Saunders and Trapp.[14]

Popular Statistical Tests Used by Otolaryngologists

Salient features of the most popular tests in otolaryngology journals[39] are listed below. Note that each test is simply an alternative way to measure error (Habit 4), not a self-contained method of data interpretation. Tests are chosen using the principles outlined in Tables 16-10 through 16-12, then analyzed with readily available software (which can also help select the best test for a specific data set).[49] Explicit guidelines are available to help authors, editors, and reviewers identify the optimal format for reporting statistical results in medical publications.[30]

The t Test

The *t* test is a classic parametric test for comparing the means of two independent or matched (related) samples of numerical data. It is also called the Student *t* test.

When interpreting a *t* test, a significant *P* value for independent samples implies a low probability that the mean values for the two groups are equal. When the samples are matched, a significant *P* value implies that the mean differences of the paired values are unlikely to be 0. Clinical importance is assessed by examining the magnitude of difference achieved and the associated 95% CI. Because valid results depend on relatively equal variances (standard deviation) within each group, a statistical test (i.e., the F test) is required to verify this assumption.

Be aware that *t* tests will produce an artificially low *P* value if the groups are small (fewer than 10 observations) or have an asymmetric distribution (one or more extreme outlying values). Instead, a nonparametric test (Mann-Whitney U or Wilcoxon rank sum test) should be used. If, however, each group contains more than 30 observations, the underlying distribution can deviate substantially from normal without invalidating results. Never use *t* tests to compare more than two groups. ANOVA is required for more than two groups.[24] When the outcome of interest is time related (e.g., cancer survival, duration of hospital stay, disease recurrence), survival analysis (discussed later in this chapter) is more appropriate than a *t* test.

ANOVA

The ANOVA tests whether the means of three or more independent groups of continuous data differ

TABLE 16-16

STATISTICAL DECEPTIONS USED IN JOURNAL ARTICLES

Deception	Problem	Solution
• Standard error is used instead of standard deviation	Range is artificially low, making data look better than they are	Always use standard deviation when summarizing data
• Small sample study results are taken at face value	Results are imprecise and would likely vary if the study were repeated; uncertainty is ignored	Determine the range of results consistent with data by using a 95% confidence interval
• Post hoc P values are used for statistical inference	Statistical tests are valid only when hypotheses are formulated before examining the data	Post hoc P values must be viewed as hypothesis-generating, not hypothesis-testing
• Some results are "significant" but there are too many P values to count in a lifetime	"Significant" results may be false positives because each P value has a 5% error rate*	Reduce the number of P values through multivariate analysis or analysis of variance
• Subgroups are compared until statistically significant results are found	If you torture the data sufficiently, they will eventually confess to something	Subgroup comparisons are valid only when all groups as a whole are significantly different
• No significant difference is found between groups in a small sample study	A significant difference may have been missed because of inadequate sample size	Be sure the authors discuss power and sample size before believing study results
• Significant P values are crafted through improper use of hypothesis tests	Small studies with asymmetrically distributed data require special methods of analysis	Don't believe results unless a nonparametric or exact statistical test was used

*Assuming that .05 is selected as the level of statistical significance.

significantly with regard to a single factor (a one-way ANOVA) or two factors (a two-way ANOVA). The ANOVA also tests whether the effect of one factor on the response variable depends on the level of a second factor (whether there is an interaction).

In the interpretation of the ANOVA, a significant P value implies a low probability that the mean values for all groups are equal. From a statistical standpoint, we say that the variance between groups is larger than the variance within each group. Note that the ANOVA provides no information on whether individual pairs of groups differ significantly. It only tests for an overall global difference. For example, when comparing 4 groups of data (A, B, C, and D), the finding "$P < .05$, ANOVA" means there is less than a 5% chance that the statement "$A \neq B \neq C \neq D$" is true; however, it says nothing about whether $A \neq B$ or $C \neq D$ or $D \neq A$, etc. Once the investigators demonstrate a significant global difference ($P < .05$) using ANOVA, they can then use multiple comparison procedures (e.g., Bonferroni adjustment, Tukey test, Newman-Keuls test, Scheffé test, Dunnett test) for individual group comparisons.

Be aware that ANOVA will produce an artificially low P value if the groups contain small samples (fewer than five observations per group, or 20 in all groups combined) with asymmetric distributions. Instead, a nonparametric test (Kruskal-Wallis ANOVA) should be used. A nonparametric test is also preferred if the

groups have unequal variance as determined by an F test. Multiple pairwise t tests cannot substitute for ANOVA. The effect is to greatly increase the odds of a false-positive result (type I statistical error).

Contingency Table

A contingency table tests for an association between two categorical variables by using the chi-square statistic. A modification, called the McNemar test, can be used for two groups of paired data.

When interpreting the results of a contingency table, a significant P value implies a significant association between the two variables whose categorical values form the rows and columns of the contingency table. However, even a very small P value provides no information about the strength of the association (effect size). Therefore, effect size can be measured with the odds ratio (two-by-two table) or by the Pearson contingency coefficient (tables with more than two rows or columns). The chi-square statistic compares the observed values for each cell (row-column intersection) with the expected values that would occur if chance alone were operating.

As with the t test and ANOVA, a contingency table's small number of samples can produce an artificially small P value. If the expected frequency for any cell is less than 5, an alternate test must be used (e.g., the Fisher exact test or the log-likelihood ratio). Beware of authors who overinterpret a "significant" chi-square result. As with ANOVA, when $P < .05$, we claim a global association between variables. We cannot specify which particular subgroups of rows and columns are or are not associated.

Survival Analysis

Survival analysis estimates the probability of an event (typically, but not necessarily, survival) based on the total period of observation and tests for associations with other variables of interest. Survival analysis permits maximum use of data from censored observations, which occur when a subject is lost to follow-up, or if the study ends before the outcome of interest has occurred.

Survival data can be interpreted in two major ways: (1) the life table method divides the time into intervals and calculates survival at each interval; (2) the Kaplan-Meier method calculates survival each time an event occurs. Both methods produce a graph (survival curve) showing the cumulative probability of the event vs total period of observation. Authors sometimes eliminate the curve, and instead give the event rates only for specific periods (e.g., 1-year, 3-year, 10-year, etc). When two or more survival curves are compared, and the P value is low, a probable association exists between time to event and the factor used to stratify the curves.

Remember that when you see a "survival cure," be sure that it has been calculated by using survival analysis (life table or Kaplan-Meier), not by simply dividing cumulative events at a given time by the total subjects still around at that time. The latter method mistreats censored observations, yielding artificially low estimates. Nor is it desirable to simply exclude from analysis all subjects not meeting some arbitrary cut-off for observation time, resulting rates may be artificially high. Whereas the life table method requires a minimum sample size of 20 uncensored observations, Kaplan-Meier analysis requires only 5 uncensored observations for valid results.

Multivariate (Regression) Procedures

Multivariate procedures examine the simultaneous effect of multiple predictor variables (generally three or more) on an outcome of interest. In contrast, t tests, one-way ANOVA, chi-square, and survival analysis examine the univariate effect of variables on an outcome one at a time. Different multivariate procedures are used depending on the measurement scale of the outcome variable (see Table 16-10).

Multivariate analysis produces a statistical model that predicts outcomes based on combinations of individual variables. The adequacy of the model as a whole is determined by the coefficient of determination (R^2), which indicates how much variability in the response variable is accounted for by the predictors and its associated P value. Each predictor variable also has an associated coefficient, whose magnitude represents the relative effect of the variable on outcome when adjusted for all the other variables in the model. A positive coefficient implies a positive association. A negative coefficient implies a negative association. When the coefficient's P value is small, the association is significant. Predictor variables should also be tested for interaction.

Always keep in mind when interpreting statistics based on multivariate procedures that biased results may occur if the data set has outliers or if variables in the model are highly correlated with each other ($r > .90$). Although a model may precisely fit the investigator's data, there is no guarantee that it will predict outcomes for subjects outside the study with equal precision. As with any statistical test, garbage in— garbage out. No degree of multivariate analysis can adjust for confounding variables that were not recorded at the start of the study.

Nonparametric Tests

Nonparametric tests consider hypotheses without requiring that the data have a normal distribution. The nonparametric equivalents of the t test, paired t test, and one-way ANOVA are the Mann-Whitney U, Wilcoxon signed rank, and Kruskal-Wallis tests, respectively (see Tables 16-10 and 16-11).

When an author uses a parametric test (e.g., t test or ANOVA), the data must be normally distributed or come from a large enough sample (about 30 or more subjects). Nonparametric tests avoid this requirement by ranking the data in each group and then comparing rank sums instead of the actual values of individual observations. Whereas the parametric tests discussed earlier in this chapter make inferences about means, nonparametric tests make inferences about medians. When there is doubt as to whether a nonparametric test is necessary, the P value should be calculated both ways—parametric and not parametric. If the results differ significantly, the nonparametric test is preferred.

Be aware that very sparse data sets are suitable neither for parametric nor nonparametric analysis. More sophisticated exact significance tests must be used. The Fisher exact test is a well-known exact procedure for two-by-two contingency tables. Exact tests for other situations require special computer software.[35]

Common Statistical Deceptions

More than a century ago, Benjamin Disraeli noted, "There are three kinds of lies: lies, damn lies and statistics."[16] Although such consummate skepticism is rarely justified, statistics can undoubtedly be misused—either by intent or through ignorance or carelessness—to produce incorrect conclusions.[2] Because most physicians are either amateur statisticians or have no recollection of statistics beyond bad memories in medical school, misuse is common. Reviews of clinical research indicate that about 50% of published articles contain statistical flaws serious enough to question the validity of the conclusions.

How does statistical misuse slip by editors, peer reviewers, and journal readers? Because of the "dazzle" phenomenon observed by Darrell Huff, author of *How to Lie with Statistics*: "If you can't prove what you want to prove, demonstrate something else and pretend that they are the same thing. In the daze that follows the collision of statistics with the human mind, hardly anybody will notice the difference."[27] Be particularly wary of the dazzling phenomena (Table 16-16) I present in the next sections.

Surgical Satisfaction Swindle

A surgeon claims a procedure is "highly effective" because 85% of patients were satisfied with results, 85% would have the surgery again, and 85% would recommend the procedure to family or friends. Unfortunately, virtually any survey achieves 80% or higher respondent satisfaction for a given question and only a few patients actually express negative views.[20] Satisfaction surveys are particularly prone to positive-response bias because they often relate more to the interpersonal skills of the surgeon and the setting in which treatment was administered than to the actual outcomes achieved. Moreover, without a comparison or control group, we cannot distinguish therapeutic effects from natural history or a placebo response.[8]

Survey results are credible only if the investigators use a previously validated instrument or perform their own validation process.[21,50] This process includes assessing: (1) test-retest reliability to ensure response stability and consistent item (question) interpretation; (2) internal consistency to determine whether allegedly similar items tap similar content domains; (3) construct validity to verify that items actually measure what they purport to measure; (4) discriminant validity to show that respondents with different levels of satisfaction or disease have measurably different survey scores; and (5) responsiveness to demonstrate that the change in survey scores before and after intervention is able to detect clinically meaningful levels of change within an individual.

Standard Error "Switcheroo"

When you see results reported as "mean value ± X," don't assume that X is the SD unless specifically stated. Sometimes X is actually the standard error (SE), a number that is always smaller than SD. Actually, SD and SE are very different. So understanding why many authors report the latter is difficult, unless they are enamored by the smaller value. When describing a set of data, SD is always preferred, because it measures how variable individual observations are within a sample.[12] If the data have a symmetric distribution, the mean ±2 SD describes about 95% of observations. In contrast, the SE is an inferential, not a descriptive, statistic. It measures how variable the mean is from one sample to another.

Consider a study of 25 patients undergoing rhinoplasty that reports a mean blood loss of 150 ± 30 ml where 30 is the SD. We now know that 95% of subjects had a blood loss of 150 ± 60 ml (assuming the data are normally distributed). To obtain the SE, we divide the SD by the square root of the sample size. In this example, the square root is 5, giving an SE 5 times smaller than the SD: 6 vs 30. The mean blood loss now is written as 150 ± 6 cc, where 6 is the SE. Obviously this "looks" better than the SD, but what exactly does it mean? It means "based on our results, if we extrapolate to the general population of rhinoplasty patients, we estimate with 95% confidence that the mean blood loss will be 150 ± 12 cc." This statement no longer describes the study data, but makes an inference about some hypothetical population. Unless the authors clearly state that this is their intent, the SD should have been used.

Small Sample Whitewash

Because medical research is costly and time-consuming, we rarely have the luxury of studying large samples. Fortunately, we can derive meaningful conclusions from small samples by estimating uncertainty (precision) with a 95% confidence interval. Remember—statistics is the art and science of dealing with uncertain data. The smaller the sample, the greater the uncertainty. Beware when authors claim their sample is "too small for statistical analysis." That's when they need it most.

For example, while perusing the bogus *Journal of Low Budget Research*, an article on an innovative new surgical procedure captures your attention. The authors operate successfully on 4/4 elephants (100% success rate) and conclude that "testing in humans is indicated based on these superb results." Do you agree? Actually, the range of results (an exact 95% binomial CI) consistent with this single experiment on four elephants is 47% to 100%! Knowing that the "true" success rate may be as low as 47%, you may now disagree with the need for human testing. Conversely, if the investigators succeeded in 40/40 elephants, the 95% CI would be 93% to 100%—a much greater level of confidence, secondary to the 10-fold increase in sample size.

Here's another way to appreciate the value of confidence limits on small samples. Imagine you are about to cross a very flimsy and tenuous-appearing bridge. Your reassuring guide states you have nothing to worry about because the first 4 travelers crossed it successfully. The statistical basis for your persistent trepidation stems from the fact that 4/4 successes is consistent with up to a 53% failure rate (as noted in the preceding paragraph). Not a very reassuring statistic to stake your life on!

Post Hoc P Values

A fundamental assumption underlying all statistical tests is that the hypothesis under study was fully developed before the data were examined in any way. When hypotheses are formulated post hoc—after even the briefest glance at the data—the basis for probability statements is invalidated. Unfortunately, we have no way of knowing at which stage in the research process a hypothesis was developed. Therefore, unless the investigators state specifically that the test was planned a priori, you should infer with caution.

As physician-friendly computer programs for statistical analysis continue to proliferate, more physicians are likely to analyze their own data. Unless the probability framework underlying hypothesis tests is understood and appreciated (Habits 3 and 4), the risk of post hoc P values will increase dramatically as they become easier to produce. When the primary research purpose is to test an a priori hypothesis, the P value will aid in statistical inference. When hypotheses are generated after the study, however, P values cannot be used to make inferences. Instead, they become a means of identifying promising associations that might form the new a priori hypotheses in a follow-up investigation.

Multiple P Value Phenomenon

P values have a momentum of their own. Once you start churning them out, it's hard to stop (especially if you have a nifty computer program that churns them out for you). When you see that a journal article or data table is chock-full of P values, realize that some "significant" P values ($P < .05$) are likely to occur by chance alone.[10] Consider, for example, a researcher who performs 20 individual hypothesis tests on a group of observations (e.g., calculates 20 P values). If we assume that the subjects studied do not differ beyond random variation, there is only a 36% chance that none of the P values will be significant! Further, the chance of getting 1, 2, or 3, significant P values is 38%, 19%, and 6%, respectively.

What accounts for the multiple P value phenomenon? The problem arises because each test is based on a cut-off of $P < .05$ as a measure of significance. The effect of performing multiple tests is to inflate this 5% error level for the study as a whole. The probability of getting at least one spurious result is $1-(1-\alpha)^n$, where α is the level of significance for each individual test (generally .05) and n is number of tests performed.

Multiple P values can arise when pairwise comparisons are made between several groups of data or when numerous hypothesis tests are applied to a single data set. When several groups are compared, ANOVA overcomes the multiple P value problem created by repeated t tests. Further, special multiple comparison tests are available with ANOVA that can search for subgroup differences, provided a global difference exists between groups. When a single data set is being studied, multivariate analysis, as I discussed earlier in this chapter, will eliminate the multiple P value problem induced by repeated univariate tests (e.g., t test, chi-square).

Selective Analysis of Results

Check for this in every study that compares three or more groups of subjects, including animal research. Authors may pluck out a few groups for pairwise comparisons and then pontificate on the "statistically significant" findings they discover. Unfortunately, this violates a basic tenet of statistics—you cannot compare subgroups of your data unless you first check for statistically significant differences between all groups considered simultaneously. For categorical data, a chi-square is first calculated for the entire contingency table. If $P < .05$, the authors can then extract subsets of the table for selective analysis, provided they adjust for multiple comparisons. For continuous data, ANOVA should be used (not multiple pairwise t tests) as described previously.

Powerless Equalities

Some authors would like to convince you that a new treatment or diagnostic test is equivalent to an established standard. In particular, support for the use of a new antibiotic or antihistamine often arises from a randomized trial claiming "no significant difference ($P > .05$)" from another drug. When interpreting these results, look not at the P value but at the statistical power. The size of the P value is pertinent only when a statistically significant result is given. Power tells you the probability that the investigators would have detected a true difference, given that one really existed. With small samples, power is usually inadequate ($<80\%$) to state confidently that the investigators didn't miss a real difference. Because very few articles calculate power, you may need to calculate it yourself (Habit 4).

Understanding Sample Size

As noted throughout this chapter, the number of observations in a data set (i.e., sample size) must be taken into account when interpreting results. Small samples may produce low precision, inadequate statistical power, and asymmetric distributions requiring nonparametric or exact techniques for proper analysis. Large samples offer high precision, but can waste resources and make results of trivial clinical importance appear statistically significant. Recognizing these problems, the American Academy of Otolaryngology—Head and Neck Surgery Foundation has made a sample size calculation a mandatory component of all grant applications for research funding. In this section, I summarize the essential concepts of sample size calculations in a nontechnical format.

A sample size calculation before beginning a study ensures that the planned number of observations will offer a reasonable chance of obtaining a clear answer at the end.[22] This is of paramount importance in animal studies, where sample size is limited by financial constraints, concerns about animal welfare, and limited laboratory space.[34] For example, a groundbreaking experiment involving 10 giraffes is of little value when a sample size of 20 is needed for adequate power or precision. Similarly, why experiment on 200 chinchillas when only 100 are adequate to test an hypothesis? Such considerations are by no means limited to basic science studies. Why devote endless hours to abstracting data from 500 patient charts when only 150 observations may be needed?

The basic ingredients needed in a statistical recipe of sample size vary slightly according to the measurement scale (see Table 16-7). Ingredients common to all scales include estimates of: (1) the smallest difference you want to be able to detect between the groups; (2) how confident you must be that any difference you detect is not simply due to chance (typically 95%–99%); and (3) how confident you must be that you can detect a difference as small as what was specified earlier (typically 80%–90%), assuming that such a difference truly exists. In addition, sample size calculations for numerical data require some estimate of the variability (variance) among observations.

Determining the minimally important difference you wish to detect is based solely on clinical judgment. When comparing categorical data, the difference of interest is between proportions or rate difference (see Table 16-8). For example, you may wish to know whether success rates for two drugs differ by at least 20% for otitis media; however, a difference of perhaps 5% may be important when treating cancer. In contrast, differences in numerical data are expressed as a difference in means. For example, you may wish to know whether a potentially ototoxic drug decreases mean hearing by at least 5 dB, or whether a new surgical technique decreases blood loss by at least 200 ml.

Outcomes measured on a numerical scale require an estimate of variance to calculate sample size. Because variance is defined as the square of the SD, we need a method to estimate SD to derive variance. If pilot data are available, some estimate of SD may already exist. Alternatively, you can "guess" the SD by realizing that the mean value ± 2 SD typically encompasses 95% of the observations. In other words, the SD of a set of measurements can be approximated as one-fourth of the range of that set of measurements. Suppose you are interested in detecting a 200-ml difference in blood loss between two procedures. Based on your clinical experience, expect that about 95% of the time you will see a difference ranging from 100 to 500 ml. Subtracting 100 from 500 and dividing by 4 gives 100 as an estimate of SD. Squaring the SD yields 10,000, which estimates the variance.

The remaining elements of a sample-size calculation reflect basic principles of statistical error (see Habit 4). Recognizing that errors are unavoidable (see Table 16-9), we specify in advance our levels of tolerance and then calculate a sample size that will accomplish this goal. Tolerating a 5% probability of type I error (false positive) is the same as being 95% certain that any difference you detect is not simply due to chance. Tolerating a 20% probability of a type II error (false negative) is the same as being 80% certain that you do not miss a true difference of the magnitude already specified (80% statistical power).

The size of the sample needed in a given study will increase when the difference of interest is small, the variance of the observations is high (applies to numerical data only, not proportions), and the tolerance for error is low. More subjects are also required to determine whether any difference at all exists between groups (two-tailed statistical test) than whether one group fares either better or worse than another (one-tailed statistical test). A two-tailed test is considered more conservative and should always be used unless it was determined a priori—before examining the data—that a one-tailed test was appropriate. A one-tailed test requires about half the sample size as a two-tailed test to show significance, and produces *P* values about half as small when applied to the data.

Sample size calculations may be performed manually,[11,22] with nomograms,[34,48] or with a computer program.[5] A computer program is optimal, because of the flexibility in seeing how different assumptions alter results. Specific formulae are required based on whether the samples are independent or related, the number of groups involved, and the measurement scale of the data. Note the similarity to selecting a statistical test (see Tables 16-10 and 16-11). When the research purpose is to demonstrate that groups are equivalent (e.g., to prove the null hypothesis), sample size requirements increase and special formulae apply.[4] Special formulae also apply to regression analysis, although a rough guide is that 10 subjects with the outcome of interest are required for each predictor variable included in the model.

PUTTING PRINCIPLES INTO PRACTICE

My goal throughout this chapter has been to convince you that effective interpretation of medical data involves much more than statistics or numerical formulae. Rather, it is a systematic process of moving from observations to generalizations with predictable degrees of certainty (and uncertainty) Every physician is involved in this process to some extent, whether a solo practitioner in a rural community or a full-time academician in a large university. Moving from observations to generalizations is the foundation for all scientific progress, a foundation that could not exist without a systematic process for interpreting data.

The seven habits listed in Table 16-1 provide a systematic framework for interpreting data, of which statistical tests are only a small part. Although Habit 4—measure error with the right statistical test—generates P values, P values are only part of the process, representing neither the beginning nor the end. We begin by verifying that the data are of sufficient quality and precision to merit statistical analysis (Habits 1–3). We end by seeking clinically significant findings that can be generalized beyond the study and are consistent with prior knowledge and experience (Habits 5–7). Obsession with P values, which has been called the "religion of statistics," may produce medical publications, but rarely achieves effective data interpretation.[47]

Every clinician need not be a statistician, but all should understand the fundamental principles of data analysis and interpretation. When understood and applied, the habits in Table 16-1 will permit intelligent, synergistic dialogue between clinicians and statisticians. Such dialogue ideally precedes any serious research endeavor because even the most elegant statistics cannot adjust for biased data or confounders that were never measured.[19] The statistician excels at analyzing data the right way, but the clinician's leadership ensures that the right data are analyzed. Further, clinical importance (Habit 5) is best determined by clinicians, not statisticians.

Hopeful that I have lit the fires of inferential desire, I will end by summarizing some good sources of fire-wood. *A Dictionary of Epidemiology* by Last[31] is an indispensable companion to reading the medical literature and understanding statistical terms. Dawson and Trapp[14] provide a delightfully palatable overview of research methodology and biostatistics in *Basic & Clinical Biostatistics*. *Making Sense of Data* by Abramson[1] is a useful self-instruction manual on association, causation, odds ratios, and other rates and measures. The essentials of research design and interpretation are discussed admirably by Troidl and others[53] in *Surgical Research* and by Hulley and others[28] in *Designing Clinical Research*. Finally, those ready to enter the brave new world of evidence-based medicine will find a warm welcome in the *Users' Guides to the Medical Literature* by Guyatt and Rennie.[25]

REFERENCES

1. Abramson JH: *Making sense of data: a self-instructional manual on the interpretation of epidemiological data*, ed 3. New York, Oxford University Press, 2001.
2. Bailar JC III: Science statistics and deception, *Ann Intern Med* 104:259-260, 1986.
3. Bentsianov B, Rosenfeld RM: Evidence-based medicine in otolaryngology journals, *Otolaryngol Head Neck Surg* 126:371-376, 2002.
4. Blackwelder WC, Chang MA: Sample size graphs for "proving the null hypothesis," *Control Clin Trials* 5:97-105, 1984.
5. Borenstein M, Rothstein H, Cohen J: *Power and precision (user's manual and software)*. Englewood, NJ, Biostat Inc, 2001.
6. Borenstein M, Rothstein H: *Comprehensive meta-analysis: a computer program for research synthesis*, vol 1.0.25. Englewood, NJ: Biostat Inc, 2000.
7. Borenstein M: The case for confidence intervals in controlled clinical trials, *Control Clin Trials* 15:411-428, 1994.
8. Brody H: *The placebo response: how you can release the body's inner pharmacy for better health*. New York, Cliff Street Books, 2000.
9. Brown GW: 2 × 2 tables. *AJDC* 139:410-416, 1985.
10. Brown GW: Errors types I and II, *AJDC* 137:58-591, 1983.
11. Brown GW: Sample size, *AJDC* 142:1213-1215, 1988.
12. Brown GW: Standard deviation standard error: which 'standard' should we use? *AJDC* 136:937-941, 1982.
13. Covey SR: *The seven habits of highly effective people*. New York, Fireside, 1989.
14. Dawson B, Trapp RG: *Basic & clinical biostatistics*, ed 3. New York, Lange Medical Books, 2001.
15. de Saintonge DMC, Herxheimer A: Harnessing placebo effects in health care, *Lancet* 344:995-998, 1994.
16. Disraeli B: *There are three kinds of lies: lies, damn lies, and statistics*.
17. Feinstein AR: Epidemiologic analyses of causation: the unlearned scientific lessons of randomized trials, *J Clin Epidemiol* 42:481-489, 1989.
18. Feinstein AR: Fraud, distortion, delusion, and consensus: the problems of human and natural deception in epidemiologic science, *Am J Med* 84:475-478, 1988.
19. Feinstein AR: Median and inner-percentile range: an improved summary for scientific communication, *J Chronic Dis* 40:283-288, 1987.
20. Finney DJ: The questioning statistician, *Stat Med* 1:5-13, 1982.

21. Fitzpatrick R: Surveys of patient satisfaction: I -important general considerations. *BMJ* 302:887-889, 1991.

22. Fitzpatrick R: Surveys of patient satisfaction: II -designing a questionnaire and conducting a survey, *BMJ* 302:1129-1132, 1991.

23. Florey C: Sample size for beginners, *BMJ* 306:1181-1184, 1993.

24. Gardner MJ, Altman DG: Confidence intervals rather than *P* values: estimation rather than hypothesis testing, *BMJ* 292:746-750, 1980.

25. Godfrey KAM: Comparing the means of several groups, *N Engl J Med* 313:1450-1456, 1985.

26. Guyatt G, Rennie D, editors: *Users' guides to the medical literature: a manual for evidence-based clinical practice.* Chicago, American Medical Association Press, 2002.

27. Hart JT, Dieppe P: Caring effects, *Lancet* 347:1606-1608, 1996.

28. Huff D: *How to lie with statistics.* New York, WW Norton and Company, 1954.

29. Hulley SB and others, editors: *Designing clinical research: an epidemiologic approach*, ed 2. Baltimore, Maryland, Lippincott Williams & Wilkins Publishers, 2001.

30. Kaleida PH and others: Amoxicillin or myringotomy or both for acute otitis media: results of a randomized clinical trial, *Pediatrics* 87:466-474, 1991.

31. Lang TA, Secic M: *How to report statistics in medicine: annotated guidelines for authors, editors, and reviewers.* Philadelphia, American College of Physicians, 1997.

32. Last JM: *A dictionary of epidemiology*, ed 4. New York, Oxford University Press, 2001.

33. Laupacis A, Sackett DL, Roberts RS: An assessment of clinically useful measures of the consequences of treatment, *N Engl J Med* 318:1728-1733,1988.

34. Light RJ, Pillemer DB: *Summing up: the science of reviewing research.* Cambridge MA, Harvard University Press, 1984.

35. Mann MD, Crouse DA, Prentice ED: Appropriate animal numbers in biomedical research in light of animal welfare considerations, *Lab Anim* 41:6-14, 1991.

36. Mehta C, Patel N: StatXact5: statistical software for exact nonparametric inference, Cambridge, MA, Cytel Software Corporation, 2002.

37. Moses LE: The series of consecutive cases as a device for assessing outcome of intervention, *N Engl J Med* 705-710, 1984.

38. Novack DH: Therapeutic aspects of the clinical encounter, *J Gen Intern Med* 2:346-355, 1987.

39. Phillips B and others: Levels of evidence and grades of recommendation. Oxford Centre for Evidence-based Medicine. *http://www.cebm.net/levels_of_evidence.asp* (cited 3/25/03).

40. Rosenfeld RM, Rockette HE: Biostatistics in otolaryngology journals, *Arch Otolaryngol Head Neck Surg* 117:1172-1176, 1991.

41. Rosenfeld RM: Clinical research in otolaryngology journals, *Arch Otolaryngol Head Neck Surg* 117:164-170, 1991.

42. Rosenfeld RM: How to systematically review the medical literature, *Otolaryngol Head Neck Surg* 115:53-63, 1996.

43. Rosenfeld RM: The 7 habits of highly effective data users, *Otolaryngol Head Neck Surg* 118:144-158, 1998.

44. Rosenfeld RM: Uncertainty-based medicine, *Otolaryngol Head Neck Surg* 128:5-7, 2003.

45. Sackett DL and others: Evidence-based medicine: what it is and what it isn't, *BMJ* 312:71-72, 1996.

46. Sackett DL: A primer on the precision and accuracy of the clinical examination, *JAMA* 267:2638-2644, 1992.

47. Sackett DL: Bias in analytic research, *J Chronic Dis* 32:51-63, 1979.

48. Salsburg DS: The religion of statistics as practiced in medical journals, *Am Stat* 39:220-223, 1985.

49. *SPSS 11.5 brief guide.* Upper Saddle River, NJ, SPSS Inc, 2002.

50. Streiner DL, Norman GR: *Health measurement scales: a practical guide to their development and use*, ed 2. New York, Oxford University Press, 1995.

51. Sutton AJ, Abrams KR, Jones DR: An illustrated guide to the methods of meta-analysis, *J Eval Clin Pract* 7:135-148, 2001.

52. Thomas DG, Gart JJ: A table of exact confidence limits for differences and ratios of two proportions and their odds ratios, *J Am Stat Assoc* 72:73-76, 1977.

53. Troidl H and others, editors: *Surgical research: basic principles and clinical practice*, ed 3. New York, Springer-Verlag Inc, 1998.

54. Young MJ, Bresnitz EA, Strom BL: Sample size nomograms for interpreting negative clinical studies, *Ann Intern Med* 99:248-251, 1983.

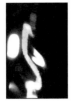

CHAPTER SEVENTEEN

PAIN MANAGEMENT IN THE HEAD AND NECK PATIENT

Peter S. Staats
Nilesh Patel

INTRODUCTION

Pain is the leading cause of health care visits and disability in the United States, costing the American people more than cancer and heart disease combined. Pain can adversely affect quality of life, and wound healing and can take on a life of its own after the pain-generating cause has been resolved. It is important, therefore, to have a rationale framework for approaching the treatment of pain.

What Is Pain?

The International Association for the Study of Pain defines pain as "an unpleasant sensory and emotional experience associated with either actual or potential tissue damage."

Acute pain is a normal and generally self-limited response to injury, including tissue degeneration, which can be considered an aging injury. Pain is defined as "chronic" when it has persisted for at least 3 months. Because of its emotional component, pain is often associated with psychological comorbidities, including depression. Chronic pain serves no useful function and leads to great disability. It is important to search for the underlying biologic aspects of pain and treat them whenever possible.

Types of pain

Somatic pain involves activation of peripheral receptors and somatic sensory efferent nerves without damage to the peripheral nerves.

Visceral pain, a poorly localized type of somatic pain, results from activation of visceral nociceptors and efferent nerves and is frequently described as deep, aching, and cramping. Although visceral pain may seem less relevant than somatic pain when assessing head and neck pain, it is important to remember that patients can experience a referred pain to the jaw or shoulder from angina or other visceral pain sources.

Myofascial pain affects skeletal muscles and can be referred or local. The presence of a trigger point in a taut band of muscle—an area where local stimulation causes referred pain—is indicative of myofascial pain, as are restricted range of motion and a local twitch response to stimulation. Trigger points develop in taut bands of muscle.

Neuropathic pain results from direct injury to the central or peripheral nervous system and is characterized by a burning sensation. It is found in postherpetic neuralgia, chronic regional pain syndrome, reflex sympathetic dystrophy, nerve injury, diabetic neuropathy, and chemical neuropathy. Neuropathic pain is further divided into the categories of sympathetically maintained pain and sympathetically independent pain. The diagnosis can be difficult to distinguish and depends on the response of pharmacologic blockade of the sympathetic nervous system. If a patient has profound relief of pain after a sympathetic blockade, the pain syndrome is said to be sympathetically mediated. If there is no relief with an appropriately performed sympathetic block of the affected area, the pain is said to be sympathetically independent.

Measurement of Pain

Unfortunately, we do not have a tool that objectively determines whether a patient has significant pain. Instead, we must rely on a number of pain scales that patients can use to describe their pain. We cannot use an x-ray or a laboratory test to determine whether someone hurts. Pain is what the patient says it is, and it is defined by the patient.[57] Asking our patients how much they hurt serves several functions. First, it defines the severity of the pain in that patient. Second, it allows us to track the success of therapy.

Numeric pain scales range from 0 to 10. Patients are asked to rate the pain, using 0 to indicate no pain and 10 for the worst pain they can imagine (Figure 17-1). Visual analog pain scales accomplish the same

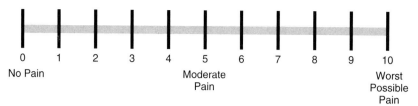

Figure 17-1. Brief pain inventory. From the Pain Research Group, Department of Neurology, University of Wisconsin—Madison.

thing with a 10 cm or 100 cm line. The far left registers "no to minimal pain," and the far right correlates with very intense pain (Figure 17-2). Other tools include a verbal descriptor, a brief pain inventory, and the CRIES assessment (for children).

Treatment of Pain

The first step in the treatment of all pain is to diagnose and treat (if possible) the root problem. All pain

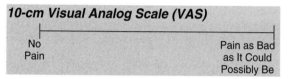

Figure 17-2. Visual analog scale. From the Agency for Healthcare Research and Quality: Acute pain management: operative or medical procedure and trauma, *Clinical Practice Guideline No. 1.* AHCPR Publication, No. 92–0032; Rockville, MD, 116–117, 1992.

treatment begins with conservative therapies (e.g., medical management and physical management) and proceeds if these therapies fail or are associated with intolerable adverse effects to neural blockade (visceral, sympathetic, sensory, spinal), the use of implantable technologies (implanted pumps or spinal cord stimulators), and neurodestructive techniques. Because pain has an emotional component, pain treatment may also involve psychological interventions.

Medical Therapies

Nonsteroidal agents. Nonsteroidal antiinflammatory drugs (NSAIDs) are used to treat mild pain associated with inflammation (Table 17-1). When added to an opioid regimen, they often permit reduction in the opioid dose. NSAIDs alter the inflammatory process by blocking expression of the cyclooxygenase (COX) enzymes that mediate production of the prostaglandins, especially PGE2, that sensitize pain afferents.

TABLE 17-1

MEDICATIONS USED IN PAIN

Class	Route	Usual Indication	Concerns	Comments
Nonsteroidal agents	• Oral • Intravenous	• Inflammatory pain	• Gastrointestinal bleeding • Platelet dysfunction • Renal dysfunction	COX-2 inhibitors appear to have a lower adverse-effect profile
Antiepileptics (neuronal stabilizing agents)	• Oral	• Neuropathic pain	• Tegretol is associated with aplastic anemia	
TCAs	• Oral	• Neuropathic pain • Depression	• Causes sedation due to anticholinergic effects	Use cautiously in patients with glaucoma, conduction abnormalities, or prostatic hypertrophy
Local anesthetics	• Oral • Local injection	• Neuropathic pain • Myofascial pain		
Botulinum toxins	• Injection	• Muscle spasm • Headache		
Opioids	• Oral • Intravenous • Intramuscular • Intrathecal • Intraventricular	• All types	• Addiction • Diversion	

Some NSAIDs (e.g., aspirin) indiscriminately block two cyclooxygenase enzymes, COX 1, which has a protective gastrointestinal role, and COX 2, which is implicated in inflammation. This distinction is not as clear-cut as was first thought, but the new "coxibs" designed to selectively block COX 2 have improved the safety profile of this class of medication.

Anticonvulsant (antiepileptic, membrane-stabilizing, or neuromodulating) agents. The "classic" antiepileptic, carbamazepine, has been widely used in the treatment of neuropathic pain associated with shooting or lanci-

nating pain and is the initial choice for many patients with trigeminal neuralgia (Table 17-2). Anticonvulsant drugs, especially gabapentin, have recently become a mainstay in the treatment of all types of neuropathic pain. The agents that fall in this class have multiple mechanisms of action and should be tried consecutively.

Tricyclic antidepressants. Tricyclic antidepressants (TCAs) also have multiple mechanisms of action and are used to treat neuropathic pain. In general, tricyclics work by decreasing the emotional depression that amplifies pain. They also decrease the reuptake

TABLE 17-2

ANTICONVULSANT AGENTS

	GABA	Glutamate & Excitatory Amino Acids (EAA)	Channels	Ectopic Impulses	Miscellaneous
I. Gabapentin	Augments transmission Increases rate of synthesis	Inhibits release	Blocks Na+ and Ca++		Stimulates 5HT release Inhibits branch chain AA transferase
Topiramate	Enhances at GABA-a receptor	Antagonizes AMPA & kainate receptors	Blocks Na+	Suppresses	Carbonic anhydrase inhibition
Lamotrigine	Decreases	Decreases release of glutamate and aspartate	Blocks voltage dependent Ca+	Suppresses	Suppresses acetylcholine
Carbamazepine		Decreases transmission	Slows recovery of voltage activated Na+ Modulates L-type Ca++	Reduces	TCA effects Antagonizes adenosine receptors
II. Phenytoin	Enhances activity		Inhibition of XXX Na+ and Ca+		May inhibit somatostatin release
Zonisamide			Blocks Na+ & T-type Ca++		Facilitates dopaminergic & serotonergic neurotransmission
Valproate	Decreases degradation, increases synthesis	Reduces cerebral EAAs			Structurally unrelated to any other anticonvulsant
Clonazepam	Increases potentiation of transmission				Structurally related to benzodiazepines May have antianxiety & antispasmodic effects

of the inhibitory neurotransmitters, norepinephrine and serotonin.

Because they have anticholinergic effects, tricyclic antidepressants must be used with caution in the elderly or in patients with comorbid disease. Care should be exercised in determining dosages for patients with cardiac conduction abnormalities, narrow-angle glaucoma, or prostatic hypertrophy.

Local anesthetics. Local anesthetics such as lidocaine have central effects but also decrease the spontaneous activity of peripheral pain generators. When applied topically or with injection, they block the transmission of ectopic impulses associated with pain. Local anesthetic injections are also used systemically to treat neuropathic pain and must be used cautiously in patients with comorbid cardiac disease.

Opioids. Patients with pain rarely become addicted to appropriately prescribed opioids, and these drugs have demonstrated efficacy in nociceptive and neuropathic pain. When possible, opioids should be administered on a time-contingent instead of a pain-contingent basis. A regimen of opioids given with nonsteroidal agents remains the mainstay of acute pain management.

Physicians and patients alike are concerned about addiction. This term is frequently confused with both physical dependence and tolerance. Addiction is an abnormal behavior pattern of drug abuse. It involves taking medications for reasons other than pain relief. Physical dependence is a normal physiologic response to chronic medical therapy and causes patients who stop receiving the drug to experience withdrawal. Tolerance necessitates taking an increasing dose to achieve the same effect.

Physical medicine and rehabilitation. Stretching techniques, including traction, massage, strengthening exercises, posture adjustment, and application of heat and cold may help correct underlying pain-generating conditions.

Neuromodulating Therapies

Neural blockade. Nerve blocks are useful for diagnosis and therapy. A diagnostic nerve block involves injecting a local anesthetic around a nerve proximal to a presumed pain-generating lesion to see whether this relieves pain. Many variables must be taken into account when interpreting the results of nerve blocks. False positives, when the pain generator is not distal to the site anesthetized, can be due to placebo response, can be the effect of systemically administered analgesics, or can be the inadvertent spread of the injected local anesthetic agents.[68] False negatives occur when the site is inadequately anesthetized or when there are multiple pain generators. Other nonspecific effects may result from improper needle placement or an unaccounted for effect of saline during a placebo test. It is, thus, inappropriate to decide that a patient's pain is psychogenic just because he or she responded to a placebo injection.

To reduce the subjective nature of the interpretation of nerve blocks, some clinicians inject a series of active agents and compare the results. This is known as the "comparative blocks" strategy. Investigation of the sensitivity and specificity of this regimen (lignocaine, bupivacaine, and saline randomly administered in masked fashion on separate occasions) compared with placebo-controlled blocks for cervical zygapophyseal joint pain (from whiplash injury) found that the comparative blocks have a specificity of 88% (causing few false-positive diagnoses) but their sensitivity is only 54%, which leads to many false-negative diagnoses.[47]

When neural blockade is used for therapy, clinicians inject local anesthetics plus steroids around the target nerves. One of the most common nerve blocks involves injecting a steroid into the epidural space. Cervical epidural blocks have been used for more than 20 years to treat chronic, benign head and neck pain.[14] Such injections are often used to treat disk herniation with nerve root injury and, when specifically directed to the transforaminal space, are thought to decrease inflammation around nerves.

Specific Nerve Blocks[60]

Trigeminal (gasserian) ganglion block: The trigeminal nerve, located in Meckel's cave, is the largest cranial nerve and provides sensation to the oral mucosa, cranial fossa, tooth pulp, gingiva, and periodontal membrane. The trigeminal ganglion block is generally reserved for cases of pain arising from a surgical procedure or when more conservative treatment fails to mitigate the pain of trigeminal neuralgia, cluster headaches, cancer pain, or pain associated with multiple sclerosis. The three percutaneous lesioning techniques, each with advantages and disadvantages, involve injection of a neurolytic solution under fluoroscopic guidance, use of an electrode for radiofrequency lesioning, or balloon compression. These blocks are associated with serious complications and must be accomplished with extreme care and attention to proper technique.

Maxillary division nerve block: The purelysensory maxillary nerve is the second division of the trigeminal nerve. Maxillary nerve blocks provide regional anesthesia for the upper jaw and are used to prevent intraoperative and postoperative pain and to treat chronic pain arising from maxillary tumors. Blockade is achieved by injection of a neurolytic solution or applying radiofrequency to induce a lesioning. Possible complications include temporary blindness, intravascular injection, and hematoma formation.

Mandibular division nerve block: The mandibular nerve, which has a sensory and motor function, is the third division of the trigeminal ganglion. Blocking of this nerve is useful in treating pain arising from treatment of a fractured mandible and from cancer of the tongue, lower jaw, or mouth floor. Using the same block technique as for the maxillary nerve results in a high degree of success with few complications.

Glossopharyngeal nerve block: This mixed motor-sensory nerve affects the stylopharyngeus muscle, the posterior third of the tongue, the palatine tonsil, and mucous membranes. A branch of this nerve transmits information that helps control blood pressure, pulse, and respiration. The proximity of the carotid artery dictates extreme care during this block to avoid profound toxicity from a misplaced injection. Indications for this block include surgery, diagnosis, conscious intubation, cancer pain, and glossopharyngeal neuralgia. These nerve blocks can be performed daily, if necessary, with reduced doses of methylprednisolone. A glossopharyngeal nerve block often severely compromises swallowing and may cause a hematoma and inadvertent dysphonia from paralysis of the ipsilateral vocal cord. Some patients develop postprocedural pain (anesthesia dolorosa) that can exceed the original pain.

Sphenopalatine ganglion block: The sphenopalatine ganglion comprises the largest neural center outside the cranial cavity and has a mixed sensory, motor, and autonomic function. Indications for this block include facial pain, cluster headaches, and migraine. After proper needle positioning, injection of a local anesthetic agent achieves a diagnostic block, and radiofrequency lesioning produces neurolysis. In some patients, stimulation-induced bradycardia may require administration of atropine to complete the procedure. Lesioning can cause transient numbness in the palate, maxilla, or posterior pharynx.

Stellate ganglion block: The stellate ganglion block is used for sympathetic denervation of the head and neck. The stellate ganglion is formed by the fusion of the inferior cervical ganglion to the first thoracic ganglion and generally extends from in front of the neck of the first rib to the space between C7 and T1. The stellate ganglion is blocked to manage pain from Raynaud's disease, arterial embolism (arm), intraarterial injection of drugs, Ménière's disease (controversial), postherpetic neuralgia in the area managed by the ganglion, complex regional pain syndrome, Sudeck's disease, and facial reflex sympathetic dystrophy. The block also provides useful diagnostic information for the management of upper extremity vascular surgery patients. Simultaneous bilateral blocks are only used as emergency treatment for a pulmonary embolism. The stellate ganglion block can be achieved with a paratracheal or anterior approach using a chemical agent or radiofrequency for neurolysis. The main complications associated with this block are pneumothorax and inadvertent intraspinal or intravascular injection. Neurolysis can also lead to Horner's syndrome. Chemical blockade can lead to hoarseness, shortness of breath, or a sensation of an obstacle in the throat.

Botulinum toxin injections. Intramuscular injection of the tiny doses of the neurotoxin botulinum toxin A is a successful short-term therapy for neurologic disorders that cause uncontrollable muscle spasm and contraction. The neurotoxin works by blocking the presynaptic release of acetylcholine. Botulinum toxin was first used therapeutically to treat strabismus and is now used to treat torticollis spasmodicus, oromandibular dystonia, blepharospasm, spasmodic dysphonia, hemifacial spasm, and infantile cerebral palsy. The efficacy of botulinum injections extends from approximately 6 weeks to several months, until neurons regenerate. Botulinum, thus, must be used long-term for chronic conditions, yet, its long-term effects are unknown.

Neurodestructive techniques. Specific techniques used to destroy nerves in the head and neck include chemical, thermal, and compression methods. Chemical neurodestruction can be accomplished with phenol or alcohol. Thermal destruction is achieved with either cold or heat. Radiofrequency lesioning to achieve facet rhizolysis is often used to treat patients whose pain is exacerbated with extension and whose imaging studies reveal facet arthropathy. Neurodestructive procedures in the spine are generally delayed until more conservative measures have failed.

Electroneuronal stimulation. In 1967, Shealy and colleagues[64] responded to the introduction of Melzack and Wall's gate control theory of pain[54] and the availability of cardiac pacemaker technology by introducing spinal cord stimulation (SCS) for the management of chronic intractable pain. Since then, the use of electrical stimulation to mask pain has been applied to ever-increasing applications with more sophisticated techniques, including the use of multi-channel systems with electrodes that can be placed percutaneously. Stimulating peripheral nerves by placing a subcutaneous electrode transversely across the base of the occipital nerve trunk at C1, for example, has been used to treat intractable occipital neuralgia with good-to-excellent results.[73] Subcutaneous implantation of electrodes has been used to stimulate greater and lesser occipital nerves, supraorbital nerves, and trigeminal nerves.

To receive SCS, a patient's pain must have an objective basis for pain and must have failed to respond to alternative therapies. Additional criteria include psychiatric clearance and no unresolved drug addition issues. SCS candidates undergo a 3- to 5-day trial before implantation to determine whether SCS will be successful (pain relief >50%) and identify the optimal frequency and duration of stimulation. If the trial is successful, an impulse-generating device is implanted subcutaneously and connected to the electrodes. The parameters are adjusted with radiofrequency telemetry.

Intrathecal/intraventricular infusion. Intrathecal infusion requires implanting a pump and catheter designed to deliver medication directly to the spine. This technique is rarely used for patients with head and neck pain. Appelgren and colleagues,[3] however, reported using intracisternal infusions of local anesthetics with dramatic reduction in head and neck pain. Catheters are placed at either C7 or T1 and threaded cephalad. Occasionally, patients with severe head pain due to cancer are treated with intraventricular morphine.[49] This approach allows clinicians to minimize the total dose delivered to control pain and, thus, reduce adverse effects.

Treatment of Acute (Postoperative) Pain

We rely on narcotics and nonsteroidal agents to treat acute pain, especially postoperative pain. Patient-controlled analgesia, a drug delivery technique that, as its name indicates, allows the patient to control some aspects of the dosing and frequency of drug delivery, is especially appropriate for use with opioids so long as safeguards are in place to prevent the patient's visitors from administering the drugs. Indeed, many of the short-acting medications that are used for chronic pain are also appropriately applied to acute pain in the postoperative setting.

HEADACHE PAIN
Etiology

Trigeminocervical complex pathophysiologies are considered the main source of headaches. Secondary causes include an identifiable pathology, infection, medication side effect, space-occupying lesions, spinal pathology, or inflammation. Headaches can be nociceptive, neurogenic, or neurohumoral. The pain of headaches results from vasodilation or muscle spasm and can be self-perpetuating. In more than 90% of patients, the primary type of head pain is migraine, cluster, or tension-type/daily headache.

Migraine
Prevalence

Migraines may affect 30 million Americans.[4] The prevalence of migraine in the United States is highest among white women at 20.4%, followed by 16.2% for black women, 9.2% for Asian American women, 8.6% for white men, 7.2% for black men, and 4.2% for Asian American men.[70]

Pathogenesis

Although the exact cause of migraine is uncertain, the results of experimental studies and the success of some migraine-specific therapies have helped define the pathology as a cervical-trigeminal-vascular disorder. Sensitization and activation of the trigeminal ganglia nerves release the calcitonin gene-related peptide and cause inflammation in the nerves serving meningeal blood vessels.

In a 1993 study on the pathogenesis of migraine, Kaube et al.[42] found that stimulating the sagittal sinus (a trigeminally innervated structure) in cats increased cervical cord activity, including expression of c-fos immunoreactivity. This allowed visualization of the neurons that likely play a role in a vascular headache such as migraine. A few years later, Goadsby and Hoskin[33] stimulated the sinuses of monkeys and mapped the resulting evoked expression of c-fos in laminae of the trigeminal nucleus and C1 dorsal horn. Because they found that the amount evoked at the C2 level was closer to the control, they concluded that C1 trigeminovascular afferents may have a specialized role in mediating the pain of migraine.

In addition, serotonin levels are higher centrally and lower peripherally during migraines. In 1993, Marcus[51] reviewed reports on the role of serotonin in migraine and concluded that changes in serotonin levels may precede the cerebral vascular dilation and muscular changes noted in both migraine and tension-type headache. Further implicating serotonin, triptans designed to activate two receptors in the 5-HT1 serotonin family, the 5-HT1B receptors that constrict meningeal vessels (reversing migraine-associated vasodilation) and the 5-HT1D receptors that may block the secretion of the trigeminal neuropeptides which may play a role in the neurogenic inflammatory response, can relieve migraine pain.[36]

Spreading oligemia has been observed in studies of cerebral blood flow during the aura phase of migraine. The time course and relationship of the changes in cerebral blood flow and the symptomatology of the migraine are as follows. As the aura phase gives way to the headache, cerebral blood flow diminishes. Depressed cortical spreading may induce neurogenic inflammation and vasodilation. This inflammation, in turn, irritates the perivascular trigeminal sensory fiber, increasing capillary permeability, vasodilation, and hypothalamic and cervical cord activation. After approximately 1 hour of headache pain, the brain becomes hyperperfused with blood. This continues for less than 2 hours beyond cessation of pain, when blood flow returns to normal.

Another hypothesis is that a "hyperexcitable" brain may be predisposed to cause an imbalance between neuronal inhibition and excitation and that this imbalance has an important role in migraine pathophysiology.[45]

As we learn more about the pathogenesis of migraine, we will be able to improve its management.

Symptoms/Diagnosis

Migraines may proceed through four phases: (1) a prodromal phase characterized by depression, irritability, and anorexia; (2) an aura phase that occurs in approximately 15% of cases, is transient and reversible, and may involve visual, somatosensory, or motor or language deficit of neurologic origin (generally, hypersensitivity to normally non-noxious stimuli, such as light or noise); (3) the headache phase marked by unilateral throbbing pain of moderate-to-severe intensity that lasts 4 to 72 hours, sometimes accompanied by nausea; and (4) a resolution phase, marked by fatigue. Migraine is never a daily occurrence, but it is a recurring syndrome.

Like all painful conditions, migraine is underdiagnosed. A pilot study indicates that as many as 96% of patients with migraine (according to the International Headache Society criteria) also have nasal symptoms and, thus, mistakenly believe they are experiecing sinus headaches.[41]

Several migraine triggers can cause pain within 12 hours of exposure, including alcohol and foods that trigger tyramine (cheese, fermented food), aspartame (diet soft drinks), monosodium glutamate (used as a flavor enhancer), phenylethylamine (chocolate), and, possibly, sinus inflammation. Additional triggers are changes in hormone levels, sleep patterns, and stress. Even a minor degree of trauma, such as whiplash,[77] concussion with subsequent normal neurologic examination,[50] or trauma causing only a brief loss of consciousness,[74] can trigger migraines.

Treatment

Migraine is an undertreated and inadequately treated syndrome because patients generally rely on over-the-counter medication, and physicians have little to guide them in prescribing for this condition.[18]

Migraine treatment can be prophylactic (including avoiding triggers), abortive (using specific or nonspe-

cific analgesics), or acute. Treatment choices include the administration of prescription or over-the-counter pharmaceuticals, physical therapy, alternative therapies, or interventional therapies (neural blockade or modulation: trigeminal blockade, C1-3 blockade, botulinum toxin A injections).

Prophylaxis. Patients who experience frequent migraines or are unable to relieve their severe migraine pain may benefit from prophylaxis.[45] The first step, eliminating or reducing exposure to triggers, can lead to a 50% improvement in 50% of intractable migraines. After that, first-line pharmacologic prophylactic treatment includes the administration of β-blockers, calcium blockers, antidepressants, or NSAIDs. The efficacy of these drugs for migraine prophylaxis was discovered by chance; their mechanism of action for this indication remains unknown.[45]

The prophylactic β-blockers include propranolol (adverse effects: hypotension, bradycardia, depression, sedation), timolol, nadolol, metoprolol, and atenolol (data suggest care in prescribing these drugs to patients with chronic heart failure or asthma). Common adverse effects of β-blockers include fatigue, depression, exacerbation of Raynaud's phenomenon, sleep disturbance, and diarrhea.

Prophylactic calcium-channel blockers include verapamil (adverse effects: hypotension, fatigue, constipation), diltiazem, nimodipine, and nicardipine (adverse effects: flushing, edema). Use of calcium-channel blockers should be avoided in patients with cardiac rhythm disorders or chronic heart failure.

Tricyclic antidepressants (TCAs), such as amitriptyline, nortriptyline, and doxepin, may be effective but their use can be limited by their adverse effect profiles.[59] Amitriptyline is one of the most anticholinergic TCAs (adverse effects dry mouth, constipation, blurred vision, and urinary retention) and nortriptyline the least. Amitriptyline also has a strong sedative effect but is least likely to cause an autonomic effect leading to orthostatic hypotension, whereas nortriptyline is most likely to. TCAs are contraindicated in patients with prolonged conduction times and should be used with caution in patients with cardiac disease.

The NSAIDs used as migraine prophylactic and abortive treatment are aspirin, naproxen, flurbiprofen, ketoprofen, and fenoprofen. As with all NSAIDs, adverse effects include analgesic nephropathy and gastrointestinal upset and bleeding.

Because these prophylactic drugs are not effective in a significant number of migraineurs, investigators continue to test the efficacy of additional pain treatments, including anticonvulsants, in preventing migraine.[9] When used to prevent and treat migraine and chronic daily headache, anticonvulsants, which are γ-aminobutyric acid agonists, are better considered "neuromodulating agents" or "neuronal stabilizing agents."[44] The use of these agents is based on the hyperexcitable brain theory of migraine pathogenesis. To date, only sodium valproate has gained approval by the U.S. Food and Drug Administration for this indication, but baclofen, gabapentin, and topiramate are under investigation and may prove to be especially useful for patients with comorbidities.[1,16,25]

A 2002 literature review concurred that divalproex sodium (valproate semi-sodium) is an efficacious migraine prophylactic. This agent dilutes cerebral arteries, but its adverse effect profile includes hepatic dysfunction thrombocytopenia, gastrointestinal upset, hair loss, and weight gain.[45] The same review noted that lamotrigine may have a role in preventing migraine-associated aura, topiramate shows promise (and additional trials are underway), and only insufficient evidence points to a role for gabapentin, magnesium, lisinopril, botulinum toxin A, tiagabine, levetiracetam, zonisamide, or petasites.[45]

Abortive therapy. The choice of abortive therapy for migraine should be based on the characteristics of the pain (severity, frequency, and associated symptoms) and on the characteristics of the patient (therapeutic history, comorbidities, etc.). Most abortive therapy is pharmaceutical, but this approach can be augmented or replaced by complementary/alternative therapies or interventional treatment.

Other nonspecific medical therapies used for abortive treatment include opioids, phenothiazines, NSAIDs, intranasal lidocaine, and steroids.[18]

Vasoconstrictors such as dihydroergotamine mesylate and other ergotamine derivatives and the triptans (selective serotonin 5-HT1B/1D agonists) are the mainstay of abortive migraine therapy. These pharmaceuticals should be used with caution in patients with coronary artery disease, primary vascular disease, and hypertension. In fact, triptans are contraindicated in patients with ischemic heart disease or symptoms consistent with ischemic heart disease; coronary artery vasospasm, including Prinzmetal's variant angina; and any other significant cardiovascular disease, including uncontrolled hypertension.

Choosing the best of the seven triptans at the best oral dose for any given patient will be difficult because the differences are small but probably clinically relevant for individual patients. One review, using the guidelines of evidence-based medicine, found that 59% of patients taking 100 mg of sumatriptan had a 2-hour improvement from moderate/severe to mild/no pain, 29% were pain free in 2 hours, and in 20% this was sustained, in 67% these results were consistent.

At least one adverse event was experienced by 13% of patients. Findings were similar but not identical (some triptans offered lower efficacy but better tolerability, for example) for sumatriptan 25 mg; rizatriptan 10 and 5 mg; eletriptan 80, 40, and 20 mg; almotriptan 12.5 mg; naratriptan 2.5 mg; and zolmitriptan 2.5 and 5 mg. The investigators noted that data suggest frovatriptan may offer substantially lower efficacy and concluded that rizatriptan 10 mg, eletriptan 80 mg, and almotriptan 12.5 mg are most likely to be consistently efficacious.[24]

Another study notes that 25% to 45% of patients suffer headache recurrence on triptans, but that almotriptan 12.5 mg is associated with a recurrence rate of just 18% to 27% while offering similar efficacy to the other triptans, 75% consistency, and tolerability similar to placebo.[17] Headache recurrence is, in fact, a major reason that patients become dissatisfied with triptans. One study of this phenomenon found that headache recurrence is lowest among triptans with the longest half-lives and greatest 5-HT1B receptor potency.[32] Tizanidine has been successfully used as an adjunct to a long-acting NSAID to treat rebound headache accompanying the discontinuation of overused acute migraine therapies.[16]

Additional analgesics used to abort migraines include rectal indomethacin; Excedrin (combination of acetaminophen, aspirin, and caffeine),[46] naratriptan, or zolmitriptan, each of which can cause flushing, nausea, esophageal spasm, or angina. The goal of these drugs is to inhibit the trigeminocervical complex and, thus, interfere with the migraine pain referral pathway. Investigators have even used intranasal capsaicin to treat migraine.[29]

Highlighting the need to find the right drug for the right patient, a study of 347 patients with migraine who self-identified as nonresponders to sumatriptan found that 36% obtained pain relief at 2 hours with a second dose of sumatriptan when the drug was masked. The group of actual nonresponders was then randomly assigned to receive 2.5 mg naratriptan vs placebo, which led to pain relief at 2 hours for 25% and at 4 hours for 42%. The placebo relieved pain in 10% at 2 hours and 20% at 4 hours.[69]

Acute therapy. When migraine is especially severe or refractory, its victims may appear in emergency rooms. Treatment options will be dictated by which pharmaceuticals the patient has recently consumed and by the associated symptoms.[34]

For acute migraine therapy, 80% efficacy can be gained with 12.5 to 37.5 mg of intravenous chlorpromazine or 10 mg of intravenous prochlorperazine.[15] However, one study showed that 16 of 28 patients treated with prochlorperazine needed rescue medication after 1 hour,[39] which is associated with a risk of hypotension, sedation, and dystonia. Other agents that are commonly administered but are only 50% to 65% effective are metoclopramide, lidocaine, transnasal butorphanol, propofol, sumatriptan (chest pressure and a sensation of heaviness are common adverse effects, and headache recurrence is as high as 40%), and intravenous valproic acid. Using dihydroergotamine or ergotamine for migraine abortive therapy is associated with a minor risk of angina, cramps, nausea, and vomiting.

Interventional therapy. Botulinum toxin type A inhibits acetylcholine release at nerve terminals and may also block parasympathetic nervous system action. In a double-blind, controlled trial of the safety and efficacy of botulinum toxin A as a migraine prophylactic, 123 patients who suffered 2 to 8 migraines per month were randomly assigned to receive injections of either 25 or 75 U botulinum A.[65] The injections occurred during a single visit and were made into various pericranial muscles. Participants kept migraine diaries for 1 month before and 3 months after the injections. In each botulinum group, the neurotoxin reduced the frequency and severity of migraines, use of migraine medication, and migraine-induced vomiting. The 75-U group, however, had a higher rate of adverse events than did the control group. Specific features of the headache (frequency, severity, etc.) may influence response.[10]

A literature review that classified this trial as negative for the 75-U group and positive for the 25-U group, the other controlled study as "partly positive," and the four open studies as negative, however, concluded that until further studies are conducted, there is insufficient evidence to recommend botulinum toxin A treatment for migraine.[22] This conclusion is echoed by other investigators who note the trials reported few significant adverse events, but more research is needed to determine the mechanism of action of botulinum toxin A in migraines as well as the optimal treatment schedule and injection sites for specific headaches.[16]

Another interventional approach is to treat moderate to severe migraines by removing the corrugator supercilii muscles, transecting the zygomaticotemporal branch of the trigeminal nerve, and repositioning the soft tissue in the temple. In a prospective study, investigators injected 25 U botulinum toxin A into each corrugator supercilii muscle of 24 female and 5 male patients. Of the 24 patients with a positive response, 22 went on to the surgical treatment. Of these, during a follow-up of 222 to 494 days, headaches were eliminated in 10 patients and considerably improved in intensity and frequency in 11. The remaining patient experi-

enced no change. These investigators concluded that the surgical approach was a success and that the botulinum injection was a reliable predictor of that success.[35]

Psychological aspects. As noted above, all pain has an emotional component, and migraine is sometimes treated with psychological interventions such as biofeedback or cognitive therapy. The placebo response also has an emotional component and, if we can expect a portion of study subjects to have an active response to a placebo, it is equally reasonable to expect a portion of study subjects to fail to respond to an active drug simply because they know they are taking part in a placebo-controlled trial. In other words, if some patients optimistically but mistakenly believe they are receiving the active drug and have a positive response to a placebo, other patients may pessimistically but mistakenly believe they are receiving a placebo and block their body's ability to have a response to the active drug. Investigators are beginning to examine this aspect of the placebo response. One such study compared the effectiveness of an active drug for migraine in trials that had a placebo control with those that did not and found a significantly lower response to the active drug in the placebo-controlled trials (61% vs 71%).[20] Findings such as these should lead investigators both to consider ways to enhance the action of migraine therapies and to develop new psychological approaches to treatment.[21]

Cluster Headache
Prevalence

Unlike migraine, cluster-type headache is uncommon, occurring in only 1 in 1000 individuals. Also unlike migraine, this headache occurs six times more often in males than females. Cycles of cluster headaches can last 1 to 4 months, and remissions range from 6 to 24 months.

Symptoms

The symptoms of cluster headache are excruciating unilateral pain involving the eye/temple/upper jaw. Attacks of pain are 15 minutes to 2 hours in duration and may occur 1 to 4 times/day. Additional symptoms include pacing the floor, lacrimation, ptosis, nasal stuffiness, and rhinorrhea.

Treatment

Prophylaxis. Verapamil (240–480 mg) is the drug of choice to prevent cluster headaches and may be combined with prednisone or 1 mg qhs Wigraine. Additional pharmaceuticals include lithium (300 mg/day divided), methysergide (2–8 mg/day). Episodic cluster headache is commonly treated with prednisone (40 mg qd tapered down every week by 10 mg).

Acute therapy. When patients with cluster headache come to the emergency room, appropriate acute therapy includes administration of oxygen 8 to 10 L/min for 10 minutes, ergotamine, DHE-45, triptans, lidocaine, or a sphenopalatine block.

Interventional therapy. In a study of the efficacy of radiofrequency lesioning of the sphenopalatine ganglion to treat and prevent cluster headache in patients refractory to pharmaceuticals, 34 of 56 patients with episodic and 3 of 10 patients with chronic cluster headache achieved complete pain relief. The remaining patients gained no relief. Eight patients had temporary postoperative epistaxis, and 11 experienced a cheek hematoma. In four patients, the maxillary nerve was partially lesioned. Hypesthesia of the palate, which occurred in nine patients, resolved within 3 months. The investigators concluded that this approach is reasonable in this population of patients.[62]

Intractable chronic cluster headaches can resolve with blockade of the trigeminal ganglion[37] or the sphenopalatine ganglion. One follow-up study found sphenopalatine ganglion neurolysis to be 60% effective in 56 patients with episodic cluster headache and 30% in 10 with chronic cluster headache.[62]

Chronic Tension-Type/Daily Headache
Prevalence

Chronic tension-type/daily headache is a relatively common condition, occurring in approximately 3% to 5% of the U.S. population and in women more often than men.

Pathophysiology

The pathophysiology of this headache type is unknown, but overactive pericranial muscles may play a role. Because chronic daily headache can be transformed migraine, new-onset daily headache, or tension-type headache,[30] achieving an exact diagnosis can be difficult.[13]

Symptoms

These headaches occur more than 15 days a month and consist of a constant band-like pain that feels like mild to moderate pressure, tightness, or dull ache. The pain is bilateral and contained in the forehead.

Treatment

Some patients benefit from psychological techniques, including strengthening exercises, self-hypnosis, cognitive therapy, and biofeedback to relax muscles.[55] Most patients can achieve adequate relief from ten-

sion-type headache with over-the-counter analgesics, such as NSAIDs. Things become more complicated for headaches that are a daily occurrence.

Prophylactic drugs for chronic daily headache include antidepressants (amitriptyline, doxepin, fluoxetine), neuromodulating agents (divalproex), ß-blockers (propranolol, nadolol, etc.), calcium-channel blockers (verapamil), and miscellaneous agents, such as methysergide.

Acute treatment relies on pharmaceutical regimens that may include tizanidine (for chronic cases or prophylaxis) or depend on augmenting standard analgesics with sedating antihistamines, antiemetics, butalbital, or opiates. Muscle relaxants may be useful for acute cases.

Regular analgesic use has been implicated as a cause of chronic headache because approximately 2% of those with daily headache use analgesics on a routine basis. In these patients, analgesic withdrawal can lead to improvement in symptoms. One study designed to shed light on this possibility examined headache history in 110 patients using daily analgesics for rheumatoid arthritis, seronegative arthritis, or miscellaneous rheumatology-related disorders and concluded that regular analgesic use in patients with a history of migraine will likely lead to chronic daily headache.[6]

The results of botulinum toxin A injections are mixed. For example, in four patients, tension-type refractory headaches improved in terms of severity, frequency, and subsequent medical interventions for control of headaches with injection of 20 U botulinum toxin A in symptomatic areas.[76] In a double-blind, randomized controlled trial involving 21 patients with acute tension headaches who received 10 pericranial injections of 20 U botulinum toxin A or saline placebo, however, no significant differences were found at 4, 6, and 12 weeks in visual analog scale pain scores, frequency and duration of attacks, analgesic use, pressure pain threshold, total tenderness score, or quality of life. These investigators concluded that peripheral mechanisms play only a minor role in the pathogenesis of tension-type headache.[61] Another double-blind, randomized controlled trial involving the injection of 100 U botulinum toxin A or 2 cc saline into temporal or cervical muscles found a 25% to greater than 50% improvement in the number of headache-free days, headache severity score, and quality of life at 3 months' follow-up in 13 treatment patients vs only 2 control subjects.[67]

Paroxysmal Hemicrania
Prevalence

Hemicrania is rare and occurs more often in women than in men.

Symptoms

As its name indicates, this is a unilateral headache. It causes excruciating pain in the ocular and frontotemporal area for 10 to 30 minutes, 10 to 30 times/day, and is provoked by certain neck movements and pressure in the upper back. Each occurrence can last up to 20 hours. Because additional symptoms include nasal congestion, conjunctival injection, lacrimation, and rhinorrhea, hemicrania is often misdiagnosed as sinus headache.

Treatment

Both hemicrania continua and chronic paroxysmal hemicrania respond to 150 to 200 mg divided doses of indomethacin. In fact, this response confirms the diagnosis: a patient may have all the symptoms of hemicrania but respond only to triptans and pizotifen, which usually work for cluster headache.[28]

Cervicogenic Headache
Prevalence

Cervicogenic headaches are common. One such headache, occipital neuralgia, results from injury to the occipital nerve caused by stress, trauma, or repetitive muscular contraction. Pain arising from the C2-C3 facet joints also generally radiates to the occiput and can be reproduced with ipsilateral rotation and extension of the cervical spine. Facet joint syndrome is difficult to diagnose because it arises from the same types of degenerative changes that show up in x-rays of asymptomatic joints. The patient's response to a nerve block helps in the diagnosis of cervical facet joint syndrome. Facet joint syndrome can be differentiated by the response to radiographically guided injections of local anesthetics into the zygapophyseal joints or around the dorsal medial branches of the posterior primary rami.

Symptoms

In 1990, Sjaastad[66] described cervicogenic headache as a variant of migraine that originates in the back of the head and spreads to the front. Pain is unilateral, of moderate severity, and, because it is triggered by neck movement, can be precipitated mechanically. He noted that occipital nerve blocks effectively stop the pain. Edmeads[19] had previously associated this phenomenon with photophobia, phonophobia, nausea, and dizziness. Cervicogenic headaches are difficult to distinguish clinically from migraine and tension-type headache.

Treatment

Treatment ranges from conservative therapy, such as massage and rest, to interventional therapy, including nerve blocks and steroid injections.

An open study with masked outcome assessment sought to determine the efficacy of manipulation therapy and exercise alone and in combination compared with controls by randomly assigning 200 patients into four groups. By 1-year follow-up, manipulative therapy and exercise therapy alone reduced the frequency and intensity of headaches and neck pain compared with control subjects. Although the combined therapy showed no significant benefit over either single therapy, 10% more of the patients in this group improved. The patients maintained the positive effects.[40]

A double-blind, randomized controlled trial examined the effects of injecting 100 U botulinum toxin A in five cervical trigger points (14 patients) vs injecting 1 mL of saline placebo (12 patients). At 2- and 4-week follow-ups, the treatment group showed a significant improvement in pain and range of motion compared with their preinjection levels, whereas the placebo group demonstrated no significant changes.[26]

A case report describes excellent but temporary results in a patient with refractory retroorbital headaches using three consecutive C2 ganglion blocks with 0.5 mL of local anesthetic administered under fluoroscopy. After the clinicians subsequently performed percutaneous radiofrequency ganglionectomy with multiple C2 lesions at 60°C for 90 seconds, the patient remained pain free throughout 4 years of follow-up.[5]

To determine the efficacy of treating intractable occipital neuralgia using percutaneous peripheral nerve electrostimulation, 13 patients had an electrode implanted transversely at the C1 level across the base of the occipital nerve trunk. With 18- to 72-month follow-ups, 12 patients reported greater than 50% pain control and required little or no medication. In the remaining patient, the symptoms resolved and the electrode was removed. The investigators concluded that electrostimulation in such cases is a reasonable therapy.[73]

Trigeminal Neuralgia
Prevalence

Trigeminal neuralgia is found more often in women than in men and generally in people over the age of 50 years.

Symptoms

Trigeminal neuralgia causes a sudden, severe pain that feels like an electric shock or stab. The pain generally affects only one side of the jaw or cheek and can last only 20 to 30 seconds or occur in rapid sequence. This pain may continue off and on for a day or several months and then might disappear only to recur months or even years later. The pain may be triggered by trivial, everyday stimuli, such as brushing teeth or touching the face.

Diagnosis

Magnetic resonance imaging (MRI) of the ganglion can be used to diagnose this condition.

Treatment

Pharmaceuticals used to treat this condition include Tegretol (carbamazepine), Dilantin (phenytoin), baclofen, clonazepam, gabapentin, and valproic acid alone or in combination.

If pain is refractory, a single percutaneous stereotactic radiofrequency rhizotomy can be effective. Barring that, patients undergo a surgical intervention.

NECK PAIN
Etiology

Biomechanical disorders are the most common cause of neck pain and can be caused by the degeneration that accompanies aging (degenerative arthritis), inflammatory diseases (rheumatoid arthritis), or trauma. This pain can also provide early warning of spinal cord compression (an emergency situation), a primary or secondary tumor, or (rarely) infection.

Additional and sometimes multiple therapies may become necessary to treat chronic or radicular neck pain.[12] As always with painful conditions, treatment begins with diagnosis and the most conservative appropriate therapies and proceeds, when indicated, to interventional therapies. Other treatments include psychological techniques (cognitive therapy), manipulative techniques, pharmaceuticals, acupuncture, massage, cervical epidural blocks (C2 ganglion, trigeminal ganglion, sphenopalatine), neuroablation (botulinum injections, radiofrequency), neuromodulation (greater occipital nerve stimulation, supraorbital nerve stimulation, gasserian ganglion stimulation), intrathecal infusion, and surgical techniques (fusion, diskectomy). In cases of systemic illnesses or spinal compression, pain and the underlying cause must be treated aggressively to prevent development of complications.

Degenerative Disk Disease

Degenerative arthritis can reduce surface cartilage in the cervical spine and/or produce bone spurs that can entangle a nerve or put pressure on a nerve root. Degenerative disk disease occurs because aging disks lose their flexibility, and the results are locally painful tears in the annulus fibrosis or herniated disks that press on nerve roots. Depending on their manifestation, degree, and location, degenerative arthritis and degenerative disk disease can be benign or can cause radiculopathy, pain that is referred to the shoulder and arm on the affected side(s) and produces a tingling sensation in fingers, hand(s), or arm(s). In severe cases, called myelopathy, degenerative disk disease can cause spinal stenosis that is sometimes manifested as weakness or difficulty with walking or coordination.

Treatment

Asymptomatic patients with degeneration should not undergo prophylactic treatment, and medical management should be tried first in patients with radiculopathy or mild myelopathy.

Many patients with radiculopathy or pronounced myelopathy, however, will have a positive outcome after a surgical intervention, even in those with severe myelopathy,[23] but especially those whose symptoms are recalcitrant through 6 weeks of management or are progressive. Cervical foraminotomy/diskectomy increases space where the nerve root exits the spinal canal by removing part of the joint that covers the nerve root and a portion of the disk, if necessary. Anterior cervical diskectomy, in which a surgeon gains access to the cervical spine through the front of the neck, is used when it is necessary to remove one or more intervertebral disks or bone spurs that are causing nerve damage. Some surgeons fill the resulting intervertebral space with a bone graft. In the presence of axial neck pain or any segmental kyphosis, fusion is also performed. In patients with posterolateral or lateral soft disk herniations, with focal osteophyte infringement, or in large patients with short necks and caudal lesions, a posterior laminoforaminotomy is often performed.[2,72]

Chronic Neck Pain

Some patients experience chronic neck pain without radiculopathy or myelopathy. Treatment can range from conservative to interventional, as seen in the following examples.

Treatment

Conservative treatment can include acupuncture and massage. In one prospective, randomized, controlled trial comparing these therapies after five treatments over 3 weeks, 56 patients received acupuncture, 60 massage, and 61 sham laser acupuncture. Compared with the massage group but not the sham group, motion-related pain significantly improved in the acupuncture group, which also had best results for all secondary outcomes. These investigators believed their results point to the short-term efficacy of acupuncture and called for studies of its long-term efficacy.[38]

A panel charged with developing evidence-based clinical practice guidelines for rehabilitation methods for neck pain identified therapeutic exercises as the only intervention offering clinically important benefits and noted that evidence is lacking for the efficacy of thermotherapy, therapeutic ultrasound, massage, and electrical stimulation.[58]

Investigators have also sought to determine the efficacy of injecting botulinum toxin A into chronically painful neck muscles. One study compared the efficacy of a single injection of high-dose botulinum toxin A vs a saline injection and found that each group of patients improved significantly in terms of pain, disability, and tolerance to trigger point pressure. The incidence of adverse events with the botulinum injections was "large," and the investigators concluded that this was not an effective single therapy.[75]

Anterior cervical diskectomy and fusion may also be performed to treat chronic neck pain without radiculopathy or myelopathy. One 53-month follow-up study involved 38 patients who had painful disk(s) proven by diskography. After the procedure, patients reported a significant decrease in pain and significant increase in function, and 30 patients were satisfied with their outcomes.[56]

Another study to assess the clinical outcome for anterior cervical diskectomy and fusion patients at an average follow-up of 4.4 years found that 82% of the 87 patients were satisfied with their outcome, and 93% reported improvement in pain.[31]

Atlantoaxial Subluxation and Basilar Invagination

Rheumatoid arthritis can cause serious problems in the relationship between C1 (the atlas vertebrae) and C2 (the axis vertebrae), including instability or a partial dislocation (atlantoaxial subluxation). When subluxation exceeds 9 mm, cord compression is likely. Rheumatoid arthritis can also cause deterioration of the joints between the base of the skull and C1-C2 to such an extent that the odontoid migrates upward and places pressure on the brain stem (basilar invagination). This can cause sudden death and may present as an untoward amount of flexion, posterior skull pain, tingling, and numbness in the fourth and fifth finger, in the medial forearm, or with neck movement.

Treatment

The KIM-STIM, an electrical stimulator that is molded to the patient's ear, fitted with multiple electrodes, and managed by the patient, is being used to treat pain associated with atlantoaxial subluxation syndrome as well as head, neck, and shoulder pain.[43]

Posterior fusion of C1-C2 is indicated for atlantoaxial subluxation when patients have neurologic abnormality, intractable pain, or vertebral artery or cord compression demonstrated on MRI. The recommended treatment for basilar invagination is neurosurgery when MRI confirms cord compression. Otherwise, patients may benefit from conservative pharmaceutical and stretching approaches (neck traction).[78]

Spinal Stenosis

Degeneration can also lead to two types of narrowing or stenosis in the cervical spine: (1) cervical spondylolysis, which occurs when the pars articulars is damaged and cannot continue to separate vertebrae, which may cause neck pain as well as arm weakness; and (2) the narrowing of the spinal canal and foramina, which occurs when the facets become inflamed from undue pressure and results in compression of the spinal cord, neuropathic symptoms, and neuropathic pain.

Treatment

Spinal stenosis is treated by decompressing the spinal cord, the nerve roots, or both, and replacing a section of the vertebra and adjacent intervertebral disks with a bone graft or metal plate (cervical corpectomy). When patients have four or more levels of stenosis, the preferred method is laminoplasty.[72]

A review was conducted of the outcome of anterior cervical corpectomy, reconstruction with allograft fibula, and placement of an anterior plate in 261 patients with spinal stenosis due to spondylosis (197 patients), postlaminectomy kyphosis (27 patients), acute fracture (25 patients), or ossification of the posterior longitudinal ligament (12 patients). Nearly half of the procedures involved two disk levels and one vertebral body; 96 involved two levels, 31 three levels, and 1 four levels. The mean follow-up was 25.7 months. The fusion was successful in 226 patients, 33 developed an asymptomatic stable or fibrous union, and 2 developed unstable pseudoarthrosis requiring reoperation. Two patients had transient unilateral upper extremity weakness, 35 developed transient dysphagia, 7 permanent dysphagia, 35 transient hoarseness, and 2 permanent hoarseness. The hardware failed in 14 patients. These investigators concluded that this procedure is effective and improves symptoms in nearly all patients.[52]

Trauma

Trauma or an accident can injure the neck through hyperextension (whiplash) or can produce fractures, dislocations, disk herniations, or an injured spinal cord (producing paralysis in extreme cases).

Treatment of Whiplash

Whiplash often leads to chronic pain in the cervical zygapophyseal joints.[8] Treatment ranges from conservative measures to neuroablation.

Bogduk et al.[11] have published widely on this condition and maintain that the evidence for efficacy of conservative measures is poor. Another group reviewed the literature to determine the efficacy of various exercise methods and concluded that moderate evidence supports early treatment with mobilizing exercise to treat acute whiplash, but no evidence supports the effectiveness of group exercise, "neck schools," or single sessions of extension-retraction exercises.[63]

Clinicians have also investigated the merits of injecting various agents. One double-blind study, for example, compared the efficacy of an intraarticular injection of 0.5% bupivacaine (n = 20) or 5.7 mg of betamethasone (n = 21). The end point was time needed to return to 50% of preinjection pain. In each group, fewer than 50% of patients had pain relief from more than a week and fewer than 20 had relief for a month, indicating that the corticosteroid injection was not effective.[7] Another randomized, controlled trial compared five trigger-point injections of botulinum toxin A in 14 patients and with saline in 12 and found that range of neck motion and subjective pain improved significantly in the treatment group compared with control subjects but the treatment only led to a trend toward improved functioning.[27]

To help establish the efficacy of percutaneous radiofrequency neurotomy for the treatment of cervical zygapophyseal joint pain, Lord et al.[48] conducted a randomized, double-blind trial, comparing percutaneous radiofrequency neurotomy involving multiple lesions using an 80°C electrode in 12 patients with a sham identical control treatment in 12 similar patients. The pain generator had been confirmed by double-blind, placebo-controlled nerve blocks using a local anesthetic. The active treatment group had a median time until pain returned to 50% of pretreatment level of 263 days vs 8 days in the control group. One control patient and 7 treatment patients were pain free at 27 weeks. These investigators concluded that multiple radiofrequency lesioning of target nerves is efficacious.

The same group reported on the use of radiofrequency neurotomy in 28 patients in whom diagnostic blocks confirmed cervical zygapophyseal pain. An initial procedure led to complete pain relief in 71% of patients. Those who failed the initial procedure did not benefit from a repeat procedure, but pain return after a beneficial initial procedure was successfully treated with a repeat neurotomy.[53]

REFERENCES

1. Agostoni A, Frigerio, Santoro P: Antiepileptic drugs in the treatment of chronic headaches, *Neurol Sci* 24(Suppl 2): S128-S131, 2003.
2. Albert TJ, Murrell SE: Surgical management of cervical radiculopathy, *J Am Acad Orthop Surg* 7:368-376, 1999.
3. Appelgren L and others: Continuous intracisternal and high cervical intrathecal bupivacaine analgesia in refractory head and neck pain, *Anesthesiology* 84:256-272, 1996.
4. Aukerman G, Knutson D, Miser WF: Management of the acute migraine headache, *Am Fam Physician* 66:2123-2130, 2002.
5. Awan S and others: Retro-orbital headaches relieved by C2-ganglion radiofrequency thermal ablation. Abstract presented to the International Spine Injection Society Meeting, 2002.
6. Bahra A and others: Does chronic daily headache arise de novo in association with regular use of analgesics? *Headache* 43:179-190, 2003.
7. Barnsley L and others: Lack of effect of intraarticular corticosteroids for chronic pain in the cervical zygapophyseal joints, *N Engl J Med* 330:1047-1050, 1994.
8. Barnsley L and others: The prevalence of chronic cervical zygapophysial joint pain after whiplash, *Spine* 20:20-25, 1995.
9. Bigal ME, Krymchantowski AV, Rapoport AM: New developments in migraine prophylaxis, *Expert Opin Pharmacother* 4:433-443, 2003.
10. Binder WJ and others: Botulinum toxin type A (BOTOX) for treatment of migraine, *Dis Mon* 48:323-335, 2002.
11. Bogduk N, Lord SM: Cervical spine disorders, *Curr Opin Rheumatol* 10:110-115, 1998.
12. Borenstein DG: Management of neck pain: a primary care approach, *Hosp Pract (Off Ed)* 33:147-154, 160, 1998.
13. Bussone G: Chronic migraine and chronic tension-type headache: different aspects of the chronic daily headache spectrum. Clinical and pathogenetic considerations, *Neurol Sci* 24(Suppl 2):S90-S93, 2003.
14. Catchlove RF, Braha R: The use of cervical epidural nerve blocks in the management of chronic head and neck pain, *Can Anaesth Soc J* 31:188-191, 1984.
15. Coppola M, Yealy DM, Leibold RA: Randomized, placebo-controlled evaluation of prochlorperazine versus metoclopramide for emergency department treatment of migraine headache, *Ann Emerg Med* 26:541-546, 1995.
16. Corbo J: The role of anticonvulsants in preventive migraine therapy, *Curr Pain Headache Rep* 7:63-66, 2003.
17. Dahlof CG and others: How does almotriptan compare with other triptans? A review of data from placebo-controlled clinical trials, *Headache* 42:99-113, 2002.
18. Diamond S, Wenzel R: Practical approaches to migraine management, *CNS Drugs* 16:385-403, 2002.
19. Edmeads J: The cervical spine and headache. *Neurology* 38:1874-1878, 1988.
20. Eikermann A, Diener H: Effect of active treatment is lower when using placebo control in clinical trials on acute therapy of migraine, *Cephalalgia* 23:344-347, 2003.
21. Evans RW: The non-nocebo response: can migraine medication efficacy be enhanced? *Headache* 43:693, 2003.
22. Evers S: Is there a role for botulinum toxin in the treatment of migraine? *Curr Pain Headache Rep* 7:229-234, 2003.
23. Falope ZF and others: Cervical myelopathy and rheumatoid arthritis: a retrospective analysis of management, *Clin Rehabil* 16:625-629, 2002.
24. Ferrari MD and others: Triptans (serotonin, 5-HT1B/1D agonists) in migraine: detailed results and methods of a meta-analysis of 53 trials, *Cephalalgia* 22:633-658, 2002.
25. Freitag F: Preventative treatment for migraine and tension-type headaches: do drugs having effects on muscle spasm and tone have a role? *CNS Drugs* 17:373-381, 2003.
26. Freund BJ, Schwartz M: Treatment of chronic cervical-associated headache with botulinum toxin A: a pilot study, *Headache* 40:231-236, 2000.
27. Freund BJ, Schwartz M: Treatment of whiplash associated neck pain [corrected] with botulinum toxin-A: a pilot study, *J Rheumatol* 27:481-484, 2000.

28. Fuad F, Jones NS: Paroxysmal hemicrania and cluster headache: two discrete entities or is there an overlap? *Clin Otolaryngol* 27:472-479, 2002.

29. Fusco BM, Barzoi G, Agro F: Repeated intranasal capsaicin applications to treat chronic migraine, *Br J Anaesth* 90:812, 2003.

30. Galego JC and others: Clinical features of episodic migraine and transformed migraine: a comparative study, *Arq Neuropsiquiatr* 60:912-916, 2002

31. Garvey TA and others: Outcome of anterior cervical discectomy and fusion as perceived by patients treated for dominant axial-mechanical cervical spine pain, *Spine* 27:1887-1895, 2002.

32. Geraud G, Keywood C, Senard JM: Migraine headache recurrence: relationship to clinical, pharmacological, and pharmacokinetic properties of triptans, *Headache* 43:376-388, 2003.

33. Goadsby PJ, Hoskin KL: The distribution of trigeminovascular afferents in the nonhuman primate brain Macaca nemestrina: a c-fos immunocytochemical study, *J Anat* 190(pt3):367-375, 1997.

34. Green MW: The emergency management of headaches, *Neurology* 9:93-98, 2003.

35. Guyuron B, Tucker T, Davis J: Surgical treatment of migraine headaches, *Plast Reconstr Surg* 109:2183-2189, 2002.

36. Hamel E: The biology of serotonin receptors: focus on migraine pathophysiology and treatment, *Can J Neurol Sci* 26(Suppl 3):S2-S6, 1999.

37. Hassenbusch SJ and others: Trigeminal cisternal injection of glycerol for treatment of chronic intractable cluster headaches, *Neurosurgery* 29:504-508, 1991.

38. Irnich D and others: Randomised trial of acupuncture compared with conventional massage and "sham" laser acupuncture for treatment of chronic neck pain, *BMJ* 322:1574-1578, 2001.

39. Jones J, Peck S, Chun E: Intramuscular prochlorperazine versus metoclopramide as single agent therapy for the treatment of acute migraine headache, *Am J Emerg Med* 14:262-264, 1996.

40. Jull G and others: A randomized controlled trial of exercise and manipulative therapy for cervicogenic headache, *Spine* 27:1835-1843, 2002.

41. Kaniecki RG: Migraine and tension-type headache: an assessment of challenges in diagnosis. *Neurology* 58(Suppl 6):S10-S14, 2002.

42. Kaube H and others: Expression of c-Fos-like immunoreactivity in the caudal medulla and upper cervical spinal cord following stimulation of the superior sagittal sinus in the cat, *Brain Res* 629:95-102, 1993.

43. Kim KH: Atlanto-axial subluxation syndrome and management of intractable headache, neck pain and shoulder pain with auricular stimulation: a clinical case report, *Acupunct Electrother Res* 26:263-275, 2001.

44. Krusz JC: Prophylaxis for chronic daily headache and chronic migraine with neuronal stabilizing agents, *Curr Pain Headache Rep* 6:480-485, 2002.

45. Krymchantowski AV, Bigal ME, Moreira PF: New and emerging prophylactic agents for migraine, *CNS Drugs* 16:611-634, 2002.

46. Lipton RB, Stewart WF, Ryan RE Jr: Efficacy and safety of acetaminophen, aspirin, and caffeine in alleviating migraine headache pain: three double-blind, randomized, placebo-controlled trials, *Arch Neurol* 55:210-217, 1998.

47. Lord SM, Barnsley L, Bogduk N: The utility of comparative local anesthetic blocks versus placebo-controlled blocks for the diagnosis of cervical zygapophysial joint pain, *Clin J Pain* 11:208-213, 1995.

48. Lord SM and others: Percutaneous radio-frequency neurotomy for chronic cervical zygapophyseal-joint pain, *N Engl J Med* 335:1721-1726, 1996.

49. Loriferne JF and others: [Cephalic cancer pain controlled by intraventricular administration of morphine and clonidine], *Ann Fr Anesth Reanim* 14:233-236, 1995.

50. Mandel S: Minor head injury may not be 'minor,' *Postgrad Med* 85:213-217, 1989.

51. Marcus DA: Serotonin and its role in headache pathogenesis, *Clin J Pain* 9:159-176, 1993.

52. Mayr MT and others: Cervical spinal stenosis: outcome after anterior corpectomy, allograft reconstruction, and instrumentation, *J Neurosurg* 96(1 Suppl):10-16, 2002.

53. McDonald GJ, Lord SM, Bogduk N: Long-term follow-up of patients treated with cervical radiofrequency neurotomy for chronic neck pain, *Neurosurgery* 45:61-67, 1999.

54. Melzack R, Wall PO: Pain mechanism: a new theory, *Science* 150:971-978, 1965.

55. Millea PJ, Brodie JJ: Tension-type headache, *Am Fam Physician* 66:797-804, 2002.

56. Palit M and others: Anterior discectomy and fusion for the management of neck pain, *Spine* 24:2224-2228, 1999.

57. Pasero C, McCaffery M: The patient's report of pain: believing vs. accepting. There's a big difference, *Am J Nurs* 101:73-74, 2001.

58. Philadelphia Panel: Philadelphia Panel evidence-based clinical practice guidelines on selected rehabilitation interventions for neck pain, *Phys Ther* 81:1701-1717, 2001.

59. Punay NC, Couch JR: Antidepressants in the treatment of migraine headache, *Curr Pain Headache Rep* 7:51-54, 2003.

60. Raj PP and others: *Radiographic imaging for regional anesthesia and pain management.* New York, Churchill Livingstone, 2002.

61. Rollnik JD and others: Treatment of tension-type headache with botulinum toxin type A: a double-blind, placebo-controlled study, *Headache* 40:300-305, 2000.

62. Sanders M, Zuurmond WW: Efficacy of sphenopalatine ganglion blockade in 66 patients suffering from cluster headache: a 12-to 70-month follow-up evaluation, *J Neurosurg* 87:876-880, 1997.

63. Sarig-Bahat H: Evidence for exercise therapy in mechanical neck disorders, *Man Ther* 8:10-20, 2003.

64. Shealy C, Mortimer J, Reswick J: Electrical inhibition of pain by stimulation of the dorsal columns: a preliminary report, *Anesth Analg* 46:489-491, 1967.

65. Silberstein S and others: Botulinum toxin type A as a migraine preventive treatment. For the BOTOX Migraine Clinical Research Group, *Headache* 40:445-450, 2000.

66. Sjaastad O: The headache challenge in our time: cervicogenic headache, *Funct Neurol* 5:155-158, 1990.

67. Smuts JA, Baker MK, Smuts HM: Prophylactic treatment of chronic tension-type headache using botulinum toxin type A, *Eur J Neurol* 6:99-102, 1999.

68. Staats PS, North RB: *Diagnostic nerve root blocks, facet blocks, and discography: a rational approach.* In Hadley M, editor: *Perspectives in neurological surgery,* vol. 7. St. Louis, Quality Medical Publishing, 1996.

69. Stark S and others: Naratriptan efficacy in migraineurs who respond poorly to oral sumatriptan, *Headache* 40:513-520, 2000.

70. Stewart WF and others: Prevention of migraine headache in the United States: relation to age, income, race, and other sociodemographic factors, *JAMA* 267:64-69, 1992.

71. Taha JM, Tew JM Jr, Buncher CR: A prospective 15-year follow up of 154 consecutive patients with trigeminal neuralgia

treated by percutaneous stereotactic radiofrequency thermal rhizotomy, *J Neurosurg* 83:989-993,1995.

72. Truumees E, Herkowitz HN: Cervical spondylotic myelopathy and radiculopathy, *Instr Course Lect* 49:339-360, 2000.

73. Weiner RL, Reed KL: Peripheral neurostimulation for control of intractable occipital neuralgia, *Neuromodulation* 2:217-221, 1999.

74. Weiss HD, Stern BJ, Goldberg J: Post-traumatic migraine: chronic migraine precipitated by minor head or neck trauma, *Headache* 31:451-456, 1991.

75. Wheeler AH, Goolkasian P, Gretz SS: Botulinum toxin A for the treatment of chronic neck pain, *Pain* 94:255-260, 2001.

76. Wheeler AH: Botulinum toxin A: adjunctive therapy for refractory headaches associated with pericranial muscle tension, *Headache* 38:468-471, 1998.

77. Winston KR: Whiplash and its relationship to migraine, *Headache* 27:452-457, 1987.

78. Yu KK and others: Nontraumatic atlantoaxial subluxation (Grisel syndrome): a rare complication of otolaryngological procedures, *Laryngoscope* 113:1047-1049, 2003.

CHAPTER EIGHTEEN

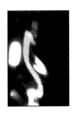

INTEGRATING PALLIATIVE AND CURATIVE CARE STRATEGIES IN THE PRACTICE OF OTOLARYNGOLOGY

Michael A. Williams
Cynda Hylton Rushton

To live in the bright light of death is to live a life in which colors and sounds and smells are all more intense, in which smiles and laughs are irresistibly infectious, in which touches and hugs are warm and tender almost beyond belief. To live in this awareness of who, what, and where I am is to live more fully than I ever dreamed possible.

William G. Bartholome, M.D.[3]

PROLOGUE

Bill Bartholome, M.D., a revered pediatrician and ethicist, describes his experience of living in the shadow of his impending death after being diagnosed with esophageal cancer in 1994. Dr. Bartholome decided to limit therapy and not to undergo some treatments that had been recommended. In doing so, he lived longer than his physicians expected and found that his life was transformed by his experiences with living and dying.

His experience was featured in the Bill Moyers PBS television series *On Our Own Terms: Moyers on Dying,* which was first aired in September 2000. His is a poignant example of many of the issues surrounding life-threatening disease, death, dying, and palliative care, as well as the challenges facing health care professionals (HCPs) of considering and balancing the benefits and burdens of proposed therapies and respecting patients' autonomy while staying involved in patients' care, even when they are dying.

INTRODUCTION

The practice of medicine and surgery is a healing art. Regardless of specialization, geographic location, or religious or cultural differences, it is safe to say that persons become physicians and nurses because of their strong desire to help patients by treating symptoms, syndromes, and disease and by alleviating pain and suffering. Compared to a century ago, our abilities to treat with medications, surgery, radiation, and endoscopic and endovascular techniques; to diagnose with detailed imaging techniques revealing anatomy, blood flow, metabolic markers of ischemia, tumor, etc.; and even to conduct emergent epidemiologic and bench research for new infectious diseases (i.e., SARS) are unimaginable! More than a century of the scientific method in basic and clinical research has brought us to cures and salvages that have changed many persons' expectations of medicine, perhaps as exemplified (rightly or wrongly) in popular entertainment (e.g., television shows such as *ER, Rescue 911,* and *Chicago Hope*) or in the portrayal of medical research in broadcast and printed media.[8]

The expectations of our patients, and our expectations as HCPs, are that *we will cure our patients*. Similarly, our academic mission is to conduct basic, translational, and clinical research and generate novel therapies to treat persons who would become impaired or die under existing standards of care.

In spite of current and future advances in medicine, several fundamental truths will always remain: (1) Medicine is a human endeavor based on trust between patients and HCPs. (2) There are illnesses beyond our capacity to treat. (3) All persons die.

In the face of these fundamental truths, physicians have often been said to have more focus on the "curing" than on the "caring" aspects of medicine. The all too often heard rhetorical question, "Why are we doing this to this patient?" is emblematic of the tension between the endeavor to cure and the recognition that almost all treatments carry burdens as well as benefits, a point that Bill Bartholome knew very well, given his experience as both a physician and a patient. The desire to cure, even when it means "pushing the envelope" of therapy is not de facto "bad," nor is it incompatible with the desire to care and to alleviate symptoms. Similarly, the aim of alleviating symptoms (palliative care) is not de facto "giving up on a patient," nor is it incompatible with the desire to cure.[23,29]

The aim of this chapter is to outline important principles and strategies for *integrating* palliative and curative care in otolaryngology–head and neck surgery (OLHNS). We start from a presumption of good will—that HCPs desire both to cure and to alleviate symptoms. We also start with the recognition that not all HCPs have been given the opportunity to learn how to integrate these aims, nor is this an issue that has been adequately covered in many medical textbooks.[19] Because we are not otolaryngology specialists, this chapter will focus more on principles rather than on specific protocols or circumstances of palliative care in otolaryngology.

IMPORTANT DEFINITIONS AND CONCEPTS
Curative and Restorative Care

Curative and restorative care involves therapies and diagnostic techniques that are specifically intended to arrest or control the pathophysiologic processes that result in a patient's disease, or to restore the structure or function lost to disease. Examples of curative care include medications, antimicrobial agents, chemotherapy, medically provided hydration and nutrition, dialysis, blood transfusion, extirpative surgery, endoscopic surgery, endovascular surgery, radiation therapy (including stereotactic radiosurgery), and administration of radiopharmaceuticals; and examples of restorative care include plastic and reconstructive surgery, prosthetic surgery (e.g., cochlear implant), hormonal therapy (e.g., thyroid replacement), and organ transplantation.

Palliative Care

Palliative care is a comprehensive approach to treating serious illness that focuses on physical, psychological, spiritual, and social needs of patients. The goal is "to achieve the best possible quality of life through relief of suffering, control of symptoms and restoration of functional capacity while remaining sensitive to personal, cultural and religious values, beliefs and practices."[28] A person does not have to be dying in order to need or to receive palliative care.

End-of-Life Care

End-of-life (EOL) care is a "subset" of palliative care that encompasses advance care planning (i.e., creating advance directives and discussing goals of care with family and HCPs, a process that should begin from the time of diagnosis of a potentially life-threatening disease); decisions to limit or withdraw life-sustaining therapies; "do not resuscitate" orders; respect for personal, cultural, and religious dying rituals; and support of patients' and families' emotional needs, including grief and bereavement. While EOL care is often provided when death is imminent, it may best be initiated when death is foreseeable.

Pain Medicine

Pain medicine has a focus on the treatment of acute and chronic pain, which includes both the unpleasant sensation that constitutes pain and the associated emotional responses. Pain specialists come from the fields of anesthesiology, psychiatry, physical medicine and rehabilitation, neurology, neurosurgery, and others, but it is the responsibility of all HCPs to address patients' pain. The American Academy of Pain Medicine defines the practice of pain medicine as a multidisciplinary approach "incorporating modalities from various specialties to ensure the comprehensive evaluation and treatment of the pain patient" and includes the treatment of pain that is a symptom of disease (eudynia) as well as the pain that is the primary disease (maldynia).[2] Although palliative care and EOL care both have a considerable focus on the treatment of pain, it is important to understand that a "pain consult" is often not sufficient by itself to attend to all the needs addressed by palliative and EOL care.

Ethics Consultation

An ethics consultation is provided either by individuals or teams assigned by a hospital the responsibility to advise patients, families, physicians, nurses, and other HCPs in circumstances when there is conflict or uncertainty regarding values used in making health care decisions for individual patients. A similar function applies to values used in making decisions for institutions or groups of patients, known as organizational ethics. The role of an ethics consultation team is not to make the decision or to dictate the patient's care plan; ethics consultations are advisory. Their role is to listen to the involved persons; to help in the communication and decision-making processes; to keep focus on the patient's values and interests; to clarify the ethical and moral aspects and boundaries of the situation; and to assist everyone involved in coming to an ethically permissible decision—and in most circumstances, there may be more than one ethically permissible decision.

Goals of Care

Goals of care can include curing disease, alleviating symptoms and improving quality of life, relieving suffering and providing comfort, and acknowledging the inevitability of dying and death while retaining hope (as Bill Bartholome did). The goals of care should be determined prospectively by discussions with the patient, or with the family or surrogates if the patient lacks decision making capacity. These discussions should include an assessment of the patient's current condition and prognosis, the risks and benefits of existing or proposed interventions, and an estimation of the effectiveness and range of outcomes of the treatment options, including palliative care. Pursuit of curative, restorative, and palliative goals of care can occur simultaneously, and often should.

PALLIATIVE CARE IMPERATIVES AND OPPORTUNITIES

In 1997, the Institute of Medicine reported that "too many dying people suffer from pain and other distress that clinicians could prevent or relieve with existing knowledge and therapies."[16] Given the extensive literature that exists and documents pain and quality-of-life measures in head and neck tumors, it is surprising and regrettable that there appears to be very little OLHNS literature that specifically addresses palliative care, as opposed to palliative surgery, radiation, or chemotherapy.[17] It would seem that the field of OLHNS possesses a large volume of data on pain and quality of life, and it is now time to move from a more passive, observational approach to these issues in research and clinical care to a more active approach that not only notes the symptoms and quality-of-life measures but anticipates and responds to them through the integration of palliative care and curative care strategies.[21] The American College of Surgeons has already undertaken a series of efforts and publications related to palliative and EOL care,[22,26,27] yet a search of the American Academy of Otolaryngology–Head and Neck Surgery Web site reveals no results for the terms *death, dying, palliative care, end-of-life care,* or their variants.[1] Thus, it appears that there is both an imperative and a significant opportunity for OLHNS clinical research and clinical care, as well as educational endeavors to more formally integrate palliative care into the practice of OLHNS.

Trust and Betrayal

Medicine is a human endeavor based on trust between patients and HCPs. Everyone wants, needs, and deserves trust in relationships. Yet trust is a complex concept with different meanings. It is emotionally provocative, both positively and negatively.[20]

However, trust can be fragile, especially under conditions of vulnerability such as illness or injury. Trust in a person (e.g., a HCP) is fostered when there is confidence that person will fulfill the expectations entrusted to them—that they will fulfill their obligations. However, a patient under the stress of illness may be less capable of extending trust, and thus the responsibility falls to the HCP to demonstrate trustworthiness, the capacity to be trusted by others, which is fostered by behaviors that are respectful and promote integrity. Especially in today's health care environment, HCPs can also be affected by stress in such a way that their capacity for trust in relationships with patients, or even other HCPs, is undermined. Trustworthy behaviors can be the expression of either conscious or unconscious choices we make, depending on our individual levels of awareness, readiness, and willingness to address trust in relationships.[20]

When persons are diagnosed with life-threatening illnesses or injuries, they may experience what they perceive as a series of major and minor betrayals. They may feel that their bodies have betrayed them, that their sense of how things work in the world has betrayed them, or even that God has betrayed them, challenging their faith. As their experiences with their illnesses progress, these patients may even experience what they sense as betrayal by family members or friends, depending on their responses to the patients' illnesses.

At times, they may experience a breach of trust by HCPs. It is not rare for physicians to encounter patients who describe their previous experiences with other physicians or institutions as unfavorable. Thus, when patients first meet health care team members, they can arrive at the encounter with an already challenged capacity to trust.

This circumstance can be disconcerting to HCPs who are trained and work in a framework in which they "expect" to be trusted by their patients from the outset. The challenge, then, is to better understand the nature of trust, trustworthiness, and betrayal and to incorporate this understanding into the HCP-patient relationship in a way that supports trust and heals the patient's sense of betrayal.

Patients come to HCPs when they are in need of their specialized expertise and may assume that HCPs will use their competency to cure the patients' ailments or injuries, improve their function, or relieve their pain and suffering, an obligation of HCP known as fiduciary responsibility.[18] Whether explicitly stated to the patient or not, the fiduciary responsibility serves as an HCP's promise to act in the patient's interest. In the HCP-patient relationship, trust is also demonstrated when an HCP regularly reviews progress, goals of care, and prognosis with the patient to ensure that the plans the HCP is pursuing are *still* consistent with the patient's wishes.

Clearly, trust of HCPs can be built or broken based on the integrity of our behaviors, but trust is also bidirectional. That is, just as patients expect that they can trust HCPs, HCPs expect that they can trust patients. For mutual trust to be fostered, a shared understanding of the meaning and conditions of the relationship will be necessary so unintentional betrayals can be avoided. In essence, it is wise to discuss obligations and expectations early in the HCP-patient relationship so as to support the trusting relationship.[20]

What is meant by *betrayal*? Betrayal is a breach of trust or the perception that a trust has been breached. Betrayals can be either intentional or unintentional. Betrayal is a natural part of both personal and professional relationships; however, it is worth considering that betrayals are best tolerated (or forgiven) in relationships that already have a strong foundation of trust.

When persons find themselves in the circumstance of being betrayed, they can question themselves, their worth, their principles and beliefs, their own trustworthiness, and their sense of belonging.[20] Betrayal can be experienced in a variety of ways, ranging from minor to major emotional responses or from mild discomfort to deep pain. A person's experiences with betrayal influences his or her future capacity for trust. In essence, persons who have experienced betrayal previously are less likely to enter into future relationships by extending their trust, which sometimes means that a physician-patient relationship that is new from the physician's relationship, and thus should be founded in trust, may be viewed from the patient's perspective with a degree of distrust.

HCPs help patients and families heal by practicing trust-promoting behaviors. These start with respectful communication, which provides the basis for shared decision making. In communication, respect is foundational. HCPs must practice humility and assume that patients are capable of understanding complex issues. This means working closely with them to clarify their intentions and to assess their preferences for involvement in decision making. Open communication about these issues decreases the likelihood of making decisions without adequate notification and involvement. It can also help prevent any breaches of confidential information to uninvolved third parties that might result in loss of resources or insurance coverage.

Respect for Persons and Autonomy

In the United States, there is a strong tradition and legal precedent for respecting the autonomy of persons with regard to their medical decisions. The underlying concept of autonomy is respect for persons. The Belmont Report, for example, describes that respect for persons incorporates (1) respect for autonomy, or self-determination, of persons with decision making capacity, and (2) protection of persons who, by virtue of impaired decision-making capacity, may not be able to express their autonomous wishes.[14]

In its broadest interpretation, "respect for persons" means recognizing another human being as sharing a common human destiny.[10] Each patient, as a person, regardless of how we as HCPs may perceive the quality of their life, must be shown consideration and regarded with deference and respect. Respect for persons not only includes respecting their choices (autonomy), but also providing them the information to make their choices (veracity, or telling the truth), which includes the obligation of HCPs to help interpret complex medical information in a way the patient and family can understand and appreciate it, and also to make recommendations for treatment based on an understanding of the values and goals of care the patient and family are using to make their choices.

A decision is not autonomous unless it is informed, uncoerced, and authentic. We would caution, however, that it can be tempting to conclude that the reason that a patient refuses our recommendation is because of a knowledge deficit, which we often try to fix by providing more knowledge. In fact, the refusal is often fully informed and represents a difference in values regarding the degree of risk and the potential to improve the patient's well-being. This places on the HCP the obligation to assess the patient's understanding of their circumstances and the rationale for the choice, as well as to offer additional information to the patient in a manner in which it is likely to be heard. In some sense, this may mean that we have to let go of our own agendas and recommendations, strive to understand "where the patient is" in regard to their illness and life, and truly meet their there by accepting the decision once we are reassured that the patient has what information, emotional and spiritual support, time, and "space" they need to make a decision.

In the course of caring for patients, differences of opinion, if not conflict, sometimes occur. Respecting another person does not mean that we must agree with their decisions, or even that we must like the person. Rather, respect requires a conscious and conscientious intention to understand, appreciate, and honor the choices, preferences, perspectives, and diversity of each person. It is usually easy to respect a patient whose wishes are in agreement with our recommendations. On the other hand, it can be challenging to respect a patient whose decision is not to proceed with a therapy or intervention that has been recommended with the belief that it is beneficial to the patient, or a patient who wishes to continue curative interventions when the HCPs believe that palliative interventions should predominate. In some circumstances, such decisions may even feel to the HCPs as if the patient is not respecting their expertise or desire to promote the patient's health and well-being, but truth be told, it's rarely about us. In most circumstances, the patient's decision is appropriately centered on the self and based more on reflection of their own experience with the illness and its treatments, as well as the patient's judgment (with rational and emotional components) regarding the benefits and burdens of the proposed therapy in the context of their goals of care.

Balancing the Benefits and Burdens of Interventions

Few medical interventions are purely beneficial. Most offer patients both potential benefit as well as potential burdens, such as pain, invasiveness, and additional physical, psychological, or spiritual burdens. The threshold for tolerating the burdens of certain therapies may change as the goals of care change, depending on the patient's responses, including physiological, emotional, and spiritual responses. For example, patients, family, and HCPs may be willing to tolerate the adverse effects of chemotherapy when cure is possible, but in the context of recurrence or inadequate response to therapy, the same burdens may no longer be acceptable and would be considered unjustified. Therefore, benefits and burdens must be weighed against one another in a constant or frequently iterative process involving patient, family, and HCPs. This approach is often described as a shared decision-making model.

Decision-making is generally easier when the benefits of the intervention far outweigh the burdens, and it becomes more complicated when the chance of a favorable outcome is less certain or expected to be of marginal usefulness, or when the nature or degree of the burden is disproportionately high. This unfavorable benefit/burden balance usually emerges as a disease progresses toward its terminal phase.

Even under the best circumstances, decisions regarding treatment occur under conditions of uncertainty because no outcome can ever be promised—only a range of potential outcomes and their likelihood can be described. If the diagnosis, complicating factors, or prognosis are unclear, there is additional uncertainty and less ability to predict the disease trajectory. Sometimes this motivates HCPs, patients, and family to pursue additional diagnostic studies or innovative therapies as they strive to reduce the degree of uncertainty, but the tradeoff is the potential for prolonged or additional burdens in the face of unlikely benefit.

A final source of uncertainty, or incongruence, is the fact that HCPs often must use short-term responses to intervention to predict whether the patient's long-term goals of care can be attained. This can be especially difficult for less-experienced members of the health care team who might not have sufficient experience following up patients through their entire illnesses, and consultation with senior HCPs can be helpful. It is wise for HCPs to disclose their sources of information (e.g., literature or experience with similar patients) and the relative strength of the information when they make recommendations regarding interventions.

Balancing benefits and burdens does not necessarily entail choosing *either* curative/restorative interventions *or* palliative interventions. In fact, the either/or approach is one that frequently results in the incorporation of palliative care measures too late in a patient's experience with illness (Figure 18-1). When curative and restorative interventions are the primary focus, and palliative care and EOL care are not discussed or incorporated, it may seem to the patient and family that the HCPs have suddenly given up on them when they're told, "There's nothing more that we can do." The fact of the matter is that most of the time the health care team is aware the patient is dying, and depending on the nature of the team and the relationships among its members, there can be conflict within the team or conflict with the family to the extent that an ethics consultation is requested. By this point, relationships can be so damaged that it is difficult to reach a resolution that is satisfactory to everyone.

An alternate approach, illustrated in Figure 18-2, is to integrate palliative care and curative/restorative care interventions from the outset of a patient's illness. This approach requires early and sensitive discussions with the patient and family about the possibility of the patient's death and a conversation about the goals of care. Ideally, in the early stages of the illness, the proportion of curative/restorative interventions is much greater than the proportion of

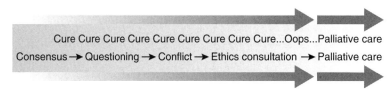

Cure Cure Cure Cure Cure Cure Cure Cure Cure...Oops...Palliative care

Consensus → Questioning → Conflict → Ethics consultation → Palliative care

Figure 18-1. This approach of palliative care often results in the patient receiving palliative care too late in the illness.

palliative interventions. As the patient's illness progresses and there is either improvement or deterioration in the condition, the proportion of these interventions should adjust accordingly. As death approaches, if a curative intervention is no longer capable of achieving the patient's goals of care, this can be discussed, and the intervention can be limited or stopped—while at the same time, palliative interventions that are achieving goals of care can be increased or added.

NEGOTIATING PLANS OF CARE

Needless to say, this type of approach requires skilled communication and negotiation between the HCPs and the patient and family. The process requires frequent conversations to reassess the patient's condition, goals of care, response to therapies, and recommendations for further treatment. It is a mistake to believe that a single conversation at the beginning of the course of treatment suffices.

The first conversation often involves breaking bad news about the patient's diagnosis. A frequently cited source for HCPs to learn skills in these conversations is Robert Buckman's book, *How to break bad news*.[5] Communicating bad news can be stressful for everyone involved, and there are often strong emotions that come forth. Once the bad news is broken, it is very common for patients and families to be so distraught that they hear nothing more of the conversation. This is natural and should most often be allowed to happen. Rather than continuing to talk, the HCP may wish to wait quietly with the patient and family as their emotions emerge. Opportunities to have the more "technical" conversation about treatment options, prognosis, etc., will arise in short order and optimally should be planned for in the process of breaking bad news. Even so, patients and families may have a hard time understanding what is said to them, and the HCP may need to restate the issues several times or over several meetings as the family seeks to understand. Attention to plain language is important, and HCPs must be particularly mindful of their tendency to use medical jargon and slang; they must consciously try to use language more appropriate to patients' and families' capacity to understand.

GENERAL AND SPECIAL PALLIATIVE CARE CONSIDERATIONS IN OLHNS
Identity

Otolaryngology–head and neck surgery is a specialty that cares for patients with diseases, injuries, and illnesses that can uniquely affect their identity and their quality of life.[4,13,15] Self-identity is often measured and manifested by appearance and recognition of the face, head, eyes, voice, and even hearing.[9,24,25] There can be intense emotional and spiritual consequences associated with disfigurement or deformity of these structures and similar beneficial consequences to plastic and reconstructive approaches to preserving or restoring these structures and the identity associated with them. Although not commonly conceived as being within the realm of palliative care, change in identity can potentially have serious consequences and most certainly is a factor in patients' decision making regarding surgery for head and neck cancer.[9] If patients fear disapproval or repulsion on the basis of appearance, smell, inability to manage secretions, or other related reasons, they may isolate themselves socially, if not physically, or may become seriously demoralized and depressed.

Loss of Function

Beyond the personal and emotional identity-related aspects of diseases affecting the structures of the head, face, and neck are important functional issues. To a certain extent, the nature of the functional loss depends on the site and type of tumor. For example, patients with laryngeal carcinoma, not surprisingly, have significant impairment of communication and vocalization, whereas patients with hypopharyngeal carcinoma have significantly impaired swallowing associated with nausea and vomiting, use of feeding tubes, and weight loss.[4,15] Other important issues include social eating, social contact, and problems with teeth, dry mouth, and mucus production.[4,15]

With specific regard to medically provided nutrition (tube feedings), it has been suggested that when cachexia is present (defined as a catabolic process often associated with tumors that actively breaks down skeletal muscle, fat, and carbohydrates despite nutritional intake), tube feedings are ineffective.[12] On

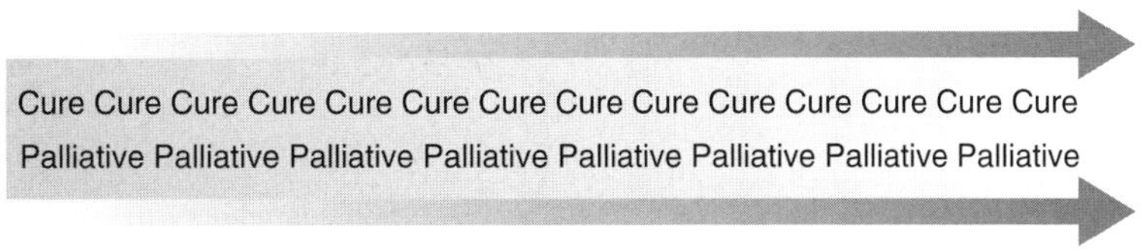

Cure Cure Cure Cure Cure Cure Cure Cure Cure Cure Cure Cure Cure Cure

Palliative Palliative Palliative Palliative Palliative Palliative Palliative Palliative

Figure 18-2. This approach of palliative care is more ideal than the one depicted in Figure 18-1 because it integrates palliative care and curative/restorative care at the outset of the patient's illness.

the other hand, if the cause of weight loss is starvation, meaning the inability to take in sufficient nutrition (as might happen with dysphagia), then tube feedings can be effective. The distinction between malnutrition and cachexia is not always easy, and it is possible that patients may initially respond to tube feedings, but later in the course of their disease become cachectic and thus unresponsive to medically provided nutrition. In this circumstance, tube feedings could be considered "futile," but the symbolic importance of feeding should not be underestimated when discussing its withdrawal with the patient or family. Indeed, even among HCPs there are varying opinions on this topic, and many consider that medically provided nutrition or hydration are not "therapies" by virtue of their strong symbolism and connection to support, love, and sustenance.

Sexual Interest and Intimacy

Long-standing relationships and intimacy can be adversely affected. Recent research on quality-of-life measures in head and neck cancer suggests that decline in sexuality or sexual interest is an outcome in 9 of 11 major categories of head and neck cancer.[4,15] This finding is somewhat surprising on first glance because the cancer may not be physiologically related to sexual function or endocrine influence on sexual function, but deeper consideration reveals that it should be nearly intuitive to understand that intimacy and sexual activities of many types involve and are influenced by the appearance and function of face, head, and neck structures.

Pain

Another important quality-of-life measure in OLHNS is pain. Quality-of-life surveys have shown differing types and intensity of pain with different tumor sites.[4,15] Bone pain, mucosal pain (mucositis), and neuropathic pain are just a few examples.[6] Different pain types and different pain sites will demand different analgesic approaches and modalities.[17]

We must strive to rarely leave a patient's pain, loss of function, or distress unaddressed. We are obliged to inquire about pain and treat it, and it is not acceptable to undertreat pain out of concern for addiction. OLHNS patients in pain may develop narcotic tolerance, but they will not develop addiction. Narcotics have virtually no ceiling effect, and the dose can be *gradually* escalated to seemingly incredible doses with no respiratory depression or sedation, although the constipation associated with diminished gastric motility should be addressed.[11]

The need for analgesia is not directly related to the imminence of death. Patients with months or years to live may have severe pain that should be addressed; thus, there is no requirement that patients must be dying before being given adequate doses of analgesics. It is widely believed that inadequate pain treatment is a reason for the requests for euthanasia or physician-assisted suicide (PAS) that physicians encounter from time to time. Although the data from Oregon's experience with PAS suggests that loss of autonomy and loss of control of bodily functions (e.g., bowel, bladder incontinence, vomiting) are the major reasons for requesting and completing PAS, it is important to recognize that over three fourths of the patients in the PAS cohort in Oregon had access to palliative care.[7] These results do not exclude the possibility that inadequately treated pain would be an important reason for patients to request PAS in a context in which palliative care is not being provided.

EPILOGUE

Four years after diagnosis, Bill Bartholome's cancer recurred with metastasis to the lungs, spine, and throat. His voice and swallowing jeopardized, he wrote about the challenges of managing the pain, symptoms, loss, and grief. Bill had symptoms of esophageal stricture that required dilation, postthoracotomy pain syndrome, dumping syndrome, and weight loss. He had palliative radiation to the spine to prevent spinal cord compression.

William G. Bartholome, MD, died August 2, 1999, at age 55, 5 years after his esophageal carcinoma was diagnosed.

ACKNOWLEDGMENT

We wish to thank Carlton Haywood, Jr., MA(c) for his assistance in researching and editing this chapter.

REFERENCES

1. The American Academy of Otolaryngology Homepage. The American Academy of Otolaryngology. 2003. Available: *http://www.aaohns.org.* Accessed June 10, 2003.
2. The American Academy of Pain Medicine: *Welcome Statement. The American Academy of Pain Medicine, 2003.* Available at: www.painmed.org. Accessed May 26, 2003.
3. Bartholome W: Living in the light of death: 2003. *Bioethics Forum Meditations* 16(1). Available at *http://www.midbio.org/bartholome.htm.* Accessed June 19, 2003.
4. Bjordal K and others: A prospective study of quality of life in head and neck cancer patients. part II: longitudinal data, *Laryngoscope* 111:1440–1452, 2001.
5. Buckman R: *How to break bad news: a guide for health care professionals.* Baltimore, Md, 1992, Johns Hopkins University Press.
6. Chaplin JM, Morton RP: A prospective, longitudinal study of pain in head and neck cancer patients, *Head Neck* 21:531–537, 1999.
7. Chin AE and others: Legalized physician-assisted suicide in Oregon: the first year's experience, *N Engl J Med* 340:577–583, 1999.

8. Diem SJ, Lantos JD, Tulsky JA: Cardiopulmonary resuscitation on television: miracles and misinformation, *N Engl J Med* 334:1578–1582, 1996.

9. Conley J: The meaning of life-threatening disease in the area of the head and neck, *Acta Otolaryngol* 99(3-4):201–204, 1985.

10. Curtin L, Chinn P, editor: *The nurse as advocate.* Rockville, Maryland, Aspen Systems, 1986.

11. Dunn GP and others: Palliative care by the surgeon: how to do it, *J Am Coll Surg* 194:509–537, 2002.

12. Easson AM, Hinshaw DB, Johnson DL: The role of tube feeding and total parenteral nutrition in advanced illness, *J Am Coll Surg* 194:225–228, 2002.

13. Epstein JB and others: Quality of life and oral function in patients treated with radiation therapy for head and neck cancer, *Head Neck* 23:389–398, 2001.

14. Ethical Principles and Guidelines for the Protection of Human Subjects of Research. The National Commission for the Protection of Human Subjects of Biomedical and Behavioral Research. U.S. Department of Health, Education, and Welfare. Protection of Human Subjects: Belmont Report—ethical principles and guidelines for the protection of human subjects of research. *Fed Regist* 44(76):23192–23197, Apr 18, 1999.

15. Hammerlid E and others: A prospective study of quality of life in head and neck cancer patients. part I: at diagnosis, *Laryngoscope* 111(4 Pt 1):669–680, 2001.

16. Institute of Medicine: Approaching death: improving care at the end of life. In Field M, Cassel C, editors: *National Academy of Sciences; Institute of Medicine Committee on Care at the End of Life.* 1997.

17. Lovel T: Palliative care and head and neck cancer, *Br J Oral Maxillofac Surg* 38:253–254, 2000.

18. McKneally MF, Martin DK: An entrustment model of consent for surgical treatment of life-threatening illness: perspective of patients requiring esophagectomy, *J Thorac Cardiovasc Surg* 120:264–269, 2000.

19. Rabow MW and others: End-of-life care content in 50 textbooks from multiple specialties, *JAMA* 283:771–778, 2000.

20. Reina D, Reina M: *Trust & betrayal in the workplace: building effective relationships in your organization.* Berrett-Koehler Publishers, 1999.

21. Richardson A, Lee L, Birchall M: Learning from patients with cancer and their spouses: a focus group study, *J Laryngol Otol* 116:1028–1035, 2002.

22. Robert Wood Johnson Foundation Office of Promoting Excellence in End-of-Life Care: executive summary of the report from the field, *J Am Coll Surg* 196:807–815, 2003.

23. Rushton CH, Williams MA, Sabatier KH: The integration of palliative care and critical care: one vision, one voice, *Crit Care Nurs Clin North Am* 14:133–140, 2002.

24. Schenck DP: Ethical considerations in the treatment of head and neck cancer, *Cancer Control* 9:410–419, 2002.

25. Sulmasy DP: Appearance and morality: ethics and otolaryngology-head and neck surgery, *Otolaryngol Head Neck Surg* 126:4–7, 2002.

26. Surgeons Palliative Care Workgroup: *Promoting excellence in end-of-life care: the American College of Surgeons, 5-12-2003.* Available at: *http://www.promotingexcellence.org/navigate/surgeons.html.* Accessed June 10, 2003.

27. Surgical Palliative Care Task Force: *The Surgeon and Palliative Care: The American College of Surgeons, 1-21-2003.* Available at: *http://www.facs.org/palliativecare/.* Accessed June 10, 2003.

28. The Task Force on Palliative Care: *Last acts: precepts of palliative care.* 1997. Chicago, Stewart Communications. Available at: *http://www.lastacts.org.* Accessed May 26, 2003.

29. Williams MA and others: Irreconcilable differences? *Crit Care Med* 31:1289–1290, 2003.

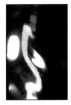

CHAPTER NINETEEN

GRAPHICS AND DIGITAL IMAGING FOR OTOLARYNGOLOGISTS

Lawrence R. Lustig
Nikolas Blevins

The ability to effectively represent visual information in novel and compelling ways has had tremendous impact in human history.[7-9] The recent emergence of the use of digital images has its history in traditional-media graphic arts, photography, and the digital computer revolution. The origin of representational drawing is said to date back to ancient Greece, when a silhouette shadow was traced and kept as a remembrance of a departing loved one (Figure 19-1). Traditional media art was refined over time, becoming more capable of capturing the likeness of the subject. In 1839, William Henry Fox Talbot presented to the Royal Society his invention to capture images on specially treated paper. Photography was born, prompting painter Paul Delaroche to proclaim, "From this day on, painting is dead."[6]

Today, the emergence of digital imaging may well present another similar revolutionary means of displaying visual information. In 1940, the world's first electronic computer, the Electronic Numeric Integrator and Computer (ENIAC) was developed. Not only did this give rise to the modern data processing industry, but it also was responsible for adding the term "computer" to our everyday lexicon.[7] One of the first digital images ever created (Figure 19-2) was produced in the mid 1950s by Russell A. Kirsch. A photograph was scanned, stored in an early computer, and the results were displayed on an oscilloscope. Much like the evolution of traditional media, digital imaging techniques have evolved, only this evolution has occurred at a tremendously accelerated pace.

Computers have integrated themselves into the very fabric of our existence. Medicine is, of course, not immune to this transformation. Computer information technologies and digital multimedia have become integrally involved in the delivery of medicine, the education of our trainees, and in the management of the business of medicine. Within our own specialty, one simply needs to browse the otolaryn-

gology journals or attend the annual meetings to see how computers have fundamentally altered the way we perform science and medicine. In addition to changing the way we practice our profession, computers have fundamentally altered the way we *communicate* our specialty—to our peers and our patients. Advances in computer hardware and software are increasingly allowing the "amateur" to create professional-appearing artwork, slides, and video. Digital presentations at national meetings are becoming increasingly common, and many physicians and scientists now render their own artwork for manuscripts, presentations, and patient education materials rather than rely on the professional medical artist or graphic designer.

The term "media" represents the myriad ways that we as humans communicate. From radio to newspapers to television, media is simply the agent of communication. The term "multimedia" has evolved from a variety of media disciplines. Nicholas Negroponte, a scientist at MIT's Media Laboratory, correctly predicted as early as 1978 the fusion of various media sources, including television broadcast, print publishing, and the computer industry.[1] Although historically this media type has remained in the "real world" of printed matter and broadcast television, recent developments in computer digitization, compression, and processing power have enabled the storage, retrieval, and manipulation of these media, including video, animation, text, and music, on everyday computers. The result has been the multimedia digital information technology revolution that is exploding around all of us.

The primary aims of this chapter are to introduce otolaryngologists to some of the fundamental aspects of digital imaging as they specifically apply to medicine. Multimedia in medicine can mean anything from adding a digitized CT scan to a discussion of a disease, to three-dimensional interactive temporal bone

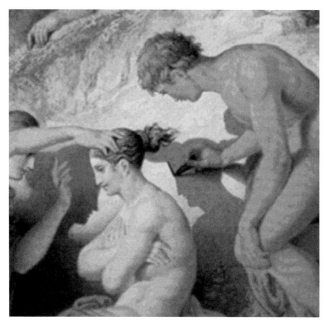

Figure 19-1. A detail from *The Invention of Drawing,* by Karl Freidrich Schinkel, 1830. Von-der-Heydt Museum, Wuppertal. Here, a shadow silhouette is traced with charcoal to serve as a remembrance of a departing loved one. Such a practice in ancient Greece is thought to represent the birth of representational drawing. (From Mitchell WJ: *The reconfigured eye: visual truth in the post-photographic era,* Cambridge, MA, The MIT Press, 1992.)

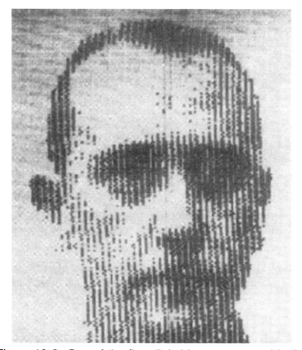

Figure 19-2. One of the first digital images, created in the early 1950s by Russell A. Kirsch. The original photograph was scanned into an early digital computer, stored, and could be displayed on an oscilloscope.

anatomy CD-ROMs. This brief review obviously cannot be a definitive text for enabling the reader to become a multimedia maven. Rather, it is intended to serve as a springboard that will hopefully encourage those who are computer literate but have thus far been resistant to make the "digital leap" to explore this fascinating, worthwhile topic.

Why should clinicians or academicians even care about multimedia and digital graphics? There are several compelling reasons. First, the ability to design one's own illustrations or artwork for a manuscript or presentation creates tremendous advantages; complex ideas or concepts do not have to be translated through an intermediate party, especially one who may not share a fundamental understanding of the topic at hand. Furthermore, the ability to design your own presentation, create your own patient handouts, and be in complete control of your own artwork is not only economically advantageous but may also create a strong sense of artistic accomplishment. Most who perform their own digital artwork do so out of sheer pleasure. However, this control does come with a price; the user, like the artist, has to assume a familiarity with the artistic medium, whether it be pencil and paper, paint and canvas, or computer software and hardware.

As any adult who has undertaken that important step toward computer literacy knows, there may be a steep learning curve. A similar learning curve may occur for those who understand basic computer functions yet would like to venture into digital imaging. Many computers and software packages often come with a frustrating set of quirks, "glitches," and design parameters that need to be explored and understood before efficient use can occur. It is this seemingly daunting challenge that prevents many in our profession from making the "digital" leap. We maintain that anyone who has mastered the art of surgery can certainly master the art of digital graphics. Like the surgical resident who learns from the experience and mistakes of those who have gone before him, it is hoped that the following discussion, garnered through the authors' experience in multimedia design, will offer some useful guideposts to make the transition to "digital" clinician both fulfilling and enjoyable.

DIGITAL BASICS
Digital Image Representation and Color Theory

The basic nature of digital images varies substantially from what we are accustomed to experiencing through our vision. The core of the difference is that between analog (continuous) and digital (discreet) information. The human eye and brain are accustomed to perceiving visual information in an analog fashion. Color gradations and contours are continuous, without any apparent divisions imposed by our visual system. Digital images, by contrast, are by definition composed of numbers with discreet values. Color and spatial information is encoded as well as possible, given a finite number of states that the numbers can represent. These differences account for both the greatest strengths and limitations of digital images.[6-9]

In a standard digital image, two-dimensional space is broken down into a Cartesian grid of points known as "picture-elements" or "pixels." Each pixel in this grid can be assigned a specific color. Then, when displayed together, this grid of pixels can represent an image. Smooth curves and color transitions can only be approximated, because the picture is no more than a series of discreet points. Close inspection or magnification of such an image will reveal the underlying grid, and further details cannot be discerned.

The amount of information present in a digital image is known as its "resolution." This is a measure of how accurately a digital image can simulate image variations with its discreet elements. Resolution can be subdivided into "spatial resolution" and "color resolution," both of which play a critical role in determining overall image quality. You can think of a digital image as a sheet of graph paper on which you can color each square a different color. Spatial resolution refers to the number of squares on the paper, and color resolution refers to the number of crayons you have at your disposal for coloring.

Spatial resolution refers to the number of pixels composing an image grid. The more pixels in a digital image, the more discreet spaces there are available to repre-

sent shape information. A grid of 600×600 pixels, for example, will represent an average image with significantly greater accuracy than a grid of 50×50 pixels (Figure 19-3). Remember that the total number of pixels in an image can increase dramatically as the grid is further subdivided. For example, a grid of 50×50 pixels contains 2500 elements, whereas a grid of 600×600 pixels grows to hold 360,000 elements. This becomes critical in considering the practical aspects of managing digital images, because the number of pixels in an image is another measure of the image's *size*, a topic that will be referred to repeatedly throughout this chapter.

Our own visual system performs a similar decomposition of the visual field. The eye breaks an image down into discreet elements on the basis of how light is cast onto the matrix of rods and cones of the retina. In the fovea, the area of the retina with greatest spatial resolution, there are as many as 150,000 such photoreceptors per square millimeter. At such high density, we perceive spatial variations to be continuous. Similarly, with high enough pixel density, we can also perceive digital images to be continuous and can overlook the grid that underlies them.

Color resolution refers to the number of discreet shades that any single pixel can represent. In the simplest case, each pixel of an image can be represented digitally as either a 1 or a 0, a single "bit," the basic numeric building block in the binary system. Such an image yields a pure black-and-white image without any shades of gray or color. However, if the spatial resolution is great enough, image clarity can still be sufficient (Figure 19-4).

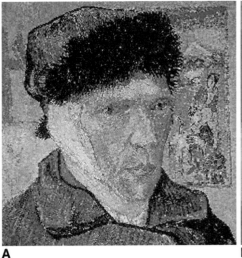 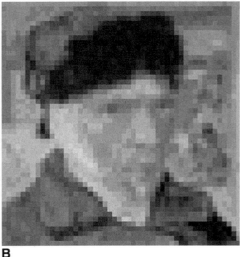

A   **B**

Figure 19-3. The effect of different spatial resolution on a digital image. Digital images are made up of discreet elements, known as "pixels." **A,** Image is composed of a 600×600 grid of pixels, whereas in **B,** the same subject is shown in a grid of 50×50 pixels. A distinct loss of information occurs as spatial resolution drops. Self Portrait with Bandaged Ear, Vincent Van Gogh, 1889, Courtauld Institute Gallery, London.

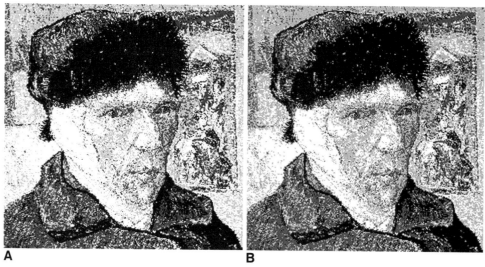

Figure 19-4. The effect of different color resolution. **A,** In the image, each pixel is represented by 1 bit, making it either black or white. **B,** In the image, each pixel is represented by 2 bits, allowing each point to be represented by one of four shades from black to white. The more bits per pixel, the better the possible color resolution. Self Portrait with Bandaged Ear, Vincent Van Gogh, 1889, Courtauld Institute Gallery, London.

If instead, 2 bits represent each pixel, you now have 2^2 or 4 crayons at your disposal. Each pixel can now represent 4 distinct shades of gray or distinct colors. Every time another bit is devoted to the pixel's color value, the number of distinct colors that spot can represent is doubled. For example, a standard "8-bit" image can be 2^8 or 256 distinct shades or colors. The human eye cannot effectively distinguish more than this number of shades of gray, and so for most purposes, no more bits need to be devoted to gray-scale images. The number of bits used to represent a color or shade is referred to as the image's "bit depth."

The digital representation of color also has its roots in physiology. The cones in the retina are the sensory cells for color information. There are cones "tuned" to be specifically more sensitive to red, green, or blue light. Any colors that we perceive are therefore varying combinations of each of these three fundamental colors. If you look closely at a color television screen, you will see that it is composed of a matrix of red, green, and blue filaments each varying in intensity independently of each other. When seen next to each other, these simulate all colors on the screen. The potential to decompose a color image into its fundamental components is even clearer in the mechanism of many projection television systems that separately project the red, green, and blue signals and have them fuse on the screen.

Digital images also use these fundamental colors as building blocks to produce all other colors. To represent the full color spectrum for most imaging purposes, each pixel is represented by 24 bits, 8 devoted to red, 8 devoted to green, and 8 devoted to blue. Each fundamental color is independently represented in one of 256 (2^8) levels of intensity. The various combinations of these levels produce more than 16 million shades of colors (2^{24}), more than sufficient to accurately produce images for most uses. The levels of red, green, and blue in an image can be thought of as being three independent images, known as *channels*, each of which has a depth of 8 bits.

When working with common computer programs that manipulate color digital images, one will find images are often referred to as being "32-bit" images. If 24 bits are sufficient to constitute "true color" as described previously, what do the additional 8 bits provide? The additional 8 bits of data represent *transparency* information for each pixel of an image. Therefore, every element of the image can have one of 256 (2^8) levels of transparency. This is useful information when combining an image with other digital pictures and determines where and how much background elements show through the foreground. This additional 8-bit channel is termed the *alpha channel*. The way in which red, green, blue, and alpha channels are combined into a final object is illustrated (Figure 19-5).

EFFICIENCY IN IMAGE SIZE

If you use digital images, why not always use the best or highest quality? The reason is that the size of an image can increase tremendously with attempts to

A. Composite Final Image

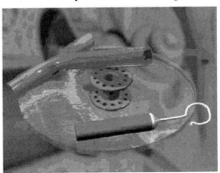

B. Red Channel   **C. Green Channel**

D. Blue Channel   **E. Transparency Channel**

Figure 19-5. Composition of a digital image. **A,** The final image represents a red piston prosthesis, a green t tube, and a blue tympanostomy tube sitting on a glass disk. The image is in 32-bit color, meaning it can be broken down into four independent 8-bit images, containing values for **B,** red, **C,** green, **D,** blue, and **E,** transparency (or alpha). The transparency channel shows how much a background image will show through. White is fully transparent, whereas black is fully solid. Although the image is gray scale, one can still understand the principles of red, green, blue, and transparency (alpha) channels that make up a final image.

add further image detail. For example, a typical digital camera may take a high-quality photograph at a spatial resolution of 1600×1200 pixels or a total of 1.9 million pixels. If this image is saved at 32-bit color resolution, it could result in an image file size of 7.7 million bytes, or 7.7 megabytes (MB). One "byte" is defined as a collection of 8 bits of data. However, if this same image is reduced in spatial resolution to 200×200 pixels in shades of gray only (8 bit, or 256 shades of gray), it would require only 40,000 bytes (40 KB), nearly 200 times smaller. Although the gray-scale image may not look quite as good as the color, such an image may be acceptable for a specific use, such as sending to a friend over the Internet.

Working with images that are too large can pose considerable difficulties in saving and manipulating files. Use of overly large images can slow a computer-based presentation to a crawl or, even worse, cause your computer to crash in the middle of a presentation. The key is to maximize the image quality for a specified purpose while maintaining workable file sizes.

What spatial resolution do you need? It depends greatly on the particular image and purpose, but some general points can be outlined. Currently, the average computer projector used in presentations shows the computer screen at no greater than 800×600 total pixels. The use of any images with spatial resolution over that is lost on such a system. Calculate the amount of the screen a particular image will be covering and adjust the size of that image accordingly. Slide printers that produce traditional optical 35-mm slides can handle much greater resolution, and the use of images up to 1600×1200 pixels can be justified in producing the most realistic look from digital photographs. In working with images for print, a good rule of thumb is to plan on about 300 pixels per inch (ppi) of finished printed image size.

HARDWARE—IS IT ALL ABOUT SPEED?

A recurrent theme throughout this chapter is the balance between file size and image quality. As the preceding discussion alludes to, trying to manipulate a large file on a computer may be difficult or even impossible. This is the primary reason that digital graphics designers are so obsessed with the concept of computer speed. For example, an average computer text file consisting of 40 pages may be only about 100,000 bytes in size, whereas an uncompressed 5×7 inch color digital image of average quality will be approximately 9 million bytes, a 90-fold difference! The larger the file size, the longer it will take a computer to complete a specific set of tasks on that file (e.g., change a color, shape, or size of an item within the image). Thus, if one is planning on performing digital imaging and graphics manipulations, computer speed becomes critical. Asking a slow computer to perform a complicated set of instructions on a large (e.g., 10 MB) file may enslave you in front of your computer screen, watching the mouse cursor turn into a "coffee cup" or "watch" for minutes on end after each incremental step. Understanding a few central concepts of computer hardware will allow you to determine whether your computer is "up to the task" of digital graphics, can be upgraded to perform sufficiently, or whether you need an entirely new system altogether.

The Computer Chip and Central Processing Unit

The most important component of the computer is the microprocessor or central processing unit (CPU). Its job is to process the steps of a computer program and send those instructions to the various components of your computer. It should go without saying that the faster your computer can perform these steps, the faster your computer will complete its task. The two main factors determining a CPU's performance are the *speed* of the chip and the *amount of data* that chip can process.

The CPU's *speed* reflects how quickly it handles a computer program's instructions, also known as clock speed, and is measured in hertz; 1 megahertz (MHz) processes 1 million clock cycles/second. However, a CPU's designated speed is not the final evaluation of a

CPU's overall performance. For example, computer chips will sometimes simplify instructions, combine common instructions, or send parallel instructions simultaneously, allowing faster processing of instructions. (An example of this is *Single Instruction Multiple Data (SIMD)* instructions used by Macintosh, which programs the most common computer tasks with fewer, simpler instructions, vastly increasing the CPU's speed.)

Over the past 30 years, fueled in large part by consumer demand for better video games, computer processing speed has grown tremendously. This was seen presciently by the Intel pioneer and cofounder Gordon E. Moore in 1965 and has since become known as "Moore's law." Moore's law has held that the number of transistors that can be etched on a single chip of silicon doubles on average every 18 months, effectively doubling the speed of the chip. Interestingly, although Moore voiced doubts about the permanence of the progression of his principle, computer design since this time has exceeded even his expectations. Current commercially available computer microprocessing speeds surpass 1 gigahertz and can perform more than 1 billion instructions per second. It is widely anticipated that within a decade, computers will be at least 25 times faster than they are at present.[5]

Hardware Upgrades

Perhaps you already own a computer that is only several years old but have already run into trouble because of your system's speed or performance. In this case, there are a variety of options available to upgrade your CPU, without having to spend more than several thousand dollars for an entirely new computer. Most computer manufacturers provide "motherboard" (CPU) upgrades, which will enable many of their older computers to function like the newer, faster models. Similarly, many personal computers have an empty microprocessor slot allowing upgrades to one of the newer chips. *Accelerators cards* are another option if you cannot wait for the next upgrade or your computer cannot accommodate an upgrade. These expansion cards simply plug into your computer and take over the processing chores for slower computers. A local or Internet computer supplier can assist you with this option.

Random Access Memory

Random access memory, or RAM, is the area of memory that your computer uses when you are first working on a file before you store the data on your computer hard disk or floppy disk (you may also think of RAM as your computer's "short-term" memory.) Most graphics and video applications are RAM-intensive, because many of the manipulations performed require a lot of processing power and memory. As a general rule, you should have three to five times your file size available in RAM. For example, when working on a 10-MB file, you should have at least 30 MB, but preferably 50 MB, RAM installed on the machine and *available* (not being used by another program). When you have an adequate CPU speed and your computer still is running quite slowly, chances are you have insufficient RAM on your computer. Fortunately, upgrading your RAM is a relatively inexpensive proposition, with a variety of third-party vendors offering RAM chips. We recommend *at least* 128 MB of RAM in your computer if you intend to begin doing your own digital graphics design, although you will find that your computer will run much quicker if you have between 256 and 512 MB of RAM. This is particularly true if you are frequently going back and forth between RAM-intensive programs and need to keep them all open at the same time.

Virtual memory is a function on some computers that will use hard disk space for extra RAM when your computer runs out of RAM during a program's operations. However, because your CPU will interact more quickly with your RAM than your hard drive, generally the use of virtual memory in many programs will slow down your computer. It is thus important to read the software designer's recommendations on the use of virtual memory.

Hard Drive

Your computer's hard drive is its main storage unit. As you enter the world of computer graphics and design, you will quickly realize that files are large and will quickly eat up your storage memory. Many people thus choose to purchase an additional hard drive(s), either for backup or additional storage. It seems that no matter how large one's hard drive is, it will inevitably get filled. Therefore, as a general rule, one should find a hard drive that is the largest and fastest that can be afforded. Hard drive speeds are measured by their "seek time," or the time it takes the drive's head to jump to a specific spot on the disk's platter, and is measured in milliseconds (ms). As expected, a faster seek time will allow your computer to retrieve data more quickly, speeding up the time it takes to open, save, and transfer files. It is recommended that at least 1 gigabyte (GB) of storage be available on your hard drive for digital imaging. Prices for external (plugs into your computer) and internal (physically located within the computer) drives have plummeted recently and should be relatively affordable. As a warning, if you plan on doing any video capture or editing, you will need a *lot* of storage, at least 20 GB but preferably much more.

If you have sufficient CPU speed and sufficient RAM on your computer but find that your computer still is not working fast, it is wise to check hard drive free space. If you are working at the maximum storage limits of your hard drive and have it filled to capacity, your computer may be running out of extra "buffer" memory. Many programs, when the amount of needed RAM exceeds what is installed in the computer, will substitute hard drive memory. If you then run out of free hard drive space, your computer will grind to an agonizingly slow pace. (A good rule of thumb is to keep at least 10% of a hard disk's space free to keep the system running smoothly).

Removable Storage and External Drives

As your collection of digitized medical images increases, you may begin to have a need for archiving your files, or you may find that you need to transport large files from home to office. In this case, it is convenient to have the ability to transport individual files or store them in smaller units rather than on a single large drive. Those nearly obsolete floppy disks, with a paltry 1.4 MB of storage space, are simply inadequate for this task when dealing with graphics files. Removable storage devices have thus become a favorite among computer users. A variety of manufacturers make newer, larger format portable "disks." Generally, they fall between 100 MB storage disks and 1000 MB (equal to 1 GB) storage disks. They function just as your old floppy drives did, with the ability to buy as many additional disks as you need. These are also an excellent, relatively inexpensive solution to freeing up badly needed space on your hard drive, if you are one of those who needs to constantly throw files away to make room for new files. It is recommended that the media purchased is the same format as your office or department, so you can easily go back and forth between systems with your files.

Recordable CD drives are increasingly becoming a standard for many computer graphics users. The disks, particularly the nonrewritable CD-R disks, are inexpensive and reliably store up to 650 MB of data. They are an outstanding solution for file backups. Rewritable disks are a bit more expensive but function like a floppy disk, allowing the user to repeatedly transfer new data onto the disk. Furthermore, most computers now have a CD-ROM drive, allowing one to easily share files with other users and computers. Other storage solutions include optical drives (often store data between 500 MB and 1 GB) and tape drives (inexpensive and slower, yet very reliable). Recordable DVD drives, with each disk able to store approximately 5 GB, are also beginning to gain in popularity. Several commercially available digital video packages for clinicians incorporate recordable DVD drives because of the huge file sizes involved with digital video capture and editing.

IMAGE INPUT DEVICES—"PERIPHERALS"

Whether for teaching residents, grand round presentations, patient handouts, or just plain fun, a creative clinician will find an image to suit their personal needs in just about any media available to them, be it video, newspapers, photographs, magazines, books, previously made slides, x-rays, CD-ROM, or the World Wide Web (WWW). The all-important step in creating a *computer* image from one of these myriad sources is digitizing the image. This digitized image will then become the template for your own creative designs. A myriad of easy-to-use and inexpensive equipment is available for this purpose. It is extremely important at this juncture to remind the reader of copyright and patent laws. Because of the ease in which existing proprietary information (text, images, video) can be digitized and altered, one must be extremely cautious when one uses existing materials. When in doubt, one should *always* consult a publisher, author, owner, or creator of the material in question.

Flatbed Scanners

Scanners are used to digitize photographs, flat art, slides, and transparent media, such as x-rays. Most scanners sold today are flatbed scanners, which resemble a small copy machine. The digitized image created by a scanner may then be saved to your computer and/or subsequently manipulated in a graphics program. Virtually any image can be scanned, as long as it can fit on top of the scanner's flat surface. Many scanners also offer attachments that will enable you to scan transparent media, such as slides and x-rays.

One of the most important points to make about scanners is that different scanners will provide different quality output, just as an inexpensive disposable camera will provide a vastly different image than a top-of-the-line 35-mm professional camera. When one uses a low-end scanner, it is much like taking a photograph with an inexpensive camera; although it may work well for text and simple images, much of the information you will want (color, depth, clarity) may be lost. In contrast, very high-end scanners are probably "overkill," offering resolutions and features that most users will never require. Flatbed scanners range in price from a hundred dollars to several thousand dollars. For someone interested in clinical images, it is highly recommended that a scanner include the ability to scan transparent media, such as slides, scans, and x-rays (Figure 19-6).

The two most important factors to consider when digitizing clinical artwork or images are its spatial resolution and its color dynamic range. Spatial resolution

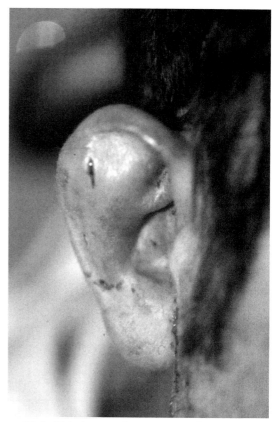

Figure 19-6. This image demonstrates the picture quality from a 35-mm color slide depicting a traumatic auricular hematoma. The 35-mm slide was scanned on a flatbed scanner with an optional transparency adapter at a resolution of 1200 ppi. The image was converted to gray scale for printing. The final size of the gray-scale image was 2.9 MB, uncompressed.

is measured in pixels per inch (ppi) or dots per inch (dpi). As described previously, digital images can be subdivided into individual color points that when taken together compose the entire image. On the computer, these points are known as "pixels," whereas on the printed page, they are commonly referred to as "dots." When considering how an image is actually printed, there are some differences between these two, but for scanning purposes, they are usually thought of as being interchangeable. The higher the pixel density, the sharper will be the image. Most scanners sold today will scan up to at least 600 ppi. As can be expected, the greater a scanner's potential spatial resolution, the greater its expected cost. Some scanners also use an "interpolation" to make the resolution appear higher. However, when a scanner interpolates, it is just adding pixels to a lower ppi image by averaging the surrounding colors and not necessarily enhancing the image sharpness. A discussion on optimizing scanning resolution is included in the following.

The color dynamic range of a scanner measures its ability to capture gradations of hue and brightness. The greater the dynamic range, the greater the veracity of the captured colors, the more accurate the picture (and of course, the more costly the scanner). Most low-end and medium-end scanners encode 24-bit color (8 bits each for red, green, and blue) and thus are able to produce more than 16 million colors (see preceding for a discussion of color resolution). For all practical purposes, this amount of information is adequate for most needs.

Slide Scanners

Because many clinicians have a huge archive of slides, slide scanners may be an ideal solution to digitize them. Optical 35-mm slides have the capacity for displaying more brightness and hue information and so have a greater color dynamic range than printed images. Thus, a scanned image from a slide will often be "clearer" than one from a photograph. Although many flatbed scanners have attachments or options for scanning slides and other transparent media, one can also purchase a scanner dedicated exclusively to slide scanning. These slide scanners tend to have superior resolution (5000 to 6000 ppi range) to typical flatbed scanners, which is needed given that the physical size of an optical slide is considerably smaller than a typical printed picture. However, a dedicated slide scanner does not have the versatility of a flatbed scanner. If superior computer resolution of slides is of paramount importance, however, a slide scanner may be an excellent solution, particularly if you have an extensive collection of archived clinical slides that need to be digitized. Many slide scanners will also provide the option for having a stack of slides scanned automatically, requiring significantly less attention during the process.

Additional Sources of Images

Digital cameras and digital video cameras are designed to capture digitized images, which then have the ability to be incorporated directly into one of a number of graphics programs for further manipulation. The advantage of this type of image is that there is no loss of quality going from one medium (i.e., photographic paper) to another (digital) inherent in scanning. A discussion of digital cameras is beyond the scope of this chapter, because they are advancing at a yearly pace, and high-end digital cameras are rapidly approaching the quality of even the best 35-mm single lens reflex (SLR) cameras. However, if one were considering beginning the digital conversion, a digital camera would be a good investment. Many professional photographic developers now offer to digitize photographic negatives in addition to providing traditional prints. For a small price, this saves you the time-consuming step of digitizing the negatives or prints yourself.

As with digital cameras, obtaining already digitized images greatly facilitates subsequent manipulations. Commercially available photo CDs are an excellent source of thousands of royalty-free, high-quality images, which you may use for your own designs. An additional source of images is the exponentially growing WWW. Virtually any image you come across while "surfing the net" can be copied and pasted into your favorite graphics program for further manipulation. However, one must be cognizant of proprietary material, and the author, designer, or publisher needs to be consulted before that image is used in a presentation or publication. Furthermore, images from the Internet are often of lower resolution to allow faster transmission and, hence, may be of insufficient quality for publications or other applications in which high-quality images are needed.

OBTAINING SUPERIOR SCANS

As a clinician, scanning images will probably be one of the most common methods used to get images from the "real" world onto your computer, such as from books or journals. Although most scanners are automated, enabling high-quality scans with the single click of a mouse button, there are a variety of techniques you can use to maximize quality and efficiency. These can be both time saving and can help optimize file sizes, which may make subsequent tasks infinitely easier. To convince yourself, compare the time it takes to alter the size of a 5-MB file vs. a 50-MB file in one of the commonly used graphics programs—the difference may run into minutes. Images that are digitized at too low a resolution, although generating a small file size, may look blurry or fuzzy. In contrast, too high a resolution may create a nearly identical equivalent of the original image but of a size so large that your computer may not be able to edit it (Figure 19-7). Thus, the trick is to optimize both image quality *and* file size.

When scanning artwork or images, it is important to keep in mind the ultimate use of that image. As a general rule, it is reasonable to scan an image at high resolution (e.g., 300 or 600 dpi for a printed image) and then reduce the resolution later as your needs become clear. It is always a good idea to archive the original high-resolution scan so that you can go back to it later if needed. Remember that the final planned size of the image is critical in deciding the resolution of the scan. For example, if you want a final printed image that will be 5 inches at 300 dpi, you will need to scan a 35-mm image at more than 1000 dpi to allow for the effect of magnification. For publications and printing on a laser printer capable of printing 300 dpi to 600 dpi, you will likely obtain good results with a

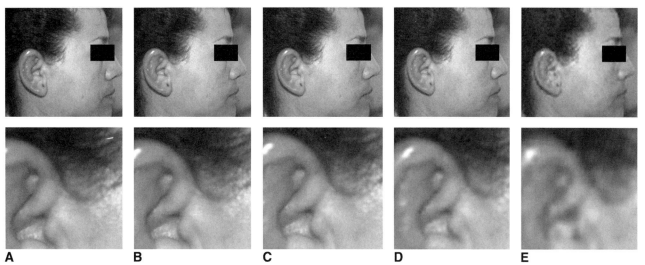

Figure 19-7. A comparison of image resolutions. The following image of a woman with auricular chondritis comes from scanning a color 35-mm slide on a standard flatbed scanner with a transparency adapter. Five different resolutions were used, including **A,** 1200 ppi, **B,** 600 ppi, **C,** 300 ppi, **D,** 150 ppi, **E,** 75 ppi. As can be seen, even a 75 ppi scan looks acceptable in the publication at the size shown on top. However, as the magnification increases (as shown below), differences become pronounced. A reasonable goal is to scan an image that will yield a spatial resolution of 300 dpi for the final desired size of the printed image.

final image with resolutions as low as 72 ppi to 150 ppi. If an on-screen digital projection is desired, one can get away with smaller scanning resolutions. For use of an image on a web site or the Internet, low-resolution scanning is perfectly adequate. Thus, experimenting and finding the appropriate medium between good resolution and reasonable size for a particular scanner is an important aspect of scanning.

As previously mentioned, the color resolution can take up a significant amount of an image's information. Thus, reducing or eliminating the "color" component of an image will significantly decrease a file's size. For equal size and resolution, a scanned gray-scale image will have a much smaller file size (8 bits) than a corresponding color one (12 or 24 bits). Nearly all color scanners give you the option of scanning at 1-bit depth for line art and text, 8-bit depth for gray-scale images, or 24-bit depth for true color images. One should scan with the option that creates the smallest file, while still picking up all the necessary information.

In addition, each scanner has a unique array of tools to manipulate the image before saving it to your computer. These options will vary with the model, make, and price of the scanner. Most medium-range scanners have a few similar options that should be used when possible. "Cropping" gives you the ability to scan only the portion of the image you want digitized, while also greatly decreasing its file size (and increasing the speed of the scan). Additional tools used to "clean" scans before saving the image to your computer include straightening and aligning the

image (e.g., if you loaded the original image at an angle) and adjusting brightness and contrast. Another important tool on most scanning software are filters that will remove the "pixilated" or printed look when scanning magazines, newspapers, and other printed matter (Figure 19-8). All these tools may be experimented with to increase the quality of your scanned image before manipulation within a graphics program. Even if your scanner does not have these tools, however, most advanced graphics programs have the ability to perform many of these tasks and more.

IMAGE MANIPULATION—ADOBE PHOTOSHOP

Many software packages are available to create and manipulate digital images. The standard for more than 10 years now has been Adobe Photoshop (Adobe Systems Inc, San Jose, Ca). Photoshop is an industrial-strength tool for virtually any purpose related to digital still images. It is impossible to cover the function or capacity of this program here, but some of its basic features are worth considering. For anyone interested in working with digital media, any effort spent learning the basics of this program will save considerable time and frustration in the future. It should be emphasized that neither the authors nor the publisher of the textbook (to the authors' knowledge) has a relationship, financial or otherwise, with Adobe Systems.

Image Acquisition and Navigation

Because Photoshop is a defacto standard for image manipulation, most flatbed scanners, slide scanners,

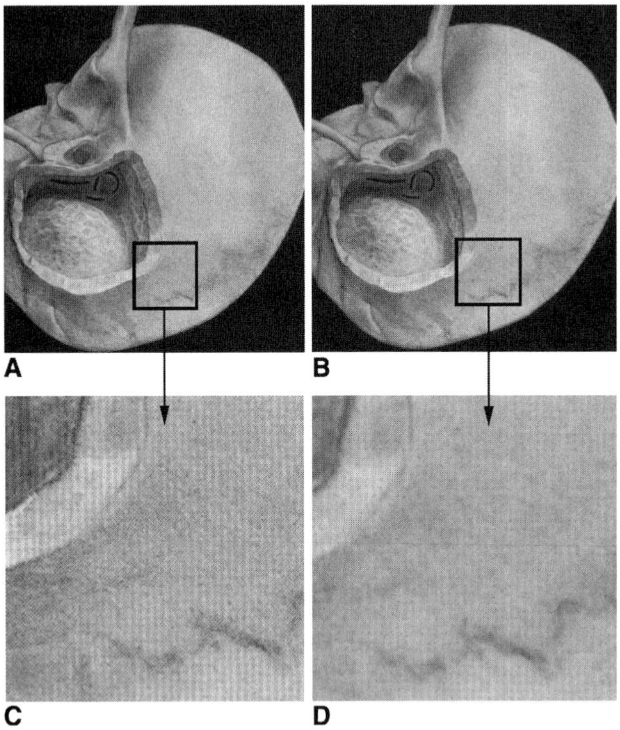

Figure 19-8. When scanning printed media, such as newspapers, books, or magazines, one will often see a repeating pattern in the digital image that was not seen in the original photograph. This is a by-product of the actual printing process. As a result, many scanners come with software that will eliminate this printed look, which uses a computer algorithm to "blur" the repeating pattern away. This figure is scanned directly from Whiting's *The Modern Mastoid Operation* (Philadelphia, P. Blakiston's Son & Co, 1905). **A,** In the original scan along the mastoid cortex, the repeating pattern of the print can be seen, particularly in **C,** the enlarged portion below. After applying the filter, the pattern largely disappears **B, D,** without noticeable loss of image quality.

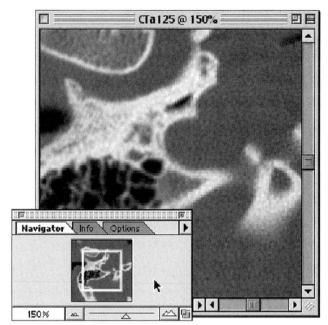

Figure 19-9. Photoshop navigation window with magnification. Within the program, an image may be displayed at various levels of magnification. The ability to efficiently navigate around an image is essential to use Photoshop effectively.

and digital cameras on the market will provide a means to easily load acquired images into the program. In addition, almost all digital images found on the Internet are in a format that can be read directly by Photoshop.

Once opened, an image is displayed in a window. The user can then change the magnification of the displayed image and focus specifically on an area of interest. Several navigation tools and a dedicated navigation window facilitate this process (Figure 19-9). In presenting the degree of magnification, Photoshop defines "100%" to be when one pixel of the image corresponds to one pixel on the computer display. Note that the standard computer display has 72 dots or ppi.

Resizing an Image

The ability to adjust the size and spatial resolution of an image is another basic function of Photoshop. Even if all you are doing is scanning images and printing

them or importing them into a computer presentation, this will be an invaluable tool with which to become familiar. Under the menu item "Image Size" from the menu, "Image" will open the window (Figure 19-10). This will allow an image to be resized to optimize its spatial resolution. Being familiar with this will prevent your files from becoming too unwieldy for storage and presentations.

Often after acquiring an image, there is extra space at the edges that may be blank or may contain extraneous information. Resizing such an image as described previously will not eliminate this, because the entire image will be resized. Photoshop provides a "Crop tool" with which a rectangle is drawn around the area of interest, and the periphery of the image is eliminated. This is another easy way to reduce the file size and eliminate distracting visual information.

Color and Tone Adjustment

Photoshop excels at providing complete control over brightness, contrast, and color correction. Most of the subtleties of these functions are beyond the needs of most users. However, a simple understanding of the tools will allow otherwise unusable scanned images to be corrected with minimal effort (Figure 19-11).

Layers

One of the most useful features of Photoshop is its ability to add successive "layers" of information to an image. These layers are analogous to acetate sheets

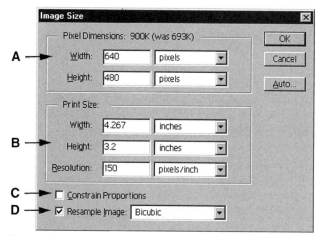

Figure 19-10. Image resizing. The image size window will allow the spatial resolution of an image to be modified. **A,** The numbers represent the total number of pixels in the image in both width and height. **B,** The numbers represent the size that the image will appear when printed on paper. These only need to be altered if the image is to be printed from Photoshop. **C,** By checking "Constrain Proportions" the ratio of height to width is fixed, preventing distortion of the image by stretching or compressing. **D,** By checking "Resample Image" the total number of pixels in **A** can be altered. If unchecked, the total number of pixels, and therefore image file size, remains fixed.

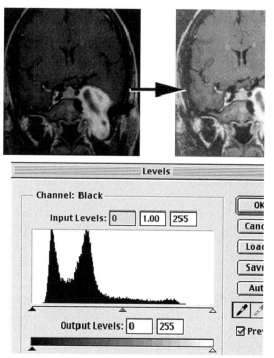

Figure 19-11. Cleaning scanned images in Photoshop. Contrast and brightness can be fine tuned with Photoshop's "Adjust levels" command. The histogram shows the frequency of pixels of a given brightness from black to white. The small triangles below the histogram can be moved to interactively change the bright, dark, and mid-tones. This is a useful way of adjusting scans that are either too dark or light to show the necessary details.

used in traditional illustration. Each sheet can contain drawing or type elements and can be individually added or subtracted without changing any information contained on the other layers. An understanding of how to add and manipulate layers will provide tremendous flexibility in experimenting with an image. For example, a label with text and arrows can be placed over an underlying image (Figure 19-12). Each element may be moved or changed independently without fear of changing the original image.

Once completed, the image can be "flattened" by pushing all the layers together into one and saving the resulting image as a smaller file, ready to be incorporated into a presentation, paper, or sent to a publisher. When working with layers, it is usually a good idea to save one version with all the layers intact ("unflattened") to allow further modifications in the future.

Selections

"Selections" are another key feature of digital image manipulation. With these, one can limit any manipulation to a specific area of the image. It is analogous to selecting a passage of text in a word processing program, only it is a group of pixels rather than characters that is being selected. A number of tools in Photoshop can help produce and modify the selection to fit almost any specific needs. The selected pixels can then, for

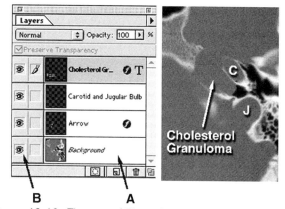

Figure 19-12. The use of Photoshop's *Layers* to label a CT scan. The layers used to form the composite image (*right*) are shown in the "Layers Palate" (*left*). **A,** Each layer contains an independent element of the final image (text, arrow, background) and can be moved, changed, or deleted without affecting the other layers. **B,** Each layer can either be hidden or viewed by clicking its associated "eye" icon.

example, be copied and pasted, modified in their contrast and brightness, deleted, or moved. Any drawing tools will only have an effect within the selection. This allows specific treatment of an area of the image without affecting the areas outside of the selection.

Adding Material to an Image

Photoshop has a complete set of tools for adding to or modifying image information. A number of painting tools are included to allow the addition of freehand shapes and lines (Figure 19-13). Each tool can be modified extensively to provide the desired effect. A line tool for adding straight lines and arrows and an eraser are also available. A "rubber stamp" tool can be used to copy one part of an image to another—a very handy feature in photo retouching, although it takes some practice to use efficiently.

Experimentation while changing an image can be hindered by the fear of creating irreparable changes. To help with this, Photoshop provides a "History" palate that records every action taken in working with an image. New users should become familiar with this early, because it allows one to go back to any previous step taken and restore the file to its previous state. The comfort that this "multiple-undo" function provides can significantly ease fears of losing previous efforts. Nonetheless, making occasional copies and backups of important files before effecting changes can save considerable frustration.

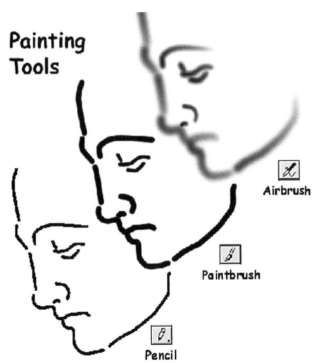

Figure 19-13. Freehand tools. A number of digital painting tools are available within Photoshop. Each tool can be modified so that a particular look can be achieved.

COMPUTER PRESENTATIONS

Once you have taken the time and energy to create your own images, the next step is getting those images into a program that will allow you to present the image in a slide presentation program. At present, the conventional standard is Microsoft's PowerPoint, although other programs also exist, each with certain advantageous features. Within PowerPoint, text is easy to work with, it is clear, and one can easily go back at a later date and change slide text, captions, or backgrounds (particularly if one has changed jobs but their slide backgrounds have not!).

To get an image into one of the presentation programs, you have two options. Either copy and paste the image directly from your favorite graphics program into the slide presentation program or save your graphics image as a file recognized by the program (e.g., TIFF, JPEG, see later for a discussion of these file types) then import the image from within the program (please consult the program manual for further instructions). Once you are within the presentation software, your image can then be resized to fit the shape of the screen, and text, arrows, and captions can be easily added directly over your image.

Equipment is now readily available to allow presentations directly from a laptop computer, eliminating the need for 35-mm slides almost entirely. This has its distinct benefits but also its limitations. A computer is much more likely to stop working than a slide carousel, and there are rarely any "compatibility" problems with 35-mm slides among various slide projectors.

Despite software and hardware advances that have made computer presentations relatively straightforward, a few precautions may help avert presentation disaster when moving to computer-projection format. First, be sure to keep your imported digital files as small as possible. The use of images that are too big can slow the time it takes to move from one slide to the next or, worse, can cause a laptop to stop functioning altogether. This is one of the many reasons that this chapter has focused so heavily on finding the appropriate median between image quality and file size. Second, make sure you store and rehearse your presentation on the computer that will be used for the presentation. It may work fine on your desktop machine but may fail on your laptop. Also, take your own computer for the presentation. You cannot be sure there will not be some conflict if relying on someone else's machine, particularly if you have complicated graphics or embedded video. Computer projection displays have improved in quality dramatically over the past several years and are standard in their attachments to laptops. Leave yourself enough time to hook up your machine, have it running, and in order by the time you are due to present. Of course, for critical material, carrying a backup of reliable, old-fashioned 35-mm slides may allow you to breathe easier. Having backup slides is always a good idea, particularly when just beginning to "go digital," when one might anticipate a computer compatibility problem, or when you are scheduled to deliver an extremely important presentation.

Take care to avoid pitfalls in computer-based presentations. Just because you can do something does not mean it will add to your presentation. Too many colors, animated transitions, flying type, and clipart will detract from your underlying message. Try to keep the material simple and use special effects *only* to highlight specific points that lend themselves to this type of treatment.

COMMON DIGITAL IMAGE FILE FORMATS AND COMPRESSION SCHEMES

A recurrent theme of this chapter has been the many methods and tricks used to *maximize* image quality while *minimizing* file size. This is a topic that is central in multimedia design and has been the impetus for the development of a variety of ways to *compress* file size for storage, transportation, and compatibility among the myriad computer systems in use. Through standardized algorithms, a computer can "code" an image so that it takes significantly less space to store the information. For example, consider an image of a black rectangle on a white background. If the resolution for this image is 640 × 480, there are more than 300,000 pixels that need to be stored to hold the information to recreate that image. However, if the computer has a way of remembering that the background is white, where the four corners of the rectangle are,

and that the rectangle is black, you could imagine the identical image could be recreated from only a few dozen bytes of information. This is the idea behind image compression, and it can be very helpful in managing digital media.

Image compression does not come without a price. Compression schemes may not store all of the information from the original uncompressed data, resulting in some loss of fidelity. These types of file formats are termed "lossy" compression formats. In contrast, "lossless" file formats compress file types without losing any fidelity. As can be expected, lossy formats generally achieve a higher degree of compression than lossless ones, at the expense of file size.

Fortunately, nearly every graphics program gives the user the option of one of a number of formats in which to save a file. The four most common graphic file formats in general use today, are TIFF, JPEG, GIF, and PNG. Each of these file formats has several distinct features. Which file type chosen for each image should ultimately depend on the intended use of the digitized file. The following discussion will focus on only the most commonly used formats. A direct comparison of these file formats is shown (Tables 19-1 and 19-2).

GIF

The GIF (graphic interchange format) format was originally developed by CompuServe in 1987 and later modified to include such features as transparency and animation. This compact file format is ideal for graphics that use only a few colors and remains a popular format for online photographs. GIF images are limited to 256 colors and can be reasonably compressed.[3] However, the GIF format has recently lost popularity

TABLE 19-1

A COMPARISON OF FILE FORMATS

Desired properties	TIFF	PNG	JPEG	JPEG	BMP	PCX	PICT	GIF
	(LOW COMPRESSION)			(HIGH COMPRESSION)				
Master archive file	++	++	+	0	+	+	+	0
Photographs	++	++	++	++	++	++	++	+
Line drawings	++	++	+	0	+	+	++	+
Files containing text	++	++	+	0	+	+	+	+
Greatest compression	0	+	+	++	0	+	0	++
Maximum compatibility	++	++	+	+	0	0	0	+
Lossy	0	0	++	++	0	0	0	++
Lossless	++	++	0	0	++	++	++	0
Internet/WWW	+	+	++	++	0	0	0	++

"++" = A highly desirable digital file format for the property listed. "+" = An acceptable choice for the listed property. "0" = This file type is the least desirable for the property listed. *Lossy* files lose data each time the file is saved, though this difference may not be noticeable. *Lossless* files maintain the integrity of the file during saving and archiving.

TABLE 19-2

REPRESENTATIVE COMPRESSION SCHEMES

File type	Original	TIFF	TIFF (+LZW)	PNG	PNG (75%)	JPG at 100% (high quality)	JPG at 75% (medium quality)	JPG at 25% (low quality)	BMP	PCX	GIF
File size (KB)	10,900	10,800	247	64	44	252	27	16	10,800	352	5

Adapted from Fulton W: *http://www.scantips.com/.*
A digital image with dimensions 7 in × 6 in (2100 × 1800 pixels) with 300-dpi resolution was saved in several file formats to compare ultimate file size. All compressions were performed in Adobe Photoshop 5.5. A comparison of file sizes shows the large discrepancy between compression schemes.

to JPEG, because JPEG files can contain up to 24-bit color and, as a result, handle photographs with truer color fidelity.

JPEG

JPEG stands for the "Joint Photographic Experts Group," experts that have been nominated by national standards bodies and industry representatives to work to produce standards for continuous-tone image coding. JPEG was designed for maximum compression of full-color or gray-scale photographs, artwork, and similar "real-world" images. Because of the method it uses to compress images, JPEG works less well for text and lettering, simple cartoons, and line drawings. JPEG is "lossy," meaning that during compression, a computer algorithm may lose some of the data embedded in the picture. However, because JPEG is designed to exploit known limitations of the human eye, taking advantage of the fact that small color changes are perceived less accurately than small changes in brightness, this is difficult to notice in many compressed files.

A useful property of JPEG is that the user can select the amount of compression desired. In other words, the user can decide on the ratio of the file size against output image quality in the compressed image. Thus, extremely small files can be created if one does not mind poor quality (for example, to post on a web page). Alternately, minimal compression can be selected, maintaining maximum image quality, although ending up with a larger file size (although still compressed, and still lossy). Because of the increasing prevalence of more powerful computers, JPEG is increasingly being used over GIF images, despite the fact that the image sizes are slightly larger. Because JPEG uses a lossy compression, *every time* the file is saved, a little more quality is lost. Therefore, most graphics artists do not recommend JPEG as an appropriate format for archiving or storing a master copy of an important image.

When creating a JPEG file in digital image manipulation software, one must select to save the image as a JPEG (or JPG) file. During the saving process, the user will be queried on the *quality* of the image to be saved or the *compression* level desired, depending on the specific program being used. The higher the quality level selected, the smaller the compression that will take place and vice versa. A good balance between size and image quality can typically be achieved with JPEG compressions in the 75% to 80% range. The user is strongly encouraged to experiment with different compression ratios, then examine the compressed image under high magnification to determine which is best for his purposes. In particular, one should pay special attention to sharply contrasted edges, such as with text letters and graphic art, because this is where JPEG compression has the most difficult time.[3]

PICT

PICT is the native graphics format used by the Macintosh Operating System (Apple Computers Inc, Cupertino, Ca). PICT is used in page layout and graphics programs and is lossless (no loss of data with compression). Because PICT is not readily suitable for exchange with Windows programs, one of its chief disadvantages in our Windows-dominated world, the authors use PICT files infrequently, despite the fact that both authors use Macintosh computers regularly.

TIFF

Tagged image file format (TIFF) files are one of the most popular and flexible of the current public domain file formats. It is the most universal format, and nearly every program on any computer will be able to read it. Because TIFF was designed by developers of printers, scanners, and monitors, it tends to integrate with these peripherals very well. Furthermore, because TIFF is lossless and loses no data with compression, it is ideal for archiving and storing master copies of images. However, as can be expected, file sizes with TIFF images are larger than comparable JPEG files, albeit with better quality images. TIFF can also incorporate additional compression (termed "LZW" compression) if desired.

PNG

Portable network graphics (PNG files, pronounced "ping"), is a newer file format that was originally intended to be the replacement for the GIF standard because of GIF's color limitations and some other patent problems. PNG supports up to 48-bit color and has reportedly excellent lossless compression. PNG compresses files by use of methods similar to the windows compression program PKZIP and also incorporates special preprocessing filters that improve its compression efficiency. These features reportedly allow PNG to achieve better compression than a comparable TIFF file by approximately 30%.[3] Most graphics applications can read the PNG format, so compatibility is currently not an issue.

BMP

BMP (Windows bit map) is another lossless compression scheme like TIFF and PNG. BMP will handle 24-bit images, but these images cannot be compressed by use of a BMP format, one of its chief limitations. BMP can compress 8-bit images but tends to be less effective with photographic images. BMP files are generally not used outside of Windows-based systems, and thus compatibility is a potential limitation of this file type.

PCX

The PCX (Windows PaintBrush) format is mentioned, because many Windows-based systems use this format. PCX is lossless like BMP, TIFF, and PNG. Like BMP images, the PCX format is generally not used except in the Windows operating system, raising potential compatibility difficulties, particularly for those who also use Macintosh computers. Furthermore, the amount of compression that the PCX format generates is limited.

CONNECTIVITY: SCSI, USB, AND FIREWIRE

The recurrent theme of computer speed throughout this chapter brings up an often overlooked aspect of the way computers "talk" to their peripheral devices such as external hard drives, scanners, or digital cameras. Depending on the type of connection a peripheral has with the main computer, download/upload speeds may be dramatically different. Furthermore, connectivity problems are a significant source of computer malfunction. It is hoped that the following brief review will clarify some of the central issues in computer connectivity.

SCSI Connections

Macintosh computers have traditionally attached their peripherals to the computer using a SCSI (Small Computer System Interface, pronounced "scuzzi") port. With this system, one can connect several peripherals in a "chain." This makes adding devices to your computer easy; you merely add to the chain. SCSI was standard in most Macintosh computers and more recent Windows machines. In contrast, the PC world uses special connections for hard drives (IDE, EIDE, ESDI), but they are not typically used for connecting peripheral devices such as scanners to the computer.

Initially, there was a single type of SCSI connection; there are now several SCSI standards. The original configuration was able to manage seven peripherals, each with its own unique identification number ("ID," numbered 0 through 6, with 7 reserved for the SCSI control board itself). The newer "wide" SCSI bus can handle 15 peripherals. Because these SCSI systems can be significantly faster than the standard connections found in many Windows-based machines, many PCs have been moving toward SCSI-type connectivity.

However, there are potential problems with SCSI connections. First, each SCSI device has to have its own unique SCSI identification number assigned; giving two peripherals the same SCSI identification number may crash the computer. Second, the last device on the SCSI chain must be "terminated." This is done by either flipping a "terminate" switch on the last device, if it has one, or by connecting a special "terminator" plug to the last device. Third, the chain cannot be longer than 6 m (19.69 feet), according to the SCSI specifications. Although that may seem like plenty of distance, if one has several peripheral devices, such as a scanner, removable disk drive, and external hard drive, the distance suddenly is not so long. Finally, one cannot add or remove SCSI devices without turning off the computer. Additional information on SCSI connectivity can be found on the official SCSI web site: *http://www.paralan.com/glos.html.*

Universal Serial Bus

Universal Serial Bus (USB) is the latest answer to the difficulties encountered by SCSI connections, as described previously, and is becoming standard in nearly all newer computers (Macintosh and Windows-based PCs). Foremost, USB connections allow the user to easily add external peripherals to the computer by simply plugging in the small, rectangular shaped connector into a USB port. USB can also support up to 127 devices by means of hubs or daisy chaining (plugging one device into another) at speeds of up to 12 MB per second, which is 10 times faster than traditional ports, although still somewhat slower than SCSI connections. One can also insert and remove USB devices while the computer is running (the so-called "plug-and-play" or "hot-swappable" feature). Virtually all peripheral computer devices sold today have optional USB connections, including mice, joysticks, keyboards, scanners, and digital video cameras.

FireWire

FireWire is a newer type of connectivity that was developed by Apple computer. It is also known as IEE1394 or i.Link on other platforms. It allows much higher speed data transfer than SCSI and USB. Like USB, it is "hot swappable," meaning one can simply plug in a FireWire device (such as a digital video camera, hard drive, Zip drive, scanner) while a computer is running and not have to shutdown and reboot the computer to access the device. Like USB, multiple FireWire devices (≤63) can be connected together in a chain, and there are no SCSI limitations or device IDs.

FireWire has become a favorite of the digital graphics and video crowd, primarily because of the very high rates of data transmission it allows, along with ability to incorporate many peripheral devices. Many new computers are able to accept FireWire devices. Older Macintosh computers (desktops and portable) and PC machines can easily be upgraded to accept FireWire devices with either a PCI card (Peripheral Component Interconnect, a local bus standard developed by Intel Corporation, standard on most desktop computers) or PCMCIA card (Personal Computer Memory Card International Association, now standard on most laptop computers). If one is considering digital video, we would strongly recommend looking further into FireWire technology, because most new devices will use this. For more information on FireWire technology, the reader is referred to Apple's web site: *www.apple.com/firewire*.

DIGITAL VIDEO—WHAT THE AMATEUR SHOULD KNOW

By now, most otolaryngologists have been to a meeting and have seen the advantages of a digitized video being seamlessly integrated into a digital slide presentation. Some may be further tempted to incorporate video into their own presentations. However, before considering taking this step, one should be warned: it can be time consuming, expensive, and complicated. However, there is no doubt that the ability to incorporate video into a presentation can take one's lectures to the next level, without worrying about switching back and forth between a videocassette player and a slide presentation. This is a wonderful example of how digital multimedia can be fully taken advantage of by the clinician.

Video and animations are a sequence of still images. When presented quickly enough, the human eye perceives these images to be in smooth motion through a phenomenon known as "persistence of vision." Therefore, the same consideration of spatial and color resolution apply to video as they do to still images. In addition, there is the significant consideration of "temporal resolution," or how many images are presented in a given time. In standard video format, the image size is best represented as a 720×486 grid with 24-bit color presented at 30 frames per second. Then, one also needs to consider the addition of synchronized sound to this. It is not surprising that computer resources are used quite rapidly in trying to capture and display this type of data. Fortunately, all these factors can be compressed, similar to methods used for still images, making the job potentially more manageable.

To begin with, one needs to understand some of the video formats that exist. The video source can be either a live video camera or video tape (analog or digital). *Composite* video gets its name from the fact that it delivers the *luminance* (Y) factor of a video image and the *chrominance* (C) factor as a "composite" of the two. Typically, the output from a standard VHS player (like the one in your home) will be a composite (or YC) signal. In contrast, *S-video* (S = separate) delivers video by separating the luminance from the chrominance, which achieves a higher resolution. *RGB* (Red Green Blue) delivers video in terms of a mix of the red, green, and blue portions of the visible light spectrum (see discussion earlier of color theory). Of the video formats, RGB video gives the best quality.[4]

Video formats are now divided into the older *analog* standards, which save the information as waveforms, and the newer *digital video* (DV) standards (by analogy, music records are analog, whereas music CDs are digital). Several common analog formats of video exist. The Beta format, developed by Sony, is still the most commonly used broadcast standard because of the excellent quality it delivers. Hi-8, also developed by Sony, is a smaller format that offers improved quality. Several Hi-8 video cameras are on the market. However, Hi-8 has largely been eclipsed by DV formats. S-VHS, commonly used in the past for educational and industrial use, is another good-quality format. Last, the VHS format is perhaps most known to the amateur, because it is used by almost all home video players. VHS has intermediate quality but is not recommended as a source for compressed digital video.

Video Capture

Capturing video can be one of the most challenging aspects of working with video, primarily because of the huge amount of data that needs to be processed.

For example, if you want to capture uncompressed video at 640 × 480 screen size (a typical size) in true 24-bit color (see bit discussion), you will be loading approximately 23 MB per second, or 1.5 GB per minute, onto your hard drive! It does not take long to realize that this amount of data will quickly use up even the largest hard drives in very little time. As a result of this huge data stream, most video capture techniques compress the video as it arrives in your desktop computer (this is usually taken care of by the video capture board).

Therefore, to capture from an analog or DV video source, one will need a capture card and a very large (at least 40 GB) hard drive capable of a high (at least 3 MB/s) sustained data rate. If it is not obvious by now, the discussion of maximizing computer speed and memory storage at the beginning of this chapter takes on critical importance during these steps. In addition, one often would like to see the video as it is being downloaded onto the computer. Because most standard video capture cards will not enable this, one may also need an additional overlay card or an external monitor if the card does not allow viewing the source while you are capturing. As this discussion is alluding to, "getting into video" can be an expensive proposition.

When considering what type of video card to get, there are several features one should be examining. One key feature is compression ratios; a lower compression ratio should be sought (e.g., 3:1), because these generally provide better quality video. One should also check whether the card will capture at a full screen size or a reduced size. In addition, one should find out whether the video card also captures sound or whether a separate sound card will be required. Cards use proprietary compression algorithms so capture quality does vary between cards. Most cards will accept YC or S-video input, whereas higher end cards will accept the higher quality RGB (such as the output from a three chip camera, where the red, green, and blue video outputs are separate). Another unfortunate feature of most capture boards is that they use their own proprietary programming code. This means that you need to have a similar board installed in any computer on which you want to play back the captured, uncompressed video.[4]

Most analog boards compress video by use of M-JPEG (also known as MPEG), which effectively produces a video stream composed of a number of still JPEG compressed images. Compression can range from 3:1 to 200:1. These compression ratios take a potentially huge video file and make it manageable. However, as with digital pictures, a higher compression ratio will degrade the quality of the video sequence.

As a general principle, to get the highest quality video always capture at the highest rate that your hardware will support. Of course, this means that you will need a very fast and large hard drive, together with a suitably fast SCSI, USB, or FireWire connection. A slow hard drive may "drop" or skip incoming video images, giving a punctuated or skipped video look.[4]

Video Editing

Once video has been captured, video editing takes over. Like manipulation of images within computer graphics software, video-editing software can be time consuming but immensely enjoyable once the learning curve has been surmounted. Fortunately, there are several software packages available to allow the amateur to edit on the computer. A discussion of their attributes is beyond the scope of this chapter, of course, and the reader is encouraged to visit corporate or independent web sites or a local computer supplier.

Once a video is produced, importing it into one of the commercially available slide presentation software programs is as easy as importing digital images. However, in contrast to digital images that are embedded in the slide file itself (and hence can "travel" with the file), only the *location* of a video image is incorporated into a slide; the actual video must be on the same computer as the slide file, so the software can find the video. Thus, when copying or transferring a digital slide presentation with embedded video, one must be sure to also copy all relevant video files.

CONCLUSIONS

The new millennium has presented vast new possibilities for multimedia creation. What was unthinkable for all but the most sophisticated supercomputers 20 years ago is now readily accomplished on most household PCs. Advancements in both computer hardware and software design will increasingly enable clinicians, even those with only rudimentary computer skills, to create fantastic documents, videos, and multimedia presentations. All it takes is the desire to make the "digital leap." It is hoped that the suggestions, tips, and recommendations offered in this chapter will provide the motivation to those sitting on the bench, waiting to enter the digital multimedia world. After all, it is those of us in the audience, on the wards, or in the examination room that will ultimately benefit from your efforts.

REFERENCES

1. Bunzel MJ: *Multimedia applications development*, ed 2, New York, McGraw-Hill, 1994.
2. Fetterman RL, Gupta SK: *Mainstream multimedia*, New York, Van Nostrand Reinhold, 1993.

3. Fulton W: *http://www.scantips.com/*.

4. Hypertech Multimedia: *http://www.hypertech.co.uk/*.

5. Markoff J: Researchers make an ultra-tiny chip, *New York Times* June 10, 2001, p 30.

6. Mitchell WJ: *The reconfigured eye: Visual truth in the post-photographic era*, Cambridge, Massachusetts, The MIT Press, 1992.

7. Tufte ER: *Envisioning information*, Cheshire, Connecticut, Graphics Press, 1990.

8. Tufte ER: *The visual display of quantitative information*, Chesire, Connecticut, Graphics Press, 1990.

9. Tufte ER: *Visual explanations*, Cheshire, Connecticut, Graphics Press, 1997.

CHAPTER TWENTY

MEDICAL INFORMATICS AND TELEMEDICINE

|| David Goldenberg
Marion Couch

INTRODUCTION

"If physiology literally means 'the logic of life,' and pathology is 'the logic of disease,' then medical informatics is the logic of healthcare."[14]

Medical informatics is a dynamic field involved with using technology and information systems to promote improved organization, management, financial analysis, security, and use of information in health care. And there are multiple levels of information systems in health care:

- Individual level: patient care decisions, physician practices, etc.
- Institutional level: institutional databases, hospital services, hospital records, etc.
- Social level: organization, finance, global management, etc.[20]

Medical informatics applies information technology to all aspects of medicine—medical research, medical education, and patient care. Broadly speaking, medical informatics has helped to develop global online communities of physicians and patients by encouraging the sharing and use of information to deliver health care and promote health. Physician-oriented Web portals tend to facilitate professional collaboration and enhance physician expertise, with the goal of raising the level of patient care. Challenging issues in medicine, such as improving patient care and safety, training physicians, and certifying physician competency, are being addressed with information technology systems. For instance, the development of common technology standards to allow the exchange of information among electronic health records, pharmacies, clinical laboratories, and medical devices can potentially result in reduced errors, saving patients' lives. The U.S. Departments of Health and Human Services, Defense, and Veterans Affairs have all endorsed the use of common standards in an effort to link vital databases together. But what comprises medical data?

MEDICAL DATA

Medical datum is defined as any single observation of a patient. A single medical datum can be defined by any of the following four elements:

- The patient (e.g., Mr. Smith).
- The parameter being observed (e.g., hemoglobin values).
- The parameter value (e.g., temperature of 100°C; profession is opera singer).
- The time of observation (e.g., 1:45 AM on 18 May 2004).

Much of health care activity actually involves the gathering, analysis, or use of this data. It has been estimated that 38% of a physician's time and 50% of a nurse's time is spent recording data in medical charts.[36] Not only the data itself, but also the circumstances under which it was obtained, are crucial to its interpretation. In other words, observation, even by the most skilled physician, cannot be accepted with absolute certainty. This leads to the issue of *uncertainty in the values of medical data*.

TYPES OF MEDICAL DATA

There is a broad range of medical data used in the practice of health care.[51] Narrative data, a large component of health care information, includes a patient's description of present symptoms and his or her responses to the physician's questions. This form of data may be handwritten by the physician in the patient's medical record, dictated, or entered directly into an electronic patient record (EPR). Often this form of data is written in cryptic shorthand and jargon known only to health care workers (e.g., "UPPP" in place of "uvulopharyngopalatoplasty").

Much of the data used in medicine takes on numeric values. This includes parameters such as vital signs and laboratory test values. The interpretation of certain numeric data, however, raises the issue of precision (i.e., how accurate is the physician's measurement of the progress of a rash?).

Data in the form of signals or tracings are very important.[51] Some of these signals are continuous, whereas others are static. The most well-known example of a contiguous signal would be an electrocardiogram. Static signal tracings include an audiogram or tympanometry.

Visual images are also a crucial type of medical data. This form of data is used because it is more precise and easier to convey to others than a textual description. Important examples of machine-generated visual data are radiologic images, digital images, and videos. These are being used by an increasing number of surgeons either for medical education or for documentation.

COMMON SET OF HEALTH CARE TECHNOLOGY STANDARDS

Documented agreements containing technical specifications that are used consistently as rules or guidelines facilitate the sharing of data between organizations and their data banks. Why is this important in medical informatics? Using the example of health education, it is clear that many shareholders in health care are involved: physician educators, publishers of content, government, health care technology vendors, learning technology vendors, industry, medical associations. Without the ability to leverage technology and share information, the complex effort of educating health care professionals will be unduly expensive and redundant. Therefore, standards for health education may include specifications for:

- Professional (health care worker or physician) profiles.
- Educational modules.
- Reporting educational/certification activities.
- Publishing content.
- Electronic medical curricula.
- Search mechanisms.
- Journal articles.

So, *standards* can be defined as a set of rules and definitions that specify how to carry out a process to make the process work more efficiently.[51] They are necessary when the potential for excess diversity impedes effectiveness. In health care, another reason for the need of standards is so that individuals, providers, and health plans can be recognized across systems. Advocates of clinical standards believe that a single format for building medical records and transmitting health care data would allow for sharing of information, especially when combating threats to public health. In informatics, standards are often developed by organizations that require a standard to carry out their principle function or by coalitions formed specifically to develop particular standards (Box 20-1).

EXCHANGING DATA/PATIENT INFORMATION
The Patient Record

Paper medical records (patient chart or medical record) are familiar to all users, but there are limitations involved with this method. It has been estimated

---

BOX 20-1

STANDARDS ORGANIZATIONS IN HEALTH CARE

Advanced Distributed Learning (ADL): An initiative funded by the U.S. Department of Defense to research and improve efficacy of online learning. Unifies best solutions by standards groups. A software model called Sharable Content Object Reference Model (SCORM) allows content to be shared across systems.

National Council on Prescription Drug Programs Script (NCPDP): An HIPAA-approved format for sending prescription information between prescribers and pharmacies.

International Organization for Standardization (ISO): A network of national standards institutes from 145 countries. Its goal is to promote the international exchange of services and information.

Institute of Electrical and Electronics Engineers (IEEE): Sets standards to allow medical devices (e.g., ventilators, monitors) to transmit data to information systems.

Logical Observation Identifier Name Codes (LOINC): A standardized format for laboratory data that allows for the exchange of test results.

Health Level 7 (HL7): The goal of HL7 is to provide a standard for the exchange of medical data among hospital computer applications such as scheduling, order entry, and documentation of patient care. HL7 is a protocol that is used to allow medical computers from different vendors to communicate with each other.

Digital Imaging and Communications in Medicine (DICOM): DICOM is an application layer network protocol for the transmission of medical images, waveforms, and ancillary information. It is controlled by the DICOM Standards Committee and is a format for retrieving information from medical imaging equipment to transfer it to physician computers or to storage systems.

Connecting for Health: Coalition of 90 or so health care organizations supporting the widespread adoption of clinical standards.

that 10% of information traditionally found in the paper record cannot be located, and 11% of laboratory tests are duplicated because the original data cannot be found.[36] Unlike loose sheets of paper, the digital information in an EPR is captured in a structured format that allows for greater accessibility and understanding of health conditions and medications. The EPR (also referred to as an *electronic medical record* [EMR]) is an electronically maintained repository of information regarding a person's lifetime health care, stored so that it is available to multiple legitimate users of the record. An EPR system adds information management tools to provide reminders and alerts, knowledge source linkages, specialized medical decision support, and analysis of aggregated data. This system provides not only safe storage for a patient's records but also computer-enhanced tools to help organize, interpret, and react to the medical data stored within; therefore, an EPR is not simply an electronic version of the paper medical record. It should be flexible and adaptable. Integrated access to all patients' data is one of the primary purposes of the EPR. The growing amount of data per patient from different sources (e.g., laboratories, imaging facilities, pharmacy outlets) make this task increasingly more complex.

Some fundamental EPR issues include clinical decision support, clinical order entry, and knowledge resources. Decision support systems may be an added adjunct to the EPR to indicate the best or most cost-effective options for further investigation and management, or to provide specific knowledge from the medical literature. These systems have a lot to offer in quality assurance and cost containment.

The online entry of orders for medications, tests, and procedures in a medical center or health care information system is known as *order entry*. Since one of the goals of any EPR is to assist clinicians in making decisions, the system should present relevant information at the time of order entry. Many queries of knowledge resources are conducted in the context of a specific patient, so the most effective time to provide access to knowledge resources is at the time a decision or order is being contemplated[15] (Figure 20-1). The EPR linked to knowledge resources can help a clinician decide whether a referral is appropriate and which tests are necessary to expedite the consultation process.[56] It may be possible to link continuing medical education to EPRs in a way that offers just-in-time learning with accreditation awarded to the physician or health care professional (Figure 20-2). Other fundamental issues for the EPR system are data entry and capture, error prevention, data display, query and surveillance systems, research, and administration.[56]

Evidence-Based Information at the Point of Care

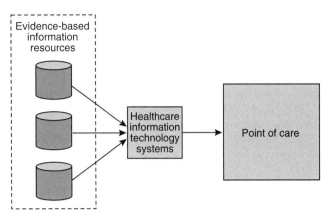

Figure 20-1. The electronic medical record can be used to effectively access evidence-based information at the point of care. Adapted from MedBiquitous.

EPR Challenges

The EPR must be able to work within the larger health care information system, and its database cannot demand to be a central repository. Unfortunately, many existing EPR systems are set up as if they are the master database, ignoring other expensive and proven systems for laboratories, registration, and billing. A good EPR system should assemble information from other systems and present it in an intuitive and consistent format, acting as a universal type interface for medical data in the form of images and text.[35]

HIPAA Regulations

The most important of all of the external forces pushing for the adaptation of EPR systems is the Health Insurance Portability and Accountability Act of 1996 (HIPAA).[36] HIPAA security rules were issued by the U.S. Department of Health and Human Services and published in the Federal Register on February 20, 2003. These rules became effective for enforcement on April 15, 2003. This act was the result of efforts by the Clinton administration and Congressional health care reform proponents to reform health care by streamlining industry inefficiencies, reducing paperwork, improving detection and prosecution of fraud and abuse, and enabling workers of all professions to change jobs, even if they (or family members) had preexisting medical conditions. These regulations have been planned to encompass electronically transmitted information, regardless of format. EPR systems are actually necessary to comply efficiently with the confidentiality and billing issues addressed by these regulations[35] (Box 20-2).

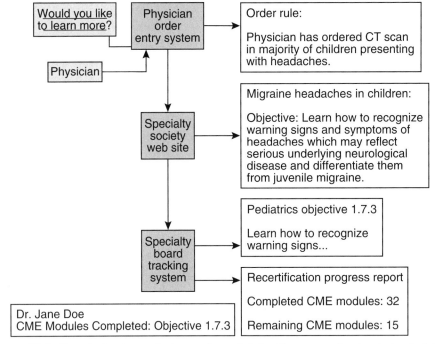

Figure 20-2. The electronic medical record can link health care professionals to decision-making information tools and opportunities for continuing medical education accreditation. Adapted from MedBiquitous.

BOX 20-2

FOUR PRIMARY OBJECTIVES OF HIPAA LEGISLATION

1. To ensure health insurance portability by eliminating job-lock due to preexisting medical conditions
2. To reduce health care fraud and abuse
3. To enforce standards for health information
4. To guarantee security and privacy of health information

HEALTH INFORMATION

Until recently, the physician was the most authoritative source of medical information. Today, the layman has access to a wide variety and quality of medical information via the Internet.[33] Fifty-two million American adults, or 55% of Americans with Internet access, have used the Web to get health or medical information. Fifty-five percent gather information on the Internet before visiting a physician.[33] Others see the Web as a good way to get a second opinion.

A study released by the American Medical Association revealed that almost half of physicians feel that the Internet has had a major impact on the way they practice medicine.[3] In 2002, two-thirds of online physicians accessed the Internet daily. Although there is still a trend for younger physicians to use the Internet more than older physicians, the percentage of older physicians using the Internet increased rapidly from the previous year. In 2001, 65% of physicians 60 years of age or older used the Internet.[3] It is not surprising that the Internet, and the enormous amount of health information available to the patient, have had a profound effect on patient's attitudes toward health care and on the patient–physician relationship. The age of information has empowered not only doctors but patients as well.

Validity of Health Information on the Web

There are a rapidly expanding number of Web sites offering health-related resources. Many sites provide reliable and valuable information, whereas others may have information that is misleading or incorrect. Much of the health information is copied from other sites and may be invalid and "rehashed." If the information is not original to that site, the original source should be clearly labeled. Medical facts and figures should have references, and opinions should be separated from information that is evidence-based. Web sites should be revised and updated on a regular basis. The source of a site's financial backing should be apparent because it can affect and possibly bias the content.

Search Engines

A search engine is a server or a collection of servers dedicated to indexing Web pages, storing the results and returning lists of pages that match particular queries. Some of the major search engines are Altavista, Excite, Hotbot, Infoseek, Lycos, Northern Light, and Webcrawler. Crawler-based search engines, such as Google, create their listings automatically.

The term *search engine* is often used generically to describe both crawler-based search engines and directories, even though these two types of search engines gather their listings in very different ways. Sites such as Yahoo are directories, not search engines. Directories or indexes are compiled manually, by user submission, and often involve an editorial selection and a categorization process.[52]

There are also two other categories of search engines: "meta" and "special interest." Meta search engines search other search engines and delete the duplicates. Special interest search engines, for example, the Internet Medical Database, search only special categories. It would be easier to find information on *otitis media* there than using Yahoo.[52] Each engine or directory has its strengths and weaknesses. Characteristics worth noting are search speed, how often the database is updated, and a site's "confidence rating" (a percentage grade given to its results).[50]

Literature Search

A literature search is a systematic and explicit approach to the identification, retrieval, and bibliographic management of independent studies.[5] The ability to perform a literature search is a necessary skill for both the researcher and the practitioner.

Computer usage has revolutionized the act of searching medical literature for research questions and determining the standard of care for practitioners. A proper literature search allows one to systematically gather together, critically appraise, and summarize research findings relating to a particular subject of interest. Until recently, literature searches were only performed by trained medical librarians. But there is in an ever increasing number of physicians performing their own searches.[23] Studies have shown that with a short period of training a clinician can attain a similar quality of search as a medical librarian.[23,35]

The quality of a literature search is traditionally assessed via search precision and recall.[34] *Precision* refers to the ratio of relevant citations retrieved to the total number of citations retrieved by a search. *Recall* refers to the ratio of relevant citations retrieved by a search to the actual number of relevant citations in the literature.[55] Exploring and selecting from the vast array of published information can be a time-consuming task, so it is important to know how to plan and carry out this work effectively. Regardless of which database is used, the researcher should take full advantage of the provided training materials to obtain

the best possible search results. Many systems provide either a user manual or an online help feature.[55] A thorough and time-efficient search should systematically go through the stages of defining the topic and choosing a specific aspect, especially if the topic is large. This cannot be overstated because the success of the search process relies on accurate formulation of the search question. It is helpful to be familiar with a special list of terms called *Medical Subject Headings,* or MeSH. MeSH is the National Library of Medicine's (NLM's) controlled vocabulary thesaurus. It consists of sets of terms naming descriptors in a hierarchic structure that permits searching at various levels of specificity. Other issues that can help improve the accuracy of one's search include limitations of publication, type, date, range, and language, as well as monitoring the results of the search as it progresses.

Electronic Health Information Resources

The NLM maintains many databases, including MEDLINE. MEDLINE is a well-known database of journal citations that covers general medicine, nursing, dentistry, health care systems, and the clinical sciences. As of the year 2002, MEDLINE contained citations to over 11 million articles from over 46,000 biomedical journals from United States and 70 other countries, dating back as far as 1966. The NLM provides free, unlimited access to MEDLINE on the Internet through a search interface known as PubMed. Entrez is a powerful and flexible search engine used by PubMed. PubMed is constantly being improved and changed. A feature called "Linkout" has been designed and added to point to additional Web-accessible resources. There are also several commercially available MEDLINE interfaces such as the one maintained by Ovid Technologies (http://*www.ovid.com*).

There are a vast number of other important medical databases. One of these is the Cochrane library, a collection of research reviews on the effect of health care interventions. It also includes DARE, the Database of Abstracts of Reviews of Effectiveness.

The National Institutes of Health (NIH) and the National Cancer Institute both maintain their own Web sites specifically for clinical trials. MDConsult from Elsevier is a useful interface for accessing full-text medical books, journals, drug information, and clinical practice guidelines (Box 20-3).

Electronic Health Information Resources in Otolaryngology

There are many otolaryngology resources available via the Internet. These include extensive Grand Rounds archives, lectures, and specialty publications. Many otolaryngology journals now provide online full-text access for subscribers. The American Academy of

---

BOX 20-3
GENERAL PROFESSIONAL MEDICAL INFORMATION AVAILABLE ONLINE

Cochrane library - *www.update-software.com/cochrane*

PubMed through links at the NLM Web site - *www.nlm.nih.gov*

PubMed directly - *www.ncbi.nlm.nih.gov/entrez/query.fcgi*

Material published before the mid-1960s through OLDMEDLINE (available through the NLM gateway) - *gateway.nlm.nih.gov/gw/Cmd*

Exerpta Medica's EMBASE (bibliographic database of 3500 journals; concentrates on drug information) - *www.embase.com*

MDConsult (Elsevier provides full-text access to approximately 40 medical textbooks, 50 medical journals, comprehensive drug information, and more than 600 clinical practice guidelines) - *www.mdconsult.com*

Clinical trials through links at the NIH - *www.clinicaltrials.gov*

National Cancer Institute - *www.cancer.gov/cancer_information* OR *http://www.cancer.gov/*

Scientific Information's Science Citation Index - *www.isinet.com/isi/products/citation/sci/*

BOX 20-4
OTOLARYNGOLOGY RESOURCES AVAILABLE ONLINE

Guide to Otolaryngology on the Internet - *www.bcm.tmc.edu/oto/others.html*

Otolaryngology *Grand Rounds* (New York Eye and Ear Infirmary) - *www.nyee.edu/page_deliv.html?page_no=46*

Otolaryngology *Grand Rounds Overviews* (Temple University School of Medicine) - *flower.aud.temple.edu/ENT/rounds/all.htm*

Otolaryngology *Grand Rounds Presentations* (University of Miami School of Medicine) - *otolaryngology.med.miami.edu/grandrounds.asp*

Dr. Quinn's Otolaryngology Grand Rounds Archive (University of Texas Medical Branch) - *www.utmb.edu/otoref/Grnds/GrndsIndex.html*

American Academy of Otolaryngology–Head and Neck Surgery - *www.entlink.net* OR *www.entnet.org/*

OTOHNS and PEDI-OTO e-mail discussion; to subscribe, send an e-mail request to *rbk@otohns.net*

Baylor College of Medicine Otolaryngology Grand Rounds Archive - *www.bcm.tmc.edu/oto/grand/grand.html*

Otolaryngology–Head and Neck Surgery (AAO–HNS) Web site features online discussion boards, patient education materials, primary care educational materials, online directories for both members and the public, practice management information, annual meeting information and registration, and a vast array of links to other otolaryngologic resources.[33] There are also a number of e-mail discussion groups (e.g., OTOHNS, PEDI-OTO) that allow otolaryngologists from around the globe to discuss professional issues on a daily basis (Box 20-4).

Informatics in Medical and Surgical Education

In a recent landmark study by the Institute of Medicine entitled "Crossing the Quality Chasm," patient safety issues were exposed.[13] The solutions for change included a project on professional education. The rationale behind the project was that health care professionals need to be better prepared to provide the highest quality and safest care possible and to function at optimum levels in an ever-evolving and increasingly complex 21st century health system.[20] Many forces were seen to be acting on medical care, including the following[20]:

- Scientific advances and new technology.
- Growing prevalence of chronic diseases.
- More reliance on teams in clinical care.
- Persistent economic exigencies.
- Legal and regulatory pressures.
- Professional discontent and shortages.
- Rising expectations for quality.
- Patient empowerment and interest group politics.

The vision of the project is that all health care professionals will be educated to deliver patient-centered care as members of an interdisciplinary team, emphasizing evidence-based practice, quality improvement approaches, and informatics. It is clear that information technology is a crucial part of educating health care professionals. What are some of the trends in online or computer-based learning?

Reusable Learning Modules

To facilitate just-in-time learning, content is thought of as "chunks of information" or "learning objects" that can be aggregated and reassembled to create the modules, or lessons, that the user desires. Modules (lessons) can then be aggregated into courses, designed to deliver just the right information that the user needs, when it is needed (Figure 20-3). If a standard format is used, the object-based content can be placed in a central repository and reused in other courses, saving resources and money.

Blended Learning

There is a growing trend toward blended learning, in which traditional learning is combined with online learning, or "eLearning." However, online learning will

WORKING WITH LEARNING OBJECTS

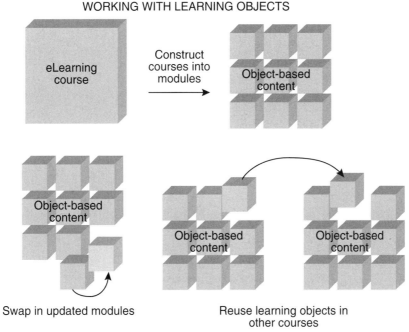

Figure 20-3. Information technology can be used to structure content into customized "learning objects" that can be aggregated and reassembled to facilitate just-in-time learning. Adapted from MedBiquitous.

never completely replace important aspects of traditional learning such as the social interactions and mentoring that occur in a more traditional setting. Training of surgical techniques can be quite a different educational process from teaching didactic courses and may be much more effectively done in a face-to-face experience. Using a combination of both forms of learning is often quite efficient.

Surgical Simulation

Many advanced teaching systems use simulation to engage the student. In otolaryngology, endoscopic sinus surgery and temporal bone surgery require a great deal of training before they can be performed adequately. Due to the complex and variable anatomy and the proximity of important structures, severe complications are possible, even for experienced surgeons. Surgical simulation and virtual reality technology can provide an excellent tool for learning or honing surgical technique.* The most complete study to date rated 10 residents in different stages of their training. Resident performance on the surgical sinus surgery simulator was evaluated, and operating room performance and surgical competency were examined. The simulator was found to be a valid training device that positively affects operating room performance.[19]

*References 9, 18, 19, 26, 27, 45, 60.

MEDICAL IMAGING INFORMATICS

Medical diagnosis and treatment often depends on the interpretation of images and is often aided by the simultaneous visualization of images by multiple clinicians, allowing them to discuss and interpret them. Therefore, the images themselves are an important part of the EPR. The movement of images along electronic media for the purpose of remote viewing, sharing, interpreting, and consulting is collectively referred to as *telemedicine.* Educational resources such as case libraries, quizzes, tutorials, and imaging atlases can provide great educational support.

One of the burdens entailed in medical imaging is the storage and retrieval of medical images. As health care delivery networks disperse, the need for remote access to images increases. This in turn creates a need for digital image capture, storage, transmission, and retrieval systems. Digital acquisition of images offers the prospect of reducing the physical space requirements, material cost, and labor invoked in traditional film handling and storage. Instead, these are handled through online digital archiving, rapid retrieval of images, and high-speed transmission of images over a variety of networks. Image storage poses a challenge because film storage requires a vast amount of digital space. Systems that possess such capabilities are known as picture-archiving and communication systems (PACS) and are becoming a common fixture in many hospitals and medical centers.[17] These systems are often incorporated in a hospital EPR. The primary requirement of a PACS is that it must acquire images in digital form either by primary digital acquisition or, less commonly, by digital scanning.[30]

Imaging in Otolaryngology

The complex nature of the upper aerodigestive system, inner ear, and head and neck region combined with the surgical nature of the profession makes otolaryngology highly dependent on useful imaging. This includes x-ray images, whether simple sinus films or three-dimensional (3D) reconstructed computed tomography (CT) images, nuclear thyroid scans and ultrasounds, and endoscopic images. Certain imaging methods are quite unique to otolaryngology.

The video otoscope (VO) provides an optoelectronically enhanced field of view of the ear that can be shared with others. The basic VO system consists of an otoscope with removable otic speculum, color video camera, high-intensity light source, and a video display monitor. Videonystagmography (VNG) is often used in the evaluation of a patient who presents with vertigo and uses the vestibular-ocular reflex to indirectly measure vestibular function. VNG tests for nystagmus using infrared light and video technology to monitor eye movements during testing.

TELEMEDICINE

Telemedicine is defined as "the use of medical information exchanged from one site to another via electronic communication for health and education of the patient or health care provider and for the purpose of improving health care,"[4] or simply "the use of telecommunications for medical diagnosis and patient care." Telemedicine is not a fad or a special area of medicine limited to fringe applications; it is rapidly becoming integrated into the practice of medicine. It holds the promise of improved health care accessibility, increased efficiency, and a more even distribution of specialized medical knowledge, especially in some remote rural, poor urban, and underserved environments.[8,21,37] An example of this is the Alaska Federal health care access network, where a small population is spread over a great distance. A high incidence of otitis media among the Alaskans has led to a sustained telehealth system. Health care professionals working with these conditions have developed a store-and-forward system using video otoscopic images. They have rendered more than 5000 store-and-forward consultations to 235 remote sites.

There is concern that telemedicine videoteleconferencing (VTC) consultations can be detrimental to doctor-patient interaction. Studies have shown that this is not the case. Telemedicine in fact represents a wider interaction system with more channels for access, inspection, and information and is perceived positively by most patients.[29]

The use of imaging and the need for consultation in our field make telemedicine quite applicable to otolaryngology.[40-42] The exact number of active telemedicine programs in otolaryngology is unknown, but one source of data is the Telemedicine Information Exchange Web site,[57] which lists 18 active programs that support otolaryngology in their telemedicine program. There are at least eight other otolaryngology programs that are not listed on the exchange. There are a number of benefits resulting from widespread acceptance of telemedicine in the field of otolaryngology, as well as other medical specialties: reduced morbidity and mortality and medical costs due to early detection of serious pathology (in this case, head and neck cancers); reduced unnecessary referrals to specialists with consequent savings to the patient and health care provider; and more efficient usage of specialist time.[25]

To date, telemedicine in head and neck oncology has been limited to remote tumor conferences and second opinions. In one study, the accuracy of such a conference was evaluated in a more objective fashion. The people attending the conference were asked to determine the tumor (TNM) classification and treatment. The patient was then presented in person to give the audience the opportunity to ask questions and perform a physical examination. In 91% of cases, the same classification and treatment plan were determined using the telemedicine simulation as in the subsequent face-to-face consultation. The researchers went on to study patient satisfaction with remote tumor conferences. Fifty-eight patients were presented to the regional tumor board via real-time telemedicine. They were compared with a group presented "face-to-face." The researchers found that patients presented by means of telemedicine were as satisfied as the patients presented face-to-face.[54]

Heneghan and others[24] conducted fiberoptic examinations on randomly selected patients. This was done in real time using three integrate service digital network (ISDN) lines at 384 kbps. Their studies found 31 of 37 patients to have a detectable pathology while only six were deemed healthy. The study clearly showed how telemedicine can be used to save lives through early detection of serious pathology.[24]

Telemedicine in otolaryngology has been used for rehabilitation purposes in a number of settings including vestibular dysfunction,[59] speech and voice therapy,[28,32] dysphagia,[39] and rehabilitation after cochlear implantation.[22] (Many of these cited works are proof-of-concept studies and projects with no clinical efficacy studies to date.[11])

Although telemedicine is used as an integrated tool during tumor conferences, the lack of palpation is a

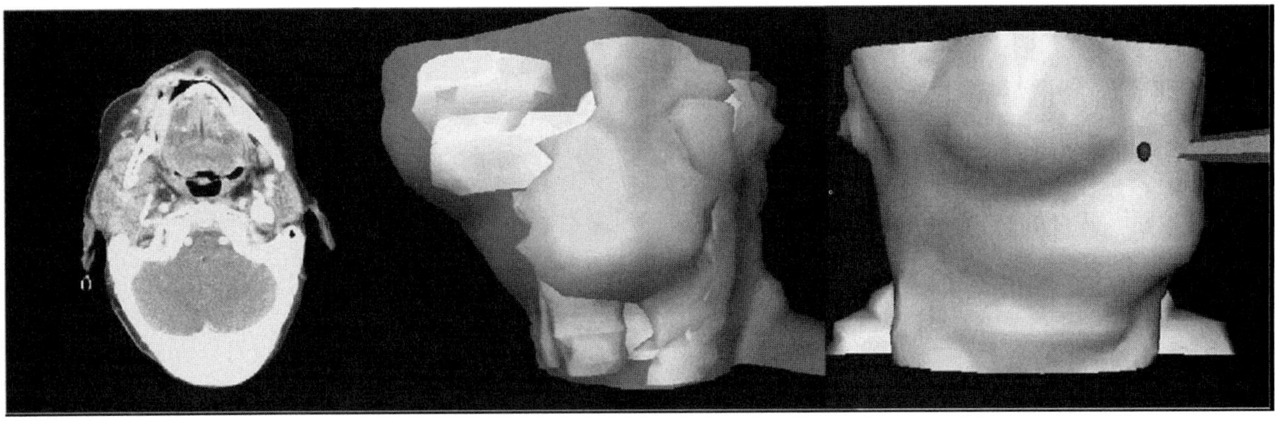

Figure 20-4. Haptic palpation of head and neck cancer patients. Panel one shows an axial CT scan with a left-sided mass. Panel two, viewed from lower left, shows a semi-transparency view; the tumor can be seen protruding from the left cheek abutting mandible. The SCM muscle is clearly viewed behind the mass. In panel three, the tumor model is visualized from the left; the haptic interface (PHANTOM desktop) is visualized as a circle and grip. From Stalfors J, Edström S, Björk-Ericsson, Mercke C and others: Accuracy of tele-oncology compared with face-to-face consultation in head and neck cancer case conferences. *J Telemed Telecare* 7(6): 338–343, 2001. To view this image in color, please go to *www.ototext.com* or the Electronic Image Collection CD, bound into your copy of Cummings Otolaryngology—Head and Neck Surgery, 4th edition.

limiting factor in its use in head and neck cancer. Stalfors and colleagues[53] developed a 3D model in VRML format. Reconstructed neck structures with high-resolution CT tactical properties were added, allow remote palpitations of the head and neck to be performed (Figure 20-4). Other areas in which telemedicine is being studied in head and neck surgery are in the postoperative monitoring of free flaps[6] and remote intraoperative frozen-section histopathologic diagnosis.[38]

There are still a number of barriers to the development of telemedicine. Lack of reimbursement is considered the major obstacle to the growth of telemedicine applications and networks.[22] As of January 2003, 18 states reimburse for some type of Medicaid telemedicine services. Private payers, particularly large integrated health systems and managed care companies, have been slow to reimburse for clinical telemedicine services until they see a better definition of their value. Licensure between states and countries is still an obstacle to the advancement of telemedicine. Many states have enacted laws specifically addressing licensure for provision of telemedicine services by out-of-state physicians, but most laws are restrictive, requiring full licensure. Some supporters of telemedicine advocate limited licensure laws, whereas others propose a national licensure. Physician acceptance of telemedicine has been slow as well. Part of this is due to a lack of validating studies of telemedicine technologies to the current standard of care.[10] Most of the available literature refers only to pilot projects and short-term

outcomes. Relatively convincing evidence of effectiveness is found in teleradiology, teleneurosurgery, telepsychiatry, and the use of electronic referral enabling e-mail consultations and VTC between primary and secondary health care providers.[43]

Security issues, while important, have been greatly overstated as a barrier to the implementation of telemedicine systems. Today, encryption, virtual private networks, and IP tunneling are solutions readily implemented and available with commercial off-the-shelf telemedicine technologies.

The implementation of telemedicine systems has been furthered by the creation of standards. These standards pertain to bandwidth, compression, and schemes used in audio, video, and the transfer of data.[31]

Bandwidth is a critical issue when practicing telemedicine (see Glossary). Two important principles of practicing telemedicine are: (1) the slowest part of the connection determines the real transfer rate; and (2) once approximately 20% of available bandwidth is used, one experiences degradation in performance[16] (Box 20-5).

Telemedicine Modalities

Diagnostic and consultative telemedicine can be basically divided into two categories: (1) store and forward and (2) interactive (real time).[1] In a store-and-forward method, the referring physician collects all relevant information and forwards it to the remote specialist (Figure 20-5). This method can ease scheduling problems for programs that cover different time

BOX 20-5

BANDWIDTH AND TELECOMMUNICATION CONNECTIONS FOR TELEMEDICINE

Data transfer: Measured in bits-per-second (bps); kilobits-per-second (Kbps) or megabits-per-second (Mbps); 56,000 bps = 56 Kbps; 1000 is often abbreviated to "K" as in "56 K"

Plain Old Telephone Service (POTS): Basic telephone service over the public telephone network; analog; most widely available telecommunication technology; used for phones, faxes and modems; suitable for audio conferencing, store-and-forward, Internet, and low-bandwidth videophone conferencing; speed = 56 Kbps; video 3 to 8 fps (compressed)

Integrated Service Digital Network (ISDN): Switchable (i.e., can be dialed like a phone) ISDN can carry information five times faster than modem via POTS; digital, so same wires better signal; each ISDN line has a capacity of 128 K (video 16 to 20 fps [compressed]); ISDN lines can be "bonded" together; 3 × 128 K = 384 K (video 28 fps [compressed])

T1 & fractional T1: Dedicated from point-to-point 24 hours a day (always connected, no need to dial); transmits data at a rate of 1.54 megabits per second (mbps) (video 30 fps [compressed]); typically available in most parts of the country; possible to purchase a fraction of a T1 line—½ T1 (768 K) or ¼ T1 (384 K) available

Internet-Based Telemedicine Connections:

Digital subscriber lines (DSL): Always on; 300 to 600 Kbps upload speeds and up to 1500 Kbps download speeds

Cable modem: Always on; speeds are not guaranteed, determined by how many users are connected on a stretch of cable at one time

Satellite: Always on; high-speed internet access available virtually everywhere in the world; sensitive to certain weather conditions

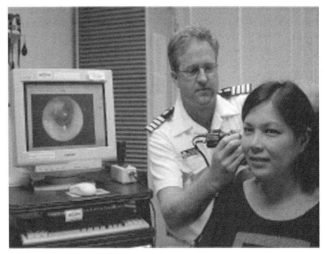

Figure 20-5. A video otoscopic examination used for store-and-forward telemedicine applications. (The authors acknowledge and thank Michael R Holtel, M.D., for kindly providing this photograph.) To view this image in color, please go to *www.ototext.com* or the Electronic Image Collection CD, bound into your copy of Cummings Otolaryngology—Head and Neck Surgery, 4th edition.

The benefits of direct interaction between the patient, referring physician, and specialist offset the increased cost and complexity of the interaction. The quality of the transmission video must be satisfactory for the diagnostic task at hand. Sclafini and colleagues[49] studied the relative strengths and weaknesses of real-time and store-and-forward teleconsultation in otolaryngology. They concluded that both real-time and delayed techniques can be used to provide relatively accurate clinical consultations. A recent study by Ullah and others[58] assessed the value of real-time consultations using low-budget equipment and connections. They used basic rate ISDN lines at 128 kbps between two rooms in a hospital. They found that even low-cost real-time telemedicine is useful and reliable for providing otolaryngologic consultation in a primary care setting.

Telesurgery

With the advent of videolaparoscopy, the surgical suite of the 19th century entered the computer age.[46] Telesurgery can be categorized into three types: (1) telerobotic surgery; (2) telepresence surgery; and (3) teleproctored or telementored surgery.

In telerobotic surgery, robots are controlled directly by the surgeon. The surgeon may stand at the side of the operating table.[2,7] At the present time, telerobotic surgical systems offer a limited selection of instruments with bulky configurations that impede many specific surgical procedures. Moreover, clinical experience with the systems is limited. Thus, telesurgery must be regarded as an emerging technology that is still in its infancy and in an early phase of feasibility testing.

zones. The store-and-forward paradigm is appropriate in many situations such as screening programs, biopsy analysis, and interpretation of radiologic scans or endoscopic images.

The interactive (real-time) consultation aims to re-create the situation in which the patient and the treating physician are both present. These consults can be performed with the patient accompanied by a preceptor (physician, physician's assistant, or registered nurse) who can carry out the necessary diagnostic procedures (e.g., otoscopic evaluation) after appropriate training. Interactive or real-time VTC is usually more complex technologically because of the dependence on strict scheduling for both parties. It is more expensive both in bandwidth and equipment.

The choice to use the store-and-forward vs the interactive method is based on a number of factors.

Telepresence projects a virtual image of the operative field to a remote site or surgical simulation.[47,48] The surgeon's hand motions are telecast to the remote operating room so that the surgeon performs the operation without actually seeing his or her patient. Telepresence thus provides a new strategy for the training of surgical residents or junior surgeons.[12]

Teleproctored (overseeing surgical procedures) or telementored (surgical instruction) surgery projects a surgeon's expertise to remote locations. Telementoring permits an expert surgeon, who remains in his or her own hospital, to instruct a novice in a remote location on how to perform a new operation or use a new surgical technology.[44] Many of these simulators incorporate haptic (forced) feedback, which allows the operator to "feel." Traditionally, surgical experience is gained through cadaver dissections and education by more experienced surgeons. The future of surgical training will surely include the use of simulators in the acquisition and maintenance of surgical skills.

Telmentored surgery is a feasible option for training residents in functional endoscopic surgery. Burgess and colleagues[12] compared conventionally proctored endoscopic sinus surgery cases with teleproctored cases, with the faculty surgeon supervising through VTC in a control room 15 seconds from the operating room. Forty-two control patients (83 sides) and 45 teleproctored patients (83 sides) were evaluated. Three teleproctored cases required faculty intervention—two for surgical difficulty, one for VTC problems. Teleproctored cases took 3.87 minutes longer per side (28.54 vs 24.67 minutes; $P < .024$), a 16% increase. This was thought to be a result of nuances of VTC proctoring. Residents had a positive learning experience, with nearly full control of the operating suite combined with remote supervision through telepresence.

CONCLUSION

The use of computers, telecommunications, and information technology in medical care, medical education, and medical research is now an integral part of our world as physicians and otolaryngologists. By creatively using this technology, we facilitate the development of the information age in the care of our patients and the education of our students.

GLOSSARY OF COMMONLY USED INFORMATION TECHNOLOGY TERMS

Analog signal: A frequency is modified in some way, such as by amplifying the strength of the signal or varying the frequency, to add information to the signal; broadcast and telephone transmission have conventionally used analog technology

Artificial intelligence in medicine: The application of artificial intelligence methods to solve problems in medicine (e.g., developing expert systems to assist with diagnosis, or therapy planning)

Bandwidth: The capacity for data transfer of an electronic communications system

Binary: A numbering scheme in which there are only two possible values for each digit: 0 and 1; also refers to any digital encoding/decoding system in which there are exactly two possible states

Bioinformatics: The science of developing computer databases and algorithms for the purpose of speeding up and enhancing biologic research; being used most noticeably in the Human Genome Project, the effort to identify the 80,000 genes in human DNA

Bit: Short for *binary digit,* the smallest unit of data in a computer

Bit rate: The number of bits that are transmitted in a given time period, usually per second; synonym for *data transfer rate*

Byte: In most computer systems, a unit of data that is eight binary digits long; the unit most computers use to represent a character such as a letter, number, or typographic symbol (related terms include *megabyte, gigabyte,* etc.)

Client server: A relationship between two computer programs in which one program, the client, makes a service request from another program, the server, which fulfills the request

Clinical decision support system: Software that taps into database resources to assist users in making decisions on care options; gives physicians structured (rules-based) information on diagnoses and treatments

Compressed video: Video images that have been processed to reduce the amount of bandwidth needed to capture the necessary information so that the information can be sent over a telephone network

Database: A collection of data organized so that its contents can easily be accessed, managed, and updated

Data mining: The comparison and study of large databases to discover new data relationships; mining a clinical database can produce new insights on outcomes, alternate treatments, or effects of treatment on different races and genders

Digital signal: Electronic technology that generates, stores, and processes data in terms of two states: positive and nonpositive; positive is expressed or represented by the number 1 and nonpositive by the number 0; thus, data transmitted or stored with digital technology is expressed as a string of 0s and 1s

Ethernet: The most widely installed local area network (LAN) technology

Evidence-based medicine: A movement advocating the practice of medicine according to clinical guidelines, developed to reflect best practice as captured from a metaanalysis of the clinical literature

Expert system: A computer program that contains expert knowledge about a particular problem, often in the form of a set of if/then rules, that is able to solve problems at a level equivalent to or greater than human experts

Frame rate: The number of frames or images that are projected or displayed per second; the higher the number of frames playing per second, the smoother the video playback appears to the user; lower rates result in a choppy playback

Full-motion video: A standard video signal requiring 6 MHz in analog format and 45 Mbps when encoded digitally

Home page: A document on the World Wide Web that acts as a front page or point of welcome to a collection of documents that may introduce an individual, organization, or point of interest

Hypertext: A method of presenting documents electronically that allows them to be read in a richly interconnected way; rather than following a single document from beginning to end, sections of each document are connected to related occurrences in other documents via hyperlinks, permitting "nonlinear" reading following concepts of interest to the reader (related terms are *hyperlink, HTML, World Wide Web*)

Hypertext markup language (HTML): The description language used to create hypertext documents that can be viewed on the World Wide Web (related terms are *HTTP, World Wide Web*)

Hypertext transfer protocol (HTTP): Communication protocol used on the Internet for the transfer of HTML documents (related terms are *HTML, World Wide Web*)

Integrate service digital network (ISDN): A system of digital phone connections. This system allows voice and data to be transmitted simultaneously using end-to-end digital connectivity

Internet: Technically, a network of computer networks; a specific global computer network that is publicly accessible and on which the transfer of HTML documents (related terms are *HTML, World Wide Web*)

Internet 2: A consortium being led by universities working in partnership with industry and government to develop and deploy advanced network applications and technologies, accelerating the creation of the next Internet

Internet protocol (IP): The method or protocol by which data is sent from one computer to another on the Internet; each computer (known as a *host*) on the Internet has at least one IP address that uniquely identifies it from all other computers on the Internet

Java: A programming language that has a modular structure so that parts of the program can be reused when necessary; can run on most computers and operating systems such as Macintosh, Windows, and UNIX systems

JavaBeans: Self-contained programs that can run on any application that understands JavaBeans specifications; can be reassembled and reused

Legacy system: Any application based on older technologies and hardware, such as mainframes, that continues to provide core services to an organization; are frequently large, monolithic, and difficult to modify, and scrapping or replacing them often means reengineering a organization's business processes as well

Local area network (LAN): A group of computers and associated devices that share a common communications line or wireless link and typically share the resources of a single processor or server within a small geographic area

Medical informatics: The theoretic and practical aspects of information processing and communication, based on knowledge and experience derived from processes in medicine and health care

Metadata: Provides a standard for describing general content to facilitate search, retrieval, and content syndication; data about data

Modulator-demodulator (MODEM): Modulates outgoing digital signals from a computer or other digital device to analog signals for a conventional copper twisted pair telephone line and demodulates the incoming analog signal and converts it to a digital signal for the digital device

Optical character recognition (OCR): Automated scanning and conversion of printed characters to computer-based text

Picture archiving and communications system (PACS): A system that acquires, transmits, stores, retrieves, and displays digital images and related patient information from a variety of imaging sources and communicates the information over a network

Portal: Originally, a gateway to Web access, a Web site that offered popular services such as e-mail, search engines, and on-line shopping; was the starting point for Web searching or "surfing;" to retain users, sites with search engines differentiated into hubs where users could find all the Web content and services that they needed; now, portals are the center for technologies that are being collectively called the *portal ecosystem*

Portlet: Access program application programming interfaces (APIs), URLs; have been the primary integration method for content, applications, and processes in portals since 1998; also known as gadgets, modules, and iViews

Universal resource locator (URL): The address for a document placed on the World Wide Web

Virtual reality: Computer-simulated environment within which humans are able to interact in some manner that approximates interactions in the physical world

Extensible markup language (XML): An open industry standard developed by the World Wide Web Consortium to facilitate the exchange of structured data over the Internet; use of XML will help eliminate barriers in communicating between different computer platforms, applications, and databases; a gradual transition from HTML to XML will be taking place over the next few years.

REFERENCES

1. Allely EB: Synchronous and asynchronous telemedicine, *J Med Syst* 19:207–212, 1995.
2. Allen D, Bowersox J, Jones GG: Telesurgery. Telepresence. Telementoring. Telerobotics, *Telemed Today* 5:18–20, 25, 1997.
3. American Medical Association: Physicians' use of internet steadily rising, *http:www.ama-assn.org.* Accessed in 2001.
4. American Telemedicine Association: Web site, *www.americantelemed.org/about/aboutata.htm.* Link JD, 2001. Accessed in 2003.
5. Auston IM, Cahn MA, Selden CR: *Literature search methods for the development of clinical practice guidelines: Agency for Health Care Policy and Research, Office of the Forum for Quality and Effectiveness in Health Care, Forum Methodology Conference.* National Library of Medicine, *http://www.nlm.nih.gov/nichsr/litsrch.html,* 1992.
6. Baldwin AJ, Langton SG: Postoperative monitoring of flaps by digital camera and Internet link, *Br J Oral Maxillofac Surg* 39:120–121, 2001.
7. Ballantyne GH: Robotic surgery, telerobotic surgery, telepresence, and telementoring: review of early clinical results, *Surg Endosc* 16:1389–402, 2002.
8. Blakeslee DB: Like it or not, telemedicine is here: making it work for us, *Arch Otolaryngol Head Neck Surg* 127:337, 2001.
9. Bockholt U and others: Realtime simulation of tissue deformation for the nasal endoscopy simulator (NES), *Stud Health Technol Inform* 62:74–75, 1999.
10. Burgess LP and others: Telemedicine in otolaryngology: implications,pitfalls,and roadblocks. *Current Opinions in Otolaryngology-Head and Neck Surgery,* 10:194–198, 2002.
11. Burgess LP, Hottel MR: Telemedicine in otolaryngology, *Otolaryngol Clin North Am* 35(6):1263–1281.
12. Burgess LP, Syms MJ, Hottel MR and others: Telemedice: teleproctored endoscopic sinus surgery, *Laryngoscope* 112(2):216–219, 2002.
13. Byrne JP, Mughal MM: Telementoring as an adjunct to training and competence-based assessment in laparoscopic cholecystectomy, *Surg Endosc* 14:1159–1161, 2000.
14. Care IoMCoQoH. *Crossing the quality chasm: a new health system for the 21st century.* Committee on Quality of Health Care in America, Institute of Medicine, editor: National Academy Press, 2001.
15. Coiera E: *Guide to medical informatics, the Internet and telemedicine.* London, Oxford University Press, 1997.
16. Covell DG, Uman GC, Manning PR: Information needs in office practice: are they being met? *Ann Intern Med* 103: 596–599, 1985.
17. Dorman T: Telemedicine, *Anesthesiol Clin North Am* 18: 663–676, 2000.
18. Dwyer SJ III: Imaging system architectures for picture archiving and communication systems, *Radiol Clin North Am* 34:495–503, 1996.
19. Ecke U and others: Virtual reality: preparation and execution of sinus surgery, *Comput Aided Surg* 3:45–50, 1998.
20. Edmond CV Jr: Impact of the endoscopic sinus surgical simulator on operating room performance, *Laryngoscope* 112:1148–1158, 2002.
21. Fineberg H: *Crossing the chasm with better medical education.* MedBiquitous Consortium Annual Conference, Baltimore, Maryland, 2003.
22. Fried MP: The challenges and potential of otolaryngological telemedicine, *Arch Otolaryngol Head Neck Surg* 127:336, 2001.
23. Goldenberg D, Wenig BL: Telemedicine in otolaryngology, *Am J Otolaryngol* 23:35–43, 2002.
24. Haynes RB and others: Developing optimal search strategies for detecting clinically sound studies in MEDLINE, *J Am Med Inform Assoc* 1:447–458, 1994.
25. Heneghan C, Stern J, Sclafani AP and others: Can tele-otolaryngology help in screening for head and neck cancer? *Telemed Today* 5:24–25, 1997.
26. Heneghan C and others: Telemedicine applications in otolaryngology, *IEEE Eng Med Biol Mag* 18:53–62, 1999.
27. Hilbert M, Muller W: Virtual reality in endonasal surgery, *Stud Health Technol Inform* 39:237–245, 1997.
28. Hilbert M, Muller W, Strutz J: Development of a surgical simulator for interventions of the paranasal sinuses: technical principles and initial prototype, *Laryngorhinootologie* 77: 153–156, 1998.
29. Hill A, Theodoros D: Research into telehealth applications in speech-language pathology, *J Telemed Telecare* 8:187–196, 2002.
30. Holtan A: Patient reactions to specialist telemedicine consultations: a sociological approach, *J Telemed Telecare* 4:206–213, 1998.
31. Horii SC: Image acquisition: sites, technologies, and approaches, *Radiol Clin North Am* 34:469–494, 1996.
32. Houtchens BA and others: Telemedicine protocols and standards: development and implementation, *J Med Syst* 19:93–119, 1995.
33. Kully D: Telehealth in speech pathology: applications to the treatment of stuttering, *J Telemed Telecare* 6 Suppl 2:S39–S41, 2000.
34. Kuppersmith R: The physician-patient relationship and the internet, *Otolaryngol Clin North Am* 35(6):1143–1147, Dec 2002.
35. Lowe HJ, Barnett GO: Understanding and using the medical subject headings (MeSH) vocabulary to perform literature searches, *JAMA* 271:1103–1108, 1994.
36. Lusk R: Update on the electronic patient record, *Otolaryngol Clin North Am* 35(6):1223–1236.
37. Lusk R, Herrmann K: The computerized patient record, *Otolaryngol Clin North Am* 31:289–300, 1998.
38. Meyers AD, Kuppersmith R: Learning objectives for telemedicine applications in otolaryngology-head and neck surgery, *Otolaryngol Head Neck Surg* 120:137–138, 1999.
39. Nordrum I, Eide TJ: Remote frozen section service in Norway, *Arch Anat Cytol Pathol* 43:253–256, 1995.
40. Pearlman ALWW: Real-time remote telefluoroscopic assessment of patients with dysphagia, *Dysphagia* 17:162–167, 2002.
41. Pedersen S, Hartviksen G, Haga D: Teleconsultation of patients with otorhinolaryngologic conditions: a telendoscopic

pilot study, *Arch Otolaryngol Head Neck Surg* 120:133–136, 1994.

42. Pedersen S, Holand U: Tele-endoscopic otorhinolaryngological examination: preliminary study of patient satisfaction, *Telemed J* 1:47–52, 1995.

43. Rinde E, Nordrum I, Nymo BJ: Telemedicine in rural Norway, *World Health Forum* 14:71–77, 1993.

44. Roine R, Ohinmaa A, Hailey D: Assessing telemedicine: a systematic review of the literature, *CMAJ* 165:765–771, 2001.

45. Rosser JC Jr, Murayama M, Gabriel NH: Minimally invasive surgical training solutions for the twenty-first century, *Surg Clin North Am* 80:1607–1624, 2000

46. Rudman DT and others: Functional endoscopic sinus surgery training simulator, *Laryngoscope* 108:1643–1647, 1998.

47. Satava RM: Nintendo surgery, *JAMA* 267:2329–2330, 1992.

48. Satava RM: Virtual reality and telepresence for military medicine, *Ann Acad Med Singapore* 26:118–120, 1997.

49. Satava RM: Virtual reality, telesurgery, and the new world order of medicine, *J Image Guid Surg* 1:12–16, 1995.

50. Sclafani AP and others: Teleconsultation in otolaryngology: live versus store and forward consultations, *Otolaryngol Head Neck Surg* 120:62–72, 1999.

51. Shortliffe EH BM: *Medical informatics.* In Shortliffe EH PL, editor: *Medical data: their acquisition, storage and use.* New York, 2000, Springer.

52. Simmonds MD: *Search engine terms.* AudetteMedia, Bethesda, Maryland, 2003.

53. The Spider's Apprentice: Search engine tips, *www.monarch.com/spidap.html.* May 2004.

54. Stalfors J and others: Haptic palpation of head and neck cancer patients: implication for education and telemedicine, *Stud Health Technol Inform* 81:471–474, 2001.

55. Stalfors JH-SL and others: Satisfaction with telemedicine presentation at a multidisciplinary tumor meeting among patients with head and neck cancer, *J Telemed Telecare* 9(3):150–151, 2003.

56. Stewart MG KR, Moore AS: Searching the medical literature on the internet, *Otolaryngol Clin North Am* 35(6):1163–1174.

57. Tang PC MC: *Computer-based patient record system.* In Shortliffe EH BM, editor: *Medical informatics.* New York, 2000, Springer.

58. Telemedicine information exchange program, *http://tie.telemed.org,* 2004.

59. Ullah R, Gilliland D, Adams D: Otolaryngology consultations by real-time telemedicine, *Ulster Med J* 71:26–29, 2002.

60. Viirre E and others: Remote medical consultation for vestibular disorders: technological solutions and case report, *Telemed J* 3:53–58, 1997.

61. Weghorst S and others: Validation of the Madigan ESS simulator, *Stud Health Technol Inform* 50:399–405, 1998.

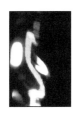

PART TWO

FACE

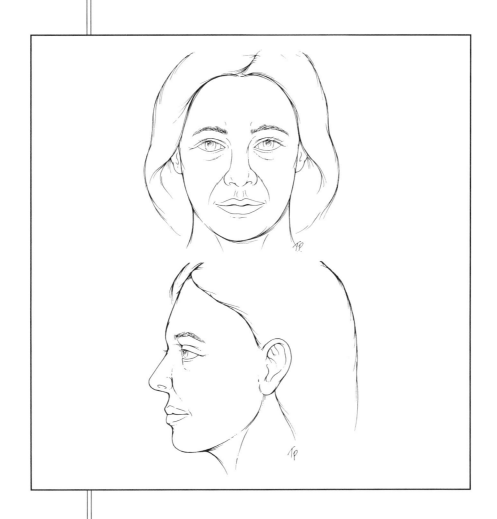

CHAPTER TWENTY ONE

AESTHETIC FACIAL ANALYSIS

Marc S. Zimbler
Jongwook Ham

INTRODUCTION

Throughout history mankind has tried to define beauty. Poets, philosophers, and artists have pondered its elusive quality while attempting to quantify that which is evident to all of us. As surgeons, however, we are required to have a more scientific approach to beauty to formulate operative plans with successful surgical outcomes. Common reference points are essential in communicating with colleagues and medical record keeping. Furthermore, we must be able to accurately define specific characteristics that deviate from the norm so that we may identify congenital anomalies and facial deformities.

As early as ancient Egypt, aesthetic facial proportions have been idealized in art. However, it was not until the Greek philosophers that the study of beauty became a formal discipline. To Plato and Aristotle beauty meant symmetry, harmony, and geometry. In the fifth century BC, the Greek sculptor Polyclitus defined perfect beauty as the mutual harmony of all parts, such that nothing could be added or subtracted. Such harmonic proportions were held to be beautiful in themselves, independent of any observer.

These ideas were later revisited by the Renaissance artists, who began to define ideal proportions for the human form. This example is nowhere more evident than in the drawings of Leonardo da Vinci and his Vitruvian man (Figure 21-1). It was da Vinci, who, through the study of anatomy, formulated ideal facial proportions and divided the profile into equal thirds (Figure 21-2). Leonardo's scientific accuracy rivaled that of Vesalius, whereas his artistic beauty remains unchallenged. Another Renaissance artist inspired by the Vitruvian notion of perfect proportions was the German printmaker Albrecht Durer. Durer used his own finger as a unit of measurement to construct a proportional system for the entire body, and in 1528 he published a four-book treatise on human proportions. Durer divided the facial profile into four equal parts and recognized that the length of the nose equals that of the ear.

The artistic cannons set forth in antiquity and during the Renaissance dominated Western art for centuries. In the twentieth century, anthropometrist Leslie Farkas[3] challenged the classical cannons by measuring the facial proportions of 200 women, including 50 models. His results concluded that some of the cannons are nothing more than artistic idealizations. Nevertheless, although social and cultural factors influence every generation's concept of beauty, the aesthetic cannons have withstood the test of time. Currently, the parameters established in the facial plastic surgery literature are based predominately on the works of Powell and Humphreys, who in 1984 crystallized this topic into a single text *Proportions of the Aesthetic Face.*[7]

ANATOMIC LANDMARKS AND REFERENCE POINTS

Facial analysis is dependent on both soft-tissue and skeletal anatomic landmarks. Soft-tissue reference points are listed in Figure 21-3 and Box 21-1. Skeletal reference points are defined by cephalometric analysis and are listed in Figure 21-4 and Box 21-2.

The Frankfort horizontal plane (Figure 21-5) is the standard reference point for patient positioning in photographs and cephalometric radiographs. The Frankfort plane is defined as a line drawn from the superior aspect of the external auditory canal to the inferior border of the infraorbital rim while the patient's gaze is parallel to the floor. A soft-tissue definition for the inferior aspect of the infraorbital rim is the point of transition between lower eyelid and cheek skin.

FACIAL PROPORTIONS

The initial assessment of the face evaluates symmetry. Symmetry is rarely perfect when comparing halves through a midsagittal plane (Figure 21-6); nevertheless, midline points should lie on the axis line. Facial width is evaluated by dividing the face into equal fifths (Figure 21-7). The width of one eye should equal one

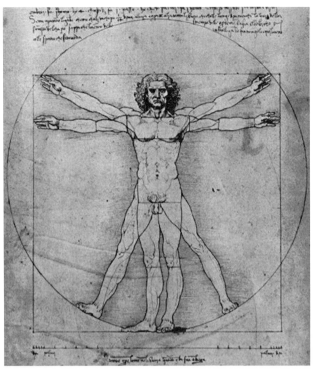

Figure 21-1. Leonardo da Vinci. The proportions of the body according to Vitruvius, ca. 1490. Pen and ink with touches of wash, over stylus 34.4 × 24.5 cm. (Courtesy of the Galleria dell' Accademia, inv.228, Venice.)

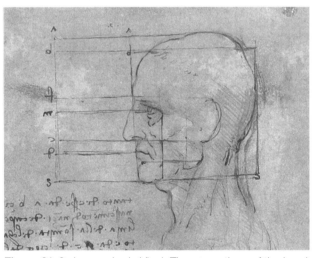

Figure 21-2. Leonardo da Vinci. The proportions of the head, ca.1490. Pen and ink over black chalk, 28.0 × 22.2 cm. (Courtesy of the Galleria dell' Academia, inv.236v, Venice.)

fifth of the total facial width, as well as the intercanthal distance or nasal base width.

Facial height is commonly assessed by one of two methods. The first method divides the face into equal thirds (Figure 21-8) as described by da Vinci. Measurements are made in the midline from the tri-

chion to the glabella, from the glabella to the subnasale, and from the subnasale to the menton. The second method excludes the upper third of the face because of common variability regarding hairline position. Measurements are made from the nasion (as opposed to the glabella) to the subnasale and from the subnasale to the menton (Figure 21-9). With this method the midface represents 43% of the height, with the lower face representing 57%.

SUBUNIT ANALYSIS

The face is divided into aesthetic units (Figure 21-10) that are further divided into subunits. The major units that are classically defined for facial analysis include the forehead, eyes, nose, lips, chin, ears, and neck. The units and subunits are based on skin thickness, color, texture, and underlying structural contour. Precise planning of surgical incisions and reconstructions require analysis of the entire unit or subunit. Incisions parallel to relaxed skin tension lines (Figure 21-11) and within unit or subunit borders result in the most favorable scars.

Forehead

The boundaries of the forehead are from the hairline to the glabella and make up the upper third of the face. The contour anatomy of the forehead is most aesthetically pleasing with a gentle convexity on profile. The nasofrontal angle (Figure 21-12) is created by a line tangent to the glabella through the nasion and intersecting with a line tangent to the nasal dorsum. The range of aesthetic measurements for this angle is from 115 to 135 degrees.

The ideal eyebrow shape follows a smooth and gently curving arc. The brow should begin medially with a slight clublike configuration and gradually taper toward its lateral end. Lateral position for a female is well above the supraorbital rim, whereas for a male it is at or close to the rim. The medial edge of the eyebrow lies on a perpendicular line that passes through the lateralmost portion of the nasal ala and approximately 10 mm above the medial canthus (Figure 21-13). In women, the highest point of the eyebrow arc is at a line drawn tangentially from the lateral limbus. However, this ideal eyebrow position can vary with fashion trends, and the highest point may actually lie anywhere from the lateral limbus to the lateral canthus. Sheen[8] describes the eyebrow arc as most pleasing when it extends as an unbroken line from the brow down to the lateral nasal tip (Figure 21-14).

Eyes

The boundaries of the orbits are in the lower third of the upper face and the upper third of the midface. The width of one eye from medial to lateral canthus should

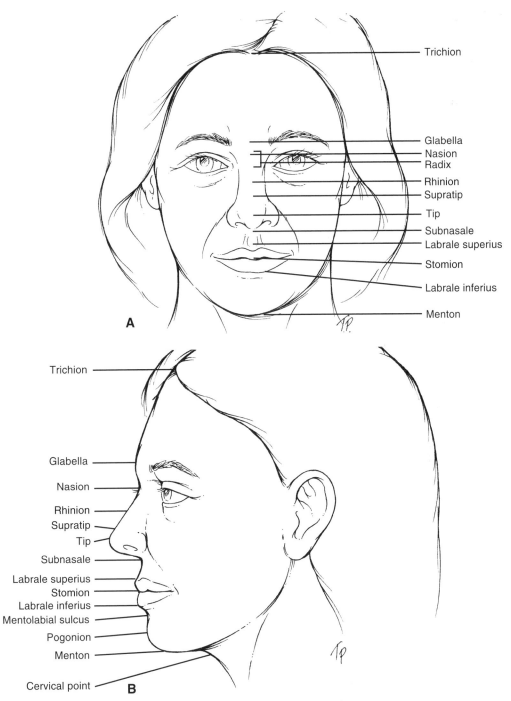

Figure 21-3. Soft tissue reference points.

equal one fifth of the facial width. The intercanthal distance should equal the width of one eye. Normal intercanthal distances for women and men are 25.5 to 37.5 mm and 26.5 to 38.7 mm, respectively. In general, the eye should be almond shaped with the lateral canthus slightly more superior than the medial canthus. The average palpebral opening is 10 to 12 mm in height and 28 to 30 mm in width. The upper lid crease is the line created by the insertion of the levator aponeurosis and orbital septum into the orbicularis oculi and dermis. The location of the crease averages approximately 11 mm from the lash line but can vary between 7 and 15 mm. The upper eyelid normally covers a small portion of the iris but not the pupil. The lower eyelid is within 1 to 2 mm of the iris on neutral gaze, with the sclera not being visible below the iris margin.

BOX 21-1
SOFT TISSUE ANATOMIC LANDMARKS

Trichion (Tr): Anterior hairline in the midline

Glabella (G): Most prominent point of the forehead on profile

Nasion (N): The deepest depression at the root of the nose; typically corresponds to the nasofrontal suture

Radix: Root of the nose, a region and not a point; part of an unbroken curve that begins at the superior orbital ridge and continues along the lateral nasal wall

Rhinion (R): Soft-tissue correlate of the osseocartilaginous junction on the nasal dorsum

Sellion: Osseocartilaginous junction on the nasal dorsum

Supratip: Point cephalic to the tip

Tip (T): Ideally, the most anterior projection of the nose on profile

Subnasale (Sn): Junction of columella and upper lip

Labrale superius (Ls): Vermilion border of upper lip

Stomion (S): Central portion of interlabial gap
  Stomion superius: Lowest point of upper lip vermilion
  Stomion inferius: Highest point of lower lip vermilion

Labrale inferius (Li): Vermilion border of lower lip

Mentolabial sulcus (Si): Most posterior point between lower lip and chin

Pogonion (Pg): Most anterior midline soft-tissue point of chin

Menton (Me): Most inferior soft-tissue point on chin

Cervical point (C): The innermost point between the submental area and the neck

BOX 21-2
CEPHALOMETRIC REFERENCE POINTS

(S) Sella: The midpoint of the hypophysial fossa

(Or) Orbitale: The most inferior point on the infraorbital rim

(P) Porion: The most superior point on the external auditory meatus

(Cd) Condylion: The most superior point on the head of the mandibular condyle

(Ar) Articulate: The point of intersection of the posterior margin of the ascending mandibular ramus and the outer margin of the cranial base

(ANS) Anterior nasal spine

(PNS) Posterior nasal spine

(A) Point A, subspinale: The deepest point in the concavity of the premaxilla

(Pr) Prosthion: The lowest most anterior point on the alveolar portion of the premaxilla

(Id) Infradentale: The highest most anterior point on the alveolar portion of the mandible

(B) Point B, supramentale: The most posterior point in the outer contour of the mandibular alveolar process

(Pg) Pogonion: Most anterior point on the bony chin in the midline

(Gn) Gnathion: A point between the most anterior (Pg) and inferior (Me) point on the chin

(Me) Menton: The lowest point on the mandible

(Go) Gonion: The midpoint at the angle of the mandible

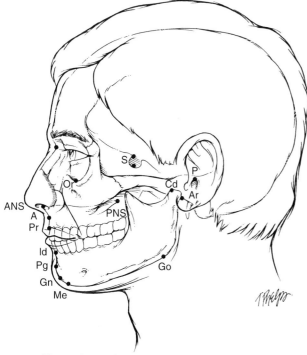

Figure 21-4. Cephalometric reference points.

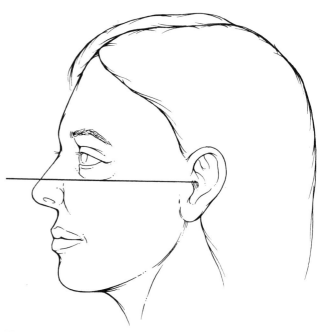

Figure 21-5. Frankfort horizontal plane. A line is drawn from the superior aspect of the external auditory canal to the most inferior aspect of the infraorbital rim.

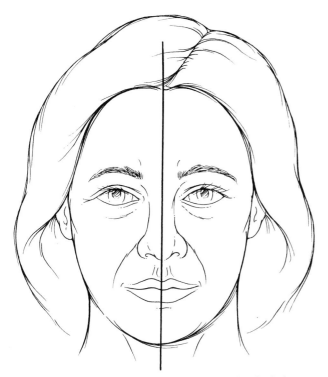

Figure 21-6. Facial symmetry through midsagittal plane.

Nose

The boundaries of the nose are within the middle third of the face. On the lateral view, the nasal starting point begins at the nasion, which ideally corresponds to the same level as the upper eyelid's superior palpebral fold (see Figure 21-3) and ends at the subnasale. Because the nose is the central and most prominent aesthetic unit of the face, it is always analyzed in relationship to other facial structures, most importantly the chin, lips, and eyebrows. The topographic subunits of the nose (see Figure 21-15) have been described by Burget[1] and are essential when planning reconstructive procedures. The borders of nasal subunits allow for scar camouflage when incisions lie along subunit margins.

Nasofacial Relationships

Powell and Humphreys[7] formulated relationships between the nose and face. They include the nasofrontal angle, nasolabial angle, nasofacial angle, and nasomental angle. The nasofrontal angle (see Figure 21-12) has been previously described in the forehead section of this chapter. The nasolabial angle defines the angular inclination of the columella as it meets the upper lip. The angle is formed between the intersection of a line tangent to the labrale superius and subnasale and a line tangent to the subnasale and the most anterior point of the columella (see Figure 21-16). This angle should measure 95 to 110 degrees

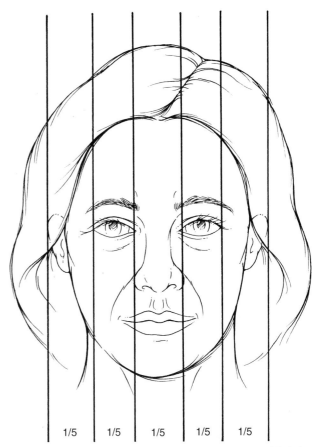

Figure 21-7. Facial width. The facial width is divided into equal fifths.

in women and 90 to 95 degrees in men. The nasofacial angle is the incline of the nasal dorsum in relation to the facial plane (see Figure 21-17). It represents the angle formed from a vertical line tangent from the glabella through the pogonion intersecting a line from the nasion through the nasal tip. This angle ideally measures 36 degrees but can vary from 30 to 40 degrees. The nasomental angle describes the angle between a tangent line from the nasion to the nasal tip intersecting with a line from the tip to the pogonion (see Figure 21-18). The range of this angle is from 120 to 132 degrees, and it can clearly be obscured if the chin or lip position is in facial disharmony.

Nasal Rotation and Projection

Nasal rotation and projection are essential measurements in determining nasal aesthetics. Tip rotation generally occurs along an arc produced by a radius based at the external auditory canal (Figure 21-19). Rotation increases along the upper portion of the arc and decreases along the lower portion. Several methods have been used to analyze tip projection and, in turn, have defined nasal length. Simons[9] measures tip

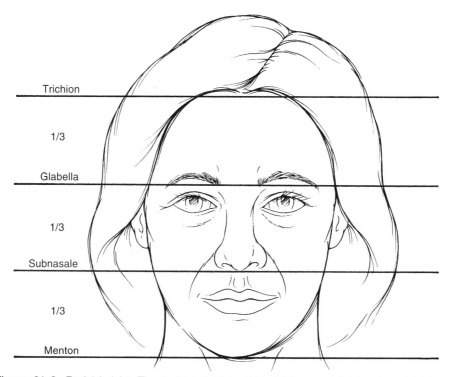

Trichion

1/3

Glabella

1/3

Subnasale

1/3

Menton

Figure 21-8. Facial height. The facial height is divided into equal thirds. From trichion to glabella, from glabella to subnasale, and from subnasale to menton.

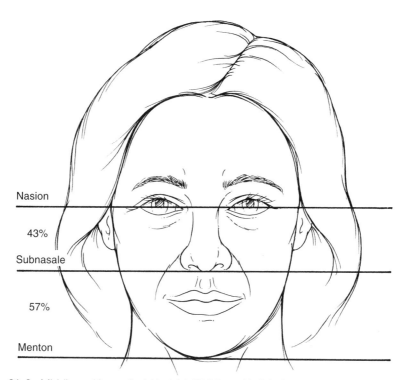

Nasion

43%

Subnasale

57%

Menton

Figure 21-9. Middle and lower facial height. Division of height is unequal and measured from the nasion to subnasale and from the subnasale to the menton.

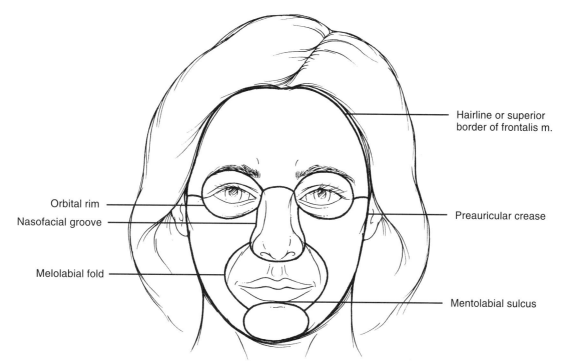

Figure 21-10. Aesthetics units of the face.

Hairline or superior border of frontalis m.

Orbital rim

Nasofacial groove

Preauricular crease

Melolabial fold

Mentolabial sulcus

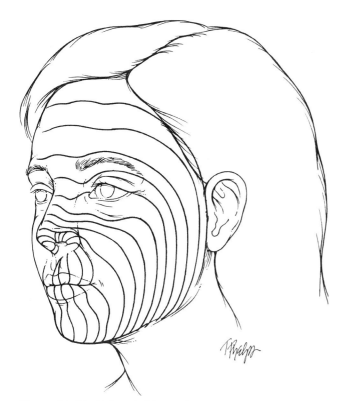

Figure 21-11. Relaxed skin tension lines (RSTL) of the face.

projection in relation to the length of the upper lip (see Figure 21-20). Nasal projection is approximately equal to the length of the upper lip, giving a ratio of 1:1.

Goode's[7] method uses a vertical line drawn from the nasion to the alar groove, a perpendicular line from the alar groove to the nasal tip, and a line from the tip back to the nasion (see Figure 21-21). The ratio comparing the length of the perpendicular line (alar groove to tip) with that of the nasal length (nasion to tip) should be 0.55 to 0.60. When these ratios are observed, the nasofacial angle is approximately 36 degrees. Crumley[2] uses a similar method and uses a 3-4-5 triangle, where the hypotenuse is the nasal length and the projection is the smallest arm of the triangle.

Alar–Columellar Complex

On lateral view, the ala-to-tip lobular complex ratio is considered optimal at 1:1 (see Figure 21-22, *A*). Columella show of 3 to 5 mm is considered acceptable (see Figure 21-22, *B*). From the basal view, the nose should be triangular in shape and divided into three equivalent units (see Figure 21-23).

Lips

The boundaries of the lips are contained within the lower one third of the face. The upper lip is measured from the subnasale to the stomion superius, whereas the lower lip and chin are measured from the stomion inferius to the menton (see Figure 21-24). The subunits of the lip are well defined (see Figure 21-25), whereas the height of the upper lip to the lower lip should have a ratio of approximately 1:2. Horizontal lip position can be determined by two separate methods. The first

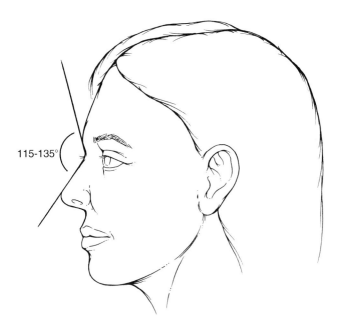

Figure 21-12. Nasofrontal angle (115–135 degrees).

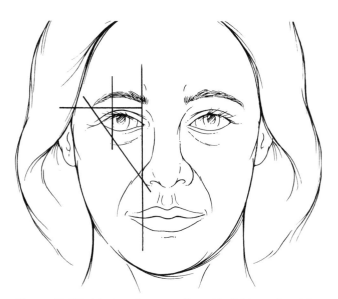

Figure 21-13. Ideal eyebrow position. Medial brow head lies along horizontal tangent with medial canthus and nasal ala. Highest point of brow arch is located above lateral limbus.

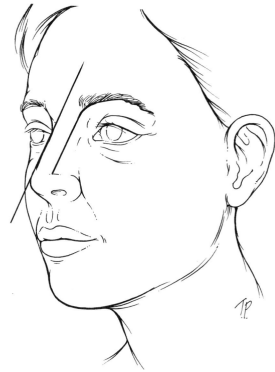

Figure 21-14. Unbroken aesthetic line form eyebrow to nasal tip.

constructs a line from the subnasale through the labrale inferius to the pogonion (see Figure 21-26). A perpendicular line through the anteriormost point of each lip defines its horizontal position. The upper and lower lip should lie 3.5 and 2.2 mm anterior to this line, respectively. The second method uses the nasomental angle to determine horizontal lip position.

The lips should fall just behind this line at a distance of 4 mm for the upper lip and 2 mm for the lower lip (see Figure 21-18).

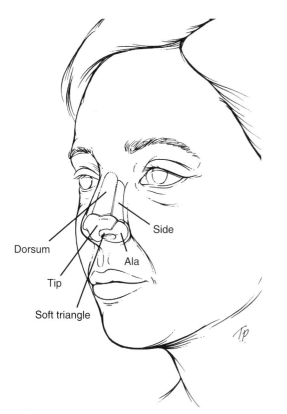

Figure 21-15. Nasal aesthetic subunits adapted from Burget.

Chin

The boundaries of the chin lie in the lower one third of the face and can be measured from the mentolabial crease to the menton. The chin is a pivotal facial unit

when analyzing the nose or neck. Most rhinoplasty analysis begins with proper chin position in relation to nasal projection and facial harmony. Gonzales-Ulloa[6] described the ideal chin position by a tangential line through the nasion to pogonion, which is almost perpendicular to the Frankfort horizontal plane (see Figure 21-27). An alternative method for analyzing chin position has already been described in the lip section (see Figure 21-26), where the mentolabial sulcus lies approximately 4 mm behind this line.

Neck

The ideal neck has a well-defined mandible from the pogonion to the angle with an acute mentocervical angle. This angle is produced by drawing a line from the glabella to the pogonion and intersecting with a line tangent from the menton to the cervical point (see Figure 21-28). The cervical point is defined as the innermost point between the submentum and neck. It is also important to evaluate chin position when analyzing the neck, because an obtuse mentocervical angle may cause the perception of poor chin projection.

Ears

The width of the ear is approximately one half its length. The ear length should approximate the length of the nose measured from the nasion to the subnasale. The superior aspect of the ear lies at the level of the eyebrow, whereas its inferior aspect is at the level of the nasal ala. The long axis of the ear is parallel to the long axis of the nasal dorsum (see Figure 21-29) and is noted to have a posterior rotation

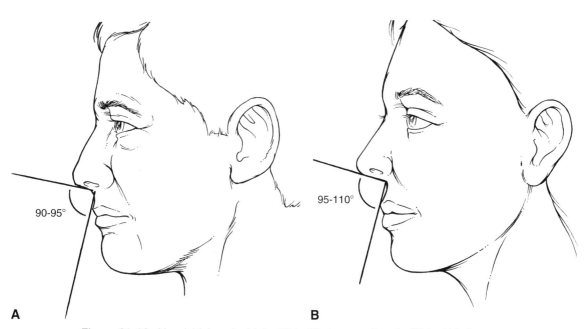

A   **B**

Figure 21-16. Nasolabial angle. Male, 90 to 95 degrees; female, 95 to 110 degrees.

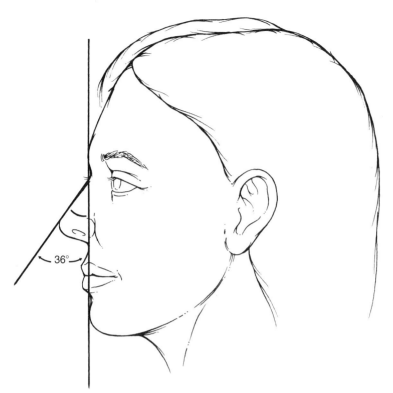

Figure 21-17. Nasofacial angle (30 to 40 degrees).

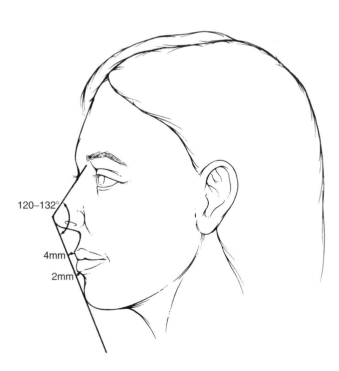

Figure 21-18. Nasomental angle (120–132 degrees). The lips should fall just behind this line at a distance of 4 mm for the upper lip and 2 mm for the lower lip.

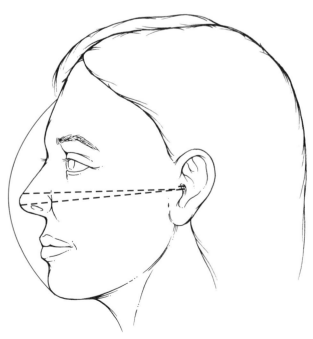

Figure 21-19. Tip rotation generally occurs along an arc produced by a radius based at the external auditory canal.

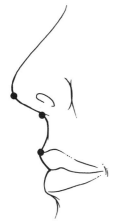

Figure 21-20. Simon's nasal projection is approximately equal to the length of the upper lip with a ratio of 1:1.

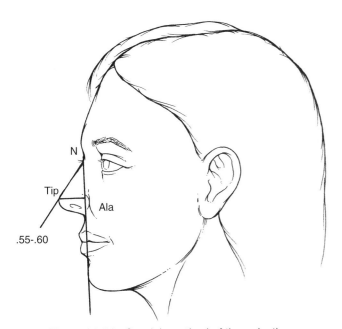

Figure 21-21. Goode's method of tip projection.

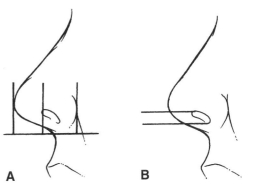

Figure 21-22. Nasal ala. Ala-to-tip lobular ratio should be 1:1. Columella shown between 3 and 5 mm.

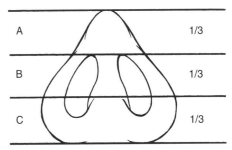

Figure 21-23. Nasal base divided into equal thirds.

Fitzpatrick[4] established skin type classification (Box 21-3), and in 1994, Glogau[5] categorized photoaged skin (see Box 21-4). Most importantly, however, in the examination of the skin is the analysis of facial rhytids. Wrinkles or rhytids originate from a wide variety of sources that can include chronologic aging, photoaging or solar damage, and skin folding secondary to loss of underlying skeletal or soft tissue support. Hyperdynamic facial lines (see Figure 21-30) are specific wrinkles that are caused by long-term facial muscle animation. Examples of these include horizontal forehead creases, crow's feet, and glabellar lines. Each line is caused by repeated underlying muscle contraction. Hyperdynamic lines should be distinguished from other facial lines such as the melolabial fold, mentolabial sulcus, and the fine crisscross wrinkling found on the cheek and under the eyelids.

COMPUTER IMAGING AND DIGITAL PHOTOGRAPHY

Technologic advances in digital photography and computer graphics have revolutionized the way many surgeons obtain and process patient photographs. The immediate availability of photographs for review and the ability to generate computer-modified images provide an easy and effective means of preoperative analysis. Routine office consultations typically include

of approximately 15 degrees from the vertical plane. The ear protrudes from the skull at an angle of approximately 20 to 30 degrees, which usually translates into a measurement of 15 to 25 mm from the helix to the mastoid skin.

Skin and Rhytids

When analyzing the face, evaluation of the skin deserves special attention. Skin texture, thickness, elasticity, and solar damage are all critical factors contributing to one's overall facial appearance. In 1988,

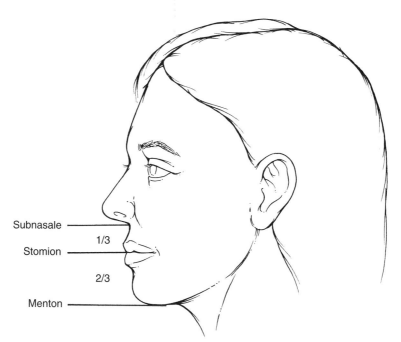

Subnasale

1/3

Stomion

2/3

Menton

Figure 21-24. Lip ratio and lower facial third.

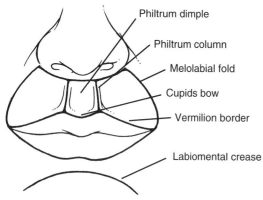

Philtrum dimple

Philtrum column

Melolabial fold

Cupids bow

Vermilion border

Labiomental crease

Figure 21-25. Lip aesthetic subunits.

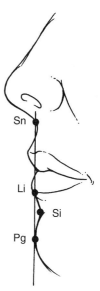

Sn

Li

Si

Pg

Figure 21-26. Horizontal lip position. Mentolabial sulcus (Si) should lie 4 mm posterior to a vertical line dropped from the subnasale through the labrale inferius (Li) and extending to the to the pogonion (Pg).

"patient imaging," which has become a vital tool toward preoperative education. It provides the surgeon an opportunity to strengthen communication with the patient regarding realistic expectations of surgical outcome. Added benefits of computer imaging also include photoarchiving and its use as an instructional tool for residents and fellows. Over the past few years, this technology has evolved from being costly, cumbersome, and slow to one that is highly efficient, user-friendly, and reasonably priced.

The essential components for a computer imaging system include a computer, an image capture device or camera, and imaging software. Computer specifications are dependent on the demands and expectations of the surgeon; however, current system requirements needed to operate high-end digital imaging software include a Pentium III processor, 256-MB RAM, a 32-bit graphics card, and a minimum of a 40-MB hard drive. Additional components that are highly recommended

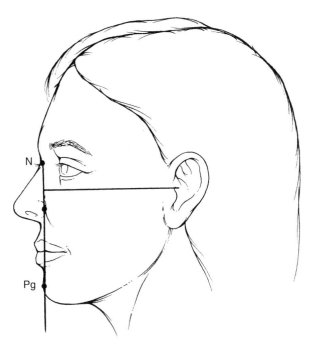

Figure 21-27. The zero meridian of Gonzalez-Ulloa. Ideal chin position is on a vertical line from the nasion (N) to the pogonion (Pg), which is perpendicular to the Frankfort horizontal.

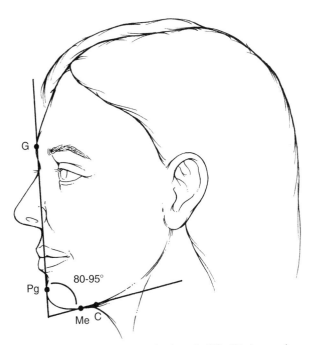

Figure 21-28. Mentocervical angle (80–95 degrees).

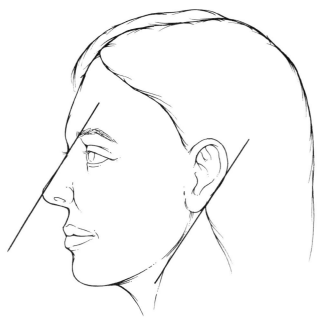

Figure 21-29. Long axis of the ear parallels the long axis of the nasal dorsum.

BOX 21-3

FITZPATRICK CLASSIFICATION OF SUN-REACTIVE SKIN TYPE

Skin type	Skin color	Characteristics
I	White	Always burns, never tans
II	White	Usually burns, tans with difficulty
III	White	Sometimes burns, sometimes tans
IV	White	Rarely burns, tans with ease
V	Brown	Very rarely burns, tans very easily
VI	Black	Never burns, always tans

BOX 21-4

GLOGAU PHOTOAGING CLASSIFICATION

Type I: No keratoses, few wrinkles, age 20 to 30, rarely wears makeup

Type II: Early lentigenes, wrinkles on animation, age 30 to 40, sometimes wears makeup

Type III: Advanced photoaging, wrinkles present at rest, age 50 to 60, always wears makeup

Type IV: Severe photoaging, severe wrinkling, age 60 to 70, makeup has minimal benefit

---

include a CD burner for archiving and storage, a graphics board, digital drawing tablet, and a high-resolution color printer.

As with 35-mm photography, the clarity of digital photography is dependent on the sophistication of the camera and its lens. The resolution of digital cameras is described in pixels, and it currently ranges up to 6.0 mega pixels. However, a camera containing 3.0 mega pixels is sufficiently suited for the demands

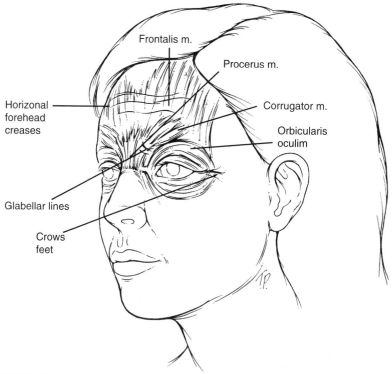

Figure 21-30. Hyperdynamic facial lines caused by repeated underlying muscle contraction.

of most medical photography. A 3.0-mega pixel image printed on 4 × 6-inch glossy photo paper is nearly indistinguishable from a conventional photograph. The Nikon Coolpix 4500 and the Canon G3 Powershot are examples of high-end consumer "point-and-shoot" cameras. These 4.0-mega pixel digital cameras cost less than $1000 and would satisfy most surgeon's needs. For a more professional look with 35-mm like quality and control, the Fuji FinePix S2 Digital Camera is a true single lens reflex (SLR) with 6.0 mega pixels (see Figure 21-31). The additional capabilities include interchangeable lenses and through-the-lens (TTL) metering. The price for advanced digital cameras has dropped dramatically over the past several years, and they can now be purchased for as little as $2000 to $3000. Lighting, background, and patient positioning are similar to conventional photography with 35-mm cameras.

Once the photograph images are downloaded onto the computer, a variety of image or graphics software may be used to open and alter images. The Mirror Suite (Image Management plus Simulation) (Canfield Scientific, Inc., Fairfield, NJ) is sophisticated but user-friendly high-end software designed for medical professionals. Image files from the camera once downloaded are automatically tethered into the Mirror Software and saved into patients' charts. The ease and

speed of image alteration lies at the heart of this sophisticated software, making patient consultations streamline and informative. Furthermore, this advanced software has the ability to measure and analyze facial angles for assistance in preoperative analysis and planning (see Figure 21-32). The cost of such commercially available systems, complete with computer, camera, and software will be several thousands of dollars. More basic systems, however, may be pieced together by a physician to maintain a more modest price point.

Computer imaging and its ability to generate altered images for patient education can be particularly helpful during the preoperative rhinoplasty consultation. Computer-generated changes are compared with preoperative images and reviewed with the patient. The surgeon must be conservative with computer-generated changes and avoid overzealous alterations. In this manner, realistic expectations are nurtured, and a common outcome concept can be reached between surgeon and patient. Computer imaging can be particularly helpful to demonstrate to the rhinoplasty patient with microgenia the added benefit of chin augmentation (see Figure 21-33). The computer-generated images assist patients in visualizing the overall improvement in facial harmony.

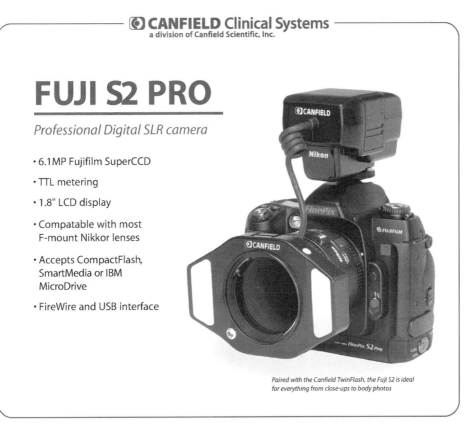

Figure 21-31. Fuji S2 pro digital SLR camera with Canfield twin flash.

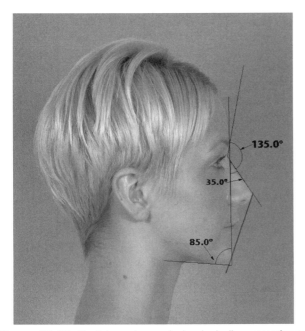

Figure 21-32. Facial angle analysis, including nasofrontal angle, nasofacial angle, and mentocervical angle. (Courtesy of Canfield Clinical Systems.)

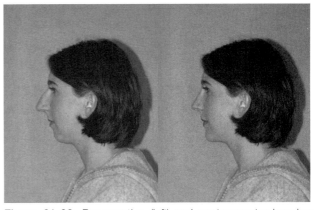

Figure 21-33. Preoperative *(left)* and postcomputer imaging *(right)* of combined rhinoplasty and chin augmentation. (Courtesy of Canfield Clinical Systems.)

REFERENCES

1. Burget GC: Aesthetic restoration of the nose, *Clin Plast Surg* 12:463, 1985.
2. Crumley RL, Lanser M: Quantitative analysis of nasal tip projection, *Laryngoscope* 98:202, 1988.
3. Farkas LG and others: Vertical and horizontal proportions of the face in young adult North American Caucasians: revision of neoclassical cannons, *Plast Reconstr Surg* 75:328, 1985.

4. Fitzpatrick TB: The validity and practicality of sun reactive skin types I through VI, *Arch Dermatol* 124:869, 1988.

5. Glogau RG: Chemical peeling and aging skin, *J Geriatr Dermatol* 2:30, 1994.

6. Gonzalez-Ulloa M: Quantitative principles in cosmetic surgery of the face (profileplasty), *Plast Reconstr Surg* 29:186, 1962.

7. Powell N, Humphreys B: *Proportions of the aesthetic face*, New York, Thieme-Stratton, 1984.

8. Sheen JH: *Aesthetic rhinoplasty*, St. Louis, Mosby, 1978.

9. Simons RL: Nasal tip projection, ptosis and supratip thickening, *Ear Nose Throat J* 61:452, 1982.

CHAPTER TWENTY TWO

RECOGNITION AND TREATMENT OF SKIN LESIONS

Ken K. Lee
Khosrow Mehrany
Neil A. Swanson

INTRODUCTION

Recognizing and treating skin lesions is an important aspect of otolaryngology–head and neck surgery. Many of the diseases that an otolaryngologist–head and neck surgeon sees can involve the skin. Whether they are a patient's chief complaint or are noted on a routine examination, skin lesions need be recognized so that proper diagnosis and management are instituted.

This chapter is structured to provide the otolaryngologist–head and neck surgeon with practical knowledge about the differential diagnosis of cutaneous tumors by the physician, including epidermal tumors, melanocytic tumors, cystic lesions, vascular tumors, and fibroadnexal tumors. Within the discussions of the various tumor categories are reviews of the preferred therapeutic options for each specific tumor. At the end of the chapter is a discussion of treatment methods and biopsy techniques commonly used by the dermatologist and cutaneous surgeon that can easily be applied by the otolaryngologist–head and neck surgeon. The details of various biopsy techniques used to establish a histologic diagnosis are stressed, because the pathologist's ability to establish a definitive diagnosis depends directly on the clinical specimen obtained for histopathologic review.

An in-depth discussion of all types of cutaneous tumors (benign and malignant) is beyond the scope of this chapter. The recognition of the three most common cutaneous malignancies will be discussed, with detailed chapters concerning these tumors to follow. The treatments of basal cell carcinoma and squamous cell carcinoma are discussed in Chapter 25; Chapter 26 details the current status of the treatment of malignant melanoma. This chapter will serve only to introduce these three tumors.

EPIDERMAL NEOPLASMS

Epithelial neoplasms of the skin can range from entirely benign to highly malignant tumors. Epidermal tumors are so common that few people go through life without acquiring at least one. A great assortment of epidermal tumors have been described, under a wide variety of names; the more common and important ones will be discussed in this chapter.[34]

Three important factors relevant to epidermal tumors should be noted. First, the epidermis in the healthy person is a relatively thin structure and is the outermost layer of the skin. Hyperproliferation of an epidermal cell results in tumors that usually appear superficially and that are often associated with scale. Dermal tumors and tumors of the cutaneous appendages (adnexal tumors) are usually deeper and, therefore, more nodular in appearance. Recognizing these differences is one general way of differentiating between the two tumor groups. The second important factor is that there are three types of lesions that occur within epidermal tumors: benign, precancerous, and cancerous. The precise nature of precancerous lesions has been debated widely, but the term persists in the literature; it refers to a group of epidermal lesions of which a small percentage can become malignant. Finally, because the epidermis is limited in the number of ways it can respond to stimuli, the clinical presentations of many tumors will be similar. Even the most experienced dermatologist often has to resort to a biopsy for the definitive diagnosis of an epidermal tumor.[41]

Seborrheic Keratoses

Seborrheic keratoses, which are very common lesions, usually begin around the fourth decade of life. They can be single or multiple and can occur anywhere on the body, with the exception of the palms and soles. Clinically, they are sharply demarcated and slightly raised, appearing as if they were stuck on the skin's surface (see Figure 22-1). Many have a verrucous surface with a soft, friable consistency; however, others

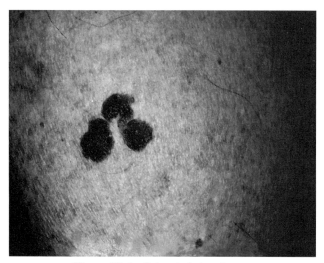

Figure 22-1. Seborrheic keratoses.

may have a smooth surface. Characteristically, all seborrheic keratoses show keratotic plugs on careful surface inspection. Their color is usually brownish to brown-black, although it can vary from flesh color to deep black. The color within the individual lesion is usually uniform. Lesions can measure from a few millimeters to several centimeters. When subjected to trauma, they can become irritated, thereby causing an inflammatory base and occasional bleeding. Occasionally, seborrheic keratoses are pedunculate, especially on the neck.[54]

The etiology of seborrheic keratoses is unknown, although they may be dominantly inherited. They are benign with no malignant potential, although the appearance of hundreds in rapid "showers" may be a sign of internal malignancy; this is the much-debated Leser-Trélat sign. The most common tumor seen in this association is colonic adenocarcinoma.[47]

In the head and neck, the most common mistaken diagnosis is melanoma; therefore, the pathologist sometimes receives a widely excised seborrheic keratosis that has been mistaken for melanoma. If the diagnosis is in doubt, a biopsy before definitive treatment should be performed.

Treatment of these lesions varies. Because these lesions are so superficial, they often can be excised flush with the skin, using any of the shaving techniques described later in this chapter. These lesions also are amenable to light liquid nitrogen freezing, which creates a subepidermal blister and allows for removal of the keratosis with the blister. Because these are truly benign lesions, the best treatment is often no treatment, unless the lesions are cosmetically disfiguring.[54]

Dermatosis Papulosa Nigra

Dermatosis papulosa nigra is a condition found in approximately 35% of black adults; its onset often occurs during adolescence. The lesions are located predominantly on the face, especially in the malar region, but they may also occur infrequently on the neck and upper trunk. They consist of small (1–3 mm), smooth, pigmented, stuck-on appearing, hyperkeratotic papules, which have the histologic appearance of seborrheic keratoses but are smaller. Most clinicians consider these papules to be a variant of seborrheic keratoses.

The treatment of dermatosis papulosa nigra is difficult because of pigmentary problems in the treatment of black skin. Options that have been tried include fine-needle electrosurgery followed by use of a small curette, light freezing with liquid nitrogen, and dermabrasion. If the lesions are few, the authors prefer the first method. Cryosurgery can produce spotted hypopigmentation in blacks and should be avoided unless other treatment modalities are not available. Dermabrasion can be of two types: using either a 2-mm wheel or a small cone or pear diamond fraise, the lesions can be removed singly, very quickly, and easily. Dermabrasion can also result in mottled pigmentation after healing, which usually will fade with time. If the lesions are multiple and confluent, total regional dermabrasion may be the treatment of choice for the best cosmetic blend.[32]

Warts (Verruca Vulgaris)

Warts are common lesions caused by the human papillomavirus (HPV), which is a deoxyribonucleic acid (DNA) virus. Warts can be classified in three ways. The traditional classification, which is based on the clinical appearance and location, is as follows: (1) verruca vulgaris, or common wart, including the filiform wart; (2) deep hyperkeratotic palmar-plantar wart; (3) superficial mosaic-type palmar-plantar wart; (4) verruca plana; (5) epidermodysplasia verruciform; and (6) condyloma acuminaturn. The second classification is based on histology. The third and most recent classification is based on the presence of several antigenic types of papilloma viruses, each with a distinct DNA genome and type-specific antigen. Serotypes have been added.[16]

The most common facial warts include common warts, flat warts (verruca plana), and filiform warts. These warts would be most commonly associated with the antigenic serotypes HPV-2 and HPV-3. Clinically, these lesions are hyperkeratotic. The filiform wart is often a pedunculate lesion occurring in isolation on the cheek, nasal tip or columella, or eyelid (Figure 22-2). Common warts can occur anywhere on the face. Flat warts usually occur in younger patients; they are small (1–2 mm), flat-topped, hyperkeratotic lesions, which can coalesce (Figure 22-3).[24]

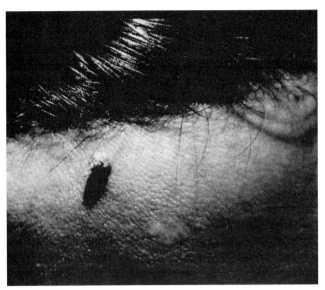

Figure 22-2. Filiform warts.

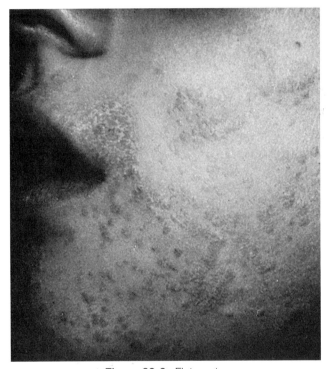

Figure 22-3. Flat warts.

Treatment of these warts is at times difficult. The filiform wart can be anesthetized at its base and excised with scissors, with the base being lightly curetted and fulgurated under low current; this approach affords the best chance for cure. Filiform warts often are too verrucous and hyperkeratotic to be effectively treated with cryosurgery. Common warts, when not too verrucous, can be treated effectively with liquid nitrogen cryotherapy, although several treatments are usually needed. Flat warts present

a difficult problem. At times, they can be effectively treated with liquid nitrogen. Perhaps the best method is to individually scrape each small wart off of the skin with a small curette, treating, when possible, all of the flat warts in an area at one time. In young children who do not tolerate surgical therapy well, one may use topical tretinoin at a concentration sufficient to produce erythema and irritation in an attempt to stimulate the body's own immunity against the wart virus. At times, avoiding treatment is best, because the vast majority of warts will spontaneously involute once the patient's immune system recognizes the virus.

Related to the poxvirus family is a group of viruses known as the molluscum contagiosum virus family (EM-2). An infection with one of these viruses appears clinically as a variable number of small, discrete, waxy, skin-colored, dome-shaped papillomas, 2 to 4 mm in diameter, with umbilicated centers (Figure 22-4). Like all viral lesions, they ultimately will involute spontaneously. Histologically, they have a classic appearance of cytoplasmic inclusion bodies, which are the so-called molluscum bodies. The best treatment is usually superficial cryotherapy or curettage, as is the case with common warts.[49] Imiquimod cream (Aldara; 3M, St. Paul, MN) has been successfully used for the treatment of warts and mollusca.

Actinic Keratoses

Actinic keratoses, which are sometimes called solar keratoses, are precancerous lesions. Studies indicate that from 5% to 20% of persons with solar keratoses will develop squamous cell carcinoma in one or more of the lesions. As the name implies, actinic keratoses

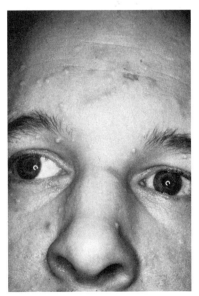

Figure 22-4. Molluscum contagiosum.

result solely from solar damage. They are seen on sun-exposed areas of the skin, usually in persons after the fourth decade of life. They are seen most commonly in fair-skinned individuals who frequently burn. Clinically, these lesions are usually erythematous with covering adherent scale and show little or no infiltration (i.e., they are very superficial) (Plate 1, A). A patient often can feel the rough, adherent scale before the lesion is clinically visible. Solar keratoses can be flesh colored or pigmented. They often do not have a sharp demarcation from surrounding skin and can spread peripherally. Occasionally these lesions develop marked hyperkeratosis, giving a clinical appearance of a cutaneous horn. On the vermillion

lip, actinic keratosis is known as solar or actinic cheilitis.

Actinic keratoses lesions are best removed and not watched. The most commonly used method for removing discrete lesions is cryosurgery. Shave excision can also be performed, but it would lead to extensive scarring in areas with numerous lesions. In persons with severe sun damage to the face or with diffuse actinic keratoses, topical 5-fluorouracil (Efudex; Valeant Pharmaceuticals International, Costa Mesa, Calif) is effective for the treatment of a region or the entire face. Imiquimod cream (Aldara; 3M, St. Paul, Minn) and topical tretinoin have also been shown to be effective. Because proper use results

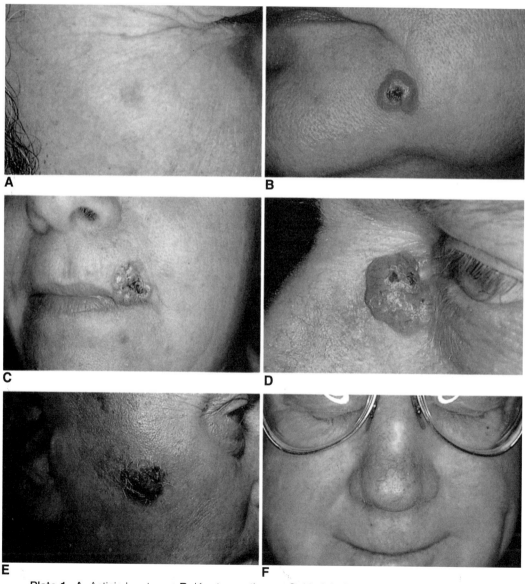

Plate 1. A, Actinic keratoses. B, Keratoacanthoma. C, Noduloulcerative basal cell carcinoma. D, Nodular basal cell carcinoma. E, Pigmented basal cell carcinoma. F, Morpheaform basal cell carcinoma.

in severe irritation, sound patient understanding and education and physician reassurance are necessary to ensure adequate compliance. A full-face dermabrasion, chemical peel, or laser resurfacing are also good methods of treatment for severe, diffuse cases.[9]

Basal Cell Carcinoma

Basal cell carcinoma is the most common malignancy in humans. It accounts for approximately 65% of all epithelioid tumors, for 20% of all cancers in men, and for 10% to 15% of all cancers in women. Depending on the study cited, approximately 86% of lesions occur initially in the head and neck, with 25% of all primary lesions occurring on the nose. Approximately 96% of recurrences are in the head and neck, with 38% being on the nose. Emmet reported that 75.5% of previously untreated basal cell carcinoma found in Australia occurred in the head and neck, 8.4% on the chest and back, and 16% on the arms and legs. When looking at recurrent tumors, Emmet found that 91% occurred on the head and neck, 7.5% on the chest and back, and 1.5% on the arms and legs. In this discussion, we will outline the epidemiology and clinical and histologic variations of basal cell carcinoma. Treatments of basal cell carcinoma and squamous cell carcinoma are addressed in detail in Chapter 25.

Basal cell carcinoma, which is more common in men than in women, is seen most frequently in individuals between the ages of 40 and 60 years. With the aging of the sunbathing generation, however, basal cell carcinomas are occurring with increasing frequency in younger people. Scandinavians and people of Celtic extraction (particularly the Irish), who frequently have Fitzpatrick Type I or Type II (sunburns easily) skin, appear to be more prone to basal cell carcinoma than those with more darkly pigmented skin.[51] Exposure to sunlight—primarily to the rays in the ultraviolet B spectrum—is the primary risk factor for basal cell carcinoma; this has been shown experimentally and reproduced clinically. The tumor is more common as one proceeds toward the equator and is also more common at high altitudes. The head and neck areas are the most common sites for basal cell carcinoma. On the head and neck, the nose is the most common site, with the nasal tip and the nasal ala being the most common locations on the nose itself; the cheeks and the forehead are the next most common sites. Basal cell carcinoma is more common on the left side of the body than on the right, perhaps because of selective sun exposure in individuals whose occupation preferentially exposes the left side (i.e., driving).[20]

Although sun exposure is the primary etiologic agent of basal cell carcinoma, other risk factors include occupation, genetic conditions, immunosuppression, and former injury. Farmers, sailors, and fishermen, because of their heavy occupationally actinic exposure, have a higher than average incidence of skin cancer. Genetic syndromes include the autosomal-dominant nevoid basal cell carcinoma syndrome and xeroderma pigmentosum. In the former, basal cell carcinomas can arise on any area of the body, with the predilection being toward sun-exposed sites, beginning at an early age and continuing throughout life. These patients also have skeletal abnormalities, including bifid ribs, jaw cysts, and frontal bossing, as well as calcified cerebra as shown on skull radiograph. Xeroderma pigmentosum, which is autosomal recessive in inheritance, is a defect in DNA repair that can result in the formation of basal cell carcinoma and other cutaneous neoplasms at a very early age, usually in response to sun exposure.

Immunosuppression (either iatrogenic or in patients with leukemias or lymphomas) has been shown to increase the incidence and aggressiveness of basal cell carcinomas. Chemical carcinogens—notably arsenic—play a tumorigenic role. The arsenic usually comes from well water that has been contaminated with arsenic, but patients with asthma, hay fever, or psoriasis may have taken arsenic as Fowler's solution. Arsenic-induced basal cell carcinomas tend to be primarily on the trunk and are accompanied by keratoses of the palms and soles, pigmentary changes, and nail changes (Mees' lines) associated with arsenic ingestion. Exposure to ionizing radiation is also an important etiologic factor; tumors can arise in areas of radiation damage, often many years after superficial radiotherapy for acne or tinea or as a depilatory at an early age. Basal cell carcinoma can arise at the edge of a scar or an area of trauma. The injury may possibly have acted as a cofactor, adding to the effect of already existing factors, such as sunlight and racial susceptibility. Smallpox vaccinations and burn scars have been associated with basal cell carcinoma.[19]

To the trained and curious eye, the clinical recognition of basal cell carcinoma is not difficult. Typically, there is a raised, nodular lesion with a smooth, clear (pearly) border and telangiectasia (Plate 1, *D*). The lesion can ulcerate and form a crust (Plate 1, *C*). A typical history involves a pimplelike lesion that bleeds and does not heal. Pruritus is a common early symptom.

Basal cell carcinoma can be pigmented (Plate 1, *E*). Even when it is pigmented, the lesion maintains the clinical features of a pearly, translucent border and telangiectasia. The superficial multicentric basal cell carcinoma is often present in the setting of actinic damage, with differing, intercommunicating extensions of tumor in a superficial histologic field.

Three forms of basal cell carcinoma are often more subtle clinically, more aggressive histologically, and more difficult to treat. Clinically, the morpheaform basal cell carcinoma (Plate 1, *F*) presents as a yellowish plaque, which develops telangiectasia, may ulcerate, and may form a sclerotic or scarlike appearance. The margins are often indistinct: Histologically, this tumor extends subclinical, fingerlike projections intradermally, which make complete excision difficult. This tumor has a scarlike, stromal matrix that gives it a very fibrous, sclerotic appearance and nature. *Recurrent* basal cell carcinoma (Plate 2, *A*) presents a varying clinical appearance, depending on the type of initial treatment. It may appear at the edge of a skin graft, within a scar created by electrosurgery, under a scar created by cryosurgery, or as a

nodule developing within a suture line. Recurrent basal cell carcinoma is often nodular and accompanied by a morpheaform or sclerotic histologic picture in the deeper portions of the tumor. This picture may represent an aggressive histologic dedifferentiation of the tumor, a factor that may partially account for its clinically aggressive behavior and resistance to treatment.[29]

The typical basal cell carcinoma that occurs in the head and neck of the middle-aged or elderly fair-skinned person is not difficult to diagnose. One must be aware, however, that this tumor has a variety of clinical appearances, can appear in young people, and can occur in areas other than the head and neck.

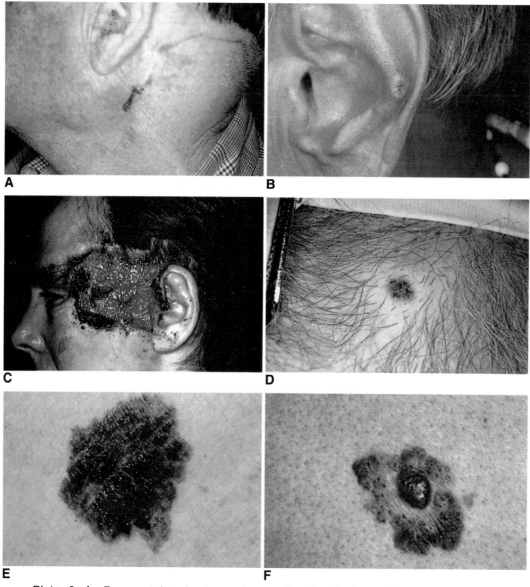

Plate 2. A, Recurrent basal cell carcinoma. **B,** Chondrodermatitis nodularis helicis. **C,** Squamous cell carcinoma. **D,** Pigmented squamous cell carcinoma. **E,** Superficial spreading melanoma. **F,** Irregular border of superficial spreading carcinoma.

Any suspicious, nonhealing, pruritic, scaly lesion—especially one that occurs in a sun-exposed area of the fair-skinned individual—should be investigated with a biopsy.

Biopsy techniques for basal cell carcinoma are simple. It has been well documented that implantation metastases from basal cell carcinoma do not occur, because the tumor needs a stroma to provide an environment in which to grow. The most appropriate technique is a medium-depth shave biopsy. The depth of the biopsy ideally should be mid-dermis; this depth gives a dermal collagen network that is amenable to any form of therapy. If a morpheaform basal cell carcinoma is suspected, the biopsy specimen often must extend deeper, perhaps through a punch or incisional biopsy. In cases of recurrent or superficial multicentric lesions or large clinical lesions, biopsy specimens should be obtained from multiple sites to assess the true clinical nature and size of the tumor. Biopsies of recurrent deep nodular lesions should be performed in an appropriate fashion to ensure an adequately deep specimen from the dermal nodule; this maneuver can be accomplished by means of an incisional biopsy or a deep-punch biopsy. As a rule of thumb, if the biopsy does not confirm the clinical opinion of basal cell carcinoma and the lesion remains suspicious, an additional biopsy of the lesion is indicated.

Chondrodermatitis nodularis helices (Plate 2, B) is an inflammatory disease of underlying helical cartilage that can mimic and be mistaken for basal cell carcinoma. The condition usually results from chronic trauma on the most protuberant portion of the ear. Surgery is the treatment of choice.[42]

Squamous Cell Carcinoma

Squamous cell carcinoma, although less common than basal cell carcinoma, is still a common neoplasm. Many of the etiologic factors are the same as for basal cell carcinoma, the most important of which is long-standing, chronic sun exposure, especially if a person has lived close to the equator or at high altitudes. Squamous cell carcinoma is more common in men than in women and is more likely to present with multiple cutaneous carcinomas. It often is found in skin adjacent to basal cell carcinomas, a fact that is indicative of similar etiologic factors for both tumors. These include actinic (solar) damage, irradiation, trauma (scars), genetic susceptibility (nevoid basal cell carcinoma syndrome and xeroderma pigmentosum), occupation, exposure to chemicals (especially arsenic), and immunosuppression.

Clinically, squamous cell carcinomas can often be separated into actinically induced squamous cell carcinomas and de novo squamous cell carcinomas. The former are the more common, arise on sun-exposed areas, and are associated with a low incidence of metastasis (<1%, in most series). The de novo lesions can be associated with some of the nonsolar etiologies for squamous cell carcinomas. Some studies suggest that de novo lesions have a higher metastatic potential (approximately 2–3%) than the actinically induced squamous cell carcinomas. The mucosal variant of the squamous cell carcinoma, seen clinically as carcinoma of the lip, has the highest metastatic potential, approaching 11% to 12% in some series; therefore, these distinctions are important in prognosis. Carcinoma of the lip is discussed in detail in Chapter 25.[26]

Squamous cell carcinoma may present clinically in any of several ways. It can present as a thick and scaly hyperkeratotic patch on the exposed surface of the body, in particular the ear, lip, or nose (Plate 2, C). The lesion may change slowly over a period of time. If the crust is removed, the base is often ulcerated and has a rolled margin. The lesion may also present as a persistent ulcer, particularly in an old scar, or as a superficial multifocal change in generally sun-damaged skin. The latter is often the most difficult lesion to diagnose, requiring several biopsies at different points. Occasionally, a squamous cell carcinoma will become a vegetative nodular lesion; this lesion often has a cystic feel and can ulcerate and progressively enlarge. Often these exophytic lesions have not invaded deeply. They all have a tendency to ulcerate and become more erosive in appearance than a basal cell carcinoma. As with basal cell carcinoma, they can become pigmented (Plate 2, D) and often appear very similar clinically to keratoacanthomas, especially when the latter are in the growth phase. However, these lesions usually grow more slowly than keratoacanthomas, thereby allowing for distinction on clinical as well as histologic grounds. When this occurs, biopsy is always indicated. The treatment of cutaneous squamous cell carcinoma, which is very similar to that of basal cell carcinoma, is discussed in depth in Chapter 25.

Bowen's disease is a variant of a squamous cell carcinoma. By definition, it is a full-thickness dysplasia of the epidermis and hence it is noninvasive; however, invasion can occur. Clinically, Bowen's disease presents as a well-demarcated, erythematous, scaly patch or plaque in sun-exposed areas. It may be very psoriasiform in nature, with psoriasis being one of the most common mistaken diagnoses. Bowen's disease carries the same etiologic implications as basal cell carcinoma and squamous cell carcinoma; it is probably the most common tumor found in patients with histories of long-term arsenic ingestion. Some studies have suggested an increased incidence of internal malignancy when Bowen's disease occurs in non–sun-exposed areas. However, reports are conflicting, and the definitive word is not in at this time.[1]

Keratoacanthoma is a rapidly growing tumor usually seen on sun-damaged skin (Plate 1, *B*). The categorization of keratoacanthoma has been controversial, but it is now thought to be a variant of squamous cell carcinoma. There are some unique features that distinguish it clinically from the common type of squamous cell carcinoma. Keratoacanthomas are characterized by a rapid proliferative phase followed by plateau, then involution. Not all keratoacanthomas, however, involute, and predicting which ones will is difficult. The involution phase can sometimes take up to one year.

Two rare clinical forms of keratoacanthomas deserve mention. The giant keratoacanthoma can reach 5 cm or more and can cause the destruction of underlying tissues. Eruptive keratoacanthomas often present as many hundreds of characteristic papules that measure 2 to 3 mm in diameter.

Keratoacanthomas can be difficult to treat. Surgical excision is the treatment of choice for most keratoacanthomas, with Mohs micrographic surgery reserved for facial lesions. Because of the involution potential of keratoacanthomas, cytotoxic agents can be used to induce involution. We favor methotrexate at a dose of 12.5 to 25 mg/mL, with approximately 0.5 to 1 cc injected into the lesion at 3- to 4-week intervals. Although complete involution may not occur, it may allow for easier surgical management by reducing the size of the tumor.

MELANOCYTIC NEOPLASMS

The melanocyte is the pigment-producing cell of the epidermis. However, many tumors of this cell line, which is embryologically from the neural crest, occur in the dermis either by migration or because crest cells fail to reach the epidermis during embryogenesis. The most common of these tumors are nevocellular nevi, and melanoma. This section discusses the clinical manifestations of melanoma and nevocellular nevi, and other tumors of melanocytes that are included in the differential diagnosis of melanoma. Chapter 26 discusses in detail the behavior and treatment of melanoma.

Malignant Melanoma

Malignant melanoma, the third most common skin cancer, is increasing in incidence throughout the world. This disease is important because it is the most lethal cutaneous neoplasm. With sophistication of the physician and patient, however, this disease can be recognized early and cured. Every effort, therefore, should be made to diagnose melanoma at its earliest stage (stage I: less than 1-mm thick). The clinical recognition of melanoma depends on four major criteria: asymmetry, border, color, and diameter—the ABCDs of melanoma. To a lesser degree, symptoms including pruritus, tingling, and bleeding are important. Changes in any of the four major criteria in connection with a preexisting mole or the continued growth of a new lesion should signal the clinician to suspect melanoma. The most significant change is one that occurs over time (weeks or months) rather than over a few days. A fairly rapid change is rarely due to malignancy but more commonly to infection or trauma.

1. *Asymmetry.* Unlike benign neoplasms, melanoma has an asymmetric shape, which means that if it could be folded, the halves would not fold evenly on each other (Plate 2, *F*). Histologically, this correlates with architectural asymmetry, which is a hallmark of melanoma diagnosis.
2. *Border.* The border of a melanoma is classically irregular and scalloped, often bending diffusely into the normal skin (Plate 2, *F*). Changes in the border of a preexisting mole are sometimes the earliest signs of transformation to melanoma, reflecting an early radial growth phase of the melanoma.
3. *Color.* Melanoma is said to be a patriotic tumor, exhibiting shades and hues of red, white, and blue. It is rarely uniform in color but often has differing hues within the same lesion (Plate 2, *E*). Blue in a lesion signifies dermal melanin; the more blue the lesion, the deeper the dermal melanin, as demonstrated by the refractile properties of the skin. One can often see shades of blue, blue-black, or blue-green within a melanoma. Red in a melanoma often indicates inflammation, and white areas indicate sites of regression.
4. *Diameter.* Melanoma is typically larger than its benign counterpart. Enlarging moles should be monitored closely or biopsied. Pigmented lesions greater than 6 mm should be scrutinized.

Changes in one or more of these important clinical criteria—as well as the other symptoms and signs—should alert one to suspect melanoma and to perform a biopsy for diagnosis.[22]

The biopsy of a melanoma is important. As will be suggested in Chapter 26, the most critical determination for judging the treatment and prognosis of stage I melanoma is the depth of invasion as defined in millimeters by Breslow or in levels by Clark.[27] The most elevated portion of a melanoma clinically is not always the deepest portion of the melanoma histologically; therefore, to give the pathologist (and thus the patient) the best chance for an accurate diagnosis and treatment recommendation, an excisional biopsy of the entire suspicious lesion should be performed. This approach allows the pathologist to step or serial section the entire specimen to determine the maximum vertical depth of the lesion. When excisional biopsy is impossible, multiple biopsies that include the most nodular area of the melanoma are the next best choice.

There are two phases of growth noted in a melanoma: a radial growth phase (centripetal growth) and a vertical growth phase. The radial growth phase involves the circumferential growth of the tumor; this type of growth is confined to the dermoepidermal junction before actual invasion. The vertical growth phase involves the invasive growth of the tumor.

The four common types of melanoma fall within a spectrum. *Lentigo maligna melanoma* occurs in the head and neck (sun-exposed areas) of elderly patients and exhibits the longest radial growth phase. This type of melanoma makes up approximately 7% of all melanomas and often carries the best prognosis. It classically begins as an irregularly pigmented, flat macule that grows very slowly over a period of several years (often a decade or more) (Plate 3, *A*). Malignant changes are evidenced by thickening and the development of discrete tumor nodules. The lesion may ultimately grow to a diameter of several centimeters because of its extensive radial growth. When it is confined to the epidermis (in situ), the lesion is

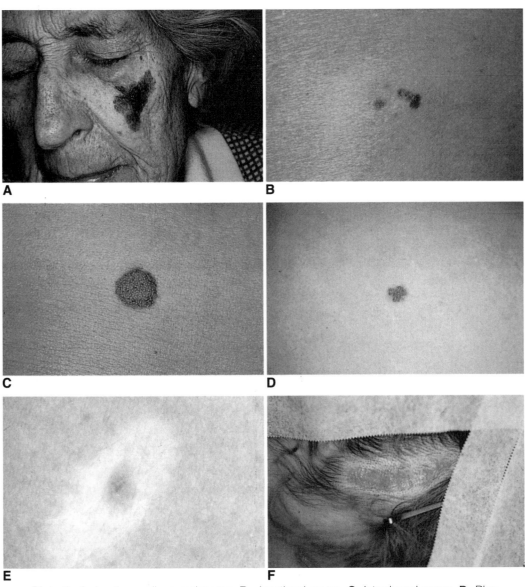

Plate 3. A, Lentigo maligna melanoma. **B,** Junctional nevus. **C,** Intradermal nevus. **D,** Blue nevus. **E,** Halo nevus. **F,** Nevus sebaceous.

called lentigo melanoma or, in older terminology, Hutchinson's freckle.

The second type in the melanoma continuum is *superficial spreading melanoma,* which is the most common form of melanoma, representing approximately 65% of cases. This tumor has variable radial and vertical growth phases, with the radial phase often existing for a period of time before nodularity and vertical growth develop. This type of melanoma occurs most commonly in the fourth and fifth decades of life, although the age is declining, as is the case with other cutaneous neoplasms, possibly because of increased sun exposure. This is the classic melanoma of multiple colors, irregular border, and nodularity (Plate 2, *E* and *F*).[40]

Next along the continuum of growth is the *acral lentiginous melanoma;* it is the most common type of melanoma seen in blacks. As implied by the name, these tumors are seen in the acral areas, including hands, feet, and oral and anogenital mucosa. These lesions make up approximately 5% to 7% of melanomas.

The last form of melanoma is *nodular melanoma,* which develops a very early vertical growth phase. It constitutes approximately 7% to 8% of melanomas and is the most invasive form. It often presents as a blue-black, polypoid, smooth surface nodule that may bleed and has a tendency toward early ulceration. By definition, it is deeply invasive, has a vertical growth phase from its inception, and is usually thicker at time of diagnosis. The prognosis of the different clinical types is the same, however, and it correlates best with the thickness of the melanoma at the time of diagnosis.[3]

Nevocellular Nevus (Mole)

Other melanocytic tumors fall into the differential diagnosis of melanoma and will be discussed in that light. They are for the most part nevocellular nevi, which are very common benign tumors that can appear shortly after birth to late in life.

Junctional Nevus

Junctional nevus is a tan to brownish macule (flat lesions) of uniform color and smooth border (Plate 3, *B*). Dots of black pigment may be present, but, unlike with melanoma, the normal skin marking are preserved. The lesion varies from a few millimeters to a centimeter or more in diameter. The melanocytes or nevus cells are located at the junction of the epidermis and the dermis (dermoepidermal junction). The lesion can occur anywhere on the body and is the nevus most commonly mistaken for melanoma. When in doubt, one should perform a biopsy of the lesion. Junctional nevi occur anytime after birth and are the common moles found in children before puberty. Their impor-

tance lies in their ability to develop into malignant melanoma, although this rarely occurs before puberty. The vast majority of junctional nevi remains benign throughout life and can evolve over time into either compound or intradermal nevi. Treatment of these nevi is often dictated by suspicion of melanoma or cosmetic reasons, and usually includes a roll shave in noncosmetic areas or a fusiform excision with closure in cosmetically important areas. Melanocytes are very cold sensitive, and a strictly junctional nevus can be removed with deep cryotherapy.

Intradermal Nevus

The intradermal nevus is the common mature mole of adults, occurring anywhere on the body but rarely on the palms and soles. It is the most common on the scalp or face in adults, varying in size from a few millimeters to several centimeters. It may be flat and smooth or raised and warty, pigmented or nonpigmented, sessile or pedunculate (Plate 3, *C*). It often contains coarse hairs, reflecting the depth within the dermis of the nevus cells. It is quite benign and rarely becomes malignant. By definition, all of the nevus cells occur within the dermis. This mole is best treated by shave excision when it is pedunculate and hairless. When it is on the head or neck and contains hair, it is necessary to excise this mole using either the punch excision technique (described later) or routine excision to remove the complete depth of the hair follicles within the nevus.[33]

Compound Nevus

The compound nevus, which is a combination of junctional and intradermal elements, is found most commonly in adults. It is a brown to black mole, usually less than 1 cm in diameter. A brown macular ring is frequently around the periphery of the lesion. It can contain hair and is often clinically indistinguishable from an intradermal nevus. Although the compound nevus, like any mole, can develop into a malignant melanoma, it usually remains benign and matures into an intradermal nevus. Treatment usually consists of shave or excision and closure. As with intradermal nevi, the choice of treatment depends on location and on the presence or absence of hair.[33]

Blue Nevus

A blue nevus may be flat or raised. These uncommon nevi present as dark blue or black hairless lesions that are less than 0.5 cm in diameter. They are usually indurated and palpable. The overlying epidermis is remarkably smooth and the outline regular (Plate 3, *D*). Blue nevi most commonly occur on the head and neck, the dorsa of the hands and feet, and the buttocks. They are more common in women than men and usually undergo very little change after their initial presentation. The treatment of these lesions is excision or observation. The excision must be deep, because the pigment often extends deep into the subcutaneous fat, thereby resulting in the deep blue color of the lesion.[46]

Halo Nevus

The halo nevus is a phenomenon usually associated with a junctional nevus in children or adolescents. Most commonly found on the back, it is often a benign-looking brown papular lesion in the center of a well-circumscribed pale white circle of depigmented skin (Plate 3, *E*). This appearance reflects the body's rejection of the nevus cells, because an inflammatory response ensues in which the melanocytes of the nevus and those of the immediately surrounding epidermis are destroyed. If left alone, these nevi will often disappear.[53]

Spitz Nevus

The Spitz nevus is also known as a juvenile melanoma or a compound melanocytoma. This rapidly growing pigmented lesion occurs principally in children, although it can occur in adults. It is usually less than 1 cm in size and is pink or red; occasionally it can be brown or black. A Spitz nevus may be soft or hard but is usually dome-shaped and can be either sessile or pedunculated. It can occur anywhere on the body and is often difficult to diagnose clinically. Its main importance is its histologic resemblance to melanoma, with even experienced pathologists having difficulty distinguishing between the two. Very few of these nevi, however, progress to malignancy. Treatment of a Spitz nevus is the same as that for an intradermal or compound nevus.[12]

Congenital Nevus

Congenital nevi are present a birth. They often are dark brown to black and contain hair, and they appear to be associated with an increased risk of the development of a malignant melanoma, especially when they are large. Most studies define "large" as lesions that are greater than 20 cm, in which case the risk of melanoma ranges from 8% to 20%. The most quoted figure is about 10%, and the highest chance of melanoma developing exists during the first two decades of life. Whether this malignant potential is due to the increased number of melanocytes or to some inherited premalignant tendency in the cells themselves is not clear. Most clinicians recommend removal during early childhood, which is often a difficult task when the lesion is very large. The treatment of choice is surgical excision, which often must be performed in stages to remove a large lesion. Dermabrasion of the lesion within the first 6 weeks of life has been proposed by some, but recent evidence suggests that such early removal is of cosmetic importance only, because a repeat biopsy of the area will show residual neural crest nevus cells.[2]

Dysplastic Nevus

Dysplastic nevus syndrome, described by Clark,[15] is also known as the B-K mole syndrome. It consists of the association of familial malignant melanoma, which often occurs in multiple lesions, with "dysplastic nevi" in both the melanoma patient and many of his or her relatives. Dysplastic nevi are usually larger than ordinary melanocytic nevi, ranging from 5 to 15 mm; they present with an irregular border and a haphazard mixture of tan, brown, black, and pink. Centrally, there is often a small, palpable component (Plate 4A). Dysplastic nevi are located on either exposed or non-exposed skin and form throughout adult life. The idea that a dysplastic nevus may transform itself into a malignant melanoma remains controversial.[18]

Solar Lentigo

Solar lentigo is not a nevocellular lesion, but it is an important entity in the diagnosis of pigmented lesions of the head and neck. Lentigo senilis commonly occurs as multiple lesions in areas exposed to sun, and it is often referred to as a solar or actinic lentigo. The lesions rarely occur before the fifth decade of life; they slowly increase in size and number; and they form in more than 90% of whites who are more than 70 years old, most commonly on the dorsa of the hands and on the face. They are not infiltrative, and they possess a uniform dark brown color and an irregular outline. Varying in size from minute to greater than 2 cm, they may coalesce to form larger lesions. Malignant degeneration does not occur. These lesions may resemble seborrheic keratoses in clinical appearance, and both conditions are referred to in lay terms as "liver spots." Lentigo senilis lesions, however, are much less hyperkeratotic than seborrheic keratoses and have no areas of follicular prominence. They are best treated with a chemical peelant such as trichloroacetic acid, with phenol, with cryosurgery using liquid nitrogen, or with a laser.[5]

Nevus Sebaceus

Nevus sebaceus is not a true nevocellular nevus. It presents clinically as a warty, pebbly, flesh-colored, hairless, well-demarcated lesion of the scalp (Plate 3, *F*); it can also present in other areas of the head and neck. Off the scalp, the lesion can be linear, closely resembling a linear epidermal nevus. The full name is "nevus sebaceus of Jadassohn." The size of this nevus varies from 0.5 cm to several centimeters. Histologically, these tumors appear in three stages. In the first few months of life, the

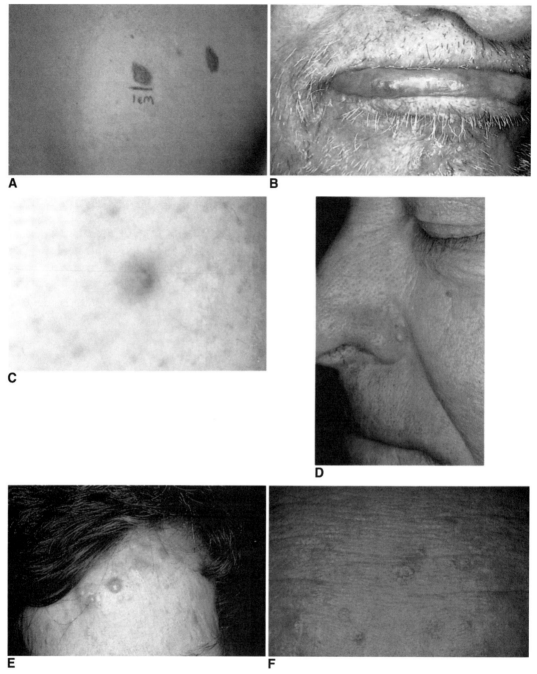

Plate 4. A, Dysplastic nevus. **B,** Venous lakes. **C,** Dermatofibroma. **D,** Fibrous papule. **E,** Cylindroma. **F,** Sebaceous hyperplasia.

sebaceous glands in the lesion are well developed. Thereafter, through childhood, the sebaceous glands in a nevus sebaceus are underdeveloped and, therefore, greatly reduced in size and number; in this phase, the diagnosis may be missed. At puberty, the lesions assume a diagnostic appearance, which is histologically characterized by the presence of large numbers of mature or nearly mature sebaceous glands and by papillomatous hyperplasia of the epidermis. During this stage, various types of appendical tumors develop secondarily within the lesion. A syringocystadenoma papilliferum has been found in 8% to 19% of lesions. Less-commonly found tumors include nodular hidradenoma, syringoma, and sebaceous epithelioma. Of primary importance is the occurrence of basal cell carcinoma in 5% to 7% of cases of nevus sebaceous; therefore, full-thickness excision of a nevus sebaceus is warranted before puberty as a preventive measure.[13]

CYSTS

Cutaneous cysts may be located either intradermally or within subcutaneous tissue. These general spherical growths contain a cavity that may be filled with fluid or contain cellular products or debris. A true cyst has an epithelial lining, whereas a pseudocyst lacks such an organized epithelium. Cysts are generally classified according to the pattern or differentiation they exhibit on histologic examination; many are difficult to differentiate clinically. As a rule, malignant degeneration is rare for all of the cysts described here.

Epidermoid Cysts

Epidermoid cysts are true cysts. The lining of these resembles that of the normal epidermis. This lining produces fully matured, keratinized cellular debris, which fills the cavity of the cyst. Epidermoid cysts are thought to originate from the follicular infundibulum of hair shafts and may arise either spontaneously or as a result of inflammation or trauma to the area. Injection of surface epidermal material to deeper dermal or subcutaneous layers as a result of penetrating trauma or the use of needles has also been postulated. These cysts are rarely found before puberty, but they have been found in all age groups after this period. If these cysts appear before puberty or in large numbers, they may be an indication of Gardner's syndrome, which is an autosomal dominant condition that predisposes the patient to intestinal cancer.

Although malignant degeneration is uncommon, epidermoid cysts can present a cosmetic problem, and, if they rupture or become infected, they may cause severe pain and scarring. Although some of these lesions will occasionally respond to intracystic injections of triamcinolone, surgical excision is the most effective treatment. It is necessary to carefully dissect and remove the entire cyst wall, because retained segments may lead to recurrent growth of the cyst.[45]

Pilar Cysts

Pilar cysts, which are also known as trichilemmal cysts or wens, are also true cysts; they are clinically indistinguishable from epidermal cysts. The tendency to form such cysts appears to be inherited as an autosomal dominant trait. The lining of the cyst differentiates in a manner analogous to that of the outer root sheath of the hair follicle; this fact allows for its differentiation from epidermal cysts. The great majority pilar cysts occur on the scalp, and they are uncommon before puberty. Multiple cysts are often present. If a pilar cyst ruptures or becomes infected, considerable pain and scarring may result. As with epidermal cysts, the best treatment is complete surgical excision.[11]

Dermoid Cysts

Dermoid cysts are rare tumors that are frequently present at birth. They may measure up to 4 cm in diameter, although they are generally less than 2 cm. They may occur anywhere, but they are most common on the face, particularly in the area of the lateral eyebrow, the orbit, and the nose. Dermoid cysts appear to result from the inclusion of embryonic epidermis within embryonal fusion planes. Histologically, these cysts are lined by an epithelium that resembles normal epidermis. They can be differentiated from epidermal cysts by their attachment to adnexal structures, which include hair, sebaceous glands, eccrine glands, and apocrine glands. Treatment is by surgical excision. If a dermoid cyst is located over the nasal root, however, care must be taken, because this tumor may be confused with a nasal glioma.[8]

Steatocystoma Multiplex

Steatocystoma multiplex, an uncommon condition, is often familial, demonstrating an autosomal dominant mode of inheritance. Although lesions can be discovered at any age, they most commonly occur shortly after puberty. The condition presents as multiple 1- to 2-cm cysts, generally located intradermally. They are most commonly found on the anterior chest, but they are also found on the face, forehead, ears, eyelids, and scalp. When punctured, these lesions exude a yellowish, oily fluid and, occasionally, hairs. On histologic examination, these cysts contain a highly corrugated wall of epithelial cells. Embedded within the wall are multiple sebaceous gland lobules, which may be partially responsible for the contents of the cyst. The mode of keratinization of the epithelial lining appears to resemble that of the outer root sheath, and indeed invaginations are often present within the cyst wall that appear similar to hair follicles. Infection with pain and subsequent scarring is a major problem associated with this condition. Treatment is disappointing because of the large number of lesions present, although individual lesions can easily be excised. On the face, cosmetically acceptable improvement has been reported with dermabrasion.[44]

Milia

Milia are small (usually 1–2 mm) cysts that differ histologically from epidermal cysts only in their small size. Clinically, they are whitish, smooth globules, most commonly seen on the face. They may arise spontaneously, but they are also frequently present as a result of trauma such as dermabrasion or burns or as a result of bullous diseases. When they arise after trauma or disease as a result of the occlusion of the pilosebaceous unit, they represent a retention cyst. Treatment is the same whether milia arise spontaneously or secondarily and is necessary only for cosmetic reasons; the lesion can easily be shelled out with a hypodermic needle or a comedo extractor. Because they may occasionally number in the hundreds, this treatment can be a considerably tedious chore.[43]

Mucous Cysts

Mucous cysts are pseudocysts, because no true lining is present; they are also called mucous retention cysts or mucoceles. These lesions are usually located on the mucous surface of the lower lip and are asymptomatic. They are generally less than 1 cm in diameter and, if superficial, may appear slightly bluish and translucent. They appear to be the result of traumatic rupture of the ducts of minor salivary glands. With leakage of the contents into the tissue, an inflammatory process ensues, with the resultant formation of granulation tissues surrounding the cystic space. Mucous cysts may resolve spontaneously or can otherwise be treated by the intralesional injection of low-dose triamcinolone (2.5 mg/mL), excision, or marsupialization.[51]

VASCULAR TUMORS

Cutaneous tumors of vascular origin may be true proliferative neoplasms, or they may be ecstatic vascular systems present in either the dermis or the subcutaneous tissue. Differentiation may be toward blood vessels, lymph vessels, or both. These tumors may be congenital or arise later in life, and most are benign. However, they may cause serious psychological or physical problems (because of impingement on important anatomic structures), or they may be markers of more serious underlying disease or syndromes. In general, these tumors can be classified histologically according to the size and nature of the vessels present. This discussion classifies the lesion as "hemangiomas vascular malformation."

Proliferative Vascular Neoplasms
Hemangiomas

Hemangiomas have classically been divided into *capillary hemangiomas* and *cavernous hemangiomas*, but it is preferable to describe them as either superficial or deep. Many contain both components. Histologically, such lesions represent capillary proliferations, although occasionally they may have cavernous spaces. Hemangiomas most often occur on the head and neck, although any portion of the skin may be affected. When first noted at or shortly after birth, they are generally macular, pink to red lesions. During the first year of life, they exhibit a rapid growth phase, and the lesions become raised, dome-shaped to polypoid, and bright red to deep purple. After the first year

of life, they enter a quiescent phase that is followed by a period of spontaneous involution. By the time the patient reaches the age of 5 years, about 50% of these lesions have spontaneously resolved; 70% resolve by the age of 7 years. If they have not involuted by the time the patient is 7 years old, they are unlikely to do so.

Although these tumors are benign, they may present significant problems to the patient if they impinge upon important anatomic structures, especially the eye or the respiratory tract. Other complications include ulceration and infection, which occur most commonly during the rapid growth phase. An uncommon complication that occurs in particularly large capillary hemangiomas with cavernous components is called the *Kasabach-Merritt syndrome*. This syndrome involves the entrapment of platelets with partial thrombosis of the capillaries, which leads to rapid consumption of the body's clotting factors. With very large lesions, this development may actually lead to the production of disseminated intravascular coagulation.

Because approximately 70% of capillary hemangiomas involute spontaneously, treatment is often not necessary. Unless the lesion is growing extremely rapidly and threatens an important anatomic structure or is ulcerating, treatment is not indicated until the patient reaches the age of at least 7 years. Rapidly growing lesions can be treated with systemic steroids. Treatment of the Kasabach-Merritt syndrome includes heparin, blood products, and systemic steroids. If a lesion fails to involute spontaneously, surgery is indicated. Cryotherapy and sclerosing agents are generally not successful, and radiotherapy is contraindicated because of long-term sequelae related to the radiation. Laser therapy, although helpful for port-wine stains, is generally not beneficial because of the depth of these lesions.[15,17]

Cherry Angiomas

Cherry angiomas are also called *senile angiomas* or *De Morgan's spots*. They may occur anywhere on the body but are most commonly found on the trunk. They usually appear during young adulthood. They are generally 1- to 3-mm, bright red, slightly raised, dome-shaped lesions. The lesions consist of multiple dilated capillaries found in the upper dermis. Cherry hemangiomas are benign and unrelated to systemic or congenital disease. Treatment is not necessary but may be desired for cosmetic reasons; these angiomas respond to both superficial electrodesiccation and laser surgery.[4]

Pyogenic Granuloma

Pyogenic granuloma, a common tumor, has several synonyms, including *granuloma pyogenicum*, *bloody wart*, and *pregnancy tumor*. It can occur at all ages, but it is most common in young children and young adults and also in pregnant women. The etiology of pyogenic granuloma is unclear, although it tends to occur at sites of trauma or infection. There may also be a hormonal factor involved, which would explain the increased incidence during pregnancy. Histologically, the lesion presents as a polypoid, lobulated mass of newly formed capillary blood vessels surrounded by an edematous stroma. An inflammatory infiltrate is generally present. Clinically, pyogenic granuloma appears as a dark red, pedunculated or dome-shaped lesion that ranges from several millimeters to centimeters in diameter; it commonly ulcerates and becomes crusted. It most commonly occurs on the distal extremities and the face, but it can present on any part of the body. Oral cavity lesions are common; the gingival is the site that is most often involved. There is frequently a collarette of epidermis around the base of the lesion. Because of their rapid and exuberant growth, these lesions are sometimes thought to be malignant. The differential diagnosis often includes malignant melanoma, Kaposi's sarcoma, metastatic carcinoma, and angiolymphoid hyperplasia with eosinophilia.

Occasionally, the lesion spontaneously resolves. Lesions associated with pregnancy frequently involute after delivery; most often, however, the lesion must be treated surgically. This treatment is easily accomplished by surgical excision or curettage with electrodesiccation.[37]

Vascular Ectasias

Vascular ectasias are actually telangiectasias or areas of vascular dilatation rather than true tumors. They may involve a significant portion of the skin and swell with time to become quite nodular. They may also cause significant problems for the patient because of secondary bleeding. These lesions may be an indication of serious underlying disease.

Nevus Flammeus

A nevus flammeus is generally present at birth, and it presents in two general forms. The first is extremely common and may be present in up to a third of newborn babies. Located on the nape of the neck, it is referred to as a *salmon patch* or *stork bite*; it may also be present on the eyelid or glabella. Eyelid lesions generally resolve within the first year of life, and the glabellar lesions also spontaneously involute but take somewhat longer. The nuchal lesions may persist into adult life, although some will spontaneously fade.

The second, less-common presentation of nevus flammeus occurs on the face and is called the port-

wine stain. This lesion is present in approximately 0.3% of newborns. Port-wine stains show no tendency to fade and in fact will generally darken and enlarge with age, becoming deeply violaceous and nodular during adult life. These lesions are generally unilateral and may follow a trigeminal distribution on the face. They may involve extensive areas of the skin of the face, as well as oral mucous membranes and conjunctival membranes. They less commonly involve other parts of the body.

Although most of these lesions represent only cosmetic problems to the patient, a small percentage may be indicators of serious underlying disease. One such disease is the Sturge-Weber syndrome (leptomeningeal nevus flammeus), in which a port-wine stain is located along the distribution of the trigeminal nerve. Patients with this syndrome may have angiomas within the meninges, with progressive calcification in these areas. Abnormalities associated with this condition include seizures (reported in patients as young as 3 weeks old but generally occurring later in infancy), mental retardation, hemiplegia, and ocular abnormalities such as glaucoma (in up to 40% of patients). Another syndrome associated with port-wine stain is the Klippel-Trenaunay-Parkes-Weber syndrome (osteohypertrophic nevus flammeus), in which hypertrophy of the soft tissues and bones of extremities is accompanied by an overlying nevus flammeus.

Histologic examination of these lesions may reveal no changes early in life. With time, however, the ecstatic or dilated vessels become more prominent. They will vary in degree of dilatation and in depth among patients. The capillaries are otherwise normal, and there may be overlying acanthosis.

Although nevus flammeus is usually an isolated cosmetic defect, its significance to the patient may be great. The natural history of these lesions is to present initially as pink or pale red patches that, with time, progress through deepening shades of red to take on a deeply violaceous hue. Also, with increasing age, the ecstatic vessels become progressively more dilated and may become nodular and protuberant. Their prominent location on the face may cause significant psychological trauma for the patient. These large nodular lesions may also tend to bleed and become crusted.

Treatment of choice is the flashlamp-pumped pulsed dye laser. With repeated treatment sessions, significant fading can occur, although only a small percentage of these nevi will resolve completely.[36]

Hereditary Hemorrhagic Telangiectasia (Rendu-Osler-Weber Syndrome)

Hereditary hemorrhagic telangiectasia is a dominantly inherited condition that affects blood vessels throughout the body. It is characterized by ectatic vessels of the skin, mucous membranes, and viscera. Often the presenting symptom is spontaneous epistaxis, which may begin during early childhood but more likely appears at puberty or during adult life. Telangiectasia generally begins around and after puberty. The superficial telangiectasia assumes three morphologic forms; the most common lesions are punctate, but they may also be linear or spiderlike. The mucous membranes are almost always involved, with lesions occurring on the nasal septum, mouth, nasopharynx, and also throughout the gastrointestinal tract. The lesions may ulcerate and frequently bleed. The condition is associated with pulmonary arteriovenous fistulas. Other viscera may also be affected, as well as the retina. Bleeding may occur from any of the vascular lesions throughout the body and may be fatal. The diagnosis is generally made when the combination of frequent hemorrhagic episodes, vascular ectasias, and a family history is recognized. Treatment is aimed at control of specific hemorrhages and of anemia, if it arises. Individual cutaneous lesions may be treated by electrocauterization and photocoagulation.[27]

Spider Angioma

Spider angioma may be present in up to 15% of healthy people. The lesions are more frequent during pregnancy, during which they occur early and increase until delivery; they generally resolve spontaneously during the postpartum period. They may also be associated with liver disease or estrogen therapy, and they tend to persist when seen in nonpregnant healthy persons. Clinically, the condition presents as a central, raised, small body that may be pulsatile. Fanning out from this central area are multiple fine telangiectases. In otherwise healthy people, the lesions are only a cosmetic problem. They may occur on mucous membranes, in which case the differentiation from hereditary hemorrhagic telangiectasia must be made. Treatment is by obliteration of the central feeding arterial, which can be accomplished with electrocautery or photocoagulation.[4]

Venous Lakes

Venous lakes present as deep blue, cutaneous nodules that occur most frequently on the face, lips, and ears of elderly patients (Plate 4, *B*). Sometimes called senile angiomas, they are composed of dilated thick- and thin-walled, otherwise normal-appearing vessels. The lesions may thrombose and involute, but frequently they persist. They are of no significance other than a cosmetic nuisance.[4]

FIBROADNEXAL TUMORS

Fibroadnexal tumors are derived from components of the deeper layers of the skin. They generally show differentiation toward the specific cell or tissue of origination and may be derived from any of the neurogenous, fibrillar, glandular, or pilar components of the dermis, as well as the subcutaneous tissue.

Acrochordon

Acrochordon (skin tag, fibroepithelial papilloma) are extremely common lesions, occurring most often during middle to late life. They are flesh colored, pedunculate tumors that are generally up to about 2 mm in diameter. They are soft and most commonly occur in flexural regions such as the axillae, the sides of the neck, inframammary areas, and the upper eyelids. The lesions are composed of mostly loose fibrous tissue (similar to that of the superficial dermis), and they are covered by a thin epidermis. No adnexal structures are present. The lesions are easily removed by simple sharp-scissors excision or light electrodesiccation.[14]

Keloids and Hypertrophic Scars

Keloids and hypertrophic scars are uncontrolled proliferative responses to trauma by the fibrous tissue of the dermis. Hypertrophic scar is a thickened scar that does not extend beyond the margins of the original injury, whereas a keloid is an exuberant growth extending beyond the borders of the initial scar. Keloids are most commonly seen in blacks. The epithelium overlying the tumor is frequently thinned and shiny, and the tumor may be tender and pruritic. The areas of predilection for keloids include the sternal area, the shoulders, and the upper back; they are also frequently seen on the earlobes after ear piercing and on the face. These tumors may be flat or extremely protuberant, dome shaped, or bosselated. They are most common in the second and third decades of life, becoming less common with age. Histologically, they present with distinctive keloidal collagen. Hypertrophic scars usually occur on sites of increased skin movement and tension; there is no racial predilection.

Treatment of keloids is very difficult. Excision of these tumors generally has resulted in regrowth. Some success has resulted from the injection of very potent corticosteroids (triamcinolone, 40 mg/mL). Pressure also seems to stimulate involution, although the pressure must be maintained daily for up to a year. Special pressure earrings can be applied to the earlobes, and Jobst body suits can be constructed. Hypertrophic scars are easier to manage, because they respond better to intralesional steroids and, over time, will usually settle down. Flashlamp-pumped pulsed dye laser has been used to improve hypertrophic scars.[7]

Dermatofibroma

The common tumors known as dermatofibromas fall into the class of fibrous histiocytomas and can occur anywhere on the body (Plate 4, *C*). They range in size up to 1 cm, and they are frequently slightly hyperpigmented and hyperkeratotic. Dermatofibromas are benign and may persist for many years, although regression is not uncommon. On microscopic examination, these tumors are composed of spindle-shaped cells arranged in a whorled fashion, with very ill-defined margins. No treatment is necessary, but, if it is desired, excision is the best approach. Some dermatofibromas may respond to cryosurgery, which may at least flatten the lesion.[21]

Dermatofibrosarcoma Protuberans

Dermatofibrosarcoma protuberans is derived from fibroblasts. It is a rare, locally invasive, malignant tumor that most commonly occurs on the trunk but may occur on the scalp, face, or neck; it seldom metastasizes. It presents as a recurrent or persistently enlarging protuberant mass, which may vary in color from flesh toned to bluish or reddish. Treatment is excision. Because incomplete removal invariably results in regrowth, microscopically controlled excision using the Mohs technique may offer a distinct advantage in the treatment of this tumor.[21]

Atypical Fibroxanthoma

Atypical fibroxanthoma is a malignant tumor that most commonly occurs on the sun-exposed areas of elderly people, where it presents as a rapidly growing nodule. A less common presentation is in persons in the third or fourth decade of life, in which case growth is less rapid. The lesion is a pink to translucent asymptomatic nodule, generally 1 to 2 cm in diameter. Ulceration is not uncommon. The nodules may be mistaken for basal cell carcinoma because of their translucent appearance, the ulceration, and their location on elderly patients.

Histologically, these lesions have a very bizarre appearance, with large and atypical epithelioid and spindle cells. Multinucleate giant cells are also present. These tumors have been misdiagnosed as several different types of malignancies, squamous cell carcinomas, and melanomas. Surgical excision is the treatment of choice.[52]

Neurofibromas

Neurofibromas are soft, dome-shaped, flesh-colored lesions that may be located anywhere on the body; they may vary greatly in size, from quite small to large pedunculate lesions. Neurofibromas are derived from the Schwann cells of cutaneous nerves. On histologic examination, they present as nonencapsulated, loose, spindeloid tumors. Solitary lesions may be easily excised.

These tumors may be indicative of the genetic neurofibromatosis syndrome, which may be associated with severe neurologic problems as well as a risk of malignant degeneration of the tumor. When a neurofibroma is found, a careful search for other manifestations, which include café-au-lait spots and axillary freckling as well as a family history, should be carried out to rule out the syndrome.[39]

Angiofibroma

Angiofibroma (adenoma sebaceum) is present as part of the genetic syndrome tuberous sclerosis. The autosomal dominant syndrome has variable expressivity; the finding of even one angiofibroma requires genetic counseling, because the patient may pass on a much more severe form of the disease to offspring. Angiofibromas present as small dome-shaped papules, 2 to 3 mm in diameter, that are flesh colored or reddish brown. They are most commonly present on the sides of the nose and the medial cheeks. The original name is a misnomer, because, on histologic examination, no sebaceous components are noted. The tumors are composed mostly of fibrous tissue, with an angioid component. When the lesions are solitary or few in number, simple excision is curative.[31]

Fibrous Papule

The fibrous papule is a common lesion, generally occurring on the nose—especially the alae—in older persons (Plate 4, *D*). However, it can also be seen on the medial cheeks. These lesions present as small, 0.5-cm, dome-shaped, flesh-colored papules. Although they are rather common, some confusion persists regarding their origin and histologic nature. They have been regarded as perifollicular fibromas, involuting melanocytic nevi, angiofibromas, or as simply the result of trauma, such as folliculitis or excoriating pimples. Histologically, the lesion presents as a papule that is composed of numerous spindle-shaped and stellate cells, with occasional multinucleate cells present. Once the lesions have grown, they are generally quite stable and may be present for years; they may be treated by excision or curettage and electrodesiccation. They are of no significance unless related to tuberous sclerosis.[35]

Trichoepithelioma

A trichoepithelioma is an uncommon entity that most often presents as small rounded nodules on the cheeks, eyelids, and nose. It appears to be dominantly inherited; however, pedigrees indicate a greater preponderance of affected females. The lesions are skin colored to slightly pink and gradually increase, with time, in both number and size. A few telangiectatic vessels may be present, and there may be a slightly translucent quality to the lesions, which may lead to confusion with basal cell carcinoma; however, the lesions rarely ulcerate. If ulceration does occur, basal cell carcinoma should be considered. The histologic appearance of these lesions also closely resembles basal cell carcinoma, and distinguishing between the two is often difficult. There are basophilic cells similar to those seen in basal cell carcinoma. The cells are arranged in masses, which may have fully keratinized centers. Abortive attempts at hair growth may also be noted, in which case differentiation from basal cell carcinoma is easy.

Occasionally the presence of a solitary lesion makes differentiation from basal cell carcinoma somewhat more difficult, and, unless definite differentiation toward hairlike structures is present, the tumor should be treated as a carcinoma. In the cases in which multiple lesions are present, treatment is difficult because of the large number of tumors. Some success has been obtained with dermabrasion of the entire affected area.[25]

Cylindroma

Cylindromas may be single or multiple. When multiple, they appear to be dominantly inherited and may literally cover the scalp, resulting in a syndrome called "turban tumors" (Plate 4, *E*). The condition affects females twice as often as males. It appears to original from apocrine glands, and the tumors may be associated with trichoepitheliomas. The tumors generally appear in adult life and are most common on the face or scalp. They present as smooth, dome-shaped, or pedunculate lesions, which may be pink to red and are firm. They grow slowly and can reach 2 to 3 cm in diameter. Histologically, these tumors are composed of nests of darkly staining epithelial cells surrounded by a narrow band of hyaline material. The solitary lesion must be differentiated from basal cell carcinoma. Surgical excision is the only treatment. When large areas of the scalp are involved, this may be quite difficult and may require grafting.[10]

Hidrocystoma

A hidrocystoma may be either eccrine or apocrine in origin. In either case, the tumor usually presents as a solitary lesion and is most frequently seen on the face. The lesion consists of translucent nodules with a firm, cystic consistency. The eccrine hidrocystoma is generally from 1 to 3 mm in diameter, whereas the apocrine may attain a diameter of 1 cm. Both may have a bluish hue. The two types are distinguishable by histologic criteria. Microscopic examination reveals differing cellular detail and secretion patterns for the two types. In either case, treatment is excision.[30]

Syringoma

Syringomas are benign tumors that originate from the eccrine sweat gland duct, and they appear more often in women than in men. Syringomas are most commonly located on the face, with the lower eyelids being the most common site. They generally occur in adolescence or early adulthood and may be eruptive or occur in crops. They present as small 1- to 5-mm papules that are usually flesh colored but may be slightly translucent or yellowish. They may resemble trichoepitheliomas, but their location and histology help to differentiate them. Histologically, these tumors appear as small nests of cystic ductal structures or as solid epithelial strands, many of which may have a characteristic tail-like projection. They are not associated with underlying abnormality. They do not tend to involute, however, and may present a cosmetic problem when located on the face. They can be treated with a pulsed ablative laser (CO_2 or erbium) or with light electrocoagulation using a fine epilating needle.[38]

Sebaceous Hyperplasia

Sebaceous hyperplasia occurs mainly on the face, particularly the forehead, and represents benign enlargement of the normal sebaceous gland (Plate 4, *F*). It is frequently called senile sebaceous hyperplasia, because it is usually seen in older persons. One or hundreds of lesions may be present. They may be from 2 to 5 mm in diameter, and there is usually a central umbilication. These lesions are soft and yellowish and must be differentiated from basal cell carcinoma. Histologically, they present as hyperplastic sebaceous lobules that are otherwise normal in appearance. They are only a cosmetic problem; solitary lesions can be easily treated with a shave excision, electrodesiccation and curettage, or cryosurgery. When the lesions are quite numerous, surgical excision is unwarranted. Therapy with system 13-cis retinoic acid has also been described.[48]

Xanthelasma

Xanthelasmas present on or close to the eyelids as soft, yellowish, irregular papules. They usually appear in middle age and can affect either sex, and they are not often associated with xanthomas elsewhere on the body. Frequently, they are an isolated finding and do not always signify elevated serum triglyceride levels, although each patient should be examined for the existence of such a systemic problem. Histologically, these lesions present as an accumulation of xanthoma cells, which are lipid-laden histiocytes. Treatment is the application of 50% to 65% trichloroacetic acid, light cautery, or excision.[6]

Lipoma

Lipomas are benign tumors that are composed of adipose tissue and that may be single or multiple. They are soft and may be lobulated or rounded and cystic in nature, and they are generally freely movable.

Except in rare syndromes, lipomas are nontender. They generally occur on the trunk, but they may also occur on the neck or any other part of the body. Histologically, they present as proliferations of normal-appearing fat cells that may be surrounded by a thin connective-tissue capsule. Single lesions present only cosmetic problems, and they are generally easily excised. Despite attaining sizes of more than 1 inch in diameter, they may often be expressed through a small, 4-mm punch hole.[23]

TREATMENT METHODS AND BIOPSY TECHNIQUES
Scalpel Surgery

The *shave biopsy* is one of the most commonly performed procedures for cutaneous lesions. It is a rapid means of removing tissue either as part of therapy or to establish diagnosis. A shave can be performed using various techniques, with the depth of the shave depending on the angle of the blade as it enters the sin. Usually a No. 15 or No. 10 Bard-Parker blade is used. One should remember that the sharpest point of the No. 15 blade is the rounded tip, whereas the No. 10 has its sharpest edge along the belly of the blade. The shave should be performed using the sharpest portion of the blade. One of the sharpest blades is the Gillette Blue Blade; it is excellent for shaving lesions. A blade breaker or hemostat can break the Blue Blade into any size or shape desired. The blade can then be held between the thumb and forefinger and flexed, thereby allowing for the performance of a superficial shave in which the blade sculpts along the contour of the surface being excised (e.g., the ala of the nose or the helix of the ear). Hemostasis can then be obtained with aluminum chloride. Monsel's solution (ferric subsulfate) should be avoided on the face or cosmetic areas because of the ability of macrophages to phagocytose the iron, thereby causing a tattoo.

The *punch*, a fixed-diameter surgical knife, is an extremely valuable tool to a dermatologist for excision or biopsy. It comes in various sizes, from 2 mm to 1 cm, with 0.5-mm increments. Punches can be purchased as disposable instruments (Baker) or as permanent, sterilizable instruments. The most common sizes used for biopsy are 3 mm and 4 mm; however, a 2-mm punch can provide a cosmetically elegant biopsy of sufficient size for the pathologist. Whenever possible, the 4-mm punch should be used. All punch-biopsy incisions should be closed.

Some tricks help with the use of a punch. By putting tension on the skin perpendicular to the anticipated line of closure (skin tension lines), one can cause the circular punch to leave an oval or ellipse for easier closure. The incision is usually closed with sutures or the recently introduced single-shot staple. A valuable trick is to use a punch to excise intradermal nevi. By selecting a punch that just fits around the nevus, one can easily excise it to the depth necessary to remove the entire lesion. Another trick, which can be used when nevi occur in areas of neutral skin tension or where skin tension lines are not obvious (e.g., the chin), is to use the punch to help determine the best lines of closure. If the surgeon uses a punch excision with no tension placed on the skin, the resulting circle will usually form itself into an oval along lines of facial expression and help in the determination of skin closure lines. Often the skin closure lines can occur at an angle that is perpendicular to what one might expect.

The *wedge excision* or biopsy, which is a variation of the fusiform excision (ellipse), can be used to remove lesions cosmetically or to perform biopsies. As a biopsy technique, it is either incisional or excisional. Whenever possible—especially when dealing with pigmented lesions—the excisional biopsy is preferred to give the pathologist the best chance for an accurate diagnosis. When the wedge procedure is performed as an incisional biopsy of a large, nodular lesion, the narrowest possible wedge (greater than the classic 3:1 length-width ratio) is made at the edge of the lesion so that one end of the wedge is through normal skin; then one side of normal skin is available through which to pass suture. This is an especially important advantage if the other side of the wedge is within friable tissue.

Scissors excision is a valuable method of cosmetically removing benign skin tumors. In the experienced hand, scissors can be used to produce an often-elegant cosmetic result very quickly. Scissors are best used on raised, pedunculate skin lesions in which the pedicle can be easily and rapidly cut with scissors. Our preference is to use fine-tipped, curved Iris or Gradle scissors. Tricks similar to those used for the shave biopsy apply to scissors excisions. Raising a bleb of anesthesia under a pedunculate lesion will allow for better access to the base. Scissors are an excellent tool around the eyelids. Often a small chalazion clamp can be placed around a lesion, thereby permitting easy excision with fine scissors. Filiform or pedunculate lesions on the eyelids can be lifted with fine forceps and then cut with curved scissors. This procedure will produce a small ellipse upon release of the eyelid skin, which will either heal by itself or with the placement of one small stitch. Scissors can also be used for biopsies of oral mucosa. Again, a chalazion clamp can be placed on the lip, or a stitch can be placed around the area of the biopsy. One can then pull up on the stitch, thus creating a tent of tissue that can be scissors excised at the base to obtain a biopsy specimen.

A curette is a valuable tool to the skin surgeon. One should have a variety of sizes of curettes available; larger curettes are used to debulk or remove larger tumors, and smaller curettes are used to do the same for small tumors or to help track small extensions of cutaneous tumors, such as basal cell carcinoma. A curette is held like a pencil, with the ring or small finger placed on the skin to anchor and stabilize the hand. Normal skin has a "gritty" feel with the curette, whereas abnormal skin or tumor often feels mushy or soft. One way to remove multiple molluscum contagiosum lesions on the face, for example, is to individually curette each small lesion (a small curette is used). If anesthesia is required, one can use either the usual local anesthetic or one of the refrigerant anesthetics, which will both induce some anesthesia in the skin and harden the lesion; hardening allows the lesion to be easily flicked off with a curette. A curette is often used in conjunction with electrosurgery.[41]

Electrosurgery

Electrosurgery is a useful way to remove small benign lesions, to assist the curette with the removal of malignant lesions, and to assist the surgeon with the obtaining of hemostasis. Most electrosurgery performed in the office requires nothing more than a Hyfrecator-like unit. This versatile instrument is easy to use because the patient does not need to be grounded, and the electrodesiccation or fulguration is at a more superficial depth than the electrocoagulation or cutting seen when a patient is grounded. Most of these electrosurgical units have two current settings. The low current is best for light electrodesiccation of benign lesions. One can also purchase a fine steel tip or place a 30-gauge needle on the standard tip; this tip can then be threaded down adnexal structures to treat benign adnexal tumors or to coagulate arterial vessels that are feeding vascular lesions. The high current setting, which is a more destructive mode, is used to burn tumor and surrounding tissue, such as during electrodesiccation or fulguration of basal cell carcinomas. Bipolar units, with the patient grounded, can be used to help sculpt lesions, such as in the case of a rhinophymatous nose.[28]

Cryosurgery

Cryosurgical removal is the treatment of choice for many lesions. Systems vary from elaborate cryospray and cryoprobe units to something as simple as a Styrofoam cup containing liquid nitrogen to be applied with a cotton-tipped applicator. The superficial use of cryosurgery destroys tumor tissue, often with excellent cosmetic results. Hypopigmentation and other sequelae can develop, however, which make the use of cryosurgery in darker skin more difficult.[28]

Chemical or Abrasive Surgery

Many superficial cutaneous lesions of the head and neck can be removed with the application of a chemical or with the use of abrasion. The chemicals most commonly used as peeling agents are trichloroacetic acid and phenol. The concentration of trichloroacetic acid used varies from 35% to 70%. Phenol is usually used as a concentrated solution (88%) or mixed as Baker's solution. These chemicals can be used to peel benign pigmented or melanotic lesions, with good success.

The most common form of abrasion is spot dermabrasion. Our favorite tool is the Bell hand engine with the diamond fraise or wire brush. The fraise can be purchased in varying sizes and shapes; small, 2-mm wheel, cone, or cylindric fraises are excellent tools for removing multiple small epithelial tumors.[28]

Laser Surgery

Laser surgery has gained tremendous popularity during the last decade. Through the principle of selective photothermolysis, the newer lasers are more specific, effective, and safer. It is beyond the scope of this chapter to review in detail all of the different cutaneous laser applications.

Vascular lesions can be effectively treated using 532 nm KTP/Nd:YAG, 585-595 nm pulsed-dye, and long-pulse 1064 nm Nd:YAG lasers. Photoaging and wrinkles are treated with the ultrapulsed CO_2 laser and erbium YAG ablative lasers. Tattoo and pigment are treated with various Q-switched lasers designed to match specifically to the pigment color. Hair can be effectively removed with long-pulsed 755 nm alexandrite, 810 nm diode, and 1064 nm Nd:YAG lasers. Further developments in laser technology will improve on the minimally invasive approach.[50]

REFERENCES

1. Alam M, Ratner D: Cutaneous squamous-cell carcinoma, *N Engl J Med* 344:979, 2001.
2. Alper JC: Congenital nevi. The controversy rages on, *Arch Dermatol* 121:734, 1985.
3. Arbiser JL: Melanoma. Lessons from metastases, *Arch Dermatol* 134:1027, 1998.
4. Aversa AJ, Miller OF 3rd: Cryo-curettage of cherry angiomas, *J Dermatol Surg Oncol* 9:930, 1983.
5. Ber Rahman S, Bhawan J: Lentigo, *Int J Dermatol* 35:229, 1996.
6. Bergman R: The pathogenesis and clinical significance of xanthelasma palpebrarum, *J Am Acad Dermatol* 30(2 Pt 1):236, 1994.
7. Berman B, Bieley HC: Keloids, *J Am Acad Dermatol* 33:117, 1995.

8. Bonavolonta G and others: Dermoid cysts: 16-year survey, *Ophthal Plast Reconstr Surg* 11:187, 1995.
9. Callen JP, Bickers DR, Moy RL: Actinic keratoses, *J Am Acad Dermatol* 36:650, 1997.
10. Cardenas AA, Norton SA, Fitzpatrick JE: Solitary violaceous nodule on the face. Dermal cylindroma (also known as cylindroma, dermal eccrine cylindroma, Spiegler's tumor, turban tumor, and tomato tumor), *Arch Dermatol* 129:498,501, 1993.
11. Carlin MC, Bailin PL, Bergfeld WF: Enlarging, painful scalp nodule. Proliferating trichilemmal tumor, *Arch Dermatol* 124:936,938, 1988.
12. Casso EM, Grin-Jorgensen CM, Grant-Kels JM: Spitz nevi, *J Am Acad Dermatol* 27(6 Pt 1):901, 1992.
13. Chun K, Vazquez M, Sanchez JL: Nevus sebaceus: clinical outcome and considerations for prophylactic excision, *Int J Dermatol* 34:538, 1995.
14. Eads TJ and others: The utility of submitting fibroepithelial polyps for histological examination, *Arch Dermatol* 132:1459, 1996.
15. Elder DE, Goldman LI, Greene MH and others: Dysplastic nevus syndrom: a phenotypic association of sporadic cutaneous melanoma, *Cancer* 46(8):1787–1794, 1980.
16. Enjolras O, Mulliken JB: Vascular tumors and vascular malformations (new issues), *Adv Dermatol* 13:375, 1997.
17. Favre M, Ramoz N, Orth G: Human papillomaviruses: general features, *Clin Dermatol* 15:181, 1997.
18. Frieden IJ and others: Guidelines of care for hemangiomas of infancy. American Academy of Dermatology Guidelines/ Outcomes Committee, *J Am Acad Dermatol* 37:631, 1997.
19. Friedman RJ and others: The dysplastic nevus. Clinical and pathologic features, *Dermatol Clin* 3:239, 1985.
20. Gailani MR, Bale AE: Acquired and inherited basal cell carcinomas and the patched gene, *Adv Dermatol* 14:261, discussion 284, 1999.
21. Goldberg LH: Basal cell carcinoma, *Lancet* 347:663, 1996.
22. Goldblum JR, Tuthill RJ: CD34 and factor-XIIIa immunoreactivity in dermatofibrosarcoma protuberans and dermatofibroma, *Am J Dermatopathol* 19:147, 1997.
23. Gross EA: Initial evaluation of melanoma. Don't stop getting that chest x-ray...yet, *Arch Dermatol* 134:623, 1998.
24. Hardin FF: A simple technique for removing lipomas, *J Dermatol Surg Oncol* 8:316, 1982.
25. Jablonska S and others: Cutaneous warts. Clinical, histologic, and virologic correlations, *Clin Dermatol* 3:71, 1985.
26. Johnson SC, Bennett RG: Occurrence of basal cell carcinoma among multiple trichoepitheliomas, *J Am Acad Dermatol* 28(2 Pt 2):322, 1993.
27. Johnson TM, Bradford CR, Gruber SB and others: Staging workup, sentinel node biopsy, and follow-up tests for melanoma: update of current concepts. *Arch Dermatol* 140(1):107–113, 2004.
28. Johnson TM and others: Squamous cell carcinoma of the skin (excluding lip and oral mucosa), *J Am Acad Dermatol* 26(3 Pt 2):467, 1992.
29. Kjeldsen AD, Vase P, Oxhoj H: Hereditary hemorrhagic telangiectasia, *N Engl J Med* 334:331, 1996.
30. Leffell DJ, Brown MD: *Manual of skin surgery: a practical guide to dermatologic procedures,* New York, Wiley-Liss, 1997.
31. Maloney ME: Histology of basal cell carcinoma, *Clin Dermatol* 13:545, 1995.
32. Masri-Fridling GD, Elgart ML: Eccrine hidrocystomas, *J Am Acad Dermatol* 26(5 Pt 1):780, 1992.
33. McGrae JD Jr, Hashimoto K: Unilateral facial angiofibromas—a segmental form of tuberous sclerosis, *Br J Dermatol* 134:727, 1996.
34. McLaurin CI: Cutaneous reaction patterns in blacks, *Dermatol Clin* 6:353, 1988.
35. Metcalf JS, Maize JC: Melanocytic nevi and malignant melanoma, *Dermatol Clin* 3:217, 1985.
36. Miller DL, Weinstock MA: Nonmelanoma skin cancer in the United States: incidence, *J Am Acad Dermatol* 30(5 Pt 1):774, 1994.
37. Nemeth AJ, Penneys NS, Bernstein HB: Fibrous papule: a tumor of fibrohistiocytic cells that contain factor XIIIa, *J Am Acad Dermatol* 19:1102, 1988.
38. Osburn K, Schosser RH, Everett MA: Congenital pigmented and vascular lesions in newborn infants, *J Am Acad Dermatol* 16:788, 1987.
39. Patrice SJ, Wiss K, Mulliken JB: Pyogenic granuloma (lobular capillary hemangioma): a clinicopathologic study of 178 cases, *Pediatr Dermatol* 8:267, 1991.
40. Patrizi A and others: Syringoma: a review of twenty-nine cases, *Acta Derm Venereol* 78:460, 1998.
41. Requena L, Sangueza OP: Benign neoplasms with neural differentiation: a review, *Am J Dermatopathol* 17:75, 1995.
42. Rhodes AR and others: Risk factors for cutaneous melanoma. A practical method of recognizing predisposed individuals, *JAMA* 258:3146, 1987.
43. Robinson JK: *Fundamentals of skin biopsy,* Chicago, Year Book Medical Publishers, 1986.
44. Rowe DE: Comparison of treatment modalities for basal cell carcinoma, *Clin Dermatol* 13:617, 1995.
45. Samlaska CP, Benson PM: Milia en plaque, *J Am Acad Dermatol* 21(2 Pt 1):311, 1989.
46. Sato K and others: Aspiration therapy in steatocystoma multiplex, *Arch Dermatol* 129:35, 1993.
47. Sau P, Graham JH, Helwig EB: Proliferating epithelial cysts. Clinicopathological analysis of 96 cases, *J Cutan Pathol* 22:394, 1995.
48. Schaffer JV, Bolognia JL: The clinical spectrum of pigmented lesions, *Clin Plast Surg* 27:391, 2000.
49. Schwartz RA: Sign of Leser-Trélat, *J Am Acad Dermatol* 35:88, 1996.
50. Sehgal VN, Bajaj P, Jain S: Sebaceous hyperplasia in youngsters, *J Dermatol* 26:619, 1999.
51. Saber AJ, Fitzpatrick TB, Mihm MC Jr.: Primary Melanoma of the skin: recognition and treatment. *J Am Acad Dermatol* 2(3):179–197, 1980.
52. Sterling JC, Handfield-Jones S, Hudson PM: Guidelines for the management of cutaneous warts, *Br J Dermatol* 144:4, 2001.
53. Tanzi EL, Lupton JR, Alster TS: Lasers in dermatology: four decades in progress, *J Am Acad Dermatol* 49:1, 2003.
54. Tran TA, Parlette HL 3rd: Surgical pearl: removal of a large labial mucocele, *J Am Acad Dermatol* 40(5 Pt 1):760, 1999.
55. Winkelmann RK, Peters MS: Atypical fibroxanthoma. A study with antibody to S-100 protein, *Arch Dermatol* 121:753, 1985.
56. Zeff RA and others: The immune response in halo nevi, *J Am Acad Dermatol* 37:620, 1997.
57. Zimmerman MC: Seborrheic keratoses, *J Dermatol Surg Oncol* 10:586, 1984.

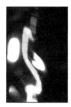

CHAPTER TWENTY THREE

THE MANAGEMENT OF HEAD AND NECK MELANOMA

Cecelia E. Schmalbach
Timothy M. Johnson
Carol R. Bradford

INTRODUCTION

The worldwide incidence of melanoma is increasing faster than any other cancer[140]; it is currently the fifth leading cause of cancer among men and the seventh leading cause among women.[79] The management of cutaneous melanoma is also one of fastest evolving fields in cancer, with promising research taking place at both the molecular and clinical levels. In fact, recent increased understanding of melanoma biology has prompted major changes in the staging classification system set forth by the American Joint Committee on Cancer (AJCC).[18] Given its association with sun exposure, melanoma is considered a preventable disease. Decreased incidence and mortality ultimately hinges upon the patient, as well as physician education, prevention, early diagnosis, and improved treatment for advanced disease.

EPIDEMIOLOGY

Despite a recent decline in the overall trends for cancer incidence and mortality, the incidence of cutaneous melanoma continues to rise faster than any other cancer.[107] On the basis of the National Cancer Institute's Surveillance, Epidemiology, and End Results Data, 54,200 new cases of invasive cutaneous melanoma were diagnosed in 2003. An additional 37,700 in situ cases were estimated that same year. For women less than 40 years old, the incidence of melanoma is second only to breast cancer.[79]

Over the past 50 years, the annual percentage change in invasive melanoma incidence has steadily increased by 4.3% each year.[107] The lifetime risk for developing invasive melanoma has climbed at an epidemic rate; it increased from 1 in 1500 individuals born in 1935 to 1 in 250 born in 1980. This trend is expected to continue at a startling rate, with 1 in 39 individuals born in 2003 projected to develop melanoma.[139]

Melanoma is the most lethal form of skin cancer. In 2003, it was responsible for an estimated 7600 deaths within the United States[107]; this estimate averages to approximately one American dying from melanoma every hour. Over the past 50 years, the annual percentage change in mortality rate has increased at a steady rate of 1.8% per year. Melanoma accounts for the second highest increase in mortality rate, especially for men over the age of 65. However, it should not be viewed as a cancer limited to the elderly. In fact, melanoma is known to afflict young adults, with 1 in 4 patients diagnosed before the age of 40.[63,139] Consequently, melanoma represents one of the leading cancer causes of lost potential life years.

Approximately 25% of all cutaneous melanomas arise in the head and neck (HN) region,[103] with more than 9000 cases diagnosed annually. A slight male predominance has been consistently reported throughout the literature.[64,123,132] The median age of diagnosis for patients with HN melanoma is 55 years.[63] However, juvenile cases account for 1.66% of HN melanoma cases, with patients as young as 4 years old being diagnosed.[60,128]

ETIOLOGY AND RISK FACTORS

Numerous environmental and genetic risk factors have been implicated in the development of cutaneous melanoma.[161] These risk factors are summarized in Table 23-1.

Risk Factors

Sun exposure is considered to be the leading cause of melanoma.[26,91] Patients with a significant history of sun exposure are at particularly high risk, especially if they experienced peeling or blistering sunburns, even during childhood.[138] Associated risk factors include blond or red hair, green or blue eyes, or fair skin consistent with Fitzpatrick skin types I through III.[65] Adults with more than 100 clinically normal-appearing nevi, children with more than 50 clinically normal-appearing nevi, and any patients with atypical or dysplastic nevi are also at risk.

TABLE 23-1

RISK FACTORS ASSOCIATED WITH CUTANEOUS MELANOMA

Environmental/Sun exposure
  Fair complexion/inability to tan
  Blue/green eyes
  Blonde/red hair
  Freckling
  Actinic keratoses
  Nonmelanoma skin cancer
  History of blistering/peeling sunburns
  Immunosuppression
  Teenage outdoor summer jobs
Genetic
  CDKN2A (p16) mutation
  Family history of melanoma
  History of prior melanoma
  Xeroderma pigmentosa
  Atypical (dysplastic) nevus
  Giant congenital melanocytic nevus

A prior history of melanoma places a patient at increased risk, with 5% to 10% of individuals developing a second primary melanoma.[82] This risk of developing a second primary is lifelong, and it can occur anywhere on the skin; therefore, long-term follow-up with a thorough total body examination is critical.

Genetics

A genetic component has also been implicated in the pathogenesis of melanoma[98]; 10% to 15% of melanoma patients report a positive family history.[133] The most common chromosomal mutation associated with melanoma involves *CDKN2A*, which is also known as p16.[87] However, the mutation only accounts for a small percentage of melanoma cases observed. Aitken and colleagues[1] estimated that *CDKN2A* mutations were responsible for only 0.2% of melanoma cases diagnosed in Australia. The genetic etiology of melanoma represents an intense area of research with future discovery.

The hereditary nature of cutaneous melanoma was also noted in the 1970s. Clark and colleagues[48] defined the *B-K mole syndrome* and named it after the two families of study. Members afflicted with this syndrome acquired large, irregular, and dysplastic nevi that were often found in sun-protected regions of the body, such as the scalp and trunk. During this time period, Lynch and colleagues[104] independently reported a familial association of melanoma among individuals with atypical nevi, which he called *familial atypical multiple mole-melanoma (FAMMM) syndrome*; today, this is called *atypical mole syndrome*.[160] Studies have

demonstrated an autosomal dominant inheritance pattern.[70] The 10-year melanoma risk in the setting of atypical mole syndrome is reported to be 10.7%, as compared with 0.62% in control patients.[107,108] Greene and others[71] approximated a 56% cumulative risk from age 20 to 59 years, with 100% of atypical mole syndrome patients developing melanoma by age 76.

Xeroderma pigmentosa is a rare hereditary disorder that is also associated with melanoma; it is inherited in an autosomally recessive fashion.[99] The fibroblasts in xeroderma pigmentosa patients have a reduced or absent ability to repair DNA that has been damaged by ultraviolet light.[49] Consequently, this disorder results in the development of multiple primary cutaneous malignancies, including melanoma, basal cell carcinoma, and squamous cell carcinoma. Individuals are usually diagnosed with their first cancer prior to the age of 10. Unfortunately, the relentless development of skin cancers—as well as other cancers—ultimately leads to death, often at an early age.

Congenital Nevi

Congenital melanocytic nevi (CMN) are present at birth or appear within the first 6 months of infancy[136]; an estimated 1% to 6% of children are born with CMN. The nevi are classified by size: Small CMN measure <1.5 mm in diameter and account for the majority of lesions; medium CMN measure between 1.5 and 19.9 mm in diameter; and large CMN, which are also called *giant congenital nevi*, measure 20 mm or greater. This large size can lead to significant cosmetic and psychosocial implications.[109]

The risk of melanoma development in small- and medium-sized CMN is similar to any other area of the skin. Melanoma development usually occurs after childhood and arises from the dermoepidermal junction, which makes early detection feasible. Routine prophylactic removal of small and medium CMN is rarely indicated in the absence of signs or symptoms indicative of malignant progression.

Conversely, giant congenital nevi carry an increased risk for melanoma, with an estimated 5% to 20% of patients going on to develop cancer.[54,28] Seventy percent of these individuals are diagnosed before the age of 10 years.[108] Melanoma can originate deep the epidermis. Consequently, diagnosis within the setting of giant congenital nevi is challenging; it may develop deep in the skin, with presentation as a more advanced primary lesion.

MELANOMA CLASSIFICATION

Several histologic subtypes of melanoma are recognized within the HN region. It is important to note that melanoma subtype does not generally influence prognosis after correcting for tumor thickness and other prognostic variables.[5] In general, *superficial spreading melanoma* is the most common type of cutaneous melanoma, and *nodular melanoma* is the second most common subtype on the skin.

Lentigo maligna (LM) is intraepidermal or in situ melanoma. Histologically, it is often seen in the background of chronic sun damage. LM is the precursor to invasive *lentigo malignant melanoma (LMM)*. The exact percentage of LMs that progress to invasive LMM remains unknown[51]; however, it is speculated that, if patients live long enough, LM will eventually progress to invasive melanoma. LM/LMM is most often found in the HN region. Traditionally, the subtype has been associated with older individuals, but the frequency in younger patients is increasing. The LM/LMM pattern warrants special comment, because this subtype is characterized by asymmetric, subclinical, and often extensive peripheral involvement of atypical junctional melanocytic hyperplasia (AJMH). Therefore, management with adequate wide margins can be challenging from both a functional and cosmetic standpoint. Additionally, amelanotic and invasive desmoplastic melanoma (see below) often arise within LM/LMM.

Desmoplastic-Neurotropic Melanoma

In 1971, Conley and others[53] described a rare subtype of melanoma comprised of spindle cells with abundant collagen. As a result of histologic features resembling fibromas, the term *desmoplastic melanoma (DM)* was introduced. Several years later, Reed and colleagues[135] noted that some DMs demonstrate a propensity for perineural and endoneural infiltration; this prompted the further subclassification of a *desmoplastic neurotropic melanoma (DNM)* variant.

DM/DNM subtypes are rare, accounting for approximately 1% of all cutaneous melanomas.[41] However, up to 75% of the lesions present in the HN region, often in the setting of LM/LMM. The clinical presentation and biologic behavior of these tumors are distinct from other cutaneous melanomas. Although amelanotic cases account for only 4% to 5% of cutaneous melanomas, up to 73% of DM/DNMs are amelanotic.[41,134] As demonstrated in Figure 23-1, the neoplasms often lack the typical ABCD criteria for melanoma (described below); they can have a difficult histologic pattern that requires interpretation by an experienced pathologist. Overall, the atypical and challenging appearance of DM/DMN is thought to result in a delay in diagnosis; this fact provides one explanation for the reason that patients with DM/DNM present with thicker, more aggressive tumors.

DM/DNM is known to be locally aggressive and highly infiltrative, and it can lead to cranial nerve and skull base involvement. Local recurrence has been reported in up to 49% of cases.[41] Explanations for this

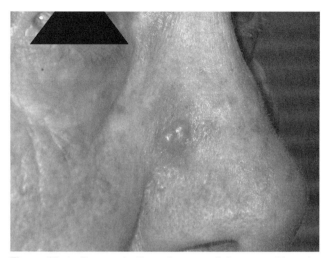

Figure 23-1. Desmoplastic melanoma of the nose. Note the amelanotic appearance and absence of typical ABCD findings associated with other melanoma subtypes. To view this image in color, please go to *www.ototext.com* or the Electronic Image Collection CD, bound into your copy of Cummings Otolaryngology—Head and Neck Surgery, 4th edition.

high rate include the association with neurotropism and the failure to recognize and adequately clear peripheral AJMH margins. Although DM/DNM demonstrates greater tumor thickness at the time of diagnosis, the 12.5% rate of regional lymph node metastasis is lower than that of other melanoma subtypes.[135]

Mucosal Melanoma

Mucosal melanoma is recognized as a distinct subtype from its cutaneous counterpart. The most common site for mucosal melanoma is the HN, with 40% to 50% of cases arising in this location.[142] However, less than 2% of all HN melanomas are mucosal in origin. Of the 84,836 melanoma cases registered in the National Cancer Database from 1985 to 1994, only 1074 (1.3%) were of the mucosal melanoma variant.[45]

Although small case numbers limit research to anecdotal reports, several common trends have been noted throughout the literature. The peak age for mucosal melanoma is during the sixth to seventh decade, which is approximately 10 to 15 years later than that of cutaneous melanoma.[25,78,106,130,142] A slight male predominance has also been reported.[78,130,153] Ethnic differences have been observed in that approximately 8.8% of mucosal melanoma cases afflict blacks and Hispanics; this is a considerable number given that less than 3% of all other melanoma variants are diagnosed among this group.[46] The relative frequency is also exceedingly high for the Japanese, for whom mucosal melanoma accounts for 7.5% of all melanoma cases in that country.[89]

Within the HN region, the most common site of origin is the nasal cavity, where the anterior nasal septum is most often involved, followed by the inferior and middle turbinates.[23,101,106,153] The second most common site is the oral cavity, where a predilection for the hard palate and maxillary alveolar gingivae has been found. A review of five major mucosal melanoma series by Batsakis and others[23] found laryngeal primary tumors to account for less than 4% of all cases. Within the larynx, the supraglottis was the most common site of origin.

The presenting signs and symptoms of mucosal melanoma directly relate to the anatomic site of origin. The majority of patients with nasal cavity primaries present with nasal obstruction and epistaxis.[23,101,153] Proptosis, diplopia, pain, and facial deformity are less common and are indicative of advanced disease. When present, the most common sign of an oral cavity tumor is a mass lesion.[101] However, oral cavity mucosal melanoma is often asymptomatic, with the cancer going undiagnosed until a neck mass develops from metastasis.[25,153] Many of the prognostic markers for cutaneous melanoma do not have correlates in mucosal sites.[142] Consequently, the cutaneous melanoma staging system set forth by the AJCC (see below) may be less applicable to mucosal melanoma. Most mucosal melanoma patients present with localized disease, with only 18.7% having regional spread detected at the time of diagnosis. The high percentage of patients with stage I disease is deceiving, because local recurrence is the major reason for treatment failure.[23] Fifty percent of patients have local recurrence, usually within 9 to 12 months of diagnosis, and the overall five-year survival rate is a dismal 10% to 20%.[23,78,106,130] Rich submucosal vasculature and lymphatics are thought to account for the aggressive behavior of mucosal melanoma.[23]

Unknown Primary

Approximately 2% to 5% of melanoma cases involve unknown primary sites.[45,46,122] Two thirds of these patients present with regional metastasis in the absence of an identifiable primary lesion or history of melanoma; the remaining third of unknown primary cases involve distant metastasis to sites such as the subcutaneous tissues, lung, and brain.[46,120,122,144]

Various theories have been proposed to explain melanoma of unknown primary origin. The identification of melanocytes and nevus cells within the lymph node capsule and visceral organ epithelium lends credence to the belief that unknown primary cases result from melanoma arising de novo at regional and distant sites.[46,85] Another clinical scenario is that the primary melanoma site undergoes complete spontaneous regression.[33,85]

Patients diagnosed with melanoma of unknown origin require a search for the primary site with a total body skin and mucosal evaluation. A history of a previous skin biopsy or skin lesion that spontaneously disappeared may be helpful. All pathology slides from previously excised lesions should be re-reviewed. The metastatic workup is identical to that of known primary cases (see below). After adjusting for tumor stage, melanoma of unknown primary origin share an overall prognosis equivalent to their counterparts with known primary sites.[46,120,122,144]

DIAGNOSTIC WORKUP
History

The majority of melanoma lesions are first detected by the patient or his or her significant other,[97,146] with less than one fourth of lesions being diagnosed during routine office physical examination. Lesions detected by a physician tend to be thinner.[146] The earliest signs for melanoma are a change in color, size, or shape of a lesion, and pruritus is the earliest symptom. Later signs; symptoms, which are usually associated with a more advanced lesion, include bleeding, ulceration, and tenderness. Patients should be questioned about a previous and family history of melanoma. Information about previous skin biopsies, sun exposure, history of blistering sunburns, tanning booth use, chronic sun exposure, and occupation should be obtained.

Physical Examination

All patients who present with a suspicious lesion warrant a full body skin examination by a physician who is experienced with skin lesions. The incidence of multiple primary cutaneous melanomas generally ranges from 5% to 8%.[24,88,82,117]

The differential diagnosis for cutaneous melanoma is broad. The American Cancer Society has published the ABCD checklist to educate both patients and physicians about the early detection of melanoma.[4] Under these guidelines, concerning signs for melanoma include the following: asymmetry in appearance; border irregularity, such as scalloped, poorly circumscribed, or ill-defined margins; color variation within a lesion, such as shades of black, red, white, or blue; and a diameter of >6 mm. Although the ABCD checklist is helpful for the identification of melanoma, it will not detect every case.[111,171] It is important to realize that a subset of cancers (e.g., amelanotic, desmoplastic, and nodular melanoma) lack the common features of the ABCDs. For this reason, a seven-point checklist developed in Europe focuses on the importance of change in the lesion.[105] Another useful screening tool is the "ugly duckling sign"[72]; any pigmented lesion that appears significantly and singularly different from other surrounding lesions should be viewed with a high index of suspicion, even if the lesion lacks the traditional ABCD criteria.

Biopsy

Any pigmented lesion that demonstrates an ABCD warning sign, has undergone change, or appears different from surrounding nevi on the body warrants histologic evaluation. Ideally, a complete excisional biopsy with a narrow 1- to 2-mm clinical margin of surrounding skin is performed. The biopsy of a potential melanoma should be considered a two-step process. The first step involves biopsy for histologic diagnosis. Pathologic review also includes microstaging of tumor depth and evaluation of other concerning features such as ulceration, mitotic rate, angiolymphatic invasion, and perineural spread.

These results then serve as the guide for the second step, which entails wide local excision (WLE). In WLE, a 0.5 to 2 cm margin of normal surrounding skin is removed, with or without sentinel lymph node mapping and biopsy (SLNB), depending on the final microstaging of the lesion. Although obtaining wider margins at the time of the initial biopsy may seem more efficient and cost-effective, clinical accuracy is uncertain, and removal of significant amounts of skin surrounding the lesion may comprise the ability to accurately stage regional lymph node basins using lymphoscintigraphy and SLNB techniques (described below).[152] Therefore, biopsy with narrow margins in a two-step fashion is advocated.

For lesions that are not amenable to excisional biopsy due to large size or anatomic location, punch biopsy or incisional biopsy through the thickest portion of the neoplasm is recommended. Superficial shave biopsy and fine needle aspiration are discouraged, because the thickness of the tumor, which dictates further diagnostic workup and treatment, cannot be obtained. It is important to realize that punch and incisional biopsies are subject to sampling error. If a diagnosis of melanoma is not rendered following a punch or incisional procedure, a repeat biopsy may be necessary.

Metastatic Workup

In an attempt to standardize staging workup for melanoma, the National Comprehensive Cancer Network (NCCN) has published guidelines.[121] The metastatic workup performed at our institution is in accordance with these guidelines and is outlined in Table 23-2.

Patients presenting with localized stage I disease simply require a thorough history and physical examination. Many physicians advocate a screening chest x-ray (CXR), because the lung is the most common site for distant metastasis.[152] Although a CXR is an inexpensive, noninvasive means for metastatic evaluation, the incidence of detecting occult pulmonary metastasis in an asymptomatic patient with stage I or II disease is exceedingly low.[9,92] Using CXR, Terhune and colleagues[157] identified only 1 of 876 (0.1%)

TABLE 23-2	
UNIVERSITY OF MICHIGAN GUIDELINES FOR CUTANEOUS MELANOMA WORKUP[84]	
Stage 0 (in situ)	History; physical examination
Stage I (<1 mm thickness)	History; physical examination
Stage I to II (1–4 mm thick)	History; physical examination *Chest x-ray optional* *Lactate dehydrogenase levels optional*
Stage III (N_0; >4 mm thick)	History; physical examination *Chest x-ray optional* *Lactate dehydrogenase levels optional*
Stage III (N^+; in transit)	History; physical examination Chest x-ray Lactate dehydrogenase levels *Other imaging studies, if clinically indicated*
Stage IV (distant metastasis)	History; physical examination Chest x-ray Lactate dehydrogenase levels *Other imaging studies, per clinical trial*

patients within this subpopulation that had occult pulmonary metastasis; however, the high false-positive rate of 15% necessitated additional and costly workups. Similarly, evidence supporting the use of other screening modalities such as computed tomography,[34,56] liver-spleen scans, magnetic resonance imaging, and bone scans for patients with limited stage I and II disease is lacking.[10,143]

CXR and screening lactate dehydrogenase (LDH) levels are both deemed optional by the National Comprehensive Cancer Network for stage II and III patients in the clinical absence of nodal disease (N0). At our institution, these studies are ordered only if the history or physical examination raises the clinician's suspicion for metastasis.[84]

Patients with stage III disease that includes clinically or radiographically suspicious lymph nodes, satellite lesions, or in-transit lesions, are at higher risk for distant metastasis. Fine-needle aspiration has been shown to be an accurate and cost-effective means of confirming metastatic melanoma within lymph nodes.[22] CXR and LDH are warranted for positive regional disease. Additional imaging studies should be ordered depending on the patient's history and physical examination. A list of concerning symptoms warranting a focused investigation of systemic metastasis is summarized in Table 23-3.[83]

Patients with known stage IV disseminated melanoma required a complete workup for systemic metastasis. In this setting, workup is often dictated by clinical trial protocols.

PROGNOSTIC FACTORS AND TUMOR STAGING

As a result of an increased understanding of cutaneous melanoma biology, the AJCC published a revised staging system in 2001.[17,18] The goal of modifying the classification system was twofold. First, the Staging Committee wanted to develop categories based on the most important independent prognostic markers for melanoma. By doing so, cohorts of patients sharing similar survival rates may become easier to identify, thereby leading to increased homogeneity in future clinical trials. To achieve this goal, reliable prognostic markers recognized throughout the literature were studied among a cohort of 17,600 melanoma patients from 13 major cancer institutions.[17] This investigation marks the largest analysis of its kind to date. The sec-

ond goal was to provide physicians with a classification system that mirrors clinical practice. For this reason, physician input related to both clinical management and research protocols was considered during the revision process.

Summary of Revisions

The new AJCC staging system for cutaneous melanoma remains founded upon the traditional tumor, node, metastases (TNM) classification system (Tables 23-4 and 23-5). Stage I and II represent localized disease, stage III is regional disease, and stage IV is reserved for distant metastatic disease. The most important predictors for survival now serve as criteria for the definition of melanoma stage and are summarized in Table 23-6. Major revisions of the staging system are outlined below:

1. *Tumor thickness* and *ulceration* are utilized in T classification, whereas level of invasion (Clark level) is only applied in the staging of thin (≤ 1 mm) T_1 lesions.
2. The *number of metastatic lymph nodes*—as opposed to the gross size of metastatic nodes—is used to define the N category.

TABLE 23-3

Review of Systems for Melanoma and Metastasis[83]

Skin/Lymphatics
  Change (i.e., size, shape, color)
  Lesion persistent pruritus
  Enlarged lymph nodes
  Mass/nodules
  Nonhealing/bleeding skin lesions
  Easy bruising
  New pigmented skin lesions
Constitutional
  Weight loss
  Malaise
  Decreased appetite
  Weakness
  Fatigue
  Fever
Respiratory
  Cough
  Hemoptysis
  Pneumonia
  Pleurisy
  Chest pain
  Dyspnea
Hepatic
  Abdominal pain
  Right upper quadrant pain

Back (scapula) pain on inspiration
Jaundice
Neurologic/Psychiatric
  Headache
  Memory disturbance
  Depression
  Focal central nervous system symptoms
  Visual disturbances
  Balance problems
  Blackouts
  Seizures
  Numbness
  Local weakness
  Paralysis
  Mood swings
Gastrointestinal
  Cramping
  Abdominal pain
  Bleeding
  Nausea
  Anorexia
  Vomiting
  Constipation
Musculoskeletal
  Bone pain (e.g., rib, spine, hip)

Adapted from: Johnson TM and others: Management of melanoma with a multidisciplinary melanoma clinic model, *J Am Acad Dermatol* 42:820, 2000.

TABLE 23-4

MELANOMA TNM CLASSIFICATION

T Classification	Thickness	Ulceration Status
T_1	≤ 1.0 mm	a: without ulceration and level II/III b: with ulceration or level IV/V
T_2	1.01-2.0 mm	a: without ulceration b: with ulceration
T_3	2.01-4.0 mm	a: without ulceration b: with ulceration
T_4	> 4.0 mm	a: without ulceration b: with ulceration
N Classification	**No. of Metastatic Nodes**	**Nodal Metastatic Mass**
N_1	1 node	a: micrometastasis* b: macrometastasis†
N_2	2-3 nodes	a: micrometastasis* b: macrometastasis† c: in transit met(s)/ satellite(s) without metastatic nodes
N_3	4 or more metastatic nodes, or matted nodes, or in transit met(s)/satellite(s) with metastatic node(s)	
M Classification	**Site**	**Serum Lactate Dehydrogenase**
M_{1a}	Distant skin, subcutaneous, or nodal mets	Normal
M_{1b}	Lung metastases	Normal
M_{1c}	All other visceral metastases	Normal
	Any distant metastasis	Elevated

*Micrometastases are diagnosed after sentinel or elective lymphadenectomy.
†Macrometastases are defined as clinically detectable nodal metastases confirmed by therapeutic lymphadenectomy or when nodal metastasis exhibits gross extracapsular extension.

3. The technique of *sentinel lymph node mapping and biopsy (SLNB)* is now incorporated into the staging system. Delineation of *occult (microscopic)* nodal metastasis vs clinically/radiographically apparent (*macroscopic*) nodal metastasis is made within the N category.
4. The *site of distant metastasis* and *LDH level* are both used in the M classification.
5. Patients with *ulcerated primary lesions* are upstaged.
6. Primary lesions with surrounding *satellite metastasis* or *in-transit metastasis* are defined as stage III regional disease.

T Classification/Localized Disease

Multivariate analysis of 13,581 patients with localized disease identified tumor thickness and ulceration as the most important predictors of outcome. Overall, tumor thickness was the most powerful prognostic indicator for this subgroup. Although tumor thickness was incorporated in the 1997 version of the staging system, the empirically based Breslow depth of 0.75 mm was used to differentiate T_1 from T_2 lesions.[31] The revised staging system now uses cutpoints of 1.0, 2.0, and 4.0 mm to delineate T stage. The new cut-points represent the best statistical fit in the correlation of tumor thickness and survival.

In the previous staging system, histologic level of invasion as represented by the Clark scale (Figure 23-2) was also used in the definition of T classification. However, the recent analysis by Balch and others[17] found the histologic level of invasion to be prognostic only for thin T_1 lesions. For tumors ≤1 mm without ulceration, invasion to Clark level II or III is considered T_{1a}, whereas invasion into the reticular dermis (level IV or V) is considered T_{1b}. With the exception of T_1 lesions, Clark level of invasion is no longer used in staging melanoma.

TABLE 23-5

Proposed Stage Groupings for Cutaneous Melanoma

	Clinical Staging*			Pathologic Staging†		
	T	N	M	T	N	M
0	T_{is}	N_0	M_0	T_{is}	N_0	M_0
IA	T_{1a}	N_0	M_0	T_{1a}	N_0	M_0
IB	T_{1b}	N_0	M_0	T_{1b}	N_0	M_0
	T_{2a}	N_0	M_0	T_{2a}	N_0	M_0
IIA	T_{2b}	N_0	M_0	T_{2b}	N_0	M_0
	T_{3a}	N_0	M_0	T_{3a}	N_0	M_0
IIB	T_{3b}	N_0	M_0	T_{3b}	N_0	M_0
	T_{4a}	N_0	M_0	T_{4a}	N_0	M_0
IIC	T_{4b}	N_0	M_0	T_{4b}	N_0	M_0
III‡	Any T	N_1	M_0			
		N_2				
		N_3				
IIIA				T_{1-4a}	N_{1a}	M_0
				T_{1-4a}	N_{2a}	M_0
IIIB				T_{1-4b}	N_{1a}	M_0
				T_{1-4b}	N_{2a}	M_0
				T_{1-4a}	N_{1b}	M_0
				T_{1-4a}	N_{2b}	M_0
				$T_{1-4a/b}$	N_{2c}	M_0
IIIC				T_{1-4b}	N_{1b}	M_0
				T_{1-4b}	N_{2b}	M_0
				Any T	N_3	M_0
IV	Any T	Any N	Any M_1	Any T	Any N	Any M_1

*Clinical staging includes microstaging of the primary melanoma and clinical/radiologic evaluation for metastases. By convention, it should be used after complete excision of the primary melanoma with clinical assessment for regional and distant metastases.
†Pathologic staging includes microstaging of the primary melanoma and pathologic information about the regional lymph nodes after partial or complete lymphadenectomy. Pathologic stage 0 or stage 1A patients are the exception; they do not require pathologic evaluation of their lymph nodes.
‡There are no stage III subgroups for clinical staging.

TABLE 23-6

Summary of the Most Important Predictors of Survival That Serve as Criteria for the 2001 AJCC Cutaneous Melanoma Staging System

Stage I and II localized disease
  1) Tumor thickness
  2) Tumor ulceration
  3) Histologic level of invasion for T_1 lesions only

Stage III regional disease
  1) Number of metastatic lymph nodes
  2) Tumor burden (microscopic vs macroscopic nodal disease)
  3) Primary tumor ulceration

Stage IV distant disease
  1) Anatomic site
  2) Elevated lactate dehydrogenase

Tumor ulceration was the second most important prognostic indicator for patients with localized disease. Ulceration is not a visible crater on gross examination, but rather a histologic diagnosis in which intact epidermis overlying the melanoma is absent. Survival rates were found to be significantly lower for all patients with ulcerated lesions as compared with their nonulcerated counterparts (Table 23-7). In fact, the survival of patients with an ulcerated tumor mirrored that of nonulcerated patients in the next highest T category; for this reason, ulceration warrants upstaging of tumors. The prognostic significance of ulceration[12] and the correlation between ulceration and mitotic rate have been reported.[11,127] Although mitotic rate was not evaluated during the revision of

the AJCC staging system, it may become an important prognostic marker in the future.

Nodal Classification/Regional Disease

Similar multivariate analysis was performed on more than 1000 melanoma patients diagnosed with lymph node metastasis. Three prognostic factors met significance at $P < .0001$: (1) number of metastatic lymph nodes; (2) tumor burden as represented by microscopic vs macroscopic disease; and (3) primary tumor ulceration. Previously, the gross diameter of metastatic nodes was used in N classification. Due to a lack of compelling evidence supporting predictive value, metastatic nodal size is no longer incorporated into melanoma staging.[35,36]

Overall, the most important predictive marker for patients with nodal metastasis was the number of positive lymph nodes; survival curves are depicted in Figure 23-3. The greatest difference in five-year survival rates was used to subclassify the N category. Patients with one metastatic node are now categorized as N_1, patients with two or three metastatic nodes as N_2, and patients with four or more nodes as N_3.

The second most important prognostic indicator for patients with regional metastasis was tumor burden. Patients identified as having microscopic nodal disease, either through SLNB or elective lymphadenectomy, were found to have a significantly better survival as compared with individuals diagnosed with macroscopic disease upon clinical or radiographic examination (Figure 23-4). This difference was so compelling that microscopic vs macroscopic nodal disease is now subclassified within the N category. In addition, the AJCC Melanoma Committee strongly recommends staging with SLNB for patients

CLARK LEVELS

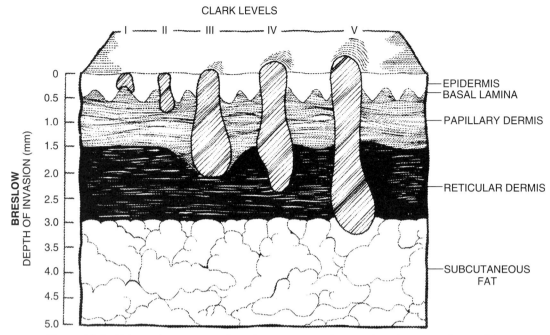

Figure 23-2. Schematic representation of cutaneous melanoma invasion according to Clark and Breslow microstaging.

with $T_2N_0M_0$, $T_3N_0M_0$, and $T_4N_0M_0$ disease before entry into clinical trials.[18] The identification of occult nodal disease will lead to accurate pathologic staging and increased homogeneity among cohorts under clinical investigation.

Ulceration continued to remain an important prognostic indicator, even in the presence of nodal metastasis. In fact, ulceration was found to be the only feature of the primary tumor that was indicative of outcome. After adjusting for regional metastasis, tumor thickness was no longer a prognostic marker ($P = .16$).

A fourth criterion now used when defining stage III regional disease is intralymphatic metastasis. The presence of satellite metastasis surrounding a primary lesion and in-transit metastasis identified between the primary melanoma and lymph node have been identified as poor prognostic indicators.[36,74] Both findings portend a prognosis similar to nodal metastasis. Under the new staging system, satellite metastasis and in-transit metastasis are classified as N_{2c} disease in the absence of nodal disease (N_0). If synchronous nodal metastasis is found in the setting of satellite or in-transient metastasis, prognosis is extremely poor. These patients are automatically upstaged to N3 disease, irrespective of the number of synchronous positive lymph nodes.

Overall 5- and 10-year survival for patients with metastatic nodal disease was 49% and 37%, respectively.[17] However, the range in survival for stage III patients was significant, ranging from 13% for patients

with ulcerated primary lesions and macroscopic disease identified in four lymph nodes to as high as 69% for patients with a nonulcerated primary tumor and microscopic disease confined to one lymph node (Table 23-8). This finding confirms previous studies that demonstrated that stage III disease represents a heterogeneous group of patients.[35,115] In addition, it highlights the critical impact on survival afforded by the early diagnosis of regional metastasis.

M Stage/Distant Metastasis

Prognostic factors for disseminated stage IV disease were studied among 1158 patients, and the most significant difference was found to be anatomic site. Patients with distant metastasis to the skin, subcutaneous tissue, or distant lymph nodes (M_{1a}) had a slightly higher survival rate as compared with patients with lung metastasis (M_{1b}). Patients with metastasis involving other visceral organs (M_{1c}) had the worst prognosis. Previous studies have also identified elevated LDH as a poor prognostic marker.[30,57,59,150] For this reason, any patient with elevated LDH and distant metastasis, regardless of site, is classified as M_{1c}. Additional studies correlated male gender, >1 metastatic site, Karnofsky performance status <80, and limited disease-free survival with a poor prognosis.[21,30]

Overall, survival for patients with distant metastasis is extremely grave, measured in months as opposed to years. The median survival time following the diagnosis of disseminated disease is only 6 to

TABLE 23-7

Survival Rates for Melanoma TNM and Staging Categories

Pathologic Stage	TNM	Thickness (mm)	Ulceration	No. + Nodes	Nodal Size	Distant Metastasis	No. of Patients	Survival ± SE 1-Year	2-Year	5-Year	10-Year
IA	T_{1a}	≤1	No	0	—	—	4510	99.7 ± 0.1	99.0 ± 0.2	95.3 ± 0.4	87.9 ± 1.0
IB	T_{1b}	≤1	Yes or level IV, V	0	—	—	1380	99.8 ± 0.1	98.7 ± 0.3	90.9 ± 1.0	83.1 ± 1.5
IIA	T_{2a}	1.01–2.0	No	0	—	—	3285	99.5 ± 0.1	97.3 ± 0.3	89.0 ± 0.7	79.2 ± 1.1
	T_{2b}	1.01–2.0	Yes	0	—	—	958	98.2 ± 0.5	92.9 ± 0.9	77.4 ± 1.7	64.4 ± 2.2
IIB	T_{3a}	2.01–4.0	No	0	—	—	1717	98.7 ± 0.3	94.3 ± 0.6	78.7 ± 1.2	63.8 ± 1.7
	T_{3b}	2.01–4.0	Yes	0	—	—	1523	95.1 ± 0.6	84.8 ± 1.0	63.0 ± 1.5	50.8 ± 1.7
IIC	T_{4a}	>4.0	No	0	—	—	563	94.8 ±1.0	88.6 ±1.5	67.4 ± 2.4	53.9 ± 3.3
	T_{4b}	>4.0	Yes	0	—	—	978	89.9 ± 1.0	70.7 ± 1.6	45.1 ± 1.9	32.3 ± 2.1
IIIA	N_{1a}	Any	No	1	Micro	—	252	95.9 ± 1.3	88.0 ± 2.3	69.5 ± 3.7	63.0 ± 4.4
	N_{2a}	Any	No	2–3	Micro	—	130	93.0 ± 2.4	82.7 ± 3.8	63.3 ± 5.6	56.9 ± 6.8
IIIB	N_{1a}	Any	Yes	1	Micro	—	217	93.3 ± 1.8	75.0 ± 3.2	52.8 ± 4.1	37.8 ± 4.8
	N_{2a}	Any	Yes	2–3	Micro	—	111	92.0 ± 2.7	81.0 ± 4.1	49.6 ± 5.7	35.9 ± 7.2
	N_{1b}	Any	No	1	Macro	—	122	88.5 ± 2.9	78.5 ± 3.7	59.0 ± 4.8	47.7 ± 5.8
	N_{2b}	Any	No	2–3	Macro	—	93	76.8 ± 4.4	65.6 ± 5.0	46.3 ± 5.5	39.2 ± 5.8
IIIC	N_{1b}	Any	Yes	1	Macro	—	98	77.9 ± 4.3	54.2 ± 5.2	29.0 ± 5.1	24.4 ± 5.3
	N_{2b}	Any	Yes	2–3	Macro	—	109	74.3 ± 4.3	44.1 ± 4.9	24.0 ± 4.4	15.0 ± 3.9
	N_3	Any	Any	4	Micro/macro	—	396	71.0 ± 2.4	49.8 ± 2.7	26.7 ± 2.5	18.4 ± 2.5
IV	M_{1a}	Any	Any	Any	Any	Skin, SQ	179	59.3 ± 3.7	36.7 ± 3.6	18.8 ± 3.0	15.7 ± 2.9
	M_{1b}	Any	Any	Any	Any	Lung	186	57.0 ± 3.7	23.1 ± 3.2	6.7 ± 2.0	2.5 ± 1.5
	M_{1c}	Any	Any	Any	Any	Other, Visceral	793	40.6 ± 1.8	23.6 ± 1.5	9.5 ± 1.1	6.0 ± 0.9
Total							17,600				

From Balch CM, Buzaid AC, Soong SJ and others: Final version of the American Joint Committee on Cancer staging system for cutaneous melanoma, *J Clin Oncol* 19: 3637, Table 3, 2001.

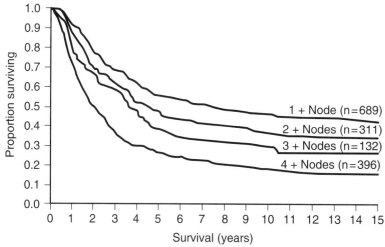

Figure 23-3. Survival curves of 1,528 melanoma patients with lymph node metastases subgrouped by actual number of metastatic lymph nodes. The correlation was significant at *P* < .0001. (From: Balch CM and others: Prognostic factors analysis of 17,600 melanoma patients: validation of the American Joint Committee on Cancer melanoma staging system, *J Clin Oncol* 19:3628, Figure 5, 2001.)

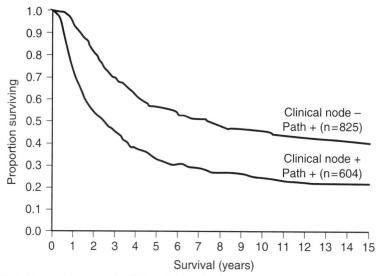

Figure 23-4. Survival curves of 1,429 patients with lymph node metastases subgrouped by presenting clinical stage. Survival rates calculated from the time of primary melanoma diagnoses were significant between the two groups (*P* < .0001). (From: Balch CM and others: Prognostic factors analysis of 17,600 melanoma patients: validation of the American Joint Committee on Cancer melanoma staging system, *J Clin Oncol* 19:3629, Figure 6, 2001.)

8 months, with a dismal 5-year survival rate of 6%.[21,30] For this reason, stage IV melanoma is not subclassified under the AJCC staging system.

Anatomic Site

Although anatomic site is not used within the formal staging system, prognostic differences have been reported.[63,66] A review of 6300 cutaneous melanomas treated at the Duke Medical Center identified the worst 10-year survival rate among HN primary tumors (54%) as compared with trunk (61%), lower extremity (71%), and upper extremity (76%) sites.[66] A 50% tumor recurrence rate has been reported for HN cutaneous melanomas.[61,62] This aggressive behavior is likely due to thicker melanoma lesions in the HN region as compared with other sites and failure to adequately remove AJMH at tumor margins, thereby causing a higher rate of local recurrence.

TABLE 23-8															
FIVE-YEAR SURVIVAL RATES FOR STAGE III (NODAL METASTASES) PATIENTS STRATIFIED BY NUMBER OF METASTATIC NODES, ULCERATION, AND TUMOR BURDEN															
	1 + NODE		MICROSCOPIC 2–3 NODES		> 3 NODES		1 + NODE		MACROSCOPIC 2–3 NODES		> 3 NODES				
Melanoma Ulceration	% ± SE	No.	% ± SE	No.	% ± SE	No.	% ± SE	No.	% ± SE	No.	% ± SE	No.			
Absent	69 ± 3.7	252	63 ± 5.6	130	27 ± 9.3	57	59 ± 4.7	122	46 ± 5.5	93	27 ± 4.6	109			
Present	52 ± 4.1	217	50 ± 5.7	111	37 ± 8.8	46	29 ± 5.0	98	25 ± 4.4	109	13 ± 3.5	104			

From Balch CM, Soong SJ, Gershenwald JE and others: Prognostic factors analysis of 17, 600 melanoma patients: validation of the American Joint Committee on Cancer melanoma staging system, *J Clin Oncol* 19: 3630, Table 9, 2001.

SURGICAL MANAGEMENT OF THE PRIMARY TUMOR
Wide Local Excision and Surgical Margins

Complete surgical excision is recognized as the standard of care for treating melanoma. However, the extent of surgical margins has previously been an issue of debate. Historically, WLE included an extensive 5-cm surrounding margin of normal tissue; this recommendation was based on an autopsy report of a patient with advanced melanoma in 1907.[73] The use of 5-cm surgical margins was routine practice until the 1970s, when Breslow and Macht challenged the concept by successfully treating 35 patients with thin melanomas using narrower margins.[32]

Two prospective, randomized trials investigating surgical margins for cutaneous melanoma have since followed. The World Health Organization (WHO) conducted an international trial in which 612 patients with thin melanomas (=2 mm) were randomized to surgical excision with 1 cm versus >3 cm margins.[166] At a mean follow-up of eight years, disease-free survival and overall survival were reported to be equivalent between the two groups.[167] For this reason, the WHO concluded that wide excision did not influence survival for patients with thin melanomas. For patients with melanomas <1 mm in thickness, the authors advocated "narrow" 1-cm margins to the muscular fascia plane.

Within the WHO trial, a subset of 245 patients had tumors measuring 1.1 to 2.0 mm in thickness. Although a difference in disease-free survival and overall survival was not observed with respect to margins, a local recurrence rate of 3.3% was reported among patients undergoing "narrow" excision. This finding prompted the Intergroup Melanoma Surgical Trial, which prospectively randomized 740 patients with intermediate-thickness (1-4 mm) melanomas to WLE with 2-cm vs 4-cm margins.[19] Local recurrence rates and 10-year survival were reported to be equivalent between the two groups. This finding led to the recommendation of a 2-cm surgical margin for patients with intermediate melanomas measuring 1.1 to 4.0 mm in thickness.

To date, there is no prospective randomized trial that has investigated the optimal surgical margin for thick melanomas. However, a retrospective study of 278 thick melanomas (>4 mm) found that surgical margins of >2 cm did not lead to a difference in local recurrence rate, disease-free survival, or overall survival as compared with margins of 2 cm.[76] Within this study, 16% of the tumors involved HN subsites.

Current guidelines for surgical margins are based on primary tumor thickness (Table 23-9). It is important to realize that these recommendations serve only as guidelines; each melanoma case must be individualized. The

TABLE 23-9

RECOMMENDED SURGICAL MARGINS FOR EXCISION OF PRIMARY CUTANEOUS MELANOMA

Tumor Thickness (mm)	Surgical Margin (cm)
In situ	0.5
<1.0	1.0
1.01–2.0	1.0–2.0
>2.0	2.0

depth of excision includes full-thickness skin and underlying subcutaneous tissue. Resection of fascia, perichondrium, and periosteum is required only in the setting of direct tumor invasion or if the surgical plane was violated during a previous biopsy.[90]

LMM warrants special comment, because it has a propensity for wide subclinical spread, which often results in positive margins.[80] Johnson and colleagues[81] and Anderson and colleagues[5] have reported on the use of the "square" procedure in the treatment of LM and LMM. This staged procedure entails complete excision of the peripheral margin with permanent section histologic evaluation of 100% of the peripheral margins surrounding the entire tumor.

Closure and Reconstruction

With the use of wide undermining, the majority of surgical sites can be closed primarily. Larger defects may require reconstruction with a split-thickness skin graft, a full-thickness skin graft, a local advancement flap, or a regional flap. The method of reconstruction will depend on the anatomic location, skin color and texture, depth of the defect, and patient and surgeon preference. The method of closure has not been shown to impact survival.[102] After clear margins have been confirmed, surgeons are encouraged to close surgical defects using the technique that they think will yield the best cosmetic result.

Melanoma of the Ear

Originally, melanoma involving the ear was thought to carry a worse prognosis than other HN sites.[62,163,169] This increased risk was attributed to rich lymphatics, complex anatomic subdivisions of the auricle, and a paucity of subcutaneous tissue between the thin auricular skin and underlying perichondrium.[38] Consequently, full-thickness excision or total auriculectomy was often advocated.

After accounting for tumor thickness, recent studies have demonstrated that melanoma of the ear carries the same prognosis as other sites.[52,152] In addition, outcome differences were not observed between auricular subsites.[38] Retrospective reviews failed to demonstrate a difference in local recurrence based on the extent of surgical excision, even when perichondrium was preserved.[52] Today, the same prognostic indicators and surgical principles of obtaining wide, clear margins for treatment of cutaneous melanoma can be safely applied to the auricular region.

SURGICAL MANAGEMENT OF REGIONAL LYMPH NODES
Therapeutic Lymph Node Dissection

The most common sites for metastasis of HN cutaneous melanoma are the cervical and parotid lymph node basins.[13,64,119] The treatment of choice for regional disease remains a therapeutic lymph node dissection (TLND) that includes draining nodal basins as well as all intervening lymphatics between the primary tumor and the site of regional disease.

The location of the primary tumor dictates the type of TLND and the need for a superficial parotidectomy. Melanomas of the anterolateral scalp, temple, lateral forehead, lateral cheek, and ear, arising anterior to an imaginary coronal plane through the external auditory canals, drain via the parotid nodal basin to the jugular lymph node chain.[40] For this reason, a superficial parotidectomy and modified radical neck dissection are both recommended. In the absence of gross tumor involvement or disruption from open biopsy or previous surgical dissection, concerted efforts should be made to preserve the spinal accessory nerve, internal jugular vein, and sternocleidomastoid muscle.[40] If the melanoma arises in a more inferior location (e.g., the chin or neck), a superficial parotidectomy is not warranted. Melanomas located on the scalp and occiput—posterior to the imaginary coronal plane through the external auditory canals—can drain to postauricular, suboccipital, and posterior triangle lymph nodes. These nodal basins are not addressed during routine modified radical neck dissection. In this situation, a posterolateral neck dissection is required.[69]

Elective Lymph Node Dissection

One of the most controversial historic debates regarding melanoma surrounded the treatment of regional nodal basins in the absence of clinical metastasis (prophylactic treatment of the N0 neck).[13,119] Prospective, randomized trials failed to demonstrate an overall survival benefit for patients undergoing elective lymph node dissection (ELND).* Therefore, ELND is no longer advocated for the routine treatment of melanoma.

---

*References 14, 16, 42, 149, 164, 165.

Sentinel Lymph Node Biopsy

SLNB is considered the method of choice for the staging of nodal basins. Appropriate patient selection is imperative. The indications for SLNB are summarized in Table 23-10. Patients with metastatic disease or who have undergone previous surgical disruption of the lymphatics or resection with wide margins are not deemed candidates.

Nodal status is currently recognized as the most important prognostic factor for melanoma patients.[18] Ten to 20% of individuals harbor occult microscopic nodal disease. In an attempt to identify this small group of patients who warranted TLND while sparing the remaining 80% of patients without regional disease the morbidity associated with a neck dissection, Morton and colleagues[114] introduced SLNB for the evaluation of patients with trunk and extremity cutaneous melanoma. The authors demonstrated that the status of the SLN accurately represented the status of the entire nodal basin from which it was obtained. SLN mapping with biopsy provides a minimally invasive means of identifying patients with occult nodal metastasis.[116] The technique is considered the best staging modality for regional disease, with the highest sensitivity and specificity of any modality currently available.

The SLN technique introduced by Morton and others has since evolved to include preoperative lymphoscintigraphy.[162] Approximately two to four hours before surgery, patients undergo intradermal injection of a radioactive colloid into the four quadrants surrounding the primary melanoma tumor. Lymphoscintigraphy is then performed. This nuclear medicine scan enables the surgeon to determine the number, location, and laterality of nodal basins at risk for metastatic disease (Figure 23-5). It is particularly helpful in the setting of midline HN melanomas, which are at risk for bilateral lymphatic drainage.

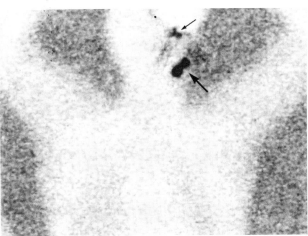

Figure 23-5. Preoperative lymphoscintigraphy is performed approximately 3 hours prior to sentinel lymph node biopsy. Approximately 2 μCi of technetium Tc-99m sulfur colloid (CIS-US, Inc; Bedford, Ma) was injected intradermally into the four quadrants surrounding the primary melanoma lesion located midline on the posterior occiput. The right posterior occiput primary lesion with an overlying shield to limit "shine-through" is denoted by the small arrow. The larger arrow points to two draining sentinel lymph nodes observed in the right posterior triangle of the neck.

Once under anesthesia, intraoperative lymphatic mapping with isosulfan blue dye (Lymphazurin 1%; Hirsch Industries, Inc; Richmond, Va) is performed.[114] Approximately 1 mL of dye is injected into the intradermal layer surrounding the primary melanoma lesion (Figure 23-6). The primary tumor and draining lymphatics are in close proximity within the HN region.

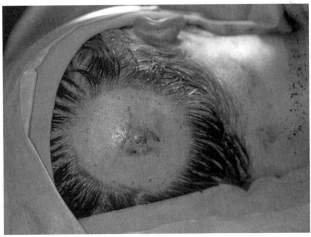

Figure 23-6. After the administration of anesthesia, intraoperative lymphatic mapping is performed using approximately 1 mL of isosulfan blue dye (Lymphazurin 1%; Hirsh Industries, Inc; Richmond, Va) injected into the intradermal layer surrounding the primary melanoma.

TABLE 23-10

UNIVERSITY OF MICHIGAN INDICATIONS FOR CONSIDERATION OF MELANOMA SENTINEL LYMPH NODE MAPPING AND BIOPSY

Breslow depth = 1 mm
Breslow depth = 1 mm in setting of adverse prognostic variables, including the following:
  Tumor extension to deep margin
  Ulceration
  Extensive regression to 1.0 mm
  Young age
  High mitotic rate[11]
  Clark level IV

Therefore, WLE of the primary tumor is performed first to reduce radioactive "shine-through," which will render the intraoperative gamma probe useless for the identification of SLNs (Figure 23-7).

Following WLE of the primary melanoma, nodal basins at risk for metastasis are evaluated for increased radioactivity using a handheld gamma probe. A 1- to 3-cm incision is made overlying the areas of increased radioactivity. A preauricular incision is recommended for SLN biopsy in the parotid region. SLNs are then identified using a combination of the gamma probe and visual cues from the blue dye (Figure 23-7). Each SLN is individually dissected from surrounding tissue. The staging procedure is considered complete when all nodal basins demonstrate minimal background radioactivity relative to the primary lesion and SLNs.

At our institution, all SLNs are sent for histologic evaluation using permanent sections. This evaluation includes serial sectioning and staining with hematoxylin and eosin (H&E). Special melanoma immunohistochemical staining for S-100 and melan-A (MART-1) are performed for all SLNs that are negative on H&E staining.

Patients with a positive SLN return to the operating room within two weeks of diagnosis for definitive TLND; patients with a negative biopsy are followed clinically. An alternative to this two-staged technique is immediate TLND on the basis of frozen section evaluation of the SLNs. However, it is important to realize

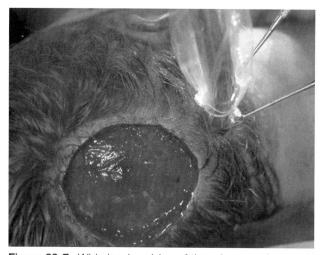

Figure 23-7. Wide local excision of the primary melanoma is performed prior to sentinel lymph node biopsy; otherwise, the close proximity of the primary lesion to the draining nodal basins within the head and neck region will cause significant radioactive "shine-through" and difficulty with the localization of the sentinel lymph node. Each sentinel lymph node is then identified using a combination of the gamma probe, which detects radioactive activity from the Tc-99m sulfur colloid, and visual cues from the isosulfan blue dye.

that the reliability of frozen sections for melanoma analysis has been questioned,[50] and permanent sections remain the gold standard.

The pathologist plays an extremely critical role in the success of the SLN biopsy. Occult lymphatic metastasis from cutaneous melanoma can be difficult to detect and warrants rigorous pathologic analysis, including serial sectioning, special immunohistochemical study when indicated, and interpretation by an experienced pathologist. Wager and others[168] reported the mean tumor volume in SLNs positive for metastatic melanoma to be only 4.7 mm³. Joseph and colleagues reported the identification of only 73% of metastatic SLNs using standard H&E staining alone. The histologic analysis of SLNs is more thorough and complete as compared with the traditional evaluation of the entire lymphadenectomy specimen, because the technique provides the pathologist with a limited number of nodes to thoroughly evaluate.[43]

SLN mapping and biopsy is a team effort involving experienced surgeons, nuclear medicine staff, and pathologists. The experience and technical skill of the surgeon is vital. A 30-case learning curve has previously been suggested[116] and may account for some of the variability observed in HN cutaneous melanoma SLN studies.[145] An experienced nuclear medicine staff is also necessary, because inappropriate administration of the radioactive tracer can also lead to "shine through." Communication with the nuclear medicine team is helpful not only for the interpretation of the lymphoscintigram but also to ensure that the appropriate lesion is mapped, because patients with melanoma often present with multiple pigmented lesions.

Recent multivariate analysis involving patients with stage I and II melanoma by Greshenwald and others[68] found the pathologic status (positive or negative for metastasis) of the SLN to be the most important prognostic factor for both recurrence and overall survival. For stage III melanoma, a survival benefit was found in patients with occult microscopic disease as compared with their counterparts who had palpable macroscopic disease (Table 23-8).[18] This survival benefit was so compelling that the AJCC has now incorporated SLN mapping into the revised staging system for cutaneous melanoma.

Although SLN mapping with biopsy has a defined role in the evaluation of cutaneous melanoma of the trunk and extremities, several questions have been posed with respect to its application in the HN region.[116] The complexity of the HN lymphatic system has caused concern surrounding the reliability of the SLN biopsy to accurately reflect the status of the entire nodal basin. The interlacing network of cervical lymphatic vessels is often deemed watershed in nature. The complexity of this lymphatic system was demonstrated by O'Brien and colleagues,[124] who reported a 34% discordance between the clinical prediction of lymphatic drainage and lymphoscintigraphy findings in 97 cases of HN cutaneous melanoma. The popularity of SLN biopsy in the HN region has also been limited by concern surrounding damage to vital structures such as the facial nerve,[58] technical difficulties,[58] and the necessity for nuclear medicine staff as well as pathologists who specialize in SLNB technique.

Our experience in staging 80 patients with HN cutaneous melanoma demonstrated that the complexity of the head and neck anatomy does not preclude the use of SLNB for the staging of cutaneous melanoma.[145] SLNB in the HN region accurately predicted the status of the nodal basin. Fourteen of 80 patients (17.5%) were identified with a positive SLN biopsy. Only 3 of 66 (4.5%) patients developed regional recurrence following a negative SLN biopsy. The 17.5% positivity rate of SLNs and the 4.5% false-negative rate both mirror the results of SLN mapping with biopsy achieved in other anatomic sites such as the trunk and extremities.[43,67] Similar success in the application of SLNB for HN cutaneous melanoma has been reported by others,[2,129] and the technique has successfully been applied in pediatric HN cases.[128]

Approximately 25% to 30% of HN cutaneous melanomas drain to lymph nodes within the parotid bed.[124,145] Potential injury to the facial nerve from SLN biopsy has led some surgeons to advocate superficial parotidectomy over the mapping procedure.[58] In our retrospective analysis, 28 of 30 (93.3%) patients draining to the parotid nodal basin successfully underwent staging using SLNB.[145] One patient required a superficial parotidectomy due to the location of the SLN deep to the facial nerve, and a second patient experienced significant bleeding from surrounding parotid tissue, which could have placed the facial nerve at increased risk. A total of 39 nodes from 28 parotid basins were removed without facial nerve injury. Continuous facial nerve monitoring for SLNB within the parotid nodal basin can be helpful when performing the biopsy with the parotid bed.

Concern has also been expressed that SLNB causes inflammation and fibrosis that could place the facial nerve at increased risk when reoperation is required to definitively treat the parotid basin in the setting of a positive SLN.[58] In our experience, all patients with a positive parotid SLN underwent a superficial parotidectomy as a subsequent procedure, without facial nerve injury. Our findings are consistent with other reports demonstrating that SLNB can reliably and safely be performed within the parotid nodal basin.[126,170]

The impact that SLNB has on overall survival remains to be determined. The answer will hopefully be provided through the multiinstitutional Sunbelt Melanoma Trial, which is currently being conducted.[113] This study is a prospective, randomized clinical trial that uses SLN staging to determine the need for adjuvant therapy. Until the results of this trial are available, McMasters and colleagues[112] provide four compelling reasons to use SLNB for the accurate regional staging of cutaneous melanoma. First, the technique provides important prognostic information to the physician and patient for guiding subsequent treatment options. Second, it helps to identify patients harboring nodal metastasis who then may benefit from early TLND.[42] Third, it identifies patients who are candidates for adjuvant treatment. Fourth, accurate regional staging enables the identification of a homogeneous population of patients for enrollment into clinical trials. Regional metastasis is the most important prognostic factor. Without accurate pathologic staging, stratification is impossible, and the results of clinical trials will remain inconsistent and difficult to interpret.

Surgical Management of Distant Metastasis

Patients with stage IV melanoma involving distant sites have an exceedingly grave prognosis. Surgical treatment has a limited role in the setting of disseminated disease. It has successfully been used as a means of palliative treatment in patients suffering from brain, lung, gastrointestinal, subcutaneous soft tissue, and distant lymph node metastasis.[172] Success of surgery in the palliative setting is heavily dependent on appropriate patient selection; it should only be considered if clearly identifiable and specific symptoms are associated with a metastatic lesion. Other considerations include surgical morbidity, expected quality of life, expected survival, and, most importantly, the patient's wishes.[3] It is imperative that the patient and his or her family understand that the goal of surgery is palliative in nature.

Several prognostic markers have been identified in patients with disseminated stage IV melanoma.[3,15] These markers are reflected in the AJCC staging system described above and should serve as guide when considering surgical resection of distant tumors. Patients with metastatic disease limited to one or two isolated sites experience a better prognosis as compared with patients with multiple metastatic lesions. A short disease-free interval is associated with an overall poor prognosis. Patients who develop distant metastasis within a year of their initial diagnosis have a poor prognosis, even when complete resection of the metastatic lesion is achieved.[3] Lastly, the anatomic site of the metastatic lesion is of importance. Patients with metastatic spread to nonvisceral sites (e.g., distant subcutaneous tissues, lymph nodes) have a better prognosis as compared to individuals with visceral metastasis. Within the group of patients suffering from visceral metastasis, individuals with pulmonary lesions experience improved survival as compared with other visceral sites.

RADIATION THERAPY

Melanoma has traditionally been classified as a radioresistant tumor.[103,159] Although adjuvant radiation has not been shown to have an impact on survival,[55] researchers at the MD Anderson Cancer Center completed a phase II clinical trial supporting the efficacy of hypofractionated radiation as an adjuvant treatment to surgery for HN cutaneous melanoma patients at high risk for local/regional recurrence.[6,7,20] Local/regional control was achieved in 88% of patients, which is an improvement over the historic control rates of 50% to 70%.[39,123] Late radiation complications were rare (3 of 174 patients) and included moderate neck fibrosis, mild ipsilateral hearing loss, and transient exposure of external auditory canal cartilage. Local/regional control is important, because recurrence can significantly impact quality of life by causing pain, wound breakdown, and socially debilitating cosmetic disfigurement.[137,148] However, no overall survival benefit has been demonstrated.

Ultimately the survival benefit achieved with adjuvant radiation therapy will be determined through the prospective, randomized phase III clinical trial (E3697) currently being conducted by the Radiation Therapy Oncology Group.[137] Until this trial is completed, most authors advocate the use of adjuvant radiation for patients demonstrating adverse prognostic markers such as neurotropism, extracapsular spread, multiple node involvement (>4), or recurrence.[8,125,154] These patients are often eligible to receive adjuvant interferon α-2b (see below). Interferon is thought to act as a radiosensitizer; therefore, it is common practice at most institutions to delay radiation until the four-week induction phase of interferon therapy is complete.[156]

On very rare occasions, primary radiation can be used to treat extensive LM or LMM in an elderly patient who is not deemed a surgical candidate.[75] Radiation therapy can also be administered as palliative treatment in patients suffering from systemic stage IV disease, especially in the setting of brain metastasis, bone metastasis, spinal cord compression, and isolated, symptomatic visceral metastasis.[8]

CHEMOTHERAPY

Melanoma is a relatively chemoresistant tumor.[37,151] A small subset of patients is thought to benefit from chemotherapy; however, a regimen that definitively has an impact on survival has not emerged. The main role of chemotherapy remains as palliative treatment in the setting of disseminated stage IV disease.

Dacarbazine (DTIC) is currently the only chemotherapeutic agent approved for the treatment of advance stage IV melanoma. Response rates following DTIC administration are modest at best, ranging from 10% to 20%.[27,77,103,110,131] This prognosis has not changed over the past 20 years, despite dedicated research efforts using a host of chemotherapeutic agent regimens. Overall, less than 5% of individuals experience a complete response with DTIC.

IMMUNOTHERAPY

Classically, immunotherapy is divided into two categories. *Specific immunotherapeutic agents* upregulate the antibody and cytotoxic T-cell immune response specifically to the patient's tumor or to known melanoma antigens; the majority of melanoma vaccines fall into this category. By contrast, *nonspecific immunotherapeutic agents* such as interferon, interleukin, and microbacterial products stimulate the host's immune system without targeting melanoma tumor antigens. These agents are often administered in concert with specific immunotherapeutic agents in an attempt to augment the immune system.[131,156]

Interferon

Despite myriad clinical trials involving adjuvant regimens, high-dose interferon α2b (INF α2b) remains the only U.S. Food and Drug Administration (FDA)-approved adjuvant treatment for stage III melanoma. It functions as a biologic response modifier; the mechanism of action includes direct antiproliferative effects, immune stimulation through the enhancement of natural killer cells, increased histocompatibility antigen expression on melanoma cells, macrophage phagocytosis, and enhanced T-cell mediated cytotoxicity.[80,147] Although all three types of interferon (INF α, INF β, and INF γ) demonstrate antitumor activity,[147] INF α2b is the only treatment that is currently approved for the adjuvant treatment of melanoma patients at high risk of recurrence after surgery.

Three large clinical trials involving adjuvant INF α2b have been conducted by the Eastern Cooperative Oncology Group (ECOG).[94–96] In brief, ECOG trial E1684 was the first study to demonstrate the efficacy of INF α2b.[94] The regimen consisted of high-dose interferon (20 million units/m²/day) administered intravenously, five days a week, for four weeks. Maintenance treatment followed and consisted of 48 weeks of subcutaneous INF α2b (10 MU/m²/day) administered three days a week. The prolonged disease-free survival rate and overall survival rate in the INF α2b arm of E1684 ultimately led to FDA approval of adjuvant high-dose INF α2b.

Although the follow-up trial E1690 failed to confirm the efficacy of high-dose INF α2b,[95] the results require careful interpretation.[112] Unlike E1684, patients enrolled in E1690 did not require pathologic staging with ELND or SLNB, nor were they stratified on ulceration. In addition, a disproportionate number of individuals from the observation arm crossed over into the INF α2b arm to receive salvage therapy for recurrent disease. Any therapeutic benefit provided to this subgroup by INF α2b went unrecognized, because the crossover patients remained in the observation arm for the purposes of statistical analysis.

The most recent and largest of the three studies, ECOG 1690,[96] once again confirmed the efficacy of high-dose INF α2b. In fact, the relapse-free and overall survival benefit observed in the high dose INF α2b control arm as compared with the GMK ganglioside vaccine treatment arm was so compelling that the Data Safety Monitoring Committee terminated the trial early.

With close follow-up, dose modification, and pharmacologic intervention, the majority of melanoma patients are able to tolerate the one-year course of INF α2b.[95,96,112,156] Almost all individuals experience flu-like symptoms (fevers, chills, malaise) during the initial treatment course. Severe and intolerable chronic fatigue is experience in 20% to 30% of patients, and an additional 2% to 10% of patients experience neurologic and psychiatric side effects, including depression, anxiety, suicidal ideation, and difficulty with cognition. Myelosuppression, thyroid dysfunction, and elevated liver enzymes require close monitoring. Contraindications include a history of myocardial infarction or dysrhythmia, liver disease, central nervous system disorders, and severe psychiatric illness.[156] Approximately 50% of patients require a dose reduction or delay as a result of these side effects. The majority of melanoma patients are willing to accept these side effects given the potential benefit of INF α2b.[93]

Although clinical trials continue to investigate alternative dosages and schedules,[44] only high-dose INF α2b is FDA approved and used as routine adjuvant therapy within the United States. All patients with regional lymph node metastasis or a primary tumor thickness of >4 mm should be informed of the option to receive postoperative INF α2b. So that the patient may make an educated decision, an objective discussion about the side effects of INF α2b and the opportunities to enroll in other clinical trials must be provided.

Interleukin 2 and Other Cytokines

Interleukin 2 (IL2) is another form of immunotherapy that is used in the primary treatment of disseminated stage IV disease. Unlike interferon, IL2 lacks direct antitumor activity and in vitro activity.[80] However, in vivo, IL2 stimulates the host's immune system by activating effector cells such as natural killer cells, monocytes, cytotoxic T cells, and helper T cells. It also induces cytokines such as IFN γ and tumor necrosis factor α.[47,80]

Rosenberg and the National Cancer Institute Surgery Branch[141] successfully used high-dose IL2 to treat 134 melanoma patients. An overall response was observed in 17% of patients, with 10% experiencing a partial response and an additional 7% experiencing complete regression. The therapeutic benefit was substantial, lasting between two and eight years.

IL2 side effects are significant and potentially lethal. Acute toxicities include myocardial infarction, arrhythmia, respiratory distress, hypotension, capillary leak syndrome, nephrotoxicity, hepatic toxicity, and sepsis.[47,100] Other toxicities include anemia, thrombocytopenia, nausea, emesis, diarrhea, myalgia/arthralgia, skin erythema, and pruritus. Only patients who demonstrate excellent cardiopulmonary health and performance status should be considered for clinical trials involving IL2.

Subsequent efforts to enhance the response to IL2 by altering the schedule and dose and by combining other therapeutic agents (e.g., lymphokine-activated killer cells) have not proved beneficial.[47,80,100,131] In addition to IL2, other cytokines have been studied alone and in combination with various chemotherapeutic agents, including IL1, IL4, IL6, and tumor necrosis factor α.[47] Again, significant therapeutic benefit has not been demonstrated.

Future Immunotherapy Investigations

Significant advances in the field of melanoma research have been achieved in recent years.[29,118,131,147,156] Intense efforts in the areas of melanoma vaccination, gene therapy, and HLA immunoprinting will likely play an important role in future research endeavors. Until therapeutic efficacy achieves that of INF α2b, all other adjuvant agents should be administered to high-risk patients only in the setting of well-designed clinical trials. Given the heterogeneous melanoma patient population, myriad immunotherapy regimens, and the limited survival of high-risk melanoma patients, multi-institutional studies with accurate clinical staging will be imperative.

FOLLOW-UP/SURVEILLANCE

The primary goals of melanoma follow-up are the early detection of local/regional tumor recurrence, the early identification of second primary tumors (including melanoma and other skin cancers), continuing patient education, and psychological support.[158] Each follow-up visit should include an inquiry into new or changing skin lesions. A review of systems (Table 23–3) as they relate to distant metastasis should be performed.[83]

A thorough examination of the skin and mucosa is required, with particular attention paid to the original melanoma site and associated draining nodal basins. Each follow-up visit should be viewed as an opportunity to re-educate patients about the ABCD melanoma warning signs and the importance of monthly skin self-examination. Sun education—including using sunscreen, avoiding peak sun hours, seeking shade, and wearing protective clothing—should be emphasized.

REFERENCES

1. Aitken J and others: CDKN2A variants in a population-based sample of Queensland families with melanoma, *J Natl Cancer Inst* 91:446, 1999.
2. Alex JC and others: Localization of regional lymph nodes in melanomas of the head and neck, *Arch Otolaryngol Head Neck Surg* 124:135, 1998.
3. Allen PJ, Coit DG: The surgical management of metastatic melanoma, *Ann Surg Oncol* 9:762, 2002.
4. American Academy of Dermatology. *Melanoma/skin cancer: you can recognize the signs* [patient handout], Evanston, Illinois, 1986, American Academy of Dermatology.
5. Anderson KW and others: Treatment of head and neck melanoma, lentigo maligna subtype, a practical surgical technique, *Arch Facial Plast Surg* 3:202, 2001.
6. Ang KK and others: Regional radiotherapy as adjuvant treatment for head and neck malignant melanoma, *Arch Otolaryngol Head Neck Surg* 116:169, 1990.
7. Ang KK and others: Postoperative radiotherapy for cutaneous melanoma of the head and neck region, *Int J Radiat Oncol* 30:795, 1994.
8. Ang KK and others: *Radiotherapy for melanoma.* In Balch CM and others, editors: *Cutaneous melanoma,* St Louis, Missouri, 1998, Quality Medical Publishing, Inc., p 389.
9. Ardizzoni A and others: Stage I-II melanoma: the value of metastatic work-up, *Oncology* 44:87, 1987.
10. Au FC and others: Preoperative nuclear scans in patients with melanoma, *Cancer* 53:2095, 1984.
11. Azzola MF, Shaw HM, Thompson JF: Tumor mitotic rate is a more powerful prognostic indicator than ulceration in patients with primary cutaneous melanoma: an analysis of 3661 patients from a single center, *Cancer* 97:1488, 2003.
12. Balch CM and others: The prognostic significance of ulceration of cutaneous melanoma, *Cancer* 45:3012, 1980.
13. Balch CM: The role of elective lymph node dissection in melanoma: rationale, results, and controversies, *J Clin Oncol* 6:163, 1988.
14. Balch CM and others: Efficacy of an elective regional lymph node dissection of 1 to 4 mm thick melanomas for patients 60 years of age and younger, *Ann Surg* 224:255, 1996.
15. Balch CM: *Surgical treatment of advanced melanoma.* In Balch CM and others, editors: *Cutaneous melanoma,* St Louis, Missouri, 1998, Quality Medical Publishing, Inc.
16. Balch CM and others: Long-term results of a multi-institutional randomized trial comparing prognostic factors and surgical results for intermediate thickness melanomas (1.0 to 4.0 mm): Intergroup Melanoma Surgical Trial, *Ann Surg Oncol* 7:87, 2000.
17. Balch CM and others: Prognostic factors analysis of 17,600 melanoma patients: validation of the American Joint Committee on Cancer melanoma staging system, *J Clin Oncol* 19:3622, 2001.
18. Balch CM and others: Final version of the American Joint Committee on Cancer staging system for cutaneous melanoma, *J Clin Oncol* 19:3635, 2001.
19. Balch CM and others: Long-term results of a prospective surgical trial comparing 2 cm vs. 4 cm excision margins for 740 patients with 1–4 mm melanomas, *Ann Surg Oncol* 8:101, 2001.
20. Ballo MT and others: Adjuvant irradiation for cervical lymph node metastases from melanoma, *Cancer* 97:1789, 2003.
21. Barth A, Wanek LA, Morton DL: Prognostic factors in 1,521 melanoma patients with distant metastases, *J Am Coll Surg* 181:193, 1995.
22. Basler GC and others: The utility of fine needle aspiration in the diagnosis of melanoma metastatic to lymph nodes, *J Am Acad Dermatol* 36:403, 1997.
23. Batsakis JG and others: The pathology of head and neck tumors: mucosal melanoma, part 13, *Head Neck Surg* 4:404, 1982.
24. Beardmore GL, Cavis NC: Multiple primary cutaneous melanomas, *Arch Dermatol* 111:603, 1975.
25. Berthelsen A and others: Melanomas of the mucosa in the oral cavity and the upper respiratory passages, *Cancer* 54:907, 1984.
26. Berwick M: *Epidemiology: current trends, risk factors, and environmental cancers.* In Balch CM and others, editors: *Cutaneous melanoma,* St Louis, Missouri, 1998, Quality Medical Publishing, Inc.
27. Biasco G, Pantaleo MA, Casadei S: Treatment of brain metastases of malignant melanoma with temozolomide, *N Engl J Med* 345:621, 2001.
28. Bittencourt FV and others: Large congenital melanocytic nevi and the risk of developing malignant melanoma and neurocutaneous melanocytosis. *Pediatrics* 106:736, 2000.
29. Bittner M and others: Molecular classification of cutaneous malignant melanoma by gene expression profiling, *Nature* 406:536, 2000.
30. Brand CU and others: Prolonged survival of 2 years or longer for patients with disseminated melanoma, an analysis of related prognostic factors, *Cancer* 79:2345, 1997.
31. Breslow A: Thickness, cross-sectional areas and depth of invasion in the prognosis of cutaneous melanoma, *Ann Surg* 172:902, 1970.
32. Breslow A, Macht SD: Optimal size of resection for thin cutaneous melanoma. *Surg Gynecol Obstet* 145:691, 1977.
33. Bulkey GB and others: Long-term spontaneous regression of malignant melanoma with visceral metastasis: report of a case with immunologic profile, *Cancer* 36:485, 1975.
34. Buzaid AC and others: Role of computed tomography in the staging of primary melanoma, *J Clin Oncol* 11:638, 1993.
35. Buzaid AC and others: Prognostic value of size of lymph node metastases in patients with cutaneous melanoma, *J Clin Oncol* 13:2361, 1995.
36. Buzaid AC and others: Critical analysis of the current American Joint Committee on Cancer staging system for cutaneous melanoma and proposal of a new staging system, *J Clin Oncol* 15:1039, 1997.
37. Buzaid AC, Bedikian A, Houghton AN: *Systemic chemotherapy and biochemotherapy.* In Balch CM and others, editors: *Cutaneous melanoma,* St Louis, Missouri, 1998, Quality Medical Publishing, Inc.
38. Byers RM and others: Malignant melanoma of the external ear. Review of 102 cases, *Am J Surg* 140:518, 1980.
39. Byers RM: The role of modified neck dissection in the treatment of cutaneous melanoma of the head and neck, *Arch Surg* 121:1338, 1986.

40. Byers RM: Treatment of the neck in melanoma, *Otolaryngol Clin North Am* 31:833, 1998.
41. Carlson JA and others: Desmoplastic neurotropic melanoma. A clinicopathologic analysis of 28 cases, *Cancer* 75:478, 1995.
42. Cascinelli N and others: Immediate or delayed dissection of regional node in patients with melanoma of the trunk: a randomized trial. WHO Melanoma Programme, *Lancet* 351:793, 1998.
43. Cascinelli N and others: Sentinel lymph node biopsy in cutaneous melanoma: the WHO Melanoma Program experience, *Ann Surg Oncol* 7:469, 2000.
44. Cascinelli N and others: Effect of long-term adjuvant therapy with interferon alpha-2a in patients with regional node metastases from cutaneous melanoma: a randomized trial, *Lancet* 358:866, 2001.
45. Chang AE, Karnell LH, Menck HR: The national cancer database report on cutaneous and noncutaneous melanoma: a summary of 84,836 cases from the past decade, *Cancer* 83:1664, 1998.
46. Chang P, Knapper WH: Metastatic melanoma of unknown primary, *Cancer* 49:1106, 1982.
47. Chapman PB, Parkinson DR, Kirkwood JM: *Biologic therapy*. In Balch CM and others, editors: *Cutaneous melanoma*, St Louis, 1998, Quality Medical Publishing, Inc.
48. Clark WH Jr and others: Origin of familial malignant melanoma from heritable melanocytic lesions: the B-K mole syndrome, *Arch Dermatol* 114:732, 1978.
49. Cleaver JE: Defective repair replication of DNA in xeroderma pigmentosum, *Nature* 218:652, 1968.
50. Cohen LM, McCall MW, Hodge SJ: Successful treatment of lentigo maligna and lentigo maligna melanoma with Mohs micrographic surgery aided by rush permanents sections, *Cancer* 73:2964, 1994.
51. Cohen LM: Lentigo maligna and lentigo maligna melanoma, *J Dermatol* 33:923, 1995.
52. Cole DJ and others: Melanoma of the external ear, *J Surg Oncol* 50:110, 1992.
53. Conley J, Lattes R, Orr W: Desmoplastic malignant melanoma (a rare variant of spindle cell melanoma), *Cancer* 28:914, 1971.
54. Consensus Development Panel: Precursors to malignant melanoma, *JAMA* 251:1864, 1984.
55. Creagan ET and others: Adjuvant radiation therapy for regional nodal metastases from malignant melanoma, a randomized prospective study, *Cancer* 42:2206, 1978.
56. Curtis AM and others: The efficacy of full-lung tomography in the detection of early metastatic disease from melanoma, *Radiology* 144:27, 1982.
57. Deichmann M and others: S100-Beta, melanoma-inhibiting activity, and lactate dehydrogenase discriminate progressive from nonprogressive American Joint Committee on Cancer stage IV melanoma, *J Clin Oncol* 17:1891, 1999.
58. Eicher SA and others: A prospective study of intraoperative lymphatic mapping for head and neck cutaneous melanoma, *Arch Otolaryngol Head Neck Surg* 128:241, 2002.
59. Eton O and others: Prognostic factors for survival of patients treated systemically for disseminated melanoma, *J Clin Oncol* 16:1103, 1998.
60. Fisher SR, Reintgen DS, Seigler HF: Juvenile malignant melanoma of the head and neck, *Laryngoscope* 98:184, 1988.
61. Fisher SR: Cutaneous malignant melanoma of the head and neck, *Laryngoscope* 99:822, 1989.
62. Fisher SR, Seigler HF, George SL: Therapeutic and prognostic considerations of head and neck melanoma, *Ann Plast Surg* 28:79, 1992.
63. Fisher SR, O'Brien CJ: *Head and neck melanoma*. In Balch CM and others, editors: *Cutaneous melanoma*, St Louis, Missouri, 1998, Quality Medical Publishing, Inc.
64. Fisher SR: Elective, therapeutic, and delayed lymph node dissection for malignant melanoma of the head and neck: analysis of 1444 patients from 1970 to 1998, *Laryngoscope* 112:99, 2002.
65. Fitzpatrick TB, Ortonne JP: *Normal skin color and general considerations of pigmentary disorders*. In Freedberg IM and others, editors: *Fitzpatrick's dermatology in general medicine*, New York, 2003, McGraw-Hill Medical Publishing Company.
66. Garbe C and others: Primary cutaneous melanoma: prognostic classification of anatomic location, *Cancer* 75:2492, 1995.
67. Gershenwald JE and others: Patterns of recurrence following a negative sentinel lymph node biopsy in 243 patients with stage I or II melanoma, *J Clin Oncol* 16:2253, 1998.
68. Gershenwald JE and others: Multi-institutional melanoma lymphatic mapping experience: the prognostic value of sentinel lymph node status in 612 stage I or II melanoma patients, *J Clin Oncol* 17:976, 1999.
69. Goepfert H, Jesse RH, Ballantyne AJ: Posterolateral neck dissection, *Arch Otolaryngol* 106:618, 1980.
70. Greene MH and others: Familial cutaneous malignant melanoma: autosomal dominant trait possibly lined to the Rh locus, *Proc Natl Acad Sci USA* 80:6071, 1983.
71. Greene MH and others: High risk of malignant melanoma in melanoma-prone families with dysplastic nevi, *Ann Intern Med* 102:458, 1985.
72. Grob JJ: The 'ugly ducking' sign: identification of the common characteristics of nevi in an individual as a basis for melanoma screening, *Arch Dermatol* 134:103, 1998.
73. Handley WS: The pathology of melanotic growths in relation to their operative treatment, *Lancet* 1:927, 1907.
74. Harrist T and others: Microscopic satellites are more highly associated with regional lymph node metastases than with primary melanoma thickness, *Cancer* 53:2183, 1984.
75. Harwood AR: Conventional fractionated radiotherapy for 51 patients with lentigo maligna and lentigo maligna melanoma, *Int J Radiation Oncol Biol Phys* 9:1019, 1983.
76. Heaton KM and others: Surgical margins and prognostic factors in patients with thick (>4mm) primary melanomas, *Ann Surg Oncol* 5:322, 1998.
77. Hill GJ and others: DTIC and combination therapy for melanoma: III.DTIC (NSC 45388) Surgical Adjuvant study COG Protocol 7040, *Cancer* 47:2556, 1981.
78. Hoyt DJ, Jordan T, Fisher SR: Mucosal melanoma of the head and neck, *Arch Otolaryngol Head Neck Surg* 115:1096, 1989.
79. Jemal A and others: Cancer statistics, 2003, *CA Cancer J Clin* 53:5, 2003.
80. Johnson TM and others: Current therapy for cutaneous melanoma, *J Am Acad Dermatol* 32:689, 1995.
81. Johnson TM and others: Usefulness of the staged excision for lentigo maligna and lentigo maligna melanoma: the "square" procedure, *J Am Acad Dermatol* 37:758, 1997.
82. Johnson TM, Hamilton T, Lowe L: Multiple primary melanomas. *J Am Acad Dermatol* 39:422, 1998.
83. Johnson TM and others: Management of melanoma with a multidisciplinary melanoma clinic model, *J Am Acad Dermatol* 42:820, 2000.
84. Johnson TM and others: Staging work-up, sentinel node biopsy and follow-up tests for melanoma: update of current concepts. *Arch Dermatol* 140:107, 2004.

85. Jonk A and others: Lymph node metastasis from melanoma with an unknown primary site, *Br J Surg* 77:665, 1990.

86. Joseph E and others: Results of complete lymph node dissection in 83 melanoma patients with positive sentinel nodes, *Ann Surg Oncol* 5:119, 1998.

87. Kamb A and others: A cell cycle regulator potentially involved in genesis of many tumor types, *Science* 264:436, 1994.

88. Kang S and others: Multiple primary cutaneous melanomas, *Cancer* 70:1911, 1992.

89. Kato T and others: Malignant melanoma of mucous membranes, *Arch Dermatol* 123:216, 1987.

90. Kenady DE, Brown BE, McBride CM: Excision of underlying fascia with a primary malignant melanoma: effect on recurrence and survival rates, *Surgery* 92:615, 1982.

91. Kennedy C and others: The influence of painful sunburns and lifetime sun exposure on the risk of actinic keratoses, seborrheic warts, melanocytic nevi, atypical nevi, and skin cancer, *J Invest Dermatol* 120:1087, 2003.

92. Khansur T, Sanders J, Das SK: Evaluation of staging workup in malignant melanoma, *Arch Surg* 124:847, 1989.

93. Kilbridge KL and others: Quality-of-life-adjusted survival analysis of high-dose adjuvant interferon alpha-2b for high-risk melanoma patients using intergroup clinical trial data, *J Clin Oncol* 20:1311, 2002.

94. Kirkwood JM and others: Interferon alpha-2b adjuvant therapy of high-risk resected cutaneous melanoma: The Eastern Cooperative Oncology Group Trial EST 1684, *J Clin Oncol* 14:7, 1996.

95. Kirkwood JM and others: High- and low-dose interferon alfa-2b in high-risk melanoma: first analysis of Intergroup Trial E1690/S9111/C9190, *J Clin Oncol* 18:2444, 2000.

96. Kirkwood JM and others: High-dose interferon alfa-2b significantly prolongs relapse-free and overall survival compared with the GM2-KLH/QS-21 vaccine in patients with resected stage IIB-III melanoma: results of Intergroup Trial E1694/S9512/C509801, *J Clin Oncol* 19:2370, 2001.

97. Koh HK and others: Who discovers melanoma? Patterns from a population-based survey, *J Am Acad Dermatol* 26:914, 1992.

98. Kraehn GM, Schartl M, Peter RU: Human malignant melanoma: a genetic disease? *Cancer* 75:1228, 1995.

99. Kraemer KH and others: Xeroderma pigmentosum and related disorders: examining the linkage between defective DNA repair and cancer, *J Invest Dermatol* 103:96, 1994.

100. Langley RGB and others: *Neoplasms: cutaneous melanoma.* In Freedberg IM and others, editors: *Fitzpatrick's dermatology in general medicine,* New York, 2003, McGraw-Hill Medical Publishing Company.

101. Lee SP and others: Mucosal melanoma of the head and neck: the impact of local control on survival, *Laryngoscope* 104:121, 1994.

102. Lent WM, Ariyan S: Flap reconstruction following wide local excision for primary malignant melanoma of the head and neck region, *Ann Plast Surg* 33:23, 1994.

103. Lentsch EJ, Myers JN: Melanoma of the head and neck: current concepts in diagnosis and management, *Laryngoscope* 111:1209, 2001.

104. Lynch HT, Frichot BC, Lynch JF: Familial atypical multiple mole-melanoma syndrome, *J Med Genetics* 15:352, 1978.

105. MacKie RM: Clinical recognition of early invasive melanoma, *BMJ* 301:1005, 1990.

106. Manolidis S, Donald PJ: Malignant mucosal melanoma of the head and neck: review of the literature and report of 14 patients, *Cancer* 80:1373, 1997.

107. Marghoob AA and others: Risk of cutaneous malignant melanoma in patients with "classic" atypical mole syndrome. A case-control study, *Arch Dermatol* 130:993, 1994.

108. Marghoob AA and others: Large congenital melanocytic nevi and the risk of developing malignant melanoma: a prospective study and review of the world literature. *J Invest Dermatol,* 104:563, 1995.

109. Marghoob AA: Congenital melanocytic nevi: evaluation and management, *Dermatol Clin* 20:4, 2002.

110. McClay EF, McClay MT: Systemic chemotherapy for the treatment of metastatic melanoma, *Semin Oncol* 23:744, 1996.

111. McGovern TW, Litaker MS: Clinical predictors of malignant pigmented lesions. A comparison of the Glasgow seven-point checklist and the American Cancer Society's ABCDs of pigmented lesions, *J Dermatol Surg Oncol* 18:22, 1992.

112. McMasters KM and others: Sentinel lymph node biopsy for melanoma: controversy despite widespread agreement, *J Clin Oncol* 19:2851, 2001.

113. McMasters KM: The sunbelt melanoma trial, *Ann Surg Oncol* 8:41, 2001.

114. Morton DL and others: Technical details of intraoperative lymphatic mapping for early stage melanoma, *Ann Surg* 127:392, 1992.

115. Morton DL and others: Multivariate analysis of the relationship between survival and the microstage of primary melanoma by Clark level and Breslow thickness, *Cancer* 71:3737, 1993.

116. Morton DL and others: Validation of the accuracy of intraoperative lymphatic mapping and sentinel lymphadenectomy for early-stage melanoma, *Ann Surg* 230:453, 1999.

117. Moseley HS and others: Multiple primary melanoma, *Cancer* 43:939, 1979.

118. Myers JN: Adjuvant immunotherapy for patients with melanoma, *Head Neck* 20:270, 1998.

119. Myers JN: Value of neck dissection in the treatment of patients with intermediate-thickness cutaneous malignant melanoma of the head and neck, *Arch Otolaryngol Head Neck Surg* 25:110, 1999.

120. Nasri S and others: Malignant melanoma of cervical and parotid lymph nodes with an unknown primary site, *Laryngoscope* 104:1194, 1994.

121. National Comprehensive Cancer Network: *Clinical practice guidelines in oncology, melanoma,* vol 1, Rockledge, Penn, National Comprehensive Cancer Network, 2002. (Visit *www.nccn.org* for recent updates.)

122. Norman J and others: Metastatic melanoma with an unknown primary, *Ann Plast Surg* 28:81, 1992.

123. O'Brien CJ and others: Experience with 998 cutaneous melanomas of the head and neck over 30 years, *Am J Surg* 162:310, 1991.

124. O'Brien CJ and others: Prediction of potential metastatic sites in cutaneous head and neck melanoma using lymphoscintigraphy, *Am J Surg* 170:461, 1995.

125. O'Brien CJ and others: Adjuvant radiotherapy following neck dissection and parotidectomy for metastatic malignant melanoma, *Head Neck* 19:589, 1997.

126. Ollila DW and others: Parotid region lymphatic mapping and sentinel lymphadenectomy for cutaneous melanoma, *Ann Surg Oncol* 6:150, 1999.

127. Ostmeier H and others: Can immunohistochemical markers and mitotic rate improve prognostic precision in patients with primary melanoma? *Cancer* 85:2391, 1999.

128. Pacella SJ, Lowe L, Bradford C: The utility of sentinel lymph node biopsy in head and neck melanoma in the pediatric population, *Plast Reconstr Surg* 112:1257, 2003.

129. Patel SG and others: Sentinel lymph node biopsy for cutaneous head and neck melanomas, *Arch Otolaryngol Head Neck Surg* 128:285, 2002.

130. Patel SG and others: Primary mucosal malignant melanoma of the head and neck, *Head Neck* 24:247, 2002.

131. Pawlik TM, Sondak VK: Malignant melanoma: current state of primary and adjuvant treatment, *Clin Rev Oncology Heme* 45:245, 2003.

132. Peralta EA, Yarington T, Glenn MG: Malignant melanoma of the head and neck: effect of treatment on survival, *Laryngoscope* 108:220, 1998.

133. Piepkorn K: Melanoma genetics: and update with focus on the CDKN2A(p16)/ARF tumor suppressors, *J Am Acad Dermatol* 42:705, 2000.

134. Quinn MJ and others: Desmoplastic and desmoplastic neurotropic melanoma: experience with 280 patients, *Cancer* 83:1128, 1998.

135. Reed JG, Leonard DD: Neurotropic melanoma: a variant of desmoplastic melanoma, *Am J Surg Pathol* 3:310, 1979.

136. Rhodes AR, Albert LS, Weinstock MA: Congenital nevomelanocytic nevi: proportionate area expansion during infancy and early childhood, *J Am Acad Dermatol* 34:51, 1996.

137. Ridge JA: Adjuvant radiation after lymph node dissection for melanoma, *Ann Surg Oncol* 7:550, 2000.

138. Rigel DS: Identification of those at highest risk for development of malignant melanoma, *Adv Dermatol,* 10:151, 1995.

139. Rigel DS, Carucci JA: Malignant melanoma: prevention, early detection, and treatment in the 21st century, *CA Cancer J Clin* 50:215, 2000.

140. Rigel DS: The effect of sunscreen on melanoma risk, *Dermatol Clin* 20:601, 2002.

141. Rosenberg SA and others: Treatment of 283 consecutive patients with metastatic melanoma or renal cell cancer using high-dose bolus interleukin-2, *JAMA* 271:907, 1994.

142. Ross MI, Stern SJ: *Mucosal melanomas.* In Balch CM and others, editors: *Cutaneous melanoma,* St Louis, Missouri, 1998, Quality Medical Publishing, Inc.

143. Roth JA and others: Radionuclide photoscanning: usefulness in preoperative evaluation of melanoma patients, *Arch Surg* 110:1211, 1975.

144. Santini H, Byers RM, Wolf PF: Melanoma metastatic to cervical and parotid nodes from an unknown primary site, *Am J Surg* 150:510, 1985.

145. Schmalbach CE and others: Reliability of sentinel lymph node mapping with biopsy for head and neck cutaneous melanoma, *Arch Otolaryngol Head Neck Surg* 129:61, 2003.

146. Schwartz JL and others: Thin primary cutaneous melanomas: associated detection patterns, lesion characteristics, and patient characteristics, *Cancer,* 95:1562, 2002.

147. Shaw PM and others: Adjuvant immunotherapy for patients with melanoma: are patients with melanoma of the head and neck candidates for this therapy? *Head Neck* 19:595, 1997.

148. Shen P, Wanek LA, Morton DL: Is adjuvant radiotherapy necessary after positive lymph node dissection in head and neck melanoma, *Ann Surg Oncol* 7:554, 2000.

149. Sim FH and others: A prospective randomized study of the efficacy of routine elective lymphadenopathy in management of malignant melanoma, *Cancer* 41:948, 1978.

150. Sirott MN and others: Prognostic factors in patients with metastatic malignant melanoma. A multivariate analysis, *Cancer* 72:3091, 1993.

151. Soengas MS, Lowe SW: Apoptosis and melanoma chemoresistance, *Oncogene* 22:3138, 2003.

152. Stadelmann WK and others: Cutaneous melanoma of the head and neck: advances in evaluation and treatment, *Plast Reconstr Surg* 105:2105, 2000.

153. Stern SJ, Guillamondegui OM: Mucosal melanoma of the head and neck, *Head Neck* 13:22, 1991.

154. Stevens G and others: Locally advanced melanoma, results of postoperative hypofractionated radiation therapy, *Cancer* 88:88, 2000.

155. Surveillance, Epidemiology and End Results. (2003). *http://seer.cancer.gov.*

156. Terando A, Sabel MS, Sondak VK: Melanoma: adjuvant therapy and other treatments, *Curr Treat Options Oncol* 4:187, 2003.

157. Terhune MH, Swanson N, Johnson TM: Use of chest radiography in the initial evaluation of patients with localized melanoma, *Arch Dermatol* 134:569, 1998.

158. Trask PC and others: Psychosocial characteristics of individuals with non-stage IV melanoma, *J Clin Oncol* 19:2844, 2001.

159. Trotti A, Peters LJ: The role of radiotherapy in the primary management of cutaneous melanoma, *Ann Plast Surg* 28:39, 1992.

160. Tsao H, Sober AJ: *Atypical melanocytic nevi.* In Freedberg IM and others, editors: *Fitzpatrick's dermatology in general medicine,* New York, 2003, McGraw-Hill Medical Publishing Company.

161. Tucker MA, Goldstein AM: Melanoma etiology: where are we? *Oncogene* 22:3042, 2003.

162. Uren RF and others: Lymphoscintigraphy in high risk melanoma of the trunk: predicting draining node groups, defining lymphatic channels and locating the sentinel node, *J Nucl Med* 34:1435, 1993.

163. Urist MN and others: Head and neck melanoma in 534 clinical stage I patients, *Ann Surg* 200:769, 1884.

164. Veronesi U and others: Inefficacy of immediate node dissection in stage I melanoma of the limbs, *N Engl J Med* 297:627, 1977.

165. Veronesi U and others: Delayed regional lymph node dissection in stage I melanoma of the skin of the lower extremities, *Cancer* 49:2420, 1982.

166. Veronesi U and others: Thin stage I primary cutaneous malignant melanoma: comparison of excision with margins of 1 or 3 cm, *N Engl J Med* 318:1159, 1988.

167. Veronesi U, Cascinelli N: Narrow excision (1 cm) margin. A safe procedure for thin cutaneous melanoma, *Arch Surg* 126:438, 1991.

168. Wagner JD and others: Lymph node tumor volumes in patients undergoing sentinel lymph node biopsy for cutaneous melanoma, *Ann Surg Oncol* 6:398, 1999.

169. Wanebo HJ and others: Prognostic factors in head and neck melanoma, *Cancer* 62:831, 1988.

170. Wells KE and others: Parotid selective lymphadenectomy in malignant melanoma, *Ann Plast Surg* 43:1, 1999.

171. Whited JD, Grichnik JM: Does this patient have a mole or a melanoma? *JAMA* 279:696, 1998.

172. Wornom IL 3rd and others: Surgery as palliative treatment for distant metastases of melanoma, *Ann Surg* 204:181, 1986.

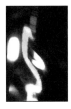

CHAPTER TWENTY FOUR

SCAR REVISION AND CAMOUFLAGE

J. Regan Thomas
Steven Ross Mobley

INTRODUCTION

The head and neck is a prominent part of the human body and can frequently be injured as a result of trauma, burns, or surgery. With superficial injuries, most facial wounds will heal with little to no scar formation. However, once the reticular dermis has been violated, some amount of residual scarring is destined to occur. Several factors that are beyond the surgeon's control can affect the final appearance of the scar, including the mechanism of injury, position of the wound, health status of the patient, the patient's skin type, and the tendency to form robust scars. Factors that are under the surgeon's control include proper realignment of wound edges, conservative debridement of injured tissues, meticulous handling of tissues during primary repair, and aesthetically favorable alignment of scars whenever possible.

After complete maturation and healing, an ideal scar should be flat and level with the surrounding skin, a good color match with the surrounding skin, narrow, parallel to the relaxed skin tension lines (RSTL) (Figure 24-1) or on the border of aesthetic facial subunits, and without straight, unbroken lines that can be easily followed with the eye (Figure 24-2).[11] Scars with aesthetically unfavorable characteristics include those that are wide, misaligned with relaxed skin tension lines or aesthetic subunits, thickened, hypertrophied or keloids (Figure 24-3).[11] The facial plastic surgeon has many options to improve, but not eliminate, these aesthetically unfavorable scars. Successful application of various treatments requires an understanding of which techniques are best indicated when performing scar revision or treating hypertrophic and keloid scars.

Successful scar revision begins with a precise analysis of both the scar and the patient's expectations. Patients often have the false perception that plastic surgery can make an existing scar invisible. The surgeon should educate the patient on the true realistic goal of surgery, which is to modify the scar to a point of maximized camouflage within the natural shadows, lines, and borders that exist within the head and neck.

INDICATIONS FOR REVISION

The surgeon should first begin with a detailed analysis of the scar. Experience has shown that many scars that are narrow, well positioned along aesthetic subunit borders, or in parallel with RSTL will continue to mature, improve, and become less noticeable over a period of 12 to 36 months.[10]

More commonly, patients will have scars that are amenable to improved surgical camouflage. Indications for scar revision include scars that are: (1) widened; (2) perpendicular to RSTL; (3) webbed; (4) pin-cushioned; (5) long and linear and misaligned with RSTL; (6) hypertrophied; (7) interrupting an aesthetic unit of the face; (8) adjacent to, but not lying within, a favorable site; or (9) causing distortion of facial features or anatomic function. Many of these scars should be considered for revision after the first 60 to 90 days of scar maturation has occurred. In fact, early revision with realignment of the scar may allow it to mature more rapidly.

Available Techniques

Numerous techniques are available when planning scar revision. This chapter has organized the available techniques into the following categories:

1. Excision
2. Expansion with excision
3. Irregularization
4. Dermabrasion
5. Steroids
6. Silicone sheeting
7. Adjunctive

EXCISION

A cardinal principle of surgery is that the best treatment of any complication is primary prevention. For

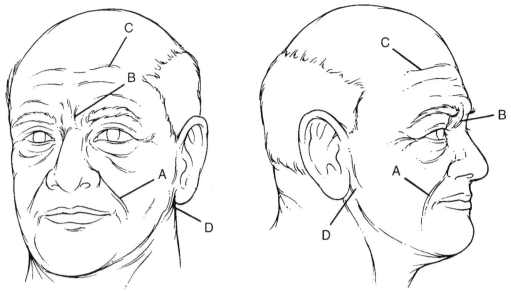

Figure 24-1. Relaxed skin tension lines and creases that can aid in scar camouflage. **A,** Nasolabial; **B,** glabellar furrows; **C,** horizontal forehead rhytids; **D,** subunit junctions (ear and cheek). (Adapted from Thomas JR, Holt GR: *Facial scars, incisions, revision & camouflage*, St. Louis, 1989, Mosby.)

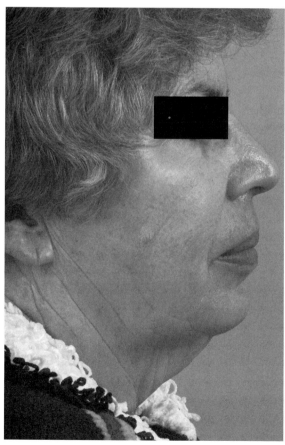

Figure 24-2. A 4-cm-long incision placed in alignment with relaxed skin tension lines and closed with multilayered closure and vertical mattress sutures.

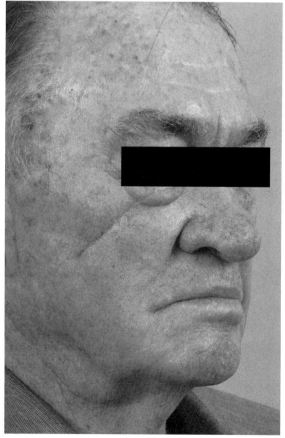

Figure 24-3. Scar on right cheek with unfavorable characteristics: depressed and not in alignment with relaxed skin tension lines. To view this image in color, please go to *www.ototext.com* or the Electronic Image Collection CD, bound into your copy of Cummings Otolaryngology—Head and Neck Surgery, 4th edition.

scar revision, this translates into the use of proper technique when closing any wound primarily. When presented with wounds that were not closed properly, reexcision with meticulous closure may be all that is needed. Reexcision should be done by use of fusiform shape with 30-degree–angled ends positioned within RSTL when possible (Figures 24-4 and 24-5). A slight vertical bevel outward from the original scar will prepare the wound edges for proper everted closure. Routine undermining of 1 to 2 cm around the periphery of the wound will allow reapproximation of the skin edges with minimal tension. The use of buried subcutaneous sutures will further decrease wound edge tension. Final eversion of the wound edges is achieved with properly placed monofilament interrupted sutures. Vertical mattress suture can also prove helpful when wound edge eversion needs to be maximized.

EXPANSION WITH EXCISION
Serial Excision

Wide scars, birthmarks, and skin grafts with poor match to surrounding tissues can all be candidates for serial excisions. In some ways, this is a variant of tis-

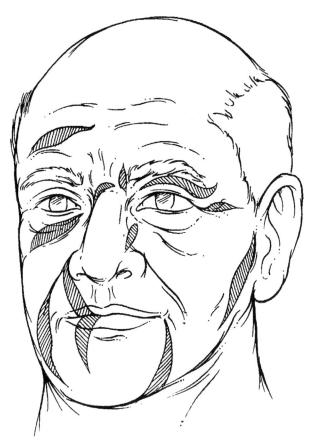

Figure 24-4. Examples of proper placement of fusiform incisions with 30-degree angled ends aligned with relaxed skin tension lines and aesthetic unit boundaries. (Adapted from Thomas JR, Holt GR: *Facial scars, incisions, revision & camouflage*, St. Louis, 1989, Mosby.)

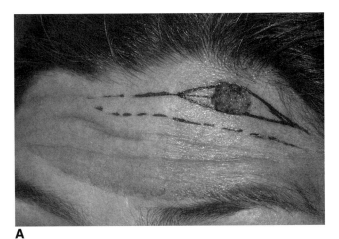

A

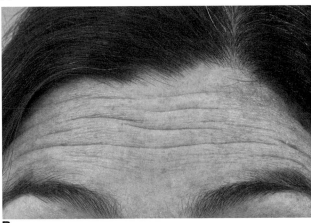

B

Figure 24-5. A, Design of fusiform closure of Mohs defect. Note the design of a longer scar in parallel with relaxed skin tension lines to achieve 30-degree angles. **B,** Same patient 1 month postoperatively. To view this image in color, please go to *www.ototext.com* or the Electronic Image Collection CD, bound into your copy of Cummings Otolaryngology—Head and Neck Surgery, 4th edition.

sue expansion in that scarred skin is excised and adjacent normal skin brought into the defect area. Like tissue expansion, this technique relies on the skin's biologic creep (ability to stretch over time) and is limited by the given amount of stretch attainable during each excision. Typically, older patients and those with increased skin laxity will require fewer excisions than younger patients with increased skin tone. As with all techniques of scar revision, the patient must be well informed as to the proposed number of excisions and must understand that serial excision can require months to years to complete.

Tissue Expansion

When treating larger scars, the best camouflage is afforded when abundant amounts of similar-appearing tissue can be brought into the repair. Tissue expansion can be a powerful tool to help create excess amounts of surrounding tissue. Tissue expanders are available in a variety of shapes and sizes. Studies on the gain of surface area afforded by the three most commonly shaped expanders have determined that rectangular expanders provide the greatest expansion at 38%, crescent-shaped expanders provide 32%, and round provide only 25%.[12] As a general rule, the base of an expander should be approximately 2.5 to 3.0 times as large as the area to be reconstructed.[1]

The effects of tissue expansion on skin have been debated. Is new skin actually produced or is the existing skin simply thinned and stretched? At present, accepted understanding on the fate of tissue layers during tissue expansion are: epidermis is thickened, melanin production increases, mitotic activity is increased, dermis is thinned (30%–50%), collagen synthesis is enhanced, hair follicle number remains unchanged, hair density decreases, muscle thins and can atrophy, and blood vessels proliferate.[6] Interestingly, epidermal changes and increased melanin production seen during expansion resolve a few months after surgery.

Implantation of the expanders must take into account the neurovascular supply and final positioning of the skin to be transferred. A second pocket is created for the injection port, which should be several centimeters away from the expansion device and in an area that is easily accessed. Expander systems with external injection ports exist and may be indicated in select patients. A 23-gauge or smaller needle is used to inject the expander. Expansion can proceed until the skin blanches or the patient complains of discomfort. Intervals between injections can be from 4 to 14 days, with two to three times per week being favorable. By properly selecting the correct expander device and understanding the preceding principles of tissue expansion, reconstruction of larger and more complex scars can be successfully achieved.

A critical point of understanding for the clinician is the temporary psychological toll that is placed on the patient undergoing expansion. Tissue expanders can cause impressive disfigurement of the head and neck, which naturally results in significant emotional stress to the patient (Figure 24-6). Repeated acknowledgment and affirmation of the patients uneasy feelings regarding the appearance of the expanders will help to support the patient throughout the expansion process. It is helpful to remind the patient that the disfigurement is temporary and that the final reconstruction will warrant the time spent dealing with the expansion devices.

IRREGULARIZATION

The human eye is more likely to perceive scars that are long, linear, and not in alignment with RSTLs and aesthetic subunits. To best camouflage these types of scars, the three most common techniques are Z-plasty, W-plasty, and geometric broken line closure

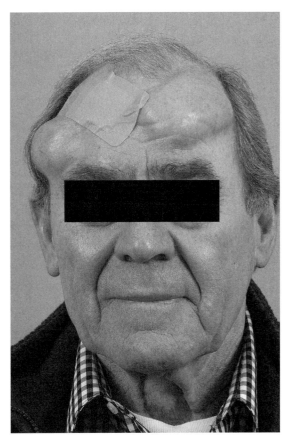

Figure 24-6. Patient midway through process of bilateral forehead tissue expansion to close a Mohs defect in forehead. To view this image in color, please go to *www. otext.com* or the Electronic Image Collection CD, bound into your copy of Cummings Otolaryngology—Head and Neck Surgery, 4th edition.

(GBLC). All three of these techniques convert linear scars to irregularized zigzagged scars that are less noticeable to the casual observer. When irregularization alone is needed, GBLC and W-plasty are the treatments of choice. However, when both irregularization and lengthening of the scar are needed, a Z-plasty technique is the technique of choice.

Z-plasty

The Z-plasty is one of the oldest and simplest techniques for scar irregularization. A "classic" Z-plasty involves the transposition of equilateral 60-degree triangles (Figure 24-7). When these triangular flaps are transposed and closed, the original direction of the scar is rotated, and the scar is lengthened by 75%. When lesser amounts of lengthening are required, a 30-degree or 45-degree Z-plasty can be used that will lengthen the scar by 25% and 50%, respectively. Longer scars may benefit from multiple Z-plasties. This can be particularly helpful when correcting scar contractures along anatomic concavities. Consecutive Z-plasties allow for the redistribution of forces more

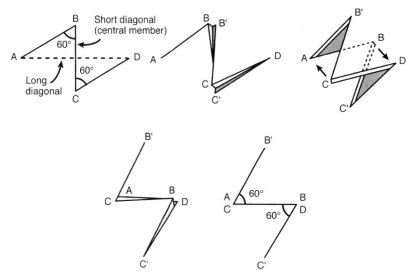

Figure 24-7. Classic equilateral triangle 60-degree Z-plasty. (Adapted from Thomas JR, Holt GR: *Facial scars, incisions, revision & camouflage*, St. Louis, 1989, Mosby.)

evenly along the entire length of the scar and also help to camouflage the scar into the surrounding RSTLs. Another common indication for multiple Z-plasties is wounds or skin flaps that have healed with a "pincushioned" appearance. Placing several small Zs around the perimeter of the wound allows interdigitation of flap with surrounding skin (Figure 24-8). The resultant interdigitated skin edge provides excellent camouflage, especially if later is treated with light dermabrasion.

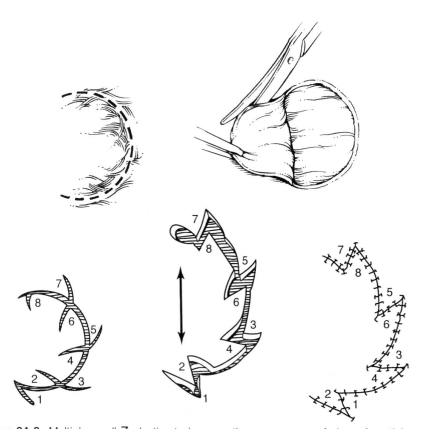

Figure 24-8. Multiple small Z-plasties to improve the appearance of circumferential or pincushioned scars. (Adapted from Thomas JR, Holt GR: *Facial scars, incisions, revision & camouflage*, St. Louis, 1989, Mosby.)

W-plasty

The most common application of W-plasty is when several W's are used in series in a technique originally described by Borge as "running W-plasty." This is a useful irregularization technique that often uses shorter limbs compared with Z-plasty and does not create lengthening of the scar.

The technique begins with the marking out of a series of consecutive triangles (W's) along the wound or scar edge. The arms should be between 5 mm and 7 mm in length, and one arm of the triangle should be drawn in parallel to the RSTL (Figure 24-9). After excision of the triangles, superficial undermining of adjacent tissues is performed, and the triangular shaped flaps are then imbricated. Care should be taken to preserve the subcutaneous scar tissue, because this can provide a stable bed for new scar healing. These wounds are also amenable to postoperative dermabrasion to further camouflage the wound.

GBLC

GBLC is an excellent technique of scar revision that creates an "irregularly irregular" scar without affecting its length. The geometry of the resultant scar is less predictable by the casual observer's eye and frequently goes unnoticed. This technique is particularly well suited to scars that traverse broad flat surfaces such as the cheek, malar, and forehead regions (Figure 24-10).

The design of a GBLC is a series of random, irregular, geometric shapes cut from one side of a wound and interdigitated with the mirror image of this pattern on the opposite side (Figure 24-11). As in running W-plasty, the length of the geometric shapes is between 5 mm and 7 mm. Similar principles of undermining and leaving deeper scar tissue in the bed of the wound are adhered to as previously described. Two-layered closure is performed, and the suture line is often reinforced with adhesive medical strips. The patient is typically seen back in 1 week for suture removal, with repeat taping of the wound edges for the next 2 weeks.

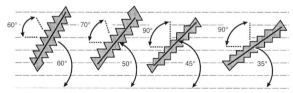

Figure 24-9. Running W-plasty with one area of triangle aligned in parallel with relaxed skin tension lines (RSTL). As scar inclination decreases, the degree of the angles should be increased to keep one arm of the triangle aligned with RSTL. (Adapted from Thomas JR, Holt GR: *Facial scars, incisions, revision & camouflage*, St. Louis, 1989, Mosby.)

DERMABRASION

Dermabrasion is a method of controlled superficial skin ablation useful for smoothing out surface contour irregularities and softening the appearance of suture lines after primary closure or irregularization. We routinely use dermabrasion as a preplanned adjunctive procedure to any irregularization scar revision procedure. Dermabrasion is best performed at the 6- to 8-week interval. There is evidence to suggest that rewounding during fibrillogenesis (i.e., 4–8 weeks after injury) may promote reaccumulation of hyaluronic acid in the wound matrix, thereby stimulating more epidermal cells to migrate and proliferate in the wound and improving the final appearance of the scar.[3]

The best candidates for dermabrasion are those with lighter complexions, because the risk of postabrasion dyspigmentation is lowest in these individuals. It is prudent to avoid dermabrasion in patients with human immunodeficiency virus or hepatitis because of the risks to personnel from airborne pathogens. The use of 13 cis-retinoic acid and its affect on healing after dermabrasion has been debated

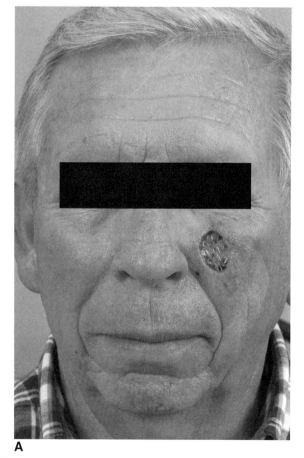

A

Figure 24-10. A, Moderate-sized Mohs defect in left cheek. To view this image in color, please go to *www.ototext.com* or the electronic Image Collection CD, bound into your copy of Cummings Otolaryngology—Head and Neck Surgery, 4th edition.
Continued

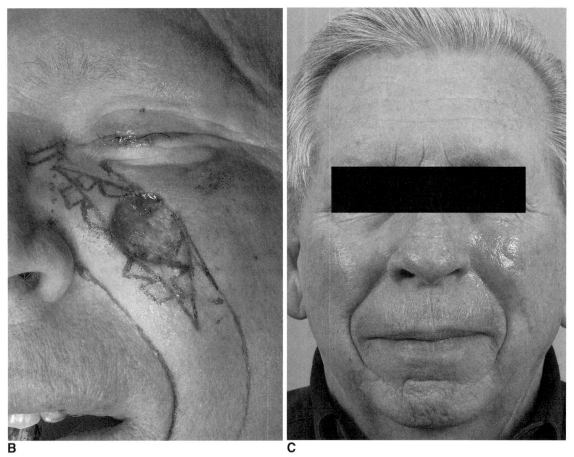

B **C**

Figure 24-10, cont'd B, Design of geometric broken line closure that is in parallel with relaxed skin tension lines. **C,** One month postoperatively. To view this image in color, please go to *www.ototext.com* or the electronic Image Collection CD, bound into your copy of Cummings Otolaryngology—Head and Neck Surgery, 4th edition.

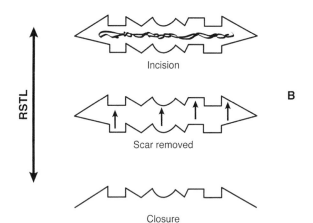

Geometric broken-line closure

Incision

Scar removed

Closure

B

RSTL

Figure 24-11. Geometric broken line closure irregularizes the scar to a less predictable pattern, further increasing camouflage. Note parts of geometric shapes in parallel with relaxed skin tension lines. (Adapted from Thomas JR, Holt GR: *Facial scars, incisions, revision & camouflage*, St. Louis, 1989, Mosby.)

in the literature. Conflicting reports exist, and until the controversy is resolved, prudence would suggest waiting 6 to 12 months before performing dermabrasion on anyone with a prior history of 13 cis-retinoic acid use.[4,9] Patients with a history of herpetic infection should be placed prophylactically on antiviral therapy. Others have advocated placing all patients on prophylactic antivirals.[32]

Diamond fraise bits are preferred, because they are easier to control and remove the skin less aggressively than wire brush fraises. The handpiece is generally held 90 degrees to the direction of wheel rotation and is advanced at right angles to the direction of wheel rotation (Figure 24-12). Preparation of the area to be dermabraded can be accomplished with local anesthesia both for nerve block and infiltration. Infiltration not only provides anesthesia but can also cause distention of the skin, which aids in the technique. Preferably, local anesthetic *without* epinephrine is used to allow for more clear visualization of capillary bleeding that is seen with dermabrasion. As

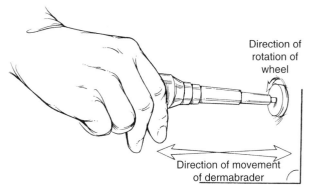

Figure 24-12. Dermabrader moved at right angles to direction of wheel rotation. (Adapted from Thomas JR, Holt GR: *Facial scars, incisions, revision & camouflage*, St. Louis, 1989, Mosby.)

one enters the superficial papillary dermis, small capillary loops are identified as pinpoint bleeding. As the papillary dermis is penetrated more deeply, small parallel strands of white-colored collagen can be appreciated. Once this is seen, dermabrasion has been taken to the appropriate depth. Preservation of the reticular

dermis with its adnexal structures will allow for the proliferation of undamaged epidermal cells across the abraded surface. The periphery of the treated area should be feathered with fine diamond fraises to allow for a smooth transition between treated and untreated areas.

Immediately after treatment an occlusive dressing such as polyethylene oxide hydrogel (Vigilon) is applied. This is left in place for 48 hours, and then the patient is instructed to keep the area moist at all times with bacitracin for the next 7 to 10 days. After that, the patient can use a thick moisturizing lotion such as Eucerin. Reepithelization is usually accomplished after 5 to 7 days, but posttreatment erythema can often take 2 to 3 months before resolution (Figure 24-13). This should be clearly communicated to the patient before the procedure. Women are usually less bothered by this, because they can begin to cover the area with make-up once reepithelization is complete.

STEROIDS

Intralesional corticosteroids can be an effective adjunct in the treatment of healing wounds, hypertrophic

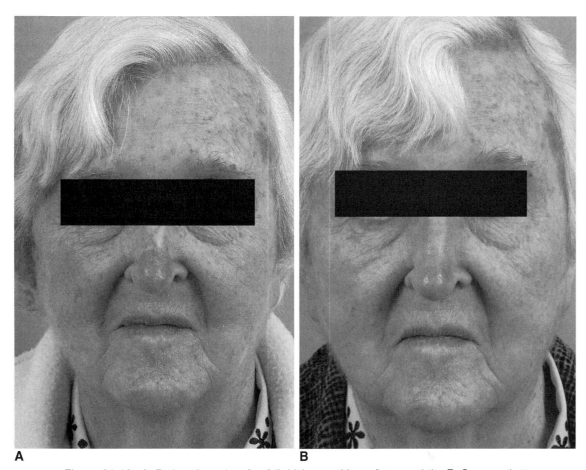

Figure 24-13. A, Patient 6 weeks after full-thickness skin graft to nasal tip. **B,** Same patient 1 month after dermabrasion of entire nasal aesthetic unit. To view this image in color, please go to *www.ototext.com* or the electronic Image Collection CD, bound into your copy of Cummings Otolaryngology—Head and Neck Surgery, 4th edition.

scars, and keloids. Steroid injections into areas of scar revision can be useful when persistent tissue edema detracts from the wound's appearance. Small doses of triamcinolone (10 mg/mL) injected into the dermis or the dermis subcutaneous junction can provide the surgeon with an ability to "sculpt" an otherwise normally healing wound and hasten the resolution of edema. For example, intralesional steroids can help to less the "pin-cushion" edema seen frequently in local flap reconstruction techniques such as bilobed flap repair (Figure 24-14). Steroids can cause hypopigmentation and telangiectasias when injected in higher concentrations into the dermis. Also, one should avoid the injection of steroids into the subcutaneous fat, because this can lead to deformity from fat atrophy. Judicious use and conservative clinical judgment are usually all that is needed to prevent these untoward events.

Topical steroids can also be used when one is trying to diminish minor wound erythema that can be a normal part of the healing process. This has an application in younger patients and those with more sebaceous skin who are prone to erythematous wounds. Also, after dermabrasion of other resurfacing procedures, short-term low-dose topical steroids can be applied after reepithelization is complete.

SILICONE SHEETING

The topical application of silicone gel sheets to the surface of keloids has shown to be beneficial to the improvement of scars. Ohmori[5] studied the effects of silicone sheeting on 46 patients with 48 keloids in all areas of the body. By use of a study-defined grading scale, he reported excellent and good results in 60% of patients and fair to poor results in 40%. Katz[2] investigated the use of silicone sheeting for both keloids and hypertrophic scars. Fifty-six percent of keloids demonstrated measurable improvement. Zero of five patients with a history of hypertrophic scarring had recurrence of their hypertrophied scars after excision and postoperative silicone sheeting. Typically, patients are encouraged to wear the silicone for a minimum of 8 to 12 hours per day and to use it for 6 to 12 months. The use of topical silicone sheets should be considered in any scar that is not ideal secondary to being slightly raised or possessing hyperpigmentation.

The biophysical properties of silicone sheeting have been studied, but still the mechanism by which silicone sheeting may improve scar healing is not well characterized.[7,8] Changes in pressure, temperature, and oxygen tension have all been studied and found to be negligible. Silicone sheeting has been shown to increase scar hydration by a more than 50% reduction in evaporation. This is postulated to cause a decrease in capillary activity and perhaps collagen deposition. It can be stated with reasonable confidence that silicone sheeting seems to have a favorable effect on wound healing and exposes the patient to little or no morbidity from the treatment.

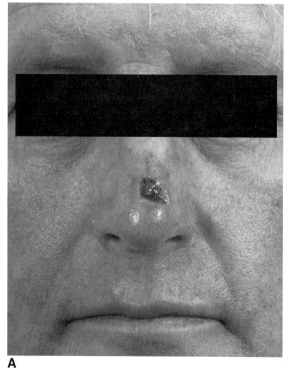

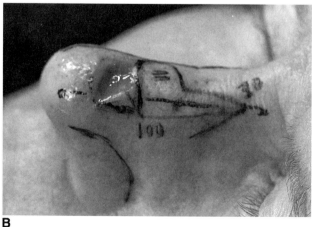

A   **B**

Figure 24-14. A, Patient with Mohs defect of nasal tip. **B,** Intraoperative photo demonstrating design of flap; note the design of the second lobe to lie within aesthetic subunits of the nose.

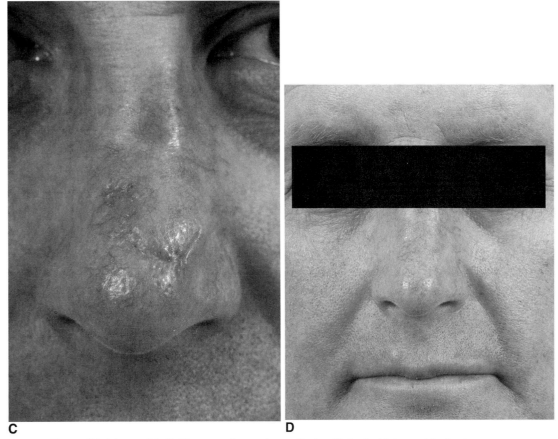

C   **D**

Figure 24-14, cont'd C, Three weeks postoperatively with typical "pin-cushion" edema seen with bilobed flaps. **D,** Three months postoperatively. Patient has received three subcutaneous injections of 10 mg/mL triamcinolone delivered 2 weeks apart. To view this image in color, please go to *www.ototext.com* or the electronic Image Collection CD, bound into your copy of Cummings Otolaryngology—Head and Neck Surgery, 4th edition.

ADJUNCTIVE PROCEDURES
Cosmetics and Hairstyling

Although not routinely thought of as part of the medical management of scar revision, cosmetics and hairstyling can play an important role in these patients. Surgeons who routinely perform scar revision are encouraged to seek out aesthetic professionals in their area that have interest in helping with the care of these patients. The physician's familiarity with these adjunctive professional services is often met with great pleasure by the patient who is eager to look normal and regain confidence in his or her appearance.

REFERENCES

1. Gibney J: *Tissue expansion in reconstructive surgery,* Presented to ASPRS annual scientific meeting, Las Vegas, Nevada, October 1984.
2. Katz BE: Silicone gel sheeting in scar therapy, *Cutis* 56:65, 1995.
3. Katz BE, Oca AG: A controlled study of the effectiveness of spot dermabrasion ("scarbrasion") on the appearance of surgical scars, *J Am Acad Dermatol* 24:462, 1991.
4. Moy R and others: *Effects of 13 cis-retinoic acid on wound healing in vivo,* Presented at the meeting of the American Academy of Dermatology, 1987.
5. Ohmori S: Effectiveness of silastic sheet coverage in the treatment of scar keloid (hypertrophic scar), *Aesth Plast Surg* 12:95, 1998.
6. Papel ID, editor: *Facial plastic and reconstructive surgery,* New York, 2002, Thieme.
7. Quin KJ: Silicone gel in scar treatment, *Burns* 13:933, 1987.
8. Quin KJ and others: Non-pressure treatment of hypertrophic scars, *Burns* 12:102, 1985.
9. Rubenstein R and others: Isoretinoin, *J Am Acad Dermatol* 15:280, 1986.
10. Thomas JR, Holt GR, editors: *Facial scars: incision, revision & camouflage,* St. Louis, 1989, Mosby.
11. Thomas JR, Prendiville S: Update in scar revision, *Facial Plast Clin North Am* 10:103, 2002.
12. van Rappard JHA, Sonneveld GJ, Borghouts JMHM: Geometric planning and the shape of the expander, *Facial Plast Surg* 5:287, 1998.

CHAPTER TWENTY FIVE

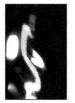
FACIAL TRAUMA: SOFT-TISSUE LACERATIONS AND BURNS

Kevin A. Shumrick
Jon B. Chadwell

INTRODUCTION

Facial soft-tissue injuries are common and have always existed.[15] Because the face is in the lead position, it is often the first recipient of any hostilities or unfortunate events. Many possible facial soft-tissue injuries exist, ranging from the uncomplicated pediatric laceration to massive disruptions with deforming sequelae. The physician should keep in mind that facial wounds consist of a physical injury and a strong psychological component; the psychological sequelae arise from the important social and self-image role physical appearance plays in our society. Additionally, the trauma of repairing a facial laceration in the emergency room may have a tremendous negative psychological effect on a pediatric patient, leaving life-long negative feelings regarding hospitals or physicians. Facial wounds that fail to achieve optimal results (with scarring or deformity) may cause self-image and self-confidence problems that may alter the patient's personality and have an impact on the course of the patient's life. This chapter provides an overview of the management of facial soft-tissue injuries and burns, and addresses effective methods for managing the physical damage and minimizing the psychological trauma.

CLINICAL HISTORY

An accurate clinical history regarding the cause of facial trauma is invaluable for completely and accurately assessing a wound and, most importantly, for planning appropriate treatment. Unfortunately, many facial injuries—particularly pediatric injuries—are not witnessed, or the patient may have an altered sensorium from the trauma or pharmacologic agents; thus, the traumatic event should be reconstructed retrospectively. Much valuable information may be lost regarding the wounding agent, the degree of contamination, and other associated injuries. Additionally, the clinician treating pediatric facial trauma should keep in mind the possibility that the facial injuries were not accidental but intentionally inflicted; it is the physi-

cian's responsibility to investigate any unusual or suspicious injuries to a child.

HISTORY OF TRAUMATIC EVENT

The history should consider the following questions: What was the mechanism of injury? Was the patient mobile, restrained, or stationary? Was the object that caused the injury mobile or stationary? Was the injury the result of blunt trauma, penetrating trauma, or both? Can the degree of energy transfer (high vs low) be estimated? Were there coincident fatalities? Were associated thermal or chemical injuries present?

ASSESSMENT OF SOFT-TISSUE INJURIES

Several types of soft-tissue facial injuries are possible, including contusions and avulsions, but the most common soft-tissue injuries are lacerations, particularly in children. Lacerations may range from simple superficial wounds that are easily repaired to injuries that involve deeper structures, including muscles, nerves, and ducts. Major lacerations that are improperly treated can leave dysfunctional and deforming sequelae. The most important factor in the treatment of any injury is proper initial evaluation and assessment, so that relevant concerns are identified and a comprehensive treatment plan is formulated.

Chart documentation is also an integral part of medical care for follow-up and medicolegal concerns. The following specifics of soft-tissue injury should be noted and documented.

Laceration Shape

A wound that is a straight laceration with clean margins can probably be closed primarily, with an acceptable result. In a stellate wound with multiple trifurcations, wound margins that are very irregular or that have adjacent devitalized tissue may have implications for management and outcome. Whereas a simple clean laceration may be repaired primarily, a complicated wound with devitalized tissue may require resources that are not available in the emergency room.

Surrounding Soft-Tissue Injury and Associated Contusion

Contusions often result in an irregular disruption of the skin with surrounding devitalized tissue; these wounds should be documented and treated conservatively. The patient (or parents) should be informed that these injuries often result in depressed scars, which may benefit from scar revision when the scar is mature.

Loss of Soft-Tissue Coverage or Lining

Although uncommon, actual loss of facial soft tissue has significant implications for wound management and eventual outcome. These injuries should be carefully documented (with photos, if possible) and the patient informed accordingly.

Injury to Structural Margins or Borders

Soft-tissue injuries involving the eyelid, nasal alar rims, auricular helical rims, and the oral stoma should be carefully examined and noted. Full-thickness injuries involving these structures have significant cosmetic and functional implications.

Penetrating Soft-Tissue Injuries

Penetrating wounds are dangerous because, although the exterior entrance point may seem relatively benign, the possibility of deeper structures being involved should be considered. A thorough physical examination should be performed to rule out the possibility of injury to a significant structure, such as a branch of the facial nerve, the parotid duct, or the lacrimal apparatus. Timely identification is important, because delay in repairing these structures can significantly decrease the chances of a successful outcome.

SPECIAL CONSIDERATIONS IN FACIAL SOFT-TISSUE TRAUMA

Although most facial soft-tissue trauma is superficial and involves only the skin and subcutaneous tissue, the treating physician should be aware of the potential for more significant injuries involving deeper structures. Because these injuries may be subtle and because younger children may be unable to voice symptoms, recognition of these injuries may be delayed and the final outcome compromised.

Facial Nerve

The status of the facial nerve should be noted and recorded on the initial evaluation of all facial trauma patients. A facial nerve deficit is commonly noted in a delayed fashion. The question then arises as to whether the deficit occurred immediately (implying a severance of the nerve, which will require repair or decompression) or on a delayed basis as a result of tissue edema (implying a contusion of the nerve, which will recover spontaneously). Additionally, during the repair of a facial laceration with local anesthesia, facial nerve deficit may be noted. If the functional status of the nerve has not been documented at the initial assessment, there will be uncertainty regarding the cause of the palsy and whether it is the result of the initial injury, induced by anesthesia (transient), or iatrogenic (during the repair). Transection of the nerve or one of its branches should be established as soon as possible, because early and accurate repair maximizes the chances of functional neural regeneration. The distal portion of a transected nerve can be stimulated for up to 72 hours after injury, which facilitates accurate the identification of the distal end of the nerve for reapproximation and repair.

Parotid Duct

Injury to the parotid (or Stensen's) duct should be considered with any deep cheek laceration or penetrating injury. Whereas an injury or transection of the duct is relatively uncommon, the morbidity of an unrecognized and unrepaired ductal injury is high and can be avoided with timely surgical intervention. The parotid duct exits the parotid gland at approximately the posterior border of the masseter muscle and then travels across the lateral border of the masseter. At the anterior border of the masseter, the duct turns medially and enters the oral cavity just lateral to the second upper molar. The facial nerve lies just lateral to the duct, and there is almost always an associated injury to a buccal branch of the facial nerve with any parotid duct injury (Figure 25-1).

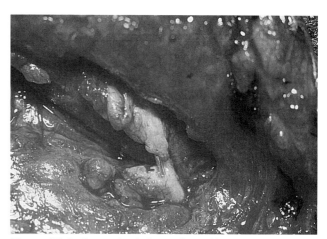

Figure 25-1. Deep cheek laceration with transection of the parotid duct. A Silastic tube has been passed intraorally, connecting the proximal and distal ends of the duct. Note the severed buccal branch of the facial nerve lateral to the duct. Both nerve and duct were repaired with 8-0 monofilament.

The most common sign of a ductal injury is saliva draining from the wound. The most direct way to confirm a ductal injury is to cannulate the duct intraorally with a lacrimal probe and use the probe to check the integrity of the duct in the depths of the wound. A laceration or transection should be repaired with fine nylon suture (8-0 or 9-0) using magnification. Some authors advocate leaving a Silastic stent in place for 7 to 10 days after repair (see Figure 25-1).

If a ductal injury is unrecognized, the patient will return with a sialocele that is often infected (Figure 25-2). Repair of the duct after the formation of a sialocele or fistula is difficult because of maceration and friability of the tissues. A salivary fistula is also possible because of injury to an ancillary duct or the parotid parenchyma. If diagnosis of a parotid duct laceration is delayed and repair is not possible or fails, or if the fistula is caused by an injured minor duct or parotid parenchyma, then conservative therapy is instituted with anticholinergics to decrease saliva output, and pressure dressings are applied with the hope that the gland will atrophy or that the ductal injury will seal itself.[17,18,22] If the fistula persists, a superficial parotidectomy may be required.

Lacrimal Apparatus

There should be a high index of suspicion for injury to the lacrimal drainage apparatus with any laceration involving the medial portion of the upper or lower eyelid in the region of the medial canthus laceration (Figure 25-3). The major sequela of a lacrimal canalicular laceration is epiphora, which may not be obvious in the acute setting because of associated pain and

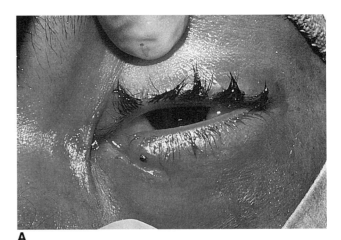

A

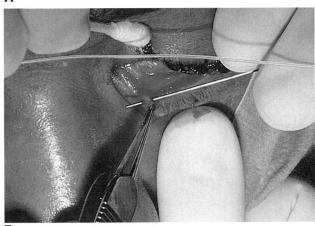

B

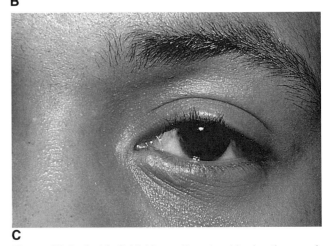

C

Figure 25-3. A, Medial lid laceration should raise the suspicion of a possible lacrimal duct injury. **B,** Documentation of lacrimal duct injury with a lacrimal probe; the duct is repaired microsurgically over a Silastic stent with 8-0 monofilament. **C,** Note there is no epiphora at 6 months postoperatively.

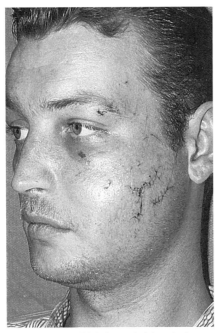

Figure 25-2. A patient with infected sialocele from a lacerated parotid duct that was not diagnosed at the time of primary repair. Treatment consisted of anticholinergics and pressure dressings. The salivary drainage stopped after 3 to 4 weeks.

edema. If a canalicular laceration or lacrimal duct laceration may be present, the lacrimal punctum and duct should be cannulated with lacrimal probes, and the laceration examined to see if they appear in the wound. A laceration should be repaired over Silastic stents, under magnification, with fine sutures (8-0).

Retained Foreign Body

The treating physician should consider the possibility of a retained foreign body in cases of penetrating injuries involving glass or wood or resulting from striking the ground (Figure 25-4). The phenomenon of debris tattooing results from particulate matter being imbedded in the dermis and not appropriately removed (Figure 25-5); typically this occurs as a result of abrasions sustained from falling and sliding along the ground or pavement. The epidermis is denuded, and dirt, stones, and other debris are implanted in the dermis. The epidermis will then resurface the wound, and the retained material will be visible externally. Once the epidermis has sealed the wound, it is virtually impossible to remove the visible debris short of full-thickness excision of the effected area (late dermabrasion has been disappointing; laser vaporization may eventually prove useful). Therefore, it is important to identify wounds with the potential for debris tattooing, because the optimum time to treat this condition is at the time of injury, when the epidermis is still open and the foreign material can be removed by scrubbing, irrigation, or dermabrasion. It is extremely difficult to achieve adequate local anesthesia for debridement of large areas of abraded tissue; these cases are probably best performed in the operating room, with general anesthesia.

REPAIR OF SOFT-TISSUE INJURIES

After ruling out injuries to associated deep structures, attention may be turned to repair of the superficial soft-tissue injury. As noted, the treating physician should meticulously remove all foreign bodies from the wound. A wound that appears grossly contaminated should be irrigated with copious quantities of saline under mild pressure. With regard to the debridement of tissue in acute wounds, it is generally accepted that the conservative removal of only obviously devitalized tissue should be performed. The specific method of repair or treatment depends primarily on the wound morphology and etiology and other relevant factors noted during the wound evaluation.

When repairing a straightforward, uncomplicated laceration, the aim should be to provide an anatomically accurate and secure repair. This aim is best accomplished with complete anesthesia, fine instruments, excellent lighting, and comfortable working conditions for the surgeon. These conditions are often not

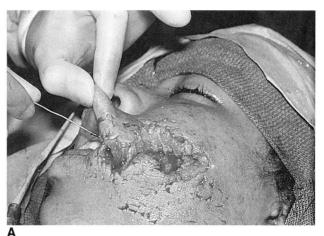

A

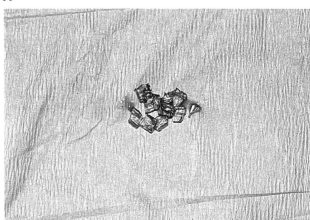

B

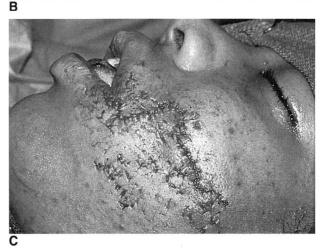

C

Figure 25-4. A, Cheek laceration from an automobile windshield. Note the lacrimal probe being used intraorally to check the integrity of the parotid duct. **B,** Glass particles removed from the wound. Automobile windshield lacerations are notorious for leaving embedded glass fragments. **C,** The results after foreign body removal and meticulous reapproximation of lacerations.

met in the usual emergency room setting, and the surgeon has a duty to the patient to ensure that the proper conditions and resources are available before

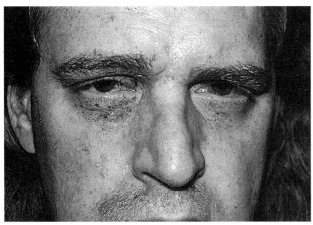

Figure 25-5. Right periocular debris tattooing after a blast injury. The epithelium has sealed the wound, thereby trapping the foreign material and making removal difficult. Note that dermabrasion of the thin eyelid skin is extremely dangerous.

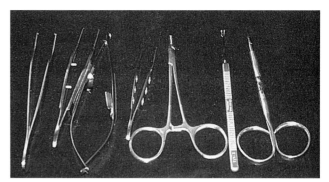

Figure 25-6. A basic set of plastic soft-tissue instruments for the emergency repair of facial lacerations.

beginning a repair. This may mean taking the patient to the operating room and using monitored sedation or general anesthesia, particularly if the patient is uncooperative.

INSTRUMENTS AND SUTURE MATERIAL

Often the physician repairing a facial wound in the emergency room is faced with the prospect of using rather crude instruments that do not lend themselves to atraumatic soft-tissue handling and optimal soft-tissue repair. Although accurate soft-tissue reapproximation may be of little consequence on the hand or trunk, scars on the face are of significant cosmetic, social, and psychological importance, and every effort should be made to minimize the visibility of a facial scar. An accurate primary repair is the first step to minimize facial scarring.

To achieve an accurate repair, the surgeon requires instruments that are commensurate with the fine work to be accomplished. The two most important instruments involved in fine suturing are a fine pair of tissue forceps and a fine-needle holder. Unfortunately, these two instruments are most commonly lacking in emergency room suture packs. Typically, the emergency room provides a thick pair of Addison toothed forceps and a long-handled, thick-jawed needle holder. These bulky instruments are inadequate for fine soft-tissue work, and every effort should be made to upgrade the available instruments, even going so far as to have plastic instruments brought from the operating room. Many facial plastic surgeons own a few key instruments and bring them to the emergency room for facial repairs (Figure 25-6). Additionally, some authors believe that wound repair under magnification (2.5× loupes) significantly enhances the final result.

The next issue to consider is that of suture material. As with instrumentation, the results achieved are directly related to the caliber of the suture material: the finer the suture, the better the results. Larger-caliber sutures significantly increase the incidence of crosshatching or a railroad-track appearance of facial scars. Additionally, large-caliber sutures do not provide as accurate skin approximation, and the quality of the final scar is compromised.

Rarely is anything larger than a 6-0 suture used on the face, especially in pediatric cases. The only time a 5-0 suture would be used is in the scalp or for a nonvisible soft-tissue surface. For skin sutures, a 7-0 monofilament suture is used. Although somewhat fine, 7-0 suture provides excellent soft-tissue approximation and does not require a microscope (although loupe magnification is helpful). Also, external nonabsorbable sutures are used only with patients who will likely return for suture removal and be cooperative. Perhaps the only thing more frustrating than performing a suture repair on an uncooperative child is trying to remove sutures from an uncooperative child. Additionally, adults who do not return for suture removal within an appropriate time will often have a worse scar (because of crosshatching or festering of the suture) than they would have if nothing had been done to the wound. Therefore, in children who may be uncooperative during suture removal or in adults whose follow-up is questionable, a 6-0 absorbing gut suture is used (Figure 25-7). This suture is different than the commonly available mild chromic sutures, which often persist longer than needed and have needles that are not ideal. Absorbing gut suture has a needle that is conducive to soft-tissue repair, and the suture will usually be gone from the wound within three to five days.

Some authors believe that absorbable subcutaneous sutures are used excessively and often inappropriately. Although the commonly available subcutaneous sutures (most of them are a variant of polyglycolic acid) are said to dissolve, they in fact elicit an inflammatory

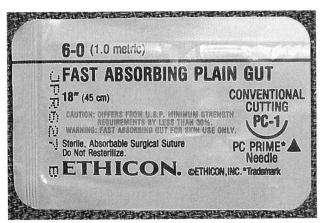

Figure 25-7. A packet of absorbing gut suture, which has a good needle for soft-tissue repair, handles easily, and is gone from the wound in 3 to 5 days. It is often the preferred suture for uncooperative children or noncompliant adults.

reaction and are broken down. This inflammatory reaction prolongs the proliferative and maturation phases of wound healing and may lead to more prominent scarring. Therefore, the least number of the finest caliber subcutaneous sutures that will adequately approximate the soft tissues should be used. Usually this entails using 6-0 or 5-0 sutures. Furthermore, muscle or fat does not have the tensile strength to effectively support a suture, and sutures placed in these tissues add little or no tensile strength to the wound and simply act as foreign bodies. The only facial tissues that will reliably support a suture with some tension are dermis and fascia that cover muscle.

Dermal sutures that are placed too superficially increase the possibility of extrusion. When subcutaneous sutures extrude, they significantly degrade the quality of the scar, and, therefore, subcutaneous sutures should be placed in the deep dermis.

ANESTHESIA FOR FACIAL LACERATIONS

The most important determinant of a positive experience for the patient and physician during the management of a facial laceration is obtaining adequate anesthesia with minimal trauma, especially in pediatric patients. In the past, the most commonly used method of obtaining anesthesia for facial laceration repair was to infiltrate the local anesthetic into the wound through a needle. Anesthetic infiltration had two negative psychological effects. First, the patient's anticipation of a needle being stuck into an open wound is enough to generate extreme anxiety, which heightens the perception of pain for any stimuli that are subsequently encountered. Second, infiltration of the local anesthetic, as expected by the patient, is painful because of the hydrostatic and chemical properties of the anesthetic. This combination of height-

ened expectation followed by painful stimuli makes anesthetic injection the most unpleasant aspect of facial laceration repair. Anesthetic injection may cause a child to become completely uncooperative on any subsequent endeavors, even if adequate anesthesia has been obtained. This hysteric response requires the placement of restraints, which further aggravate the child; the following repair is an ordeal for all involved. If the physician can achieve anesthesia of the wound without inflicting additional anxiety or pain, the suture repair is usually fairly simple. To minimize the pain of anesthetizing facial lacerations, TAC (tetracaine 0.5%, adrenaline 1:2000, and cocaine 11.8%)[5] anesthesia has been developed and effectively used in the management of facial lacerations.[2,25]

TAC anesthesia is applied topically into a facial wound and usually obviates the need for injected anesthetics. The primary advantage of TAC anesthesia is that the patient never experiences pain. If the physician can avoid creating pain for the patient initially, even small infants can be sutured without requiring restraints such as the papoose board.

A variant of TAC called LAT (lidocaine 4%, adrenaline 1:2000, and tetracaine 1%) makes use of lidocaine instead of cocaine.[12] Ernst and others[12] reported that LAT seemed to better control pain than TAC and that the cost per dose for LAT was $3 vs $35 for TAC. Because the chance for systemic toxicity with LAT is small and the potential for abuse is low, LAT may become the topical anesthesia of choice.

TECHNIQUE OF TETRACAINE, ADRENALINE, AND COCAINE ANESTHESIA

The application of TAC anesthesia is straightforward. The wound can be briefly cleaned, but no attempt should be made to perform a complete scrubbing, because children may interpret this as being potentially painful. It is necessary to remove any clots from the wound so that the solution has a chance to diffuse into the surrounding tissue. The TAC solution comes in 3-mL vials; some have found that the simplest way to apply TAC solution is to place it in a medicine cup, use sterile cotton-tipped applicators to absorb the solution, and then place the applicators directly into the wound (Figure 25-8). The applicators should then be completely saturated with the TAC solution (Figure 25-9). Once the applicator is in the wound, it is generally changed every four to five minutes to ensure that the concentration of the TAC solution is maximal within the wound. It generally takes seven to 12 minutes for the TAC solution to become effective. However, the duration to achieve anesthetic effect can vary; perhaps the most reliable sign is the presence of a ring of blanching around the wound margin, which indicates that the solution has moved out into the

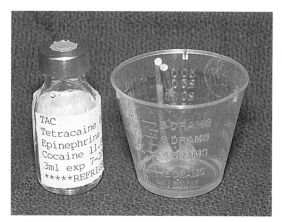

Figure 25-8. Tetracaine, adrenaline, and cocaine (TAC) in a 3-mL vial. TAC is often applied with cotton-tipped applicators, but dental pledgets can also be used.

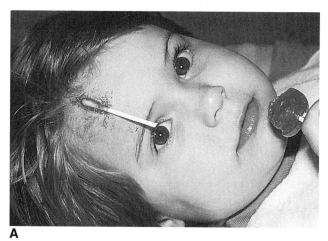

A

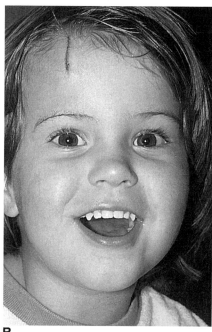

B

Figure 25-9. A, Tetracaine, adrenaline, and cocaine–soaked applicator in wound. The patient has not been hurt and is easily distracted from the suturing. **B,** The final result. Note the faint blanching around the wound, which signifies that the solution has taken effect.

surrounding tissues and has now become effective (see Figure 25-9B). Once this blanching has occurred, the anesthetic has taken effect, and repair can begin.

INDICATIONS AND CONTRAINDICATIONS OF TETRACAINE, ADRENALINE, AND COCAINE ANESTHESIA

TAC anesthesia has been used for lacerations involving the entire face and head and neck region. However, TAC is probably contraindicated in several areas. Because TAC contains cocaine, a major concern regarding its use is the possibility of systemic absorption of cocaine sufficient to cause toxic symptoms. The fact that TAC is mixed with a vasoconstrictor lessens the possibility of a systemic dose. There have been instances of toxic symptoms, but they occurred when TAC was used around mucosal membranes. The proposed explanation for the increased toxicity of TAC when used on mucous membranes is that, because of the high blood flow in mucosal membranes, enough of the cocaine is picked up to cause systemic symptoms. Therefore, it is generally recommended that TAC anesthesia not be used on significant mucosal lacerations of the lips or nose. Additionally, because of its vasoconstrictive effect, TAC should be used with care in end-arterial situations, such as the tip of the nose or ear or when pedicled flaps of tissue are encountered.

In addition, TAC administration will cause a positive urine or blood test for cocaine.[1] Although this is rarely of concern in children, it may cause significant difficulty for adults undergoing routine drug testing.

MINIMIZING PAIN WITH INJECTABLE ANESTHETICS

TAC anesthesia has been extremely effective, and many pediatric patients have been managed with it as the only anesthesia. However, TAC anesthesia is not advised for lip lacerations that extend onto the mucosa, lacerations in which a flap has been raised, or lacerated areas in which the vascularity is in question. Additionally, TAC anesthesia may not be available in all emergency rooms, particularly at smaller community hospitals. In these situations, the physician may need to use the standard injectable anesthetic. Injection of a local anesthetic is painful; however, most of the pain associated with local anesthetic injection is not from the injection procedure but from the chemical properties of the anesthetic. Specifically, the pH of most commercially available anesthetics is in the range of 4.0; this acidic pH causes most of the stinging encountered with local anesthetic injection. If the anesthetic solution is buffered so that the pH is increased to the physiologic range, the pain of the local injection considerably diminishes. Neutralization of the anesthetic solution may be achieved by mixing sodium bicarbonate with the local anesthetic solution. Generally, 1 mL of 8.4% sodium bicarbonate is mixed with 9 mL of 1% lidocaine with 1:100,000 epinephrine, which will raise the pH to approximately 7.0. Sodium bicarbonate solution is available in multiple-use bottles or may be obtained from the pharmacy in single-use vials for injection on emergency resuscitation carts (Figure 25-10). The cost of a sodium bicarbonate vial is approximately $2. If a 10-mL injection is not needed, a proportional solution may be used (e.g., 0.5 mL sodium bicarbonate with 4.5 mL local anesthetic). Using this buffered anesthetic solution with a fine needle (27 or 30 gauge) can significantly diminish—and often eliminate—the pain of local anesthetic injection. If done properly with concealment of the needle, slow injection technique, and some form of distraction, the anesthesia can be administered with little or no discomfort to the patient.

However, buffered local anesthetic solution should be used with caution, because the duration of effective anesthesia is lessened by neutralizing the solution. The treating physician can expect at least 30 to 45 minutes of substantial anesthetic effect, which should be sufficient for most uncomplicated facial lacerations.

VASOCONSTRICTORS IN LOCAL ANESTHETICS

Although the vascular supply of the facial skin is probably the best of the entire body, thereby necessitating the addition of a vasoconstrictor to the lidocaine, vasoconstrictor use may be inappropriate in some situations. In particular, vasoconstrictors should probably be avoided when the pedicle-type blood supply is limited (e.g., injury to the tip of the nose or ear, an avulsion type injury in which a pedicled flap of skin has been raised). In these types of injuries, consideration should be given to using a solution with a reduced concentration of epinephrine (e.g., 0.5% lidocaine with 1:200,000 epinephrine), using a plain anesthetic without epinephrine, or performing the repair under regional or general anesthesia.

MANAGEMENT ISSUES WITH COMPLICATED WOUNDS
Soft-Tissue Contusions

Blunt trauma often presents with an associated stellate laceration resulting from the skin being caught between the striking object externally and the facial skeleton internally. In these situations, the skin is actually ripped rather than cut, giving rise to widespread surrounding tissue disruption. These wounds often do poorly from an aesthetic standpoint, even with the most meticulous repair (Figure 25-11). Scars that result from these injuries are irregular, often widen, and tend to become depressed. Initial treatment should be directed at obtaining as accurate a repair as possible (Figure 25-12). As a general rule, extensive débridement should not be performed at the time of primary repair because of the difficulty in assessing what tissue will be important for the final outcome. When the wound has fully matured (in at least 6 months or, ideally, 1 year), a scar revision may be considered.

Soft-Tissue Avulsions

Actual loss of soft tissue represents one of the most difficult wound management situations. If soft tissue is available, it is not unreasonable to try and reattach it as a full-thickness graft (Figure 25-13). Some authors believe that hyperbaric oxygen may facilitate the survival of these grafts. Adjunctive treatment might include some form of anticoagulation or platelet inhibition. If the portion of tissue is large with identifiable blood vessels (e.g., scalp, ear), microvascular reattachment may be considered. If the reattached portion survives long enough to develop venous stasis, surgical leeches have been used with some success to provide temporary venous decompression until the

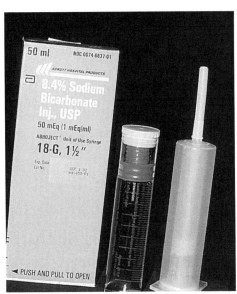

Figure 25-10. Commonly available vials of 8.4% sodium bicarbonate, which may be used for buffering local anaesthetics. One mL of sodium bicarbonate is mixed with 9 mL of 1% lidocaine and 1:100,000 epinephrine to achieve a pH of approximately 7.0.

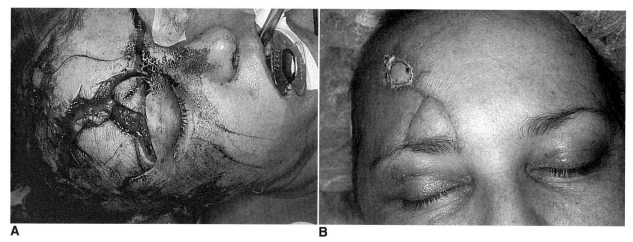

A **B**

Figure 25-11. A, Severe facial contusion resulting from a train-auto accident. Soft-tissue disruption extends beyond the borders of the laceration. This wound has a prognosis for an aesthetic outcome. **B,** The result at 6 months. Note the loss of skin centrally, the depressed scar, and the "pin cushioning" of the triangular segment of skin above the brow.

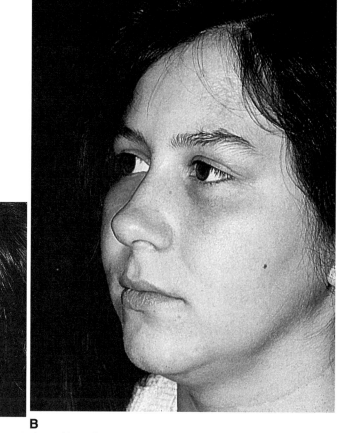

A **B**

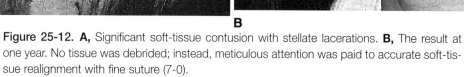

Figure 25-12. A, Significant soft-tissue contusion with stellate lacerations. **B,** The result at one year. No tissue was debrided; instead, meticulous attention was paid to accurate soft-tissue realignment with fine suture (7-0).

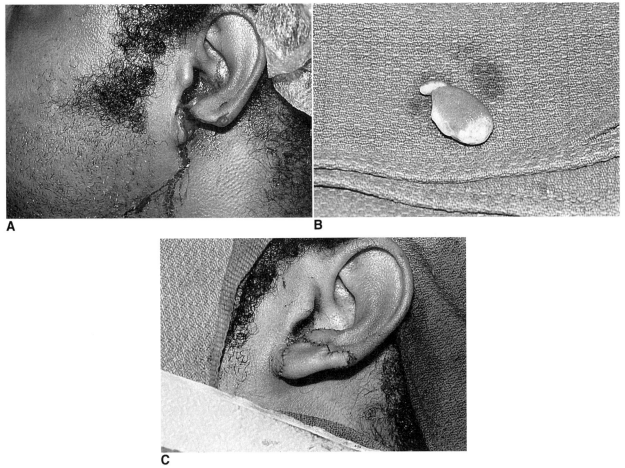

Figure 25-13. A, Human bite to the ear, with avulsion of the lobule. **B,** Recovered lobule before replantation. **C,** Replanted lobule. The patient was managed with antibiotics and hyperbaric oxygen, with complete survival of the lobule.

peripheral circulation reestablishes itself.[6] If the avulsed tissue is not available, the surgeon should manage the wound in its absence. If the defect is not too wide, an attempt at primary closure with undermining can be considered (Figure 25-14). However, if excessive tension on the wound distorts anatomic landmarks (e.g., lip, eyebrow), it is probably best to allow the wound to granulate and heal by secondary intention, with a revision when the wound is stable (Figure 25-15).

No matter how tempting, split-or full-thickness skin grafting is indicated in few situations (except perhaps massive tissue loss or third-degree burns) (Figure 25-16). Placement of a skin graft in situations where soft tissue has been avulsed or lost stops the secondary healing of the wound (which can be helpful in closing a wound) and almost always provides a poor tissue match. This is particularly true in cases in which full-thickness skin and subcutaneous tissue has been lost. For situations in which there has been loss of skin and subcutaneous tissue, placement of a skin graft—even a full-thickness one—will result in a poor tissue match and leave a noticeable contour defect. It is usually best to allow these wounds to stabilize and plan a local or regional flap repair with facial skin that matches the skin surrounding the wound.

Lacerations Involving a Margin or Border

Special consideration should be given to any laceration that extends through an anatomic margin or border because of the aesthetic and functional importance of these junctional structures. Aesthetically, the eye is attracted to discrepancies in facial lines and contours, and a misaligned margin or border will immediately be noticed. Technically, these structures are somewhat more demanding to repair, because they have an internal and external surface, both of which may be involved with the laceration. If an optimal repair is to be performed, all three layers (internal, middle, and external) should be completely and accurately

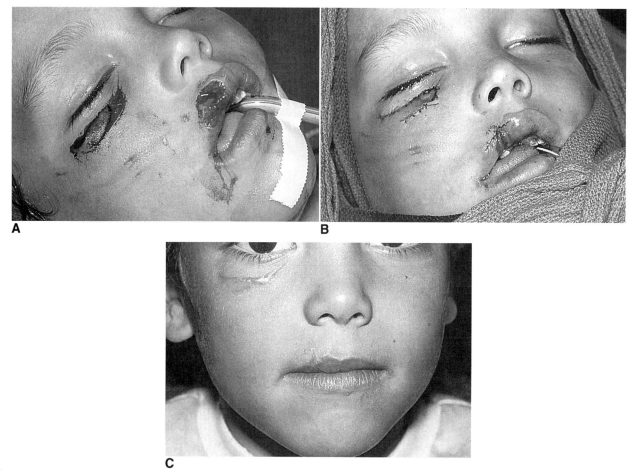

Figure 25-14. **A,** Avulsion of a portion of the upper lip secondary to a dog bite. **B,** Because only a moderate portion was missing, soft-tissue undermining and closure was performed. **C,** The results at 1 year, showing an acceptable lip scar.

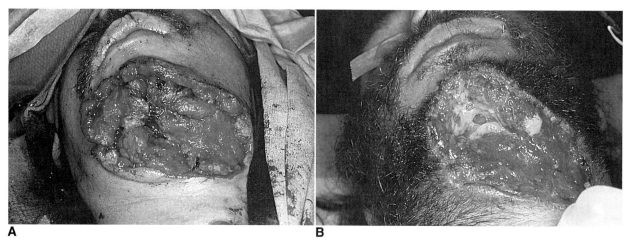

Figure 25-15. **A,** Massive soft-tissue loss secondary to a shotgun blast. **B,** The wound is stable and beginning to granulate; it is now ready for wide undermining and closure.

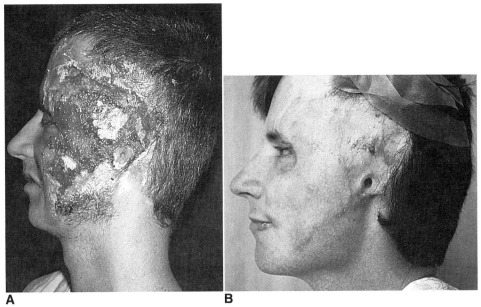

Figure 25-15, cont'd C, The wound is closed without the need for flaps or skin grafts. **D,** An acceptable chin scar 4 months after closure.

Figure 25-16. A, Massive abrasion injury of the left side of the face, with loss of the auricle. **B,** Because the defect was large and relatively superficial, it was skin grafted. No attempt was made to reconstruct the auricle.

realigned. In particular, if the internal surface of the laceration is not repaired, the wound contraction associated with secondary wound healing may cause distortion of the external surface or margin. The sites that merit special attention include the following.

Vermilion Border of the Lip

The smooth line of transition between the pale, external, cutaneous lip skin and the red mucosa is a critical facial landmark, and any malalignment, even as small as 1 mm, will be quite noticeable (Figure 25-17). With any lip repair, the vermilion border should be a primary focus of attention, and the continuity of the border should be accurately realigned first to ensure that repair of the rest of the lip structures will not distort the vermilion border (Figures 25-18, and 25-19). With the vermilion border aligned and stabilized, the rest of the lip layers (inner mucosal, muscular, and cutaneous) are repaired in the standard fashion. Generally the inner mucosa is closed loosely with 4-0

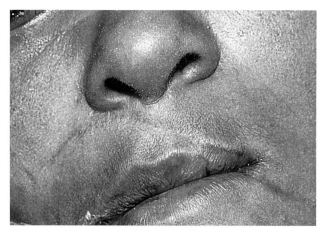

Figure 25-17. A poorly aligned vermilion border distorts the lip contour.

plain gut sutures, the muscular layer with 6-0 polyglycolic acid, and the external skin and mucosa with a fine monofilament (7-0).

Nostril Margin

Lacerations involving the margin of the nostril need to be accurately repaired to ensure that unsightly notching does not occur. Additionally, in the medial portion of the nostril and superior columella, the lower lateral cartilages are quite close to the margin and relatively superficial. If a coincident laceration of the lower lateral cartilage is not recognized and repaired, the likelihood is high that the nose will shift and twist as the forces of healing put stress on the ipsilateral nose and as the ends of the lower lateral cartilage slip over one another (Figure 25-20). If the inner mucosa is not repaired, the contraction resulting from secondary wound healing may cause superior retraction of the nostril margin. Because the nose is aesthetically important and secondary repair of the complications is so difficult, significant lacerations that involve the nostril margin are often best repaired in the operating room. The principal of a three-layer closure is followed, with the exception that a laceration of the lower lateral

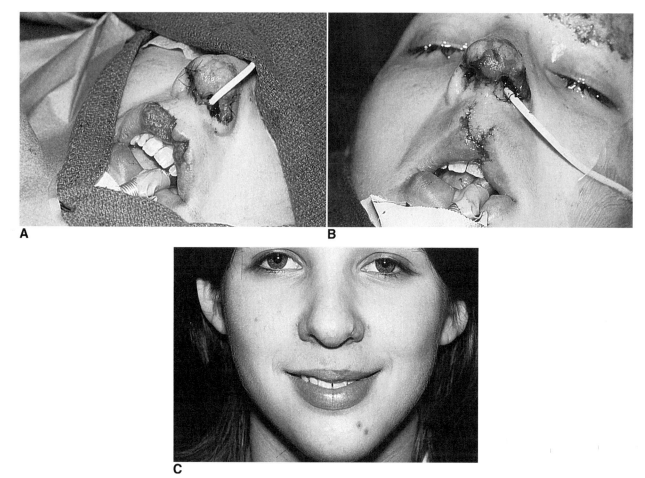

Figure 25-18. A, Upper lip laceration and avulsion. **B,** Closure with meticulous attention to reestablishing the continuity of the vermilion border. **C,** The result at 1 year postoperatively. Note that, if the vermilion border is reestablished, the rest of the lip will adjust to regain normal symmetry.

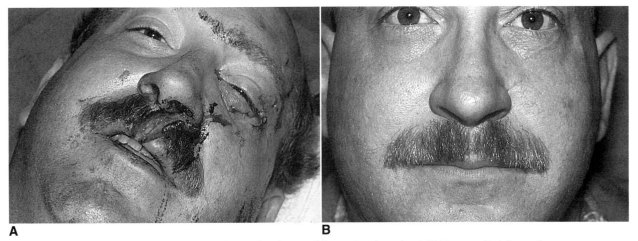

A   **B**

Figure 25-19. A, Upper lip laceration from striking a steering wheel. **B,** The result at 6 months after repair following the principles of accurate vermilion border realignment and three-layer closure.

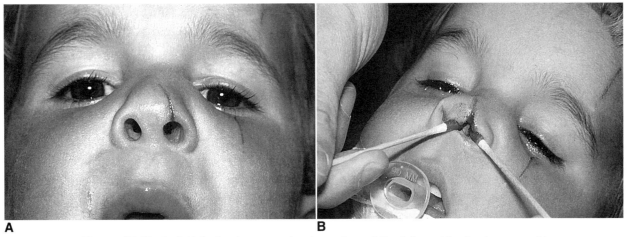

A   **B**

Figure 25-20. A, Initially benign-appearing laceration of the left nostril of a two-year-old patient. **B,** However, further investigation shows a full-thickness injury with a laceration of the lower lateral cartilage. A three-layer closure with reapproximation of the cartilage was performed.

cartilage is identified and repaired with 5-0 or 6-0 clear monofilament nylon to impart some permanent strength to the wound (Figure 25-21).

Auricular Helical Rim

Lacerations of the helical rim that traverse the two skin surfaces and the cartilage require a three-layer repair with accurate reapproximation of the auricular cartilage, as is done for the nose, to avoid notching. The cartilage is repaired by placing 5-0 or 6-0 clear monofilament through the perichondrium and cartilage. The skin is repaired with a 6-0 or 7-0 monofilament (Figure 25-22).

Eyelids

Although laceration or injury of the globe is a primary concern (and should be ruled out with appropriate ophthalmologic consultation or examination), other structures may be involved with eyelid trauma and should be considered. With upper eyelid lacerations, the surgeon should consider the possibility of injury to the levator palpebrae, which could cause ptosis of the upper lid if not repaired. The lacrimal gland may be involved with lacerations of the lateral portion of the upper lid and may be mistaken for orbital fat. There are reports of the lacrimal gland being excised under the mistaken assumption that orbital fat was

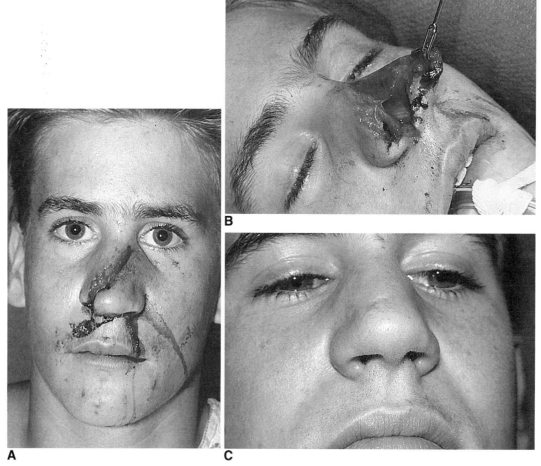

Figure 25-21. **A,** Full-thickness nasal injury from a boat propeller. **B,** Because this injury is extensive, it is best repaired in the operating room under general anesthesia. Mucosal and cartilaginous lacerations were accurately realigned. **C,** The result at 1 year after repair. Note the continuity of the nostril margin and the integrity of the nasal skeleton support.

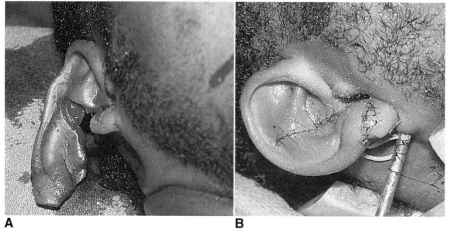

Figure 25-22. **A,** Full-thickness knife wound of the right auricle. **B,** After three-layer closure, with accurate reapproximation of skin and cartilage.

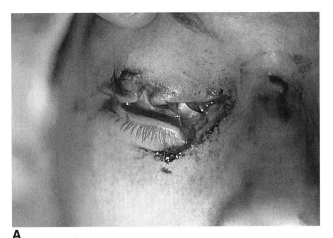

A

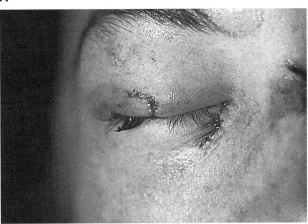

B

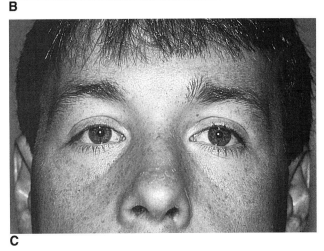

C

Figure 25-23. **A,** Full-thickness lacerations of upper right and lower lids. **B,** After three-layer repair of lacerations. **C,** The result at 6 months after repair, showing good continuity of lid margins.

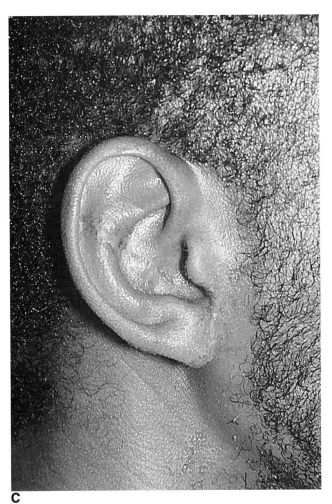

C

Figure 25-22, cont'd C, Follow-up at 6 months showing normal auricular contour.

being debrided. In the lower eyelid, the possibility of a laceration to the lacrimal system should be considered with any medial lid laceration (Figure 25-23). In the upper and lower eyelids, special concern should be given to lacerations that involve the lid margin (see Figure 25-23). If lacerations involving margins elsewhere on the face are improperly repaired, unsightly notching may occur. Briefly, repair of a lid margin laceration involves a three-layer closure with a fine plain gut suture (6-0 or 7-0) on the conjunctival side (to avoid irritation of the scleral conjunctiva), a fine absorbable suture in the tarsal plate, and a fine monofilament on the external surface.

FACIAL BURNS
General Comments

Burns are a separate category of soft-tissue facial injuries. Although the term *burn* implies a thermal injury, other causes are cold or freezing temperatures, electrical current, chemicals, or ionizing radiation.

Regardless of the cause, the common histologic picture of a burn is that of widespread cell death in the affected tissue. Cell death typically extends from the external skin surface internally for a variable depth. In fact, burns are classified on the basis of the depth of extension of cell death into the soft tissue and are referred to as first-, second-, or third-degree burns.

First-degree burns are defined as a superficial injury involving just the epidermis. They result in pain and redness but little significant tissue damage, and they heal without scarring.

Second-degree burns extend into the dermis for a variable distance. The identifying features of a second-degree burn are pain (often severe), erythema, and blistering (Figure 25-24). Second-degree burns will reepithelialize spontaneously and generally have limited scarring (unless they are deep into the dermis). A deep second-degree burn may be converted to a full-thickness injury by improper wound management or infection.

Third-degree burns extend through (or nearly through) the full thickness of the dermis and destroy all of the adnexal structures, which are the source of epithelial regeneration, blood vessels, and nerve endings. Severe third-degree burns can extend through the dermis into the subcutaneous tissue and can even involve bone. Clinical evaluation of third-degree burns is deceptive regarding the severity of this type of injury. By definition, in a third-degree burn, blood vessels and nerves are destroyed, so there is no bleeding, inflammation, blistering, or pain in the area of full-thickness injury, although pain may occur in surrounding areas with just partial-thickness injury (Figure 25-25). Pricking a third-degree burn with a needle elicits no bleeding or pain. The initial relatively benign appearance of a third-degree burn belies the serious nature of this injury. Because the full thickness of the dermis has been

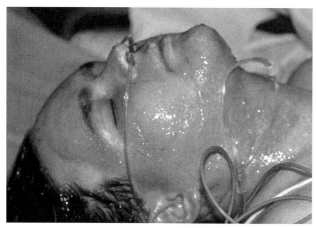

Figure 25-24. A patient with second-degree burns of most of the face, sparing the upper forehead. Note the redness and blistering of the skin, which indicate that it is still viable. To view this image in color, please go to *www.ototext.com* or the Electronic Image Collection CD, bound into your copy of Cummings Otolaryngology—Head and Neck Surgery, 4th edition.

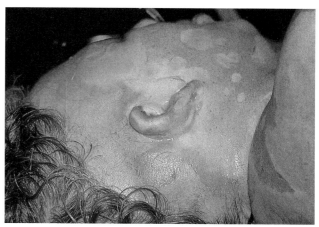

Figure 25-25. Second-and third-degree burns juxtaposed. Note the gray, leather-like appearance of the third-degree burns of the cheek skin as compared with the second-degree injury of the postauricular skin. To view this image in color, please go to *www.ototext.com* or the Electronic Image Collection CD, bound into your copy of Cummings Otolaryngology—Head and Neck Surgery, 4th edition.

lost, there is no possibility of regeneration or reepithelization of this portion of skin (as there is in a second-degree burn). A third-degree burn of the skin results in an eschar that will eventually slough or require débridement, thus leaving a full-thickness wound that can only heal by secondary wound contraction (which invariably causes severe hypertrophic scarring).

Acute Treatment

The major concern with the acute treatment of facial burns relates to making sure that systemic life-threatening issues are addressed. Third-degree burns of any size are serious and may be fatal with as little as 20% of the body surface burned. Formerly, the major cause of death in burn patients was "burn shock" resulting from massive extravascular fluid shifts. With modern physiologic monitoring and improved replacement fluids, mortality from burns has been steadily decreasing over the past several decades.

Respiratory Concerns
Types of Respiratory Burns

Any patient with a significant facial burn should be considered to have a possible coincident burn of the respiratory system. Although most patients with inhalation injuries have extensive burns (>50% of the body surface), Cudmore and Vivori[8] pointed out that it is possible to sustain severe damage to the larynx and lungs from the inhalation of hot fumes and gases without there being any significant degree of body-surface injury.[7,19,24]

Three major factors should be kept in mind when considering the cause of inhalation burn injury: (1) hot, dry gas; (2) steam; and (3) smoke. These three byproducts of combustion are often found together in a fire, but each produces a distinct injury to the respiratory tract.

Hot, dry gas primarily affects the nasal cavity, nasopharynx, oropharynx, and supraglottis. These structures absorb most of the heat, and little damage is done to the glottis, subglottis, trachea, or lung parenchyma. The protective effect of this rapid dissipation of heat is enhanced by the anatomic barrier of the vocal cords and the reflex closure of the cords to heat stimulus.[21]

Steam, on the other hand, with its superheated water vapor, has 4000 times the heat-bearing capacity of air. The large amount of latent heat released during steam condensation overwhelms the cooling capacity of the upper air passages, and thermal burns may result down to the level of the bronchioles. More commonly, steam burns are confined to the subglottis and trachea, with severe subglottic stenosis a frequent sequela.

Smoke inhalation produces a chemical injury to the respiratory tract that usually affects the entire airway and pulmonary tissue. The effects of smoke inhalation may be confined to the epithelial lining, or they may be systemic, as they are with carbon monoxide and cyanide. This chemical toxicity causes intense inflammation and edema of the upper airway and larynx. In the trachea, the mucosa sloughs and denudes the cartilages. The cilia are paralyzed, and debris accumulates, with plug and cast formation. The alveoli also are damaged, with loss of surfactant and increased capillary permeability. The result is atelectasis and a picture similar to adult respiratory distress syndrome. Finally, the damaged airways are susceptible to infection, with the development of bronchopneumonia several days later.

Symptoms of Inhalation Injury

Burns that occur in confined areas or with steam or other superheated gases should raise concern about the possibility of inhalation injury. Common symptoms of inhalation injury are a sensation of choking, a metallic taste in the mouth, dizziness, wheezing, hoarseness, odynophagia, dysphagia, coughing, and increasing respiratory difficulty. Typically, an inhalation injury has an evolving nature, and careful attention should be paid to the development of new symptoms or a changing physical examination.

Physical Signs of Inhalation Injury

Physical findings that suggest an inhalation injury include facial burns, particularly around the mouth or

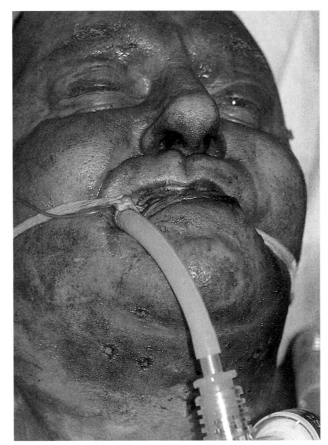

Figure 25-26. A patient with third-degree burns over most of the face. Note the singed nasal vibrissae and soot around the nostrils, which indicate that this patient inhaled hot gases and smoke. Patients with these findings are at high risk for burns of the respiratory tree. To view this image in color, please go to *www.ototext.com* or the Electronic Image Collection CD, bound into your copy of Cummings Otolaryngology—Head and Neck Surgery, 4th edition.

nose; singed nasal vibrissae; soot in the nasal cavities or oropharynx; and swelling and hyperemia of the nasal or oropharyngeal mucosa (Figure 25-26). Laryngeal findings depend on the nature and extent of the injury and may vary with time. With direct thermal injuries to the larynx as a result of dry heat, hyperemia and moderate to marked firm edema of the larynx are present. Bronchoscopy often shows soot-stained sputum and mucus plugs, edema, and necrosis of mucosa. Wheezing, rales, or rhonchi present on admission or developing later are also signs of respiratory tract injury and should prompt further investigation.

Inhalation injury to the respiratory tree is diagnosed almost exclusively by history and physical examination. Hypoxemia, hypercapnia, and increased carboxyhemoglobin levels are laboratory indicators that should prompt further clinical investigations. The most reliable test to detect early inhalation injury to the larynx, subglottis, and trachea is endoscopy, usually with a flexible bronchoscope.

Treatment of Inhalation Injuries

With regard to the treatment of inhalation injuries to the larynx and subglottis, some basic tenets exist: (1) be aware of the possibility of an inhalation injury in any burn patient, particularly in patients who were burned in a confined area with facial burns or soot around the nose; (2) the laryngeal injury may not immediately manifest itself and may evolve over 6 to 12 hours, with eventual respiratory obstruction; and (3) oxygen through nasal prongs or a face mask, a cool mist, and systemic rehydration are generally agreed on. Corticosteroid use is controversial, but the trend appears to avoid their routine use in inhalation injury.

Finally, what is the best way to manage respiratory obstruction in inhalation injury? This complicated issue depends, to a large extent, on the overall status of the patient. Sataloff and Sataloff[21] detailed general guidelines for dealing with pediatric inhalation burn injuries. Patients with extensive burns and coincident inhalation injury are best managed with intubation. Patients with generalized lower respiratory tract inhalation injury that does not affect the larynx are best managed with intubation. Patients with severe upper airway obstruction and laryngeal burns are best managed with tracheotomy to avoid the additional trauma of an endotracheal tube. Patients with severe facial burns sparing the neck, with or without inhalation injury, are often best managed with tracheotomy. Tracheotomies are best avoided in patients with significant coincident neck burns because of the adverse wound healing of burns in the presence of a tracheotomy, and the potential for pulmonary sepsis from the infected burn eschar. Obviously, these guidelines are general, and treatment should be tailored to the patient's situation and needs.

Definitive Treatment

A generally accepted treatment principle for facial burns is that the sooner burns of the face and neck are sealed by spontaneous reepithelization or skin graft, the better will be the ultimate cosmetic and functional outcome. Complete closure of the wound should be accomplished by the third or fourth week after the injury. If a burn spontaneously heals within 10 to 14 days, there will usually be little scarring, and the skin quality will be good. However, if healing has not taken place by two weeks, the chances of unsatisfactory hypertrophic scarring increase dramatically. Therefore, at approximately 10 days, the wound is assessed with regard to its ability to heal spontaneously. If it is determined that healing will be significantly delayed, the burn eschar is tangentially excised until viable tissue is reached, and the wound is skin grafted. While awaiting eschar excision and grafting, a major source of potential morbidity lies with colonization and superinfection of the eschar. In the past, a major cause of burn sepsis was the heavily infected eschar having direct access to the bloodstream through the adjacent viable tissues. Topical antimicrobial agents have significantly reduced the dangers of eschar superinfection, and the most commonly used preparation is silver sulfadiazine applied twice daily.

When planning skin grafts to the face, it is important to consider the unit theory of facial reconstruction by Gonzalez-Ullola[13,14] and replace entire facial units (i.e., perioral region, cheek, forehead, nose) rather than just portions of a unit. Failure to follow the unit concept of facial reconstruction will result in a patchwork appearance with diminished aesthetic results. As a general rule, the thicker the skin graft, the closer the results will be healthy to skin color and texture, but full-thickness skin grafts create more donor site morbidity; therefore, split-thickness grafts of 0.015 to 0.035 inches are the most common alternative.

Postgrafting care is directed at avoiding scar contracture through vigorous physical therapy, splints, and pressure garments. A major source of long-term facial burn morbidity is hypertrophic scarring with scar contracture and distortion of anatomic structures such as the neck, lip, eyelid, and nostril margin. Pressure garments and anatomically contoured acrylic splints are beneficial for keeping hypertrophic scars soft and thin and for lessening scar contracture. However, no technique will completely rehabilitate a severely burned face, and long-term management with various techniques (skin grafts, contracture releases, local flaps, possibly free microvascular flaps, and cosmetic camouflage) at an experienced institution is required for maximum patient benefit.[20]

Special Considerations
Eyelids

With thermal injuries to the periorbital region, direct injury to the eye is rare, but there may be severe long-term ocular sequelae. The major concern in patients with eyelid burns is the maintenance of adequate corneal covering. Corneal exposure typically does not occur until the initial periorbital swelling subsides and scar contracture begins to occur, with ectropion formation. Treatment consists of early eschar removal and skin grafting (thick split-thickness grafts for the upper lids and full-thickness for the lower lids), with meticulous attention paid to corneal lubrication using ointment and appropriate ophthalmologic consultation. Tarsorrhaphy, once routinely recommended, is now reserved for difficult cases with a high chance of corneal ulceration.[7]

Ears

Because of their exposed position and thin skin, ears are often severely injured in any major facial burn. Of all burns of the face, 90% involve the ears.[11,16] Conservatism is the best course of therapy in the acute care of the burned ear. Previously, a major source of morbidity in burned ears was progressive chondritis caused by infection of the exposed cartilage, which led to the admonition of early radical debridement and closure of all ear burns, regardless of size. With the addition of topical antimicrobials, the complication of progressive chondritis has virtually disappeared. The presently recommended treatment is the liberal use of silver sulfadiazine, continuous conservative débridement, and grafting when a suitable recipient bed is available.

Reconstruction of the ear depends on the type of deformity, but classically the ear periphery is most affected and the concha the least. With moderate injuries involving the helical rim, conchal transposition has proved useful.[9] More severe injuries may require rib grafts with temporoparietal fascial flaps or a prosthesis.[3,23]

Oral Commissure Burns

A characteristic pediatric burn is of the oral commissure from an electric current. These injuries occur most commonly in children who are between two and three years old. Typically, oral commissure burns result from the child biting an electric cord, thereby causing an arc of electric energy at the oral commissure, where the cord was in contact with the lip. Because this injury results from the electric current passing through the tissue rather than from heat applied to the skin surface, the initial injury may seem limited, but progressive necrosis becomes evident over the next 36 to 48 hours. Because of the difficulty in distinguishing viable from nonviable tissue, early debridement and primary closure is generally not recommended. Instead, it is advocated that the wound be treated conservatively with topical antibiotics and progressive gentle debridement. Earlier literature attached considerable importance to the possible complication of delayed hemorrhage from the labial artery when the eschar separates, but several large recent series have had a 0% incidence of this complication.[4,10]

Treatment of the resultant oral commissure deformity is somewhat controversial. For some time, oral splints were routinely advocated, but Donelan[10] and Canady[4] question the benefits of splints and believe they may do some harm. Presently the consensus appears to be to treat the wounds conservatively until the scar matures and softens, and then to perform the definitive repair with one of various commissureplasties.

REFERENCES

1. Altieri M, Bogema S, Schwartz RH: TAC topical anesthesia produces positive urine tests for cocaine, *Ann Emerg Med* 19:577, 1990.
2. Anderson AB and others: Local anesthesia in pediatric patients: topical TAC versus lidocaine, *Ann Emerg Med* 19:519, 1990.
3. Brent B: Auricular repair with autogenous rib cartilage grafts: two decades of experience with 600 cases, *Plast Reconstr Surg* 90:355, 1992.
4. Canady JW, Thompson SA, Bardach J: Oral commissure burns in children, *Plast Reconstr Surg* 97:738, 1995.
5. Cannon RC, Chouteau S, Hutchinson K: Brief communications: topically applied tetracaine, adrenalin, and cocaine in the repair of traumatic wounds of the head and neck, *Otolaryngol Head Neck Surg* 100:78, 1989.
6. Chalain T, Jones G: Replantation of the avulsed pinna: 100 percent survival with a single arterial anastomosis and substitution of leeches for a venous anastomosis, *Plast Reconstr Surg* 95:1275, 1995.
7. Constable JD: *Thermal injuries of the head and neck*. In Stark RB, editor: *Plastic surgery of the head and neck*, ed 1, vol 1, New York, 1987, Churchill Livingstone, 275–281.
8. Cudmore RE, Vivore E: Inhalation injury to the respiratory tract of children, *Prog Pediatr Surg* 14:173, 1981.
9. Donelan MB: Conchal transposition flap for postburn ear deformities, *Plast Reconstr Surg* 83:641, 1989.
10. Donelan MB: Reconstruction of electrical burns of the oral commissure with a ventral tongue flap, *Plast Reconstr Surg* 95:1155, 1990.
11. Dowling JA, Foley FD: Chondritis in the burned ear, *Plast Reconstr Surg* 42:115, 1968.
12. Ernst AA and others: LAT (lidocaine-adrenaline-tetracaine) versus TAC (tetracaine-adrenaline-cocaine) for topical anesthesia in face and scalp lacerations, *Am J Emerg Med* 13:151, 1995.
13. Gonzalez-Ulloa M: A quantum method for the appreciation of the morphology of the face, *Plast Reconstr Surg* 34:241, 1964.
14. Gonzalez-Ulloa M and others: Preliminary study of the total restoration of the facial skin, *Plast Reconstr Surg* 13:151, 1954.
15. Gore R: The dawn of humans: neandertals, *National Geographic* 189:2, 1996.
16. Hammond JS, Ward CG: Burns of the head and neck, *Otolaryngol Clin North Am* 16:679, 1983.
17. Levine CL, Berger JR, Lazow SK: Parotid salivary fistula secondary to external pin fixation: case report, *J Craniomaxillofac Trauma* 2:20, 1996.
18. Parekh D and others: Posttraumatic parotid fistulae and sialoceles. A prospective study of conservative management in 51 cases, *Ann Surg* 209:105, 1989.
19. Phillips AW, Cope O: Burn therapy: III. Beware the facial burn, *Ann Surg* 156:759, 1962.
20. Rose EH: Aesthetic restoration of the severely disfigured face in burn victims: a comprehensive strategy, *Plast Reconstr Surg* 96:1573, 1995.
21. Sataloff DM, Sataloff RT: Tracheotomy and inhalation injury, *Head Neck Surg* 6:1024, 1984.
22. Tachmes L and others: Parotid gland and facial nerve trauma: a retrospective review, *J Trauma* 30:1395, 1990.
23. Tjellstrom A: Osseointegrated implants for replacement of absent or defective ears, *Clin Plast Surg* 17:355, 1990.
24. Trunkey DD: Inhalation injury, *Surg Clin North Am* 58:1133, 1978.
25. White WB, Iserson KV, Criss E: Topical anesthesia for laceration repair: tetracaine versus TAC (tetracaine, adrenaline, and cocaine), *Am J Emerg Med* 4:319, 1986.

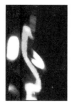

CHAPTER TWENTY SIX

MAXILLOFACIAL TRAUMA

ǁ Robert M. Kellman

INTRODUCTION

The term *maxillofacial trauma* (or *craniomaxillofacial trauma*, as it might be better described, since the anterior wall and floor of the anterior cranial fossa are included in these injuries) is generally used to refer to the injuries of the facial skeleton, and the management of these injuries is sometimes thought of as *facial orthopedics*. As in this text, soft tissue injuries are often discussed separately. However, accurate repositioning of fractured skeletal fragments has major implications for facial aesthetics and soft tissue redraping as well as a significant impact on critical functions such as vision and mastication. Positioning of incisions and the extent of various surgical exposures can influence the final appearance of the face and the function of facial structures like the eyelids, lips, and nose. Therefore, the proper management of maxillofacial trauma requires a comprehensive approach. These injuries should be addressed by practitioners who are familiar with the various ramifications of skull base, orbital, facial, sinus, dentoalveolar, and airway injuries and, most importantly, by those willing to collaborate when necessary with other specialists who may have overlapping areas of expertise. For example, combined facial and anterior skull base injuries are frequently best approached jointly by a neurosurgeon and a craniomaxillofacial surgeon as opposed to the use of separate, independent, and even staged management. Although this chapter can only scratch the surface of many of the complex and controversial aspects of craniomaxillofacial trauma management, it will always assume a comprehensive approach to these often complex and challenging injuries.

The management of facial injuries has evolved significantly during the past two decades. The evaluation of craniomaxillofacial injuries has changed dramatically with the advent of computerized tomography (CT), which has improved dramatically during this interval. Modern CT scanners are exceptionally fast and offer high enough resolution to allow dependable and accurate reconstruction in multiple planes and in three-dimensional (3D) imaging. These advances have added greatly to the surgeon's preoperative understanding of the nature of the injuries.

Borrowing from the revolutionary techniques of congenital craniofacial surgery pioneered by Paul Tessier, wider exposures have been possible, and visible scars have been minimized. Wider access has led to a better understanding of common fracture patterns and their management, and, as might be expected, taking advantage of the experience gained from extended access approaches, surgeons are now trying to perform the same complex surgeries using less invasive techniques.[58] Most recently, these have been improved by taking advantage of the additional visualization offered by endoscopic assistance.*

Bone repair techniques have evolved as well from the frequent use of interosseous wire repairs and Adams suspension wiring[1] to the common use of rigid fixation with plates and screws. Many early mandibular fixations used large plate with large diameter screws,[39,57,94,95] and these repairs have progressed more recently to the frequent use of smaller ("miniplating") techniques as advocated by Michelet[69] and Champy and colleagues[6-8] (and more recently, Ellis[18]). Microplates and even absorbable plates have been advocated for the repair of mid and upper facial as well as cranial fractures and osteotomies. Progress in understanding the biomechanical principles involved in facial fracture repair has resulted in more dependable repairs, both from the standpoint of the technology and in its application. In addition, while not yet widely available, advanced intraoperative imaging techniques allow for more dependable and accurate restoration of the complex 3D facial skeletal architecture.[45,100]

---

*References 9, 11, 36, 38, 49, 50, 91, 102.

Advances in implant technology, particularly the wide use of titanium mesh, plates, and screws, have led to better biocompatibility.[79] Porous polyethylene implants seem to be well tolerated in the orbit (at least so far), and such implants along with the advent of hydroxyapatite cements have provided a wider variety of options for craniofacial reconstruction. Finally, secondary (late) repair of unsatisfactory results has progressed as well, providing more options for the unfortunate patient with a poor outcome due either to an untreated injury or suboptimal initial repair. This chapter will focus primarily on management, including evaluation and primary repair, with mention of complications and the treatment of unsatisfactory late outcomes.

ANATOMY, PHYSIOLOGY, AND PATHOPHYSIOLOGY
General

While form and function are the underpinnings of facial anatomy, and generally speaking form is important for function, the facial architecture is also critically important aesthetically. Knowledge of facial skeletal anatomy is necessary for understanding the mechanisms and patterns of facial injuries as well as the approaches to their repair. Anatomic depictions are available in many anatomy texts and atlases; the focus herein will be on aspects relevant to injury and repair.

The "face" can be arbitrarily divided into sections, each including bony anatomic structures and associated visceral and soft tissue entities. From superior to inferior, the frontal bones are generally considered the "upper third" of the face. The maxillae, zygomas, and orbits compose the "middle third" or "midface" which may include the nose; or the nose and nasoethmoid complex may be separately considered as the "central face." The mandible is generally considered the "lower third," although of course the vertical (posterior) portions of the mandible extend superiorly to the skull base, which is well above the lower third.

Upper Third

The frontal bone forms the contour of the forehead. Displaced fractures can create various deformities, the most common of which is a central forehead depression (Figure 26-1). The frontal bone forms the junction between the cranium and the face, and it relates to several visceral structures, the most critical of which is the brain. The typically paired frontal sinuses, when present (approximately 85% of the time), are housed completely within the frontal bones (Figure 26-2). Frontal bone fractures may involve only the anterior sinus walls, in which case the fractures are significant only for sinus function and cosmesis; or

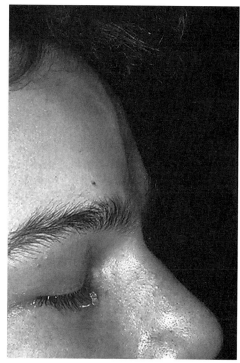

Figure 26-1. Lateral view of a patient with a depressed central frontal fracture. To view this image in color, please go to *www.ototext.com* or the Electronic Image Collection CD, bound into your copy of Cummings Otolaryngology—Head and Neck Surgery, 4th edition.

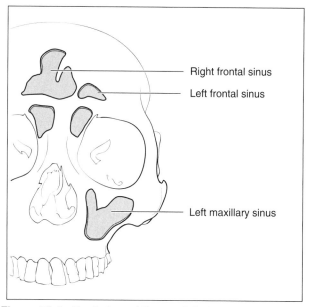

Figure 26-2. Front view of the craniofacial skeleton demonstrating the presence of the frontal sinuses within the frontal bone. (From *Grant's Atlas of Anatomy* with permission.)

they may involve the posterior wall of the sinus(es) or extend beyond the sinus(es), in which case they are true skull fractures and become neurosurgical concerns as well. The supraorbital rims and roofs are also part of the frontal bones, which are therefore also related to the orbits, and fractures can thus affect orbital and ocular functions. Inferiorly in the midline, the glabella portion of the frontal bone relates to the superior extent of the nasal bones. This thick glabellar bone protects the underlying frontal outflow tracts and the cribriform plates that house the branches of the olfactory nerves. The supraorbital and supratrochlear nerves pass through notches or foramina in the supraorbital rims and can be injured here from trauma and, more commonly, as a result of surgical manipulation.

Middle Third

The middle third includes the zygomas, orbits, and maxillae, as well as the nose (which together with the anterior medial orbits forms the central face). The anterior projection of the zygomas, the malar eminence or "cheekbone prominences," are important determinants of facial projection and contour. The posterolateral projections, the zygomatic arches abut the temporal bones posteriorly and provide the attachments for the masseter muscles superiorly. The superior and medial projections of the zygoma contribute to the lateral and inferior orbital rims and the inferolateral orbital walls. Displacement of this portion of the zygoma can significantly alter the position of the globe in the orbit. The inferomedial extension of the zygoma extends from the inferior orbital rim and broadly contacts the maxilla forming the important lateral buttress of the midface (Figure 26-3). While the superior, medial, and inferior orbital rims extend anterior to the globe, the lateral rim, which is comprised primarily of the zygoma, is situated near the equator of the globe (Figure 26-4).[75] Therefore, minor changes in the position of the zygoma can have a significant impact on the anteroposterior position of the globe. Thus, enophthalmos is a common complication of inadequately repaired or unrepaired zygomatic fractures.

The maxillae extend from the zygomas laterally to the nasal bones medially, forming the medial portions of the infraorbital rims and anterior orbital floors and the supports for the nasal bones. They also form the pyriform apertures and house the nasolacrimal ducts. The maxillary dentition is important for mastication, and proper repositioning of the maxillae after trauma is critical to the recreation of a functional occlusion between the maxillary and mandibular teeth. Superomedially, the anterior lacrimal crest is formed by the maxillary bone. Fractures of this area often lead to malpositions of the medial canthal ligaments, which can result in telecanthus, an unsightly cosmetic deformity.

The maxilla also contains the infraorbital nerve, the terminal branch of V2 that provides sensation to the medial cheek, lateral nose, upper lip, and upper gingiva and teeth (Figure 26-5). Fractures can compromise this nerve and care must be taken to both preserve it and, if necessary, decompress it when repairing these fractures. The maxillae also house the maxillary sinuses, which drain into the middle meati of the nose, lateral to the middle turbinates. Injury to the outflow tracts is uncommon, but preexisting obstruction may contribute to infection.

The nasal bones form the bony nasal projection and support the upper lateral cartilages that form the internal nasal valves. Due to their prominent position in the middle of the face, the nasal bones are the most frequently fractured bones in the human body. Restoration of nasal function is important for breathing and olfaction, which also may have a significant impact on taste. The nasal bones are also cosmetically important, and suboptimal restoration of nasal contour is usually quite apparent. The nasal bones are supported by the frontal processes of the maxillae, which are anterior projections of the maxillae superomedially. Failure to identify fractures in this area can lead to unsatisfactory results of nasal fracture reductions.

The orbits are complex bony structures with structural contributions from multiple facial and skull bones. In addition to the frontal, zygomatic, and maxillary contributions discussed previously, the lacrimal bone sits behind the maxillary bone medially (Figure 26-6). The maxillary bone and the lacrimal bone together form the lacrimal fossa, which houses the lacrimal sac. The strong anterior (maxillary bone) and posterior (lacrimal bone) lacrimal crests provide the sites of attachment of the components of the medial canthal ligaments. Note that the medial canthal ligaments have three components: an anterior, posterior, and superior attachment (Figure 26-7). The thin lamina papyracea of the ethmoid bone completes the medial orbital wall. The palatine bone makes a small contribution posteroinferiorly. The posterior lateral orbit is provided by the greater wing of the sphenoid, and the solid optic canal bone is contributed by the lesser wing of the sphenoid. The optic canal sits posteromedially behind the medial wall, where it is generally protected from all but the most severe of injuries. Note that the optic foramen is actually directed toward the lateral orbital rim rather than directly anteroposterior. The important "orbital apex" includes the area lateral to the optic canal through which cranial nerves III, IV, V, and VI pass to enter the orbit, which is considered part of the superior orbital fissure. When pressure from an injury (or tumor, abscess, or hematoma) causes dysfunction in these nerves, it is called *superior orbital fissure syndrome* and requires urgent surgical intervention.[26,99]

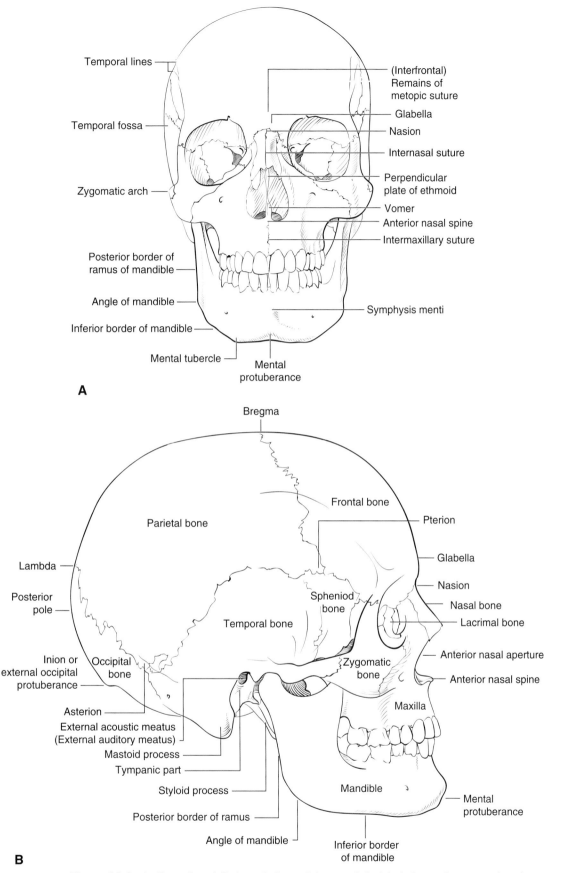

Figure 26-3. A, Frontal and B, lateral view of the craniofacial skeleton demonstrating the broad attachment of the zygomatic bone to the maxilla extending from the infraorbital rim inferolaterally. (Redrawn from Grant JCP: Grant's Atlas of Anatomy, Baltimore, 1972, Williams & Wilkins. Used with permission.)

605

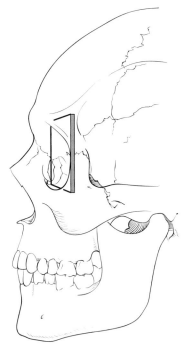

Figure 26-4. Schematic representation of axis of the globe extending from the lateral orbital wall to the lacrimal bone. The entire lateral wall is behind the axis of the globe, whereas only a portion of the floor is so situated. (Redrawn from Pearl RM: Treatment of Enophthalmos, Clin Plast Surg 19(1), 1992.)

Familiarity with the complex shape of the orbital walls is important for repair. The position of the globe is determined by the orbital shape and contents. The best way to prevent globe malpositions is to restore the natural shape of the orbit and ensure that orbital fat that has escaped through fractures is returned to the orbit. Although the orbital floor is gently concave inferolaterally, it tends to be more convex medially and becomes significantly convex posteriorly behind the equator of the globe (see Figure 26-6). Familiarity with this anatomy will increase the likelihood of proper repair after injury.

It is also important to understand the proper terminology associated with injuries. The term *blowout fracture* implies that the orbital rims have remained intact, whereas one or more walls of the orbit, typically the floor (although the medial wall is also commonly affected) has/have fractured. It also has implications for the mechanism of injury, which is a force transmitted by a blunt impact through the globe to the surrounding walls. Also note that floor fractures can damage the infraorbital nerve, which runs through the floor of the orbit.

The midfacial structures are paired, and the central bones are joined in the midline. The nasal bones and maxillae are joined vertically, and the palate forms the inferior horizontal bridge between the two maxillae. The upper horizontal bridge is formed by the anterior cranial base. There are horizontal connections across the nasal bones, but these are not straight across because the nasal bones are situated on a line superior to the infraorbital rims and posteriorly across the sphenoid. The relationships between the various bones are important not only when considering normal anatomy and its reconstitution but also for understanding how facial architecture distributes biomechanical forces, which is important for the repair of fractured structures.

The concept of the *central face* comes into play only in the presence of injury and refers to injury in which the trauma to the solid nasal root is transmitted posteriorly, resulting in a telescoping injury. This has variously been called a *nasoorbital fracture, fracture of the ethmoids,*[15] *nasoethmoid complex* (NEC) *fracture,* and more recently, *nasoorbitalethmoid* (NOE) *fracture.* It is an important fracture clinically, but it takes on even greater significance when used as a paradigm for understanding how facial fractures occur and how the face is designed to provide maximum protection for structures important for the survival of the human organism.

Although the nose is important for airway, smell, and cosmesis, it is less critical to human survival than vision or cerebral function. The solid glabellar and nasal root bones not only protect the underlying cribriform plate, they also take the first impact to the central face. Because the nasal bones and frontal processes of the maxillae are backed up by the thin laminae papyracea of the ethmoid bones, these latter provide little support and crumple, thereby allowing the nasal bones to telescope posteriorly while dissipating the shock wave into the ethmoid sinuses. The optic nerves are suspended in cushioning orbital fat anterior to the optic foramen and more posteriorly are protected by the thick bone of the lesser sphenoid wings once they enter the bony canal. Thus, the medial orbits form a "crumple zone" to protect the globes and optic nerves in most central facial traumas.

This same concept can be applied to other aspects of facial skeletal anatomy. The globes tend to be protected in direct blunt trauma by the thin bones of both the orbital floors and the medial walls. The globes are relatively round and suspended in fat so that most blunt traumas are transmitted to the thin orbital floors and medial walls, explaining why blowout fractures are much more common than globe ruptures. Similarly, the face itself functions as a shock absorber for the cranial cavity, so that the frequency and severity of brain injury can be limited. Finally, this theory provides an explanation for the presence of the paranasal sinuses that offers a survival advan-

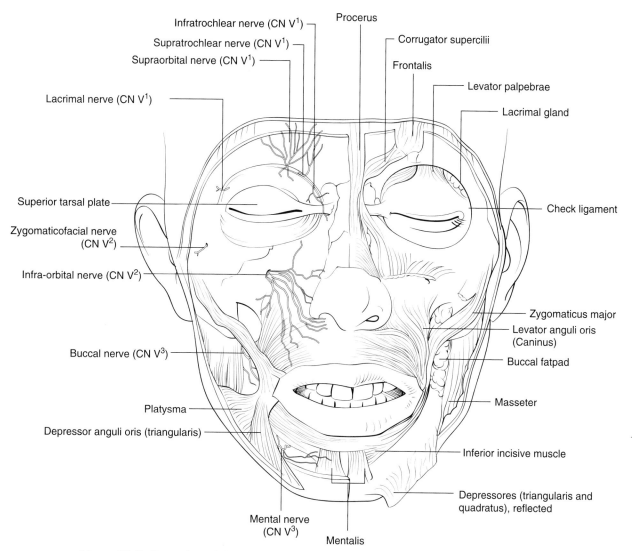

Infratrochlear nerve (CN V¹)
Supratrochlear nerve (CN V¹)
Supraorbital nerve (CN V¹)
Lacrimal nerve (CN V¹)
Superior tarsal plate
Zygomaticofacial nerve (CN V²)
Infra-orbital nerve (CN V²)
Buccal nerve (CN V³)
Platysma
Depressor anguli oris (triangularis)
Mental nerve (CN V³)
Mentalis
Procerus
Corrugator supercilii
Frontalis
Levator palpebrae
Lacrimal gland
Check ligament
Zygomaticus major
Levator anguli oris (Caninus)
Buccal fatpad
Masseter
Inferior incisive muscle
Depressores (triangularis and quadratus), reflected

Figure 26-5. Front view of the partially dissected face. The infraorbital nerve is seen exiting the infraorbital foramen. (Reproduced with permission from *Grant's Atlas of Anatomy,* #470.)

tage—that is, the sinuses serve as a crumple zone for the face, allowing the energy to be dissipated before it reaches the eyes and brain. Thus, the entire facial architecture has evolved by design to provide survival protection for critical organs (Table 26-1).

Lower Third

The mandible is generally considered the lower third of the facial structure. It contains the mandibular dentition, which of course interfaces with the maxillary dentition for mastication. Unlike the middle third, which is fixed to the skull, the mandible is mobile and swings, hinged to the skull base in two bilaterally symmetrical attachments. The hinges occur at the tem-

poromandibular joints (TMJs), which are true arthrodial joints that both swing and slide. The conformation of the mandible, a somewhat horseshoe-shaped bone hinged in two places to the same solid entity, the skull, makes it well designed to absorb impact forces rather than transmitting them to the solid middle fossa floor, and therefore multiple mandible fractures due to a single impact force are not uncommon. (Mandibular trauma causing injury to the skull base can occur, and the condylar head of the mandible has even rarely traversed the glenoid fossa, which houses the articular cartilage of the joint and entered the middle fossa, but such injuries remain rare and reportable.[46]) The condylar head of the mandible is housed within the

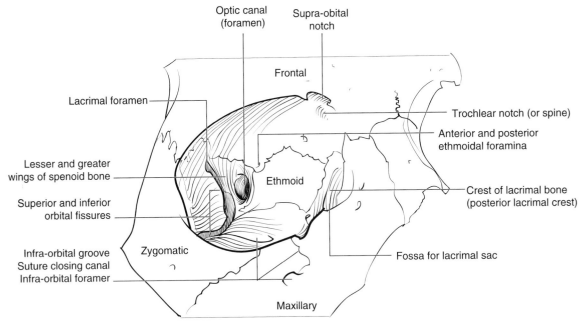

Figure 26-6. Bony orbital anatomy demonstrating the contributions of multiple bones. (Reproduced with permission from Zide and Jelks).

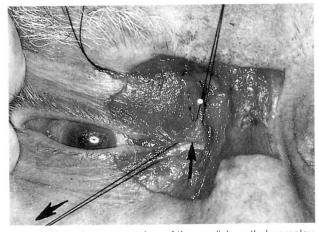

Figure 26-7. A cut-away view of the medial canthal complex. In this view, a suture near the nose is around the superior component and the suture pulling laterally is around the anterior component which has been severed. The posterior component is running behind the anterior component and is fixing the medial structures to the posterior lacrimal crest. (Reproduced with permission from Zide, Jelks: *Surgical anatomy of the orbit,* p 45).

TABLE 26-1

FACIAL ARCHITECTURE

Facial Crumple Zone	Area Protected
Medial orbital wall	Optic nerve, globe
Orbital floor	Globe
Maxillary sinus	Globe, middle cranial fossa
Ethmoid sinus	Globe, optic nerve, anterior cranial fossa, middle cranial fossa
Frontal sinus	Anterior cranial fossa
Sphenoid sinus	Carotid arteries, cavernous sinuses
Face as a whole	Cranial cavity
Condylar necks of mandible	Middle cranial fossae

TMJ and is connected to the vertical ramus by the relatively thin and weak condylar neck. This weak area of the bone seems to give way easily when a contralateral impact is applied, and fractures of this "neck" area are generally called *subcondylar fractures,* indicating that they occur below the TMJ. A central impact to the mentum will, not uncommonly, result in bilateral subcondylar fractures. The condylar neck extends inferiorly into the vertical ramus, which is also relatively thin compared with the tooth-bearing body and symphyseal regions of the bone. However, fractures of the vertical ramus (other than extensions of subcondylar fractures) are relatively uncommon, presumably due to the protective effects of the muscular sling provided by the muscles of mastication, all of which attach to aspects of the vertical rami. The powerful masseter muscle attaches broadly to the inferolateral surface of the ramus whereas the pterygoids attach to the medial surface. The temporalis attaches to the coronoid process, a superior extension of the anterior ramus. The angle region of the mandible occurs at the posterior extent of the tooth-bearing region and is a common area for fracture. Fractures here extend from the thick, tooth-bearing area in the third molar region posteroinferiorly into the much thinner bone of the ramus. The presence of the third molar tends to thin the bone superiorly, and tension of the muscle sling may also splint the area creating a natural break point. Fractures in this region are particularly difficult to stabilize, and repairs have traditionally resulted in the highest rates of complications (see below). As might be predicted, the mandible is thickest in the tooth-bearing areas. The anterior portion from canine to canine is referred to as the *symphyseal region* or *symphysis* (sometimes arbitrarily divided into symphysis in the midline and parasymphyseal regions on either side of the midline), and from canine to angle the body of the mandible contains the two premolar (bicuspid) and three molar teeth.

Another unique aspect of mandibular anatomy is the presence of the inferior alveolar nerve. A branch of the third division of the trigeminal nerve, it enters the mandible at the lingula and travels beneath the tooth roots that it supplies, exiting the mental foramen as the mental nerve generally in the region of the first bicuspid tooth. It is important to keep in mind, when repairing mandibular fractures, that the mental foramen does not generally represent the most inferior position of the nerve, and this must be considered when placing hardware on the mandible in the body region behind the mental foramen.

A common classification scheme for mandible fractures uses the terms *favorable* and *unfavorable*[98]; however, since this scheme has no impact on management, it will not be addressed here. It is also important to be familiar with the changes that take place in the mandible with age and tooth loss. When people lose teeth, the normal stresses on the bone are significantly altered, and bone remodeling tends to result in atrophy of the alveolar portion of the bone. The tooth-bearing portions of the mandible atrophy from the top down, bringing the inferior alveolar nerve closer and closer to the oral surface; in extreme cases, it can even rest on top of the bone. In addition, atherosclerosis of the inferior alveolar artery occurs, limiting the blood supply to the thin atrophic bone.[4] This has significant implications for repair of these fractures.

Fractures of alveolar segments, tooth fractures, and tooth avulsions are beyond the scope of this chapter.

Knowledge of basic dental anatomy and familiarity with normal and common abnormal occlusal relationships are important for anyone treating fractures in the tooth-bearing facial bones. Therefore, these topics will be reviewed here. The normal adult complement is 32 teeth, with eight in each quadrant of the maxilla and mandible. Common numbering of these in the United States is from 1 to 32, starting from the right maxillary third molar (#1) counting toward the left with the left maxillary third molar being #16, the left mandibular third molar #17, and ending with the right mandibular third molar as #32. (Pediatric and European systems will not be discussed here.) The dental surfaces contain cusps for chewing and grooves between these cusps, and in multicusp teeth these are identified by their positions: mesial (toward the incisors), distal (toward the posterior mandible or maxilla), buccal (toward the cheek), and lingual (toward the tongue). Occlusion is complex and has many aspects, but a normal molar relationship has been defined by Angle (as cited by Wilson and Hohmann[106]) as the "mesio-buccal cusp of the maxillary first molar sitting within the mesio-buccal groove of the mandibular first molar." This is Angle's class I. When the maxillary molar is more anterior (chin generally relatively retruded) it is class II, and when the maxillary molar is more posterior (chin relatively pronathic) it is Angle's class III. The maxillary arch should be wider than the mandibular, and when the maxillary buccal cusps fall lingual to the mandibular buccal cusps, it is a crossbite on that side. Similarly, anteriorly, the maxillary teeth should extend anterior to the mandibular teeth, and this is defined as a *normal overjet*. The maxillary incisors should also overlap the mandibular incisors vertically, defined as a *normal overbite*[44] (Figure 26-8).

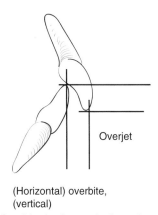

Overjet

(Horizontal) overbite, (vertical)

Figure 26-8. Overbite is the vertical overlap of the maxillary incisors over the mandibular incisors. Overjet indicates the horizontal extension anteriorly of the maxillary incisors forward of the mandibular incisors. (Redrawn from Bailey BJ: *Atlas of Head & Neck Surgery—Otolaryngology,* ed 2, Philadelphia, 1998, Lippincott-Raven.)

EVALUATION AND DIAGNOSIS
Physical Examination

Although the CT scan has become the workhorse of maxillofacial trauma diagnosis, there are still important aspects of facial injuries that are best assessed by means of a good physical examination. The importance of this sometimes lost art must be emphasized.

First and foremost, the initial assessment must address the ABCs and any other potentially life-threatening injuries. Facial trauma may be associated with primary airway injuries to the larynx or trachea, or the airway may be secondarily obstructed by swelling of the oral cavity or pharynx or by blood. Establishing a safe airway may require intubation or tracheotomy, and the status of the cervical spine must always be considered. When bleeding is not severe, use of a fiberoptic endoscope may allow intubation without manipulation (extension) of the neck. Other options include use of the lighted stylet and retrograde intubation or temporary airway stabilization using the laryngeal mask airway. When necessary, a cricothyroidotomy may be performed although, if possible, a tracheotomy is preferred.

Most severe bleeding will be from the nose and sinuses and can be managed by tamponade with packing. Laceration of the internal carotid artery in the skull base may require immediate angiography and balloon occlusion above and below the tear, although these injuries are rarely compatible with survival. Of course, neurologic injuries should be evaluated by the neurosurgeons because these may be life threatening as well.

Although not a life-threatening concern, visual status should always be evaluated as soon as possible because progressive loss of vision usually indicates increasing intraorbital pressure or optic nerve injury, and early intervention will be needed if there is to be any hope of salvaging vision.

The quality of the physical examination of the facial structures will vary depending on the amount of time that has transpired since the injury, the amount of swelling that has developed, the presence of hematoma, and the presence of treatment-related devices such as packing, tubes, cervical collars, etc. The general facial appearance should be assessed first, looking for penetrating injuries and lacerations as well as the possibility of foreign bodies. Facial nerve function should be evaluated in each division, and the possibility of cerebrospinal fluid (CSF) leakage, otorrhea, or rhinorrhea should be considered if there is any fluid discharge. If the patient is able cooperate, a thorough evaluation of cranial nerve function should be performed. When lacerations are present, sterile examination of the wound may yield information about the status of the underlying bone. In particularly severe injuries, for example, if

brain is herniating through the wound, this should be deferred to surgery.

Upper Third

In the upper third of the face, the forehead is evaluated for sensation and motor function. In some cases, fractures may be visible as depressions (see Figure 26-1) or palpable as step-offs, although typically these fractures are more readily seen on CT scans.

Middle Third

As noted in the "Anatomy" section, the middle third of the face houses numerous structures. Functionally, the most important of these are the eyes. Vision should be assessed as soon as possible because progressive visual loss demands emergency management. A light shined in the eye will evaluate pupillary response, even in an unresponsive patient. Failure of the pupil to respond can indicate injury to the afferent system (optic nerve) or efferent system (cranial nerve III and/or ciliary ganglion), or it could indicate a more serious intracranial condition. This must be immediately evaluated by both the neurosurgeon and the ophthalmologist. Of course, a CT scan is imperative to assess the nature and extent of injuries. Other significant though less serious dysfunctions include gaze limitation with or without diplopia. Forced duction testing is performed by anesthetizing the conjunctiva and then manually manipulating the globe in all directions with forceps. An applanation tonometer can also be used to see whether there is an increase in pressure when the patient looks in the direction of gaze limitation (an increase in pressure of 4 mmHg or more is indicative of entrapment).[42] The position of the globe should be assessed both in its anteroposterior position (enophthalmos vs proptosis) as well as its vertical position. The Hertel exophthalmometer is a good tool for measuring globe position when the lateral orbital rims are not displaced. Otherwise, devices that measure relative to the external auditory canal (Naugle) should be used.[88] Enophthalmos may also be identified clinically, either by recognizing the more posterior position of the globe or sometimes by the deepening of the upper lid crease and elongation of the upper lid. Schubert[89] recommends measuring the anteroposterior distance from the globe to the upper brow with the patient in the supine position because it will be increase in the presence of enophthalmos.[89] Chemosis and subconjunctival hemorrhage as well as periorbital ecchymosis are telltale signs of orbital injury. Although not universally accepted, regardless of the findings, if a periorbital fracture is identified, this author believes that ophthalmologic evaluation should be performed before repair because subtle injuries such as retinal tears can be a contraindication for surgery.

Zygomatic malposition may be visible or palpable, although if there is a large amount of swelling present, it may be obscured. The same is true of nasal fractures. The nasal septum must be visualized because septal hematomas must be drained before they result in necrosis of the septal cartilage. A careful nasal examination may also reveal trauma to the upper lateral cartilage with resultant loss of nasal valve support. Note that cheek and lateral nasal numbness (V2 injury) may be the only indication of the zygomatic fracture and should alert the clinician to obtain a CT scan.

Telescoping fractures of the nasal, lacrimal, and ethmoid bones (so-called NEC or NOE fractures) require careful evaluation of the medial canthal relationships, and even with close study they can still be missed. When the canthal ligament is fully avulsed (which is uncommon) or when the bone to which it attaches is completely detached (more common), the medial canthal ligament gets slowly pulled away from its natural position. It tends to displace laterally, anteriorly, and inferiorly, although the displacement may take place very gradually and be missed during the acute phase. Careful assessment includes measurement of the horizontal palpebral widths and the intercanthal distance, as well as the distance between the nasal dorsal midline and each medial canthus. The two sides should be equal, and the intercanthal distance should be approximately equal to each horizontal palpebral width—the two of which should of course be equal. It has also been described as one half the interpupillary distance[33] (Figure 26-9). A loss of nasal dorsal height and development of epicanthal folds are other telltale signs. Finally, direct traction on the medial canthi should be performed to test the firmness of the attachment. A bimanual examination performed with an instrument in the nose and a finger over the medial canthal area as advocated by Paskert and Manson[73] may also be attempted. Evaluation of the lacrimal collecting system is generally reserved for surgery.

Displaced or mobile fractures of the maxillae are generally assessed at the level of the dentition. A change in the patient's preinjury occlusion is indicative of a fracture in one or more of the tooth-bearing bones. Of course, evaluation starts at the teeth themselves, which will alter the occlusion if displaced. Excluding loose teeth, the teeth are carefully evaluated for mobility of the alveolar segments to which they are attached. Motion of an entire midfacial segment indicates midfacial fracture, most of which will occur at the maxillary level, even when more superior fractures are present. Pure craniofacial separation at the Le Fort III level in the absence of lower midfacial (maxillary) fractures is an extremely rare occurrence. More important than identifying the level of a midfa-

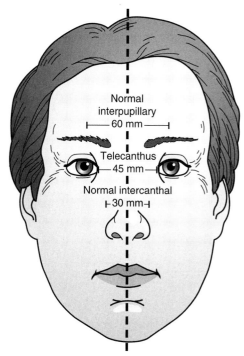

Figure 26-9. Metric relationship of normal and abnormal intercanthal distances to interpupillary distance in traumatic telecanthus. (Redrawn from Holt JR, Holt GR: *Ocular and orbital trauma.* Washington, D.C., 1983, American Academy of Otolaryngology–Head and Neck Surgery Foundation.)

cial fracture on clinical examination is finding evidence of its presence, which will indicate the need for repair as well as careful study of the CT scan to identify all levels involved. Generally, if the teeth and alveoli are intact, grasping the maxilla at or above the incisors and gently rocking back and forth will identify motion relative to either the nasal root or the skull above it. Note that the absence of motion does not ensure that the bones are not fractured because impacted segments may not be mobile. The presence of an anterior open bite is also suspicious, although subcondylar mandible fractures may produce the same finding. Examination of the palate may also reveal evidence of fracture, and it is not uncommon to find mucosal tears along the paths of palatal fractures.

Lower Third

The mandible should be evaluated for sensitive areas, mucosal tears along the gingiva, and of course mobility of fragments. Foreshortening of a vertical ramus, deviation to that side, premature contact of the molars, and an anterior open bite can all be indications of a subcondylar fracture. Bilateral subcondylar fractures may show only the anterior open bite and bilateral premature molar contact when they are present. It is important to assess sensation in the mental nerve distribution because postoperative numbness is not uncommon, and unless it is documented preoperatively, it will be difficult to determine whether it was due to the injury or the surgery. The patient's teeth should be assessed for fractures and other injuries such as intrusions, subluxations, and avulsions. Unless the facial plastic/head and neck surgeon is comfortable managing these, a dental consultation should be obtained.

X-Ray Evaluation

With some exceptions, the CT scan has replaced other forms of x-ray imaging for the assessment of craniomaxillofacial injuries. With the high availability of modern high-speed, high-resolution CT scanners, most maxillofacial trauma surgeons have abandoned plain x-rays of middle and upper third facial bones, even as a screening tool. The numerous overlapping shadows make it easy to miss fractures that would be found on a CT scan, and the presence of a fracture would certainly mandate a CT scan. The exception here is for simple nasal fractures ("simple" meaning without evidence of involvement of other facial bones) that are routinely assessed using plain x-rays— although even these may be unnecessary because they have little effect on management. Another exception is the use of the 6-foot anteroposterior Caldwell view for creation of a template for use in creating an osteoplastic frontal sinus bone flap.

In general, the plane of the CT (axial vs coronal) does make a difference in how effectively selected fractures are visualized.[53,54] In a series of studies, fractures were created in fresh cadaveric heads, and these were scanned using various protocols. Dissections were then carried out to correlate the CT findings and also to see which planes of orientation yielded not only the best primary CT data but also the best 3D reconstructions. It was found that axial orientation was best for visualizing most frontal fractures as well as NOE fractures and the zygomatic arches and vertical orbital walls. Coronal orientation was better for the orbital roofs and floors and the pterygoid plates. In general, as would be predicted, vertical structures were better seen on axial scans and horizontal structures were better seen on coronal scans. It was also found that scans performed at a resolution of less than 1.5 mm should not be used to make 3D reconstructions because the "fill-in" algorithms used by the computer programs created too many misrepresentations. In general, although 3D reconstructions create an overview picture that may help the surgeon visualize the overall facial architecture, it should be borne in mind that they contain potential inaccuracies that are not present in directly obtained scans.

Upper Third

For frontal fractures, a high-resolution axial CT gives good information about the anterior and posterior walls (Figure 26-10). However, it should be noted that in the presence of posterior wall fractures, it is impossible to determine the significance of soft tissue density inside the sinuses. When the posterior wall is displaced (regardless of the degree of displacement), and there is soft tissue density within the sinus, I recommend that the inside of the sinus be visualized (either directly or endoscopically) (see section entitled "Management"). (We have had more than one experience in which placement of an endoscope in a sinus with minimal displacement of the posterior wall and no CSF leakage revealed brain tissue herniating into the sinus.) Displaced anterior wall fractures that require repair are commonly found on CT, even when there is no clinical evidence of cosmetic deformity. Fractures extending into the floor of the anterior fossa are best evaluated with a high-resolution CT scan.

Middle Third

Simple orbital floor blowout fractures are best assessed via coronal CT scanning. However, if there is suggestion of extension into the medial wall, an axial scan (or a high-quality reconstruction from a 1.0- or 1.5-mm coronal scan) should be obtained as well (Figure 26-11). In addition, for accurate orbital assessment, Warren Schubert[89] has recommended creating a parasagittal reconstruction in the plane of the optic nerve (which actually traverses the orbit from posteromedial to anterolateral, so it is not in a true sagittal plane).

Accurate assessment of orbital wall displacement allows the surgeon to anticipate the amount of enoph-

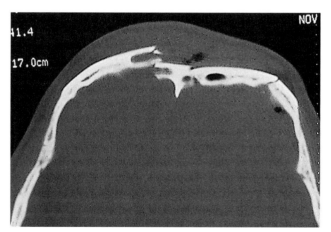

Figure 26-10. Axial CT demonstrates markedly displaced anterior and posterior walls of the frontal sinus. To view this image in color, please go to *www.ototext.com* or the Electronic Image Collection CD, bound into your copy of Cummings Otolaryngology—Head and Neck Surgery, 4th edition.

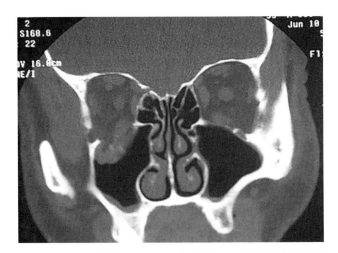

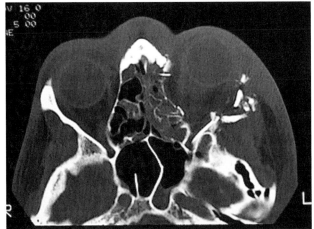

Figure 26-11. **A,** A coronal scan clearly demonstrating a complete blowout fracture of the right orbital floor. **B,** An axial scan demonstrating a medial orbital blowout fracture. To view this image in color, please go to *www.ototext.com* or the Electronic Image Collection CD, bound into your copy of Cummings Otolaryngology—Head and Neck Surgery, 4th edition.

thalmos that is likely to result if the fractures are not repaired.[65,73,84] This not only helps determine the extent of orbital repair that will be necessary but also whether repair is required at all. CT evaluation of the optic canal and orbital apex take on critical significance in the presence of cranial neuropathies related to these areas. Obviously, visual loss due to trauma mandates immediate analysis of orbital CT scans when possible because a reversible injury causing constriction of the orbital apex may be identified.[26,99]

Although zygomatic fractures can be visualized on plain films, accurate assessment of displacement is best analyzed on CT scans. The status of the arch can of course be evaluated on plain films (so-called

bucket-handle views). However, although this may be adequate for simple zygomatic arch fractures (without involvement of the malar portion of the zygoma), most zygomatic fractures involve complex 3D alterations in position as well as involvement of the lateral and inferior orbital walls and are best assessed with CT scans. The axial CT will demonstrate shifts in the position of the zygomatic arch that may be otherwise missed in high-impact trauma in the anteroposterior direction. Careful comparison to the contralateral arch is very important as is a familiarity with the normal shape of the zygomatic arch, which is more flattened anteriorly and does not therefore represent a true convex arch. Careful analysis of the left and right arches seen in Figure 26-12, *A* and *B,* shows the difference between two otherwise normal-seeming arches. Figure 26-12, *C,* shows the two together, and it of course becomes quite clear that one must be abnormal.

Displacement of maxillary fractures is typically well demonstrated on axial scans. These scans also show fractures through the pterygoid plates that help define the presence of Le Fort type fractures. However, the horizontal components of these fractures were in fact best displayed on coronal scans (and as might be expected, on 3D reconstructions from the coronal scans).[55]

Lower Third

For the mandible, unlike the middle and upper thirds of the face, most surgeons prefer plain x-rays, or more commonly panoramic tomography, and often both as the imaging techniques of choice. Several studies[13,66] have found x-rays better than CT scans, although 3.0-mm slice resolution was used in these studies. Wilson and colleagues[104] suggested that the addition of axial CT in 39 patients with mandible fractures revealed two parasymphyseal fractures and 15 cases of comminution or displacement that had been missed on panoramic tomography. However, the CT also missed posterior mandibular fractures, so that both were required to maximize information. However, 3- to 5-mm slice resolution was used, and this might account for the poor sensitivity of the CT scans in their series. In a subsequent study using high-resolution helical CT (1-mm slice resolution), the sensitivity for the CT scans was 100% whereas that for panoramic tomography was 86% (seven fractures missed in 6 of 12 patients).[105] Considering the cost disparity between panoramic tomography and CT scanning, it is unclear whether the standard of care for mandibular evaluation will change. Lee and others[50] have suggested that coronal CT scanning with 3D reconstruction is the procedure of choice for assessing the position of the proximal fragment in

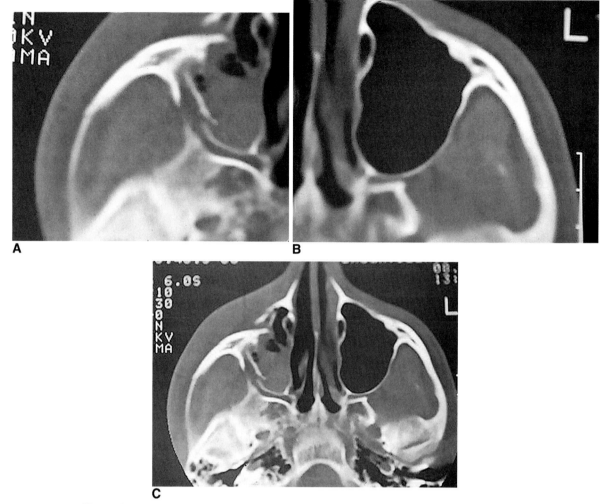

Figure 26-12. A, The right zygomatic arch in the presence of a trimalar (tripod) fracture. While it appears grossly intact on this view, this is in fact not the normal contour of the arch. The shape here is too much of a "true arch," which is not the actual natural shape. **B,** The left zygomatic arch on the same patient has the more normal appearance with the anterior portion of the arch being relatively flat followed by the convexity of the posterior portion. **C,** The two arches together, demonstrating that the abnormal contour on the right side of the patient (left side of the figure) is the result of the zygomatic fracture.

subcondylar fractures of the mandible. Furthermore, they recommend a postoperative scan to ensure that the reduction is accurate after endoscopic repair. This is certainly a more expensive approach than the Towne's view x-ray that is typically used to view the position of the condylar fragment. Additional experience will ultimately determine the most appropriate studies.

CLASSIFICATION SCHEMA

Numerous classification systems have been developed and reported for the various fractures that occur in the facial skeleton. Such systems are useful for communication between physicians and are valuable for docu-

mentation purposes, particularly statistical analyses, but they should also be useful for treatment planning. Unfortunately, many classification schemes fail to meet one or more of these criteria. A brief summary of some of the more widely used systems will be reviewed.

Upper Third

In the frontal area, classification schemes have focused on the involvement of the frontal sinuses, and these systems have been treatment oriented. The most useful classification was presented by Stanley and Becker,[101] since it predicts the likelihood of disruption of the frontal sinus drainage passages. They separated frontal sinus fractures into linear horizontal and linear vertical and comminuted anterior and posterior walls, with and without NEC or supraorbital rim fractures. Of interest was the finding that whenever an NEC or a supraorbital rim fracture occurred in combination with comminuted fractures of either the anterior or posterior frontal sinus walls, a ductal injury was predicted. This scheme has been modified by Gonty and others,[28] but interestingly, in the commentary on this paper written by Stanley,[96] it is suggested that even his own classification system is not all that useful clinically. Numerous other classification systems have been suggested, but they offer little to the planning of the treatment approach.

There are also classification schemas designed to predict the incidence of CSF rhinorrhea after anterior skull base trauma. The most useful of these, which is also somewhat intuitively predictable, was reported by Sakas and colleagues,[87] who found that the more centrally located the fracture in the skull base and the more severe the fracture, the greater the likelihood of CSF leakage.

Middle Third

Numerous classification systems have been created for addressing the multiple fractures that occur in the middle third of the face. Although not always applicable, the most important system is that developed over 100 years ago by Rene Le Fort.[51] It was developed artificially through an analysis of the facial fracture patterns that were seen in cadavers that were traumatized by being dropped from a height. The Le Fort I fracture, or horizontal maxillary fracture, occurs above the level of the maxillary dentition, separating the alveoli and teeth from the remaining craniofacial skeleton. It of course crosses the nasal septum, and posteriorly it completes the fractures through the posterior maxillary walls and pterygoid plates. The Le Fort II fracture, or pyramidal fracture, starts on one side at the zygomaticomaxillary buttress, crosses the face in a superomedial direction (fracturing the inferior orbital rim and orbital floor), traverses the medial orbit, and crosses the midline at the nasal root or through the nasal bones, and then travels inferolaterally across the contralateral side of the facial skeleton, creating a pyramid-shaped inferior facial segment that is separated from the remaining craniofacial skeleton. Like the Le Fort I, Le Fort II fractures the nasal septum, the posterior maxillary walls, and the pterygoid plates. The Le Fort III fracture, or complete craniofacial separation, occurs at the level of the skull base, separating the zygomas from the temporal bones and frontal bones, crossing the lateral orbits and medial orbits, and reaching the midline at the nasofrontal junction and violating the nasal septum and pterygoid plates (Figure 26-13). Although many fractures seen clinically do not

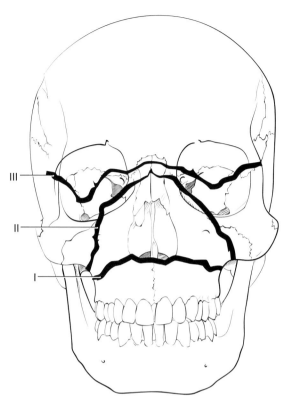

Figure 26-13. Le Fort I fracture is a horizontal fracture that separates the bone containing the maxillary dentition from the remainder of the craniofacial skeleton. The Le Fort II fracture is a "parametal" fracture that extends across the maxilla through the infraorbital rim and orbital floor up through the medial orbital wall and across the nasal root area, then across similarly the other side. The LeFort III fracture is the true craniofacial separation that includes fractures of the zygomatic arches and frontozygomatic areas, then crosses the lateral inferior and medial orbits and is completed across the nasal root. Note that all Le Fort fractures cross the nasal septum and pterygoid plates.

fit precisely into this classification scheme, it has stood the test of time, and it does prove useful for communication and treatment planning. To use the scheme for documentation purposes, it is helpful to more specifically describe the nature of the particular fractures in each case. For example, a pure Le Fort III fracture is probably a rare occurrence, yet many surgeons will describe an injury by the most severe level encountered and then describe the additional components.

Numerous classification schemes have been used to describe NOE fractures. The system that is probably the most useful for treatment planning is that described by Markowitz and others[66] (Figure 26-14). In this scheme, a type I fracture occurs when a large central fragment containing the medial canthal ligament is freed from the surrounding bone. It is repaired by rigidly fixing this central fragment in place. In a

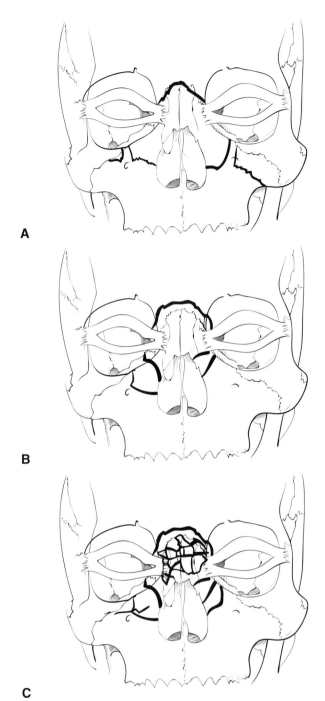

A

B

C

Figure 26-14. Naso-orbital ethmoid fractures have been classified as Type I, Type II, and Type III by Markowitz and others.[66] Type I fractures include a solid central segment to which the medial canthus is attached. Type II injuries are more comminuted than Type I but still leave a central segment to which the medial canthus is intact. In Type III injuries, the bone is shattered and there is no solid bone to which the medial canthal tendon is attached. (Redrawn from Markowitz BL and others: Management of the medial canthal tendon in nasoethmoid orbital fractures: the importance of the central fragment in classification and treatment. *Plast Reconstr Surg* 87(5):843–853, 1991.)

type II fracture, there is significant comminution, but the fragment containing the medial canthal ligament is still repairable. However, transnasal fixation of this fragment or the tendon is still necessary. In type III injuries, the tendon is either detached or attached to an unusable fragment. It must be freed and directly repaired with transnasal fixation. This description shows how a useful classification not only describes the injury but helps in the planning of the repair.

Lower Third

Mandibular fractures are for the most part classified by the anatomic region in which they occur as well as by their severity. Severity typically includes simple, comminuted, or avulsive (bone loss) fractures. The mandible is also categorized as dentulous, edentulous, or atrophic edentulous. Historically, a common classification has separated "favorable" from "unfavorable" fractures. In fact, these descriptions are no longer considered helpful in determining the treatment plan, and they certainly offer no documentation or communication advantages. They are thus of historical significance only.

MANAGEMENT
General

Once the injuries have been identified, a management plan should be developed. As noted above, appropriate consultations should be made, and, when necessary, the consultants should be included in the process so that the management plan is comprehensive. A piecemeal approach increases the likelihood of a less than ideal outcome and should therefore be avoided.

It is generally accepted that since most maxillofacial injuries are considered contaminated due to communication with the nose, sinuses, oral cavity, or a combination thereof, antibiotic treatment should be initiated at the time the patient initially presents. A prospective study by Chole and Yee[12] demonstrated some benefit of this approach. Typically, antibiotics that cover oral organisms such as penicillins, cephalosporins, or clindamycin are selected. It is unclear how long administration should be continued, but these medications are generally given until at least 24 hours after surgery, although they are sometimes given for longer periods.

An issue that has generated strong opinions is that of the timing of surgery. Early reviews of mandible fractures suggested that delay in treatment increased the likelihood of infection.[3] However, since the advent of routine prophylactic antibiotic therapy, this does not seem to be true. Many surgeons have suggested that surgery should be delayed until swelling resolves so that facial asymmetries can be better assessed.

However, because fractures are assessed using CT scans, this is probably not a relevant concern, particularly since extensive soft tissue exposures recreate the soft tissue swelling anyway. More recent and cogent arguments have suggested that reinsulting the soft tissues after the acute inflammatory phase has resolved may result in a less pliable and resilient soft tissue envelope and less satisfactory healing and outcomes, although this remains more theoretic than proven. Certainly, logic seems to suggest that early intervention to restore the hard and soft tissues to their normal anatomic positions would be beneficial. However, it is not uncommon for other considerations to intervene, particularly in severe trauma where the stabilization of the patient with life-threatening injuries takes priority. Thus, the level of urgency remains an individual decision.

SURGICAL ACCESS

There is little doubt that the frequent use of extended access approaches[30,64] has led to a better understanding of fracture patterns and the complexities of reduction and fixation. Combined with the use of rigid fixation techniques and the liberal use of bone grafts,[29] repair of the facial skeleton has become more dependable, and the need for postsurgical maxillomandibular fixation (MMF) and tracheotomy has been minimized (Kellman & Schilli). However, there are also disadvantages to these wide exposures, and facial asymmetries may be seen in the presence of excellent skeletal reduction. These have been attributed to problems with soft tissue healing and redraping, leading surgeons to look for more limited access approaches that will still allow for correct bony repositioning.[61]

An additional challenge in craniomaxillofacial surgery is the inability to make incisions directly over most fractures, since unacceptable scars and facial nerve injuries would result. Incisions are carefully planned to take advantage of sites that are either well hidden or transmucosal, or those in which the scar can be adequately camouflaged. Frequently, however, this requires extensive undermining and elevation as well as significant intraoperative retraction, all of which can lead to soft tissue changes that result in a less than ideal outcome. These issues must be carefully considered when planning surgery, keeping in mind that it is sometimes wiser to extend an incision than to damage the soft tissues with overzealous retraction.

Upper Third

Today, the workhorse of frontal and supraorbital rim exposure is the coronal incision. Generally speaking, this incision will be less obtrusive even in the bald or balding male than the bilateral brow ("butterfly" or "gull-wing" incision). (The exception might be a unilateral brow incision in the patient with bushy eyebrows or in the presence of a significant laceration.) In a patient with hair, irregularizing the incision with a *running* "w" or a wavy line[24] prevents the scar from parting the hair and therefore makes the scar virtually unnoticeable. However, a straight incision seems to be less visible on the bald scalp (Figure 26-15).

Shaving the hair is not required, although creating a hairless strip makes it easier to keep hair out of the wound during surgery and wound closure. (Some neurosurgeons favor a complete shave when an intracranial injury is present.) When full exposure of the zygomas is required, the incision typically begins in the preauricular crease and extends superiorly above the auricle and over the top of the head to the contralateral auricle. The incision may curve anteriorly

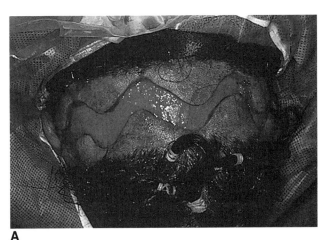

A

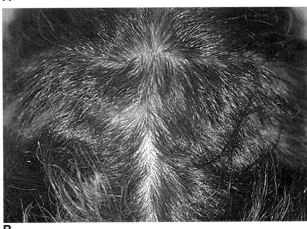

B

Figure 26-15. **A,** A coronal incision broken up by irregularization. **B,** Even when the hair is relatively short, the irregularization of the incision allows it be well hidden beneath the hair. To view this image in color, please go to *www.ototext.com* or the Electronic Image Collection CD bound into your copy of Cummings Otolaryngology—Head and Neck Surgery, 4th edition.

over the central scalp to shorten the skin flap, which allows the flap to flip more easily. When zygomatic exposure is not needed, the incision starts above the auricle. When a long pericranial flap is needed (for anterior fossa repair or frontal sinus obliteration), the incision should not violate the pericranium. The skin can then be elevated posteriorly over the pericranium, which is then incised more posteriorly and elevated with the anterior skin flap, thus creating a long, anteriorly based pericranial flap for later use (Figure 26-16).

As the flap is elevated anteriorly, care must be used to avoid injury to the temporal (frontalis) branches of the facial nerve. This can be accomplished by either elevating directly against the temporalis fascia or incising the superficial layer of the deep temporal fascia at the temporal line of fusion and continuing elevation beneath this layer. If the latter is done,[Au11] it is critical that the fascia be resuspended at the time of closure to prevent desuspension of the midfacial soft tissues. The supraorbital and supratrochlear nerves are encountered as the flap is elevated to the supraorbital rims. When the supraorbital nerve passes through a notch, it is easily elevated inferiorly with the flap, although care must be used to avoid injuring it. When the nerve passes through a true foramen, the inferior lip of the foramen must be fractured (using an osteotome, curette, or other bone-biting instrument) to allow the nerve to move inferiorly with the flap. Orbital fat may herniate around the nerve. Elevation of the superior orbital periosteum from the orbital roof requires elevating first in a superior direction once over the rim, since there is typically an overhang

of 3 to 7 mm. (Failure to recognize this can result in elevation directly into the orbital tissues.) The periosteum tends to be very adherent at the nasofrontal suture, and sharp elevation may be needed here. Elevation to this level provides wide access to the upper third of the face. Elevation of this flap can also be continued inferiorly in the midline for exposure of the nasal bones, medial orbital walls, and frontal processes of the maxillae; elevation laterally provides exposure of the zygomatic arches and most of the zygomatic bones and lateral orbital walls.

Middle Third

There are numerous options available to the surgeon for approaching the middle third of the facial skeleton, and selection of incisions based on the access needed to properly repair a particular injury, the ability to camouflage scars on the patient, and the surgeon's individual experience. Zygomatic fractures are generally repaired at more than one site, often necessitating more than one surgical exposure. As noted above, the zygomatic arches are well exposed via the coronal incision. A simple arch fracture, however, may be accessed via a Gillies' incision, which is made within the temporal hairline and elevated beneath the temporalis fascia (over the temporalis muscle, since the fascia inserts on the arch, while the muscle passes beneath the arch), allowing an instrument to be passed with assurance beneath the arch for elevation; or it may be similarly approached using a transmucosal incision in the gingivobuccal sulcus intraorally. The frontozygomatic area (lateral orbital rim) can be accessed in several ways, and the facial plastic sur-

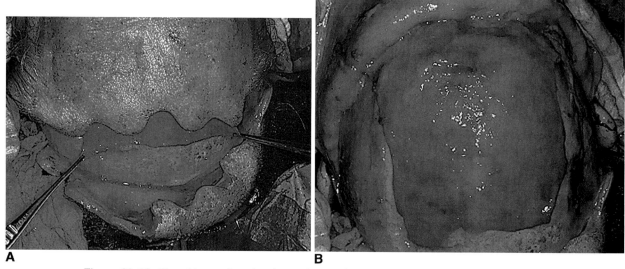

A　　　　　　　　　　　　**B**

Figure 26-16. The skin can then be elevated posteriorly over the pericranium, which is then incised more posteriorly and elevated with the anterior skin flap, thus creating a long, anteriorly based pericranial flap for later use. To view this image in color, please go to *www.ototext.com* or the Electronic Image Collection CD bound into your copy of Cummings Otolaryngology—Head and Neck Surgery, 4th edition.

geon must select the most appropriate incision for the individual situation. The lateral upper lid incision (sometimes described as the "upper lid blepharoplasty incision") is commonly used today (Figure 26-17) because it tends to hide well in the upper lid crease; it is replacing the lateral brow incision, which, although still considered quite acceptable by many, not infrequently leaves a noticeable scar.

The lateral rim can also be reached through a lower lid conjunctival incision when the incision is extended laterally and a canthotomy is performed. However, an unacceptable amount of retraction can sometimes be required when this approach is used. The orbital floor, on the other hand, is well exposed via the transconjunctival incision through the lower lid. This can be performed using either a preseptal or a postseptal approach, and each has its advantages and disadvantages. Whichever approach is used, care must be used to avoid injury to the orbital septum because scarring in this layer tends to lead to postop-

erative lower lid malpositions. Extending these incisions to include a lateral canthotomy and skin incision allows wider exposure, particularly for placement of large grafts and for exposure of the medial and lateral orbits. The orbital floor can also be explored via transcutaneous incisions through the lower lid, including the subciliary and the lower lid crease incisions. The infraorbital incision has for the most part been abandoned due to limited access and excessive, prolonged lower lid swelling (except when there is already a significant laceration present). The medial orbit can be explored via a coronal incision, a transconjunctival incision (transcaruncular or retrocaruncular) or a cutaneous incision similar to an external ethmoidectomy approach. (Note that whenever a lower lid incision has been used, it is wise to place a Frost stitch at the end of the procedure and leave it in place for 24 to 48 hours. It is placed through the lower lid and taped to the forehead; it stretches the lower lid and may decrease the likelihood of lower lid malposition [Figure 26-18].)

The lower portion of the middle third (i.e., the anterior maxillary walls, including the pyriform apertures, the frontal processes, and the zygomaticomaxillary junction) are best approached transorally by incising the mucosa of the gingivobuccal sulcus. Care must be taken to avoid elevating bone fragments in the flap and to avoid injury to the infraorbital nerves. This incision will allow elevation superiorly to the infraorbital rims. Additional exposure can be obtained by using the midfacial degloving approach, although this does add the risk of nasal stenosis because the mucosa of the nasal vestibule is incised circumferentially in this approach. Palatal exposure is generally obtained through lacerations that occur along fracture

A

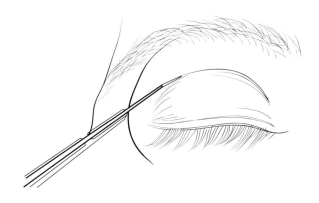

B

Figure 26-17. The upper lid blepharoplasty incision provides excellent access to the lateral orbital rim and lateral orbit. (Redrawn with permission from Bailey BJ, Calhoun KH: *Atlas of Head & Neck Surgery—Otolaryngology,* Philadelphia, 2001, Lippincott William & Wilkins.)

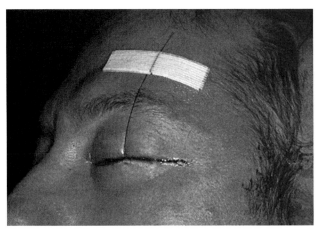

Figure 26-18. The platysma is incised two fingerbreadths below the mandible to minimize the risk to the facial nerve. To view this image in color, please go to *www.ototext.com* or the Electronic Image Collection CD bound into your copy of Cummings Otolaryngology—Head and Neck Surgery, 4th edition.

lines. A U-shaped palatal flap can also be elevated for wide palatal exposure.

Lower Third

The mandible can be exposed either transmucosally or transcutaneously. Early concerns that intraoral exposures would lead to higher infection rates have not proved true in large experiences.[60] Virtually all areas of the mandible can be reached via transoral incisions. The symphyseal region is easily exposed using an incision that is placed 5 to 10 mm below the gingival margin, thereby leaving enough free mucosa for easy wound closure. Body fractures can be similarly exposed. Care must be used to avoid injury to the mental nerve as it exits the mandible and enters the soft tissues to supply sensation to the overlying skin. The angle region is best exposed using an incision that begins at the inferior portion of the anterior ramus of the mandible. This is extended over the oblique line and carried below the gingival margin of the posterior molars. Finally, the vertical ramus and subcondylar regions are exposed using the vertical portion of this last incision and extending it superiorly. Exposure of the subcondylar region is enhanced with the aid of endoscopes.[38,49,50]

Extraoral incisions add the risk of a visible scar as well as the possibility of injury to the mandibular ramus of the facial nerve. On the other hand, for anterior body fractures, the risk of injury to the mental nerve may be decreased. The symphysis is best approached using a submental incision. The posterior body, angle, and even the subcondylar regions are best approached using a submandibular incision. To aid bone exposure and minimize retraction, the incision can be made one fingerbreadth or less below the mandible and elevated inferiorly superficial to the platysma. The platysma is incised two fingerbreadths below the mandible to minimize the risk to the facial nerve (Figure 26-19). The anterior body is more difficult to reach transcutaneously because the relaxed skin tension lines cross the mandible and risk injury to the facial nerve. This area is probably best approached by combining a submental incision with an anterior submandibular incision and connecting them via a "Z" to minimize the scar. The ramus and subcondylar regions can be approached via the submandibular incison and elevation between the masseter muscle and the bone. Alternatively, a retromandibular incision can be used as advocated by Ellis and Zide[22] (Figure 26-26). A preauricular incision can be used, but this may increase the risk of injuring the main trunk of the facial nerve, and if a preauricular approach is used, a

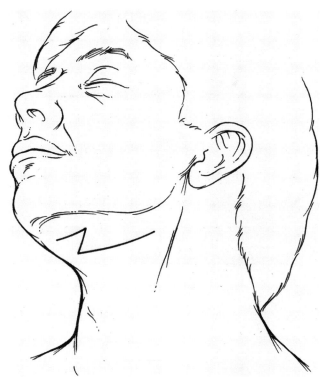

Figure 26-19. The mid body is difficult to reach through an external incision. The direction of the submental incision is different than the direction of the submandibular incision. Sometimes greater length can be obtained by combining these two incisions in a Z-plasty fashion.

facial nerve dissection should be considered for protection of the facial nerve.

BONE HEALING

A cursory introduction to bone healing will be included here from the standpoint of the interaction between repair techniques and the way that bone tends to heal. In general, like other injured tissue, bone tends to heal. The process begins almost immediately after injury with the development of a fracture hematoma. Subsequent ingrowth of vessels brings fibroblasts and other progenitor cells. There is a differentiation to chondroblasts, and these lay down fibrocartilage and chondroid matrix, which lead to early stabilization and provide the substrate for the development of osteoid. With differentiation into osteoblasts, osteoid is deposited, and this results in callus formation. It is helpful to think of callus as nature's fixation device because callus is deposited until motion ceases at the site of the fracture. Once motion ceases, delicate osteons each with their own vessels can grow across the fracture, resulting in the

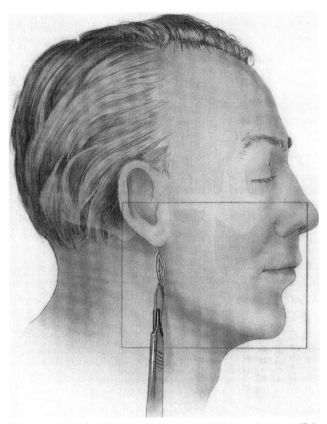

Figure 26-20. Vertical incision just posterior to the mandible through skin and subcutaneous tissue to the depth of the platysma muscle. (Reprinted with permission from Ellis E III, Zide MF: *Surgical Approaches to the Facial Skeleton,* Philadelphia, 1994, Lippincott Williams & Wilkins, p 143.)

bridging of the fracture by new bone and thus full stabilization and healing.[78,79] Once the fracture is bridged by bone, the bone form can then be remodeled to match its function according to Wolff's law, which says that bone remodels according to the forces acting on it. This results in a recreation of proper form to match function. This process tends to be very effective for long bone healing.

Unfortunately for the craniomaxillofacial surgeon, Wolff's law fails to account for two key needs of the facial skeleton: aesthetics and dental function. Thus, allowing facial bones to heal on their own tends to result in both significant cosmetic deformities and compromised masticatory function, which can also have significant implications for nutrition. Although the tooth-containing bones will indeed remodel in response to the forces that act on them, they will not remodel to recreate a proper and functional occlusal relationship between the maxillary and mandibular dentition. It is therefore critical that these fractures be managed in a way that will guide the healing

process to recreate both satisfactory form and proper function.

There are two aspects to consider in performing these repairs. One is as noted the proper realignment of the bones to recreate aesthetic form and occlusal function. The other is methodologic and refers to the type of fixation accomplished, rigid fixation, which is designed to maximize the amount of stability created at the time of repair in the hopes of minimizing callus formation, infection, and any shifting in the surgical positioning. *Rigid fixation* refers to the use of devices (typically plates and screws) that fix the positions of the bones firmly enough to prevent motion of the fragments, even in the presence of functional loading. When properly accomplished, this type of fixation minimizes the development of callus (which can be cosmetically deforming), minimizes infection, and allows for immediate function, thereby avoiding the need for MMF.

Bone healing via the differentiation cascade described above has been referred to as "indirect" or "secondary" bone healing to distinguish it from so-called direct or primary bone healing, which only occurs when there is no motion across the fracture line.[78] It appears that the bridging of a bony gap by bone can only occur in the absence of motion across that gap. The more motion is present, the greater the amount of callus will be needed to stabilize the fragments so that healing by bone can eventually occur. Conversely, the more stable a repair is (and thus the less motion is present), the less callus will form and the greater is the likelihood that bone will directly bridge the fracture and heal the injury. It of course follows that when callus is unable to stabilize a fracture, bone will never form; the fracture remains bridged by fibrous tissue, thus forming a fibrous union (alternately known as a "nonunion," a "fibrous nonunion," or a "pseudoarthrosis") (see section entitled "Complications"). To accomplish a stable repair, it is necessary to understand the biomechanics of the facial skeleton, and even more important, it is critical to use this understanding when applying fixation. Otherwise, motion will tend to occur when the repair is loaded in function, and complications are then more likely to occur.

BIOMECHANICS OF THE FACIAL SKELETON

The forces acting on the facial bones are extremely complex and not fully elaborated as yet.[85] However, the current level of understanding has provided enough information to guide rigid repair techniques that will result in a rather high success rate. On the other hand, disregarding these principles will likely result in higher than acceptable complication rates.

As discussed above, the facial form is designed to support its function and also to serve as a buffer to protect more critical organs from traumatic injury. Areas that support function must have strength along the paths of force. In the midface, these have been variously called "pillars" and "buttresses," and these areas support the facial architecture during the powerful acts of biting and chewing.[63,85,98] It is particularly important to reestablish these buttresses when they have been fractured. Furthermore, these buttresses are separated by areas of weakness, which seem to facilitate their acting as crumple zones. The mandible provides support to the dentition during biting and chewing. Since this bone swings from the cranium, forces generated when a bolus of food is compressed between the teeth result in a fulcrum effect that generates tension and compression zones in various areas (Figure 26-21). These must be considered when repairing fractures because the repairs must overcome both the forces exerted by muscular contraction and the forces created by particular functions such as chewing.

Upper Third

In the upper third, the anterior wall of the frontal sinus is thin because it merely provides cover to the sinus itself, and there are no significant forces acting on this area. This can be considered when planning the repair. So long as the bones are held in position, a satisfactory outcome should result. On the other hand, the supraorbital rims and the frontal bones lateral and superior to the frontal sinuses are thicker, providing protection for the orbital contents and the anterior fossa contents, respectively. It requires more force to fracture these bones, and they are therefore more likely to be impacted and difficult to reduce. Still, there are no significant functional forces acting on these bones.

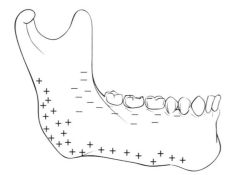

Figure 26-21. The mandible provides support to the dentition during biting and chewing. Since this bone swings from the cranium, forces generated when a bolus of food is compressed between the teeth result in a fulcrum effect that generates tension and compression zones in various areas.

Middle Third

The middle third is of course more complex. The so-called pillars or buttresses function to accept the high forces of mastication without fracturing. These "vertical" buttresses have been described as lateral and medial on each side, as well as posterior vertical[Au15] (Figure 26-22). The lateral buttress passes from the molar regions superiorly along the zygomaticomaxillary suture, through the solid malar eminence, and up along the lateral orbital rim and the frontozygomatic suture into the frontal bone. The medial buttress passes from the canine region superiorly along the solid bone that borders the pyriform aperture, then superiorly along the solid frontal process of the maxilla into the frontal bone. As Rudderman and Mullen[85] point out, the goal of repair is to reconstruct "load paths" so that the bone can once again support the loads for which it was designed. In the middle third of the face, this requires reestablishment of these four

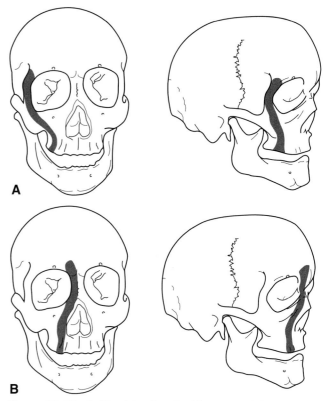

A

B

Figure 26-22. A, The lateral vertical buttress of the midface extends from the frontal bone along the frontozygomatic area and down across the strong bone of the zygomaticomaxillary area. **B,** The medial vertical buttress extends from the frontal bone across the frontonasal region and down across the nasomaxillary junction, encompassing the thick bone of the pyriform aperture.

vertical buttresses that support the impact forces of mastication. There is an additional posterior vertical buttress that transmits forces via the pterygoid plates to the skull base, but little attention is paid to this buttress since we do not have access to repair it.

The horizontal buttresses of the midface serve as the connectors across the vertical buttresses. These occur at the palate, incompletely across the central face from malar eminence to malar eminence along the infraorbital rims (incomplete because this horizontal strut is incomplete across the pyriform aperture), and across the frontal bar. These buttresses are primarily important to the facial surgeon for reestablishing the correct facial architecture. There is also the third dimension from anterior to posterior, and the only reconstructable buttress in this direction passes from the temporal root of the zygomatic arch anteriorly to the malar eminence on each side.

The zygoma forms an important attachment for the powerful masseter muscle. To support the function of this muscle, the bone needs to be solidly attached; yet to crumple, it also has to be able to give way in response to a traumatic force. The multiple attachments of the zygomatic "tripod" make this possible. Whether it is considered a tripod or quadrapod matters little; what is important is the nature of its attachments. The malar eminence is quite solid, but its attachments to the surrounding bone are less so. The zygomatic arch is quite thin, as is the inferior orbital rim. The lateral orbital rim is quite solid, and it is not uncommon for zygomatic fractures to be hinged from this attachment. The attachment to the remainder of the maxilla is broad (and continuous with the inferior orbital rim, thereby allowing the *tripod* nomenclature to make sense). Although the broad bony attachment between the zygoma and maxilla is relatively solid vertically to support the forces of mastication, it is actually thin bone that gives easily to a more horizontally or obliquely directed force. Repair requires stabilization of the zygoma in three dimensions. Traditional repairs focused on the most solid fixation point, and it was not uncommon for zygomatic fractures to be repaired with a single wire at the frontozygomatic fracture. The validity of this repair was called into question years ago,[37] and more recent data have suggested that multiple fixation points are required to maintain the 3D position of the zygoma against the strong masseteric pull.[14] More recent repair techniques have focused on the zygomaticomaxillary buttress because this is usually the mobile area, rather than fixing the hinge point, which tends to be the frontozygomatic area.

The bony orbit serves as a support for the orbital contents. Thus, for the orbit, the only biomechanical concerns are the reconstitution of the orbital shape for proper positioning of the orbital contents. This ensures proper globe position, which is necessary both cosmetically and functionally. The orbital reconstruction must be strong enough to support the orbital contents.

The central facial area includes the attachments for the medial eyelids and the projection of the nose. The medial eyelids are attached by the medial canthal ligaments to the solid lacrimal crests. When these are disrupted, the tendons are pulled laterally (as well as anteriorly and inferiorly), and the horizontal length of the eyelids is shortened. This needs to be reconstructed adequately to withstand the constant lateral tension of the lids. Otherwise, an unsightly appearance is likely, and poor function of the lacrimal collecting system may result as well. Reconstitution of the nasal bones is important both for nasal function and cosmesis.

Lower Third

As noted above, while the dental portions of the mandible occupy the lower third, the vertical rami of the mandible will be included in this discussion as well. The normal adult mandible is a strong, solid bone that contains the mandibular dentition. Numerous muscles attach to the mandible, and forces are developed across the bone when these muscles contract, even in the absence of mastication. (This is important because forces continue to act across the mandible when a patient is in MMF.) The mandible supports the tongue and the hyoid, structures important for swallowing and airway function. However, the most significant forces across the mandible are developed during mastication, and the forces acting on a given area of the mandible will vary depending on the location of a food bolus between the teeth.

Early explanations of mandibular biomechanics assumed a simple beam with forces along the top of the beam always creating tension zones superiorly (toward the alveolar surface) and compression zones inferiorly. This concept was introduced in Europe almost simultaneously by Spiessl[94] in Switzerland and Champy[7,8] in France. Interestingly, however, these two maxillofacial surgeons developed two entirely different repair techniques to overcome these forces, and two competing schools of thought developed as a result. Those who followed Spiessl and the Arbeitsgemeinschaft fur Osteosynthesefragen (AO) used compression-plating techniques to repair most mandible fractures, and those who followed Champy used "miniplating" techniques. Today, it has become apparent that there is room for both of these concepts, and it is more important to understand the biomechanics of fracture repair and to select a particular technique that has the highest likelihood of success in a given situation.

In the simple beam model, a fracture of the mandibular body will be distracted superiorly (the tension zone) and compressed inferiorly (compression zone) when a force is applied to the dental surfaces anteriorly (e.g., chewing a bolus between the incisors) (Figure 26-23). In this situation, controlling the tension zone results in a maintenance of reduction. Furthermore, when a force is applied by chewing anteriorly with the tension zone controlled, the compressive force in function will be distributed across the length of the fracture. Once this is clearly understood, a variety of repair options become available to the head and neck surgeon. However, certain limitations created by the unique aspects of mandibular anatomy must first be overcome. These are the presence of tooth roots within the bone and the presence of the inferior alveolar nerve within the bone. Because it is important to preserve these structures uninjured, certain areas of the mandibular bone become unavailable for the placement of fixation appliances. Both Champy and Spiessl came to the same conclusions regarding the need to control the tension zones without injuring vital structures, but they solved the problem of avoiding the teeth and nerves in different ways. Champy chose to control the tension zone with small (thus the name *mini*) plates that are positioned carefully between the tooth roots and the inferior alveolar nerve using screws that pass through only one bony cortex, thereby minimizing the risk to the teeth and nerve should the placement be imperfect. Spiessl shunned the use of these small plates with monocortical screws and instead used a well-placed arch bar across the dentition to control the tension zone and a larger

compression plate using bicortical screws placed below the inferior alveolar nerve to maximize the amount of stabilization. The larger, compressive fixation was believed to be necessary since it was being placed in a position that was actually biomechanically disadavantageous. However, using this approach, it is absolutely critical that the tension zone be controlled first; otherwise, the compression plate on the inferior mandible will actually distract the alveolar portion of the fracture. Ultimately, as it became clear that both of these techniques had high success rates, the battle between the schools of thought dissolved, and it is now clear that so long as biomechanical principles are properly followed, high success rates should be expected.[35]

Unfortunately, not all aspects of mandibular function follow this simple beam model. There are also irregularities of the mandibular bone that make some areas more potentially unstable than others. There appears to be greater potential for torque and rotational motion in the symphyseal region, so that when using miniplates, two are required to obtain a stable fixation in this area. A single miniplate appears to be adequate along the mandibular body, so long as the patient does not chew on the side of the fracture during the healing period. The angle region presents some particular problems, and it is the region in which the highest number of complications has always been noted.[34,51] The angle region has thick bone superiorly and thin bone posteroinferiorly. There is often a tooth in the thick superior bone, and its presence can weaken the bone, but extracting this tooth (which may be unavoidable in some cases) tends to weaken the area even more. Furthermore, there is no dentition behind the fracture, so an arch bar lends no support to the repair. The complexity of forces acting on this area adds another challenge. It was first noted by Kroon and others[47] that depending on where a bolus of food was placed along the mandibular dentition, the location of the compression zones and tension zones at the angle actually varied so much that the inferior area could change from compression to tension and vice versa. (Rudderman and Mullen[85] confirmed this finding for other areas of the mandible as well.) The repair of the angle area remains quite controversial, but most authors agree that though more difficult, time consuming, and demanding to apply, the larger, longer, mandibular reconstruction plates will offer the most dependable repairs and the highest overall success rates.[19,34]

On the other hand, the desire to use easier and simpler techniques has resulted in a pushing of the envelope, and Ellis has recently advocated the use of a single 1.3-mm miniplate placed intraorally along the oblique line of the mandible as adequate fixation for

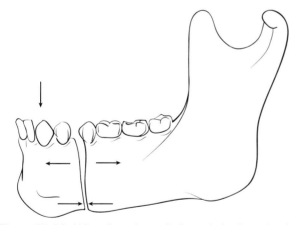

Figure 26-23. When force is applied anteriorly along the dental surface, the posterior portion of the mandible was held in place by the mandibular musculature. This results in the generation of a compressive force along the inferior border while the superior border is distracted (an area of tension). (Redrawn from Kellman RM, Marentette LJ: *Atlas of Craniomaxillofacial Fixation,* New York, 1995, Raven Press.)

mandibular angle fractures.[77] A more recent report by Fox and Kellman[23] suggests that when using miniplating techniques to repair mandibular angle fractures, two miniplates are best (and they should probably be 2.0 mm), as has been previously suggested by Levy and colleagues[52] and Kroon and others.[47]

Another very important aspect of mandibular biomechanics is the role that the vertical ramus plays in establishing facial relationships. When the midface is shattered, the vertical rami of the mandible become the only determinant of the correct facial height. Therefore, it is critical that these buttresses of facial height be reestablished before attempting to reposition the crushed midfacial bones.

FRACTURE REPAIR

The key to fracture repair is an understanding of the biomechanical principles just described, along with the various aspects of evaluation and access outlined above. Applying all of these principles should allow the surgeon to analyze the injuries, plan the repair, and execute it. The following description will address some of the controversies and sequencing issues that the surgeon will face in managing these patients.

Note that most repairs today are performed using titanium plates and screws, although a variety of absorbable plates and screws are used as well. These are generally polyester polymers containing polylactic acid, polyglycolic acid, or a variety of mixtures of these and a few other polymers. They degrade primarily via hydrolytic scission, and their byproducts are for the most part well tolerated by the human body. However, there is certainly no contraindication to the use of stainless steel wires when needed, and repairs using such wires have certainly stood the test of time.

Occlusion

First and foremost, in any maxillofacial trauma that involves tooth-bearing segments, it is essential that the proper occlusal relationship be reestablished. This is important for the restoration of normal masticatory function. The occlusal relationship between the maxillary and mandibular dentition also determines the relationship between the bones of the lower central face. Direct alignment of bone fragments virtually always takes second place to alignment of the occlusion. This is particularly true when the middle third of the face is collapsed because the mandibular height is used to reestablish facial height, and the occlusion is a key component of the relationship between the mandible and the maxilla.

Occlusion is best reestablished using arch bars, which are pliable metal bands with hooks for wires or rubber bands that are wired directly to the teeth. The most common arch bar in this country is the Erich arch bar. Other options include Ivy loops, although these only stabilize a few teeth rather than the entire dental arch. They also do not provide tension banding across the mandibular dental arch. A variety of other options are available as well. A recent innovation has been the use of screws for MMF. Although these can be placed quickly and easily, they offer several disadvantages, the most common of which is the frequent penetration of tooth roots when placing them[2] (Figure 26-24). All arch bars tend to pull the dentition lingually; however, the more inferior and buccal positioning of the screws when screw-MMF is used tends to increase this tendency.

Once arch bars have been placed, they can be used to hold the patient in MMF. This is done by placing wires or rubber bands between the hooks on the upper arch bar and those on the lower arch bar. After rigid fixation of all of the facial fractures has been completed, the MMF can be released, but the arch bars should be kept in place in case training elastics are needed during the healing period. Note that MMF will not correct a malocclusion that is the result of rigid fixation of fragments in suboptimal positions; only replating the fragments will correct such malpositions. MMF may also be needed for the management of unfixed fractures, such as subcondylar fractures of the mandible.

Upper Third

A number of algorithms have been published regarding the management of frontal fractures, particularly frontal sinus fractures. Although each has its merits, they tend to be somewhat complicated. Instead, a more simplified approach is presented here. The key issues in frontal sinus trauma relate to two fundamental questions: (1) Is exploration necessary? (2) Is obliteration necessary? The answers require the use of surgical judgment, but certain guidelines are logical.

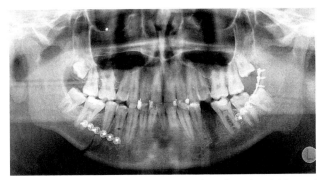

Figure 26-24. Although screws can be placed quickly and easily, they offer several disadvantages, the most common of which is the frequent penetration of tooth roots when placing them.

Keep in mind the purposes of the bone repair. The anterior wall needs to be repaired for cosmetic reasons. The posterior wall needs to be managed to protect the anterior cranial fossa. The sinus outflow tracts must function to drain the sinuses, or the sinuses must be obliterated; otherwise chronic infection will result. Thus, pure anterior wall fractures that do not extend into the nasofrontal ducts are repaired for cosmetic purposes only. These should be explored if they are significantly depressed, since even in the absence of acute deformity they are likely to lead to deformities when the swelling resolves. The smallest plates available are generally used, and absorbable plates may work well in this area as well because there are little or no force demands on the repair. Comminuted fragments can be pieced together and "lagged" with single screws to a plate that bridges the defect, or small fragments can be pieced together with small plates or wires. Use of the endoscope may allow repair of selected anterior wall fractures with minimal incisions. These techniques are currently in their infancy, and they are likely to become more prevalent as new instruments are developed to simplify the procedures. When the ducts are involved but the posterior wall is intact, judgment allows more than one option. Frontal sinus obliteration is always acceptable, but it is also reasonable to allow the sinus to function and see what happens. If the sinus becomes obstructed and acute or chronic sinusitis develops, the sinus can be opened endoscopically, or obliteration can be carried out at a later date.[93] In the absence of posterior wall injury, nothing should be lost by this approach (so long as appropriate follow-up of the patient can be ensured).

The presence of posterior wall injury complicates the questions. A nondisplaced posterior wall fracture that does not demand exploration for ductal injury or for anterior wall displacement can be observed. However, if the posterior wall is displaced, it is difficult to determine the status of the dura and the underlying brain. In the absence of apparent ductal injury, it is still wise to consider trephination and transcutaneous endoscopy because unexpected herniation of brain into the sinus has been observed using this approach. (The dictum about a wall width of displacement has little meaning in this regard.) In the absence of posterior wall displacement, and with no soft tissue abnormalities associated with such a nondisplaced fracture, it is unclear that obliteration is mandatory, even in the presence of ductal injuries. Careful follow-up including interval CT scans will demonstrate whether aeration of the sinus ensues. If chronic obstruction persists, obliteration should be carried out. The choice of obliteration technique includes several options, and most seem to work. Fat has certainly withstood the test of time, as has bone and even leaving the sinus empty (after careful obstruction of the ducts with fascia) to allow for osteoneogenesis.[27,31,83,86,92] Numerous complications have been encountered using hydroxyapatite cements,[25,68] but in one series using it in combination with live pericranial flaps, no complications were seen.[76] The cements do offer the unique advantage of contourability, so they can be used to repair the frontal contour in the presence of severe comminution or bone loss of the anterior wall (Figure 26-25).

Finally, the option of obliteration via cranialization (i.e., the complete removal of the posterior sinus walls) is reserved for cases in which the posterior walls are severely comminuted. Donald[16,17] uses this technique extensively whenever the posterior wall of the frontal sinus is involved in trauma. On the other hand, Schultz[90] actually believes that obliteration of the frontal sinuses is never necessary. If the sinus is to be obliterated anyway, it seems logical that the additional layer of the posterior wall adds another barrier between the contaminated nasal cavity and the anterior fossa and should be reconstructed and preserved if possible.

Cerebrospinal Fluid Rhinorrhea

In the presence of severe trauma with fractures of the anterior fossa, CSF rhinorrhea is not rare and can occur via the frontal sinuses or through the cribriform plate, ethmoid sinuses, or sphenoid sinuses. Large defects should be repaired at the time of facial fracture repair. Small defects should be identified endoscopically and can usually be repaired using this approach. Careful examination of defects is important because a transient leak may have stopped as a result of herniated brain, and late complications such as meningitis or death can occur if these are left untreated.[56]

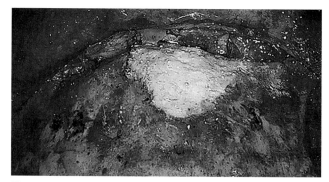

Figure 26-25. The anterior frontal sinus wall was unilaterally severely comminuted in this patient. The sinus was therefore obliterated using hydroxy apatite cement, which was simultaneously used to create a satisfactory contour. To view this image in color, please go to *www.ototext.com* or the Electronic Image Collection CD, bound into your copy of Cummings Otolaryngology—Head and Neck Surgery, 4th edition.

Skull Base Disruption

In the presence of severe disruption of the anterior skull base, brain injury and CSF rhinorrhea are common. The best way to address these injuries is in collaboration with the neurosurgeons. The presence of brain injuries will often lead to delays in management of the facial fractures and can actually increase the risk of meningitis. There is evidence that the longer a CSF leak persists, the greater is the risk of meningitis.[70,87] Therefore, earlier intervention may decrease the risk of such complications. The use of the transglabellar subcranial approach may allow for earlier intervention because it allows more direct access to the anterior fossa floor without the need for significant retraction of the frontal lobes.[41,80–82] It also allows direct visualization of the cribriform area without disarticulating it completely, so that many anterior fossa floor injuries may be repaired without completely sacrificing olfaction. The anterior fossa may be segregated from the nasal and sinus cavities, and the facial fractures can be repaired earlier, hopefully leading to better outcomes in these severely injured patients.[41]

Middle Third

Fractures that involve tooth-bearing segments are first stabilized at the level of the occlusion. Horizontal fractures above the occlusal level (Le Fort I) are repaired by reestablishing the four vertical buttresses, two medial and two lateral. Most surgeons repair these fractures using 1.5- to 2.0-mm "L" and "J" plates (Figure 26-26), although other combinations and sizes can be used as well. It is important to ensure that two screws are placed on either side of each fracture plated, although more can certainly be placed so long as tooth roots are not violated. The key is to fix these in the direction of the forces of mastication so that chewing will not be likely to disrupt the repair.[85]

When the palate is fractured, it is important to ensure that the teeth have not rotated around the palatal fracture, which would result in lingual or buccal version of the teeth and a significant malposition of the bone fragments. In cases of severe disruption, particularly when alveolar segments are fractured or the mandible is similarly disrupted, a palatal splint may be needed to stabilize the dentition in the proper position. The palate can be repaired directly with a plate, or it can be stabilized along the premaxillary area if the occlusal stabilization is adequate to prevent rotation (Figure 26-27).

Maxillary fractures at the Le Fort II level are similarly stabilized using 1.5- to 2.0-mm plates, again ensuring that at least two screws are placed on either side of each fracture plated (Figure 26-28). A plate can be placed along the infraorbital rim to stabilize the upper portion of these fractures. Otherwise, when

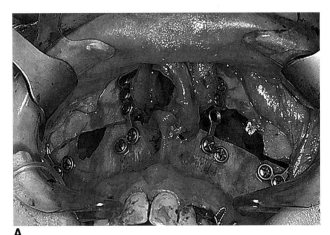

A

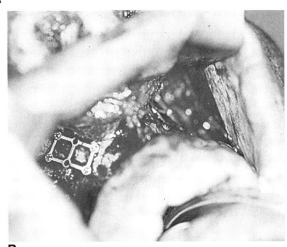

B

Figure 26-26. A, This is an example of a planned Le Fort I osteotomy repaired using "L" and "J" plates. **B,** An alternative repair using 1.0-mm box plates. The geometric shape of these plates adds additional strength to the repair. To view this image in color, please go to *www.ototext.com* or the Electronic Image Collection CD bound into your copy of Cummings Otolaryngology—Head and Neck Surgery, 4th edition.

accessed, the nasal root should be rigidly fixated using very small plates (Figure 26-29). It is critically important to be certain that the midface is not impacted and rotated superiorly before fixing the bones in place. Although MMF is applied first, it is actually possible to pull the patient into what appears to be good occlusion even though the midface is impacted; the mandibular teeth are pulled by the MMF toward the superiorly rotated maxilla, pulling the mandibular condyles out of the glenoid fossae. A patient can even remain in what appears to be good MMF for a full 6 weeks or longer, and when the MMF is released, the mandible returns to its neutral position revealing a significant anterior open bite. It is therefore important to recognize this at the time of surgery so that the midface can

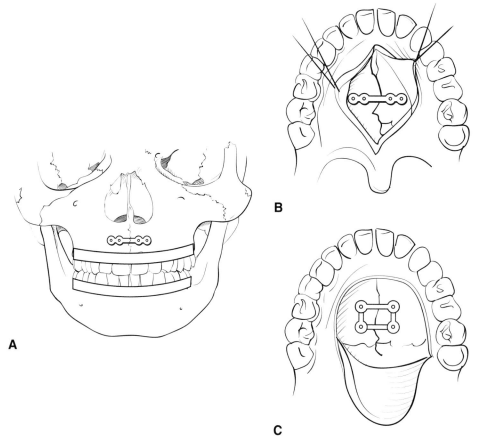

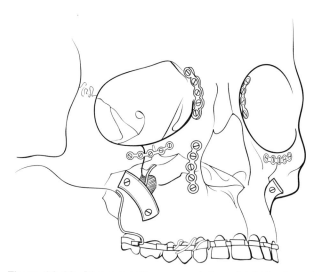

B

C

Figure 26-27. A, This demonstrates the repair of a split palate by the placement of a plate across the fracture in the anterior maxilla. **B,** This demonstrates direct placement of a plate along the palatal fracture. **C,** Similar to **(B),** this demonstrates the use of a "box plate" to lend greater stability to the palatal fracture repair. (Redrawn from Bailey BJ, Calhoun KH: *Atlas of Head & Neck Surgery–Otolaryngology*, Philadelphia, 2001, Lippincott William & Wilkins.)

Figure 26-28. Diagrammatic representation of rigid fixation of LeFort I and II level fractures with miniplates. Note that the right maxillary defect is repaired with a bone graft. The bone graft is lagged to the bone on either end so that the bone graft itself functions as the rigid fixation device. (Redrawn from Kellman RM, Marentette LJ: *Atlas of Craniomaxillofacial Fixation*, New York, 1995, Raven Press.)

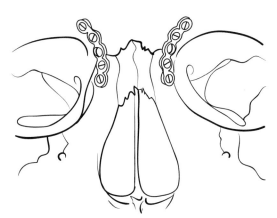

Figure 26-29. Diagrammatic representation of repair of the nasal frontal region with small plates and screws. (Redrawn from Kellman RM, Marentette LJ: *Atlas of Craniomaxillofacial Fixation*, New York, 1995, Raven Press.)

be properly rotated downward into the correct position. If it is severely impacted, the Rowe midfacial disimpacters may be required to mobilize the midface and bring it down into its proper position. It is interesting to note that, for many years, surgeons were more concerned about the possibility of facial elongation due to MMF pulling on unfixed maxillary fractures than they were about midfacial rotation and foreshortening. Therefore, the mainstay of treatment was Adams suspension wiring, in which the upper arch bar was wired to the zygomatic arches (or frontal bones when the zygomas were fractured) to prevent facial elongation; unfortunately, this treatment probably aggravated midfacial rotation and led to foreshortening and anterior open bite formation in many patients. With the advent of extended access approaches and routine exposure and fixation of midfacial fractures, this problem was recognized and is now carefully avoided. Similarly, with the availability of rigid fixation techniques, the use of halos for external fixation of midfacial fractures has become extremely uncommon. Nonetheless, familiarity with such techniques is of value in understanding the variety of surgical options.

Although the areas between the buttresses are not particularly important for structural support, the buttresses themselves are. Therefore, when bone is deficient along these buttresses, it should be replaced. A defect less then 5 mm in a single buttress can probably be safely bridged with a plate. Otherwise, defects should be bridged using bone grafts from another site. Split calvarium is a common source of bone graft material. It can be stabilized under a plate, or it may be used as a biologic plate and fixed to the bone at each end using lag screws (Figure 26-26).

The amount of stabilization (and, therefore, the amount of surgical exposure) required for fixation of zygomatic fractures can vary depending on the amount of instability and comminution of the fractures. Manson[62] has suggested the severity of the injury is determined by the amount of energy transmitted to the bone at the time of injury. Of course, this is implied by the injury, so it is the severity that is actually analyzed in planning the repair. However, for minimally displaced fractures, the zygoma tends to hinge at the frontozygomatic area and repair may require only percutaneous reduction, and it may pop into place and stay or it may need only a sublabial exposure and fixation along the zygomaticomaxillary area. When greater force causes the injury, there tends to be comminution at the zygomaticomaxillary area, making this an inadequate point of reference for reduction. A lower lid exposure will allow alignment of the infraorbital rim, as well as later exploration of the orbital floor if needed. Access to the lateral orbit is also

particularly helpful because alignment of the zygoma with the greater wing of the sphenoid in the lateral orbit tends to be a dependable landmark for proper bony reduction. With more severe impacts, marked comminution may make it more difficult to be assured that the zygoma has been properly repositioned. A coronal incision allows full exposure of the entirety of the zygomatic arches. When the contralateral zygoma is intact, it serves as a good frame of reference. Otherwise, even wide exposure may not ensure accurate repositioning of the zygoma. Intraoperative radiography can be useful in this regard. The arch position can be checked using fluoroscopy.[45] However, although not commonly available, intraoperative CT scanning certainly provides the most accurate assessment of bone position. Otherwise, a postoperative scan may indicate the need for revision surgery. Finally, it is important to keep in mind that although most orbital floor defects can be evaluated on preoperative CT scans, a potential orbital floor defect may not be visible. This occurs when the zygoma is severely impacted into the orbital space. After disimpaction of the zygoma, a previously absent orbital floor defect that requires repair may be present. Failure to look for this can result in unanticipated enophthalmos postoperatively. An endoscope placed into the maxillary sinus provides a minimally invasive way to assess the orbital floor in this situation. It is also important to repair the orbital rims before addressing the orbital walls because the rim position will affect the globe position and the overall shape of the orbit.

The orbit itself needs to be restored as closely as possible to its preinjury shape. This requires a familiarity with the normal orbital contours. A skull in the operating room may be helpful in this regard, and some surgeons even place a skull into a clear sterile bag and bend orbital wall implants on it. It is important to recognize the convexity on the orbital floor medially behind the equator of the globe. Failure to reconstitute this will create a tendency toward enophthalmos. It is also important to fill in significant defects in the medial wall for the same reason. Any trapped orbital tissues must be released into their normal positions in the orbit, and forced duction testing should be performed before and after all maneuvers in the orbit. The orbital wall contours can be reconstructed with autologous materials or with alloplastic materials, and each option has its particular advantages and disadvantages. Split calvarial bone is readily available, but it is very rigid and cannot be bent to shape.[40] Molding requires cutting the bone and plating pieces together in different shapes. Split rib is more pliable and can be bent to shape, but it undergoes greater resorption. For small defects, nasal septal cartilage or bone and the front face of maxillary bone have been used successfully. After release of the inferior rectus, a crack in the orbital floor can be covered with fascia or gelatin film. Titanium is easily moldable, but there is concern about the growth of fibrous tissue into holes in the material, although there are no actual reports of this being a problem. Porous polyethylene has become popular in the last few years for the repair of orbital floor defects, and it is replacing previously used materials that had variable extrusion rates. Most surgeons place orbital implants directly via transconjunctival and transcutaneous lid incisions, although recently the successful placement of these implants via the maxillary sinus using endoscopic assistance has been reported.[10,36] Note that enophthalmos generally needs to be slightly overcorrected to compensate for the swelling that develops during the surgical procedure itself. Hypophthalmos (inferior eye position), on the other hand, should not be overcorrected because overcorrection in this direction is more likely to persist.

Nasoorbital ethmoid fractures (i.e., NOE, NEC) are among the most difficult to repair. Simple fractures in which the medial canthal ligaments remain attached to a significant, solid piece of central bone (type I) are repaired by stabilizing the solid piece of bone to the surrounding skeleton with plates. This must be properly positioned and fixed, or it will slowly lateralize, resulting in a significant deformity over time. Repair of the more severe type II and III injuries is a bit more controversial, and some argue for maintenance of any ligamentous attachments to bone, whereas others recommend focusing on the ligaments themselves.[41,79–81] With the ligaments exposed (generally via a coronal incision), a permanent suture or wire is passed through the ligament and the suture is passed through the area of the posterior lacrimal crest (which may or may not be present), behind the nasal bones, through the nasal septum, and out the same area on the contralateral side (using extreme caution to avoid injury to the contralateral globe), where it may be fixed either to the contralateral frontal bone (around a screw, through a plate hole, or through a hole in the supraorbital rim) or to the contralateral medial canthal ligament. A broad retractor (a sterilized teaspoon can be used) should cover and protect the contralateral globe during passing of wires or sutures from one side to the other. If this latter approach is used, tightening the wire fixes both medial canthal ligaments together. If the suture is fixed to the frontal bone, the same procedure must be repeated for the contralateral medial canthal ligament (assuming it is also damaged) (Figure 26-30).

Great care must be used to ensure proper positioning and fixation of the canthal ligament. When identification of the medial canthal ligament is difficult, a

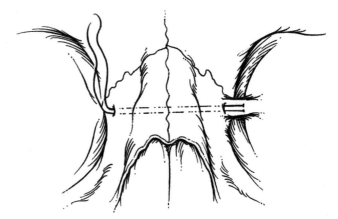

Figure 26-30. A diagrammatic representation of a suture passing through the left medial canthal ligament and then through the lacrimal bone behind the nasal root. It is then fixed to the contralateral frontal bone. This allows appropriate tension to be placed on the medial canthal ligament for proper repositioning. (Redrawn with permission from Bailey BJ, Calhoun KH: *Atlas of Head & Neck Surgery—Otolaryngology,* Philadelphia, 2001, Lippincott William & Wilkins.)

hemostat may be placed in the caruncle and pushed medially. When the area is examined from the deep surface, the ligament should be approximately in the area of the bulge created by the hemostat (Figure 26-31). (Obviously, great care must be used to avoid corneal injury when using this technique.) If the ligament is not fixed medially, it will slowly lateralize over time, resulting in unsightly telecanthus, malposition of the caruncle, horizontal shortening of the lids, and potential lacrimal dysfunction. It is also important to make certain that the full nasal dorsal height is reestablished, and bone grafts should be used if necessary. Failure to do so tends to exaggerate any appearance of telecanthus and increases the likelihood of developing epicanthal folds. Some surgeons advocate the placement of percutaneous supporting plates against the overlying nasal skin to recreate the natural concavity in this area. It is unclear at this time if these are actually necessary. Note that while these are passed transnasally, these are not the same as the old percutaneous repairs of NOE fractures, which in fact should not be used to repair these fractures because they are for the most part ineffective.

Lower Third

The basic principles of mandibular fracture repair have been discussed above in the section discussing biomechanics. The repair of particular fractures will be discussed more specifically here. In the dentate mandible, the first priority is the reestablishment of the proper occlusal relationship of the teeth. As noted, a good arch bar will not only aid in this effort, it will

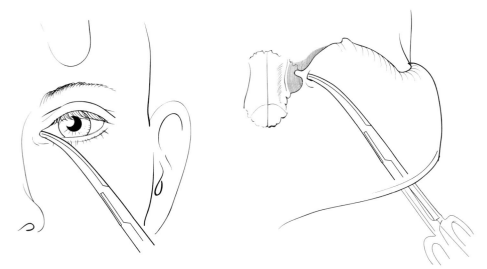

Figure 26-31. With the ligaments exposed (generally via a coronal incision), a permanent suture or wire is passed through the ligament and the suture is passed through the area of the posterior lacrimal crest (which may or may not be present), behind the nasal bones, through the nasal septum, out the same area on the contralateral side (using extreme caution to avoid injury to the contralateral globe), where it may be fixed either to the contralateral frontal bone. (Redrawn from Bailey BJ, Calhoun KH: *Atlas of Head & Neck Surgery–Otolaryngology*, Philadelphia, 2001, Lippincott William & Wilkins.)

also provide a good tension band across the alveolar portion of the fracture. Sometimes, a badly displaced fracture will make arch bar application more difficult. In this situation, an intraoral incision that exposes the fracture will allow preliminary reduction of the fracture and aid in the proper positioning of the arch bar. If placement of the arch bar is begun at the fracture site, and successive wires are placed alternately on either side of the fracture, a tight tension band can be well applied to hold the fracture in reasonable approximation. (Note that there are some surgeons who are repairing simple mandible fractures without the aid of arch bar fixation of the occlusion, but this approach is not currently recommended.) The proper occlusal relationship between the maxillary and mandibular dentition should then be determined, and wires are generally used to hold the patient in MMF while the fracture is repaired.

There are a variety of treatment options for most fractures, and a familiarity with the basic principles of fracture repair will allow the surgeon to select a preferred method for any given fracture. First, a familiarity with "load-sharing" and "load-bearing" repairs will help determine what options are available for the repair of a particular mandible fracture. A load-sharing repair depends on the integrity of the underlying bone, and the fixation appliance is positioned so as to ensure that the forces in function are borne by the bone itself. Thus, as discussed above, a small plate across the tension zone will ensure that the solid bone is pushed together in function so that it shares the load with the fixation appliance. Miniplate fixation, compression plate fixation, and lag screw fixation all represent load-sharing repairs and require adequate bone contact to succeed.

On the other hand, when the bone is inadequate to share the load with the fixation appliance, as is seen when bone is too thin and atrophic, fractures are significantly comminuted, or there is bone loss, the repair has to bear the load across the repaired area, and thus a load-bearing repair is needed. This requires a repair that is strong enough to bear the load that is applied to the particular area in function, and thus a fairly long and strong plate is required. Until recently, 2.7-mm plates and screws were used for most load-bearing mandibular repairs; however, a strong 2.4-mm titanium mandibular reconstruction plate appears to be adequate in most instances. Note that to successfully accomplish a load-bearing repair in the mandible, a minimum of three and preferably four solidly held bicortical screws should be placed in the bone on each side of the weak (defective) area.[32] It should also be apparent, therefore, that a load-bearing type of reconstruction plate can be used as a "fall-back" technique for any fracture because, if it is strong enough to support a defect, it should be strong enough to repair any fracture. This is consistent with the finding noted above that a mandibular reconstruction plate (MRP) provides the most dependable repair of mandibular angle fractures.[19,34]

If the MRP can be used as a fall-back technique for any fracture, the obvious question that arises is why it is not recommended for all fractures. The answer is technical. Since the plate is larger, and because it requires multiple bicortical screws over a long distance, it is more difficult to place. It is a stronger plate, which makes it harder to bend; it is longer, which requires more surgical exposure; and the screws have to be bicortical, which means they have to be placed along the inferior border of the mandible, which often requires external incisions, particularly in the more posterior portions of the mandible. Furthermore, improper placement of a bicortical screw will result in undesirable complications.

When using a reconstruction plate, the option of a design that locks the head of the screw to the plate should be considered. Various devices have been developed, including those in which the screw heads were threaded and expandable, and after placement an insert screw was placed that expanded the screw head so that it was fixed to the plate. More recent designs use a threaded screw head that tightens (locks) directly into the plate. A particular advantage of such designs is that they may allow for imperfect bending of the plate without disturbing the fracture reduction because the screw stops when the head is fully engaged in the plate hole, rather than continuing to tighten and pulling the bone to the less than ideally bent plate. However, the use of this type of plate should not be considered a substitute for proper bending.

External fixation is also an option, although it is less stable than a rigidly placed reconstruction plate. This technique requires externally placed pins, which leave scars around the pin sites and increase the risk of infection. Like an MRP, the more fixation points placed, the greater the stability obtained.

Note that whenever there is an oblique fracture (i.e., when the bone splits obliquely so that the two fragments overlap rather than abut each other), lag screw fixation is recommended with or without plate fixation. Lag screws are placed so that the first cortex functions as a washer, and when the screw is tightened, the two cortices are compressed together. This is accomplished most easily by overdrilling the first cortex, rather than requiring special screws with unthreaded portions. At least two screws are required to prevent rotation around the first one, and three provide a more secure fixation.

In the symphyseal region, when a load-sharing repair can be used, there are a number of options available to the maxillofacial surgeon. Because the

bone is curved, there is a solid cortex on either side of the fracture that is accessible to screws. Therefore, lag screw fixation can be applied. When this is performed, it is recommended that two screws be used, and although it is not critical, it is probably better if the head of each screw comes in from the opposite side of the fracture (Figure 26-32). It is also possible to use two miniplates, with a minimum of two screws on each side of the fracture through each miniplate. It is recommended at this time that 2.0-mm screws be used. Once a good tension band arch bar (or miniplate) has been applied, a bicortical compression plate along the inferior border of the mandible is also an option.

In the body region, a single miniplate is generally believed to be adequate, so long as the patient does not chew on the side of the fracture during the healing period. A tension band arch bar (or miniplate) can also be combined with a bicortical compression plate along the inferior border.

The angle region is more complex, and, as expected, the choice of repair technique is more controversial. The use of a tension band plate and a compression plate, while once advocated by proponents of AO technique,[94,95] is no longer recommended.[34] In fact, current AO philosophy recommends using either a miniplate technique or a reconstruction plate (load-bearing repair). However, the best miniplate approach remains controversial as well. Champy[6,7] recommends a single 2.0-mm miniplate placed along the oblique line of the angle region. The patient is then instructed not to chew on that side for 6 weeks. Kroon and others,[47] on the other hand, performed studies that demonstrated the changing location of the tension zone and therefore recommended using two miniplates at the angle. Levy and colleagues[52] reviewed

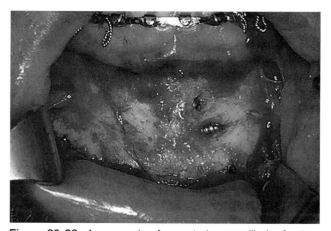

Figure 26-32. An example of an anterior mandibular fracture repair using two lag screws. To view this image in color, please go to *www.ototext.com* or the Electronic Image Collection CD, bound into your copy of Cummings Otolaryngology—Head and Neck Surgery, 4th edition.

their experience using a single miniplate at the angle and compared the results to those patients who had two miniplates placed at the angle. There was a significant difference in the outcomes, with the two miniplate group experiencing a 3.1% infection rate, compared with a 26.3% infection rate when a single miniplate was used. Fox and Kellman[23] reported an infection rate of 2.9% in 72 patients using two 4-hole, 2.0-mm miniplates to repair angle fractures. Conversely, Ellis and Potter report a low major complication rate using a single 1.3-mm miniplate along the oblique line.[77] However, major complications were arbitrarily defined as requiring a return to the operating room, so that some complete failures did not count as major complications because they were managed in the office. Finally, Niederdellmann and Shetty[71] advocate a lag screw technique for mandibular angle fractures, but this is a difficult technique and should not be attempted unless the surgeon has extensive experience with these techniques.

The amount of fixation required for mandibular ramus fractures is less clear, but it is probably wise to consider two 2.0-mm miniplates for such fractures.

The management of subcondylar fractures remains the most controversial, and many surgeons treat almost all of these with MMF, although there are some who advocate routine open reduction for these fractures. It is of course interesting that the "closed reduction" has been so well accepted for so many years, since in fact it is really "closed treatment" and not reduction at all. MMF is used to train the mandible to return to its preinjury occlusion, and, combined with physiotherapy, a satisfactory outcome is in fact typical. However, if x-rays are obtained at the completion of a period of closed reduction, the position of the condylar fragment is not likely to be altered. Patients seem to do reasonably well in spite of this, most of the time. If this approach is selected, it is recommended that the MMF be released after 10 to 14 days so that physiotherapy can be initiated early. Some surgeons recommend no MMF, treating the patient instead with immediate physiotherapy. If the patient develops a malocclusion, the surgeon has the option of replacing the MMF (usually using training elastics) or of reconsidering open reduction. On the other hand, it is not clear that patients do much better when a true open reduction is accomplished, and this fact, combined with the traditionally significant risk of facial nerve injury (which is indeed a major complication), has led to the acceptance of closed treatment. Most surgeons have accepted the classic indications for open reduction reported by Zide and Kent in 1983[108] including the following: (1) condylar displacement into the middle fossa; (2) inability to obtain reduction; (3) lateral extracapsular displacement of the condyle; (4) invasion by a foreign body. Of course, the relative indications they offered are more frequent, including: (1) bilateral condylar fractures in an edentulous mandible when no splint is available; (2) condylar fractures when splinting is not recommended; (3) bilateral condylar fractures along with comminuted midface fractures; (4) bilateral condylar fractures associated with gnathologic problems. In truth, recent prospective studies have suggested that patients actually do better after open reduction than closed treatment.[20,21,72,107] The key issue is whether the unacceptable complication of facial nerve paralysis can be lowered to an acceptable level to justify routine open reduction of these fractures. In recent years, the introduction of endoscope-assisted transoral repair of these fractures seems to be changing the paradigm somewhat.[10,38,48–50] Unfortunately, although the overall success rate is high and the complication rate exceedingly low, the endoscopic repair of subcondylar fractures remains a challenging technique with a steep learning curve, and it requires specialized instrumentation to facilitate its performance.[38] However, as greater experience is obtained, it is not unlikely that it will become a more commonplace technique, and more subcondylar fractures will likely be opened, reduced, and rigidly fixed.

Note that although the focus has been on open reduction, in fact there is still a place for closed reduction of mandible fractures as well. *Closed reduction* refers to the use of MMF as the sole treatment for selected mandible fractures. Generally speaking, closed reduction using 4 to 6 weeks of MMF is reserved for fractures within the line of dentition that are nondisplaced. The teeth have to be adequate to support a solid arch bar, and the patient has to be willing to cooperate with the period of MMF. The patient must also be carefully observed for any signs of movement of the fragments, and if the bone is shifting or if signs of infection appear, open reduction should be considered.

The issue of teeth in the line of mandibular fractures has evolved significantly over the last several decades. Before the routine use of antibiotics, the presence of a tooth in the fracture line was associated with a high incidence of infection and even osteomyelitis.[5] Dental extraction would minimize these complications, although they were still not rare. More recent reviews have still noted a higher incidence of infection when a fracture occurs through or around a tooth, but extraction no longer decreases the already lower infection rate. Thus, there does not appear to be an indication to extract an otherwise healthy tooth, so long as it is not interfering with the reduction. On the other hand, an abscessed or infected tooth in the line of fracture should be extracted. Note that in the region of the angle, the third molar contributes significantly to the cross-sectional area of the bone, and extracting it tends to destabilize the fracture and its repair.[34] Iizuka and Lindqvist[34] actually found that a higher complication rate resulted when these teeth were extracted at the time of repair of angle fractures. They therefore recommend that the angle fracture be stabilized before the extraction using a load-bearing repair.

Edentulous Mandible

The edentulous mandible presents two particular problems. One is the absence of teeth, which as noted above are important to the proper reestablishment of the occlusal relationship, and this in turn is critical to proper masticatory function. The other consideration is the amount of mandibular atrophy that is typically seen in edentulous mandibles.

The occlusion is important both for function and for proper repositioning of the bone fragments. Therefore, if there is a denture available, it should be used as a splint to ensure proper realignment of the bones. In addition, functional repositioning is important even in the absence of teeth because improper positioning can make prosthetic rehabilitation more difficult or even impossible, and even when a prosthesis can be constructed, the stress on the TMJ can lead to additional problems for the patient.

Mandibular atrophy is an even bigger problem because it has traditionally led to unacceptably high complication rates. A common misconception is that since the mandible is small, only a small plate is required to repair it. In fact, the forces on the mandible continue to be large, and the small amount of bone available means that there is limited bone-to-bone contact for healing, and the thin bone does not provide enough support to adequately share the load with small fixation plates. Thus, the atrophic mandible is a contraindication to a load-sharing repair. To minimize the complication rate, a load-bearing repair must be used, and this requires long, strong plates with multiple fixation points using bicortical screws. Because this approach has been used, the success rate for bone healing in these difficult fractures has risen dramatically.[59]

Pan-Facial Fractures

When broken down into its individual parts, each of the fractures described above is quite reparable. However, when all or most of the facial skeleton is fractured, it is much more difficult to recreate the correct 3D shape and to properly reposition the fractured fragments. Of course, logic dictates that reconstruction should be performed from the known to the unknown, which might also be stated as working from the stable to the unstable. In fact, with the exception of the occlusion, which should be established first to

whatever extent is possible, the reconstruction actually develops from the periphery toward the center. Using this approach, the typically more solid cranial areas are first repaired so that they can help form the template for repositioning of the zygomas. The facial height is reestablished by completing the reconstruction of the mandible, so that the mandibular teeth can serve as the template for the repositioning of the maxillary dental arches. Tooth loss and bone comminution may mandate the use of prosthetic splints, and there should be no hesitation to have these made. Note that in panfacial fractures open reduction of subcondylar fractures, particularly bilateral subcondylar fractures, becomes an essential component of the repair because the mandibular ramus height is a critical guide to the overall facial height. The lower maxilla can then be stabilized to the repositioned zygomas above and the mandibular dentition below. Once the maxillae have been repositioned and reconstructed, attention can be turned to the central face, that is, the nose and nasal-ethmoid complex region (NOE fractures). Finally, after the facial architecture has been reestablished, the orbital walls are reconstituted. If this has been performed successfully, a postoperative CT scan should confirm a reasonably normal facial skeletal architecture.

COMPLICATIONS

The most common complication is failure to obtain an ideal reduction. When this involves tooth-bearing bones, a malocclusion will result. If it is minimal and can be resolved with occlusal grinding, reoperation may be unnecessary, but this is up to the discretion of the surgeon and the patient. If the malocclusion is more significant, reoperation is indicated. When a closed reduction technique has been used, a malocclusion can be corrected by adjusting the MMF. However, if rigid fixation has been applied, only removing the plates and repositioning them will repair a malposition. When the bone heals in the incorrect position, a malunion results. The term *malunion* implies that healing has in fact occurred (as opposed to nonunion). In other areas of the face, malunions will usually lead to facial asymmetries. In the orbit, globe malpositions may result, the most common of which is enophthalmos. When the orbital floor has been inadequately reconstituted, it is not uncommon to see hypophthalmos as well. These deformities generally mandate reexploration and placement of additional graft material. Failure to adequately repair NOE fractures will lead to telecanthus; however, this may not be recognizable initially, and the deformity may become apparent later when repair is more difficult.

Nonunion is a more serious complication. It is not common in the mid and upper face, but it is unfortunately not rare in the mandible. It is usually associated with motion at the fracture site, although it may be associated with an infected tooth. When fracture fragments are mobile, the motion interferes with bone healing and seems to predispose to the development of infection. Once infection develops, failure to stabilize the fracture and treat the infection can lead to osteomyelitis. This results in bone loss and typically results in an infected nonunion. As a result of bone loss, even if the infection resolves, the defect will likely heal with fibrous tissue rather than bone. This also occurs when an injury results in bone loss. There is a race between bone growth and fibrous ingrowth. If the fibrous tissue wins, the bond that forms between the bone fragments is not solid, and therefore motion persists between the fragments. This has been called a *pseudoarthrosis* because the movement of the bones around the fibrous union acts as a false joint. It has been variously also called a *nonunion*, implying that the bone has not healed across the area, or a *fibrous nonunion*. If the bone is stabilized across a fibrous nonunion either using prolonged MMF or a rigid fixation device, the bone may still bridge the gap and heal. In the presence of osteitis, it is important to débride any devitalized bone in addition to treating the infection with antibiotics.

Multiple soft tissue complications occur as well. The most common, of course, is scarring. However, a significant problem after extended open access approaches is a droop of the midfacial soft tissues. This can be prevented by proper resuspension of the soft tissues before wound closure. Lower lid malpositions such as ectropion or entropion can result when lower lid incisions are used. Care should be used to avoid injury to the orbital septum as well as excessive retraction during the bony repair. A Frost stitch left in place for 1 to 2 days postoperatively may decrease the occurrence of this problem. It is also recommended that the lower lid be massaged by the patient multiple times daily beginning after the first week postoperatively to help break up any developing scar contracture. Suture fixation of the nasal alae subcutaneously may prevent alar base widening after use of the midface degloving approach. Also, as noted above, irregularization of the coronal incision allows it to hide more gracefully within the hair.

Related structures may be injured as well, typically as a result of the trauma, although these can occur as a result of the surgery as well. Most feared, of course, are brain and ocular injuries. Great care must be exercised when exploring the orbit. Surgical injury to branches of the trigeminal nerve is not uncommon. The supraorbital and sutpratrochlear nerves are at risk when elevating the coronal flap inferiorly over the supraorbital rims. The infraorbital nerves are at risk when exposing

the maxilla via the sublabial approach, as well as via the lower lid approach. Finally, the mental nerve is vulnerable during mandibular exposure, and its predecessor, the inferior alveolar, nerve is particularly vulnerable during drilling and screw placement in the mandibular body and angle regions. The facial nerve is at risk during multiple facial exposures, and great care should be exercised to avoid injuring this important structure. The lacrimal collecting system may be injured from the trauma, but it can also be injured during surgery. If its continuity is in question, cannulation of the canaliculi and stenting are recommended. Injury to the extraocular muscles or their nerves can result in diplopia, even in the absence of entrapment.

Finally, the issue of secondary, revision, or delayed fracture repair represents an entire field of advanced maxillofacial trauma management. It relies heavily on the techniques of craniofacial surgery and orthognathic surgery. As in primary repair, the most critical part is careful assessment via clinical evaluation and CT scanning, followed by careful planning of these complex and difficult procedures. Sometimes prefabricated prostheses can be created to assist in the reconstruction. Even with extensive planning and precise execution, the limitations of the soft tissue envelope may preclude obtaining an ideal result.

FUTURE DIRECTIONS AND NEW HORIZONS

Of course, it is impossible to predict exactly how the problems discussed above will be managed in the future. However, some of the new technologies currently being used can provide some insight into the directions in which developments are going. The recent introduction of endoscopes into facial trauma management has already altered the way some surgeons manage mandible and orbital fractures, and some are already adapting these techniques to more complex fractures, such as zygomatic fractures[9] and frontal fractures, and even a variety of maxillofacial osteotomies.[103] The development of better CT-based planning and navigational technology may well result in the more frequent use of percutaneous techniques for the repositioning of facial bones.

Constantly improving distraction technology will not only allow for better correction of congenital deformities, but it will also allow for repair of secondary traumatic defects as well as primary reconstruction of traumatically induced defects.

Advances in understanding of biomechanical principles will allow for continued refinement of fixation appliances and their placement. Improvements in resorbable technology may lead to the routine use of

---

*References 10, 36, 38, 48, 49, 82.

such materials in the repair of many if not all facial fractures. Currently, one of the intrinsic problems with resorbable materials is that they break down faster when the stresses acting on them are greater. This makes them less useful for fractures in high stress-bearing areas. Hopefully, such problems will be overcome with new materials.

Finally, bone replacement materials and glues are currently under intense study. Combined with proteins that modulate bone healing, it may not only become possible to repair bones more effectively, but the technology of reconstruction and guided healing may allow for controlled repair and reshaping of the facial skeleton.

REFERENCES

1. Adams WM: Internal wiring fixation of facial fractures, *Surgery* 12:523–540, 1942.
2. Alpert B: AO Advanced Course, Tucson, Arizona, February 2003.
3. Anderson T, Alpert B: Experience with rigid fixation of mandibular fractures and immediate function, *J Oral Maxillofac Surg* 50:555–560, 1992.
4. Bradley JA: Age changes in the vascular supply o the mandible, *Br Dent J* 132:142–144, 1972.
5. Bradley RL: Treatment of the fractured mandible, *Am Surg* 31:289–290, 1965.
6. Champy M and others: Osteosynthesis using miniaturized screw-on plates in facial and cranial surgery, *Ann Chir Plast* 22:261–264, 1977.
7. Champy M and others: *The Strasbourg mini plate Osteosynthesis.* In Krüger E, Schilli W, Worthingon P, editors: *Oral and maxillofacial traumatology,* vol 2, Chicago, 1986, Quintessence Publishing.
8. Champy M and others: Osteosyntheses mandibulaires selon la technique de Mechelet. I. bases biomecaniques, *Rev Stomatol Chir Maxillofac* 77:569, 1976.
9. Chen CT and others: Application of endoscopies in zygomatic fracture repair, *Br J Plast Surg* 53:100–105, 2000.
10. Chen CT and others: Endoscopically assisted mandibular subcondylar fracture repair, *Plast Reconstr Surg* 103:60–65, 1999.
11. Chen CT and others: Endoscopically assisted reconstruction of orbital medial wall fractures, *Plast Reconstr Surg* 103: 714–720, 1999.
12. Chole RA, Yee J: Antibiotic prophylaxis for facial fractures: a prospective, randomized clinical trial, *Arch Otolaryngol Head Neck Surg* 113:1055–1057, 1987.
13. Creasman CN and others: Computed tomography versus standard radiography in the assessment of fractures of the mandible, *Ann Plast Surg* 29:109–113, 1992.
14. Davidson J, Nickerson D, Nickerson B: Zygomatic fractures: comparison of methods of internal fixation, *Plast Reconstr Surg* 86:25–32, 1990.
15. Dawson RLG, Fordyce GL: Complex fractures of the middle third of the face and their early treatment, *Br J Surg* 41:254, 1953.
16. Donald PJ: Frontal sinus ablation by cranialization: report of 21 cases, *Arch Otol* 108:142–146, 1982.
17. Donald PJ, Bernstein L: Compound frontal sinus injuries with intracranial penetration, *Laryngoscope* 88:225–232, 1978.
18. Ellis E III: Outcomes of patients with teeth in the line of mandibular angle fractures treated with stable internal fixation, *J Oral Maxillofac Surg* 60:863–866, 2002.
19. Ellis E III: Treatment of mandibular angle fractures using the AO reconstruction plate, *J Oral Maxillofac Surg* 51:250–254, 1993.
20. Ellis E III, Simon P, Throckmorton GS: Occlusal results after open or closed treatment of fractures of the mandibular condylar process, *J Oral Maxillofac Surg* 58:260–268, 2000.
21. Ellis E III, Throckmorton G: Facial symmetry after closed and open treatment of fractures of the mandibular condylar process, *J Oral Maxillofac Surg* 58:719–728, 2000.
22. Ellis E, Zide MF: *Surgical approaches to the facial skeleton.* Philadelphia, 1995, Williams and Wilkins.
23. Fox AJ, Kellman RM: Mandibular angle fractures: two-miniplate fixation and complications, *Arch Facial Plast Surg* 5:464–469, 2003.
24. Fox AJ, Tatum SA: The coronal incision: sinusoidal, sawtooth, and postauricular techniques, *Arch Facial Plast Surg* 5:259–262, 2003.
25. Friedman CD and others: Hydroxyapatite cement, II: obliteration and reconstruction of the cat frontal sinus, *Arch Otolaryngol Head Neck Surg* 117:385–389, 1991.
26. Funk GF, Stanley RB, Becker TS: Reversible visual loss due to impacted lateral orbital wall fractures, *Head Neck* 11:295–300, 1989.
27. Gerbino G and others: Analysis of 158 frontal sinus fractures: current surgical management, *J Cranio-Maxillofac Surg* 28:133–139, 2000.
28. Gonty AA, Marciani RD, Adornato DC: Management of frontal sinus fractures: a review of 33 cases, *J Oral Maxillofac Surg* 57:372–379, 1999.
29. Gruss JS, Mackinnon SE: Complex maxillary fractures: role of buttress reconstruction and immediate bone grafts, *Plast Reconstr Surg* 78:9–22, 1986.
30. Gruss JS and others: The role of primary bone grafting in complex craniomaxillofacial trauma, *Plast Reconstr Surg* 75:17–24, 1985.
31. Hardy JM, Montgomery WW: Osteoplastic frontal sinusotomy: an analysis of 250 operations, *Ann Otol Rhinol Laryngol* 85:523–532, 1976.
32. Haug RH: Effect of screw number on reconstruction plating, *Oral Surg Oral Med Oral Pathol* 75:664–668, 1993.
33. Holt GR, Holt JE: Occipital and orbital trauma, *AAO-HNSF Manual.* Washington, DC, 1983.
34. Iizuka T, Lindqvist C: Rigid internal fixation of fractures in the angular region of the mandible: an analysis of factors contributing to difference complications, *Plast Reconstr Surg* 91:265–271, 1993.
35. Iizuka T and others: Infection after rigid fixation of mandibular fractures: a clinical and radiologic study, *J Oral Maxillofac Surg* 49:585–593, 1991.
36. Ikeda K and others: Endoscopic endonasal repair of orbital floor fracture, *Arch Otolaryngol Head Neck Surg* 125:59–63, 1999.
37. Karlan MS, Cassisi NJ: Fractures of the zygoma, *Arch Otolaryngol* 105:322–327, 1979.
38. Kellman RM: Endoscopically assisted repair of subcondylar fractures of the mandible: an evolving technique, *Arch Facial Plast Surg* 5:244–250, 2003.
39. Kellman RM: Repair of mandibular fractures via compression plating and more traditional techniques: a comparison of results, *Laryngoscope* 94(12 Pt 1):1560–1567, 1984.
40. Kellman RM: Safe and dependable harvesting of large outer-table calvarial bone grafts, *Arch Otolaryngol Head Neck Surg* 120:856–860, 1994.

41. Kellman RM: Use of the subcranial approach in maxillofacial trauma, *Facial Plastic Surg Clin North Am* 6:501–510, 1998.

42. Kellman RM, Bersani T: Delayed and secondary repair of posttraumatic enophthalmos and orbital deformities, *Facial Plast Surg Clin North Am* 10:311–323, 2002.

43. Kellman RM, Schilli W: Plate fixation of fractures of the middle and upper face, *Otolaryngol Clin North Am* 20(3):559–572, 1987.

44. Kellman RM, Tatum SA: *Complex facial trauma with plating.* In Bailey BJ, editor: *Head and Neck Surgery–Otolaryngology.* Philadelphia, 2001, Lippincott-Raven.

45. Kobiena BJ and others: Portable fluoroscopy in the management of zygomatic arch fractures, *Ann Plast Surg* 40:260–264, 1998.

46. Kroetsch LJ and others: Traumatic dislocation of the mandibular condyle into the middle cranial fossa: report of a case, review of the literature, and a proposal management protocol, *J Oral Maxillofac Surg* 59:88–94, 2001.

47. Kroon F and others: The use of miniplates in mandibular fractures, *J Craniomaxillofac Surg* 19:199–204, 1991.

48. Lauer G, Schmelzeisen R: Endoscope-assisted fixation of mandibular condylar process fractures, *J Oral Maxillofac Surg* 57:36–39, 1999.

49. Lee C and others: Endoscopic subcondylar fracture repair: functional aesthetic, and radiographic outcomes, *Plast Reconstr Surg* 102:1434–1443, 1998.

50. Lee C and others: Minimally invasive approaches to mandibular fractures, *Facial Plast Surg Clinc North Am* 9:475–487, 2001.

51. Le Fort R: Etude experimentale sur les fractures de la machoire superieure, *Rev Chir Paris* 23:208, 360, 479, 1901.

52. Levy FE and others: Monocortical miniplate fixation of mandibular angle fractures, *Arch Otolaryngol Head Neck Surg* 117:149–154, 1991.

53. Levy RA, Kellman RM, Rosenbaum AE: The effect of computed tomographic scan orientation on information loss in the three-dimensional reconstruction of tripod zygomatic fractures, *Invest Radiol* 26:427–431, 1991.

54. Levy RA and others: Assessing whether the plane of section on CT affects accuracy in demonstrating facial fractures in 3-D reconstruction when using a dried skull, *Am J Neuroradiol* 12:861–866, 1991.

55. Levy RA and others: Facial trauma and 3-D reconstructive imaging: insufficiencies and correctives, *Am J Neuroradiol* 13:885–892, 1992.

56. Lewin W: Cerebral spinal fluid rhinorrhea in closed head injuries, *Br J Surg* 42:1–18, 1954.

57. Lindqvist C and others: Rigid internal fixation of mandibular fractures: an analysis of 45 patients treated according to the ASIF method, *Int J Oral Maxillofac Surg* 15:657–664, 1986.

58. Longaker MT, Kawamoto HK: Enophthalmos revisited, *Clin Plast Surg* 24:531–537, 1997.

59. Luhr HG, Reidick T, Merten HA: Results of treatment of fractures of the atrophic edentulous mandible by compression plating: a retrospective evaluation of 84 consecutive cases, *J Oral Maxillofac Surg* 54:250–254, 1996.

60. Luhr HG and others: *Comparative studies between the extraoral and intraoral approach in compression-osteosynthesis of mandibular fractures.* In Hjorting-Hansen E, editor: *Oral and maxillofacial surgery: proceedings from the 8th International Conference on Oral and Maxillofacial Surgery*, Chicago, 1985, Quintessence Publishing Co, pp 133–137.

61. Manson PN: Computed tomography use and repair of orbitozygomatic fractures, *Arch Facial Plast Surg* 1:25–26, 1999.

62. Manson PN: Dimensional analysis of the facial skeleton: avoiding complications in the management of facial fractures by improved organization of treatment based on CT scans, *Probl Plast Reconstr Surg* 1:213–237, 1991.

63. Manson PN, Hoopes JE, Su CT: Structural pillars of the facial skeleton: an approach to the management of Le Fort fractures, *Plast Reconstr Surg* 66:54–61, 1980.

64. Manson PN and others: Midface fractures: advantages of immediate extended open reduction and bone grafting, *Plast Reconstr Surg* 76:1–12, 1985.

65. Manson PN and others: Studies on enophthalmos: II. the measurement of orbital injuries and their treatment by quantitative computed tomography, *Plast Reconstr Surg* 77:203, 1986.

66. Markowitz BL and others: Management of the medial canthal tendon in nasoethmoid orbital fractures: the importance of the central fragment in classification and treatment, *Plast Reconstr Surg* 87:843–853, 1991.

67. Markowitz BL and others: Prospective comparison of axial computed tomography and standard and panoramic radiographs in the diagnosis of mandibular fractures, *Ann Plast Surg* 42:163–169, 1999.

68. Mathur KK, Tatum SA, Kellman RM: Carbonated apatite and hydroxyapatite in craniofacial reconstruction, *Arch Facial Plast Surg* 5:379–383, 2003.

69. Michelet FX, Deymes J, Dessus B: Osteosynthesis with miniaturized screwed plates in maxillofacial surgery, *J Maxillofac Surg* 1:79, 1973.

70. Mincy JE: Posttraumatic cerebrospinal fluid fistula of the frontal fossa, *J Trauma Inj Infect Crit Care* 6:618–622, 1966.

71. Niederdellmann H, Shetty V: Solitary lag screw osteosynthesis in the treatment of fractures of the angle of the mandible: a retrospective study, *Plast Reconstr Surg* 80:68–74, 1987.

72. Palmieri C, Ellis E III, Throckmorton G: Mandibular motion after closed and open treatment of unilateral mandibular condylar process fractures, *J Oral Maxillofac Surg* 57:764–775, 1999.

73. Parsons GS, Mathog RH: Orbital wall and volume relationships, *Arch Otolaryngol Head Neck Surg* 114:743–747, 1988.

74. Paskert JP, Manson PN: The bimanual examination of assessing instability in naso-orbitoethmoidal injuries, *Plast Reconstr Surg* 83:165–167, 1989.

75. Pearl RM: Treatment of enophthalmos, *Clin Plast Surg* 19:99–111, 1992.

76. Petruzzelli GJ, Stankiewicz JA: Frontal sinus obliteration with hydroxyapatite cement, *Laryngoscope* 112:32–36, 2002.

77. Potter J, Ellis E III: Treatment of mandibular angle fractures with a malleable noncompression miniplate, *J Oral Maxillofac Surg* 57:288–292, 1999.

78. Rahn BA: Direct and indirect bone healing after operative fracture treatment, *Otolaryngol Clin North Am* 20:425–440, 1987.

79. Rahn BA: Theoretical considerations in rigid fixation of facial bones, *Clin Plast Surg* 16:21–27, 1989.

80. Raveh J, Redli M, Markwalder TM: Operative management of 194 cases of combined maxillofacial-frontobasal fractures: principles and surgical modifications, *J Oral Maxillofac Surg* 42:555–564, 1984.

81. Raveh J, Vuillemin T, Sutter F: Subcranial management of 395 combined frontobasal-midface fractures, *Arch Otolaryngol Head Neck Surg* 114:1114–1122, 1988.

82. Raveh J and others: Management of combined frontonaso–orbital/skull base fractures and telecanthus in 355 cases, *Arch Otolaryngol Head Neck Surg* 118:605–614, 1992.

83. Rohrich RJ, Hollier LH: Management of frontal sinus fractures: changing concepts, *Clin Plast Surg* 19:219–232, 1992.

84. Rubin PAD, Bilyk JR, Shore JW: Management of orbital trauma: fractures, hemorrhage, and traumatic optic neuropathy. Focal points, *Am Acad Ophthalmol* 12:1, 1994.

85. Rudderman RH, Mullen RL: Biomechanics of the facial skeleton, *Clin Plast Surg* 19:11–29, 1992.

86. Sailer HF, Gratz KW, Kalavrezos ND: Frontal sinus fractures: principles of treatment and long term results after sinus obliteration with the use of lyophilized cartilage, *J Cranio-Maxillofac Surg* 26:235–242,1998.

87. Sakas DE and others: Compound anterior cranial base fractures: classification using computed tomography scanning as a basis for selection of patients for dural repair, *J Neurosurg* 88:471–477, 1998.

88. Schmitz JP and others: The use of the Naugle orbitometer in maxillofacial trauma, *J Cranio-Maxillofac Trauma* 5:13–18, 1999.

89. Schubert W: AO Advanced Course, Tucson, Arizona, February 2003.

90. Schultz RC: Frontal sinus and supraorbital fractures from vehicle accidents, *Clin Plast Surg* 2:93–106, 1975.

91. Shumrick KA, Ryzenman JM: Endoscopic management of facial fractures, *Facial Plast Surg Clin North Am* 9:469–474, 2001.

92. Shumrick KA, Smith CP: The use of cancellous bone for frontal sinus obliteration and reconstruction of frontal bony defects, *Arch Otolaryngol Head Neck Surg* 120:1003–1009, 1994.

93. Smith TL and others: Endoscopic management of the frontal recess in frontal sinus fractures: a shift in the paradigm? *Laryngoscope* 112:784–790, 2002.

94. Spiessl B, editor: *New concepts in maxillofacial bone surgery*. New York, Springer-Verlag, 1976.

95. Spiessl B: *Stable internal fixation*. In Mathog RH: *Maxillofacial trauma*. Baltimore, Maryland, 1984, Williams & Wilkins.

96. Stanley RB: Management of frontal sinus fractures: a review of 33 cases, *J Oral Maxillofac Surg* 57:380–381, 1999.

97. Stanley RB: *Pathogenesis and evaluation of mandibular fractures*. In Mathog RH: *Maxillofacial trauma*. Baltimore, Maryland, 1984, Williams & Wilkins.

98. Stanley RB Jr.: Reconstruction of midface vertical dimension following LeFort fractures, *Arch Otorhinolaryngol* 110:571, 1984.

99. Stanley RB Jr.: The temporal approach to impacted lateral orbital wall fractures, *Arch Otolaryngol Head Neck Surg* 114:550–553, 1988.

100. Stanley RB Jr.: Use of intraoperative computed tomography during repair of obitozygomatic fractures, *Arch Facial Plast Surg* 1:19–24, 1999.

101. Stanley RB, Becker TS: Injuries of the nasofrontal orifices in frontal sinus fractures, *Laryngoscope* 97:728–731, 1987.

102. Strong EB, Buchalter GM, Moulthrop THM: Endoscopic repair of isolated anterior table frontal sinus fractures, *Arch Facial Plast Surg* 5:514–521, 2003.

103. Troulis MJ, Perrott DH, Kaban LB: Endoscopic mandibular osteotomy, and placement and activation of a semiburied distractor, *J Oral Maxillofac Surg* 57:1110–1113, 1999.

104. Wilson IF and others: Contribution of conventional axial computed tomography (nonhelical), in conjunction with panoramic tomography (zonography), in evaluating mandibular fractures, *Ann Plast Surg* 45:415–421, 2000.

105. Wilson IF and others: Prospective comparison of panoramic tomography (zonography) and helical computed tomography in the diagnosis and operative management of mandibular fractures, *Plast Reconstr Surg* 107:1369–1375, 2001.

106. Wilson K, Hohmann A: *Applied dental anatomy and occlusion*. In Mathog RH: *Maxillofacial trauma*. Baltimore, 1984, Williams & Wilkins.

107. Worsaae N, Thorn JJ: Surgical versus nonsurgical treatment of unilateral dislocated low subcondylar fractures: a clinical study of 52 cases, *J Oral Maxillofac Surg* 52:353–360, 1994.

108. Zide MF, Kent JN: Indications for open reduction of mandibular condyle fractures, *J Oral Maxillofac Surg* 41:89–98, 1983.

CHAPTER TWENTY SEVEN

RECONSTRUCTION OF FACIAL DEFECTS

‖ Shan R. Baker

INTRODUCTION

Skin cancer is the most common cancer of humans, and most skin cancers occur on the face. The incidence of squamous cell carcinoma, basal cell carcinoma, and melanoma is increasing, perhaps because of the depletion of the ozone layer or other environmental factors not yet determined. Most cutaneous malignancies are managed surgically, leaving skin defects that require reconstruction. Skin cancers, birth defects, and injuries as a result of trauma and burns require that surgeons be skilled in the repair of facial defects. This chapter addresses the management of many types of facial defects, primarily those resulting from ablation of cutaneous malignancies. However, the principles of local flap design and tissue movement can be readily applied to the reconstruction of all forms of facial defects.

Most facial defects result from ablation of cutaneous malignancies, and most cases can be repaired by primary wound closure or with a local cutaneous or musculocutaneous flap. Because the topic of facial reconstruction is extremely broad and complex, this chapter discusses only local flaps and grafts in the repair of facial cutaneous defects with the occasional appropriate reference to the repair of skeletal deficiencies. Other publications better address the use of regional flaps in facial reconstruction.[5,7,12]

The face can be divided into aesthetic facial units, which include the forehead, cheeks, eyelids, nose, lips, auricles, and sometimes the scalp. Reconstruction of some of these areas of the face are discussed elsewhere in this textbook. A multitude of different flaps and grafts can be used to repair a given facial defect; thus, several techniques for repair of a given aesthetic facial unit are discussed. The algorithm in Figure 27-1 displays an approach for analyzing and developing a management plan for surface defects of the face and neck. The selection of a specific flap depends on the location and size of the defect and the intrinsic properties of the flap. Larger defects of the face and

neck may be difficult to resurface with local flaps without considerable impairment in form or function. In such circumstances, the surgeon should select a regional flap or skin graft that might be aesthetically less pleasing but will provide a functional repair. These decisions are determined by clinical judgment. The greater the experience of the surgeon, the better will be the clinical judgment.

CLASSIFICATION OF LOCAL FLAPS

Several methods are used to classify cutaneous flaps[3,16]: (1) by arrangement of their blood supply (e.g., random vs arterial); (2) by configuration (e.g., rhomboid, bilobe); (3) by location (e.g., local, regional, distant); and (4) by the method of transferring the flap. Local cutaneous flaps are designed immediately adjacent to or near the location of the defect. When classified by method of transfer (Box 27-1), local flaps are divided into pivotal, advancement, and hinged categories. A fourth method of tissue movement is microsurgical, although this method does not apply to local flaps. Most local flaps are moved, in reality, through a combination of pivoting and advancement. For example, most pivotal flaps are aided in tissue movement by using the intrinsic elasticity of the flap through stretching (advancement). Thus, surgeons often speak of combined mechanisms of tissue movement, such as advancement rotation flap. For classification purposes, however, the major mechanism of tissue transfer should dictate the term given to describe a particular flap, unless both mechanisms are of approximately equal importance, in which case the terms describing both mechanisms should be used.

PIVOTAL FLAPS

The three types of pivotal flaps are rotation, transposition, and interpolated (see Box 27-1). All pivotal flaps are moved toward the defect by rotating the base of the flap around a pivotal point. Except with island axial flaps, which have been skeletonized to the level

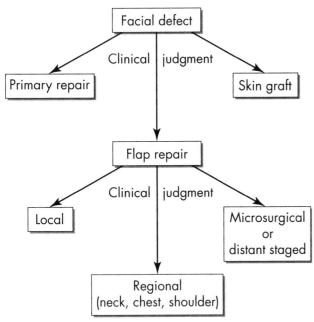

Figure 27-1. Skin defect repair.

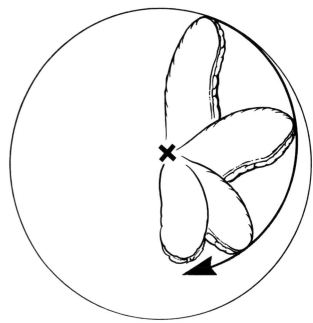

Figure 27-2. The effective length of a pivotal flap moving through an arch of 180 degrees is reduced 40%. (Adapted from Gorney M: *Tissue dynamics and surgical geometry.* In Kernakian DA, Vistnes LM, editors: *Basic concepts of reconstructive surgery*, Boston, 1977, Little, Brown.)

BOX 27-1

LOCAL FLAPS CLASSIFIED
BY TISSUE MOVEMENT

Pivotal flaps
   Rotation
   Transposition
   Interpolated
Advancement flaps
   Pedicle
   Bipedicle
   V-Y
Hinged flap

---

of the nutrient vessels, the greater the degree of pivot, the shorter is the effective length of the flap (Figure 27-2). This is because the pivotal point is fixed in position and the base of the flap is restricted when pivoting around this point because of the development of a standing cutaneous deformity (dog ear). A pivotal flap should be designed to account for this reduction in effective length as it moves through the pivotal arc, which may be as much as 40% with an arc of 180 degrees.

Rotation Flaps

Rotation flaps are pivotal flaps that have a curvilinear configuration. They are designed immediately adjacent to the defect and are best used to close triangular defects (Figure 27-3). Rotation flaps are usually random in their vascularity but, depending on the

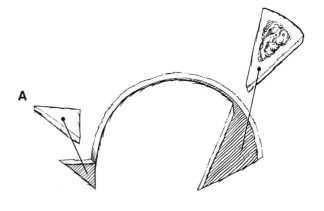

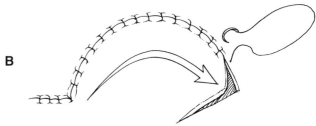

Figure 27-3. **A,** Rotation flaps are pivotal flaps with curvilinear configuration. Removal of a Burow's triangle can facilitate repair of the donor site. **B,** Standing cutaneous deformity will form at the base of the flap. Triangle-shaped defects use a portion of this redundant tissue. (From Baker SR, Swanson N: *Local flaps in facial reconstruction.* St. Louis, Mosby, 1995.)

position of the base of the flap, may be axial. Because a rotation flap has a broad base, its vascularity tends to be reliable. When possible, the flap should be designed to be inferiorly based, which promotes lymphatic drainage and reduces flap edema. Rotation flaps are useful in repairing medial cheek defects located near the nasofacial sulcus or nasal sidewall. The curvilinear border of the flap can often be positioned along the infraorbital rim, which represents an important border of aesthetic units (eyelid and cheek). Positioning the incision for the flap along this border enhances scar camouflage.

Large rotation flaps are particularly useful for reconstruction of sizable posterior cheek and upper neck defects. Large medial, inferiorly based rotation flaps are a flexible means of transferring large amounts of tissue from the remaining cheek and upper cervical regions. Incisions for the flap are placed in a preauricular crease and can extend for some distance along the anterior border of the trapezius muscle to facilitate rotation of upper cervical skin toward the area of the posterior cheek. A Z-plasty at the base of the flap facilitates closure of the secondary defect. Chin reconstruction can often be readily accomplished with rotation flaps, occasionally using two flaps to optimize the use of the aesthetic border of the submental crease to camouflage incisions. Smaller rotation flaps can also be used for repair of defects located in the glabellar area. Because rotation flaps are less dependent than most on tissue elasticity for movement, they are particularly useful for scalp defects in which the skin is quite inelastic. In addition, curvilinear configuration of rotation flaps adapts well to the spherical shaped cranium. Thus, scalp defects in general are best reconstructed with one or more rotation flaps. A rotation scalp flap must be quite large relative to the size of the defect, with the width of the pedicle being twice the width of the defect.[19]

Rotation flaps have relatively few disadvantages. The defect itself should be somewhat triangular or should be modified by removal of additional tissue to create a triangular defect. The configuration of the flap creates a right angle at the distal tip, and the surgeon should take care in positioning the tip so that it is not subjected to excessive wound tension and vascular compromise. As with all pivotal flaps, a rotation flap may develop a standing cutaneous deformity at the base that may not be easily removed without compromising the vascularity of the flap. Thus, a second-stage removal of the deformity may be necessary.

Transposition Flaps

In contrast to rotation flaps, transposition flaps have a linear axis (Figure 27-4). Both are pivotal flaps moving around a pivotal point. A transposition flap can be

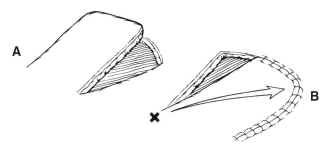

Figure 27-4. A, Transposition flaps have a linear configuration. **B,** The greatest line of wound closure tension is between the pivotal point and the most peripheral point of the flap. (**A,** Adapted from Baker SR, Swanson N: *Local flaps in facial reconstruction*, St. Louis, Mosby, 1995.)

designed similar to a rotation flap so that a border of the flap is also a border of the defect. However, it may also be designed with borders that are removed from the defect, with only the base of the flap contiguous with the defect. The ability to construct a flap at some distance from the defect with an axis that is independent of the linear axis of the defect is one of the greatest advantages of transposition flaps. This advantage enables the surgeon to recruit skin at variable distances from the defect, selecting areas of greater skin elasticity or redundancy. In addition, the ability to select variable sites for harvesting a flap ensures that the donor site scar by its location and orientation will best be camouflaged.

Transposition is the most common method of moving local flaps into skin defects of the head and neck. Transposition flaps, elevated in a multitude of sizes, shapes, and orientation, are usually of random blood supply but may occasionally be axial or compound. A transposition flap is a reconstructive option for small- to medium-sized defects in most configurations or locations, thus making it the most useful local flap in head and neck reconstruction. Although it is recommended that the length of random cutaneous transposition flaps not exceed three times their width, this ratio is not very applicable to such flaps designed on the face and scalp. More important than this ratio are the location and the specific orientation of a transposition flap. The abundant vascularity of the skin of the face and scalp often enables the development of flaps that exceed the 3:1 ratio. An example is the inferiorly or superiorly based melolabial transposition flap, in which its linear axis is directly above and parallel to the linear axis of the angular artery. Although the flap is rarely elevated as a true axial flap incorporating the angular artery, many small peripheral branches of the artery are probably included in the base of the melolabial flap, accounting for its dependability even when designed as a lengthy flap.

Interpolated Flaps

The interpolated flap is a pivotal flap that has a linear configuration, but it differs from transposition flaps in that its base is located at some distance from the defect (Figure 27-5). Thus, the pedicle should pass over or under intervening tissue. If the pedicle passes over intervening tissue, the flap should subsequently be detached in a second surgical procedure. This is perhaps the greatest disadvantage of these flaps. On occasion, the pedicle can be deepithelialized or reduced to subcutaneous tissue only and brought under the intervening skin as an island flap to allow a single-stage reconstruction.

Common interpolated flaps used in the repair of facial defects are the vertically oriented midforehead flaps, which include median and perimedian flaps.[1] These flaps are highly effective in reconstruction of the midface because of their excellent vascularity and because their skin color and texture superbly match the skin of the nose. The high success rate, reliability, and popularity are primarily the result of a dependable axial blood supply. Based on the supratrochlear artery and its anastomoses to surrounding vessels, midforehead flaps are axial flaps with excellent vascularity that can be transferred without delay. The excellent vascularity allows for the incorporation of cartilage or

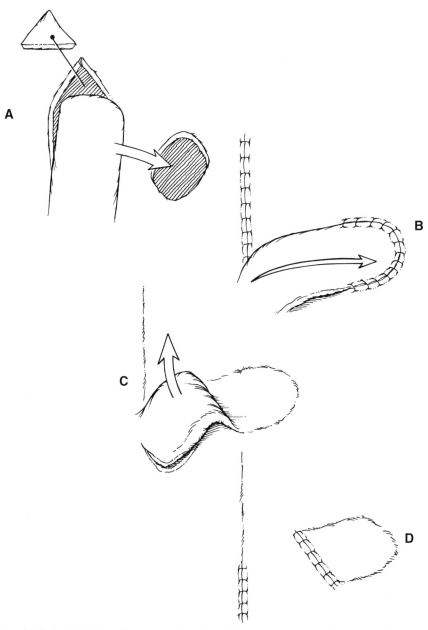

Figure 27-5. Interpolation flaps are pivotal and have a linear configuration. The pedicle passes over intervening tissue and requires subsequent division.

tissue grafts, which can then act as support structures or lining tissue for nasal reconstruction. Careful removal of muscle and subcutaneous fat from the distal portion of a midforehead flap makes it thin, pliable, and easily contoured to fit any defect of the midface. The frontalis muscle and fascia are included with the distal flap when more stiffness and bulk are required to fit defects of greater depth.

The close proximity of forehead skin to the midface provides a source of skin with excellent color and texture match to the central face. Modern use of the midforehead flap has been expanded beyond nasal reconstruction to include any soft tissue defect of the midface that the flap can be designed to reach.[6] Defects of the medial canthal region, upper and lower eyelids, medial cheek, melolabial region, and upper lip can be repaired with midforehead flaps. These flaps can also be used in combination with other flaps for the reconstruction of complex facial defects; for example, a midforehead flap can be combined with a scalping flap for total nasal reconstruction.

ADVANCEMENT FLAPS

Advancement flaps have a linear configuration and are moved into a defect by being stretched forward. These flaps depend on the elasticity of the tissue of the flap (primary movement) and tissue adjacent to the defect (secondary movement) to achieve wound closure. Tissue transfer is achieved by moving the flap and its pedicle in a single vector. Advancement flaps can be categorized as single or unipedicle, bipedicle, or V-Y. Bipedicle advancement flaps are used primarily for repair of large defects of the scalp; the flap is designed adjacent to the defect and advanced into the defect perpendicular to the linear axis of the flap. This leaves a secondary defect, which usually should be covered with a split-thickness skin graft. As a consequence, bipedicle flaps are rarely used for reconstruction of the face and neck.

Pedicle Advancement Flap

A unipedicle advancement flap is created by parallel incisions that allow the tissue to "slide" in a single vector toward a defect (Figure 27-6). The movement is in one direction, and the flap advances directly over the defect. As a consequence, the flap should be developed adjacent to the defect, and one border of the defect becomes a border of the flap. Repair with an advancement flap involves primary and secondary tissue movement. In primary movement, the incised flap is pushed or pulled forward by stretching the skin. Secondary movement of surrounding skin and soft tissue immediately adjacent to the defect occurs in a direction opposite the movement of the advancing edge of the flap. This secondary movement may

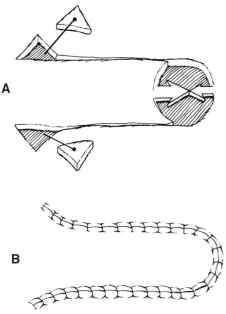

Figure 27-6. **A** and **B,** A pedicle advancement flap is created by parallel incisions, which allow a tissue to slide in a single vector toward the defect. Secondary movement of surrounding skin immediately adjacent to the defect occurs in a direction opposite the direction of the flap. (Adapted from Baker SR, Swanson N: *Local flaps in facial reconstruction*, St. Louis, Mosby, 1995.)

help in repair by providing less wound closure tension, or it may be detrimental, displacing nearby facial structures.

Complete undermining of the advancement flap, and of the skin and soft tissue around the pedicle, is important to enhance tissue movement. Standing cutaneous deformities are created with all advancement flaps and may require excision. Excision of standing cutaneous deformities (Burow's triangles) may also facilitate movement of the flap. Unlike the pivotal flap, in which a single-standing cutaneous deformity should be dealt with at the base of the flap, deformities develop on both sides of the base. However, they may be excised anywhere along the length of the flap and not necessarily near the base. Selection of the best location for excising tissue is based on where it can be placed within relaxed skin tension lines or long aesthetic borders. Bilateral Z-plasties performed at the base of the flap often eliminate or reduce the need for excision of standing cutaneous deformities. Occasionally, if the flap is sufficiently long, standing cutaneous deformities can be subdivided into multiple smaller puckers of tissue that need not be excised but merely can be "sewn out" by sequentially suturing the flap lengths in one half. On the face, pedicle advancement flaps work especially well in the forehead (particularly in the vicinity of the eyebrow), helical rim, upper and lower lips, and medial cheek. Mucosal advancement flaps are also useful for vermilion reconstruction. Bilateral advancement flaps are commonly used to close large defects, resulting in H- or T-shaped repairs, depending on the configuration of the defect (Figure 27-7). Repair in this manner is often referred to as an *H-plasty* or *T-plasty*. In both cases, advancement flaps are designed on opposite sides of a defect and advanced toward each other, each responsible for reconstructing a portion of the defect. In such cases, standing cutaneous deformities are often excised partly in the area of the defect and partly along the linear axis of the two flaps. The two flaps harvested from either side of the defect do not necessarily have to be of the same length. The length of each flap is determined primarily by the elasticity and redundancy of the donor resource.

A special type of pedicle advancement flap is the island advancement flap. A segment of skin is isolated as an island while protecting the subcutaneous tissue and blood supply. The geometric shape of the cutaneous island may vary but is frequently triangular. As the flap advances toward the recipient site, the donor area is closed in a simple V-Y manner. This flap is particularly useful in the repair of medium-sized defects of the medial cheek near the alar base.

V-Y Advancement Flap

The V-Y advancement flap is unique in that the V-shaped flap is not stretched toward the recipient site but advances by recoil or by being pushed rather

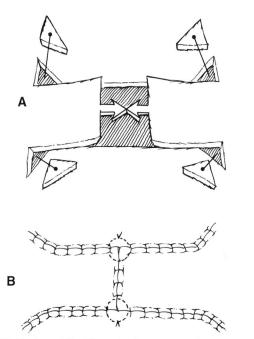

Figure 27-7. **A** and **B,** Bilateral advancement flaps with excision of Burow's triangles.

than pulled toward the defect. Thus, the flap is allowed to move into the recipient site without any wound closure tension. The secondary triangular donor defect is then repaired by advancing the two edges of the remaining donor site wound toward each other. In so doing, the wound closure suture line assumes a Y configuration, with the common limb of the Y representing the suture line resulting from closure of the secondary defect.

V-Y advancement is useful when a structure or region requires lengthening or release from a contracted state. The technique is particularly effective in lengthening the columella in the repair of cleft lip nasal deformities in which a portion or all of the columella is underdeveloped (Figure 27-8). A V-Y advancement flap is elevated, recruiting skin from the midportion of the lip between the philtral ridges. The length of the columella is augmented by advancing the flap upward into the base of the columella. The secondary donor defect is approximated by closing the remaining lip skin together in the midline. V-Y advancement is also helpful in releasing contracted scars that distort adjacent structures, such as the eyelid or vermilion. An example is the correction of an ectropion of the vermilion caused by scarring (Figure 27-9). The segment of distorted vermilion is incorporated into the V-shaped flap and advanced toward the lip to restore the natural topography of the vermilion-cutaneous junction. The skin edges on both sides of the secondary defect are then advanced toward each other and sutured. The suture line becomes the vertical or common limb of the Y configuration.

Y-V Advancement Flaps

Y-V advancement flaps differ from V-Y advancement flaps in that a Y-shaped incision is made initially. In contrast to the V-Y design in which the V-shaped flap recoils or is pushed toward the area for supplementation, in the Y-V design, the flap is pulled or stretched toward the area for supplementation. The flap augments the area of the common limb while reducing the triangular area. Y-V advancement flaps are indicated in circumstances in which the surgeon wants to decrease the redundancy of an area by moving tissue away from the site. Occasionally, relocating a free margin of a facial structure using a Y-V flap can be useful to improve symmetry.

HINGE FLAPS

Cutaneous hinge flaps, sometimes referred to as *trap door, turn-in,* or *turn-down* flaps, have a unique method of tissue movement. These flaps can be designed in a linear or curvilinear shape with the pedicle based on one border of the defect. The flap is dissected in the subcutaneous plane and turned over

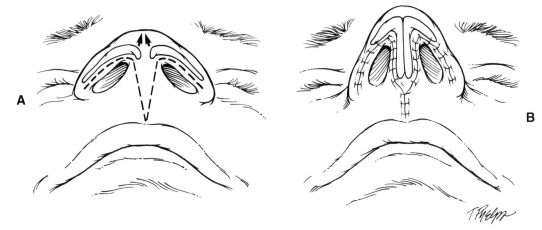

Figure 27-8. **A** and **B,** A V-Y advancement flap augments columellar length.

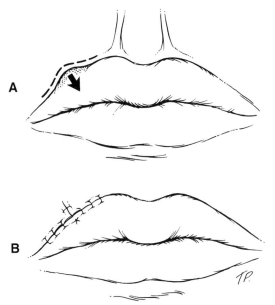

Figure 27-9. **A** and **B,** A V-Y advancement flap corrects ectopian of vermilion. (Adapted from Baker SR, Swanson N: *Local flaps in facial reconstruction*, St. Louis, Mosby, 1995.)

onto the defect like a page in a book. The epithelial surface of the flap is turned downward to provide internal lining for a facial defect that requires external and internal lining surfaces. The exposed subcutaneous surface of the hinge flap is covered by a second flap. Thus, hinge flaps are always used with another flap or graft that provides the external coverage of the defect. The vascular supply of hinge flaps is derived from the soft tissue border of the defect that it is designed to repair. As a consequence, such flaps have limited and often restricted vascularity. Survival of hinge flaps can be improved if they are used when the wound margin of the defect is well healed rather than freshly created. Because the pedicle of the hinge flap is along a border of the defect, the flap should be elevated in such a way that, as flap dissection proceeds toward the base of the flap, the plane of dissection becomes deeper; thus, the base is thicker than the distal portion of the flap. This technique enhances the vascularity of the flap by increasing the likelihood of including more nutrient vessels within the pedicle.

Hinge flaps are commonly used for repair of full-thickness nasal defects in which the remaining adjacent nasal skin is sufficient to develop a hinge flap for internal nasal lining. Hinge flaps can also be used to close mature sinofacial and salivary fistulas anywhere in the upper aerodigestive tract. Hinge flaps consisting of subcutaneous tissue, and sometimes muscle without overlying skin, can be used to fill in contour deficits.[17] Hinged flaps consisting of nasal mucosa (with or without attached septal cartilage) are frequently used for internal lining in the repair of full-thickness nasal defects. These mucosal flaps are axial and do not require a thick base to ensure adequate vascularity.

DEFECTS OF THE NOSE

Skin cancer most frequently occurs on the nose; thus, reconstructive surgeons should be familiar with several methods for repairing nasal defects using local flaps. Burget and Menick[14] have elevated reconstructive rhinoplasty by emphasizing the importance of replacing deficient nasal tissue with similar tissue. For example, defects of the internal nasal lining are replaced with hinged or bipedicle advancement mucosal flaps harvested from the remaining nasal lining. Missing cartilage or fibrofatty tissue giving contour to the nose is replaced with septal or conchal cartilage, positioned and sculpted to replicate the missing skeletal support as closely as possible. Thinning and contouring the cartilage grafts should be emphasized so that they replicate the exact topography of the contralateral cartilage if present, or the form that can be expected in an ideally shaped nose. Burget and

Menick[14] also emphasized the aesthetic advantages of isolating nasal defects as a separate entity from any extension of the defect onto the cheek or lip, repairing each aesthetic unit with independent flaps. This maintains scars in borders between major aesthetic units and prevents distortion or obliteration of these borders while maximizing scar camouflage. Within the nasal aesthetic unit, subunits can be identified, including the dorsum, nasal sidewalls, ala, tip, and columella (Figure 27-10). When a surface defect involves greater than 50% of the surface area of the subunit, resurfacing of the entire subunit with a flap usually provides a better aesthetic result by hiding scars along borders of the subunits.[14]

The nasal ala is a common site of nasal defects resulting from removal of skin cancers. If not repaired properly, distortion of the alar margin and partial collapse of the external nasal valve occur with compromise of the airway. Too often in the past, the alar facial sulcus and nasal alar crease have been violated by transposition flaps harvested from the medial cheek to repair alar defects. When this occurs, a completely natural-appearing border between the cheek and the ala and nasal sidewall is extremely difficult to restore. For this reason, the author prefers to use interpolated flaps from the cheek, the pedicle of which crosses over, but not through, the alar facial sulcus. The pedicle may consist of skin or subcutaneous tissue only, and is detached from the cheek 3 weeks after the initial transfer to the nose.[8] This interval allows the surgeon to aggressively defat and sculpt the distal flap at the time of flap transfer and again at the time of pedicle detachment and flap inset. On detachment of the flap, the patient has a completely natural-appearing alar facial sulcus and nasal alar crease (provided the defect does not extend into the crease) because no incisions or dissections have been made in these regions.

Usually, resurfacing of the entire ala is preferred, removing any remaining skin. Full-thickness defects are reconstructed by restoring the internal nasal lining deficit with a vascularized vestibular skin or mucosal flap. Full-thickness defects of the ala with a vertical height of 1.5 cm or less can use a bipedicle mucosal flap for internal lining (Figure 27-11). The flap is created by making an extended intercartilaginous incision from the nasal dome to the lateral floor of the vestibule. The vestibular skin is mobilized inferiorly, and the inferior edge is sutured to the inferior border of the nasal vestibular skin defect. If the vestibular skin defect extends to the alar rim, then the inferior aspect of the flap used is sutured to the edge of the cutaneous flap used to provide external coverage of the defect. The flap is attached to overlying cartilage grafts placed to provide structural support by horizontal mattress sutures placed through the cartilage and bipedicle flap. The donor site for the flap is repaired with a thin full-thickness skin graft harvested from the standing cutaneous deformity removed when closing the donor site of the interpolated cheek flap.

After reconstruction of the internal nasal lining defect with a bipedicle mucosal flap, the next step is to completely replace all missing nasal cartilage with free cartilage grafts harvested from the nasal septum or, preferably, from the auricle. If the inferior edge of the lateral crura has been removed, the missing cartilage should be replaced with a free cartilage graft, and additional grafts should be placed along the alar margin inferior to the position of the original lateral crus. This prevents notching or upper contraction of the alar rim. Likewise, when the fibrofatty tissue of the lateral portion of the alar lobule is missing, it should be replaced with free cartilage grafts because this tissue, although not rigid, provides structural support and contour to the lobule. If the surgeon depends strictly

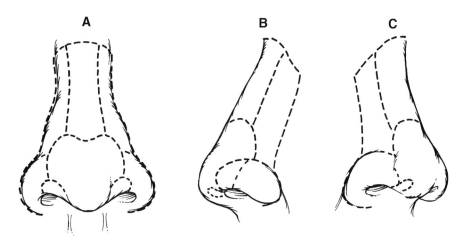

Figure 27-10. A through **C,** Nasal topographic aesthetic units. (Adapted from Baker SR, Swanson N: *Local flaps in facial reconstruction*, St. Louis, Mosby, 1995.)

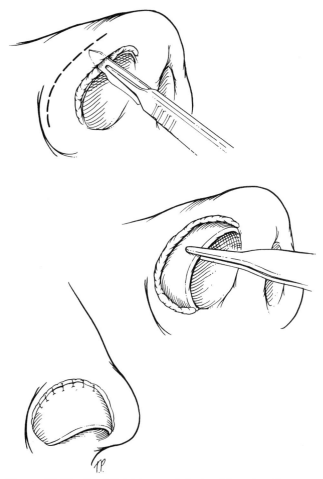

Figure 27-11. For full-thickness defects of the ala with a vertical height of 1.5 cm or less, one can use a bipedicle mucosal advancement flap for internal lining. The donor site is closed with a thin full-thickness skin graft. (Adapted from Baker SR, Swanson N: *Local flaps in facial reconstruction*, St. Louis, Mosby, 1995.)

on a skin flap to replace the fibrofatty tissue in the alar lobule, less structural support is provided and scar contracture causes an unnatural appearance, usually with some notching of the alar rim and partial collapse of the external nasal valve.

Once the structural support for the alar lobule has been secured, a cheek flap is planed to resurface the lobule and cover the restored skeletal support. A template is fashioned to exactly represent the size and shape of the surface defect. This template is used to design a superiorly based melolabial interpolated flap. The flap should be designed so that the medial border falls in the melolabial sulcus. The flap is elevated in a subcutaneous plane and may be lifted on a skin and subcutaneous fat pedicle or based on a subcutaneous pedicle only. A subcutaneous pedicle is preferred in nonsmokers because the flap can transpose more easily and reduces the amount of skin to be removed

from the upper melolabial fold, thus maintaining better facial symmetry. The flap donor site is closed primarily by undermining the skin of the cheek. The standing cutaneous deformity that occurs with advancement of the cheek skin medially is excised, and a portion is used as a full-thickness skin graft to cover the donor site of the intranasal mucosal flap. The interpolated flap is transposed over the alar facial sulcus, and the distal two thirds of the flap is thinned appropriately so that the flap will drape over the cartilage grafts in a manner that replicates the contour of the alar lobule and alar nasal crease. This may require thinning of the flap to the level of the dermis in the area along the alar rim to restore the delicate topography of the rim. When the defect involves the alar rim and internal nasal vestibular skin, the inferior border of the flap is sutured to the inferior border of the bipedicle mucosal flap used to replace the missing internal nasal lining. The proximal third of the interpolated flap is left with an ample amount of subcutaneous tissue to enhance flap vascularity. At the time of pedicle detachment, the proximal portion of the flap to be inset is defatted and contoured.

The main advantage of the melolabial interpolated flap is that it does not violate the aesthetically important alar facial sulcus. It also minimizes distortion of the melolabial fold because the skin removed from the cheek is skin located at the inferior aspect of the fold where greater skin redundancy is present. Using a subcutaneous pedicle, only a small amount of skin from the upper melolabial fold is discarded as a result of a small-standing cutaneous deformity in that area during closure of the donor site.

When tissue defects extend into the alar facial sulcus, the task of restoring this area of complex topography to its natural appearance (i.e., symmetrical to its counterpart) is difficult. When confronted with this problem, the surgeon often prefers to reconstruct the medial cheek and alar facial sulcus component of the defect with an advancement cheek flap and reconstruct the alar lobule with a separate cheek or forehead interpolated flap (Figure 27-12). This allows each flap to reconstruct the independent aesthetic units of the nose and cheek, and it places the junction of the borders of the two flaps along the restored alar facial sulcus. When such defects are reconstructed with a single transposition cheek flap, partial or complete obliteration of the alar facial sulcus occurs, and it should be restored through additional operations. This usually involves multiple surgical procedures and only limited success.

Surface defects of the nasal tip, columella, sidewalls, and dorsum are best repaired with paramedian forehead flaps, although partial loss of the columella may be repaired with a single or bilateral superiorly based melolabial interpolated flap. If the defect involves more than 50% of the surface area of an aesthetic subunit, the remaining skin should be removed and the entire subunit of the nose resurfaced. As with reconstruction of the ala, all missing cartilage should be replaced. Auricular cartilage is an excellent source for replacing missing lower lateral cartilage, whereas septal cartilage is most useful for replacing upper lateral cartilage. Full-thickness defects require unilateral or bilateral septal mucosal flaps for repair of the internal lining (Figure 27-13). Burget and Menick[14] showed that the entire mucosal lining of the nasal septum can be mobilized as a hinge flap based anteriorly on the caudal septum and nourished by the septal branch of the labial artery. This hinge flap is turned laterally across the nasal passage to provide lining to the lateral nasal wall. When greater lining deficits (e.g., the entire length of the sidewall) are present, a second mucosal flap from the contralateral side is developed. In contrast to the ipsilateral flap, the contralateral flap is hinged on the dorsal septum and is nourished by the anterior ethmoid artery (see Figure 27-13). Thus,

the lining for a heminasal defect is supplied inferiorly by an ipsilateral hinge septal mucosal flap based on the superior labial artery and superiorly by a contralateral septal mucosal hinge flap based on the anterior ethmoid artery. A permanent septal fistula remains. Although crusting can occur for several months, the large septal fistula is rarely symptomatic. The ipsilateral mucosal flap crosses the nasal passage in such a way that it blocks the airway, and should be detached from the caudal septum to restore a patent nasal passage. This maneuver is accomplished using local anesthesia 3 weeks after initial transfer. The excellent vascular supply of these mucosal flaps provides a well-vascularized recipient site to support free cartilage grafts of all sizes. The grafts are sandwiched between the mucosal flap internally and the interpolated forehead or cheek flap externally and thus have a dual source of vascularization.

In repair of full-thickness central nasal defects of the tip or dorsum, a composite turnout flap consisting of septal cartilage with attached mucosa on either side is developed. Its base is centered in the region of the

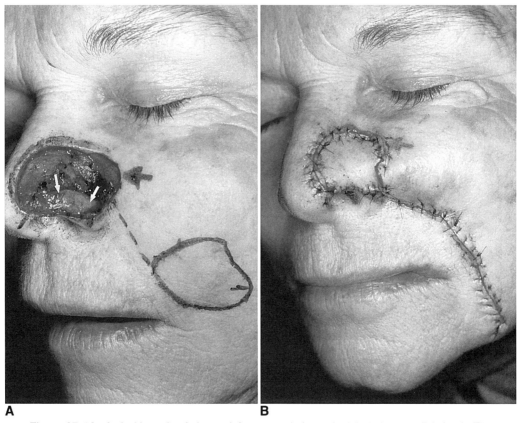

A **B**

Figure 27-12. **A,** A skin and soft tissue defect extends from alar lobule into medial cheek. The cheek advancement flap is designed to repair cheek defect. Separate subcutaneous pedicle transposition flap is designed to resurface the alar lobule after placement of auricular cartilage graft (arrows) along the missing alar margin. **B,** Two flaps are in position.

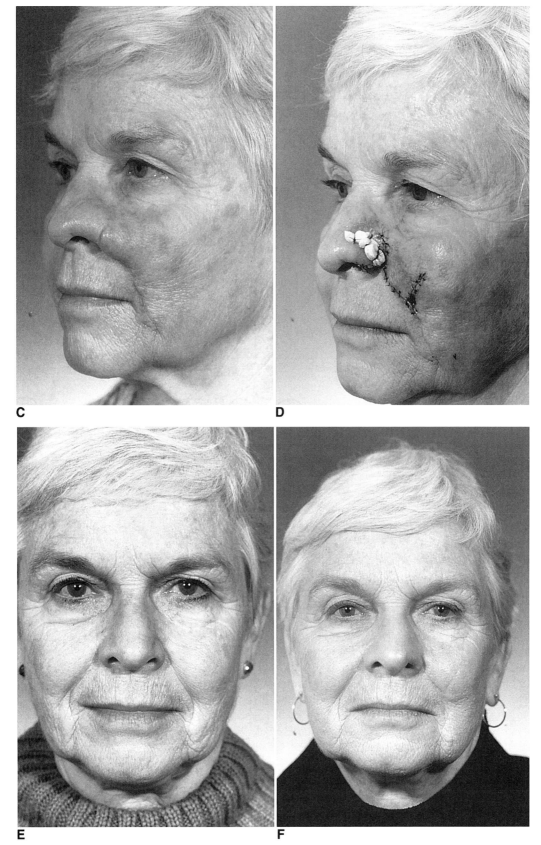

Figure 27-12, cont'd C and D, Three weeks after transfer of transposition flap, the pedicle is separated and the distal flap is sculptured to reconstitute the alar nasal crease. The standing cutaneous deformity from the cheek advancement flap is removed in the melolabial sulcus. E and F, Preoperative (E) and 1 year postoperative (F) view. Harvesting the transposition cheek flap from jowl area reduces asymmetric fullness of the melolabial folds.

Continued

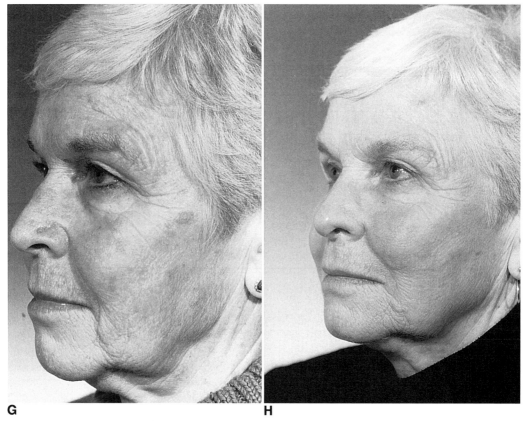

G   **H**

Figure 27-12, cont'd G and **H,** Preoperative **(G)** and 1-year postoperative **(H)** view. The reconstituted alar nasal crease simulates original crease by aggressively debulking flap at the time of inset.

nasal spine and upper lip and contains both septal branches of the superior labial arteries. A flap of appropriate dimensions is outlined and incised with a right-angle knife or scissors. Such flaps may include bone and extend from the nasal floor inferiorly to the level of the medial canthi cephalically and posteriorly to include portions of the perpendicular plate. To allow rotation, the septal mucoperichondrial leaves are separated from the septal cartilage near the nasal spine and a triangular-shaped piece of septal cartilage at the level of the inferior septal angle is removed (Figure 27-14). This maneuver permits the flap to rotate up and out to reach the tip and dorsum. The flap is designed overly wide and long to create an excess of mucosa and cartilage. As the flap pivots into position, its distal end passes over the exposed remnant of the nasal bones or missing dorsal septum and locks into position. The extra lining is peeled downward as bilateral hinge flaps, which extend laterally to line the dorsal nasal vault and tip. Cartilage grafts are placed on top of these flaps to restore missing dome cartilage in the case of central tip defects or to restore nasal bridge in the case of dorsal defects. A paramedian

forehead flap provides the external surface cover to complete the reconstruction (Figure 27-15).

Paramedian forehead flaps are the preferred local flap for resurfacing most large nasal defects. The flap can be dissected under local or general anesthesia. The base of the pedicle is placed in the glabellar region centered over the supratrochlear artery on the same side as most of the nasal defect. The origin of the supratrochlear artery is consistently found to be 1.7 to 2.2 cm lateral to the midline and corresponds usually to a vertical tangent of the medial aspect of the brow. The vessel exits the orbit by piercing the orbital septum and passing under the orbicularis oculi muscle and over the corrugator superciliary muscle. At the level of the eyebrow, the artery passes through orbicularis and frontalis muscle and continues upward in a vertical direction in a subcutaneous plane. The pedicle of the flap may be as narrow as 1.2 cm. A narrow pedicle provides greater effective length with less standing cutaneous deformity than a broader pedicle (Figure 27-16). An exact template of the defect is used to design the paramedian forehead flap, which is centered over the vertical axis of the supratrochlear

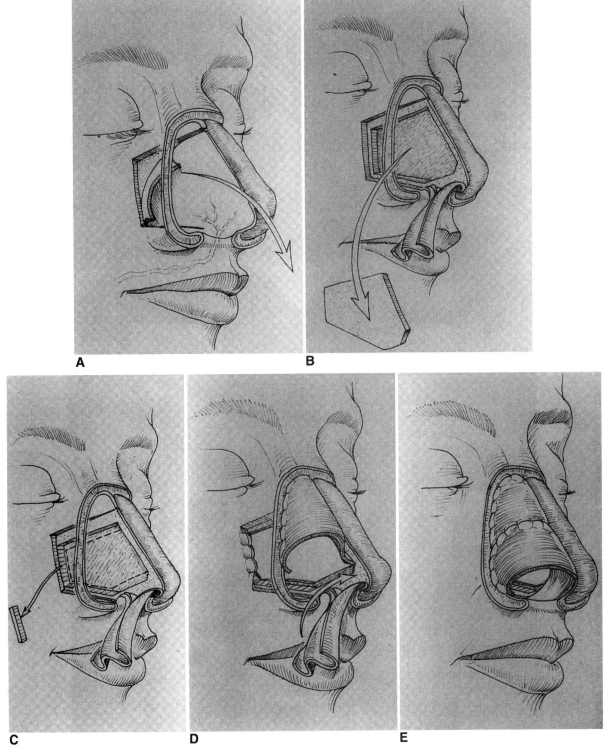

Figure 27-13. A and **B,** Ipsilateral hinged flap can be used to restore internal lining of full-thickness nasal sidewall defects with a vertical height of 2.5 cm or less. In such instances, exposed septal cartilage is removed to allow septum to heal by second intention. **C** through **E,** For defects greater than 2.5 cm in vertical height, a second contralateral septal mucosal hinged flap is required to supplement ipsilateral flap.

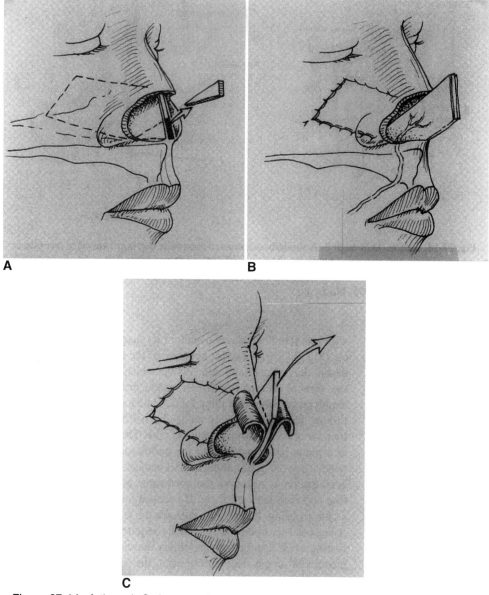

A

B

C

Figure 27-14. A through **C,** A composite pivotal septal flap is used to replace structure and internal lining for central defects of the tip and dorsum.

artery. If adequate length necessitates extending the flap into hair-bearing scalp, turning the flap obliquely along the hairline will prevent transfer of hair-bearing skin to the nose. The flap is elevated in a plane just superficial to the periosteum of the frontal bone. To avoid injury to the arterial pedicle, blunt dissection near the brow separates the corrugator muscles from the flap and facilitates mobility. If necessary, incisions can be extended below the brow to enhance the length of the flap. Adequate flap mobilization usually requires complete sectioning of the corrugator superciliary muscle to achieve free movement of the flap. Before inset, the flap is sculptured and contoured to fit the depth, breadth, and height of the defect by

removal of all or some of the muscle and subcutaneous tissues from the distal portion of the flap. When necessary, all but 1 mm of the fat beneath the dermis can be removed. It may be necessary to resect a portion of the dermis along the edge of the flap so that the thickness of the skin flap matches the adjacent nasal skin. Only the distal three-fourths of the flap required for reconstruction is sculptured; the proximal one-fourth is left thick and is debulked at the time of pedicle detachment 3 weeks later. Donor site closure is accomplished by undermining the forehead skin in the subfascial plane from the anterior border of one temporalis muscle to the other. Several parallel vertical fasciotomies 2 to 3 cm apart may be necessary to

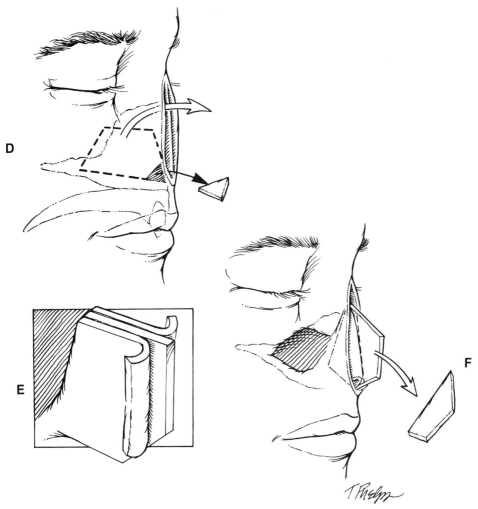

Figure 27-14, cont'd D through **F,** A similarly constructed composite flap can be used to reconstruct internal lining and skeletal support for the nasal dorsum. (Adapted from Baker SR, Swanson N: *Local flaps in facial reconstruction*, St. Louis, Mosby, 1995.)

achieve primary closure of the wound. Any portion of the donor site that cannot be closed primarily should be left to heal by second intention, keeping the open wound moist at all times. Healing by second intention usually results in an acceptable scar but may take several weeks for complete healing. When necessary, the scar can be revised later. Three weeks after the initial flap transfer, the pedicle is divided under local anesthesia. The dorsal skin above the defect is undermined for approximately 1 cm. The portion of the transposed skin flap that was not thinned at the time of flap transfer is now thinned appropriately. For skin-only nasal defects that extend to the rhinion, the flap should be aggressively thinned to the level of the dermis to reduplicate the thin skin that is normally found in this area. Deep layer closure is not necessary because closure should not be under any tension. The base of the pedicle is returned to the donor site in such a way as to create the normal intereyebrow

distance (see Figure 27-16). Care should be taken to maintain the muscular component of the proximal pedicle that is returned so that a depression between the eyebrows does not occur. Any excess pedicle should be discarded rather than returned to the forehead above the level of the eyebrows.

DEFECTS OF THE LIP

The lips play a key role in deglutition, formation of speech, and facial expression. Reconstruction offers a unique challenge to the surgeon. Few other sites require such attention to precise details of form and function. Over the past several years, emphasis has been placed on reconstructing the aesthetic units of the lip or even the aesthetic subunits. For the upper lip, these are the filtrum and the two lateral segments. This principle can be applied in repairing smaller-sized defects of the lip and frequently obviates the need to borrow tissue from the cheek.

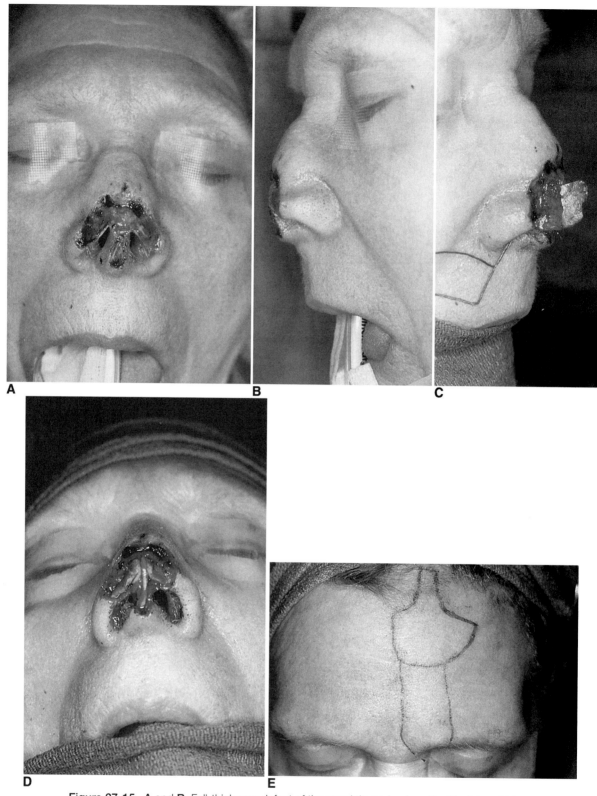

Figure 27-15. A and **B,** Full-thickness defect of the nasal tip and columella. Medial and intermediate crurae of lower lateral cartilages are absent. **C,** Composite pivotal septal flap turned outward to provide structure and mucosa for reconstruction. Bilateral hinged septal mucosal flaps have been turned downward to provide internal lining to the missing nasal tip. **D,** Septal cartilage from the composite flap replaces medial crura whereas auricular cartilage grafts replace dome cartilage bilaterally. **E,** The paramedian forehead flap is designed to resurface the nasal tip and columella.

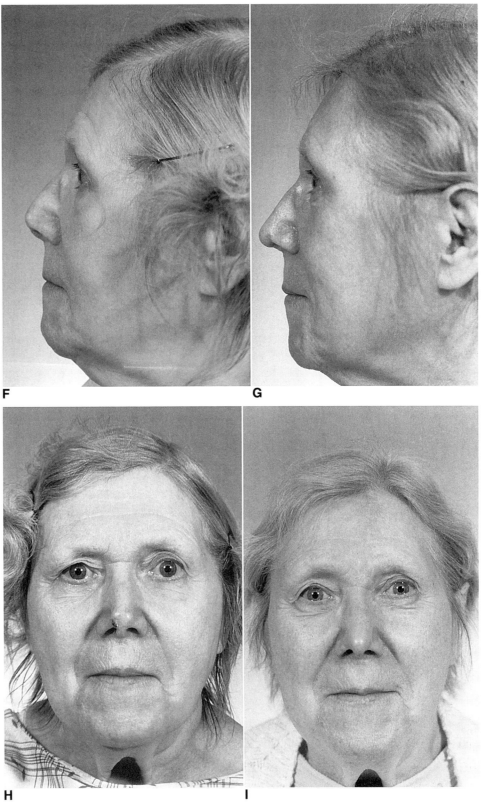

Figure 27-15, cont'd F and **G,** Preoperative **(F)** and 1-year postoperative **(G)** profiles show enhanced tip projection after reconstruction. **H** and **I,** Preoperative **(H)** and 1-year postoperative **(I)** views show restored tip definition and shape.

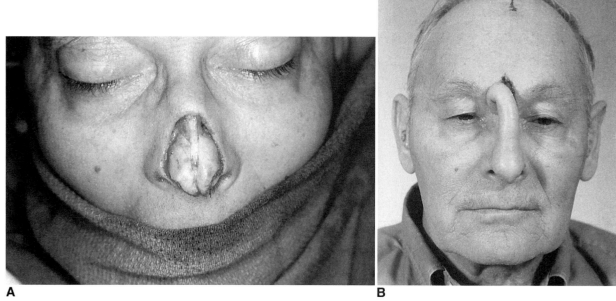

A   **B**

Figure 27-16. A and **B,** Paramedian forehead flaps are preferred for resurfacing large skin defects of the nasal tip or dorsum. A narrow pedicle enhances effective flap length.

Surgical procedures used to reconstruct the lip after tumor ablation may be classified as[2]: (1) those that use remaining lip tissue; (2) those that borrow tissue from the opposite lip; (3) those that use adjacent cheek tissue; and (4) those that use distant flaps. The first two categories enable the reconstruction to remain within the aesthetic units of the lips and, when possible, are the preferred method of surgical management. The algorithms displayed in Figures 27-17 and 27-18 provide a helpful approach to reconstruction of the lip for defects that are full thickness or that represent loss of skin and muscle.[2] This approach categorizes the size of lip defects into those less than one-half the width of the lip, those between one-half and two-thirds of the lip, and those greater than two-thirds of the lip width. The edges of the defect immediately retract, so the defect size is measured *before* excising the lesion. Defects less than one-half the lip width can usually be managed by primary wound closure or by using smaller local flaps confined to an aesthetic subunit of the lip (Figure 27-19). In the lower lip, a wedge excision should not be carried below the mental line unless necessary for tumor removal. A W-plasty at the mental line allows for rectangular excision. Lateral advancement flaps may be required when the defect base is broad. The W-shaped configuration maximizes the conservation of tissue and prevents an unsightly pointed chin, which occurs when the incision is extended below the mental crease. Primary closure should be in four layers: mucosa,

muscle, deep dermal, and skin. Care is taken to perform a precise approximation of the "white line" at the vermilion border on either side of the defect.

Primary wound closure of defects near the midline of the upper lip can be facilitated by excising a crescent of cheek skin in the perialar region to increase flap advancement. This method is similar to that described by Webster.[21] Perialar skin excision allows advancement of the remaining lip segments medially and lessens wound closure tension after primary wound repair.

Reconstruction of defects from one-half to two-thirds of the lip usually requires lip augmentation. Closure can be most readily achieved by a full-thickness pedicle flap from the opposite lip (lip switch flap) or from the adjacent cheek. The Karapendzic flap[18] may also be effective in closing medium-sized defects of the lip and, in some instances, may provide better functional results than other denervated flaps. This technique consists of circumoral incisions through the skin and subcutaneous tissue, encompassing the remaining portions of the upper and lower lips.[5] The orbicularis oris is mobilized and remains pedicled bilaterally on the superior and inferior labial arteries. Adequate mobilization enables primary closure of the defect by rotating portions of the remaining lip tissue into the defect. The advantage of the Karapendzic flap is that it restores a continuous circle of functioning orbicularis muscle to maintain oral competence. However, because no new tissue is recruited to aid in the reconstruction of the

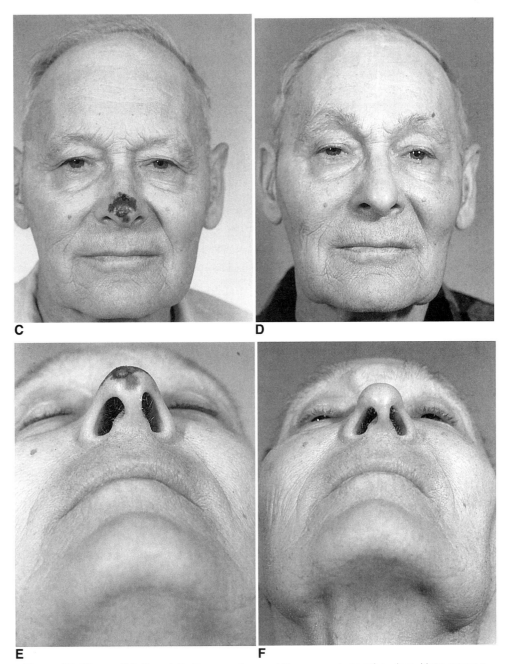

Figure 27-16, cont'd C and **D,** Preoperative and 2-year postoperative view. Note symmetry of medial brows after detachment of the pedicle. **E** and **F,** Preoperative and 2-year postoperative view.

lip, microstomia may be a problem. Also, the circumoral incisions can be unsightly. Patients 60 years of age or older often develop laxity of the oral stoma following a Karapendzic flap and do not require commissuroplasties to correct the microstomia.

Local flaps are preferable to regional flaps for closing defects of less than two-thirds of the lip width because of the close skin color, the similar texture, and the availability of mucous membrane for internal lining. Defects located away from the commissure are best closed with an Abbé flap consisting of a full-thickness flap from the opposite lip pedicled on the vermilion border and containing the labial artery.[4] Estlander[15] devised an operation for closure of a lower lip defect near the commissure of the mouth. Since the original description of the Abbé and Estlander

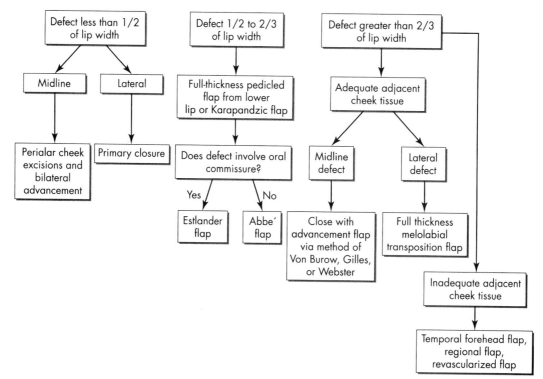

Figure 27-17. Correction of upper lip defects.

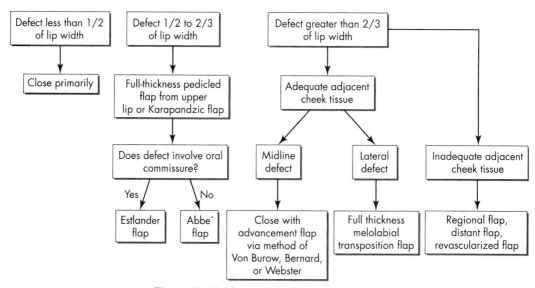

Figure 27-18. Correction of lower lip defects.

flaps, the operations have been modified to accommodate surgical defects located anywhere in the upper or lower lip.

The Abbé and Estlander flaps should be constructed so that the height of the flap equals the height of the defect. The width of the flap should be approximately one-half that of the defect to be reconstructed; however, when the entire filtrum is missing, the width of the flap should equal that of the filtrum. This will restore the total aesthetic subunit, which is preferable cosmetically and functionally. The pedicle should be made narrow to facilitate transposition and should be positioned near the center line of the recipient site. The secondary defect should be closed in four layers with accurate approximation of the vermilion border.

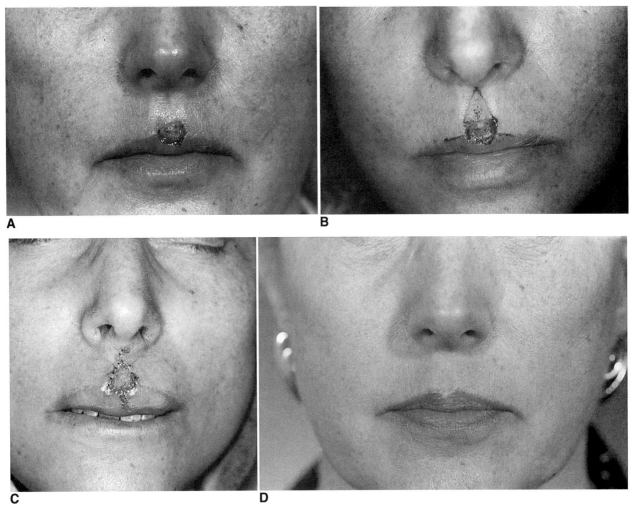

Figure 27-19. A, A small skin defect confined to the philtral aesthetic subunit. **B,** A V-Y musculocutaneous island pedicle flap is designed within the subunit. **C,** Flap advancement. **D,** The 7-month postoperative view.

The pedicle of the Abbé flap crosses the oral stoma and can be severed in 2 to 3 weeks. During the interval between transfer of the flap and the division of the pedicle, the patient is maintained on a liquid or soft diet that does not require excessive chewing. It is essential to ensure precise approximation of the vermilion border at the time of pedicle severance.

The superiorly based Estlander flap may be modified from its original description so that the flap lies within the melolabial sulcus (Figure 27-20).[10] This provides better scar camouflage of the donor site and, at the same time, allows easy rotation of the flap into the lower lip defect. The Estlander flap causes oral commissure distortion, or microstomia, which can be corrected with a secondary commissuroplasty when desired.

Defects greater than two-thirds of the width of the lip and some smaller lateral defects are best recon-

structed by using adjacent cheek flaps in the form of advancement or transposition flaps. Massive or total lip defects are best reconstructed by using regional or distant flaps or vascularized microsurgical flaps. Large defects of the upper lip can be reconstructed by transferring bilateral crescent-shaped perialar cheek tissue downward and medially (Bruns flaps). If wound closure tension is excessive, an Abbé flap can be added in the midline.[10]

Similarly, midline lower lip defects can be closed by full-thickness advancement flaps as described by Bernard,[13] Webster[21] or Gilles. These techniques may require excision of additional triangles in the melolabial sulcus to allow advancement of the cheek flaps. Triangular excision should follow the lines of the sulcus and should include only skin and subcutaneous tissues. The underlying muscle is mobilized to form a new commissure. The mucous membrane is separated

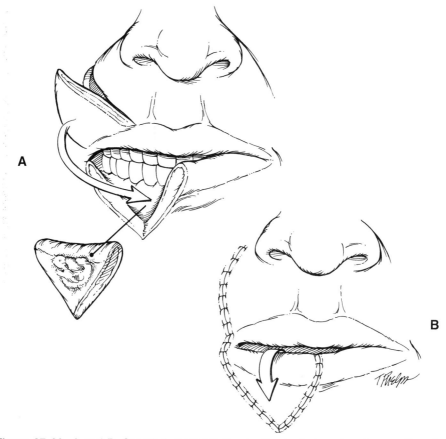

Figure 27-20. **A** and **B,** Superiorly based Estlander flap is designed so the resulting donor site scar lies within or parallel to melolabial sulcus. Mucosal advancement assists in correcting discrepancies in vermilion vertical height of flap and recipient site. (Adapted from Baker SR, Swanson N: *Local flaps in facial reconstruction*, St. Louis, Mosby, 1995.)

from the muscle and advanced outward to provide a vermilion border. Incisions are made in the gingival buccal sulcus as far posterior as the last molar tooth, if necessary, to allow proper approximation of the remaining lip segments without excessive wound closure tension.

Melolabial transposition flaps consisting of skin and subcutaneous tissue or full-thickness flaps consisting of skin, subcutaneous tissue, and mucosa can be useful in reconstructing lip defects as large as three-fourths of the width of the lip.[11] Large skin-only defects of the lateral lip are repaired nicely with melolabial flaps; however, keeping with the principles of maintaining borders between aesthetic units, some surgeons prefer to repair defects that extend from the lip onto the cheek with two separate flaps (Figure 27-21). A large rotation flap from the remaining lip segment is useful for repairing skin-only defects of the upper lip that extend into the cheek. The cheek component of the defect is then repaired by a separate transposition or advancement cheek flap. This places nearly all the scars in the melolabial sulcus while maintaining the integrity of the border between the lip and cheek aesthetic units.

Adjacent cheek tissue may not be applicable or sufficient for reconstruction of near-total defects of the lip. In such cases, regional flaps can be used for reconstruction. Excisions of the lower lip, chin, and anterior section of the mandible for carcinoma often require such flaps for reconstruction.

The temporal forehead flap designed as a bipedicle advancement or unipedicle interpolation flap can be used for total upper lip reconstruction, but the unsightly secondary deformity precludes its common use. The flap may be lined with a full-thickness skin or mucosal graft. In males, hair-bearing scalp can be incorporated to provide hair growth for scar camouflage.

Several regional flaps are used for repair of large defects of the upper and lower lip. Other publications describe the use of regional flaps in lip reconstruction.[7]

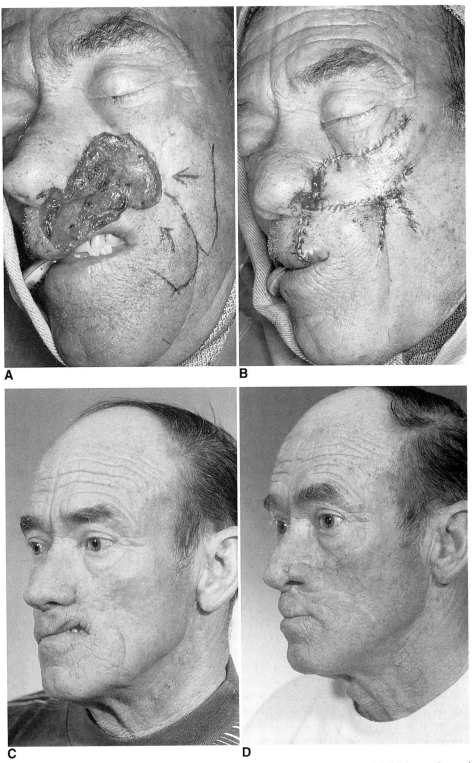

Figure 27-21. **A** and **B,** Extensive skin defect of upper lip and cheek. A full-thickness loss of the alar lobule is present. Repair of cheek and lip defects are planned with flaps harvested from separate aesthetic units of the face. Repair of the alar defect is delayed. **C** and **D,** Preoperative **(C)** and 1-year postoperative view **(D)**. The alar lobule was reconstructed with a hinged septal mucosal flap, auricular cartilage graft, and paramedian forehead flap.

Continued

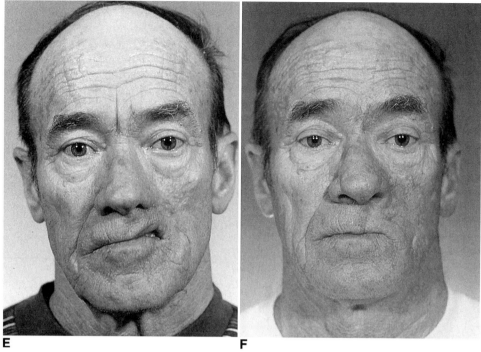

E　　　　　　　　　　　　　**F**

Figure 27-21, cont'd E and **F,** Preoperative **(E)** and 1-year postoperative view **(F).**

RECONSTRUCTION OF CHEEK DEFECTS

Relative to the nose and lip, repair of cheek defects is less complex and is usually best accomplished with transposition or advancement flaps. Rhombus-shaped and other transposition flaps are very versatile and can be used anywhere in the cheek for small- to medium-sized defects. Particular attention should be placed in designing flaps for repair of defects near the lips or eyelids. For rhombus-shaped flaps, the orientation should be designed so that the area of greatest wound closure tension is away from these structures so as not to cause distortion. Rhombus-shaped flaps are a type of transposition advancement flap. This flap is useful when the defect has a shape of a rhombus with angles approximating 120 and 60 degrees. Success of the flap depends on adjacent areas of redundant skin. These areas should lie adjacent to the 120-degree angle of the rhombus. The flap is designed by extending a line of the rhombus straight out from the point of the 120-degree angle. The length of this line should equal the length of the side of the rhombus. At the end of this line, a second line is extended parallel to the side of the defect and is of the same length. The flap is dissected in the subcutaneous plane and requires wide undermining of the entire area of the flap and defect. The flap is transposed and sutured into position. The donor site is closed primarily and represents the area of greatest wound closure tension. Usually a standing cuta-

neous deformity should be excised to complete the repair.

A bilobed flap represents a double transposition flap that has a single pivotal point and is useful in repairing larger cheek defects (Figure 27-22). The axis of the two lobes is dependent on where the resource of tissue is located and, as such, may be separated by a few degrees up to 180 degrees. The greater the separation, the greater the standing cutaneous deformity between the two lobes. Large bilobed flaps are useful for the repair of central and lateral cheek defects recruiting tissue from the remaining preauricular and infraauricular areas. Depending on the location of the defect, the first lobe may be designed as much as 20% smaller than the defect. It may be made even smaller when a great deal of advancement of the defect margins is possible or desirable. The second lobe that is used to repair the donor site of the first lobe is usually constructed 20% smaller than the first lobe. In general, the major advantage of a bilobed flap is the ability to recruit redundant tissue from two independent areas to assist in the repair of the defect. The major disadvantage of the flap is the extensive undermining that is required and the extensive linear scar that is created. When the incision lines do not fall within relaxed skin tension lines, the scars may not be favorable. Bilobed flaps for repair of cheek defects should be based inferiorly, and the standing cutaneous deformities should be excised in such a way that the

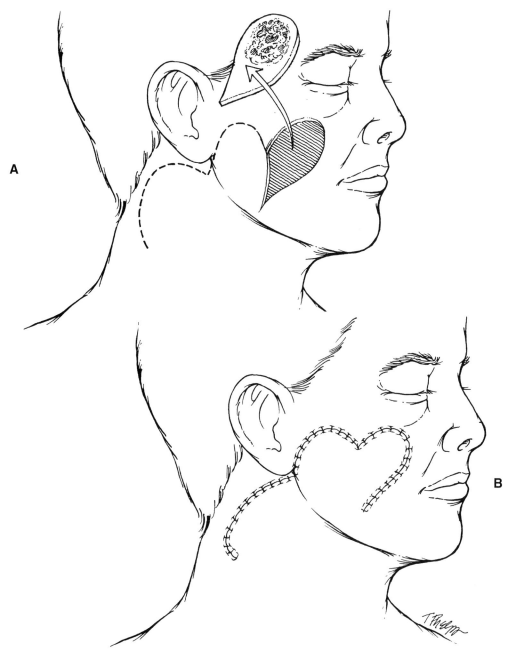

Figure 27-22. A and **B,** Bilobed flaps represent a double transposition flap with a single pivotal point. (Adapted from Baker SR, Swanson N: *Local flaps in facial reconstruction*, St. Louis, Mosby, 1995.)

resulting scars are parallel to or lie within natural skin creases.

Rotation flaps are useful for repairing medial cheek defects in the vicinity of the border between the nasal sidewall and the cheek. The curvilinear border of the flap can often be positioned along the infraorbital rim, which represents an important aesthetic boundary. By positioning the incision for the flap along this border, the surgeon can enhance scar camouflage. When possible, the margin of the rota-

tion flap should extend above the level of the lateral canthus to reduce the risk of lower lid retraction (Figure 27-23). It may also be helpful to suspend the flap to the periosteum of the lateral orbital rim. Despite these precautions, lower lid retraction is not an uncommon sequela when a rotation flap is used to repair large medial cheek defects in elderly patients, who frequently have lax lower eyelids. Large rotation flaps are particularly useful for the reconstruction of sizable defects of the posterior cheek and upper

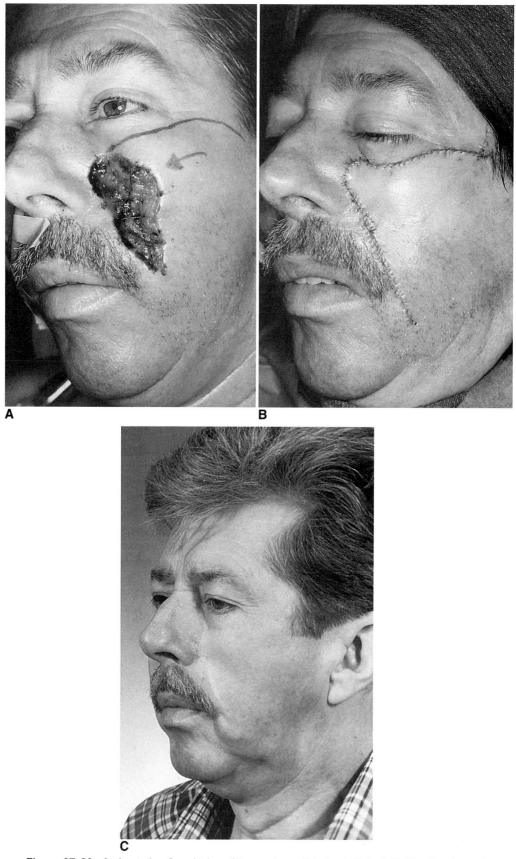

Figure 27-23. A, A rotation flap designed to repair medial cheek defect. **B,** The flap in position. The border of the flap extends above the level of the lateral canthus. **C,** The 7-year postoperative view.

neck. Large inferiorly based rotation flaps provide a flexible means for transfer of large amounts of skin from the remaining cheek and upper cervical skin.[3] Incisions for the flap are placed in a preauricular crease and can extend to the level of the clavicle or below along the anterior border of the trapezius muscle to facilitate rotation of the upper cervical skin toward the posterior cheek area. To enhance the vascularity to such flaps, it is advantageous to dissect the flap beneath the superficial musculoaponeurotic system in the cheek and beneath the platysmal muscle in the neck. A sub-superficial musculoaponeurotic system dissection in the face allows the placement of a great deal of tension on the flap without compromise of the skin vascularity. However, care should be taken to not injure the mandibular branch of the facial nerve (Figure 27-24).

Advancement flaps are dependent on the elasticity of the skin for successful repair. Many cheek defects can be closed or greatly reduced in size by simply advancing the defect margins and closing as much of the defect as possible within relaxed skin tension lines. Advancement flaps can be designed so that the incisions fall within natural skin creases of the cheek. To follow this principle, incisions used to form the border of the flap usually should diverge slightly,

rather than remaining completely parallel. It is usually necessary to remove bilateral standing cutaneous deformities near the base of the flap. This should be accomplished in such a way that the resulting scar lies within relaxed skin tension lines. As an alternative, two bilateral Z-plasties at the base of the flap reduce or eliminate the standing cutaneous deformities. Advancement flaps work well for medial and central cheek defects.

V-Y advancement flaps are particularly useful for repair of small- and medium-sized skin defects of the medial cheek near the alar facial sulcus. This technique is useful for younger patients in whom there is a lack of redundant facial skin and in patients who have considerable subcutaneous facial fat ("chipmunk cheeks") (Figure 27-25). The flap is designed in a triangular configuration with the surface area of the flap 1.5 to 2 times the surface area of the defect. The skin of the flap is isolated as an island on a subcutaneous pedicle by incising through skin around the perimeter of the flap. The subcutaneous pedicle is then dissected, flaring away from the margins of the flap. Incisions should be made through the fat down to the level of the facial musculature. This deep dissection provides the mobility of the flap, enabling it to be advanced 2 to 3 cm. This mobility is enhanced by

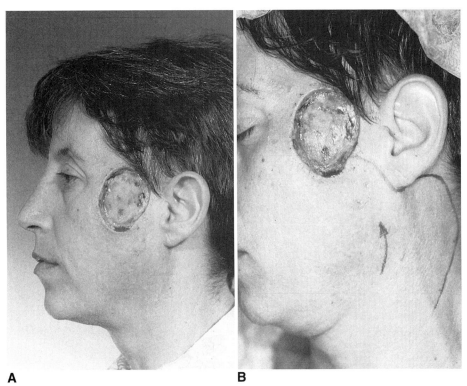

A　　　　　　　　　　　　　　**B**

Figure 27-24. A, A large cheek defect in a 40-year-old female smoker. No redundant cheek skin is available because of the patient's age. **B,** A bilobed cheek and neck flap designed for repair. *Continued*

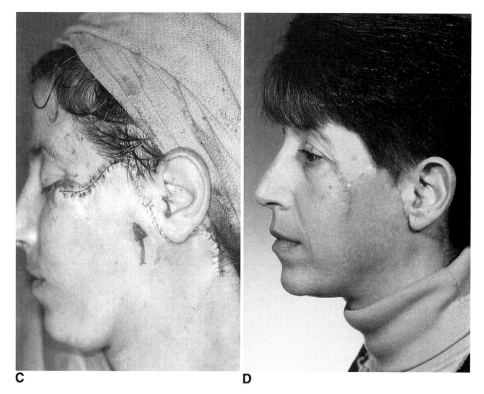

C   D

Figure 27-24, cont'd C, The flap is transferred. The flap was dissected beneath the superficial musculoaponeurotic system, which allowed great wound closure tension without compromise of skin vascularity. **D,** The 3-month postoperative view.

undermining the proximal and distal fourth of the flap just deep to the skin. The peripheral margins of the donor and recipient site should also be undermined for 2 cm in the subcutaneous plane to provide for secondary tissue movement and easy closure of the donor site. The flap is advanced and sutured in the recipient site first, followed by layered closure of the donor site.

A disadvantage of the V-Y subcutaneous advancement flap is that not all of the incisions used to harvest the flap fall within relaxed skin tension lines. However, when appropriately selected, the flap has many advantages. A major advantage is the limited dissection required compared with other techniques. Thus, there is minimal dead space with a concomitant reduced risk of the development of hematoma and seroma. Another major advantage is that no standing cutaneous deformity develops and, therefore, no tissue is discarded. The flap is harvested from the jowl area, where facial skin is most redundant and, as a consequence, there is minimal or no deformity of the melolabial fold and sulcus.

Most skin defects of the cheek can be repaired with primary closure, transposition, or rotation flaps. Transposition flaps tend to be very useful and are usu-ally harvested from adjacent cheek skin, but they can be developed in the upper neck to resurface larger defects in the lower cheek. Melolabial transposition flaps are best designed as a superiorly based flap (Figure 27-26). This design allows the recruitment of redundant skin in the lower medial face for construction of the flap. Such flaps can be used for small- to moderate-sized defects of the upper, middle, and lower medial aspect of the cheek. Positioning the base of the flap near the alar facial sulcus enhances the vascularity of the flap by including the numerous perforating vessels that extend into the subcutaneous tissue from the facial artery. Superiorly based transposition flaps are excellent for repairing defects of the medial and lateral aspect of the cheek. The flap is designed so that the medial border of the flap lies in the melolabial sulcus whenever possible. The width of the flap is dependent on the size of the defect and the quantity of donor site resource. The larger the flap or the greater the arc of pivot, the larger the standing cutaneous deformity. Excision of standing cutaneous deformities of the cheek can be accomplished at the time of flap transfer or delayed for a second stage; however, some excision of the standing cutaneous deformity is nearly always necessary because it will not completely absorb by itself.

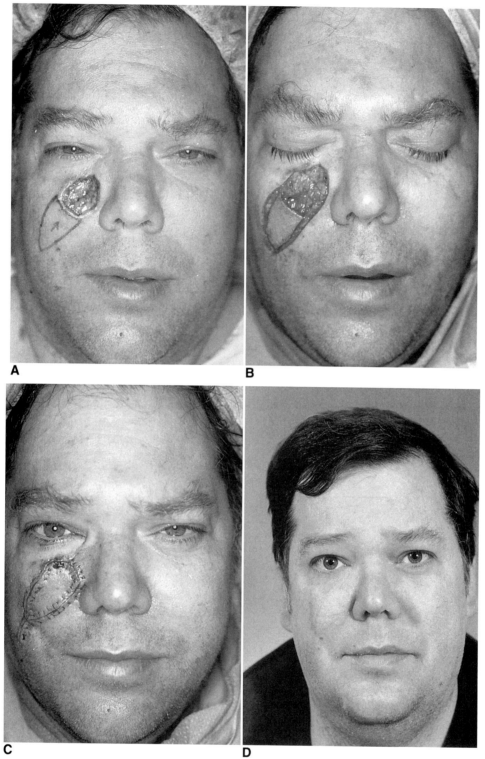

Figure 27-25. **A,** The V-Y advancement flap designed to repair medial cheek defect. **B,** The flap is based on the subcutaneous pedicle. **C,** The flap is positioned in a recipient site. **D,** The 5-month postoperative view.

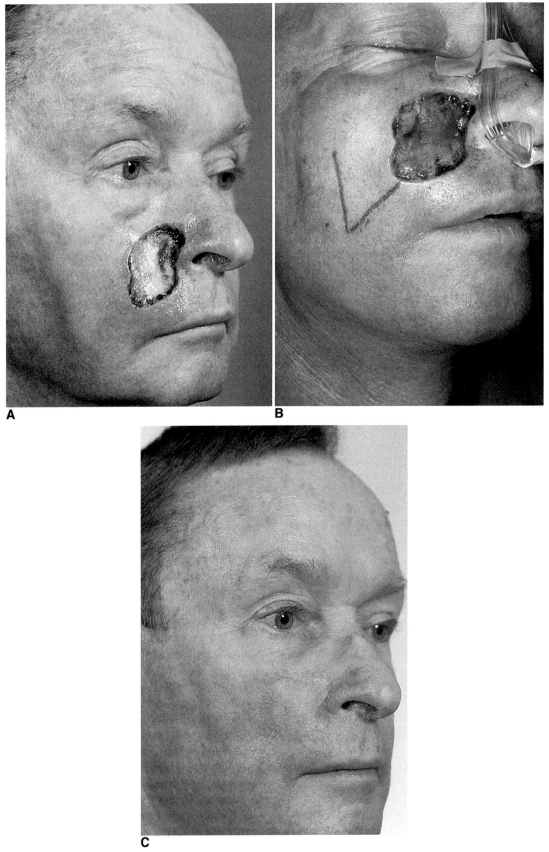

A

B

C

Figure 27-26. A, A large medial cheek defect. **B,** A superiorly based transposition flap designed for repair. **C,** The 2-month postoperative view.

FOREHEAD DEFECTS

Reconstruction of defects of the forehead should accomplish the following goals[20]: (1) preservation of frontalis muscle function; (2) preservation of sensation of the forehead skin; and (3) placement of scars within aesthetic borders or the horizontal furrows of the forehead. The forehead aesthetic unit is defined by junctional lines with the frontal scalp superiorly, the temporal scalp and temple laterally, and the eyebrows and glabella inferiorly. The forehead can be divided into aesthetic subunits, which include median, paramedian, and lateral temple.[20] The median is in the midline of the forehead. The paramedian extends from midline to a vertical axis above the pupil, and the lateral temple extends from the paramedian border to the temporal hair line laterally. Siegle[20] noted that when planning repair of forehead defects, aesthetic goals include the following: (1) maintenance of eyebrow symmetry; (2) maintenance of natural-appearing temporal and frontal hairlines; (3) the hiding of scars; when possible, along hairlines or eyebrows; (4) the creation of transverse instead of vertical scars whenever possible (except in the midline forehead); and (5) the avoidance of diagonal scars.

Primary wound repair of defects of forehead skin are often possible in older persons and in those with sun-damaged skin. Deep horizontal furrows may provide extra skin for reconstruction. When primary closure is not possible, the use of single or multiple local flaps is preferred over skin grafts because of the poor aesthetic result from the use of skin grafts. When a local flap is not possible, healing by second intention is often less deforming than a skin graft. For midline forehead defects, healing by second intention often produces a very acceptable aesthetic result, particularly when the defect is located in the superior aspect of the forehead. Should the scar not be acceptable, a later scar revision usually provides an excellent result.

Defects of the central third of the forehead can be repaired in a vertical axis with a predictably pleasant aesthetic result. This is probably caused by the natural dehiscence or attenuation of the frontalis muscle in this portion of the forehead. Larger midline defects closed in a vertical orientation can result in large standing cutaneous deformities, which may be excised with use of a W-plasty within glabellar creases (Figure 27-27). An M-plasty superiorly may also be necessary to eliminate a standing cutaneous deformity at the hairline. M-plasty and W-plasty techniques reduce the overall vertical length of the closure scar. This type of repair allows extensive undermining in the subfascial plane to facilitate closure without compromise of motor or sensory function of the forehead.

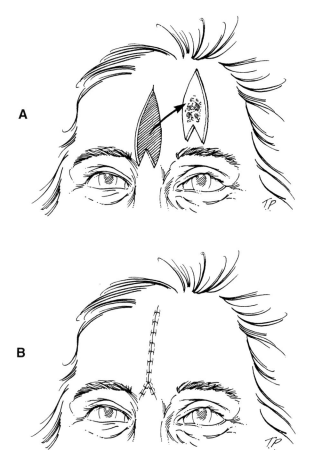

Figure 27-27. A and **B,** Closure of large midline forehead defects are often facilitated by W-plasties inferior or M-plasties superior to the border of the defect. (Adapted from Baker SR, Swanson N: *Local flaps in facial reconstruction,* St. Louis, Mosby, 1995.)

In general, vertical-oriented primary repairs, rotation flaps, and transposition flaps are to be avoided in the repair of paramedian forehead defects because they often result in vertical scars.[20] Vertical scars in the lateral two-thirds of the forehead on either side are usually wide and quite noticeable. Such scars should be avoided whenever possible and revised with a geometric closure when present. Median and paramedian forehead defects can be reconstructed with unilateral or bilateral advancement flaps, keeping most of the resulting scars oriented horizontally.

The lateral forehead represents a transition in topography from the convexity of the median and paramedian forehead to a flat lateral forehead, which continues into a slightly concave temple. The slightly concave nature of the temple makes this region of the forehead particularly good for healing by second intention. The enhanced elasticity of lateral forehead skin compared with more centrally located skin allows more reconstructive options.

Primary wound closure is also often feasible with orientation of the repair parallel to the forehead skin creases, which become curvilinear as they arc downward toward the cheek. These lines are excellent locations for placement of incisions. The location of the temporal hairline and the brow dictate the orientation and size of advancement, rotation, and transposition flaps in this area. The surgeon should take particular care in the lateral forehead area when dissecting such flaps because of the vulnerability of the frontal branch of the facial nerve. Advancement and advancement rotation flaps are perhaps most useful for repair of lateral forehead defects (Figure 27-28). Usually bilateral advancement flaps are preferred over single flaps, with the greatest advancement achieved from the more elastic laterally based flaps.

A variation of advancement flaps for repair of medium-sized defects of both the lateral and paramedian forehead is the O-T or A-T repair. This method consists of extending horizontal incisions along both sides of the defect within relaxed skin tension lines or along the border of the brow or temporal hairline. The two flaps are dissected in the subcutaneous plane and advanced toward the triangular or circular defect (Figure 27-29). Standing cutaneous deformities are resected when necessary from within the brow or are eliminated by the rule of halving the wound closure. If necessary, the standing cutaneous deformity that results from the pivotal portion of the flap movement can be removed by enlarging the defect itself. The final wound closure takes the configuration of a T-shaped repair. Thus, circular defects closed in this manner are referred to as an *O-T repair* and triangular defects (A-shaped) are referred to as an *A-T repair*. These techniques camouflage scars, except for those along the central vertical wound closure line.

Rotation flaps are very useful in reconstructing medium and large lateral forehead defects. A unilateral rotation flap, based inferiorly and laterally and designed so that its curvilinear incision follows the margin of the temporal hairline, is an excellent method of reconstructing lateral forehead defects that are close to the hairline. The curvilinear incision can be designed to incorporate hair-bearing scalp to bring hair into the reconstructed area if some of the temporal tuff has been lost.[20] The standing cutaneous deformity that inevitably forms with such a flap can be removed inferiorly in the crow's feet to camouflage the scar.

The most effective technique for reconstruction of the forehead usually involves one or more advancement flaps. Despite the relative inelasticity of forehead skin, the use of advancement flaps is preferred because they produce the most favorable cosmetic result. However, the surgeon should be aware that many skin defects of the forehead can be successfully managed by allowing the wound to heal by secondary intention. This often gives a cosmetic result that is comparable with that of flap repair when the appropriate forehead site is selected. An ideal location

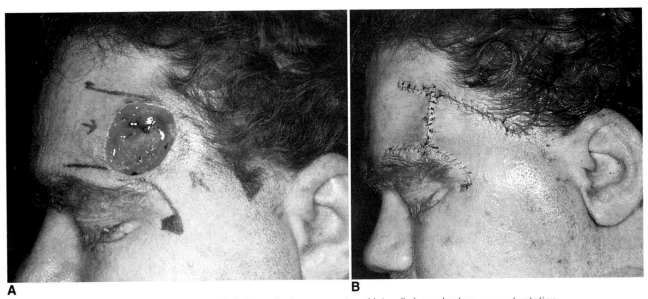

A   **B**

Figure 27-28. A, The medially based advancement and laterally based advancement rotation flap designed to repair lateral forehead defect. **B,** The flaps advanced. A standing cutaneous deformity of the laterally based flap is removed in periocular rhytid.

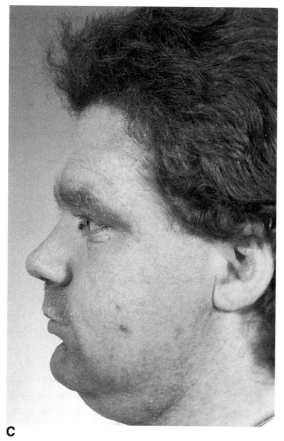

C

Figure 27-28, cont'd C, The 6-month postoperative view.

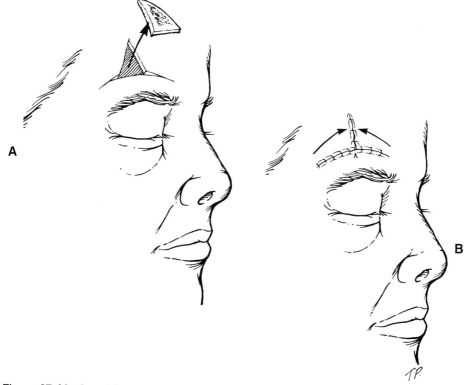

A

B

Figure 27-29. A and **B,** A T-shaped repair of a lateral forehead defect. (Adapted from Baker SR, Swanson N: *Local flaps in facial reconstruction*, St. Louis, Mosby, 1995.)

for healing by secondary intention is high on the forehead well away from the brow, in the central or lateral third of the forehead.

Tissue expansion enables the surgeon to reconstruct sizable forehead defects, which in the past could be repaired only with skin grafts. Controlled, prolonged tissue expansion can be used to reconstruct very large forehead defects by expansion of the remaining forehead skin over 6 to 12 weeks. Reconstruction is achieved by direct advancement of the expanded skin or used in combination with other scalp, cheek, or temple skin flaps. The disadvantages of tissue expansion include the fact that it is a two-staged procedure and considerable deformity of the forehead is present during the expansion process. These disadvantages are far outweighed by the excellent results that can be achieved with tissue expansion in the repair of very large defects of the forehead.[9]

REFERENCES

1. Alford EL, Baker SR, Shumrick KA: *Midforehead flaps.* In Baker SR, Swanson NA, editors: *Local flaps in facial reconstruction,* St. Louis, 1995, Mosby.

2. Baker SR: *Lip reconstruction.* In Holt GR, Gates GA, Mattox DE, editors: *Decision making in otolaryngology,* Burlington, Ontario, 1983, Mosby.

3. Baker SR: Local cutaneous flaps in soft tissue augmentation and reconstruction in the head and neck, *Otolaryngol Clin North Am* 27:139, 1994.

4. Baker SR: *Malignancy of the lip.* In Gluckman J, editor: *Otolaryngology,* ed 3, Philadelphia, 1988, WB Saunders.

5. Baker SR: *Options for reconstruction in head and neck surgery.* In Cummings CW and others, editors: *Otolaryngology—head and neck surgery: update 1,* St. Louis, 1989, Mosby.

6. Baker SR: *The orbit and midface.* In Soutar DS, Tiwari R, editors: *Excision and reconstruction in head and neck cancer,* New York, 1994, Churchill Livingstone.

7. Baker SR: Regional flaps in facial reconstruction, *Facial Plast Surg* 23:925, 1990.

8. Baker SR, Johnson TM, Nelson BR: The importance of maintaining the alar facial sulcus in nasal reconstruction, *Arch Otolaryngol Head Neck Surg* 121:617, 1995.

9. Baker SR, Johnson TM, Nelson BR: Technical aspects of prolonged scalp expansion, *Arch Otolaryngol Head Neck Surg* 120:431, 1994.

10. Baker SR, Krause CJ: *Cancer of the lip.* In Suen JY, Myers EN, editor: *Cancer of the head and neck,* New York, 1981, Churchill Livingstone.

11. Baker SR, Krause CJ: Pedicle flaps in reconstruction of the lip, *Facial Plast Surg* 1:61, 1983.

12. Baker SR, Swanson NA: Regional and distant skin flaps in nasal reconstruction, *Facial Plast Surg* 2:33, 1984.

13. Bernard C: Concer de la levre inferieure opéré par un procédé nouveau, *Bulletin et memoirs de la société de chirugic* 3:357, 1853.

14. Burget GC, Menick FJ: *Aesthetic reconstruction of the nose,* St. Louis, 1993, Mosby.

15. Estlander JA: Eine methods aus der einen Lippe Substanzverlustre der Onderen zu Ersetzen, *Arch für Klin Chir* 14:622, 1872.

16. Grabb WC, Myers MB: *Skin flaps,* Boston, Little Brown, 1975.

17. Johnson TM and others: Utility of the subcutaneous hinge flap in nasal reconstruction, *Dermatol Surg* 3:459, 1994.

18. Karapandzic M: Reconstruction of lip defects by local arterial flaps, *Br J Plast Surg* 27:93, 1974.

19. Panje WR, Minor LB: *Reconstruction of the scalp.* In Baker SR, Swanson NA, editors: *Local flaps in facial reconstruction,* St. Louis, 1995, Mosby.

20. Siegle RJ: *Reconstruction of the forehead.* In Baker SR, Swanson NA, editors: *Local flaps in facial reconstruction,* St. Louis, 1995, Mosby.

21. Webster JP: Crescentic peri-alar cheek excision for upper lip flap advancement with a short history of upper lip repair, *Plast Reconstr Surg* 16:434, 1955.

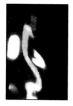

CHAPTER TWENTY EIGHT

HAIR RESTORATION: MEDICAL AND SURGICAL TECHNIQUES

|| Benjamin M. Loos
|| Sheldon S. Kabaker

INTRODUCTION

Throughout history, powerful cultural symbolism has been associated with hair—both its length and its loss. An individual's hair plays an important role in his or her overall appearance. Framing the face, hair helps to draw the observer to the focus of the face: the eyes. Hair also conveys nonverbal clues about an individual's age and personality. Long, luxuriant hair is associated with youthfulness and physical attractiveness. Balding, thinning, and graying hair signifies maturity and advanced age.

As a result, hair restoration has long been considered an integral part of facial rejuvenation. Scalp hair loss—alopecia—can dramatically affect an individual. In fact, alopecia has been associated with significant changes in self-image, psychological well-being, and even success in career.[6] Hair loss draws attention to the forehead, the scalp, and the shape of the head and distracts the viewer from the central face and eyes. Hair loss can be a source of tremendous patient concern and anxiety. Subsequently, individuals invest considerable time and money in seeking treatment.

Unfortunately, neither gender escapes the difficulties associated with hair loss. In women, greater distress may be associated with even minimal hair loss, because alopecia in women is a less common and accepted problem.[6] Although alopecia is the result of several different processes, the most common cause remains androgenetic alopecia (AGA). In men, AGA is characterized by the classic hereditary male-pattern baldness. In women, it manifests as a diffuse thinning with an intact anterior hairline, although occasionally a male-pattern type of hair loss can occur. AGA affects more than half of the male population and up to 40% of women over the age of 70.[5,15]

Aging and hair loss are dynamic processes. Therefore, the goal of treatment should be to create and maintain an appearance that remains natural over time. In recent years there has been an explosive growth in techniques for the management of alopecia. New advances in both medical and surgical treatments have been developed and modified to achieve more natural-appearing and undetectable hair restoration. Current medical therapies provide powerful treatment options that arrest hair loss and, in some patients, provide hair regrowth. Advanced surgical techniques such as follicular-unit hair transplantation have replaced the traditional procedures such as plug grafts, scalp reductions, and rotational flaps to become the state of the art in terms of inconspicuous hair restoration. The goal of this chapter is to provide an overview of the pathophysiology, the evaluation, and the current medical and surgical management of hair loss.

PATHOPHYSIOLOGY

The average scalp has approximately 100,000 to 150,000 hairs.[1] Each hair contains both a matrix that is located below the dermis and a visible hair shaft (see Figure 28-1). The matrix lies beneath the dermis in the subcutaneous fat at the base of the hair follicle and contains rapidly dividing cells that migrate superiorly into the zone of keratinization. In this zone, cells undergo a process of dehydration and chemical change that results in the formation of the hair shaft, which is a dense mass of dead keratinized cells. As more cells are added to the base of the follicle, the shaft is displaced superiorly, and the hair shaft grows to become visible at the surface.

The formation of hair is a cyclical process that has periods of growth, involution, and rest. The majority of hair follicles in the scalp (approximately 90%) are in the growth, or *anagen*, phase. For the scalp, this growth phase lasts approximately 1000 days and is longer in women than in men. The next stage is the *catagen* or involutional phase, in which less than 1% of the hair follicles are present at a given time. This stage is quite short and lasts for less than two weeks for scalp hair. Entry into this stage is random in

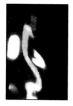

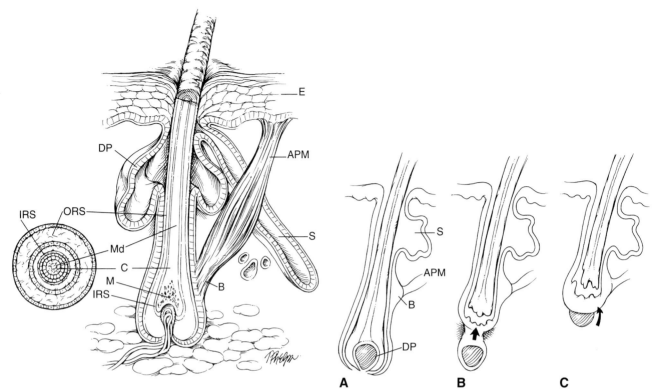

Figure 28-1. Anatomy of the hair follicle and the different phases of the hair cycle: **A,** anagen; **B,** catagen; and **C,** telogen. Structures labeled include the *arrector pili muscle (APM),* bulge *(B), cortex (C), dermal papilla (DP), epidermis (E), inner root sheath (IRS), matrix (M), medulla (Md), outer root sheath (ORS),* and *sebaceous gland (S).* Panel A adapted from Bennett RG: *Anatomy and physiology of the skin.* In Papel ID, editor: *Facial plastic and reconstructive surgery,* ed 2. Papel, New York. 2002, Thieme, p 11. Panels B and C modified from Cotsarelis G, Sun TT, Lavker RM: Label-retaining cells reside in the bulge area of pilosebaceous unit: implications for follicular stem cells, hair cycle, and skin carcinogenesis, *Cell* 61:1329, 1990, as reprinted in Stough DB, Haber RS, editors: *Hair replacement: surgical and medical.* St Louis, 1996, Mosby, p 222.

humans in contrast with some animals, which have seasonal variations (e.g. molting). The remaining 5% to 10% of hair follicles are in the resting, or *telogen,* phase. This stage last approximately 3 to 4 months and, during this phase, there is no active hair growth.[1] At the end of the telogen phase, the hair shaft is extruded and shed; up to 100 hairs are shed as a result of this process each day. The cycle begins again with the anagen phase. Androgens play an essential role in regulating hair growth. At puberty, androgens increase the size of the follicles in the beard, chest, and extremities while decreasing the follicles' size in the bitemporal region, thereby reshaping the anterior hairline.[41]

Androgenetic Alopecia (AGA)

There are various etiologies of hair loss. AGA—or male-pattern baldness—is the most common cause in both genders (Table 28-1). AGA eventually affects 60% to 80% of white men and can begin as early as puberty.

In fact, approximately 20% of men note some hair loss at puberty, and the number increases sequentially with each decade. For example, by 30 years of age, 30% of white men have noted baldness, and, by 50 years of age, approximately 50% to 60% demonstrate alopecia.[15] In women, the onset is typically later, with 40% of women 70 years old or older demonstrating alopecia.[5]

The incidence of AGA varies among ethnic groups. The black population, the incidence is approximately one fourth of that of white men.[46] Japanese men have a similar incidence of AGA as compared with black men during the earlier years, but the incidence increases to one third that of whites as age advances.[47] In Chinese men, AGA is rare before age 40.[15] In all groups of patients, the incidence and severity of AGA increase with age.

The development of AGA is dependent on several factors. In a study of identical twins, Hamilton showed that the extent and development of AGA depended on the interaction of three factors: androgens, genetic

TABLE 28-1

VARIOUS ETIOLOGIES OF ALOPECIA

Diffuse hair loss	Focal hair loss
Nonscarring	Nonscarring
Androgenetic alopecia	Androgenetic alopecia
Alopecia areata	Alopecia areata
Anagen effluvium	Trichotillomania
Congenital hypotrichosis or atrichia	Traction alopecia
Hair shaft abnormalities	Hair shaft abnormalities
Syphilis	Tinea capitis
Telogen effluvium	Syphilis
Thyroid disorders	
Postpartum	Scarring
Postmenopause	Lacerations
Drug induced	Postsurgical
Iron deficiency	Burns
Malnutrition	Radiation
Physiologic stress	Neoplasms
Psychological stress	Discoid lupus erythematosus
	Sarcoidosis
	Dermatomyositis
	Lichen planopilaris
	Scleroderma variant morphea
	Temporal arteritis
	Bacterial folliculitis
	Herpetic infections

predisposition, and age.[15] The interaction of several genes (polygenic) and certain environmental factors influence the expression of hair loss.[2,25] It is most important to note that androgens play a critical role in the development of hair loss. No expression of baldness occurs in the absence of circulating androgens.

Hair follicles on the scalp are genetically predisposed to be either sensitive or resistant to androgenic factors that inhibit hair growth. Autograft studies have demonstrated this genetic predisposition. For example, hair follicles from the occipital scalp that are immune to androgens were transplanted to the bald frontal scalp and continued to grow. These findings established the concept of donor dominance and the basis for successful hair-graft transplantation.[39]

Various androgens variably affect different regions of hair growth. Testosterone influences axillary and pubic hair growth, whereas dihydrotestosterone (DHT) affects beard growth and scalp hair, specifically the development of AGA.[42] In addition, a hair's sensitivity to androgens may change over time; this accounts for the effect of age, puberty, and possibly environment.

Extensive hair loss in men is not necessarily a reflection of an overall increase in testosterone. Two enzymes play critical roles in AGA (Figure 28-2). The 5-alpha reductase enzyme is responsible for the

metabolism of testosterone into DHT, which is the androgen that is most directly associated with the inhibition of hair growth and AGA. The cytochrome P-450 aromatase enzyme also has an important role in the hormonal pathway. Aromatase metabolizes testosterone into estradiol and androstenedione into estrone.[45] A decrease in aromatase consequently increases the amount of testosterone that will be metabolized into DHT via the 5-alpha reductase pathway. Therefore, AGA is mediated by increased 5-alpha reductase activity and by the lack of aromatase enzyme in specific regions of the scalp, thereby resulting in higher levels of DHT.

The end result of this androgen-mediated process in the development of AGA is the miniaturization of susceptible hair follicles. The follicles become progressively smaller in size and have shorter periods of growth so that coarse, terminal hairs progress through a thinner, more lightly pigmented intermediate phase before they are replaced by fine vellus hairs (see Figure 28-3).[34] In women, this process may advance beyond the stage of vellus hairs to produce a bald scalp that is completely free of hair.

Other Etiologies

Although androgenetic alopecia is the most common cause of hair loss, a variety of other etiologies should

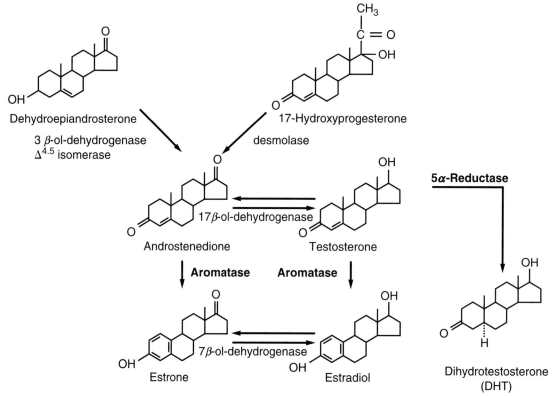

Figure 28-2. The androgen metabolic pathway within the skin. Both 5-alpha reductase and aromatase have significant roles in androgenetic alopecia. From Stough DB, Haber RS, editors: *Pathophysiology of androgenic alopecia,* St Louis, 1996, Mosby, p 11.

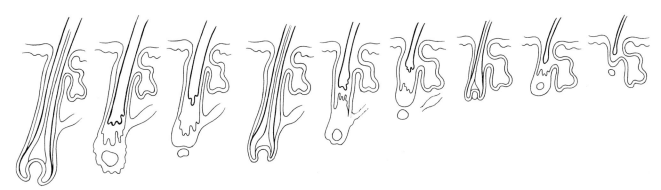

Figure 28-3. Miniaturization of the hair follicle in androgenetic alopecia. Hair grows for shorter periods of time, becoming smaller, finer, and lighter as it approaches the vellus stage. From Stough DB, Haber RS, editors: *Pathophysiology of androgenic alopecia,* St Louis, 1996, Mosby, p 9.

be considered in the patient's evaluation (Table 28-1). Alopecia manifests as either a focal or diffuse process and can be associated with or without scarring. Scarring can directly injure the hair follicle and lead to focal alopecia. Scarring alopecia is typically seen in patients with traumatic injuries such as lacerations, burns, and radiation as well as with selective connective tissue dis-eases, including discoid lupus erythematosus, lichen planopilaris, dermatomyositis, and sarcoidosis.[11] If only the hair shaft is damaged, alopecia will be temporary, because the underlying follicular apparatus will con-tinue to grow new hair. If the follicle, including the matrix, is completely destroyed, the loss of hair will likely be permanent. Traumatic, nonscarring alopecia may also occur as a result of externally applied traction with certain hairstyles (e.g., cornrows, hair weaves).

Infectious etiologies should be considered in cases of focal alopecia. *Staphylococcus aureus, Streptococcus,* and syphilis are associated with folliculitis and furuncles, which can possibly result in scarring and permanent alopecia. Tinea capitis is a fungal infection that results in focal, nonscarring alopecia and is diagnosed with a Wood's light or a potassium hydroxide preparation of a hair sample.[11]

Diffuse, nonscarring alopecia is often associated with telogen effluvium in which diffuse hair shedding occurs as hairs precipitously shift from the growth phase to the resting phase. Telogen effluvium is a physiologic response to a variety of stressors including hormonal or systemic conditions and a broad range of medications. Hypothyroidism, hyperthyroidism, postpartum, and postmenopause are frequently seen as manifesting with diffuse alopecia.[13] Categories of drugs that may result in temporary hair loss include chemotherapy agents, anticoagulants, anticonvulsants, thyroid replacement, beta-blockers, tricyclic antidepressants, and oral contraceptives.[13] Patients with malnutrition—specifically with deficiencies in protein and essential minerals such as zinc and iron—may have poor hair growth and develop alopecia. Finally, patients undergoing severe physiologic (e.g., with acute and chronic systemic illness) or significant psychological stress can suffer from temporary hair loss.[13]

Focal or diffuse alopecia can also result from alopecia areata. Alopecia areata is an autoimmune disease that affects almost 2% of the population and typically manifests as small round patches of hair loss without evidence of scarring.[41,44] The hair loss ranges in severity from small areas of alopecia that spontaneously regrow to persistent, extensive patches. The extent of loss can include the complete loss of all scalp hair (alopecia totalis) or all hair on the body (alopecia universalis).[41] Inflammation may play a role by stimulating cytokines and growth factors, which retard hair growth.[10]

PATIENT EVALUATION

When evaluating a patient with hair loss, a detailed history and physical examination are mandatory for the proper diagnosis and treatment of the underlying etiology. Focused questioning should center on the hair loss' onset, progression, location, and other associated conditions that affect the skin, joints, and thyroid gland. Past medical history and medications need to be reviewed. Family history can also play an important role in predicting the probable progressive pattern of future hair loss in androgenetic alopecia.

For the majority of women with AGA, extensive hormonal evaluation is not necessary. Testing total

testosterone, dehydroepiandrosterone, and prolactin levels is warranted if any of the following conditions associated with androgen excess are present: hirsutism, severe cystic acne, irregular menses, infertility, virilization, or galactorrhea. Measuring thyroid-stimulating hormone levels may be helpful if thyroid abnormalities are suspected. A complete blood count and iron studies should also be considered for a woman who has heavy or long-lasting menses.[41]

Examination of the scalp skin should include evaluating the pattern of hair loss as well as any skin lesions that are indicative of infection or malignancy. Hamilton[15] published the first useful classification of AGA in 1951; Norwood's[32] modification has become the standard system of classification used by hair restoration surgeons. This complete classification system includes seven categories (Figure 28-4). The anterior hairline is altered with bitemporal recession occurring first, followed by balding of the vertex. As a more uniform frontal recession progresses posteriorly, the entire frontoparietal region eventually bears only inconspicuous vellus hair. The inferior occipital and temporal scalp are spared, resulting in the classic hair fringe.

Female-baldness patterns can be similar to those seen in men, and, in these patients, the Norwood classification system can be used. However, female alopecia more often consists of a diffuse thinning in an oval area on top of the scalp. In 1977, Ludwig classified AGA in females into three stages (Figure 28-5).[29] In Grade I, only perceptible thinning of the hair occurs at the vertex, while a thin band of more dense hair from 1 to 3 cm in width is retained at the hairline. More advanced stages correlate with an increase in hair loss on the vertex and a progressive thinning of the anterior hairline.

PATIENT COUNSELING

The initial consultation of a patient with hair loss must foster open communication and trust. Often these patients suffer from an altered body image and insecurity about their physical appearance. The patient must understand that the goal is not necessarily to restore his or her previous head of hair but rather to remove the appearance of baldness by recreating hairlines and increasing hair density (Figure 28-6).

Hair restoration surgery is a calculated risk. Although family history and age at the time of presentation may give the surgeon some feel for the possible course of hair loss, these factors are by no means always predictive. In cases of AGA, it should be impressed upon the patient that the natural progression of alopecia is usually relentless and often unpredictable. Ideally, management should allow for changes in the hair pattern with an ever-increasing bald area and a decreasing supply of permanent hair as

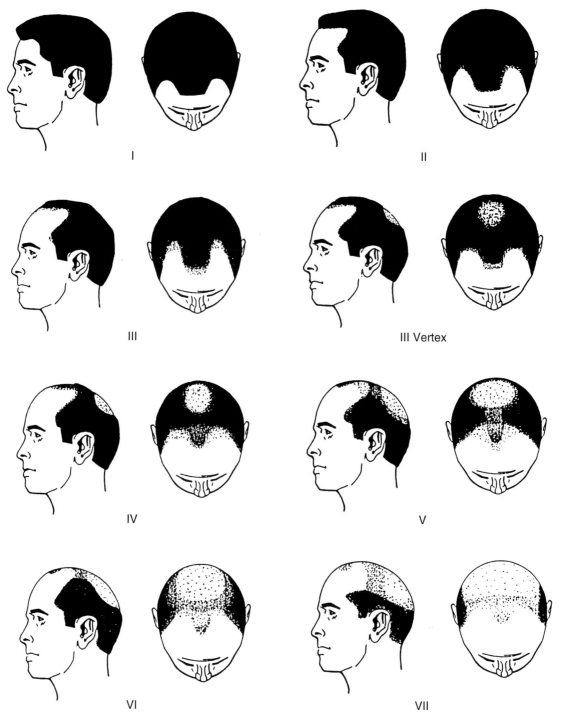

Figure 28-4. Norwood classification of the most common types of male-pattern baldness. From Norwood OT: Male pattern baldness: classification and incidence, *South Med J* 68:1359, 1975. Courtesy of Charles C. Thomas, Publisher, Ltd, Springfield, Illinois.

the patient ages. As a result, the physician should evaluate the patients' subjective expectations and provide realistic options and outcomes. As with any facial plastic surgical procedure, photodocumentation of physical findings, specifically the hair loss pattern, needs to be done in a consistent manner.

MEDICAL MANAGEMENT

Before considering a surgical approach to a patient's alopecia, any treatable etiologic factors should be eliminated. Endocrinopathies associated with hair loss should be appropriately managed. Scalp infections need to be properly diagnosed and treated. Autoimmune

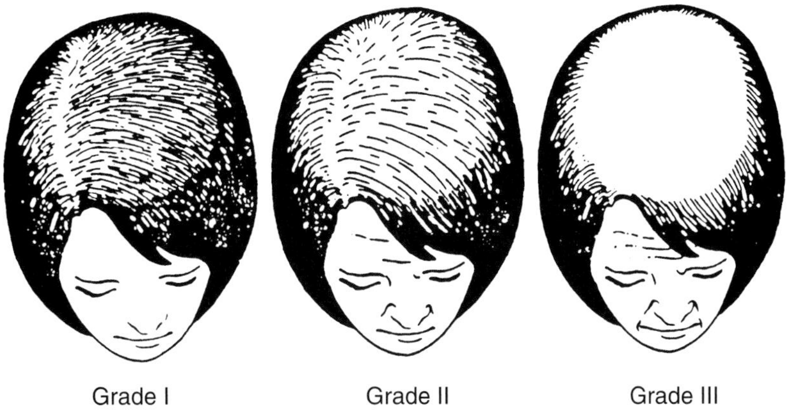

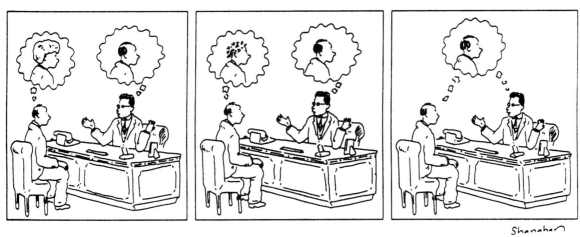

Grade I   Grade II   Grade III

Figure 28-5. Ludwig classification of female-pattern baldness. From Montagna W, Parakkal PF: *The structure and function of the skin*, ed 3. New York, Academic Press, 1974. To view this image in color, please go to *www.ototext.com* or the Electronic Image Collection CD, bound into your copy of Cummings Otolaryngology—Head and Neck Surgery, 4th edition.

Figure 28-6. The initial consultation must foster the open discussion of realistic and obtainable goals. From Quinlan P: *The Consultation*, p. 29. To view this image in color, please go to *www.ototext.com* or the Electronic Image Collection CD, bound into your copy of Cummings Otolaryngology—Head and Neck Surgery, 4th edition.

conditions such as alopecia areata, lichen planopilaris, and lupus erythematosus can benefit from corticosteroid therapy delivered either topically, orally, or intralesionally.

Numerous topical and oral treatments for androgenetic hair loss claim hair regrowth. Only two therapies, topical minoxidil (Rogaine) and oral finasteride (Propecia), have been clinically proven to be effective for preventing further hair loss and promoting future growth. Both drugs affect the hair-growth cycle via different mechanisms of action and result in an increase in existing hairs' length and diameter.

Minoxidil

Topical minoxidil is a piperidinopyrimidine derivative vasodilator that possesses trichogenic properties. Topical minoxidil is available in two strengths (2% and 5%) and is applied topically to the scalp twice daily. Minoxidil is safe for both men and women for the treatment of androgenetic hair loss. Originally used as an oral antihypertensive medication, minoxidil acts as a potassium-channel agonist, thereby resulting in a reduction in cytoplasmic-free calcium. The relevance of this unique cellular mechanism to hair growth is unclear. Various theories have postulated that hair growth is due to several mechanisms at the cellular level: 1) decreased activity of epidermal growth factor; 2) increased angiogenesis as a result of the up-regulated expression of vascular endothelial growth factor; and 3) increased activation of prostaglandin endoperoxide synthase-1.[26,31,33]

In several clinical trials, applying topical minoxidil (2%) twice daily resulted in dense hair regrowth on the vertex scalp in less than 5% of patients, while 25% to 30% of patients demonstrated moderate hair regrowth over one year.[7,35,38] In patients for whom significant hair regrowth did not occur, minoxidil did appear to stop or significantly slow the progression of

AGA.[43] The results in women with AGA have been similar to those seen in men. Unfortunately, maintenance of the regrowth is dependent on continued use of minoxidil. When the treatment is discontinued, the hair gained is lost, and the hair that should have been shed during the treatment period will follow within three to four months. For those who continue its use, a peak effect is reached at approximately one year, with a subsequent slow decline in regrowth.[36,37]

Adverse reactions associated with topical minoxidil are primarily limited to irritant dermatitis or folliculitis (3%–5%) and allergic contact dermatitis (<1%).[35] Modifying treatment to include a lower concentration and less frequent application may alleviate these reactions. Increased hair growth (hypertrichosis) outside of the area of application (e.g., eyebrows, face, ears, arms, beard) has been reported, more commonly in women. The reason is unclear, but its occurrence is possibly the result of the inadvertent transfer of the topical solution.[8,34] Patient compliance is also an issue with topical minoxidil given its oily consistency and twice-daily application.

Finasteride

Finasteride (Propecia) is a type 2 5-alpha reductase inhibitor that results in the suppression of circulating DHT, the hormone that directly affects AGA. Finasteride has no affinity for the androgen receptor and therefore does not interfere with the actions or effects of testosterone.

In studies of males between the ages of 18 and 41 with mild to moderate hair loss, 1 mg of finasteride was administered daily for 24 months. After 12 months, 48% to 65% of patients maintained or increased their hair counts, primarily on the vertex and anterior midscalp. After 24 months, the number of patients that responded increased to 66% to 80%.[20,28,40] A 5-year controlled clinical trial demonstrated that 65% of men taking finasteride maintained or improved their hair count as compared with hair counts taken at the start of the study, whereas men taking placebo continued to lose hair. In addition, a reviewing of standardized clinical photographs, showed 90% of men on finasteride were rated as having no further visible hair loss as compared with baseline vs 25% of patients on placebo.[21] As is the case with minoxidil, patients need to be on continued therapy to preserve the renewed hair growth. Recent studies have noted a possible synergistic response with the combination therapy of minoxidil and finasteride.[9,22,49]

Adverse effects of finasteride are limited to decreased sexual libido, erectile dysfunction, and decreased ejaculate volume; these adverse effects were reported in 0.8% to 1.8% of patients in the treatment group taking finasteride. Interestingly, the placebo group also reported the same adverse effects in 0.4% to 1.3% of patients. These problems resolve with discontinued therapy. By the end of the fifth year, the incidence of side effects was 0.3% or less among men taking finasteride. Other recent other studies have also found no significant difference in sexual function between treated patients and age-matched control males[48]; these findings are consistent with the experience of many clinicians. In addition, finasteride has been shown to lower a patient's prostate-specific antigen (PSA). Therefore, with older men, a new baseline level should be obtained after approximately four months of therapy. Finasteride is limited to male patients because of its teratogenic effects during pregnancy.

SURGICAL MANAGEMENT

Surgical options for alopecia range from individual follicular-unit hair graft transplantation to scalp reductions and axial flap transfers. The goals of surgery are to create a natural-appearing hairline and to increase scalp coverage. Prediction of future hair loss needs to be factored into the surgical planning. In addition, the patient must be informed that usually three to four grafting sessions may be required to recreate a substantial anterior hairline and an increase in hair density. During the initial consultation, it is extremely unlikely, despite many marketing claims to the contrary, for hair restoration to be completed in one operative session.

Follicular-Unit Hair Transplantation

Hair transplantation with hair grafts has been modified over the last two decades to become the established method of choice for hair restoration. Earlier grafting techniques depended on harvesting 4-mm round punch grafts, which evolved into 3- to 6-hair minigrafts and single-hair micrografts. The principal problems with the larger grafts have been related to the unnatural creation of a "doll's-hair" or "toothbrush" appearance that is the result of circumferential contracture and compression of the hair follicles during wound healing (Figure 28-7).

Micrografts were primarily reserved for the transition zones (e.g., the anterior hairline), because these individual hairs blend naturally. Micrografts are too small to provide substantial density in more posterior areas. Nonetheless, micrografts have evolved into the concept of follicular-unit grafts. Follicular units are naturally occurring groups of one to four terminal hairs.[4] All of the support structures, including sebaceous glands, subcutaneous fat, and a circumferential band of collagen around the follicle, are left intact. The final result is a more natural look as compared with micrografts, which consist of multiple, partial,

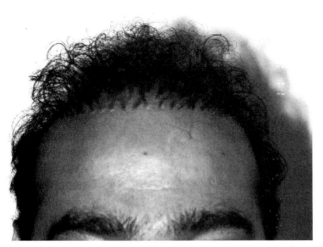

Figure 28-7. The classic "doll's hair" appearance results from circumferential contracture and compression of the hair follicle after placement of 4-mm punch grafts. To view this image in color, please go to *www.ototext.com* or the Electronic Image Collection CD, bound into your copy of Cummings Otolaryngology—Head and Neck Surgery, 4th edition.

or complete follicular units along with intervening skin (Figure 28-8). The ideal candidates for transplantation have minimal contrast between hair color and skin color, an adequate donor area, and are old enough that future hair loss is more likely to be predictable.

Preoperative Evaluation

During the preoperative evaluation of the patient, specific attention should be given to planning the anterior hairline. The lowest point of the hairline, called the trichion, frames the face. In terms of dividing the face into proportional vertical thirds, the distance between the trichion and the glabella should equal the distance between the glabella and the subnasale (see Figure 28-9). However, in patients with significant hair loss and regression, the newly created hairline should be placed higher for a more aesthetically acceptable appearance. The hairline design should have some degree of frontotemporal recession while augmenting a dense frontal forelock. The natural hairline does not abruptly start on the forehead; instead, a 0.5- to 1-cm "feathering" transition zone exists and needs to be recreated using fine, single-hair, follicular-unit grafts. The balding vertex should be addressed thoughtfully given that hair loss will progress in this region in a circumferential manner. Donor grafts may provide some coverage, but they may be insufficient in number to adequately cover these areas during the patient's lifetime.

Other planned recipient regions can be marked out on the scalp in a grid pattern of 1-cm² dimensions (see Figure 28-10). By creating a grid pattern over the recipient sites, the surgeon is able to ensure a uniform distribution, hair grafts during their placement.

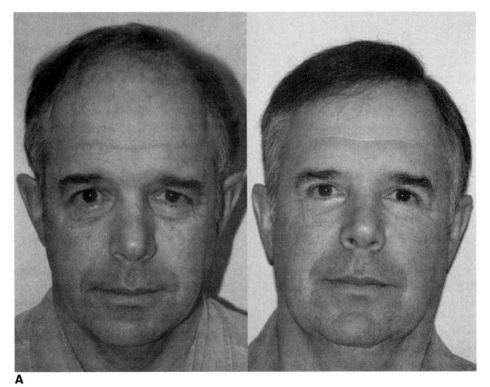

A

Figure 28-8. A, Preoperative and **B,** postoperative photographs after three sessions of follicular-unit hair transplantation using approximately 1500 grafts per session. To view this image in color, please go to *www.ototext.com* or the Electronic Image Collection CD, bound into your copy of Cummings Otolaryngology—Head and Neck Surgery, 4th edition.

Continued

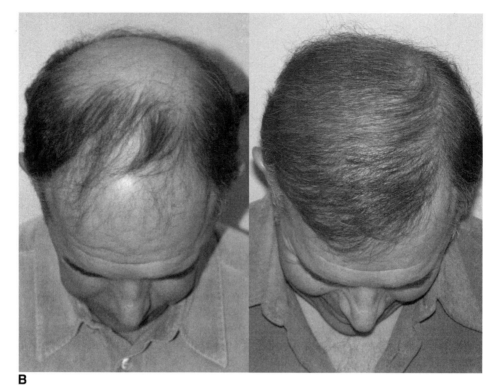

B

Figure 28-8, cont'd.

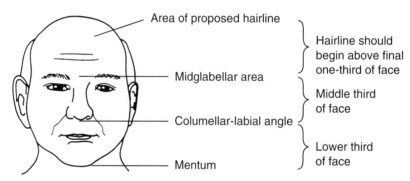

Figure 28-9. The anterior hairline, or trichion, should generally begin 6 to 8 cm above the glabella, in accordance with the rule of thirds of facial analysis. Its exact placement may need to be higher to create a more aesthetically acceptable appearance in the setting of significant hair loss and regression. From Stough DB, Haber RS, editors: *Hair replacement: surgical and medical.* St Louis, Mosby, 1996, p 170. To view this image in color, please go to *www.ototext.com* or the Electronic Image Collection CD, bound into your copy of Cummings Otolaryngology—Head and Neck Surgery, 4th edition.

In addition, the estimated number of grafts needed is calculated by multiplying the measured recipient area by the goal in graft density, approximately 20 to 40 units per square centimeter.

An assessment of the donor reserves should also be completed during the preoperative evaluation. The donor reserves are harvested within the predicted fringe margin of the scalp. The fringe margin extends from each temporoparietal region to the midoccipital scalp over the inion, which is the most prominent point on the posterior skull. The hair follicles within the hair fringe are relatively resistant to the effects of DHT and tend to persist, even in extensively bald individuals.

Specifically, the scalp in the donor region needs to be evaluated in terms of donor hair density and laxity. The number of follicular units in the midoccipital portion of the donor area of a typical white male is 100 units per square centimeter.[16] In terms of estimating donor site hair density, approximately 100 units per square centimeter can be used as a rough guide, and accounts for follicles in the telogen phase.[3]

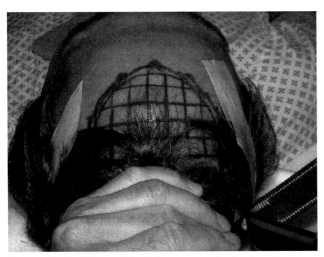

Figure 28-10. The recipient sites are marked out on the scalp in a grid pattern of 1 cm². To view this image in color, please go to *www.ototext.com* or the Electronic Image Collection CD, bound into your copy of Cummings Otolaryngology—Head and Neck Surgery, 4th edition.

A donor strip of scalp is generally 0.8 to 1.5 cm wide by 8 to 30 cm long and marked off in 1-cm intervals (Figure 28-11). If a prior session was previously performed, the scar should be included in the subsequent donor strip. If the scalp has been stretched from previous procedures, the follicles will be spaced out further apart, thus resulting in a decrease in hair density. Furthermore, the less laxity the scalp has, the more likely that the closure will be more difficult and that it will possibly lead to a widened scar. In such

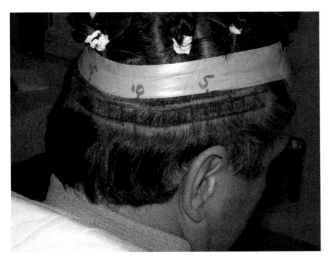

Figure 28-11. The donor strip is marked off within the hair fringe, where the hair follicles are relatively resistant to the effects of dihydrotestosterone. To view this image in color, please go to *www.ototext.com* or the Electronic Image Collection CD, bound into your copy of Cummings Otolaryngology—Head and Neck Surgery, 4th edition.

cases, a donor strip of less width and greater length should be taken.

Operative Procedure

After the appropriate donor site is located, the surrounding hair is kept away from the surgical field using either tape or elastic bands. The donor area is shaved with a mustache trimmer, leaving a few millimeters of hair growth to assist in the fashioning and placement of the grafts (Figure 28-11).

The procedure is performed with the patient in a sitting position in a standard examination chair. After cleansing the scalp with an antiseptic solution, the donor and recipient areas are anesthetized with 10 to 20 mL of 1% lidocaine with 1:100,000 epinephrine. Forty milligrams of triamcinolone are added to 10 mL of the local anesthesia for the infiltration of the recipient site. This infiltration is theorized to assist in minimizing postoperative swelling and telogen effluvium, which is the temporary hair loss that results from local trauma during surgical manipulation. Preoperative oral sedatives, inhaled nitrous oxide, or intravenous sedation may be used to decrease the discomfort associated with initial local anesthesia infiltration. Twenty to 150 mL of diluted lidocaine solution (approx 0.1%) is infiltrated using a three-inch, 22-gauge needle inserted into the subcutaneous layer of the donor strip via a tumescent technique. This infiltration assists with tissue dissection and minimizes bleeding.

The donor strip is harvested with a No. 10 scalpel blade in a single strip. Care is taken to cut parallel to the hair shafts to preserve intact hair follicles. Some surgeons advocate the use of a multibladed (usually four to seven blades) knife to create strips of narrower widths; in our experience, more hair follicles are inadvertently injured with this technique. The strip of scalp is excised at a level just below the hair follicles within the subcutaneous fat layer (Figure 28-12). Bleeding vessels are occasionally coagulated or sutured if needed, particularly if the occipital vessels are transected. The incision is closed in a running fashion using 3.0 Prolene suture placed at half the depth of the surrounding hair follicles. Undermining or deep closure is usually not performed, because closure is achieved with the use of modified towel clamps to pull the skin edges together and provide adequate tissue creep.

The donor strip is passed off of the field to the hair technicians for further sectioning. Using 10× binocular magnification, the strip is dissected into individual vertical slivers of one follicular-unit thickness using countertraction and a No. 10 scalpel blade (Figure 28-13, *A*). The dissection is made carefully in a line parallel to the follicle, but the follicular epithelium is left intact. Under magnification, these slivers of

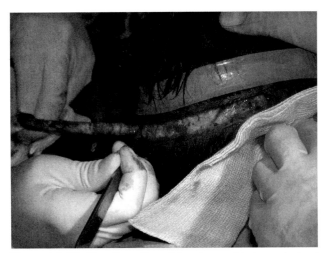

Figure 28-12. The dissection of the donor strip is carried out within the subcutaneous fat layer, below the hair follicles. To view this image in color, please go to *www.ototext.com* or the Electronic Image Collection CD, bound into your copy of Cummings Otolaryngology—Head and Neck Surgery, 4th edition.

follicular units are dissected transversely into individual grafts that contain one to three hairs, depending on the natural follicular-unit makeup (Figure 28-13, *B*). During their dissection, the grafts are kept moist on Telfa pads in saline-filled Petri dishes.

The graft recipient sites or incisions are made with specific attention given to the surrounding natural hair growth in terms of proper hair direction and angulation from the scalp. Incisional slits are made with a 1.3- or 1.5-mm Minde sharp point blade (Medical

Sterile Products, Rincón, Puerto Rico) or one of various other types of needles and miniature blades, including the NoKor needle (Becton Dickinson & Co, Rutherford, NJ) (Figure 28-14). The smaller incisions are primarily placed at the anterior hairline and in the "feathering" transition zone to allow for the placement of smaller grafts of single hairs; larger slits are made further back for larger grafts that provide additional hair density. A similar "feathering" transition zone can also be created posteriorly toward the vertex.

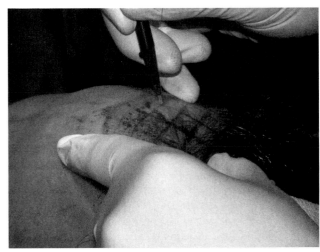

Figure 28-14. The incisions at the recipient sites are made with 1.3- or 1.5-mm Minde blades in the same direction and angulation from the scalp as the surrounding hairs. To view this image in color, please go to *www.ototext.com* or the Electronic Image Collection CD, bound into your copy of Cummings Otolaryngology—Head and Neck Surgery, 4th edition.

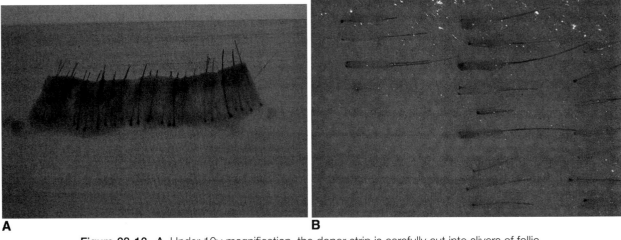

A   **B**

Figure 28-13. A, Under 10× magnification, the donor strip is carefully cut into slivers of follicular units. **B,** These are dissected into individual follicular-unit grafts that contain one to three hairs. To view this image in color, please go to *www.ototext.com* or the Electronic Image Collection CD, bound into your copy of Cummings Otolaryngology—Head and Neck Surgery, 4th edition.

The depth of the slit incisions should be made to accommodate most of the graft's length.

The actual placement of the grafts requires meticulous manipulation as they are placed into the individual slits. Using fine-pointed forceps, the grafts are individually placed within the recipient slits, with attention given to proper orientation and angulation. One set of forceps is used to open the slit, while a second set places the graft into the opening (Figure 28-15). The grafts are gently grasped by the surrounding fat so that the hair follicle is not injured. An alternative technique is to place a graft immediately after creating a slit; this is called the "stick and place" technique. Before the placement of the grafts, the recipient areas can be reinjected with small amounts of 2% lidocaine with epinephrine 1:15,000 to enhance anesthesia and vasoconstriction. No more than 2 cc is injected via a 30-gauge needle at any one time.

At the completion of the procedure, the scalp and the recipient sites are cleansed with 1.5% hydrogen peroxide or saline spray to remove crusted blood. Antibiotic ointment is applied to the closed donor incision, and no surgical dressing is applied. Postoperative care includes oral antibiotics for three days, pain medication, and frequent light spraying of the scalp with 1.5% hydrogen peroxide (approximately every hour while awake for 24 to 48 hours postoperatively). The patient is allowed a light shower and shampoo after 72 hours.

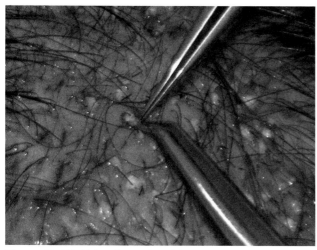

Figure 28-15. Using fine-pointed forceps, the grafts are individually placed within the recipient slits, with attention given to proper orientation and angulation. One set of forceps is used to open the slit, while a second set is used to place the graft into the opening. To view this image in color, please go to *www.ototext.com* or the Electronic Image Collection CD, bound into your copy of Cummings Otolaryngology—Head and Neck Surgery, 4th edition.

The patient can expect crusting at the grafted sites and occasional scalp and forehead edema and ecchymosis after the operation. Nonetheless, the patient can often return to normal daily activities within one day while wearing a loose-fitting cap or by styling existing hair to cover the expected crusting. After 10 to 14 days, the donor site suture is removed, and most patients should have no visible signs of the procedure.

Follicular Unit Extraction (Fue)

In the past 2 years, there has been an increasing interest in harvesting follicular unit grafts individually so as not to have a linear scar in the donor site as occurs in standard strip harvesting. The technique seems similar to the old punch graft technique in that a small sharp punch (usually 1 mm in diameter) is used on a shaved donor site to cut around a follicular unit. Done under loupe magnification or with an operating microscope, the cut goes through the dermis and just barely into the subcutaneous fat. The encircled follicular unit is then grasped with a fine forceps and teased out with a small dissecting needle. The follicular unit is extracted, trying not to damage it or the surrounding follicles. Transplanting to the recipient area is directed into pre-made slits or by a "stick and place" method. At present, some surgeons are doing this particularly tedious and costly technique on only those patients who think in the future they might want to shave their head or who are fearful of having any scars. Whether or not this technique becomes frequently performed will depend on leaders in the field developing efficiency and economy in its use.

Complications

Complications from follicular-unit transplantation are uncommon. Poor results can be due to inappropriate hairline placement. A hairline placed too low is often done in accordance with a patient's requests; this result should be avoided with careful preoperative evaluation and consultation. In addition, telogen effluvium (temporary hair loss) may occur in both donor and recipient regions as a result of the surgical manipulation of the adjacent hairs. The patient must be informed of this possibility before undergoing the procedure, and he or she need to be reassured that hair regrowth is expected in approximately three months, along with the growth of the transplanted hairs. Epidermal cysts and ingrown hairs can develop; these require unroofing with a needle tip. Temporary or permanent hypoesthesia is possible, primarily in the regions that are adjacent to the harvested donor strip. Scarring is usually minimal. However, some donor site incisions—primarily in the temporoparietal regions—may widen with time, most likely from significant scalp tension. Graft survival may decrease slightly during subsequent sessions as a result of scarring and altered vascularity at the recipient sites.

Scalp Reductions

In the past, scalp reductions were used extensively to minimize or eliminate areas of alopecia by excising bald portions of the scalp after subgaleal undermining. The amount of scalp excision was proportional to its inherent elasticity. Numerous shapes of excisions have been used to excise the balding areas of scalp. These designs include an ellipse, a Y, a crescent, and a horse-shoe. They are individualized on the basis of the patient's pattern of hair loss (see Figure 28-16).

Additional bald scalp excision can be achieved with the use of tissue expanders or scalp extenders. The expander or extender is placed in the subgaleal plane approximately 6 weeks before the scalp reduction. In scalp expansion, serial injections of saline via the percutaneous port will result in a progressive increase in scalp surface area. Scalp extension depends on the inherent elastic recoil of the implanted extender device to give tissue creep to adjacent areas of hair-bearing scalp.

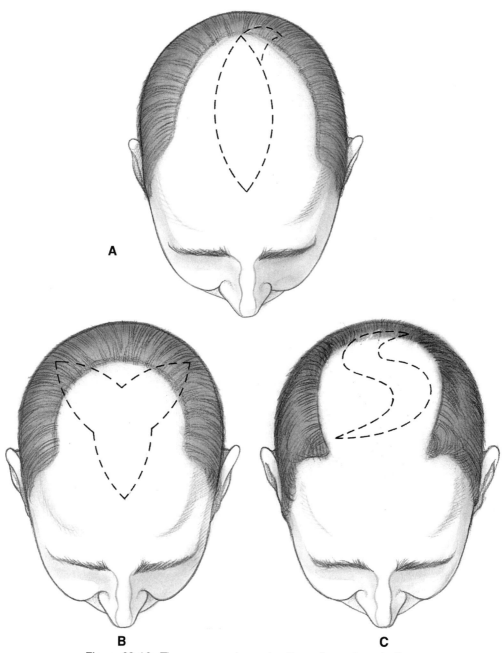

A

B

C

Figure 28-16. Three commonly used patterns for scalp reduction.

For some patients (especially females), an anterior hairline advancement with excision of pretrichial skin is an excellent option for the treatment of a high hairline and a prominent forehead. The advancement can be performed in conjunction with a browlift procedure that addresses the corrugator and procerus muscle groups. An irregularly trichophytic incision made perpendicular to the hair follicles facilitates hair growth through the resulting scar, and careful wound closure with proper skin eversion ensures inconspicuous healing. Preliminary scalp expansion may be needed in patients with minimal scalp laxity and in those who need more than 3 cm of advancement (see Figure 28-17).

Complications

Although effective for the removal of areas of baldness, reductions have created their own unique set of problems: misdirected hair, severely decreased hair density, elevated hairlines, detectable scars, and, most notably, the posterior vertical "slot" defect (Figure 28-18).

Perhaps the most noticeable of these complications is related to the misdirected hair from repetitive scalp reductions. Normally, temporoparietal hair points directly down toward the ears and exits the scalp at an acute angle; mid-scalp hair grows in a frontal direction

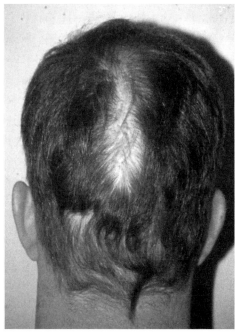

Figure 28-18. The posterior vertical "slot" defect after serial scalp reductions. Note the misdirected hair.

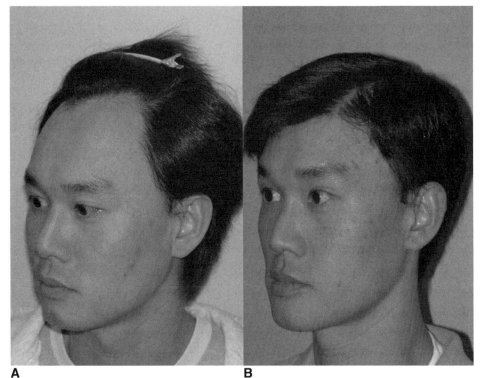

A　　　　　　　　　　　　　　**B**

Figure 28-17. A, Preoperative and **B,** postoperative photographs of a patient with a high hairline who underwent an anterior hairline advancement after scalp expansion with a tissue expander.

and with a more perpendicular angle from the scalp. When both superior aspects of the fringe are brought together in the midline with scalp reduction, the hair direction becomes noticeably divergent in this region, which creates an unnatural appearance.

The vertical or "slot" defect is created in the posterior occiput by closing an elliptical resected area into an elongated scar. This unfavorable scar can be corrected by excising the scar and using a series of three anteriorly based rotational flaps as described by Frechet.[14] Using these flaps, hair direction is reoriented so that hair grows inferiorly, thereby covering the incisions (see Figure 28-19). Although many results have been less than satisfactory, modified scalp reductions still have a role in hair restoration that has a specific goal of alopecia reduction rather than elimination. Modified scalp reductions are performed on select patients, often in conjunction with hair grafting.

Flap Procedures

Large delayed temporoparietal-occipital (TPO) pedicle flaps are unique and involved procedures

that can create complete hairlines of great density in a short period of time (see Figure 28-20). Originally described by Juri,[18] the TPO pedicle flap essentially recreates the anterior hairline with hair-bearing scalp from the temporoparietal hair fringe region, which is resistant to androgenetic alopecia.[19] Although it does achieve its primary goal, the TPO flap is an exacting procedure that requires three staged surgeries in addition to a highly motivated patient with frontal baldness, stable crown coverage, and good hair density and laxity in the donor region.

The pedicle of the axial TPO flap is centered over the posterior branch of the superficial temporal artery, which usually runs superiorly through the midportion of the sideburn and curves posteriorly. Because of the large flap length-to-width ratio and the random blood supply at the distal portion of the flap, Juri[18] described two delay procedures for vascular preconditioning of the flap. The first delay procedure is the creation of a bipedicled flap with posterior circulation that is provided by the perforating branches

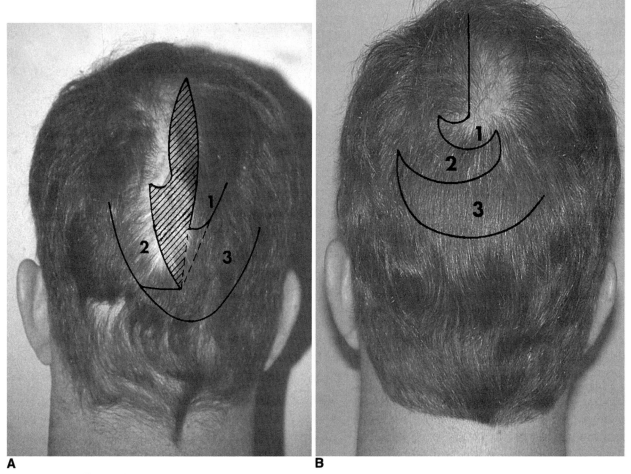

A   **B**

Figure 28-19. A, The Frechet triple flap repair for the correction of the vertical "slot" defect, and **B,** the postoperative result.

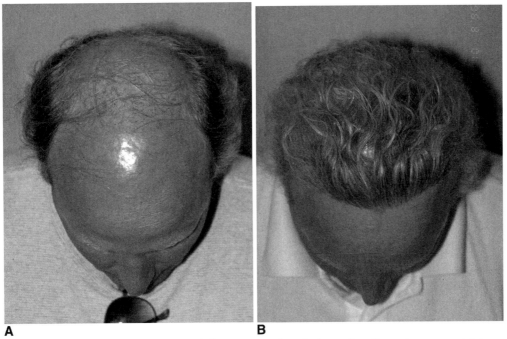

A **B**

Figure 28-20. A, Preoperative and **B,** postoperative photographs after a temporoparietal-occipital (or Juri) flap.

of the occipital artery. One week later, the posterior bridge of scalp is transected and stapled closed in a brief second procedure. The need for delaying these large flaps has been challenged, and the operation has been performed with only one or no delay.

The third stage involves the actual flap transfer and is performed one week after the second delay (Figure 28-21). The flap is elevated in the subgaleal plane. A slightly irregular hairline incision is made, and it is beveled posteriorly at about a 45-degree angle to the scalp. Extensive undermining of the scalp, neck, and postauricular region is necessary to facilitate closure with minimal tension. The leading edge of the flap is deepithelialized and sutured to the contralateral side of the forehead. A second TPO flap can be performed months after the initial flap transfer for additional posterior coverage. However, closure problems as a result of subsequent decreased scalp laxity become more of a concern.

Complications

Complications associated with the TPO or Juri flap include postoperative swelling and ecchymosis; a persistent dog-ear deformity at the proximal side of the flap, with a blunted temporofrontal angle; widened temporal scars; and occasional necrosis of the distal end of the flap. If distal flap necrosis delayed healing

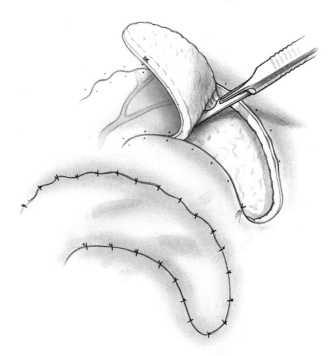

Figure 28-21. The temporoparietal-occipital or Juri flap.

and antibiotics are recommended, followed by possible revision surgery.

Of further concern is the aesthetic result in terms of progressive alopecia and misdirected hair growth.

After a successful flap procedure, further hair loss can result in an unnaturally dense anterior hair zone with an extensively bald vertex. This undesirable effect can be camouflaged by combing the hair straight back or with a hairpiece system. Nonetheless, the results are generally not consistent with the current philosophy of inconspicuous hair restoration. Consequently, given its complexity and possible disadvantages, the TPO flap has largely been abandoned as an option for hair restoration for typical AGA. It is of note that bilateral nondelayed flaps from the temporal regions have also been used to recreate the anterior hairline. These flaps are mentioned only to be avoided given their accentuated problems with misdirected hair and hairline asymmetry.

Reconstructive Procedures

All of the principles and techniques described in this chapter also apply to alopecia resulting from prior surgical procedures, trauma, and radiation. Again, the surgeon must be attentive preoperatively to proper positioning of the hairline and the surrounding hair direction to achieve the most aesthetically pleasing results. Limited alopecia may be treated as a modified scar revision or with local rotational or advancement flaps. More extensive areas of alopecia may require serial scalp reductions, often after tissue expansion.

Follicular-unit hair transplantation is used as a separate modality or in conjunction with other procedures to further enhance coverage and camouflage scalp scarring. Specifically, follicular-unit hair transplantation has been successfully implemented in cases of unfavorable scarring after procedures such as rhytidectomy, browlift, or craniotomy.[12] For example, altered hairlines with stepoff deformities in the temporal and occipital areas can occur in rhytidectomies with poorly designed incisions or after skin necrosis. These cases can be successfully corrected with follicular-unit hair grafting (see Figure 28-22). Furthermore, alopecia associated with the loss of eyebrow hair, eyelashes, and facial hair (i.e., beard and mustache) can be similarly treated, with good success.[23]

Alternative procedures may be required in cases of more extensive scalp loss, such as after scalp avulsion with loss of viable tissue or significant scalp resection for malignancy. If the underlying pericranium is intact, a split-thickness skin graft may be used. This approach is preferred in cases that involve high rates of cancer recurrence, given the fact that the thin graft will allow for enhanced monitoring. For larger scalp defects, a superficial temporoparietal fascia flap, a trapezius myocutaneous rotational flap, a latissimus dorsi muscle or radial forearm microvascular free-flap

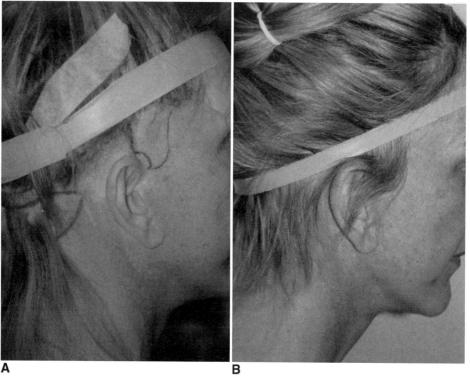

A   **B**

Figure 28-22. Alopecia after rhytidectomy. **A,** Notice the loss of the temporal tuft of hair, the altered occipital hairline, and the visible scars. **B,** Patient's appearance 6 months after two sessions (520 grafts and 400 grafts, respectively) of follicular-unit hair transplantations.

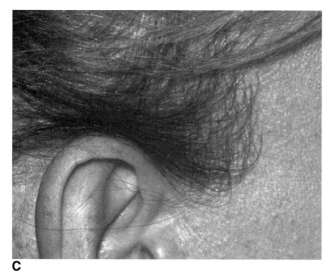

C

Figure 28-22, cont'd C, Close-up showing hair growth in the temporal region.

can provide well-vascularized tissue for proper soft tissue coverage.[30]

Nonsurgical Hair Restoration

Modern artificial hair systems or additions can augment surgical hair restoration or serve as a substitute. Although these options are often associated with negative images, current designs in hair systems can provide a natural appearance and remain virtually undetectable. Devices include hair weaves, partial hairpieces, and complete wigs. The fibers used consist of human hair, synthetic fibers, or combinations of both. Custom designs are generally integrated with the patient's own hair or hairline to create a natural appearance while the patient remains comfortable. Improved fixation techniques involving either the scalp or the surrounding hair can accommodate a wide variety of lifestyles.

ALTERNATIVES AND FUTURE TREATMENT OPTIONS

Various new avenues are being explored in surgical hair restoration. Synthetic hair grafts were originally introduced in Japan by Yamada and Fukuta in 1972,[50] and they remain an accepted alternative treatment for alopecia in many countries. The synthetic hair consists of polyethylene terephthalate, which is the same material used in the suture fiber Prolene (Ethicon, Johnson & Johnson, Somerville, NJ) with a thin coating of amorphous silver added for its antibacterial properties.[50] Disadvantages include the constant risk of infection and progressive scarring as a result of a chronic foreign body reaction. In addition, the hair fibers have an unnatural appearance on close inspec-

tion, and monthly follow-up visits and frequent graft replacements are necessary.[27] Given that no independent clinical studies have shown that synthetic grafting is safe, the U.S. Food and Drug Administration has never approved its use in the United States.

Research has also focused on follicle regeneration and its possible implications in the field of hair transplantation. Studies have demonstrated that horizontal sectioning of a hair follicle across its perifollicular sheath will result in two portions that will continue to grow.[24] One follicular-unit hair graft could possibly be fashioned into two or more viable grafts, thereby dramatically increasing the number of available donor grafts. Ultimately, current investigations into the potential of cloning hair follicle stem cells may revolutionize hair restoration by providing an unlimited supply of donor grafts.

SUMMARY

Although an extensive list of causes of alopecia exists for both men and women, the most common type remains AGA. Advances in medical therapy (e.g., finasteride) have been relatively successful for selectively targeting the underlying processes of hair loss. For those patients who require significant hair coverage, follicular-unit hair transplantation has become the gold standard surgical method for providing a patient with a natural-appearing hairline and the illusion of a full head of hair. Other surgical options (e.g., scalp reductions, large flaps) should remain in the surgeon's armamentarium for select patients and situations. Future advances are focused on hair restoration at the cellular level in terms of maximizing both remaining follicles and aesthetic results. Overall, the treatment of alopecia should be viewed as having an integral role in appearance enhancement and facial rejuvenation as well as in improving a patient's self-image and quality of life.

REFERENCES

1. Abell E: *Embryology and anatomy of the hair follicle.* In Olsen EA, editor: *Disorders of hair growth: diagnosis and treatment.* New York, 1994, McGraw-Hill, p 1–19.
2. Bergfeld WF: Androgenetic alopecia: an autosomal dominant disorder, *Am J Med* 98(Suppl 1A):95S, 1995.
3. Bernstein RM, Rassman WR: Follicular transplantation: patient evaluation and surgical planning, *Am Soc Dermatol Surg* 23:771, 1998.
4. Bernstein RM, Rassman WR: The logic of follicular unit transplantation, *Dermatol Clin* 17:277, 1999.
5. Birch MP, Messenger JF, Messenger AG: Hair density, hair diameter, and prevalence of female pattern hair loss, *Br J Dermatol* 144:297, 2001.
6. Cash TF: The psychological consequences of androgenic alopecia: a review of the research literature, *Br J Dermatol* 141:398, 1999.
7. De Villez RL: Topical minoxidil therapy in hereditary androgenetic alopecia, *Arch Dermatol* 121:197, 1985.

8. DeVillez RL: *Drug therapy.* In Stough DB, Haber RS, editors: *Hair replacement: surgical and medical.* St Louis, 1996, Mosby, p 375–382.
9. Diani AR and others: Hair growth effects of oral administration of finasteride, a steroid 5α-reductase inhibitor, alone and in combination with topical minoxidil in the balding stumptail macaque, *J Clin Endocrinol Metab* 74:345, 1992.
10. Domnitz JN, Silvers DN: Giant cells in male pattern alopecia—a histologic marker and pathogenic clue, *J Cutan Pathol* 6:108, 1976.
11. Elston DM, Bergfeld WF: *Cicatricial alopecia and other causes of permanent alopecia.* In Olsen EA, editor: *Disorders of hair growth: diagnosis and treatment.* New York, 1994, McGraw-Hill, p 285–313.
12. Epstein JS: Hair transplantation in women: treating female pattern baldness and repairing distortion and scarring from prior cosmetic surgery, *Arch Facial Plast Surg* 5:121, 2003.
13. Fiedler VC, Hafeez A: *Diffuse alopecia: telogen hair loss.* In Olsen EA, editor: *Disorders of hair growth: diagnosis and treatment.* New York, 1994, McGraw-Hill, p 241–255.
14. Frechet P: A new method for correction of the vertical scar observed following scalp reduction for extensive baldness, *J Dermatol Surg Oncol* 16:640, 1990.
15. Hamilton JB: Patterned loss of hair in men: types and incidence, *Ann N Y Acad Sci* 53:708, 1951.
16. Headington JT: Transverse microscopic anatomy of the human scalp, *Arch Dermatol* 120:449, 1984.
17. Johnson TM and others: Histology and physiology of tissue expansion, *J Dermatol Surg Oncol* 19:1074, 1993.
18. Juri J: Use of parieto-occipital flaps in the surgical treatment of baldness, *Plast Reconstr Surg* 55:456, 1975.
19. Kabaker SS: Juri flap procedure for the treatment of baldness. Two-year experience, *Arch Otolaryngol* 105:509, 1979.
20. Kaufman KD and others: Finasteride in the treatment of men with androgenic alopecia, *J Am Acad Dermatol* 39:578, 1998.
21. Kaufman KD and others: Long-term (5-year) multinational experience with finasteride 1 mg in the treatment of men with androgenic alopecia, *Eur J Dermatol* 12:38, 2002.
22. Khandpur S, Suman M, Reddy BS: Comparative efficacy of various treatment regimens for androgenetic alopecia in men, *J Dermatol* 29:489, 2002.
23. Kim JC, Choi YC: *Hair transplantation of the eyelashes and eyebrows, special categories.* In Stough DB, Haber RS, editors: *Hair replacement: surgical and medical.* St Louis, 1996, Mosby, p 216–218.
24. Kim JC, Choi YC: *Hair follicle regeneration after horizontal resectioning—implications for hair transplantation. Selected topics in hair replacement.* In Stough DB, Haber RS, editors: *Hair replacement: surgical and medical.* St Louis, 1996, Mosby, p 358–363.
25. Küster W, Happle R: The inheritance of common baldness: two B or not two B?, *J Am Acad Dermatol* 11:921, 1984.
26. Lachgar S and others: Minoxidil upregulates the expression of vascular endothelial growth factor in human hair dermal papilla cells, *Br J Dermatol* 138:407, 1998.
27. Lepaw MI: *Critique of synthetic hair grafting. Selected topics in hair replacement.* In Stough DB, Haber RS, editors: *Hair replacement: surgical and medical.* St Louis, 1996, Mosby, p 357–358.
28. Leyden J and others: Finasteride in the treatment of men with frontal male pattern hair loss, *J Am Acad Dermatol* 40:930, 1999.
29. Ludwig E: Classification of the types of androgenic alopecia (common baldness) occurring in the female sex, *Br J Dermatol* 97:247, 1977.
30. Lutz BS and others: Reconstruction of scalp defects with free flaps in 30 cases, *Br J Plast Surg* 51:186, 1998.
31. Michelet JF and others: Activation of cytoprotective prostaglandin synthesase-1 by minoxidil as a possible explanation for its hair growth-stimulating effect, *J Invest Dermatol* 108:205, 1997.
32. Norwood OT, Shiell RC: *Hair transplant surgery.* Springfield, Illinois, 1984, Charles C. Thomas.
33. Ohtsuyama M, Morhashi M: *Minoxidil sulfate effect on internal calcium of cell in the epidermis and epidermal appendages.* In Van Neste D, Randall V, editors: *Hair research for the next millennium.* Amsterdam, The Netherlands, 1996, Elsevier Science, p 471–480.
34. Olsen EA: *Androgenetic alopecia.* In Olsen EA, editor: *Disorders of hair growth: diagnosis and treatment.* New York, 1994, McGraw-Hill, p 257–283.
35. Olsen EA: Treatment of androgenetic alopecia with topical minoxidil, *Res Staff Phys* 35:53, 1989.
36. Olsen EA, DeLong ER, Weiner MS: Long-term follow-up of men with male pattern baldness treated with topical minoxidil, *J Am Acad Dermatol* 16:688, 1987.
37. Olsen EA and others: Five year follow-up of men with androgenetic alopecia treated with topical minoxidil, *J Am Acad Dermatol* 22:643, 1990.
38. Olsen E and others: Topical minoxidil in early male pattern baldness, *J Am Acad Dermatol* 13:185, 1985.
39. Orentreich N: Autografts in alopecia and other selected dermatological conditions, *Ann N Y Acad Sci* 83:463, 1959.
40. Physicians' circular for Propecia. West Point, PA, 1997, Merck.
41. Price VH: Treatment of hair loss, *N Engl J Med* 341:964, 1999.
42. Price VH: Hormonal control of baldness, *Int J Dermatol* 15:742, 1976.
43. Price VH: Rogaine (topical minoxidil) in the management of male-pattern baldness and alopecia areata: summary, *J Am Acad Dermatol* 16:749, 1987.
44. Safavi KH and others: Incidence of alopecia areata in Olmstead County, Minnesota, 1975 through 1989, *Mayo Clin Proc* 70:628, 1995.
45. Sawaya ME, Hordinsky MK: The anti-androgens: when and how they should be used, *Dermatol Clin* 11:65, 1993.
46. Setty LR: Hair patterns of the scalp of a white and negro male, *Am J Phys Anthropol* 33:49, 1970.
47. Takashima M, Iju, Sudo M: *Alopecia androgenica—its incidence in Japanese and associated conditions.* In Orfanos CE, Montagna W, Studen G, editors: *Hair research status and feature aspects.* Berlin, 1981, Springer-Verlag, p 287–293.
48. Tosti A, Piraccini BM, Soli M: Evaluation of sexual function in subjects taking finasteride for the treatment of androgenetic alopecia, *J Eur Acad Dermatol Venereol* 15:418, 2001.
49. Walsh DS, Dunn CL, James WD: Improvement in androgenetic alopecia (stage V) using topical minoxidil in a retinoid vehicle and oral finasteride, *Arch Dermatol* 131:1373, 1995.
50. Yamada S, Fukuta K: *Synthetic hair grafting. Selected topics in hair replacement.* In Stough DB, Haber RS, editors: *Hair replacement: surgical and medical.* St Louis, 1996, Mosby, p 345–357.
51. Young JW and others: Cutaneous immunopathology of androgenic alopecia, *J Am Osteopath Assoc* 91:765, 1991.

CHAPTER TWENTY NINE

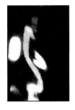

MANAGEMENT OF AGING SKIN

|| Stephen W. Perkins
|| Timothy G. Gillum

INTRODUCTION

As the general population ages, interest in maintaining a youthful appearance is at an all-time high. People are seeking more avenues for facial rejuvenation, and with the explosion of the information age, physicians are presented with a more educated consumer. This demand has promoted tremendous growth in the cosmetic industry, with numerous over-the-counter products available to "reverse aging changes." Similarly, there has been an increase in medical cosmeceutical products and technologic advances producing more resurfacing options for the consumer. As a result, a growing number of patients are visiting their cosmetic surgeons, estheticians, and dermatologists requesting the latest options to reverse aging skin changes. This chapter will focus primarily on chemical peels in facial resurfacing but will also discuss other rejuvenation topics in the management of aging skin, including the following:

• Histologic changes of aging skin.
• Patient evaluation and classification.
• Chemical peels.
• Dermabrasion.
• Laser resurfacing.
• Nonablative resurfacing.
• Microdermabrasion.
• Medical/topical skin care regimens.

HISTOLOGIC CHANGES OF AGING SKIN

The first scholarly report on phenol chemical peels, including the formula and technique, was written by Brown and others.[14] Brown described the histologic changes that were induced including laminated collagen in the epidermis, with fibrous strands consistently paralleling the newly formed epidermis.

Later, Kligman and colleagues[31] studied the skin taken from Baker and Gordon's facelift patients who had chemical peels 1½ to 20 years earlier. First, they described histologic changes of non-peeled skin.

These aging skin changes were typical of actinic exposure with a loss of orderly differentiation in the epidermis and degeneration of the elastic network, along with some mottled pigmentation and lymphocytic infiltration. There was a decrease in collagen amounts as well as disordered degeneration of the dermal fibers, a flattening of the dermal-epidermal junction, and multiple actinic keratoses with atypia seen. The number of melanocytes was increased in this actinic skin, but they were unevenly distributed and contained variable amounts of melanin.

The skin of patients who had undergone a previous chemical peel showed a new band of dermis 2- to 3-mm-thick just beneath the epidermis and lying on top of the old elastotic dermis. The epidermis had returned to orderly cellular differentiation without irregularities or microscopic actinic keratoses. Although there was an abundance of melanocytes present containing some fine, evenly distributed melanin granules, there appeared to be impaired melanin synthesis with a generalized bleaching effect, or *hypopigmentation*. Lentigines were not seen. Further, the epidermal-dermal matrix was composed of thin, compact, parallel collagen bundles arranged horizontally in contrast to the usual wavy pattern. Elastotic fibers had actually regenerated, forming a network of fibers paralleling the new collagen. Finally, the lymphocytic infiltration was diminished compared with that of untreated skin. Kligman and colleagues[31] felt that the dermal reconstruction lasted about 20 years based on their study. They further concluded that chemical peel reduced the development of new neoplasms. The laying down of a band of new connective tissue can adequately account for the effacement of the wrinkles seen clinically. The skin is smoother, fuller, and tighter. Stegman[57] and Litton and colleagues[37,38] showed the chemical peel solution penetrating deeper in the dermis of actinically damaged skin than nonactinically damaged skin. Hayes and Stambaugh[27] demonstrated that during the first 2 to 5 days of a chemical peel there is epidermal necrosis, edema, and homogenization with the lymphocytic infiltration all the way into the reticular dermis.[26] At 2 weeks, new collagen formation had begun. Stegman,[57] Alt,[1] and Brody and Alt[11] have illustrated that there is deeper penetration of phenol with occlusion than with nonocclusion. According to Beeson and McCollough,[5] this is apparently true but not necessarily desired.

Litton and others[38] agreed with Kligman and colleagues[31] that the rate of appearance with precancerous and early cancerous lesions of photoaged skin was decreased after a phenol chemical peel.

Brodland and Roenigk[7] showed that the trichloroacetic acid (TCA) destroys the epidermis and upper dermis and further showed that the new epidermis migrated from the cutaneous adnexa beneath the destroyed tissue. This is similar to phenol peel. Histologically, the atypical clones of keratinocytes are removed and replaced by normal epidermal cells.

PATIENT EVALUATION, CLASSIFICATION, AND SELECTION

The actual process or technique of chemical peels (and other resurfacing modalities) is relatively easy to learn. However, it takes a great deal of experience with many different types of patients to learn the wide variation in skin types and how these respond to peel solutions.[12] It also takes a great deal of experience to predict the way in which each area of the face will respond to light or deep resurfacing in an individual patient, and how one can influence the method of application used. Careful selection of the appropriate patients for resurfacing is the first and most important consideration. According to McCollough and Hillman,[43] "The ideal patient is a thin-skinned female with fair complexion and fine rhytids."

Fitzpatrick[20] described types of actinically damaged skin ranging from type I to type VI (Table 29-1). Brody[9] stated that Fitzpatrick types I through III patients are suitable for a chemical peel. He describes the ideal patient as a light-complected person of Celtic or Northern European descent with skin types I or II.[13]

The Glogau classification system[45] was created in 1994 and provides an objective assessment of the degree of photoaging, categorizing the patient's skin damage into mild, moderate, advanced, or severe (groups I–IV) (Table 29-2). Patients in category I are often young with minimal photoaging and are best managed with a superficial peel in conjunction with a good medical skin care program. Patients in category II or III are candidates for medium-depth peels in addition to long-term medical therapy as with retinoids or alpha-hydroxy acids. Category IV photoaging patients are best treated with medium or deep chemical peels, ablative lasers, or dermabrasion, in conjunction with long-term medical skin care regimens.

There are several aesthetic and therapeutic indications for chemical peels and resurfacing (Box 29-1).

Today's facial plastic surgeon must be aware of the aesthetic and therapeutic indications of facial resurfacing to effectively rejuvenate aging skin. Additionally, treating a patient based on his or her Fitzpatrick skin type and Glogau aging characteristics is essential to select the best type and depth of facial resurfacing.

CONTRAINDICATIONS

There are a few relative contraindications to chemical peels in addition to some absolute contraindications (Table 29-3). In the past, a history of herpes simplex virus was a contraindication to chemical peel.[17] With the advent of antiviral drugs, however, acyclovir (Zovirax) or valacyclovir (Valtrex) can be effectively used as preventative or therapeutic intervention. Telangiectasias are relative contraindications in that they become more apparent after chemical peels or laser resurfacing. Confirmed malignant lesions should not be treated with chemical peels unless they are very superficial basal cell carcinomas. Nevoid or nevus lesions may become darker or actually stimulated to grow, and port-wine stains, hemangiomas, and neurofibromatoses are not effectively treated with chemical peels. Contraindications include the presence of hepatorenal disease or cardiac disease (for phenol peels), unless approved by an appropriate specialist. True documented allergies to an agent are obvious contraindications, and dressings should be

TABLE 29-1

FITZPATRICK SUN-REACTIVE SKIN TYPES I TO VI

Type I	Fair-skinned, blue or hazel eyes, blond or red hair
	Always burns, never tans
Type II	Fair-skinned; blond, red, or brown hair
	Usually burns, tans less than average
Type III	Fair-skinned, largest group of U.S. citizens
	Sometimes burns mildly, tans about average
Type IV	Still considered white-skinned
	Rarely burns, tans more than average and with ease
Type V	Intermediate-colored skin; that is, Asian, Latin, Indian
	Brown skin
Type VI	Black-skinned persons
	Never burns

TABLE 29-2

GLOGAU CLASSIFICATION OF PHOTOAGING GROUPS

Group I Mild	Group II Moderate	Group III Advanced	Group IV Severe
Little wrinkling or scarring	Early wrinkling; mild scarring	Persistent wrinkling or moderate acne scarring	Wrinkling: photoaging, gravitational, and dynamic
No keratoses	Sallow color with early actinic keratoses	Discoloration with telangiectasias and actinic keratoses	Actinic keratoses with or without skin cancer or acne scars
Typical age, 28 to 35 years old	Typical age, 35 to 50 years old	Typical age, 50 to 65 years old	Typical age, 60 to 75 years old

BOX 29-1

INDICATIONS FOR FACIAL RESURFACING

Aesthetic Indications
Fine facial rhytids
Atrophic changes in skin caused by excessive sun exposure
Spotty or splotchy hyperpigmentation
Chataigne skin (sailor's or farmer's skin)
Multiple actinic and solar keratoses
Superficial acne scarring
Melasma
Excessively wrinkles skin
After blepharoplasty or face-lift

Therapeutic Indications
Multiple actinic, seborrheic, and solar pigmented keratoses
Superficial basal cell carcinomas
Lentigo maligna lentigines
Melasma (discoloration of skin caused by pregnancy)

*Data from McCollough and Hillman,[43] Farber and colleagues,[18] and Litton and colleagues.[38]

TABLE 29-3

BRODY'S RELATIVE AND ABSOLUTE CONTRAINDICATIONS TO CHEMICAL PEELS

Relative Contraindications
Darker skin type (Fitzpatrick IV, V, and VI)
Keloid formation by history
History of herpes infections
Cardiac abnormalities
History of previous facial irradiation
Marked quantity of vellus hair present
Unrealistic patient expectations
Physical inability to perform quality postoperative care
Telangiectasias
Anticipation of inadequate photo protection because of job, vocation, or recreation

Absolute Contraindications
Significant hepatorenal disease
HIV-positive patient
Significant immunosuppression (i.e., hypogammaglobulinemia)
Emotional instability or mental illness
Ehlers-Danlos syndrome
Scleroderma or collagen vascular diseases
Recent isotretinoin (Accutane) treatment (within 6–12 months before)

latex free in sensitive patients. Patients who are unstable psychologically should not be treated with any resurfacing modality, particularly because the postoperative care may require intense patient involvement, education, and understanding.

CHEMICAL PEELS
Patient Selection and Education

Patients requesting rejuvenation of aging skin via chemical peels must have a realistic understanding of potential outcomes, limitations, and postoperative care. The process begins with preconsultation written materials to educate the patient on chemical peels. Often, a patient will assume a rhytidectomy will remove wrinkles or chemical peels will replace a "mini-facelift," therefore education is key. It is imperative that the physician help the patient understand that chemical peel is a technique that rejuvenates sun-damaged skin and reduces other effects of aging, giving a more youthful appearance.

During consultation, the surgeon must determine whether the patient wears makeup routinely and whether the patient's lifestyle indicates heavy sun exposure.[44] Female patients who are unwilling to wear makeup or males who are generally not able to use makeup to cover postoperative hypopigmentation are not good candidates for this procedure. Those patients who are unwilling to decrease their sun exposure are likewise poor candidates for chemical peel because the procedure does in fact reduce their melanin protection.

Litton and colleagues[38] believe it is imperative that the patient has appropriate motivation and expectations to achieve a successful result. The patient must have a clear understanding of the postoperative discomfort, appearance, and care that will follow. He or she must understand that preexisting large pores will remain unchanged, and that telangiectasias may appear to be more prominent. Informed consent about the risks and benefits is essential. At the end of the consultation, high-quality photographic documentation is obtained and should be standardized using reproducible measures. Acne scarring will be notoriously under- or overdemonstrated, depending on the lighting or flash used, therefore the clinician should adjust the setup to accurately reflect the patient's true skin appearance. This is the only objective way that the surgeon can later determine whether he or she is achieving satisfactory results. Standard preoperative workup and medical clearance is obtained, dependent on the patient's preexisting health status. If a phenol chemical peel is to be used, special attention must be given to cardiac, liver, and kidney function in the preoperative medical workup. Any impairment of liver or kidney function could slow the excretion of phenol, potentially increasing the bloodstream concentration and leading to cardiac irregularities or even death.

Prepeel Preparations

Before any resurfacing procedure, considerations must be taken to optimize the patient's final aesthetic outcome. The preoperative consultation is used to assure that the patient is adequately prepared for the day of the chemical peel. Considerations such as a positive history of herpetic outbreaks should warrant appropriate prophylaxis. In patients with no preceding history of fever blisters who are undergoing a medium or deep peel, we have found that Valtrex is an appropriate prophylaxis at 500 mg PO bid starting the day before the peel and continuing through the 10th to the 14th day. For patients with a known history of herpetic outbreaks, we have found that prophylaxis with acyclovir at 800 mg PO qid over the same period, until reepithelialization is complete, is more effective at preventing outbreaks.

To achieve optimal results, patients must adhere to a skin care regimen in both the preoperative and postoperative periods. Patients undergoing medium or deep chemical peels are best pretreated with tretinoin (Retin A or Renova) on a nightly basis starting 2 to 4 weeks before the peel. The use of retinoic acid before chemical peels, dermabrasion, or laser resurfacing speeds epidermal healing and enhances the effects of the procedure. Retinoic acid also increases the depth of a chemical peel by decreasing the thickness of the stratum corneum. Its use is restricted during the postoperative period until reepithelialization is complete and maturization of the skin has occurred. This takes approximately 3 months.

In darker-skinned individuals, Fitzpatrick type III or greater, the use of 4% to 8% hydroquinone gel in the preoperative and postoperative periods may reduce the incidence of hyperpigmentation. It is also necessary to use hydroquinone when peeling for the treatment of pigmentary dyschromia (i.e., melasma) in patients of any skin type. Hydroquinone blocks the enzyme tyrosinase from developing melanin precursors for the production of new pigment in the epidermis during the healing phase.

All patients undergoing medium to deep facial resurfacing procedures must minimize sun exposure in the postoperative period. This is even more important in patients taking estrogens and those with preexisting pigmentary disturbances. Wearing sunblock with a sun protection factor (SPF) of 30 or greater is recommended during the first 9 to 12 months after a peel.

Chemical Peel Agents
Superficial Peels

Depending on the surgical goal, the appropriate agent is selected for each individual patient. Histologically, superficial peels extend down into the level of the stratum granulosum and papillary dermis. Such depth is good for treating mild photoaging (Glogau I and II), melasma, comedonal acne, and postinflammatory erythema. Multiple peels are usually required for a maximal result, ranging from six to eight peels on a weekly basis or every other week. A nice "refreshing of the skin" is achieved; however, it is important to note that *multiple superficial peels do not equate to the results of a medium or deep chemical peel.*

Several chemical agents fall into the superficial peel category. These agents include low concentrations of glycolic acid; 10% to 20% TCA; Jessner's solution (resorcinol, 14 g; salicylic acid, 14 g; lactic acid, 14 mL; ethanol, 100 mL); tretinoin; 5-fluorouracil (5-FU); and salicylic acid, a beta-hydroxy acid. The depth of the peel achieved with each of the above agents will vary depending on the concentration of agent used, the duration of the application, and the number of times the agent is applied. During application, there may be a mild stinging followed by a level I frosting, defined as the appearance of erythema and streaky whitening on the surface.[45] Regular washing with a mild cleanser and the use of routine moisturizers and sunscreens is all that is needed after the procedure. Superficial peels usually cause mild erythema and desquamation, with a healing time varying from 1 to 4 days, depending on the strength of the chemical agent.

Medium-Depth Chemical Peels

A medium-depth peel is one in which the injury extends through the epidermis to the papillary dermis in a single setting. In the past, 50% TCA was the standard medium-depth peeling agent, but it has been abandoned with time because of a high rate of complications including pigmentary changes and scarring. Currently, a combination of agents or modalities are used for medium-depth resurfacing. The most common agents include a combination of 35% TCA with Jessner's solution, 70% glycolic acid, or carbon dioxide (CO_2) laser. Phenol 88% by itself will give a medium-depth peel. The senior author prefers to use phenol 88% for chemical exfoliation of the lower eyelid. It produces more consistent results than CO_2 laser resurfacing without the temporary lower eyelid–tightening effect. Current indications for medium-depth chemical peels include moderate photoaging (Glogau II), actinic keratoses, pigmentary dyschromia, mild acne scarring, and blending of other resurfacing modalities (i.e., deep peels or lasers).

Monheit has demonstrated the use of Jessner's solution before the application of TCA as a synergistic combination. Jessner's solution effectively destroys the epidermal barrier by breaking up individual keratinocytes, allowing deeper and more even penetration of the 35% TCA. This technique is useful for the improvement of mild to moderate photoaging. There is minimal risk of pigmentary or textural complications, and this combination softens fine rhytids and freshens sallow, atrophic skin. Collagen remodeling and thickening occurs over a 3- to 4-month period, with continued improvement in rhytid effacement and texture quality of aging skin. Deep furrows, however, are not eliminated with this medium-depth combination alone. The Jessner's solution +35% TCA combination has been shown as effective as topical 5-FU chemotherapy in removing grossly visible and clinically undetectable actinic keratoses, with less morbidity and the positive effect of antiaging. This combination of agents is also used to blend resurfacing procedures with the surrounding skin. For example, patients who have undergone dermabrasion, CO_2 laser resurfacing, or deep chemical peels in an isolated region (e.g., perioral or periorbital) may develop a sharp line of demarcation or hypopigmentation when compared to nontreated skin. In these instances, use of Jessner's solution +35% TCA on the surrounding nontreated skin helps to blend the treated area into its surroundings.

Technique: Medium-Depth Peels

The medium-depth Jessner's +35% TCA peel is performed with the patient under intravenous sedation as necessary as an isolated procedure. The burning sensation is typically short-lived, therefore short-acting drugs are sufficient. Five to 15 mg of diazepam plus 1 to 2 mg of hydromorphone hydrochloride (Dilaudid) is typically sufficient. Nonsteroidal antiinflammatory drugs or aspirin can also be given within the first 24 hours to relieve pain and inflammation. A fan to cool the patient is also helpful.

The skin must first be cleansed of all residual oils, debris, and excess stratum corneum before the application of any peels (Figure 29-1). The patient's face is vigorously scrubbed with acetone using 2×2-cm gauze pads folded on a hemostat. Thorough degreasing is necessary for even penetration of the peeling solution. Uneven or splotchy peels are typically caused by residual oils on the stratum corneum from inadequate degreasing.

Once adequate preparation and cleansing of the skin has been completed, the Jessner's solution is evenly applied with cotton pads or gauze. On application, a faint frosting will appear within 1 minute within a background of mild erythema. The frosting is much less obvious than that seen when using TCA, and this portion of the peel is not uncomfortable for the patient.

After the Jessner's solution has dried, 35% TCA is evenly applied using cotton pads or swabs. It is important to note that the amount of TCA delivered to the skin surface is dependent on the number of applications, the degree of saturation (volume of solution), the amount of pressure applied to the skin, and contact time with the peel solution. Larger areas are treated first with cotton pad applicators including the

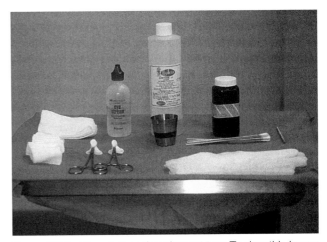

Figure 29-1. Chemical peel equipment tray. To view this image in color, please go to *www.ototext.com* or the Electronic Image Collection CD, bound into your copy of Cummings Otolaryngology—Head and Neck Surgery, 4th edition.

forehead, bilateral cheeks, nose, and chin. Then, using cotton swabs, the perioral area and eyelids are treated, coming within 1 to 2 mm of the lower eyelid margin. An assistant should always be on standby with sterile eye wash for irrigation in case the surgeon inadvertently spills any peel solution into the eye. The white frost should appear within 30 seconds to 2 minutes after application of the TCA peel (Figures 29-2 and 29-3). Before re-treating an area, however, one should wait at least 3 to 4 minutes to ensure that the frosting has reached its peak before determining for asymmetry. Additional applications can then be added with caution, as the depth of peel and potential complications are proportional to the volume of chemical applied.

The white frosting seen after a peel indicates the process of keratocoagulation, the completion of the chemical reaction. A level II or III frosting is a sufficient end point of a medium-depth peel. Level II frosting is defined as a white coat frosting with a background of erythema. Level III frosting is a solid white enamel frosting with no background of erythema, indicative of penetration into the reticular dermis. Such level III peeling should be limited to areas of thicker skin and heavy actinic damage. Sensitive areas such as thin eyelid skin and bony prominences (which have a high propensity for scarring) should be limited to a level II frosting.[45]

An immediate burning sensation is felt with the application of the TCA peel, but this begins to dissipate with the onset of frosting and is typically resolved by the time of discharge. Cool saline compresses offer symptomatic relief for a peeled area and are used over the entire face after completion of a peel. On comple-

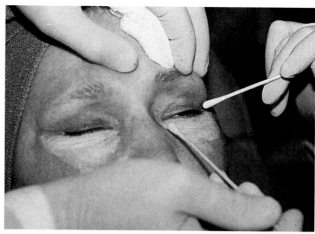

Figure 29-3. Medium-depth 35% TCA chemical peel; treatment of eyelid area. To view this image in color, please go to *www.ototext.com* or the Electronic Image Collection CD, bound into your copy of Cummings Otolaryngology—Head and Neck Surgery, 4th edition.

tion of the peel, a brawny, dusky erythema will progress over the first 12 hours. Mild to moderate edema soon follows and can be severe over the thin eyelid skin and forehead regions. As the edema begins to resolve, dark crusts appear that peel off during the subsequent 5 to 7 days to reveal a new, erythematous epithelium. The redness will soon fade to a pink color that resembles a sunburn and can typically be camouflaged with makeup by the 10th day after the peel. A formal makeover with a makeup artist within the esthetics department is a valuable experience for the patient once he or she has reepithelialized on day 10. The patient can begin using sunscreens as tolerated. He or she should wait at least 3 months before resuming regular aesthetic skin care services such as superficial chemical peels or microdermabrasion. Cleansing facials can begin as early as 4 to 6 weeks after the peel. Repeat medium-depth chemical peel should not be performed for at least 1 year. Several studies have demonstrated microscopic improvement of collagen thickness progressing over a 6- to 13-month period (Figure 29-4).

The medium-depth peel is a widely accepted resurfacing modality that has a broad range of applications for the management of aging skin. If the above measures and precautions are followed, an excellent safety profile will be maintained.

Deep Chemical Peels

Resurfacing techniques that penetrate or wound the midreticular dermis are classified as deep chemical peels. Patients with Glogau group III or IV photodamage may require deep chemical peeling. The classic chemical compound is the Baker's solution that consists of the following[2]:

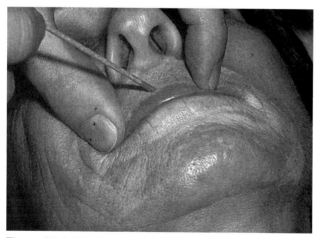

Figure 29-2. Medium-depth 35% TCA chemical peel; treatment of perioral area. To view this image in color, please go to *www.ototext.com* or the Electronic Image Collection CD, bound into your copy of Cummings Otolaryngology—Head and Neck Surgery, 4th edition.

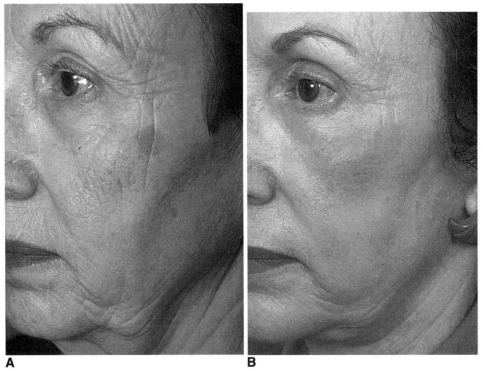

Figure 29-4. A, Pre-treatment medium-depth chemical peel. **B,** Post-treatment medium-depth chemical peel. To view this image in color, please go to *www.ototext.com* or the Electronic Image Collection CD, bound into your copy of Cummings Otolaryngology—Head and Neck Surgery, 4th edition.

Phenol 88%	3 mL
Septisol	8 drops
Croton oil	3 drops
Distilled water	2 mL

This depth can also be achieved with a 50% or greater TCA peel; however, the high risk of scarring and pigmentation problems have resulted in a trend away from these concentrations.

Phenol itself is carbolic acid (C_6H_5OH), an aromatic benzene-ring hydrocarbon formed from coal tar.[34,38,43] At concentrations greater than 80%, carbolic acid is a keratocoagulant precipitating the surface protein, thus preventing further penetration of the peel solution. Phenol produces an extremely rapid denaturization and irreversible coagulation.[37] Further penetration of the phenol is prevented when the keratin protein binds to the phenol, creating large molecules that cannot penetrate further. McCollough and Hillman[43] state that if the concentration of phenol is less than 50%, it becomes keratolytic, interrupting sulfur bridges in the keratin layer, and can then produce deeper penetration and more destruction than desired. Therefore, as one decreases the concentration of phenol, the depth and therefore wounding of tissue becomes more severe.

The croton oil included in the formula is composed of glycerides of several acids and can be very irritating to the skin. Because of its inflammatory characteris-

tics, it induces more collagen formation.[38,43] Recent studies have demonstrated that croton oil is the key ingredient, creating the significant depth of wounding.[28] Some surgeons vary the depth of Baker's solution peeling by using one, two, or three drops of croton oil. Soap in the solution acts as a surfactant, reducing surface tension and enhancing the penetration of the waxes and cholesterol esters of phenol. Septisol (hexachlorophene and alcohol) is a partial astringent that helps remove the stratum corneum and plays the role of a surfactant. The addition of distilled water produces the desired concentration of phenol between 50% and 60%. The mixture of ingredients is freshly prepared and must be stirred vigorously before application because of its poor miscibility.

The two main variations in deep chemical peeling with Baker's phenol solution included occlude vs nonoccluded. Occlusion of the peeling solution with tape increases its penetration, creating injury to the midreticular dermis. Classically, this technique has been used for deeply lined, "weather-beaten" faces, but it should only be used by the experienced surgeon due to the higher risk of complications such as delayed healing, prolonged erythema, and late hypopigmentation. The unoccluded technique as modified my McCollough and Langsdon[44] involves more cleansing of the skin and the application of more peel solution. This enhances the efficacy of the solution without penetrating as deeply as in the occluded peel. Both methods are reliable resurfacing tools for the rejuvenation of advanced to severe photoaged skin.

Patient selection is crucial with deep chemical peeling. These patients must be informed and willing to undergo a greater degree of morbidity and the higher potential for textural changes and pigmentary disturbances. They must accept the possibility that they will always need to wear makeup and use protective sunscreen.

Phenol itself is cardiotoxic and undergoes both hepatic and renal elimination. Standard preoperative workup must include a complete blood cell count; liver function tests; serum urea nitrogen, creatinine, and electrolyte determinations; and a baseline electrocardiogram. Any patient who has a history of cardiac arrhythmias or is taking medications that are potentially arrhythmia precipitating may not be a good candidate for Baker's phenol peeling. Additionally, patients with poor renal or hepatic function are poor candidates.

Technique: Deep Chemical Peels

Patient preparation and education before a deep chemical peel procedure is important. Preoperative prescriptions should be given at the time of scheduling. Preoperative antibiotics such as cephalexin (Keflex) (500 mg bid) are started 24 hours before the procedure and continued for 1 week. Patients are offered a sedative to help them sleep the night before the procedure. Patients are given 5 mg of diazepam (Valium) PO 1 to 2 hours before the peel. All makeup, including mascara, eyeliner, eye shadow, and lipstick, is to be removed before arrival at the surgery facility. The face is washed twice with Septisol and rinsed thoroughly after each washing. PhisoHex or pHisoDerm should not be used because they leave a residue on the skin[44] that may interfere with the penetration of the phenol. Brody and Alt[11] believe in treating the skin with retinoic acids (Retin A) immediately before the peel to stimulate skin healing and to remove more of the stratum corneum. This, however, only pertains to a medium-depth chemical peel and should not be used before a Baker's solution chemical peel.

A deep Baker's peel is a time-consuming procedure that must be performed in a properly suited facility. The patient is given a preoperative sedative (diazepam), antinausea medication (promethazine), and a prokinetic agent (metoclopramide; e.g., Reglan). An intravenous line is introduced and approximately 500 to 1000 mL of Ringer's lactate solution is administered. The patient is then moved to the operative or procedure room where full cardiovascular monitoring is commenced, including checks of blood pressure and oxygen saturation. The patient is given a narcotic med-

ication to offset the burning sensation, typically 1 or 2 mg of Dilaudid. Additional midazolam (Versed), usually 1 to 2 mg, is given for sedation and as an amnestic agent at this time. Sensory nerve blocks are then administered with injections of bupivacaine (Marcaine) 0.05% with 1:200,000 epinephrine solution. The regional blocks include the supraorbital, infraorbital, incisive foramen, and mental nerves, as well as infiltration of the lower eyelids and preauricular area. This spares the patient the typical 4 to 6 hours of postoperative burning discomfort. An additional liter of saline is given over the course of the procedure.

The face is divided into six aesthetic subunits including the forehead, perioral region, bilateral cheeks, nose, and periorbital region. First, thorough scrubbing with acetone soaked 2 × 2-inch gauze is applied to each region. Baker's solution is then applied with a cotton-tipped applicator to each region with feathering performed at the periphery of the peeled area, especially in the regions of the hairline, jawline, and overlap of regions by 5 mm. There is a minimum of 15 minutes between the treatment of each cosmetic area, totalling 60 to 90 minutes for the entire procedure. This allows for the renal clearance of phenol from the circulatory system. Death from arrhythmia has been reported when phenol is applied to the full face in a short period of time. Frosting occurs rapidly, therefore less solution is used compared with TCA peels. The solution should be applied in the direction of relaxed skin tension lines. A prominent white frost should be obtained immediately on application of the solution in each area, which rapidly changes to a zone of intense erythema extending 1 to 2 cm beyond the area treated with solution. It is therefore important to peel across this band of erythema when peeling the next region to avoid skipping areas.

When peeling the perioral area, one must apply the phenol solution with a slanted-cut wooden applicator so that the solution to reaches the bottom of each individual rhytid. The lip is then stretched to spread out the rhytids while the solution is applied with a very wet cotton-tipped applicator. One needs to obtain a white frost that is carried 2 to 3 mm across the vermilion border. When treating the lower eyelid, it is important to use a semidry applicator rolled once across the skin. The lower eyelids need to be treated to within 1 to 2 mm of the ciliary margin. On the upper eyelid, one must be very judicious about treating below the supratarsal fold, and most surgeons do not breach this boundary.

Application of the peeling agent creates an immediate burning sensation that lasts for 15 to 20 seconds and then resolves. After 20 minutes, the pain returns and lasts from 6 to 8 hours; then it typically resolves. The combination of Marcaine nerve blocks and narcotics usually makes the procedure very well tolerated by the patient.

Phenol Toxicity

Phenol is essentially toxic to all cells. It is absorbed through the skin into the bloodstream, and therefore must be excreted rapidly. The cardiac, hepatic, and renal systems are all affected by toxic doses of phenol (between 8 and 15 g for adults). Systemic toxicity is first suggested by central nervous system (CNS) stimulation, including tremors, hyperreflexia, and hypertension. After this, CNS depression occurs with respiratory failure, hypotension, and cardiac arrhythmias ensuing rapidly. Cardiac signs of toxicity develop in the following order: (1) tachycardia, (2) premature ventricular contractions, then (3) atrial fibrillation.[25] In Gross'[25] study, the average time from application of phenol to the onset of arrhythmias was 17.5 minutes, and most patients had 50% of the face covered at one time. Therefore, to prevent such toxicity, volume loading with intravenous fluids before, during, and after phenol peeling will enhance excretion in patients with normal liver and renal function. Many authors including Botta and colleagues[6] recommend maintaining a fluid load to force diuresis with 20 mg of furosemide given 10 minutes before the application of phenol. Controversies exist over the use of plasma expanders (i.e., colloids). Therefore, phenol should be avoided in patients with renal disease because they may not excrete it rapidly enough to avoid direct cardiac toxicity. Waiting as much as 20 to 30 minutes between treatment of each area and not peeling more than 50% of the face at one time minimizes the risk of phenol toxicity in most patients. Postoperative cardiac monitoring is necessary for a minimum of 30 minutes after the procedure, and personnel trained in advanced cardiac life support must be immediately available in the recovery unit.

Postoperative Care Routine

Postoperative care includes administration of an analgesic such as oxycodone (Percocet) or hydrocodone and acetaminophen (Lortab). Patients should minimize activity and rest until the next morning's office visit. Cool compresses can be applied in addition to their Aquaphor ointment or petroleum jelly. The patient will need assistance and is not allowed to drive or take care of himself or herself the day of the peel. A postoperative instruction booklet is given to the patient that discusses the expectations of marked edema, moderate temperature elevation to 99°F to 100°F, occasional nausea, and moderate discomfort. The morning after surgery, the patient is instructed to wash or rinse the face without soap using tepid tap water five or six times per day, followed by the appli-

cation of Aquaphor in an "icing on cake" fashion. Alternately, Eucerin cream or bacitracin ointment can be applied, however antibiotic sensitivity may develop with time. The patient is given 10 mg of dexamethasone (Decadron) IV intraoperatively and methylprednisolone (Medrol Dose Pack) postoperatively to reduce swelling. The patient is encouraged to take 1000 to 2000 mg/day of vitamin C as well as a multivitamin and to continue the antibiotic prophylaxis for 4 to 5 days postoperatively.

The patient is asked to return to the office on the third postoperative day to assure the physician that the wound is being cleaned as instructed. It is this time that allows the physician to intervene early if the wound has been neglected or if superficial infection has become a problem, such as with *Pseudomonas* infection, which can create a deeper injury. The patient often requires further education regarding the importance of his or her involvement in removing the desquamating skin and crust. The patient is then again evaluated in 3 to 4 days to observe the amount of wound healing and residual crusting. After 7 to 10 days, the patient can begin to apply makeup if epithelialization is complete. A makeup artist should be available and camouflage techniques should be provided to instruct the patient how to cover the pink/red areas. Generally, a mint green base is used before the foundation is applied to neutralize the red. Additionally, a brand-name hypoallergenic moisturizer is recommended for use once or twice daily.

The use of sunscreens and sun avoidance is critically important. Sunscreen with an SPF of 30 or greater is advised. The patient is not allowed any direct sun exposure for 6 weeks and is told to minimize sun exposure for up to 6 months.

To reduce the possibility of hyperpigmentation, estrogens should be withheld 4 weeks before the peel and for at least 6 to 8 weeks postoperatively. As the erythema is fading, pigmentation abnormalities are possible, and estrogen may increase the risk of this abnormality.

At our facility, nonfluorinated hydrocortisone (Hytone cream 2.5%) is recommended for 2 or 3 weeks after reepithelialization to decrease the erythema and the hypersensitivity that is common. The patient often complains of intense pruritus during the early recovery period, and Pramosone 2.5% steroid cream (pramoxine hydrochloride and hydrocortisone) with an antipruritic agent can be helpful. During the day, the patient may benefit from a nonsedating antihistamine such as desloratadine (Clarinex) or fexofenadine (Allegra), and may require hydroxyzine (Atarax) or diphenhydramine (Benadryl) at night to decrease the sensation of itching. Hypnotics such as temazepam (Restoril) or zolpidem tartrate (Ambien) may be necessary for sleep.

Although some surgeons begin the administration of retinoic acid (Retin A) as soon as epithelialization has occurred, we prefer to wait at least 3 months after the peel before giving the patient Retin A, and we then use it only if the patient desires it.

The patient returns for an office visit at 2 weeks and again 6 weeks later for evaluation of the early development of splotchy hyperpigmentation. Collins[15] recommends the use of hydroquinone gel almost routinely for 2 to 4 months as a prophylactic regimen against this condition, especially in darker-skinned persons Fitzpatrick type III or greater. If splotchy pigmentation develops, a combination of Retin A, hydroquinone (Eldoquin Forte), and triamcinolone (Aristocort) may provide an improvement. The patient is seen again at the 3-month, 6-month, and 1-year period postoperatively. Photographs are taken at each session (Figure 29-5).

Chemical Peel Complications

It is important to recognize the expected sequelae that accompany healing with chemical peels, as opposed to true complications. The following represent sequelae of chemical face peeling:

1. Pigmentary changes
   a. Hyperpigmentation
   b. Hypopigmentation
   c. Depigmentation (rarely, and in isolated areas)
2. Persistence of rhytids
3. Prolonged erythema
4. Persistent texture change of skin
5. Hypertrophic subepidermal healing
6. Milia
7. Skin pore prominence
8. Increased prominence of telangiectasias
9. Darkening and growth of preexisting nevi

Pigmentation changes are by far the most common phenomenon seen with chemical peels, and these predominantly occur as hypopigmentation. These areas are most obvious in transition zones between peeled and nonpeeled areas, which can be minimized with the feathering technique described earlier. Splotchy pigmentation can either be hypopigmentation or hyperpigmentation and is increased with exposure to sun or the use of systemic estrogens. This sequela is most commonly seen during the first 3 months of healing. Brody[9] notes that pigmentary changes rarely occur in Fitzpatrick type I and II patients, but in type III and IV patients there are frequently prominent lines of demarcation. Type V and VI patients will usually develop hyperpigmentation that may resolve over 18 to 24 months; however, most surgeons will not peel this population (Asian, Latin, or Indian) due to the risk of

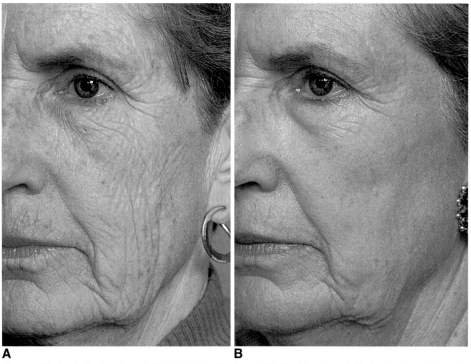

A   **B**

Figure 29-5. A, Pretreatment, Baker's chemical peel. **B,** Posttreatment, Baker's chemical peel. To view this image in color, please go to *www.ototext.com* or the Electronic Image Collection CD, bound into your copy of Cummings Otolaryngology—Head and Neck Surgery, 4th edition.

irregular coloration postoperatively. Retin A 0.1% and Eldoquin Forte 4% mixed with Aristocort 0.1% should be applied at the onset of early hyperpigmentation and continued for 2 to 3 months after the peel.

Unfortunately, persistent rhytids or wrinkles are relatively common after peeling, especially if they were prominent before the peel. McCollough and Brody believe that waiting 3 to 6 months is appropriate before repeating a chemical peel. We often touch up rhytids of the vermilion border and perioral area with dermabrasion between 3 and 6 months. Repeeling rhytids before the 2-month mark can result in severe hypopigmentation and subepithelial hypertrophic scarring. Prolonged erythema should be expected with early repeeling.

Complications of chemical peels include, but are not limited to, the following:

1. Skin infection
    a. Herpes simplex virus
    b. Pseudomonas organisms
    c. Staphylococcus/Streptococcus organisms
    d. Candida organisms
2. Lower eyelid ectropion
3. Cardiac arrhythmias
4. Renal failure
5. Laryngeal edema[32]
6. Toxic shock syndrome[40]
7. Facial scarring
8. Poor patient–physician relationship

Infections are uncommon, but herpetic breakouts can almost be expected if appropriate antiviral prophylaxis is not given (e.g., Valtrex 500 mg PO bid or Zovirax 800 mg PO tid starting 2 to 3 days before the peel). For patients with a strong history of herpetic outbreaks, at least 2 weeks of antiviral therapy should be administered after the peel. For patients who do undergo a herpetic outbreak despite prophylaxis, we have found that Zovirax dosed at 4.0 g/day is most expedient at clearing the infection. Superficial infection with *Pseudomonas, Staphylococcus,* or *Streptococcus* species is rare and can usually be attributed to poor postoperative wound care. *Candida* infections can occur, which will delay epithelialization. These should be treated with topical nystatin cream. Prolonged ointments after chemical peel may promote folliculitis and acne, especially in patients with a prior history. These conditions may become secondarily infected with *Staphylococcus* or *Streptococcus* species and should be treated with the appropriate oral antibiotic, in addition to topical clindamycin phosphate (Cleocin T) gel.

In summary, chemical peels are an effective and extremely satisfactory procedure with which every facial plastic surgeon should be familiar. Careful patient selection and education are crucial to both the patient's final result and his or her satisfaction. Learning the chemical peel technique is only a small part of the overall process; postoperative care and close patient follow-up are equally as important. Understanding these principles and knowing how to treat the sequelae or complications of chemical peels will allow the surgeon and patient to achieve a satisfactory result in facial skin rejuvenation, in addition to establishing a positive long-term relationship.

DERMABRASION

Facial dermabrasion is an effective technique in skilled hands. It dates back to 1905, when Kronmayer[35] used rotating burrs for removal of various skin lesions, and was modernized in the late 1940s by Kurtin[36] with the development of the wire brush technique. Although discussed here for the management of aging skin, dermabrasion is most commonly used for the treatment facial scars induced by acne, trauma, varicella, or surgery, in addition to removal of superficial skin lesions. However, dermabrasion is a time-tested technique for the removal of wrinkles, especially in the difficult to treat perioral and vermillion regions.

Dermabrasion is a mechanical method using abrasive surfaces to remove the epidermis and create a wound in the papillary or reticular dermis. This subsequently causes the stimulation of type I and III collagen and formation of a fresh new layer of skin. An excellent cosmetic improvement is seen, and the collagen continues to thicken over a 12- to 18-month period, further enhancing a youthful appearance. Sun-damaged cells, superficial scars, and premalignant lesions are removed and replaced with the epithelialization process, enhancing the final aesthetic outcome.

Patient Selection and Consultation

Facial scars and skin lesions can be improved but not entirely eliminated by dermabrasion techniques. The treatment of rhytids and photodamage may only improve by 50% to 80%, especially in the perioral region. Similarly, bad acne scars are only expected to improve by 30% to 40% or less. This point must be stressed during the initial patient consultation for both patient and physician satisfaction. The patient must accept a 10- to 14-day healing time with a relatively intense postoperative wound care regimen. The patient should be educated on the amount of anticipated drainage, swelling, discomfort, and bruising in addition to a period of prolonged erythema lasing up to 8 to 12 weeks. The risks and benefits should be covered during the consultation period with a witnessed informed consent form signed. Preoperative and postoperative photographs are very important for documentation, although acne scarring may be difficult to photograph without proper lighting techniques.

Careful patient selection is important to the final outcome of dermabrasion resurfacing. Patients with a history of prior skin resurfacing tend to have a less dramatic result with dermabrasion and are at a slightly higher risk of hypopigmentation and complications. A minimum of 12 months is recommended before a second dermabrasion procedure to allow for maximal improvement of scars and completion of the healing process. Scars or wrinkles on the neck should not be treated with dermabrasion due to the high risk of hypertrophic scarring and depigmentation caused by a significant decrease in adnexal structures and a much thinner dermis.

Patients with a history of acne should be under complete medical control before any dermabrasion resurfacing techniques. The use of isotretinoin (Accutane) within a 6-month period is a contraindication to dermabrasion due to the increased risk of scarring because this medicine decreases the number of pilosebaceous units required for adequate healing.[30,50,51] Some dermatologists recommend waiting a full year after the end of Accutane administration before facial resurfacing. Dermabrasion is also contraindicated in patients with deficient healing capacities, collagen vascular disorders, and a personal history of keloids.

Equipment

Equipment for dermabrasion techniques varies from handheld manual units, to sterile sandpaper, to high-speed machines. Modern electrical dermabrasion machines are compact and easy to use, and they gener-ate rotational speeds up to 33,000 rpm. The handpiece accepts various tips that allow site- and lesion-specific treatment for the patient (Figure 29-6). Additionally, the rotation of direction is reversible, making the approach to anatomic sites safer and enabling access for either a right- or left-handed surgeon.

Dermabrasion is performed with either a wire brush, diamond fraise, or serrated wheel placed into the handpiece unit. The wire brush attachment is a wheel with rigid stainless steel wires protruding from its circumference. The wire brush is very efficient at tissue removal, often achieving the desired depth with only one pass. It therefore has a narrow margin of error and is preferred by more experienced surgeons. The microlacerations created by the wire brush are believed to improve the final result of the procedure because the papillary or outer reticular dermis is wounded and subsequent collagen formation stimulated. The skin surface must be frozen when using the wire brush to achieve efficient abrasion and to maintain the surface topography. This technique also decreases the risk of gouging the skin, and free margins of the lip must also be approached with care because it is easy to catch the margin and create an intraoral tear.

The diamond fraise attachment consists of a wheel or cone studded with diamond chips of various degrees of coarseness. The coarser the unit, the deeper the skin penetration achieved, and the finer diamond fraises are used more as a "polishing" or blending tool. The diamond fraise is the safest and easiest dermabrasion unit to use, but is also the slowest. The use of the diamond wheel/burr also requires little or no cryogen spray, which is unique among the dermabrasion attachments.

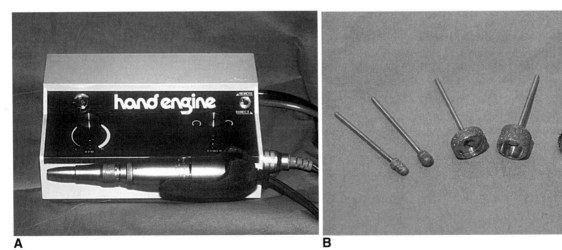

A **B**

Figure 29-6. A, Electrical dermabrasion machine. **B,** Various tips for use with electrical dermabrasion machine handpiece. To view this image in color, please go to *www.ototext.com* or the Electronic Image Collection CD, bound into your copy of Cummings Otolaryngology— Head and Neck Surgery, 4th edition.

Technique

Dermabrasion at our facility can be performed with the patient under intravenous sedation, or with "twilight anesthesia" as an isolated procedure. The patient receives 10 to 20 mg of Valium PO before the procedure. Cardiovascular monitoring is used, and the patient is administered 3 mg of Versed and 1 mg of Dilaudid before regional blocks. The local blocks are performed with bupivacaine 0.25% and epinephrine 1/200,000 and include the supraorbital, infraorbital, and mental foramen for full-face dermabrasion. This technique, in conjunction with the use of refrigerant spray (Frigiderm), allows for a pain-free experience for most patients.

The face or region of concern is treated in 1- or 2-square-inch segments. These areas are blocked off by a 4 × 4-inch gauze pad before application of the refrigerant spray, which avoids inhalation or ocular injury. Once the skin has been chilled, a 10- to 12-second period of dermabrasion is allowable until further freezing is required. Overzealous use of the refrigerant spray should be avoided, however, because tissue damage and focal skin necrosis is possible. The dermabrasion handpiece should be held firmly and pulled only in a plane perpendicular to the plane of rotation (Figure 29-7). One should avoid rotary or back-and-forth motions because this may increase the risk of gouging the skin and causing deeper injury. Use of the wire brush requires minimal pressure because the steel wires cause numerous microlacerations, whereas the diamond fraise requires significantly more pressure. Adequate depth of treatment is determined by observing the skin surface. Stripping off the epidermis will reveal a slightly gray papillary dermis. In the midpapillary dermis, multiple small punc-

tate bleeding points are seen and represent the dermal capillary loops. The border between the papillary and reticular dermis is marked by a slightly yellow color signifying the sebaceous gland lobules. As the midreticular dermis is approached, larger but fewer bleeding points appear and the surface becomes coarser. Care must be given as one proceeds deeper than this level because the risk of scarring significantly increases.

It is best to begin the dermabrasion process centrally near the nose and work outward toward the cheeks (begin in the dependent areas to avoid pooling of blood in the upcoming region). In the perioral areas, special care must be given to holding the lip taut and keeping the direction of rotation away from the mouth to avoid significant laceration (Figure 29-8). One must always stay parallel to the skin's surface when performing dermabrasion. Dermabrasion should also be carried out in facial units and carried to, but not across, the jawline, hairline, and orbital rims. Untreated areas are then peeled with the appropriate chemical agent such as Jessner's solution plus 35% TCA or phenol 88% to the lower eyelids. This allows for better blending of pigmentation and avoids discrete areas of hypopigmentation. One should never dermabrade the neck due to the high risk of scarring and pigmentation difficulties.

Postoperative Care

The regional nerve blocks given during the onset of the dermabrasion procedure typically last for 6 to 8 hours, and a narcotic script is provided to control delayed pain. Wet gauze is applied to the dermabraded regions immediately after the procedure for about 5 minutes, and after this most bleeding has usually subsided. Xeroform gauze is applied topically to all

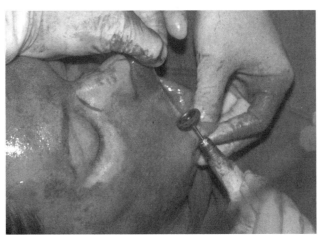

Figure 29-7. Proper technique for use of dermabrasion handpiece. To view this image in color, please go to *www.ototext.com* or the Electronic Image Collection CD, bound into your copy of Cummings Otolaryngology—Head and Neck Surgery, 4th edition.

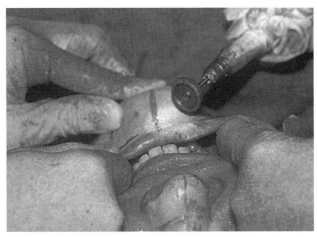

Figure 29-8. Proper technique for performing dermabrasion in the perioral area. To view this image in color, please go to *www.ototext.com* or the Electronic Image Collection CD, bound into your copy of Cummings Otolaryngology—Head and Neck Surgery, 4th edition.

areas of dermabrasion, not a silicon-based (Silon) mask. The xeroform dressing is allowed to dry overnight before moisturization and lubrication are begun. Using tepid water or saline-soaked gauze, the clinician cleanses the sites of dermabrasion of all serum and crusting all the way down to the visible gauze fibers, and a fresh coat of Aquaphor or bacitracin is applied topically 4 to 6 times daily. Alternatively, if Silon was applied, it would be removed on the third postoperative day, at which point lubrication would begin. The administration of a Medrol Dose Pack is usually started on the day of the procedure, and the patient continues to take antibiotic and antiviral prescriptions started on preoperative day 1. When epithelialization begins, the xeroform gauze starts to separate and can be trimmed progressively. Complete reepithelialization has occurred by the seventh to tenth day, and a session with a makeup artist is provided for the patient to teach him or her more about camouflage techniques. Strict adherence to sun avoidance or the use of sunscreen with an SPF of 30 or greater is discussed with the patient because serious pigmentation problems can be caused by early sun exposure. Patients with prolonged erythema are given Hytone cream 2.5% topically bid. Patients with signs of hyperpigmentation or know melasma are given topical hydroquinone 4% or 8% to be applied nightly. Most patients can return to work by the seventh to tenth postoperative day with a light covering of makeup; however, such cosmetics should be avoided before complete reepithelialization because as contact dermatitis and further infection may follow (Figure 29-9).

Complications

Acne outbreaks are a common complication of dermabrasion, especially in patients with a previous his-tory. The breakouts can be minimized with the preoperative use of tetracycline in high-risk patients. Active breakouts respond to tetracycline plus topical Cleocin T gel. Other common complications include milia formation at the site of dermabrasion. This can be avoided or treated with the use of tretinoin therapy. The use of a sloughing pad or sponge (Buf-Puf) to lightly abrade the surface of these lesions is helpful. Deep pore cleansing facials and extractions are also helpful and can be performed by an aesthetician. Prolonged erythema beyond 4 weeks should be treated with a topical steroid such as Hytone cream 2.5% to avoid pigmentary problems or scarring. Subepithelial hyperplasia should be injected with triamcinolone steroid (Kenalog-10), to avoid potential scarring. Another uncommon complication is postoperative infection. The most common microorganisms include *Staphylococcus aureus,* herpes simplex virus, and *Candida* species.[21] The prompt use of the appropriate antibiotic, antiviral, or antifungal agent should be sufficient for treatment, and often poor cleansing is the culprit for infection. Additionally, some hypopigmentation is seen quite often after dermabrasion.[46]

Dermabrasion is therefore a longstanding, reliable method for rejuvenation of aging skin with predictable and reproducible results. The equipment is inexpensive and simple to operate; however, technique is very important to obtain the best results. Recent studies have shown that dermabraded skin in the perioral region has identical cosmetic results when compared to CO_2 laser but heals in half of the time with less postoperative erythema and morbidity.[22,29] Additionally, dermabrasion for lip rhytids tends to be more effective and predictable as a single treatment compared with CO_2 laser or chemical peel. Therefore, an understanding

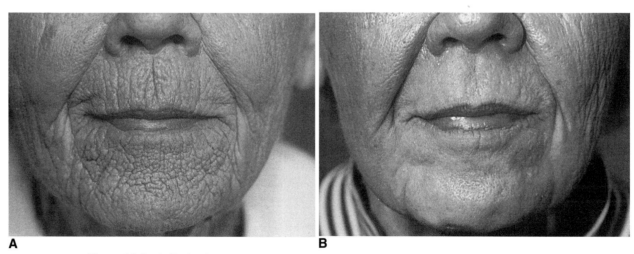

A   **B**

Figure 29-9. A, Perioral dermabrasion: preoperative view. **B,** Perioral dermabrasion: postoperative view. To view this image in color, please go to *www.ototext.com* or the Electronic Image Collection CD, bound into your copy of Cummings Otolaryngology—Head and Neck Surgery, 4th edition.

of and an ability to perform dermabrasion techniques should be in the armamentarium of all facial plastic surgeons because it serves as an excellent and diverse tool for facial resurfacing.

LASER RESURFACING

Laser skin resurfacing has become more popular over the past several years and is an important modality in rejuvenation of the aging face. Many surgeons have turned to laser resurfacing instead of dermabrasion due to the higher risk of bloodborne pathogens when performing dermabrasion. Although numerous lasers exist, the primary lasers used for facial resurfacing today are the pulsed carbon dioxide (CO_2) and erbium:yttrium-aluminum-garnet (Er:YAG) lasers. The practice of combining these lasers is also gaining popularity.[24] Laser resurfacing can also be combined with the use of chemical peels or dermabrasion when clinically indicated. Additionally, laser skin resurfacing is commonly combined with other surgical procedures such as endoscopic browlifts, facelifts, and transconjunctival blepharoplasty. The physician should become aware of the unique properties of these resurfacing lasers to best treat his or her patients' aging skin needs.

CO_2 Laser

Energy of the pulsed CO_2 laser is produced in the 10,600-nm spectrum. Approximate tissue ablation of the CO_2 laser is 50 to 100 μm with collateral thermal conduction reported between 30 and 50 μm. Laser facial resurfacing is excellent for treating light- to medium-depth rhytids. The pulsed CO_2 laser is particularly good for treating perioral vertical furrows, periocular crow's feet, glabellar rhytids, and diffuse actinic damage and aging spots. Additional uses of the CO_2 laser include removal of superficial lesions and scars down to the epidermal-dermal junction.

There are a variety of pulsed CO_2 lasers available (Figure 29-10). The laser energy is delivered through a flexible waveguide handpiece to the targeted area in a geometric pattern that varies in size and is easily adjustable. The UltraPulse Encore CO_2 laser (Coherent, Inc.) has a randomization pattern feature (*cool scan*) that prevents the "postage-stamped" mark on the patient's skin. The operator selects the energy density (i.e., fluence) and power in millijoule that determines the depth of tissue ablation. The microprocessor will calculate the peak power in watts based on the above settings and the spot size delivered. Standard settings for a patient undergoing initial full-face resurfacing for moderate aging and photodamage ranges from 80 to 90 mJ and a density of 4 or 5 with the largest rectangular spot size at our facility (ranging from 46 to 60 W). A second pass over regions with

more photoaging will typically be set at 20 mJ less than the first pass and at a density setting of 4. The deeper passes are used to treat the base of the furrow, using the principle of dermal remodeling with subsequent collagen thickening. The edges of the wound are also blended with that of nondamaged skin, giving a more uniform appearance after healing (Figure 29-11). Depending on the depth of treatment required,

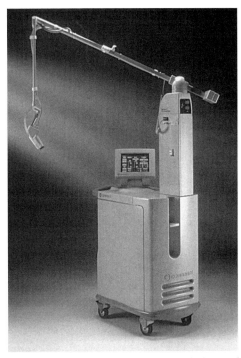

Figure 29-10. Pulsed CO_2 laser. To view this image in color, please go to *www.ototext.com* or the Electronic Image Collection CD, bound into your copy of Cummings Otolaryngology—Head and Neck Surgery, 4th edition.

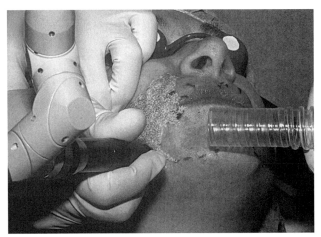

Figure 29-11. Example of blending of wound edges with that of nondamaged skin during CO_2 laser treatment. To view this image in color, please go to *www.ototext.com* or the Electronic Image Collection CD, bound into your copy of Cummings Otolaryngology—Head and Neck Surgery, 4th edition.

the clinician can pass superficially to the upper papillary dermis (denoted by pink), to the upper reticular dermis (denoted by gray), or to the deepest recommended midreticular level (seen as chamois-brown with pinpoint bleeding). Care must be given when treating the thin eyelid skin, and most operators recommend only one pass in this region.

Er:YAG Laser

The technique of facial resurfacing using the Er:YAG laser is similar to that of the CO_2 laser, except there is no coagulative necrosis with less tissue interaction. Therefore, one can overlap pulses by 10%, which must be avoided when using the CO_2 laser secondary to thermal damage. Due to less tissue damage, the classic skin color changes involved in CO_2 laser surgery are not seen, however a useful depth indicator when using the Er:YAG laser is pinpoint bleeding, which occurs at the level of the papillary dermis. This high-powered laser transforms the superficial skin into particulate matter, therefore a smoke evacuator and laser that masks filter 0.1-µm particles is recommended in addition to laser eyewear. Some authors recommend the combined use of the CO_2 laser with the Er:YAG laser for optimum postoperative healing. The first pass is performed using the CO_2 laser for primary resurfacing. The Er:YAG laser is then used to clean up the zone of thermal necrosis created by the CO_2 laser which would otherwise turn into persistent erythema. The favorably heated deeper dermis remains, and the fibroblasts have been stimulated to secrete neocollagen.[33] Usually two to three passes are required, using the Er:YAG laser with this technique. The study by Utley and colleagues[60] showed that one pass with the Er:YAG laser penetrated 20 µm, vs 62.5 µm with the CO_2 laser.

Postoperative Laser Care

A post-laser occlusive dressing (silicone based Silon) is used for the first 3 to 4 days. The use of an occlusive dressing is less painful for the patient, prevents crusting seen with the exudative phase, and promotes moist reepithelialization (Figure 29-12). Once this dressing is removed on postoperative day 4, the patient is instructed on wound care. This regimen includes cleansing the entire face (or resurfaced region) using saline and 4 × 4-inch gauze four to five times daily down to pink-healing skin, followed by a generous layer of Aquaphor. If required, dilute acetic acid soaks are used for increased removal of serum exudates. Additionally, appropriate antibacterial agents (e.g., bacitracin ointment) or antifungal agents are used if clinically indicated and are typically a sign of inadequate cleansing. Once reepithelialization has

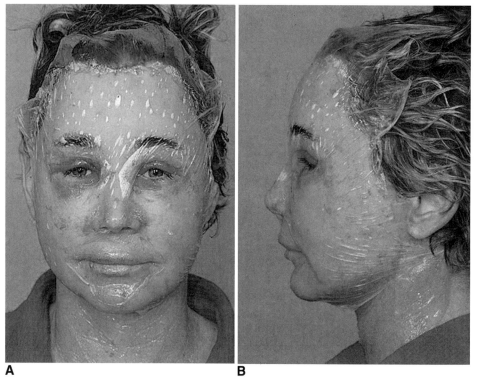

A   **B**

Figure 29-12. A, Post-laser occlusive (Silon) dressing: frontal view. To view this image in color, please go to *www.ototext.com* or the Electronic Image Collection CD, bound into your copy of Cummings Otolaryngology—Head and Neck Surgery, 4th edition. **B,** Post-laser occlusive (Silon) dressing: lateral view.

occurred, by the seventh to 10th day, a makeup session with an aesthetician or makeup artist should be offered to teach important camouflage techniques during the period of postoperative erythema. A good waterproof sunscreen with an SPF of 30 or greater is recommended for a minimum of 6 to 12 months postoperatively to minimize discoloration issues and to maximize healing (Figures 29-13 and 29-14).

Postoperative laser complications are the same as discussed in terms of chemical peel procedures, and therefore frequent and meticulous postoperative visits and patient evaluation cannot be overemphasized. Additionally, "hot spots" often seen with CO_2 laser treatment will benefit from hydrocolloid (DuoDerm) occlusive dressings during the early healing periods. These should be changed every 24 to 72 hours until reepithelialization has occurred.

In general, facial resurfacing using the CO_2 laser requires a longer "downtime" of 7 to 10 days with prolonged erythema up to 3 to 4 months compared with the Er:YAG laser, which tends to involve a healing time of 4 to 5 days with short-lived erythema. However, the CO_2 laser produces a true skin-tightening result with improved elasticity, rhytid removal, and long-term results than the Er:YAG laser.[60] Although the pulsed CO_2 laser and Er:YAG laser are the most popular ablative resurfacing lasers available at present, technology is rapidly advancing, and one must stay current with such advances to be competitive in today's market. Additionally, nonablative resurfacing lasers and technologies are gaining more popularity and *may* surpass conventional laser use due to the minimal downtime and post-laser care required for the patient. However, to date, none of these lasers are able to treat significant rhytids and photoaging, even with a series of four to six treatments.

AESTHETICIAN'S ROLE IN THE MANAGEMENT OF AGING SKIN

The role of the esthetician in facial rejuvenation and skin care is rapidly expanding. The esthetician has numerous options and skills available that do not

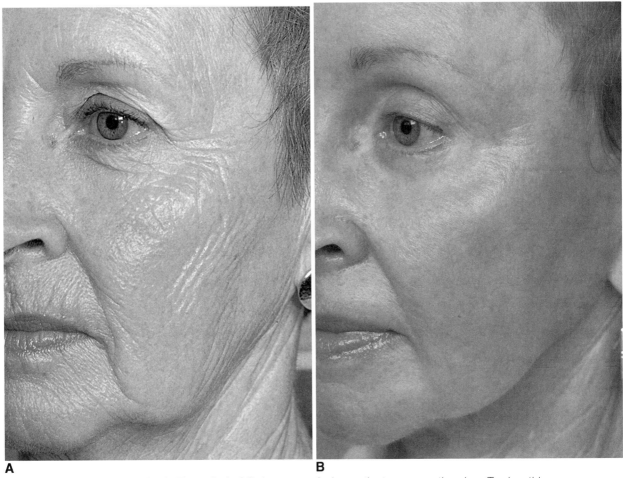

A   **B**

Figure 29-13. A, Example 1, CO_2 laser resurfacing patient: preoperative view. To view this image in color, please go to *www.ototext.com* or the Electronic Image Collection CD, bound into your copy of Cummings Otolaryngology—Head and Neck Surgery, 4th edition. **B,** Example 1, CO_2 laser resurfacing patient: postoperative view.

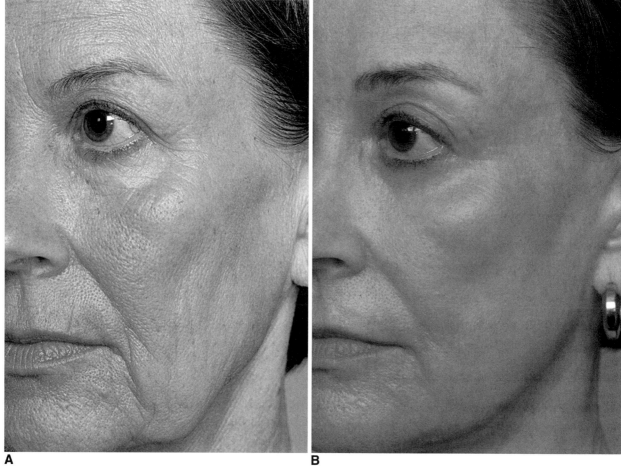

A   B

Figure 29-14. A, Example 2, CO_2 laser resurfacing patient: preoperative view. To view this image in color, please go to *www.ototext.com* or the Electronic Image Collection CD, bound into your copy of Cummings Otolaryngology—Head and Neck Surgery, 4th edition. B, Example 2, CO_2 laser resurfacing patient: postoperative view.

require sedation or direct physician supervision to improve skin quality. Such interventions include:

• Nonablative resurfacing.
• Microdermabrasion.
• Superficial chemical peels.
• Medical skin care regimens.
• Intense pulsed light "laser" treatment of facial dyschromia.

NONABLATIVE FACIAL RESURFACING

As technology improves, new devices are being introduced to the marketplace at a stunning pace as options for nonablative facial rejuvenation. Some of the more popular devices include the IPL (Intense Pulsed Light) therapy, neodymium (Nd) YAG laser system (Cool Touch, Roseville, Ca), ThermaCool TC system (Thermage, Hayward, Ca), and other ultrasound or radiofrequency units. Although the subject is too lengthy to discuss each novel modality in detail, these

technologies have a similar goal in common. This goal is to stimulate the deeper papillary and reticular dermis to thicken and generate new, healthy collagen while maintaining an intact epidermis that requires little downtime for healing. Such collagen stimulation can occur by intense light therapy, radiofrequency waves or coblation, specific thermal energy delivery, or focused laser wavelengths. Typically, multiple treatments are required for improved rhytid removal and skin texture quality, usually over a 4- to 12-week interval. Advantages of the nonablative techniques include avoiding the potential complications of deeper peels and lasers such as hypopigmentation, prolonged erythema, and hypertrophic scarring. The disadvantages of these new technologies are mostly in the long-term results. Many investigators feel that the nonablative devices show modest improvement in wrinkles, at best, which is likely a result of collagen homogenization. This clinical improvement requires 3 to 6 months to appreciate, and such results are often short lived.[23] With further clinical trials and improving technology, however, these less invasive alternatives to facial rejuvenation may predominate in the near future.

MICRODERMABRASION

Microdermabrasion is a popular noninvasive technique performed by estheticians for facial rejuvenation. The term for this procedure is actually a misnomer because the controlled injury created by this process is actually to the epidermis. Microdermabrasion uses the abrasive action of small particle microcrystals (i.e., aluminum oxide, sodium chloride, or sodium bicarbonate) to wound the epidermis, coupled with suction to remove any skin debris. An inflammatory response is stimulated within the epidermis and results in the formation of a new stratum corneum within 3 to 5 days. Some authors believe that repeated microdermabrasion treatments not only increase the thickness of the outer epidermis after a 6-week period, but may even stimulate fibroblasts and new collagen deposition in the superficial papillary dermis.[52]

Typically, a series of treatments are required to achieve the desired resurfacing results (6 to 10 treatments), followed by a maintenance program every 4 to 6 weeks. The patient's skin surface will feel smoother with a firmer texture reported. Microdermabrasion is best used for epidermal conditions including fine rhytids, dyschromia, superficial scarring (e.g., acne), and actinic keratosis. Microdermabrasion techniques are best complimented with a daily medical skin care program. As the process histologically removes the stratum corneum, the penetration of the topical medications is enhanced, yielding a more desired outcome. Patient satisfaction is typically good after a full series of microdermabrasion treatments because there is minimal discomfort with little recovery or downtime.

Contraindications to microdermabrasion treatments are relative but should include open herpetic lesions, bleeding disorders, active inflammatory rosacea, open wounds or sores, vascular lesions, warty growths, or sunburned skin. Although active acne regions can be covered individually with small tape, widespread active acne should be viewed as a contraindication.

After each microdermabrasion session, the patient should expect several hours of increased pinkness or redness and sensitivity to the skin (occasionally days with deeper treatments). With the stratum corneum disrupted, the skin requires more moisturization and sun protection. A sunblock with zinc oxide, titanium oxide, or an SPF of 30 or greater is recommended for the first week after each treatment.

Patients will note increased skin tightness for the first 12 to 24 hours, with a corresponding decrease in fine wrinkles. Some peeling of the skin may be noted 48 to 96 hours after a treatment session; this can be reduced or avoided with the use of a strong moisturizer. Makeup can be reapplied within minutes of a treatment, and medical skin care programs can be resumed within 48 hours.

SUPERFICIAL CHEMICAL PEELS

Although medium and deep chemical peels require a physician's expertise and patient sedation, lighter chemical peels can be performed by the esthetician as an excellent skin maintenance program. These treatments are often combined with other techniques such as microdermabrasion for improved efficacy. The following are common superficial peels used routinely for skin rejuvenation and maintenance:

- Glycolic acid 20% to 70%.
- TCA peels 10% to 30%.
- Resorcinol 20% to 30%.
- Jessner's solution.
- Alpha-hydroxy acid.
- Retinoic acid.
- Enzymatic peels.

Superficial peels effectively slough the outer epidermis (stratum corneum), improving skin texture by producing a thicker epidermal layer. Additionally, superficial skin lesions and dyschromias are treated by these peels. Precautions to avoid sun exposure should be taken for at least 72 hours after a peel, and patients with sensitive skin should avoid hydroxy acid and retinoid products for 24 to 48 hours after the procedure.

MEDICAL SKIN CARE REGIMENS

"Anti-aging" and "wrinkle cream" products have flooded the market over the past few years, often making false promises regarding potential facial rejuvenation outcomes. The majority of these products are not approved by the U.S. Food and Drug Administration nor are they supported with clinical prospective trials. It is therefore imperative we use medical skin care maintenance programs for our patients that are both safe and efficacious.

Retinoids are derivatives of Vitamin A and are most commonly prescribed as tretinoin. Tretinoin has been proven effective through numerous double-blind studies for treating mild to moderate photodamaged skin. Available tretinoin products include Renova, Retin A, MicroRetin A, and Avita. Daily application of these topical creams has been shown to improve fine wrinkling, surface roughness, hyperpigmentation, and sallowness[61] over a 6- to 12-month period. Tazarotene cream, a tretinoin receptor derivative, has been shown to improve fine wrinkling, mottled hyperpigmentation, lentigines, elastosis, pore size, irregular depigmentation, tactile roughness, and coarse rhytids in a 12-month multicenter randomized trial.[47] Tretinoin induces type I procollagen formation, thickens the epidermis, reduces melanin content, increases glycosaminoglycans and stimulates angiogenesis, giving a "rosy" appearance to the skin. Histologically, tretinoin-treated skin is more stable due to increased anchoring fibrils and decreased activity of collagenase enzyme. Tretinoin can also reduce UV-induced collagen destruction and therefore helps prevent photodamage.[19] Adverse effects include mild to moderate dryness, skin irritation, peeling, and photosensitivity, therefore protection from sun exposure is important.

Alpha-hydroxy acids have long been used in skin care products and have a proven level of safety as adjunctive therapy in photodamaged skin, melasma, hyperpigmentation, acne, and rosacea. Although their exact mechanism of action is unknown, alpha-hydroxy acids function by thinning the stratum corneum, promoting epidermolysis, dispersing basal layer melanin, and increasing collagen synthesis within the dermis.[59] Alpha-hydroxy acids are often used in combination with retinoids and other antioxidants for maximum clinical benefit.

Beta-hydroxy acids contain salicylic acid and have similar properties to alpha-hydroxy acids. Beta-hydroxy acids are also antiinflammatory in nature and are often less irritating than their alpha counterparts.

N6-furfuryladenine (Kinerase, ICN Pharmaceuticals) is a plant-growth factor that is good for patients with very sensitive skin who cannot tolerate retinoids and alpha-hydroxy acids. In a large, 6-month uncontrolled study, use of N6-furfuryladenine led to a significant reduction in skin roughness (63%) and to smaller reductions in hyperpigmentation (32%) and fine wrinkles (17%).[47] Further double-blind studies are warranted.

Numerous "anti-aging" creams and products are being investigated at present. Considerable interest has been given to the antioxidants such as vitamins C and E applied topically to protect or reverse photoaging. Initial results of high-dose vitamin C proved to be a prooxidant causing oxidative DNA damage, however the use of vitamin C esters has been promising in terms of effectively reducing photodamage. Further investigation and trials are warranted in the realm of topical antiinflammatory, antioxidant, cytokine, and growth factor creams to prove their long-term clinical efficacy and safety records.

In summary, the management of aging skin is a very important topic in today's society for which facial plastic surgeons play a predominant role. It is imperative to remain current with the latest technologies because the patient's expectations and knowledge base are rapidly increasing in the Internet age. One should maintain a diverse repertoire of options in his or her armamentarium for the management of aging skin, where patient selection and education will ultimately provide the best clinical outcome and patient satisfaction.

REFERENCES

1. Alt TH: Occluded Baker-Gordon chemical peel: review and update, *J Dermatol Surg Oncol* 15:980, 1989.
2. Baker TJ, Gordon HL: The ablation of rhytids by chemical means: a preliminary report, *J Fla Med Assoc* 48:451, 1961.
3. Baker TJ, Gordon HL, editors: *Chemical face peeling*. In *Surgical rejuvenation of the face*. St. Louis, 1986, Mosby–Year Book.
4. Baker TJ, Gordon HL, Stuzin JM: Chemical peel: a change in routine, *Ann Plast Surg* 23:166-169, 1989.
5. Beeson WH, McCollough EG: Chemical face peeling, *J Dermatol Surg Oncol* 11:10, 1985.
6. Botta SA, Straith RE, Goodwin HH: Cardiac arrhythmias in phenol face peeling: a suggested protocol for prevention, *Aesthetic Plast Surg* 12:115, 1988.
7. Brodland DG, Roenigk RK: Trichloracetic acid chemexfoliation (chemical peel) for extensive premalignant actinic damage of the face and scalp, *Mayo Clin Proc* 63:887, 1988.
8. Brody HJ: The art of chemical peeling, *J Dermatol Surg Oncol* 15:918, 1989a.
9. Brody HJ: Complications of chemical peeling, *J Dermatol Surg Oncol* 15:1010, 1989b.
10. Brody HJ: Variations and comparisons in medium depth chemical peeling, *J Dermatol Surg Oncol* 15:953, 1989c.
11. Brody HJ, Alt TH: *Cosmetic surgery of the skin: principles and techniques*. In Coleman WP, editor: *Chemical peeling*, Philadelphia, 1991, BC Decker.
12. Brody HJ, Hailey CW: Medium-depth chemical peeling, *J Dermatol Surg Oncol* 12:1268, 1989.
13. Brody HJ, Hailey CW: Medium-depth chemical peeling of the skin: a variation of superficial chemosurgery, *Adv Dermatol* 3:205, 1986.
14. Brown AM, Kaplan LM, Brown ME: Phenol-induced histological skin changes: hazards, technique, and uses, *Br J Plast Surg* 13:158, 1960.
15. Collins PS: Trichloracetic acid peels revisited, *J Dermatol Surg Oncol* 15:933, 1989.
16. Dmytryshyan JR: Chemical face peel complicated by toxic-shock syndrome, *Arch Otolaryngol* 109:170, 1983.
17. Farber GA: *Chemical peeling*. In Burks JW, editor: *The treatment of certain cosmetic defects and diseases of the skin*. Springfield, Ill, 1979, Charles C. Thomas.
18. Farber GA, Collins PS, Scott MW: Update on chemical peel, *J Dermatol Surg Oncol* 10:559, 1984.
19. Fisher GJ, Talwar HS, Lin J, Voorhees J: Molecular mechanisms of photoaging in human skin in vivo and their prevention by all-trans retinoic acid *Photochem Photobiol* 69:154-7, 1999.
20. Fitzpatrick TB: The validity and practicality of sun-reactive skin types I-VI, *Arch Dermatol* 124: 869, 1988.
21. Fulton JE Jr: The prevention and management of post-dermabrasion complications, *J Dermatol Surg Oncol* 17:431, 1991.

22. Gin I and others: Treatment of upper lip wrinkles: a comparison of the 950 microsec dwell time carbon dioxide laser to manual tumescent dermabrasion, *Dermatol Surg* 25:468-73, 1999.

23. Goldberg DJ: Nonablative dermal remodeling: does it really work? *Arch Dermatol* 138:1366-8, 2002.

24. Greene D and others: In vivo model of histologic changes following treatment with the superpulsed CO_2 laser, erbium:YAG laser, and blended lasers: a 4 to 6 month prospective histologic and clinical study, *Lasers Surg Med* 27:362-72, 2000.

25. Gross BG: Cardiac arrhythmias during phenol face peeling, *Plast Reconstr Surg* 73:590, 1984.

26. Hayes DK, Berkland ME, Stambaugh KS: Dermal healing after local skin flaps and chemical peel, *Arch Otolaryngol Head and Neck Surg* 116:794, 1990.

27. Hayes DK, Stambaugh KS: Viability of skin flaps subjected to simultaneous chemical peel with occlusive taping, *Larngoscope* 99:1016, 1989.

28. Hetter GP: An examination of the phenol-croton oil peel: part 1. Dissecting the formula, *Plast Reconstr Surg* 105:227, 2000.

29. Holmkvist KA, Rogers GS: Treatment of perioral rhytids: a comparison of dermabrasion and superpulsed carbon dioxide laser. *Arch of Dermatol* 136:725-31, 2000.

30. Katz BE, MacFarlane DF: Atypical facial scarring after isotretinoin therapy in a patient with previous dermabrasion, *J Am Acad Dermatol* 30:852, 1994.

31. Kligman AM, Baker TJ, Gordon HL: Long-term histologic follow-up of phenol peels, *Plast Reconstr Surg* 75:652, 1985.

32. Kline DR, Little JH: Laryngeal edema as a complication of chemical peel, *Plast Reconstr Surg* 71:419, 1983.

33. Koch RJ, Cheng E: Quantification of skin elasticity changes associated with pulsed carbon dioxide laser skin resurfacing, *Arch Facial Plast Surg* 1:272-275, 1999.

34. Koopman CF Jr.: Phenol toxicity during face peels, *Otolaryngol Head and Neck Surg* 90:383, 1982.

35. Kronmayer E: Die Heilung der Akne Durch in Nevus Norbenlases Operaionsverfahren: Das Stanzen, *Illustriert Monatsschrift Arzlich Polytechnisch* 27:101, 1905.

36. Kurtin A: Corrective surgical planning of skin, *Arch Dermatol Syhilol* 68:389, 1953.

37. Litton C: Chemical face lifting, *Plast Reconstr Surg* 29:371, 1962.

38. Litton C, Sachowicz EH, Trinidad GP: Present day status of the chemical face peel, *Aesthetic Plast Surg* 10:1, 1986.

39. Litton C, Trinidad GP: Complications of chemical peeling as evaluated by questionnaire, *Plast Reconstr Surg* 1981:738, 1981.

40. LoVerme WE and others: Toxic shock syndrome after chemical face peel, *Plast Reconstr Surg* 80:115-118, 1987.

41. Maibach HI, Rovee DT: Epidermal wound healing, Chicago, 1972, Mosby-Year Book.

42. Mandy SH: Tretinoin in the preoperative and postoperative management of dermabrasion, J Am Acad Dermatol 15:870, 1986.

43. McCollough EG, Hillman RA Jr: Symposium on the aging face, *Otolaryngol Clin North Am* 13:353, 1980.

44. McCollough EG, Langsdon PR: *Dermabrasion and chemical peel: a guide for facial plastic surgeons.* In McCollough EG, Langsdon PR, editors: *Chemical peel.* New York, 1988, Thieme Medical Publishers.

45. Mendelson JE: Update on chemical peels, *Otolaryngol Clin North Am* 35:57, 2002.

46. Niechajev I, Ljungqvist A: Perioral dermabrasion: clinical and experimental studies, *Aesthetic Plast Surg* 16:11, 1992.

47. Phillips TJ and others: Efficacy of 0.1% tazarotene cream for the treatment of photodamage: a 12-month multicenter randomized trial, *Arch Dermatol* 138:1486-1493, 2002.

48. Rappaport MJ, Kramer F: Exacerbation of facial herpes simplex after phenol face peels, *J Dermatol Surg Oncol* 10:57, 1984.

49. Reiman P: Non-Rx extract adjunct slows photoaging without irritation, *Dermatol Times* 5:22, 1999.

50. Roenigk HH Jr. and others: Acne, retinoids, and dermabrasion, *J Dermatol Surg Oncol* 11:396, 1985.

51. Rubenstein R and others: Atypical keloids after dermabrasion of patients taking isotretinoin, *J Am Acad Dermatol* 15:280, 1986.

52. Rubin MG, Greenbaum SS: Histologic effects of aluminum oxide microabrasion on facial skin, *J Aesthet Derm Cosmet Surg* 1:237-239, 2000.

53. Spira M: Treatment of acne scarring by combined dermabrasion and chemical peel, *Plast Reconstr Surg* 60:38, 1977.

54. Spira M, Gerow FJ, Hardy SB: Complications of chemical face peeling, *Plast Reconstr Surg* 54:397, 1974.

55. Stagnone JJ: *Chemical peeling and dermabrasion.* In Epstein E, Epstein E Jr, editors: *Skin surgery,* Philadelphia, 1987, WB Saunders.

56. Stagnone JJ: Superficial peeling, *J Dermatol Surg Oncol* 15:924, 1989.

57. Stegman SJ: A comparative histologic study of the effects of three peeling agents in dermabrasion of normal and sun damaged skin, *Aesthetic Plast Surg* 6:123, 1982.

58. Truppman ES, Ellenby JD: Major electrocardiographic changes during chemical face peeling, *Plast Reconstr Surg* 63:45, 1979.

59. Tung RC and others: alpha-Hydroxy acid-based cosmetic procedures: guidelines for patient management, *Am J Clin Dermatol* 1:81-8, 2000.

60. Utley DS, Koch RJ, Egbert BM: Histologic analysis of the thermal effect on epidermal and dermal structures following treatment with the superpulsed CO_2 laser and the erbium: YAG laser: an in vivo model, *Lasers Surg Med* 24:93-102, 1999.

61. Weinstein GD and others: Topical tretinoin for treatment of photodamaged skin: a multicenter study, *Arch Dermatol* 127:659-665, 1991.

62. Weis J and others: Topical tretinoid improves photoaged skin: a double blind vehicle controlled study, *JAMA* 259:527, 1988.

CHAPTER THIRTY

RHYTIDECTOMY

|| Shan R. Baker

HISTORICAL PERSPECTIVE

In 1907, Miller[30] published the first medical book ever written on the subject of cosmetic surgery. Thus was born the surgical field of aesthetic surgery. Around this same time, perhaps as early as 1901, the first rhytidectomy was performed and took the primitive form of excising skin and repairing the wound without undermining the facial skin. Early facelift techniques were probably developed by German surgeons, but by 1906, American surgeons were beginning to adopt and improve the techniques of facelifting. By 1926, surgeons were using coronal incisions for forehead lifting and were developing methods of dealing with the double chin. By the 1930s, facelift surgery had attained a level of sophistication that inspired no major innovations until after World War II, when the development of antibiotics and improved anesthesia provided safer elective surgery. Before the World War II, aesthetic surgery was looked on by organized medicine with disfavor, believing that it was not warranted because of associated risks. By 1960, this attitude had changed somewhat. The greater affluence of the middle class and changing attitudes helped spawn a renewed interest in rhytidectomy. However, it was not until the 1970s that significant innovations in facelifting were introduced. This was initiated by the work of Skoog,[33] who reported dissecting beneath the superficial fascia of the face. Before 1974, rhytidectomy had consisted of a simple subcutaneous dissection of facial and cervical skin with or without suture suspension of the underlying superficial fascia. Skoog demonstrated that an advancement flap dissected beneath the superficial fascia, later to be named the superficial musculoaponeurotic system (SMAS), while leaving the overlying skin attached, could improve the jaw line better than a subcutaneous dissection of the skin. Skoog's discovery that enhanced results were possible from dissecting deeper than the conventional subcutaneous plane ushered in a renaissance for rhytidec-

tomy, and today surgeons are in the midst of this renaissance. Skoog's report created considerable interest in the superficial facial fascia and led to the 1976 report by Mitz and Pyronie.[24] This and subsequent studies showed that the SMAS is a fibromuscular fascial extension of the platysmal muscle that arises superiorly from the fascia over the zygomatic arch and is continuous in the inferior cheek with the platysma. Throughout this chapter when the term SMAS is referred to, the reader should understand that this structure consists of a fibrous layer of connective tissue in the mid-face but has more consistency in the inferior cheek, where it consists of the platysmal muscle. This is particularly true over the tail of the parotid gland and anterior to the gland. The distribution of the facial nerve is deep to the SMAS[24] (Figure 30-1). Presumably, the function of the SMAS is to transmit to the facial skin the activity of the facial mimetic musculature.

Surgeons familiar with the subcutaneous facelift began incising the SMAS superficial to the parotid gland and creating a rotation advancement SMAS flap. Other surgeons made incisions through the SMAS anterior to the parotid gland and dissected beneath the platysma, creating a musculocutaneous advancement flap, which was suspended posterosuperiorly to the fascia of the parotid gland. Some excised a strip of SMAS and reapproximated it rather than dissecting beneath it. Although the SMAS flap dramatically improved the jowl, it did not improve the melolabial fold of the mid-face. The mid-face can be defined as that portion of the cheek that encompasses the area between the lower eyelid and the level of the oral commissure.

Yousif and others investigated the anatomy of the melolabial fold and found that the fold resulted from descent of the anterior cheek fat and overlying attached skin.[36] With aging, the cheek fat of the mid-face descends inferomedially (Figure 30-2). This

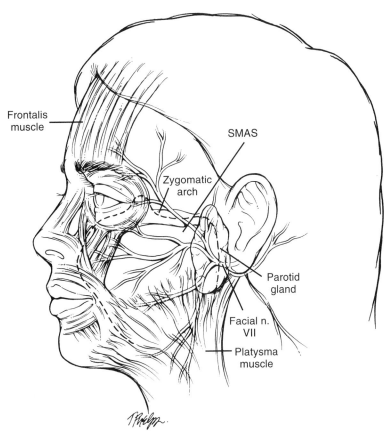

Figure 30-1. The superficial musculoaponeurotic system (SMAS) is a fibromuscular fascial extension of the platysmal muscle that arises superiorly from the fascia over the zygomatic arch and is continuous in the inferior cheek with the platysmal muscle. The facial nerve lies deep to the SMAS and innervates the mimetic muscles of the forehead and midface from the ventral aspect of the muscles.

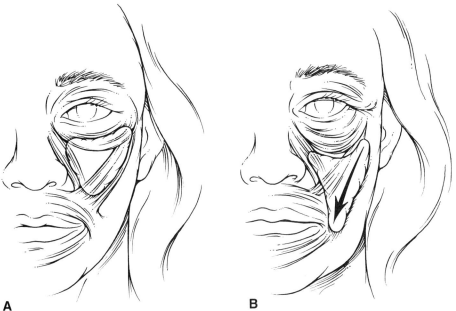

A   **B**

Figure 30-2. A, Aging causes inferomedial descent of the cheek fat, which increases the melolabial fold and deepens the melolabial crease. **B,** The orbicularis muscle of the lower eyelid stretches and descends inferolaterally, causing lower lid retraction and scleral show.

tissue migration has the effect of enhancing the melolabial fold and deepening the melolabial crease. At the same time, the orbicularis muscle of the lower eyelid stretches and descends inferolaterally. This movement causes the margin of the lower eyelid to move below the inferior limbus, which, in turn, produces scleral show. The junction between the cheek and lower eyelid descends below the orbital rim, causing skeletonization of the inferior bony orbital rim and, in some patients, the development of a nasojugal groove. On the basis of the anatomic changes of the lower eyelid and mid-face that occur from aging, it eventually became evident that rejuvenation of the mid-face required elevation and fixation of the mid-facial soft tissues and correction of the redundant orbicularis muscle of the lower eyelid by excision or repositioning of the muscle superomedially.

The SMAS is essentially a fascial extension of the platysmal muscle beneath the cheek fat of the mid-face.[5,12,34,36] Traction placed on the SMAS is not transmitted to the melolabial fold and as a consequence does not ameliorate the fold. This is because the SMAS is effectively anchored by the bony origins of the mimetic muscles it envelops, especially the zygomatic major muscle in the region of the body of the zygoma. This point of fixation prevents the upward lateral displacement of a sub-SMAS rhytidectomy flap and the flattening of the melolabial fold. This finding led to the realization that a sub-SMAS dissection must release the investments of the SMAS to the zygomatic musculature to move the SMAS and the overlying cheek fat upward, thereby improving the melolabial fold and the appearance of the mid-face.[6] The deep-plane rhytidectomy perfected by Hamra extended a sub-SMAS dissection of the inferior cheek superiorly, cutting through the SMAS peripherally, and releasing it from its investment of the zygomatic muscles, so that the SMAS and the overlying skin and subcutaneous tissues could be advanced upward.[14] This release was accomplished by transitioning from a sub-SMAS plane in the inferior cheek to a supra-SMAS plane in the superior medial cheek (Figure 30-3). The dissection extended medially beyond the melolabial fold, totally releasing all SMAS attachments to the dermis of the upper lip and creating a thick musculocutaneous flap composed of skin, subcutaneous fat of the cheek, and the platysma. Hamra subsequently modified the deep plane rhytidectomy by including the orbicularis oculi in the rhytidectomy flap and termed it a composite rhytidectomy.[15] Owsley[26] showed that by dissecting medially from the malar eminence to the lateral upper lip just superficial to the SMAS in the plane immediately above the orbicularis oculi, zygomaticus, and levator muscles, the cheek fat could be suspended superiorly, restoring a youthful appearance

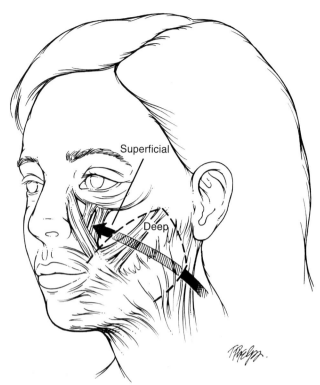

Figure 30-3. The deep-plane rhytidectomy described by Hamra[20] extended a sub-superficial musculoaponeurotic system (sub-SMAS) dissection of the inferior cheek superiorly, cutting through the SMAS peripherally, thus releasing the SMAS from investments to the zygomatic muscles, so that the SMAS and overlying skin and cheek fat could be mobilized upward. This release was accompanied by transitioning from a deep (sub-SMAS) plane in the inferior cheek to a superficial (supra-SMAS) plane in the superior medial cheek.

to the mid-face and effacing the melolabial fold. He showed that a sub-SMAS dissection was not at all necessary to improve the mid-face. Owsley's approach is often referred to as an extended supra-SMAS rhytidectomy.

From the preceding discussion, it is apparent that advancement of the cheek fat superolaterally is necessary to improve the mid-face, whereas a sub-SMAS dissection with mobilization of a composite flap of platysma and overlying skin is beneficial for correcting the jowl. Dissection beneath the SMAS of the inferior cheek is readily accomplished with blunt dissection once the SMAS has been incised. However, shifting the dissection to a more superficial plane as one extends superiorly from beneath the platysma of the lower cheek to a plane superficial to the SMAS superior and anterior to the zygomatic major muscle in the superomedial cheek is tedious and must be performed sharply. By necessity, the surgeon must make a transition from one surgical plane to another and risk injury to the zygomatic branch of the facial nerve.

In addition, to mobilize the ptotic cheek fat upward in the mid-face, a lengthy anterior dissection over the convexity of the zygoma is necessary. The convexity often prevents direct visualization of the dissection.

The knowledge gained from the clinical and anatomic studies performed in the mid and late 70s enabled continued refinement of sub-SMAS and extended supra-SMAS dissection techniques, culminating in the early 1990s. Emerging in parallel with these surgical approaches was the development of a different concept for rejuvenating the mid-face accomplished by a subperiosteal dissection. In 1980, Tessier[35] demonstrated that undermining the periosteum of the superior and lateral orbital rim allowed elevation of the soft tissues of the forehead and eyebrows, with improved results compared with previous techniques for forehead lifting. In 1988, Psillakis and others[28] reported on a subperiosteal rhytidectomy technique that involved detachment of all periosteum from the bony orbital rims, upper maxilla, zygoma, and nose. After this detachment, the soft tissues of the forehead, lateral canthus, mid-face including the melolabial folds, and to some degree the jowls were lifted to reestablish a more youthful relationship with the underlying facial skeleton. Because of troubling temporary forehead paralysis from trauma to the temporal branch of the facial nerve (6.7%), the authors advocated restricting subperiosteal dissection of the zygomatic arch to the anterior third to reduce the risk of injury. Ramirez and others[29] modified the subperiosteal facelift described by Psillakis permitting significant improvement in the safety and clinical results. They released the periosteum from the entire zygomatic arch by dissecting deep to the temporalis fascia. The temporalis fascia was then used as a lifting and anchoring element of the entire cheek and perioral soft tissues (Figure 30-4). The surgical approach by Ramirez and others showed improved mid-face suspension by complete subperiosteal undermining of the mid-facial bones. The suspension seemed to have the same influence on the melolabial fold as the deep-plane facelift, that is, elevation of the ptotic cheek fat to a more youthful position with effacement of the fold.

The subperiosteal approach had the advantage of rejuvenating the mid-face without placing unnatural tension on the skin in the temporal area. This tension is necessary when using an extended supra-SMAS or deep-plane rhytidectomy to pull the cheek fat with the overlying skin upward. In contrast, the subperiosteal approach placed traction on the periosteum to maintain repositioning of the mid-face tissues. It

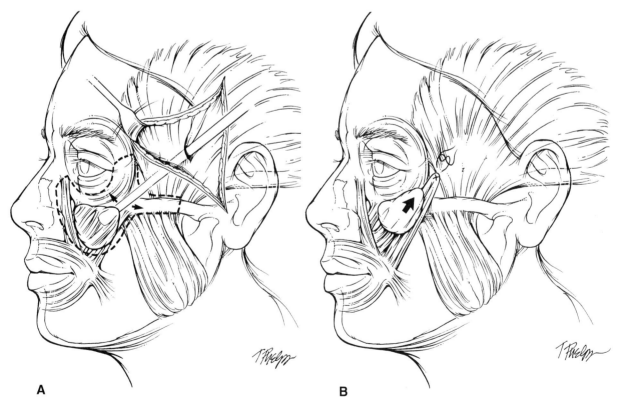

A   **B**

Figure 30-4. **A,** Subperiosteal mid-facelift accomplished through transtemporal approach. Periosteum is released from the maxilla and zygoma and all or portions of the zygomatic arch. **B,** Periosteum of zygoma suspended to temporalis fascia to lift soft tissues of mid-face.

also did not require a long cheek flap extending anteriorly beyond the convexity of the zygoma as called for by the deep-plane and extended supra-SMAS facelifts. The extensive release of the periosteum away from the zygoma and maxilla allowed better elevation of the upper lip and corner of the mouth by moving the origin of the zygomatic musculature to a higher position on the zygoma. This effectively "shortens" the zygomatic musculature, which lifts the oral commissure upward, producing a more pleasant shape to the mouth. This maneuver cannot be accomplished with sub-SMAS or extended supra-SMAS dissections. Finally, in individuals with early facial aging, the subperiosteal approach through endoscopic techniques offered a method of lifting the face without skin excisions and the resulting preauricular scar.

The subperiosteal facelift described by Ramirez and others[29] is technically difficult, because it requires a temporal approach, which is considerably removed from the body of the zygoma and the anterior maxilla where the mid-face soft tissues are attached. As with the deep-plane rhytidectomy, visibility anterior to the convexity of the zygoma is limited, and it may be necessary to perform some dissection blindly. Because the temporal approach by itself presented difficulties with detachment of the periosteum from the maxilla, surgeons turned to other approaches. The most popular of these was transorbital access to the mid-face achieved by performing a lower lid blepharoplasty by use of a transcutaneous or transconjunctival approach. Through the blepharoplasty incision, the periosteum was released from the maxilla and zygoma and the soft tissues of the mid-face suspended either to a periosteal cuff at the inferior bony orbital rim or to the temporalis fascia in the anteroinferior aspect of the temporal fossa.[13,18,19,27] A major drawback of the transorbital route was not infrequent problems of lower lid retraction or even ectropion. This complication occurs from trauma to the orbicularis oculi and subsequent scar contracture. Some surgeons recommended concomitant lateral canthoplasty or at the very least canthopexy to reduce this risk. Other surgeons avoided this risk altogether by combining a transtemporal and transoral approach and not performing any dissection of the mid-face through the lower eyelid. The transtemporal approach was used to elevate the periosteum from the zygomatic arch and the superior aspect of the zygoma. The transoral approach was used to free the periosteum from the maxilla and inferior aspects of the zygoma. This combined approach had the advantage of allowing the surgeon direct access for performing a subperiosteal dissection of the entire mid-face under direct vision without the need of an endoscope. It also avoided the risk of lower eyelid retraction or ectropion.

Whether superior movement of the mid-face soft tissues is accomplished by a subperiosteal or by an extended supra-SMAS dissection, the goal is to produce a dramatic lifting of mid-face tissues. Proponents of the extended supra-SMAS approach argue that the periosteum does not stretch with age and, thus, a subperiosteal approach repositions the origin of the zygomatic musculature to a more superior and abnormal position. This may have the effect of giving an excessive horizontal width to the mid-face. Considerably more postoperative facial edema is associated with this approach compared with the transfacial supra-SMAS dissection. Another disadvantage of a subperiosteal dissection is that most approaches call for elevation of the periosteum from the anterior portion of the zygomatic arch, placing the temporal branch of the facial nerve at risk.

Proponents of the subperiosteal approach point to the safety of keeping all of the soft tissue, including the facial nerve above the plane of dissection. There is less risk of injury to the zygomatic and buccal branches of the facial nerve with the subperiosteal approach compared with the deep-plane or extended supra-SMAS facelift. There is no disruption of the blood supply to the skin of the mid-face, because the plane of dissection is beneath all of the major blood supply to the face. There is no need for a lengthy skin flap lifted from the preauricular area or for a blind dissection of soft tissues of the mid-face. Although not part of the discussion in this chapter, it has become apparent that the aging changes in the lower periocular area are maximally rejuvenated when mid-facelifting is performed in conjunction with orbicularis oculi repositioning to a more superior and medial position.[15] Repositioning of the ptotic orbicularis muscle is most easily accomplished by performing a subperiosteal mid-facelift. Transfacial supra-SMAS midfacelifts do not reposition this muscle. Table 30-1 summarizes the advantages and disadvantages of the various approaches to lifting the mid-face.

Recently, suture suspension of the soft tissues of the mid-face has been promoted, because it avoids the need for a subperiosteal or a supra-SMAS dissection of the mid-face and thus many of the complications associated with these techniques.[20,31] Sasaki and Cohen[31] described a simple and adjustable long-lasting percutaneous suture elevation technique to reposition the cheek fat of the mid-face in a superolateral vector. Through a puncture incision just lateral to the alar base and within the melolabial crease, a permanent suspension suture is looped through a 3-x 8-mm GorTex anchor patch to suspend the cheek fat in a direction perpendicular to the melolabial crease. A second suspension suture is identically passed through another puncture incision in the melolabial crease

TABLE 30-1

DISSECTION PLANES OF MID-FACELIFTING

	Advantages	Disadvantages
Subperiosteal	1. Does not require preauricular incision/skin flap 2. Does not impair vascular supply of facial skin 3. Avoids risk to zygomatic branch of VII nerve 4. Lifts orbicularis oculi of lower eyelid 5. Some lifting of oral commissure	1. Increases horizontal width of face 2. Risk to temporal and buccal branches of VII nerve and infraorbital nerve 3. Greater postoperative edema
Supra-SMAS	1. Does not reposition zygomatic musculature 2. Avoids risk to temporal and buccal branches of VII nerve 3. Less postoperative edema	1. Long preauricular cutaneous flap 2. Reduces skin vascularity of face 3. Risk to zygomatic branch of VII nerve 4. Does not lift orbicularis oculi

1 cm below the first (Figure 30-5). This second suture has a trajectory parallel and below the first to broaden the repositioning vectors on the cheek fat. The sutures are positioned to loop around the fat of the melolabial fold. One arm of the loop passes through the deep aspect of the fat and the other arm in a more superficial subcutaneous plane. Both arms attached to Keith needles extend to the subcutaneous fat 1 cm lateral to

the posterior border of the bony orbital rim at the level of the lateral canthus. These sutures are then inserted through a 4 x 4-mm GorTex anchor, which is sutured to the temporalis fascia 1 cm posterior to the temporal hairline. Although this technique seems to give lasting improvement greater than 2 years, by itself it does not reposition the orbicularis oculi. It is too early in the use of suture suspension to know

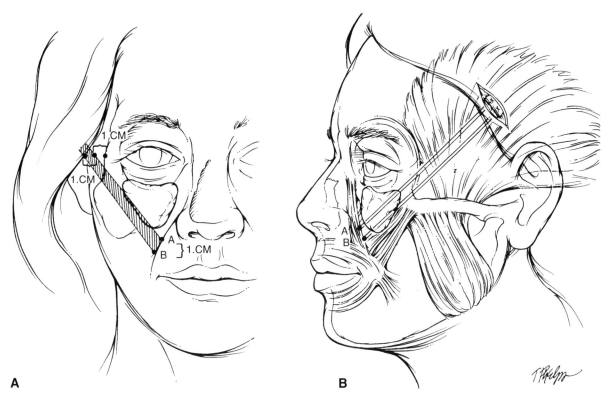

A

B

Figure 30-5. Suture suspension of cheek fat. Two sutures spaced 1 cm apart are looped around the cheek fat of the mid-face and secured to the temporalis fascia behind the temporal hairline. Sutures are placed through puncture sites within the melolabial crease at points A and B.

whether it will provide results that are as aesthetically desirable or as long lasting as supra-SMAS and subperiosteal mid-facelifts.

The extreme interest in developing new surgical approaches to rhytidectomy and to refining those techniques over the past two decades has resulted in considerable improvement in surgical results. This has taken the form of a more natural and youthful restoration of the face by together lifting forehead, mid-face, and lower face. This approach produces a more harmonious balance of the upper and lower portions of the face than was possible before the introduction of mid-facelifting techniques. Added to this has been the emphasis by some surgeons on restoring tissue volume to the face with autogenous fat injections.[8] One can conclude that the most favorable results in facelifting will likely occur when the lower cheek is rejuvenated by dissecting beneath the SMAS to create an advancement flap together with the lifting of the cheek fat of the mid-face posterosuperiorly.

ANATOMY
SMAS

The pertinent anatomy of the face when considering lower facelifting relates to the sensory and motor nerves of the face, the platysma, and the superficial muscular aponeurotic system. The platysma is a rhomboidal subcutaneous sheet of muscle. It extends from the lower cheek to the level of the second rib. The muscle crosses the entire length of the mandible and accounts for the mobility of the skin along the jaw line. It continues above the lower cheek as a superficial aponeurotic fascia, which invests the muscles of facial expression located in the mid-face, including the orbicularis oculi, the levators of the upper lip including the zygomatic major and minor muscles, and the orbicularis oris (see Figure 30-1). Although the platysma covers the inferior aspect of the parotid gland, it rapidly dissipates and becomes fascia over most of the gland. The muscles, together with the fascia, are known as the superficial muscular aponeurotic system or SMAS. The only bony attachment of the platysma is the most anterior fibers, which are attached to the lower border of the anterior mandible. Other anterior fibers decussate with the opposite platysma. The degree of decussation is variable and may extend inferiorly to the level of the thyroid cartilage.[7] There are three basic variations of the medial decussations of the platysma. In type I, medial fibers interdigitate 1 to 2 cm below the mentum (75% of cases). In type II, the interdigitation extends to the level of the thyroid cartilage (15%). In type III, fibers remain completely separated along the entire length of the two muscles (10%).[7] Laxity of the platysma in the anterior neck accounts for the paramedian vertical bands that

extend from the mentum to the mid or lower neck observed with aging. The anterior borders of the platysma are firmly attached to the deep cervical fascia in the region of the hyoid bone. Therefore, the vertical bands observed in the aging neck are not the medial borders of the muscles but rather lateral pleats caused by laxity of the muscle.[22] The SMAS represents a fascial extension of the platysma that arises superiorly from the fascia over the zygomatic arch and is continuous in the inferior cheek with the platysma. Posteriorly, the SMAS fuses with the fascia overlying the sternocleidomastoid muscle, but it is a distinct layer superficial to the parotid fascia. Anterosuperiorly, the SMAS invests the facial mimetic muscles of the mid-face (i.e., orbicularis oculi, zygomatic major/minor, levator labii, superioris). Anteriorly, the SMAS invests the superficial portions of the orbicularis oris and gives off fibrous septi that insert into the dermis along the melolabial crease and upper lip.

Facial Nerve

The facial nerve emerges from the substance of the parotid gland in the form of several branches and remains deep to the SMAS (see Figure 30-1). Anterior to the parotid gland in the lower cheek the branches are also deep to the masseter fascia covering the masseter muscle. A potential space exists between the SMAS and the masseter fascia and enables the surgeon to safely dissect in an avascular plane beneath the SMAS and above the masseter fascia to prevent nerve injury. This is only true in the inferior cheek. The SMAS invests the mimetic muscles of the mid-face. Branches of the facial nerve traverse the SMAS to enter the deep aspect of these muscles. The deep-plane and composite rhytidectomy, as described by Hamra, involves a dissection in the inferior cheek beneath the platysma and SMAS but above the fascia of the masseter muscle. The dissection transitions to a tissue plane immediately superficial to the SMAS in the mid-face[14,15] (see Figure 30-3). This transition prevents inadvertent injury to the facial nerve and allows release of the SMAS from its attachment to the zygomatic musculature.

The temporal branch of the facial nerve is the most superficial branch and, as a consequence, may be injured during rhytidectomy. The nerve exits the superior aspect of the parotid gland beneath the SMAS. It crosses the junction of the anterior one third and posterior two thirds of the zygomatic arch frequently in the form of two or more branches. Above the arch the nerve travels in the temporoparietal fascia and enters the ventral aspect of the lateral frontalis muscle and superior portions of the orbicularis oculi (see Figure 30-1). Dissection in the area of the zygomatic arch and lateral temporal region during a combined forehead lift and facelift usually requires two planes of dissection. The forehead lift is usually accomplished by dissecting in the temporal area below the temporoparietal fascia. At the same time, the facelift dissection is performed in the subcutaneous plane so that the temporal branch remains between the two dissecting planes.

Another branch of the facial nerve that is susceptible to injury during rhytidectomy is the marginal mandibularis branch. This nerve exits the substance of the inferior parotid gland and extends along the ventral aspect of the platysma 1 or 2 cm below the body of the mandible (see Figure 30-1). Thus, when dissecting beneath the platysma in the inferior cheek, it is prudent to remain above the inferior border of the mandible to prevent injury to the nerve. Anterior to where the facial artery crosses the mandible, the nerve is above the inferior border of the mandible as it passes through the platysma to lie beneath the depressor anguli oris. Because the nerve is superficial to the platysma in this region, it is susceptible to injury during suction-assisted liposculpturing in the region of the lower anterior jowl. The marginal mandibular nerve supplies the muscles covering the surface of the chin.

The zygomatic branch of the facial nerve extends in a trajectory along a line drawn from the tragus through the most lateral projection of the zygoma (malar eminence) where the zygomatic major muscle rises. It provides innervation to the orbicularis oculi through multiple branches. The interconnecting rami make permanent paralysis of the nerve unlikely from dissecting in the periocular region during facelift surgery. Sometimes a branch of the zygomatic division extends superficial to the zygomatic major muscle to innervate the inferior medial orbicularis oculi. This branch is susceptible to injury during supra-SMAS mid-facelifting as the surgeon dissects the cheek fat away from the underlying zygomatic major muscle. Injury to this branch may cause mild synkinesis of the lower eyelid during facial animation.

The buccal branch of the facial nerve exits the anterior parotid gland onto the surface of the masseter muscle deep to the masseter fascia. The nerve passes superficial to the buccal fat pad of Bichat. The nerve is at risk for injury when dissecting beneath the SMAS during deep-plane rhytidectomy or from removing fat from the mid-face. It may also be injured during subperiosteal mid-face dissections during release of the periosteum from the inferior aspect of the zygoma and zygomatic arch. Injury to this nerve can result in sagging of the upper lip on the affected side from paralysis of the zygomatic major and minor muscles, levator labii, and superioris alaeque nasi, all supplied by branches of the buccal nerve.

Sensory Nerves

Several sensory nerves are important in rhytidectomy. The greater auricular nerve is the most common nerve injured in facelifting because of its superficial location in the upper neck. The nerve passes around the posterior border of the sternocleidomastoid muscle 6.5 cm below the external auditory canal. The external jugular vein is parallel and .5 cm anterior to the axis of the nerve at this point (Figure 30-6). The nerve extends upward under the fascia of the muscle to innervate the auricle and periauricular areas. It is vulnerable to injury as it passes over the sternocleidomastoid muscle, because it is not protected by a platysma–SMAS layer, and there is little subcutaneous fat superficial to the nerve.[32] Suture suspension of the SMAS to the mastoid fascia can result in a compression injury of the greater auricular nerve. This may result in painful postsurgical neuralgia. Suture suspension of the SMAS to the fascia covering the sternocleidomastoid muscle must be performed with great care. Sutures should only penetrate the fascia of the muscle to prevent encircling branches of the nerve.

Another sensory nerve in the vicinity of the greater auricular nerve that may be injured when dissecting in the neck is the lesser occipital nerve. This nerve runs 1 cm posterior and parallel to the greater auricular nerve just superficial to the cervical fascia. The nerve innervates the superior and posterior one third of the auricle. If the postauricular facelift flap is dissected at the fascia level rather than in the subcutaneous plane, the lesser occipital nerve may be injured.

The zygomaticofacial nerve is a small sensory nerve that may exit as two separate sensory nerves through small foramens on the lateral aspect of the zygoma. When two nerves are present, they are known as the zygomatic facial and zygomatic temporal nerves. These nerves provide sensory innervation to the skin of the malar eminence and the anteroinferior aspect of the temple. Disruption of these nerves during subperiosteal dissection of the mid-face can result in permanent numbness over the malar eminence, although reinnervation of the area usually occurs with time.

Injury to the infraorbital nerve may occur during subperiosteal mid-facelifting. This nerve exits the infraorbital foramen, which is 1 cm below the inferior bony orbital rim along a line drawn vertically through the mid-pupil and the second mandibular premolar.[32] This nerve provides sensory innervation to the lower eyelid, medial cheek, lateral nose, and upper lip.

SURGICAL APPROACHES

Although there are a multitude of variations in performing a rhytidectomy of the lower face and upper neck, they may be divided into four categories according to the tissue planes used for dissection.

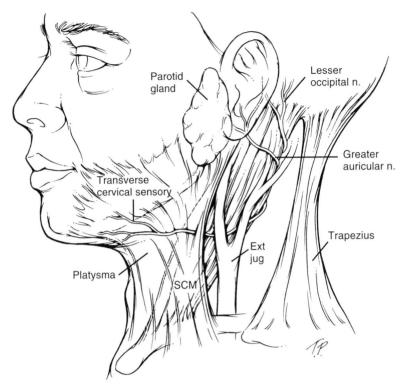

Figure 30-6. Anatomic relationship of greater auricular nerve to sternocleidomastoid muscle, external jugular vein, and lesser occipital nerve.

These include subcutaneous, sub-SMAS, supra-SMAS, and subperiosteal (Table 30-2).

Subcutaneous Rhytidectomy

All approaches except the endoscopic facelift without preauricular or postauricular incisions call for some subcutaneous dissection of the facial skin. The postauricular skin flap is always elevated in the subcutaneous plane. Likewise, the preauricular skin must be dissected in the subcutaneous plane for variable distances before incisions can be made through the SMAS. Typically, the skin of the upper neck is also elevated in the subcutaneous plane or immediately superficial to the platysmal muscle (preplatysmal). Dissection may continue forward in the neck to the midline. The extent of anterior dissection in the subcutaneous plane of the face depends on the surgeon's preference and may be influenced by the degree of facial skin laxity. In the past, there have been controversies concerning the benefits of long-flap vs short-flap rhytidectomies. A benefit of dissecting to the lateral bony orbital rim in the temple is that it releases the skin from the underlying orbicularis oculi. This helps to improve the crow's feet and also assists with redistribution of the vertically advanced preauricular skin flap. Once a skin flap has been elevated, the exposed SMAS can be imbricated by folding it on itself by use of sutures to suspend it to the periparotid fascia. The subcutaneous facelift with imbrication of the SMAS is still the most common surgical approach used by plastic surgeons, comprising 23% of facelift procedures performed.[21] It is probably the safest approach from the standpoint of risk of facial nerve injury but has the disadvantages compared with other techniques of shorter long-term improvement of the jowl and no correction of the mid-face.

SMAS-Rhytidectomy

The sub-SMAS dissection of the lower face is another common surgical approach performed by approximately 20% of facelift surgeons.[21] This may take the form of elevating an SMAS flap limited to the area over the parotid gland (25% of surgeons) or extending the SMAS flap anterior to the parotid gland. The SMAS flap is then suspended posterosuperiorly. Neither of these approaches lifts the mid-face, but they markedly improve the jowl. When an SMAS flap is dissected from the parotid fascia, it is frequently referred to as an SMAS rhytidectomy. Dissecting beneath the SMAS anterior to the parotid gland and then transitioning to a supra-SMAS plane and dissecting all of the cheek fat with attached overlying skin away from the zygomatic musculature as described by Hamra is known as a deep-plane rhytidectomy[14] (see Figure 30-3). Later,

TABLE 30-2

SURGICAL APPROACHES TO MID-FACELIFTING

Surgical Approach	Plane of Dissection	Advantages	Disadvantages
Transfacial	Supra-SMAS	1. Avoids risk to temporal and buccal branches of VII nerve 2. Less postoperative edema	1. Preauricular incision and long skin flap 2. Requires some blind dissection 3. Does not lift orbicularis oculi
Transtemporal	Subperiosteal	1. No preauricular incision 2. Concomitant lateral brow lift	1. Risk to temporal and buccal branches of VII nerve 2. Requires endoscope 3. Poor access to periosteal dissection of maxilla
Transorbital	Subperiosteal or supraperiosteal	1. Direct access for dissection and suspension of mid-face 2. More vertical vector for suspension of mid-face soft tissues	1. Risk to buccal branch of VII nerve 2. Risk to infraorbital nerve 3. Risk of lower lid retraction/ectropion
Transoral	Subperiosteal	1. Direct access for dissection of mid-face 2. Ease in elevating periosteum of maxilla	1. Risk to buccal branch of VII nerve 2. Does not provide access for suspension of mid-face tissues 3. Greater risk of infection 4. Risk to infraorbital nerve
Combined	Subperiosteal; usually transoral combined with transtemporal or transorbital	1. Direct visualization of entire dissection 2. Ease of suspension of mid-face tissues	1. More postoperative edema 2. Greater risk of infection if transoral route used

Hamra added to this dissection a supraperiosteal dissection of the superior aspect of the mid-face through a lower eyelid incision. This biplane dissection was termed a composite rhytidectomy by Hamra.[15] Nine percent of facelift surgeons perform a deep plane or composite rhytidectomy.[21]

A variation of the sub-SMAS dissection is a strip SMASectomy described by Baker.[1] This technique consists of excising a strip of SMAS along a line that extends from the angle of the mandible to the lateral malar eminence. Usually, a 2- to 4-cm wide strip of SMAS is excised, depending on laxity. Much of this excision is anterior to the parotid gland. No anterior dissection beneath the SMAS is performed. The SMAS is reapproximated, advancing the mobile SMAS and platysma posterosuperiorly to the junction of the SMAS fixed to the periparotid fascia. Approximately 20% of facelift surgeons use the technique of SMASectomy.[21] It has the advantage of simplicity but does not address the mid-face.

Supra-SMAS Rhytidectomy

The term supra-SMAS usually refers to dissection just superficial to the SMAS in the mid-face. All subcutaneous dissections in the preauricular area are also supra-SMAS. However, remaining just superficial to the SMAS as the limits of the dissection are extended anteriorly beyond the parotid gland toward the mid-face requires a deeper dissection than is required for a standard subcutaneous facelift. Because the SMAS invests the mimetic muscles of the mid-face, a supra-SMAS dissection requires a forward dissection immediately superficial to these muscles. This results in a thick cutaneous flap consisting of the cheek fat and the overlying attached facial skin. The dissection is usually carried to the upper lip to release all of the dermal attachments of the SMAS to the melolabial crease. This extreme anterior dissection is commonly referred to as an extended SMAS rhytidectomy or an extended supra-SMAS rhytidectomy. The cutaneous flap is then suspended under considerable tension posterosuperiorly to the fascia overlying the zygoma and parotid gland. The primary purpose of the extended supra-SMAS rhytidectomy is to displace superiorly the cheek fat of the mid-face. This corrects the ptotic cheek fat that occurs in the mid-face with aging and softens the melolabial fold.

The main disadvantage of the extended supra-SMAS rhytidectomy is the long preauricular skin flap resulting from a lengthy anterior dissection. This creates a potentially large dead space where hematomas can collect. A dissection beyond the convexity of the zygoma may require some blind dissection or at least impair the exposure available to the surgeon. In addition, remaining above the SMAS throughout the dissection does not provide as much improvement of the jowl compared with developing a SMAS flap of the inferior cheek. Approximately 20% of facelift surgeons perform the extended supra-SMAS rhytidectomy.[21] The advantage of the deep-plane facelift compared with the supra-SMAS lift is that the inferior cheek is dissected in a sub-SMAS plane, creating an advancement flap, whereas the mid-face is dissected in a supra-SMAS plane. The sub-SMAS dissection in the lower face provides long-term correction of the jowl.[16]

Subperiosteal Rhytidectomy

Subperiosteal rhytidectomy refers to the lifting of the cheek tissues by dissecting in the subperiosteal plane over the maxilla and zygoma. The procedure usually includes an endoscopic subperiosteal forehead lift as well. All of the soft tissues of the mid-face are lifted, including the elevators of the lip, the zygomatic major and minor, and often the orbicularis oculi. The fundamental difference between the subperiosteal mid-facelift and the transfacial supra-SMAS facelift is the superior displacement of these muscles (see Figure 30-4). The extended supra-SMAS and deep-plane rhytidectomy only elevate the cheek fat and skin and not the muscles of the mid-face. Subperiosteal mid-facelifts do not significantly correct the jowl and have no influence on the upper neck. Another disadvantage of a subperiosteal mid-facelift is the tendency to increase the horizontal width of the face by displacing the origin of the zygomatic major muscle to a more superior and lateral position. However, in most patients this has the pleasing effect of enhancing the malar eminence.

There are four surgical approaches used to perform subperiosteal mid-facelifting: transtemporal usually using an endoscope, transorbital through a lower eyelid or transconjunctival incision, transoral through an upper gingival buccal incision, and combined using two or more of the previously listed approaches. Regardless of the approach, it is necessary to release the periosteum from the lateral and inferior bony orbital rim and from the entire zygoma and maxilla.

The temporal approach is accomplished through an incision behind the hairline in the temple. An endoscope is frequently used to perform a dissection beneath the temporoparietal fascia of the anterior lateral scalp. Transition is then made to a subperiosteal plane as dissection continues inferiorly over the zygoma and zygomatic arch. Subperiosteal dissection

also proceeds medially in the mid-face, releasing the soft tissues from their attachment to the maxilla. This necessitates limited dissection onto the upper portion of the masseter muscle. A disadvantage of the transtemporal approach is the difficulty releasing the periosteum from the medial maxilla because of insufficient exposure even when an endoscope is used.

The transorbital route has the advantage of direct access to the mid-face with less need for the use of an endoscope. Through this approach, the subperiosteal dissection is accomplished under direct vision, and the mid-face soft tissues are suspended either to the superior orbital rim or to the anteroinferior temporalis fascia (Figure 30-7). Some surgeons perform a supraperiosteal dissection of the mid-face through a lower eyelid incision. A disadvantage of the transorbital approach is temporary distortion of the lateral canthal area from bunching of redundant soft tissue. Another disadvantage is the risk of lower eyelid retraction or ectropion.

The transoral approach is not often used by itself but is combined with transorbital or transtemporal incisions to create a combined surgical approach.[3,4] This enables the periosteum to be easily stripped from the inferior aspects of the maxilla and zygoma from the oral access. The remaining periosteum is then elevated from the superior aspect of the zygoma and

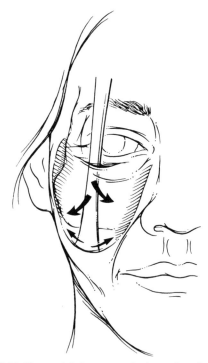

Figure 30-7. Transorbital approach to subperiosteal mid-facelift. The subperiosteal dissection is accomplished under direct vision, and the mid-face soft tissues are suspended to the superior orbital rim or the anteroinferior temporalis fascia.

from the anterior zygomatic arch through an orbital or temporal access. The advantage of this combined approach is ease of dissection and direct visualization without the need for an endoscope. The main disadvantage is the potential risk of wound infection because of exposure of the dissection to bacteria in the oral cavity. Table 30-2 summarizes the surgical approaches to the mid-face and the advantages and disadvantages of each. Only 2% of facelift surgeons generally perform subperiosteal facelifting, and of those, approximately half use an endoscope.[21]

SURGICAL TECHNIQUES

Regardless of the surgical approach used to perform a rhytidectomy, the goals are the same. These include: (1) preserve motor and sensory innervation of the face; (2) modify cervical fat if excessive; (3) tighten the SMAS and platysma; and (4) redrape cervical and facial skin and trim excess. This chapter has discussed

many of the approaches used to achieve these goals and listed many of the advantages and disadvantages of each surgical approach. This section will address more technical aspects of facelifting.

Incisions

Factors that influence the configuration of the facelift incision include gender, hairline, hairstyle, a history of previous facelift surgery, and the redundancy of facial and cervical skin. In the temporal area, the classic incision is one that extends above the auricle into the hair curving upward and forward to end 1 or 2 cm above the level of the eyebrow. More than half of facelift surgeons also add to this incision a horizontal incision beneath the temporal tuff of hair to facilitate removal of vertically elevated facial skin without raising the temporal hairline to an abnormal height.[21] This horizontal incision is often referred to as a sideburn incision and facilitates removal of a great deal of

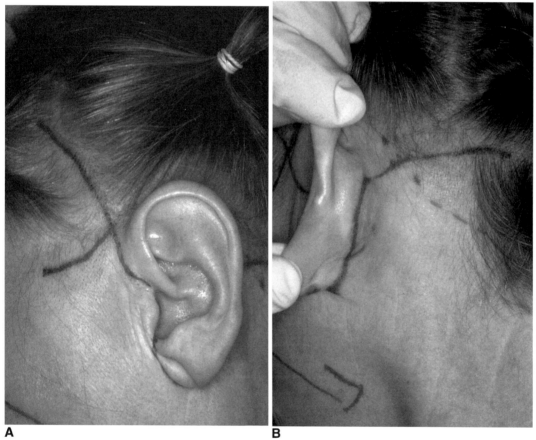

A   **B**

Figure 30-8. Female facelift incision. **A,** The incision begins in the hair above the auricle. A horizontal incision beneath the temporal tuft of hair is usually performed. The preauricular incision follows the curve of the root of the helical crus and then continues posterior to the tragus. **B,** The retroauricular incision is 2 mm anterior to the postauricular sulcus. At the level where the helix meets the hairline (*dotted line*) the incision crosses the postauricular skin to the scalp. The scalp incision curves slightly inferiorly. To view this image in color, please go to *www.ototext.com* or the Electronic Image Collection CD, bound into your copy of Cummings Otolaryngology—Head and Neck Surgery, 4th edition.

excess facial skin. Only 13% of facelift surgeons use a prehairline incision in the temple.[21] The disadvantage of creating a permanent and often noticeable scar anterior to the temporal hair tuft prevents most surgeons from using this incision. The preauricular incision follows the curve of the root of the helical crus to the level of the tragus (Figure 30-8). The incision may then continue posterior to the tragus or in the pretragal crease to the inferior aspect of the earlobe. A retrotragal incision is preferred by 57% of facelift surgeons.[21] The advantages of the retrotragal incision are that this portion of the incision is hidden behind the posterior border of the tragus. It should only be used in women. In men, this technique will result in the tragus being covered with hair-bearing skin. Disadvantages of the retrotragal incision include obliteration of the pretragal crease and scar contraction that can pull the tragus forward, causing an unnatural visibility of the external auditory canal. These problems can be prevented to some degree by thinning the portion of skin flap that will lie immediately anterior to the tragus and trimming the flap so that there is a slight redundancy of skin of the flap covering the tragus. This latter technique ensures that wound closure tension will not occur in this area.

The incision around the earlobe is designed so the lobe is detached from the skin flap, with a 2-mm cuff of facial skin at its base. This ensures the preservation of the sulcus between the lobe and the facial skin and reduces the risk of developing satyr ears.

In the woman, the retroauricular incision is designed 2 to 3 mm anterior to the postauricular sulcus on the medial surface of the auricle. Placement here allows for the possibility of some posterior migration of the retroauricular scar, so that the scar will remain hidden by the auricle. The posterior scalp incision extends from the retroauricular incision across the postauricular sulcus at the level of the tragus or where the helix meets the hairline. This straight line from the auricle to the hair-bearing scalp can be modified by making a small superiorly based triangular flap in the mastoid area. This dart of skin helps prevent straight-line scar contracture and subsequent development of a hypertrophic scar. The scalp incision should be directed into the hair, curving slightly inferiorly and parallel to the postauricular hairline. The incision should not be made along the inferior border of the postauricular hairline except under unusual circumstances because of the visibility of the resulting scar. The retroauricular incision may be limited only to a short vertical incision behind the ear in younger patients with only mild elastosis. In such patients, neck dissection may not be necessary and so the skin does not need to be elevated from the postauricular area.

In men, facelift incisions are modified from that described for women. The temple incision remains unchanged, but the sideburn incision is usually not necessary, because the temporal hair tuft is continuous with the facial hair (Figure 30-9). Retrotragal incisions are not used. The preauricular incision should be curvilinear following the root of the helical crus and then transition into the pretragal crease. The retroauricular incision is also occasionally modified by placing the mastoid incision more inferior than is done in women. This design is used when there is a great deal of cervical skin laxity that will require excision. The more inferiorly located incision reduces the height of the hair-bearing flap behind the ear and the need for shaving in the superior postauricular sulcus.

Submentoplasty

Ellenbogen and Karlin[9] have established five visual criteria that the eye translates as a youthful profile of the neck: (1) distinct inferior mandibular border from mentum to angle with no jowl overhang, (2) slight subhyoid depression at the apex of the cervicomental angle (This depression on profile gives the impression of a thin and long neck.), (3) visible thyroid cartilage convexity, (4) distinct visible anterior border of the sternocleidomastoid muscle in its entire length from mastoid to sternum, and (5) cervicomental angle between 105 and 120 degrees. This translates into a 90-degree angle between the axis of the sternocleidomastoid muscle and a line drawn tangent to the submentum in an anteroposterior orientation[9] (Figure 30-10). An inferiorly positioned hyoid, excessive submental fat, laxity of the platysma (anterior bands), and microgenia can all contribute to blunting of the cervicomental angle.

Anterior bands that develop near the mid-line of the neck with age are the result of elastosis and sagging of the platysmal muscles. When banding is mild, they can be eradicated by developing a platysmal flap posteriorly near the angle of the mandible and advancing this flap posterosuperiorly over the parotid gland. Another less effective method is to suture-suspend the lateral border of the muscle below the angle of the mandible to the fascia of the mastoid and sternocleidomastoid muscle. In the past, surgeons advocated partial or complete horizontal division of the platysmal muscle 5 or more centimeters below the mandible to achieve a greater posterior advancement of the muscle flap and better topographic delineation between the neck and the lower jaw. This practice has been abandoned because of unnatural contours and deformities that develop in the neck as a result of this technique.

When managing platysmal bands, the most effective method, with greatest longevity of results, is to

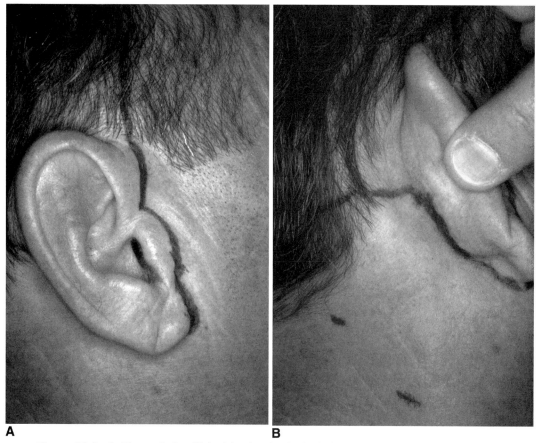

Figure 30-9. A, The male facelift incision begins in the hair-bearing scalp above the ear and follows the curve of the root of the helical crus. It then transitions into a pretragal crease. **B,** The retroauricular incision is positioned in the depths of the postauricular sulcus. To view this image in color, please go to *www.ototext.com* or the Electronic Image Collection CD, bound into your copy of Cummings Otolaryngology—Head and Neck Surgery, 4th edition.

correct the deformity anteriorly where it is located. This is accomplished by performing a submentoplasty. A submentoplasty is indicated if the patient has excessive fatty deposits in the submental area, marked elastosis of neck skin, or platysmal banding. The author performs a submentoplasty with or without posterior neck dissection in a manner described by Hamra.[14] A submentoplasty is required in most patients having rhytidectomy and typically is the first stage of a rhytidectomy. A 2.5-cm curvilinear incision is made just anterior to the submental crease (Figure 30-11). A flap consisting of skin and all of the fat superficial to the platysmal muscle is elevated in a preplatysmal plane. This dissection extends to the level of the superior aspect of the thyroid cartilage and laterally for 6 cm on either side of midline. In the paramedian position, the platysmal muscles are bluntly undermined in a vertical direction from the mandible to the level of the thyroid cartilage and then cross-clamped and incised. The muscle between the two incisions is resected. The amount of muscle resected

depends on redundancy. Sufficient muscle should be removed so that when the borders of the two platysmal muscles are brought together, a tautness is created. Before suturing the muscles together, any excess subplatysmal fat is resected under direct vision. The incised borders of the platysmal muscles are then approximated with interrupted sutures, burying the knot beneath the muscles. Any excess fat elevated with the submental skin is removed with scissors under direct vision (Figure 30-12). Other surgeons prefer to use suction-assisted liposculpturing to modify the submental fat instead of direct excision with scissors. Sixty percent of facelift surgeons perform direct excision of submental fat, whereas only 27% perform suction-assisted lipectomy.[21] Perhaps the reason for the popularity of direct excision is that a greater amount of subcutaneous fat can be removed with greater ease and accuracy by direct excision compared with the use of a suction cannula. Because the skin of the neck is attached to the platysmal muscle, wide undermining of the skin in the submental area is necessary to

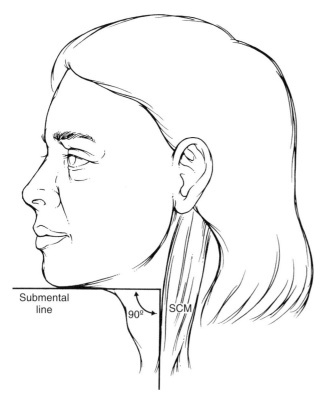

Figure 30-10. The youthful neckline has a cervicomental angle of 105 to 120 degrees. This translates into a 90-degree angle between the axis of the sternocleidomastoid muscle and the submental line.

prevent bunching of the submental skin when the platysma is advanced medially. This is the greatest disadvantage of a submentoplasty as described.

Some surgeons prefer to perform a horizontal incision of the platysma extending laterally from its anterior border for variable distances at the level of the thyroid cartilage. The two platysmal muscles are then sutured together in the midline without excision of muscle tissue. The horizontal incision is believed by some to create a more acute cervicomental angle. Transecting the muscle and midline suturing is performed by 40% of surgeons, whereas 21% perform vertical incision and resection of the platysmal redundancy and midline suturing.[21]

The advantage of resecting redundant platysmal muscle is the elimination of the excess muscle and subplatysmal fat rather than attempting to imbricate the redundancy. By resecting muscle and advancing the platysma medially toward the midline, the surgeon is addressing the deformity at its origin and is advancing tissue in the same direction as the gravitational forces on the neck. In contrast, posterior suspension of the platysma near the angle of the mandible is removed from the area of deformity and moves tissue against gravitational pull. Posterior suspension of the cervical platysma is frequently prone to early recurrence of banding.

Even with the direct approach of correcting banding by performing a surgical excision of muscle redundancy, the anterior neck is the weak link of facelifting. Relaxation of skin and platysma occurs here first before other areas of the face and neck. Mild recurrent banding and skin laxity of the submentum may be observed as soon as 6 months after facelifting. This may be related to the increased tissue creep observe in the SMAS located in the neck compared with the

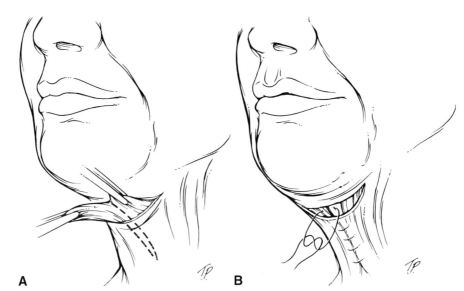

A   **B**

Figure 30-11. A, The skin and fat of the submental area are widely undermined in the preplatysmal plane. Redundant platysmal muscle is resected in a vertical orientation. **B,** The skin flap is thinned of excessive fat, and the borders of the platysmal muscles are approximated.

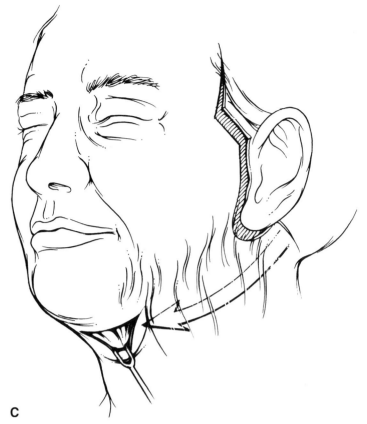

C

Figure 30-11, cont'd C, Depending on cervical skin laxity, it may be necessary to connect the submental dissection with a posterior dissection, so that the entire upper cervical skin is freed from the platysma.

SMAS in the cheek.[17] Patients should be counseled that anterior neck laxity and melolabial folds are the two regions of the face that are most difficult to completely correct with rhytidectomy.

Mid-Facelift

If a subperiosteal mid-facelift is to be performed, this is accomplished before dissecting SMAS flaps. A sub-SMAS dissection does not improve the mid-face. For this, a subperiosteal mid-facelift is performed through a combined transoral and transtemporal approach. A bilateral subperiosteal mid-face dissection is accomplished under direct vision with a headlight and tissue retractor. A 2-cm upper gingival buccal incision is made, and with the use of a periosteal elevator, a complete detachment of the periosteum from the face of the maxilla is accomplished including release from the pyriform aperture, nasal sidewall, the entire infraorbital bony rim, and zygomatic eminence (Figure 30-13). Care is taken to observe and preserve the infraorbital nerve. From the zygoma, the dissection is carried inferiorly over the anterior masseter for 2 cm, releasing the soft tissue from its attachment to the anterior tendinous aspect of the muscle. This maneuver detaches the masseteric cutaneous ligaments, allowing upward advancement of the platysma in the

region of the jowl.[26] Subperiosteal dissection of the superior aspect of the zygoma is accomplished through a temporal scalp incision. Dissection in the temple begins in the subgaleal plane proceeding forward and downward toward the zygoma (Figure 30-14). Two centimeters above the zygomatic arch an incision is made through the temporalis fascia, and dissection continues just superficial to the temporal fat pad to the level of the medial aspect of the zygomatic arch. An incision is then made through the periosteum along the superior border of the arch, and the periosteum is raised off of the arch. Dissection of the subperiosteal plane continues anteriorly to connect with the dissection plane created from the transoral approach. The periosteum is also elevated off the frontal process of the zygoma to free the periosteum from the entire lateral orbital bony rim. Once all of the soft tissue of the mid-face has been freed from its bony attachment to the maxilla and zygoma, the tissue is suspended with sutures placed between the periosteum over the malar eminence and the temporalis fascia (Figure 30-15). This suspension is placed under considerable tension. Marked upward movement of the soft tissues is noted, often resulting in exposure of the upper incisors (Figure 30-16). Suspension of the mid-face soft tissues is always performed before

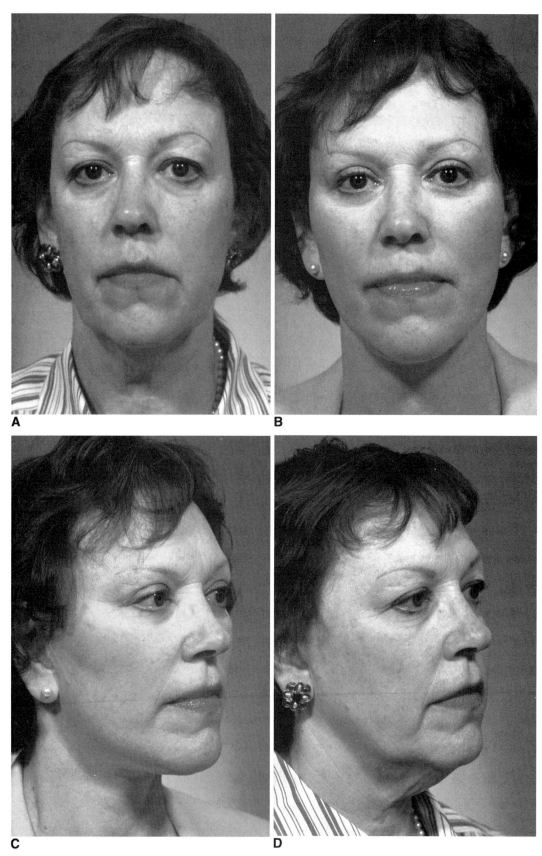

Figure 30-12. Preoperative and 18 months postoperative views after rhytidectomy with sub-mentoplasty as described in text. To view this image in color, please go to *www.ototext.com* or the Electronic Image Collection CD, bound into your copy of Cummings Otolaryngology—Head and Neck Surgery, 4th edition.

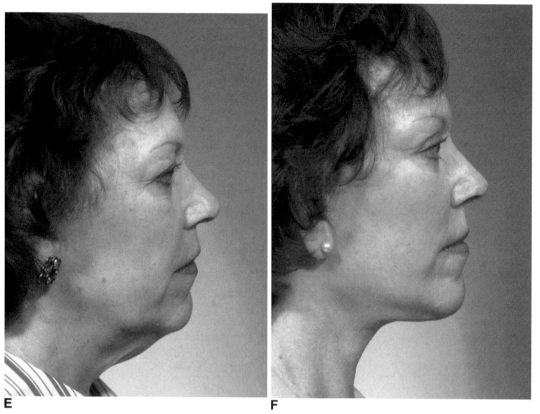

Figure 30-12, cont'd.

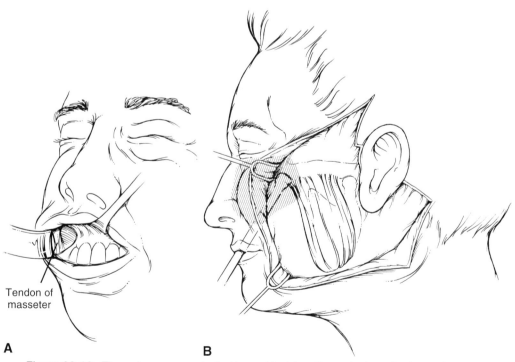

Tendon of
masseter

A   B

Figure 30-13. Through an upper gingival buccal incision, the periosteum is elevated from the face of the maxilla and lower portion of the zygoma. From the zygoma, the dissection is carried inferiorly over the anterior masseter tendon. (Courtesy of Archives of Otolaryngology.[14])

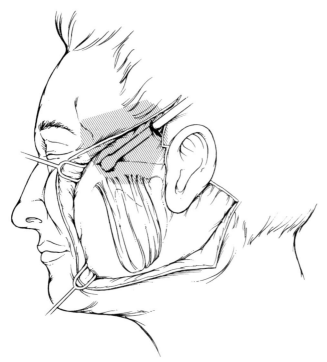

Figure 30-14. Subperiosteal dissection of the superior aspect of the zygoma is accomplished from above through a temporal incision.

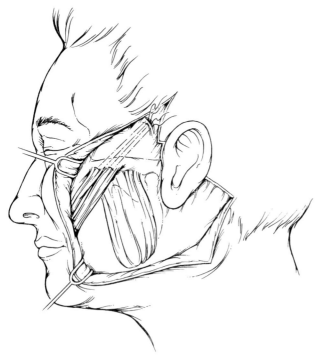

Figure 30-15. The mid-face soft tissues are suspended with sutures placed between the periosteum of the zygoma and the temporalis fascia.

suspension of the SMAS flap. Subperiosteal mid-facelifts reposition the ptotic cheek fat to a more youthful position. They also lift the orbicularis muscle of the lower eyelid and restore the relationship between the lower eyelid and the cheek observed in youthful faces (Figure 30-17).

Skin Flap Elevation

The extent of skin undermining varies with each patient and the surgical approach used (Figure 30-18). When a sub-SMAS dissection is performed, the facial skin may be left attached to the underlying SMAS or may be separated from the portion of the SMAS dissected as a flap. Leaving the skin attached to the SMAS helps to preserve the integrity of this structure and facilitates an easier sub-SMAS dissection. It also provides more substance for suture suspension of the SMAS flap. The depth of dissection varies in each

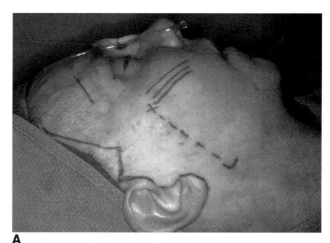

A

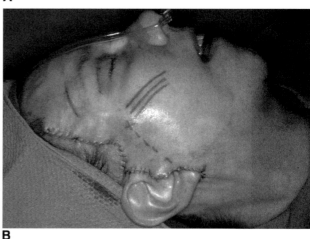

B

Figure 30-16. A, Before suspension of the mid-face. **B,** After subperiosteal dissection of the mid-face and suspension to the temporalis fascia. Note: Marked upward movement of the mid-facial soft tissues with exposure of upper incisors. To view this image in color, please go to *www.ototext.com* or the Electronic Image Collection CD, bound into your copy of Cummings Otolaryngology—Head and Neck Surgery, 4th edition.

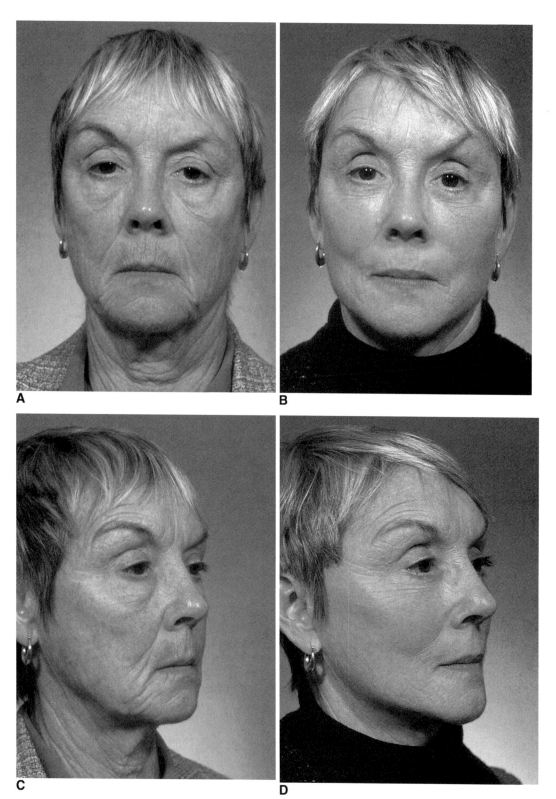

A

B

C

D

Figure 30-17. Preoperative and 1 year postoperative views after blepharoplasty and rhytidectomy with subperiosteal mid-facelift. The patient had a left direct brow lift and dermabrasion of the perioral area. Preoperative views show ptosis of the mid-face with skeletonization of the inferior bony orbital rim. The junction between the cheek and lower eyelid is displaced inferiorly. Postoperative views show elevation of the cheek fat of the mid-face and a youthful repositioning of eyelid and cheek tissues. The vertical height of the lower eyelid (i.e., from lid margin to lid–cheek junction) has been shortened as a result of mid-facelifting. To view this image in color, please go to *www.ototext.com* or the Electronic Image Collection CD, bound into your copy of Cummings Otolaryngology—Head and Neck Surgery, 4th edition.

Continued

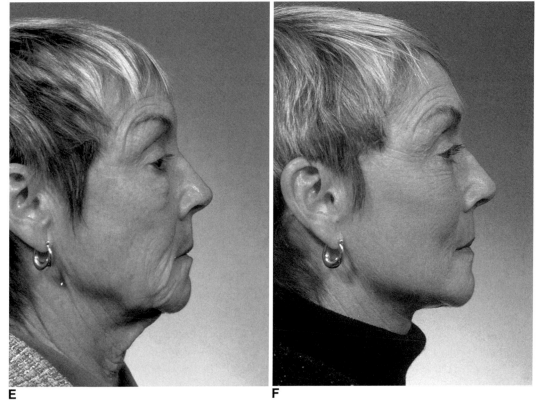

E

F

Figure 30-17, cont'd.

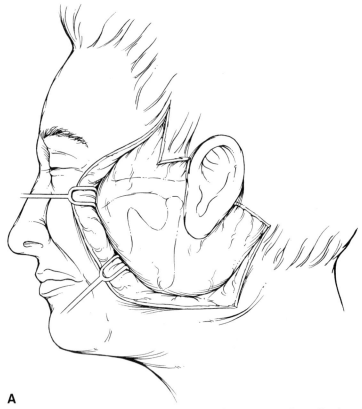

A

Figure 30-18. Typical extent of skin undermining in subcutaneous plane. To view this image in color, please go to *www.ototext.com* or the Electronic Image Collection CD, bound into your copy of Cummings Otolaryngology—Head and Neck Surgery, 4th edition.

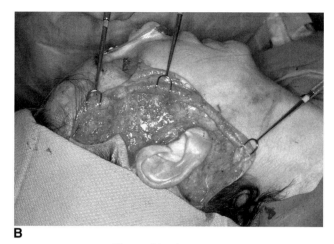

B

Figure 30-18, cont'd.

region of the face. The posterior scalp is elevated below the hair follicles transitioning to a more superficial subcutaneous plane under the postauricular skin. Over the sternocleidomastoid muscle, the dissection must be very superficial, remaining above the fascia of the muscle to avoid injury to the greater auricular nerve. Anterior to the sternocleidomastoid muscle, the neck skin is dissected either in the subcutaneous plane or immediately superficial to the platysma. The preplatysmal plane is preferred by the author, because it enables the surgeon to accurately remove excessive fat from the cervical skin flap.

In the temple, the dissection may be in the subgaleal plane or below the hair follicles in the deep subcutaneous plane. The subcutaneous plane of dissection is preferred to the subgaleal approach because greater lifting is possible of the skin lateral to the eye. If the subcutaneous plane is used, the dissection should transition to a more superficial level under the temple skin anterior to the hairline.

Over the parotid gland in the preauricular area, dissection is accomplished in the subcutaneous plane. The anterior extent of the dissection varies with the surgical approach used. The author extends the dissection forward to a line extending from the lateral canthus to the angle of the mandible (Figure 30-19). The dissection does not extend beyond this line so as to leave the facial skin attached to the underlying SMAS. In individuals with marked laxity of the cervical skin or who require liposculpturing, a posterior neck dissection in the relatively avascular preplatysmal plane is carried forward from the upper sternocleidomastoid muscle to the mid-line. Lifting the cervical fat with the skin enables the surgeon to remove fat from the flap selectively and evenly under direct vision with scissors or a liposculpturing cannula. After the posterior neck dissection is completed, an incision is made through the SMAS from the malar

eminence to the angle of the mandible (Figure 30-20). The upper third of the incision is undermined 2 cm to allow a cuff of SMAS for suturing. The lower two thirds of the incision is undermined in the subplatysmal plane. The dissection is carried forward beneath the jowl, remaining above the inferior border of the mandible and deep to the platysma. This is accomplished with ease, primarily by blunt dissection, because the SMAS–platysma is separated in this region from the masseter muscle and buccal fat by a layer of loose areolar tissue between the platysma and the masseter fascia (Figure 30-21). The dissection must remain superficial to the masseteric fascia, because the facial nerve lies deep to the fascia. Before advancement of the SMAS, the cervical skin flap is liposculptured by removing excessive subcutaneous fat from the cervical skin flap (Figure 30-22). The SMAS flap is suspended posterosuperiorly after suspension of the mid-face if a subperiosteal mid-facelift has been performed. Sutures are placed through the ventral aspect of the elevated platysma of the inferior cheek and secured to the posterior incised border of the SMAS. This causes marked posterosuperior advancement of the SMAS flap, the advance border of which overlaps the parotid gland and is secured to the preauricular parotid fascia with a second series of suspension sutures (Figure 30-23). The SMAS flap is often advanced to within 2 cm of the earlobe and, on occasion, may require excision and discarding of redundant SMAS and platysmal muscle. The advancement produces a short skin flap in this area.

Skin Trimming

On completion of skin undermining and suspension of the SMAS and the mid-face (if mid-facelifting has been performed), final hemostasis is performed. There has been recent interest in the use of fibrin sealants in facelifting to reduce postoperative bleeding. Applications of these substances assist with hemostasis and cause rapid adherence of the skin flap to the underlying platysma and SMAS. Its use may also enable the surgeon to trim a greater amount of facial skin without increasing wound closure tension. Disadvantages of fibrin sealants are cost of the material and problems with seroma formation if the sealant is not applied evenly, carefully, and rapidly. The use of fibrin sealants in an elective surgical procedure raises an ethical consideration, because the material is derived from pooled blood products. Fibrinogen, thrombin, and factor VIII, all present in fibrin sealants, are isolated from human plasma. Therefore, there is a theoretical risk of transmission of hepatitis B and C viruses, human immunodeficiency virus, and human T-cell leukemia/lymphoma virus type I or II from human blood products.[25]

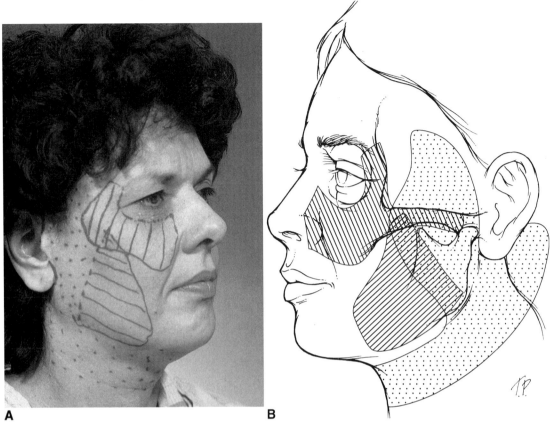

A　　　　　　　　　　　　　　　　　**B**

Figure 30-19. **A,** Topographic display of the limits of dissection planes used by author. Stippled area represents subcutaneous or preplatysmal dissection. Vertical lines represent sub- periosteal dissection. Horizontal lines represent sub-superficial musculoaponeurotic system (sub-SMAS) dissection. To view this image in color, please go to *www.ototext.com* or the Electronic Image Collection CD, bound into your copy of Cummings Otolaryngology—Head and Neck Surgery, 4th edition. **B,** Diagram showing limits of subperiosteal and sub-SMAS dissection.

Skin trimming is accomplished in two steps. The first is placement of two key tension sutures, one imme- diately above the auricle in the scalp and the other midway along the horizontal segment of the posterior scalp incision. This is accomplished by placing the skin flap under traction while it is overlapping the auri- cle. The flap is split to the point where the flap meets the temporal scalp incision at the level of the superior auricular sulcus, and one of the two key tension sutures is placed. Traction is then placed on the postauricular skin flap, and the flap is split to the point where it meets the posterior scalp incision (Figure 30-24). The second tension suture is placed at this point. Traction on the skin flap and securing the position of the flap with the key sutures determines the degree of lifting. Use of SMAS flaps as described earlier in this chapter assists with the posterosuperior advancement of the skin flap and reduces the need for as much tension on the key sutures for the same degree of skin advance- ment compared with not using such techniques[10] (Figure 30-25).

The temporal scalp flap is trimmed so there is no wound closure tension. To prevent upward migration of the temporal tuft of hair, a horizontal sideburn inci- sion beneath the tuft is usually performed to facili- tate excision of vertical lifted skin excess (Figure 30-25). The preauricular skin is then trimmed so there is no wound closure tension. When trimming the skin beneath the earlobe, it is important to leave a slight degree of redundancy of the skin flap so it will lift the lobe upward slightly. This will ensure that as the scar contracts in this area and drifts inferiorly, the earlobe will not be pulled down, resulting in loss of the sulcus between the lobe and cheek skin. This technique eliminates the risk of developing a satyr's ear deformity. The postauricular skin flap is pivoted slightly anteriorly on the earlobe as necessary to realign the postauricular hairline. The postauricular flap is then trimmed conservatively to minimize wound closure tension. It is especially important to have no wound closure tension in the area of the supe- rior apex of the mastoid skin incision because of the

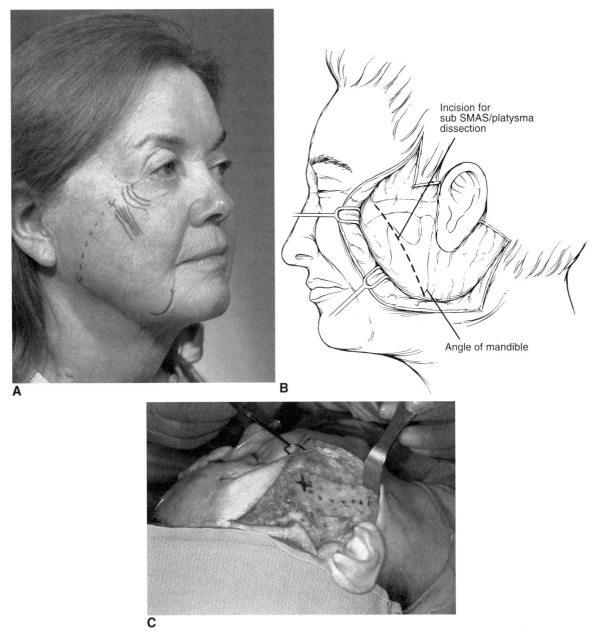

Figure 30-20. A and **B,** Dotted line indicates incision line through superficial musculoaponeurotic system (SMAS). **C,** Intraoperative view of SMAS incision. (Courtesy Archives of Otolaryngology.[14])
To view this image in color, please go to *www.ototext.com* or the Electronic Image Collection CD, bound into your copy of Cummings Otolaryngology—Head and Neck Surgery, 4th edition.

thin skin in this area. Hypertrophic scars occur most commonly at this point.

Drains may be inserted through separate incisions in the postauricular scalp and tunneled to the area of the neck dissection where they are positioned in the dependent portion of the wound. Wound closure is accomplished by approximating the subcutaneous tissues of the scalp incisions with absorbable suture and staples for the skin. The skin incisions anterior and posterior to the ear do not usually require subcutaneous sutures. A simple running cutaneous suture is

all that is required. A compression dressing of the surgeon's choice is then used.

The patient is seen the day after surgery. Dressings and drains (if used) are removed. Careful examination of the skin flap is performed to evaluate skin vascularity. All areas are inspected for the presence of a hematoma. A light compression dressing is reapplied, and the patient is asked to return the next day for a second examination. On the second postoperative day, all dressings are removed, and the patient is allowed to shower and shampoo the hair. The patient

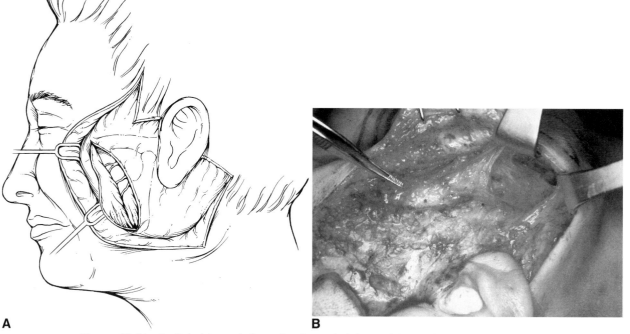

Figure 30-21. A, Subplatysmal dissection is carried forward beneath the jowl, remaining above the inferior border of the mandible. **B,** The dissection plane is in the avascular loose areolar tissue plane between the platysma and the mesenteric fascia. To view this image in color, please go to *www.ototext.com* or the Electronic Image Collection CD, bound into your copy of Cummings Otolaryngology-Head and Neck Surgery, 4th edition.

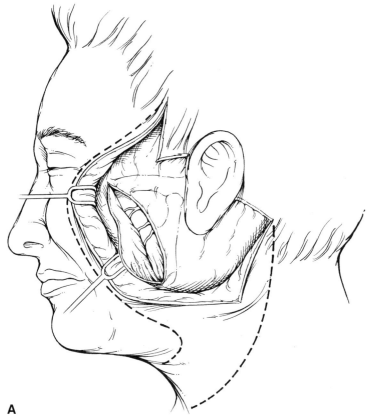

A

Figure 30-22. A and **B,** After dissection and before suspension of the superficial musculoaponeurotic system flap. The cervical skin flap is trimmed of any excessive subcutaneous fat. This may be accomplished with scissors or with a liposculpture cannula.

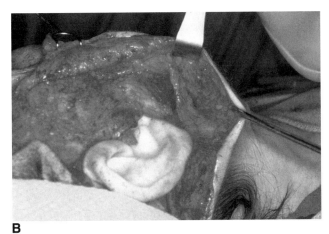

B

Figure 30-22, cont'd. B, Intraoperative view showing separate dissection planes for the cervical skin flap and the platysma. To view this image in color, please go to *www.ototext.com* or the Electronic Image Collection CD, bound into your copy of Cummings Otolaryngology—Head and Neck Surgery, 4th edition.

is seen on the fifth postoperative day for suture removal and the seventh postoperative day for removal of scalp staples. If all wounds are healing well, patients return 2 and 4 weeks after surgery for examination of their wounds. Photographs are performed 3 months postoperatively. By this time, most of the facial edema from mid-facelifting has subsided (Figure 30-26).

COMPLICATIONS

All surgical procedures are associated with potential complications. The goal is to minimize the frequency and severity of complications. Modern techniques such as sub-SMAS rhytidectomies and mid-facelifting are associated with certain complications rarely observed with subcutaneous rhytidectomies.

Hematoma

The most common perioperative complication of rhytidectomy is hematoma, which occurs in 1% to 10% of patients and may be a major or minor collection of blood beneath the skin flap. Major and expanding hematomas usually occur within 24 hours of surgery and are heralded by increasing facial edema, bruising, and pain. Hypertension predisposes to this risk, and hematomas occur more frequently in men. Other factors related to hematoma are recent ingestion of aspirin, nonsteroidal antiinflammatory drugs, high doses of vitamin E, and certain herbal health supplements. Major hematomas require immediate wound exploration, evacuation of blood, and control of hemorrhaging. If not detected and treated within a few hours, there is risk of skin flap necrosis and subsequent scarring of the periauricular skin (Figure 30-27). Minor hematomas of 2 to 10 mL of blood may not be detected until the first dressing change. These

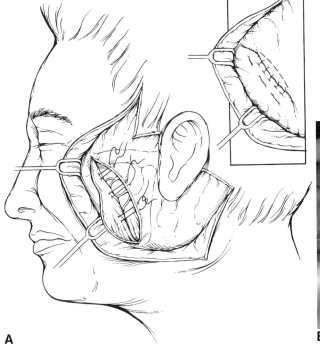

A

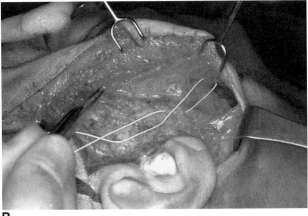

B

Figure 30-23. A and **B,** Sutures are placed through the ventral aspect of the elevated platysma of the inferior cheek and secured to the posterior incised border of the superficial musculoaponeurotic system (SMAS).

Continued

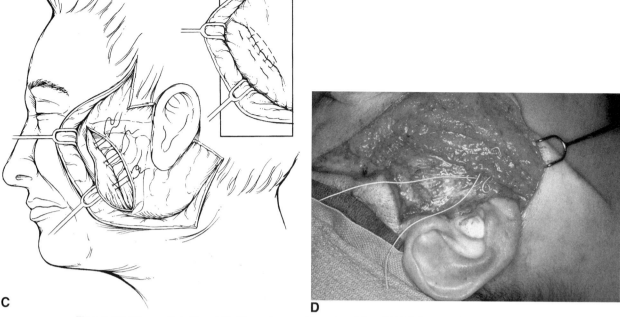

C

D

Figure 30-23, cont'd C and **D,** The advanced border of the SMAS flap overlaps the parotid and is secured to the fascia with a second series of suspension sutures. (Courtesy of Archives of Otolaryngology.[14]) To view this image in color, please go to *www.ototext.com* or the Electronic Image Collection CD, bound into your copy of Cummings Otolaryngology—Head and Neck Surgery, 4th edition.

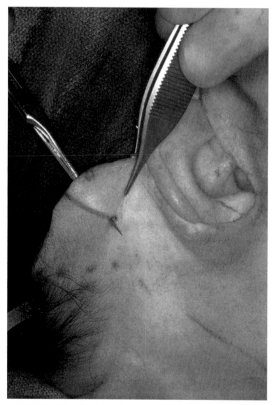

Figure 30-24. Dart incision is made through posterior skin flap to place key scalp suspension suture. To view this image in color, please go to *www.ototext.com* or the Electronic Image Collection CD, bound into your copy of Cummings Otolaryngology-Head and Neck Surgery, 4th edition.

occur most frequently in the infraauricular and postauricular region of the neck and can be evacuated in the office. Inserting a sterile slender suction device through the postauricular incision line enables complete evacuation of the blood. A compression dressing is applied to the neck, and the area is examined again in 24 hours. Typically, a small residual collection of blood is present and can be removed by percutaneous aspiration with a syringe attached to an 18-gauge needle. Seromas beneath the facial or cervical skin are usually apparent 5 to 7 days postoperatively and can similarly be treated with percutaneous aspiration.

Skin Flap Necrosis

Skin flap necrosis is associated with untreated major hematomas. It may also occur from ischemia related to the use of tobacco, certain systemic medical conditions, injury to the subdermal plexus during flap dissection, or closing the facelift incisions under excessive wound closure tension. Use of tobacco products increases the risk of flap necrosis by a factor of 12. To see any benefit of cessation of tobacco use, the patient must stop all tobacco products (including nicotine skin patches) for a minimum of 2 weeks before and after surgery.

Conservative treatment of a skin slough is recommended (Figure 30-28). Typically, epithelialization of the affected area will occur. If flap necrosis is full thickness, subsequent healing may result in a hypertrophic scar. Partial thickness necrosis may heal with little or no visible sign of scarring or with a hypopigmented scar, depending on the depth of tissue necrosis (Figure 30-29).

Nerve Injury

When performing a rhytidectomy, the most common nerve injury is to the greater auricular sensory nerve and occurs in 1% to 7% of rhytidectomies. Damage to this nerve results in loss of sensation over the inferior half of the ear. Injury to the nerve can be prevented by a superficial dissection of the skin over the sternocleidomastoid muscle. The neck skin is firmly adherent to the muscle below the earlobe, and hydrodissection by injecting local anesthetic beneath the skin along the vertical axis of the muscle helps facilitate dissection of the skin flap. If the

nerve is inadvertently injured, it should be repaired with 10-0 nylon perineural sutures placed under magnification. Like the greater auricular nerve, the lesser occipital nerve and the spinal accessory nerve may be injured during elevation of the postauricular skin flap. These nerves are positioned considerably deeper than the greater auricular nerve, and injury to these structures is rare.

Injuries of motor nerves during rhytidectomy may result in complete paralysis of a facial nerve branch or mild paresis. The incidence of motor nerve injury ranges from .3% to 2.6%.[2] The most commonly affected nerves are the temporal and marginal mandibular branches of the facial nerve. The temporal branch is particularly prone to injury when combining forehead and facelifting (Figure 30-30). Above the zygomatic arch, the nerve travels in the temporoparietal fascia. To avoid injury when dissecting in the temple and lateral orbital areas, the plane of dissection for the lateral portion of the forehead lift is in the subgaleal

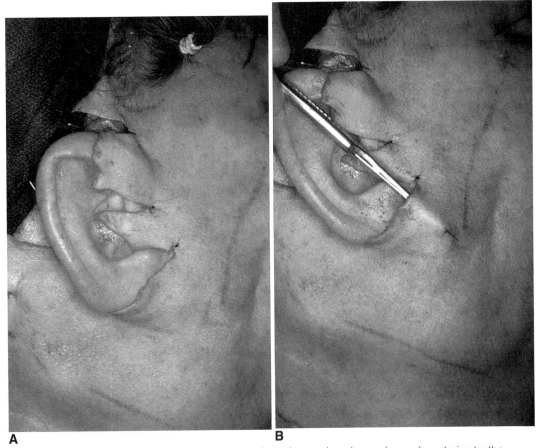

A   **B**

Figure 30-25. **A,** Key suspension sutures have been placed superior and posterior to the auricle. Dart incisions are made through the preauricular flap immediately above and below the level of the tragus, and sutures are placed. **B** and **C,** Dart incision is made to liberate earlobe. **D,** Skin flap is trimmed so that there is minimal wound closure tension. Sideburn incision has been made to spare excision of temporal hair tuft. To view this image in color, please go to *www.ototext.com* or the Electronic Image Collection CD, bound into your copy of Cummings Otolaryngology—Head and Neck Surgery, 4th edition.

Continued

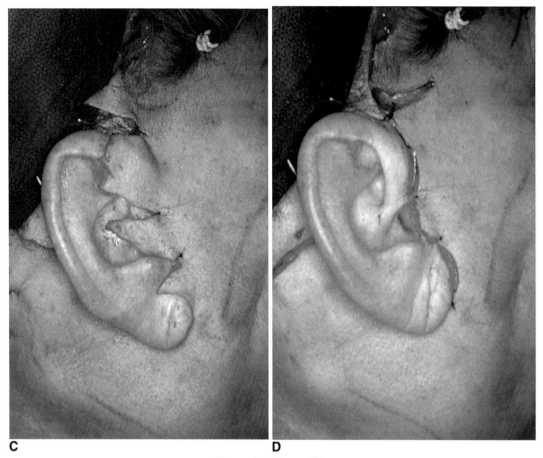

C   D

Figure 30-25, cont'd.

plane below the temporoparietal fascia. The facelift dissection anterior to the hairline in the temple is in the superficial subcutaneous plane. So, there are two planes of dissection overlapping in the lateral orbital and temporal region.

Dissection beneath the lateral border of the platysma below the angle of the mandible is at risk for causing injury to the marginal mandibular nerve, because the nerve is located immediately beneath the muscle in this region (Figure 30-31). Surgeons who develop a posterior platysmal flap in the superior aspect of the neck to correct platysmal laxity must take care to remain just ventral to the muscle during dissection.

The buccal branch of the facial nerve may be injured when performing mid-facelifting (Figure 30-32). This is most likely to occur with subperiosteal dissection rather than supra-SMAS dissection of the mid-face. Release of the periosteum from the inferior border of the zygoma necessitates dissection over the masseter muscle tendon in the vicinity of the buccal nerve.

Mid-facelifting also increases the risks of injury to the zygomatic branch of the facial nerve. The zygomatico-facial and infraorbital sensory nerves are also at risk for injury during mid-facelifting (see discussion on mid-facelifting). Fortunately, injury to motor nerves during rhytidectomy does not usually lead to permanent paresis in most cases. When injury does occur, in most cases it probably represents neuropraxia from traction, heat injury from electrocautery, or needle injury.

Scars

Hypertrophic scars occasionally occur in the retroauricular incision. This is most often observed in that portion of the incision extending from the postauricular sulcus to the scalp. The skin is thin in this, the apex of the mastoid skin, and even moderate wound closure tension may precipitate scar thickening. Fortunately, if scar hypertrophy occurs, it usually responds rapidly to serial injections with intralesional injections of triamcinolone in a concentration of 10 mg/mL. Hypertrophic scars occurring in the preauricular and temple incisions are exceedingly rare. Wound closure tension and subsequent scar contracture of the incisions around the earlobe may produce a variety of deformities, including displacement of the earlobe, obliteration of the sulcus between earlobe and cheek, and downward traction causing a satyr ear. These problems are best avoided by carefully trimming the skin flap beneath the earlobe, so there remains a slight redundancy of flap skin. This redundancy of skin provides a safety against scar contracture and subsequent downward migration of the earlobe. Mild traction deformities of the earlobe can be corrected as soon as 6 months after facelift by direct excision of the scar, creating a rounded lobule, and closing the triangular-shaped defect primarily. This in essence represents a V-Y advancement of the earlobe. For more severe deformities, repair should be delayed for 1 year from the time of the facelift and requires wide undermining of the inferior periauricular cheek skin, so that the area of the excised scar can be moved behind the ear and closed in the postauricular sulcus by advancement of the infraauricular skin.

Hair Loss

Hair loss is more common adjacent to temple incisions than postauricular scalp incisions. This may occur even when the dissection is performed well below the level of the hair follicles and is known as tel-ogen effluvium. In such circumstances, hair regrowth will occur within 6 months. Electrocautery in the vicinity of the hair follicles and excessive wound closure tension may cause permanent hair loss. This may require excision of the scalp devoid of hair. Micrografting of the area of alopecia is an alternative.

Distortion of the natural hairline may occur if the postauricular flap is not pivoted anteriorly sufficiently to realign the hairline. Stair stepping of the postauricular hairline is more difficult to prevent when there is marked advancement of the cervical skin during rhytidectomy. The temporal hair tuft may be elevated to an unnatural height when trimming the facial flap in the temple (Figure 30-33). This deformity can be completely prevented by the use of a horizontal sideburn incision beneath the tuft to facilitate trimming of the vertically lifted facial skin.

Parotid Injury

Injury to the parotid gland parenchyma is likely to occur more frequently than in the past because of the popularity of SMAS flaps and sub-SMAS dissections.

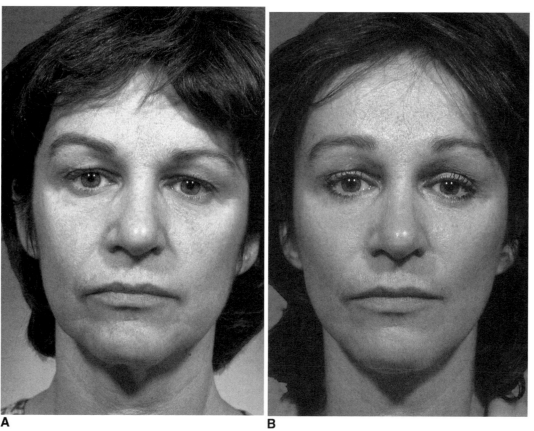

A **B**

Figure 30-26. Preoperative and 6 months postoperative views of patient undergoing endoscopic forehead lift, lower lid blepharoplasty, and rhytidectomy with subperiosteal mid-facelift. To view this image in color, please go to *www.ototext.com* or the Electronic Image Collection CD, bound into your copy of Cummings Otolaryngology—Head and Neck Surgery, 4th edition.

Continued

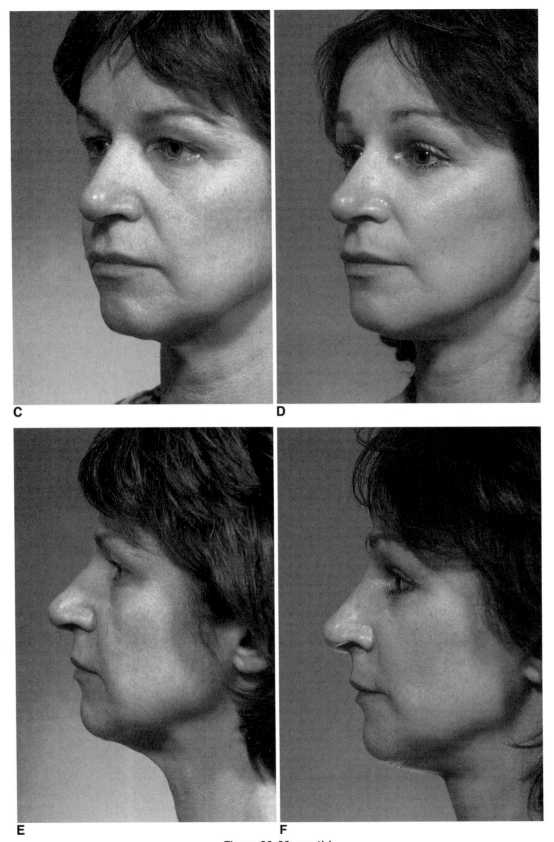

C
D
E
F

Figure 30-26, cont'd.

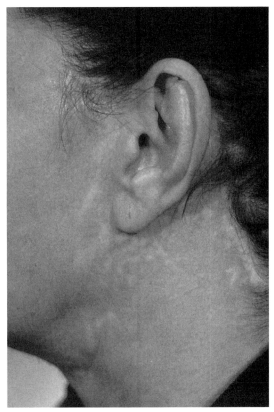

Figure 30-27. Periauricular scarring subsequent to skin necrosis resulting from hematoma that was not detected until 2 days after surgery. To view this image in color, please go to *www.ototext.com* or the Electronic Image Collection CD, bound into your copy of Cummings Otolaryngology—Head and Neck Surgery, 4th edition.

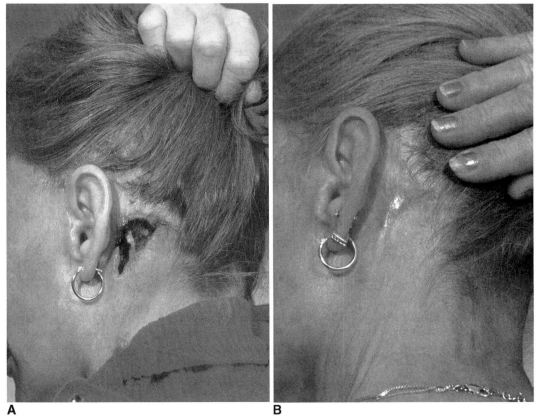

A   B

Figure 30-28. A, Postauricular skin slough after rhytidectomy. **B,** Conservative treatment led to healing with modest scar formation. To view this image in color, please go to *www. ototext.com* or the Electronic Image Collection CD, bound into your copy of Cummings Otolaryngology—Head and Neck Surgery, 4th edition.

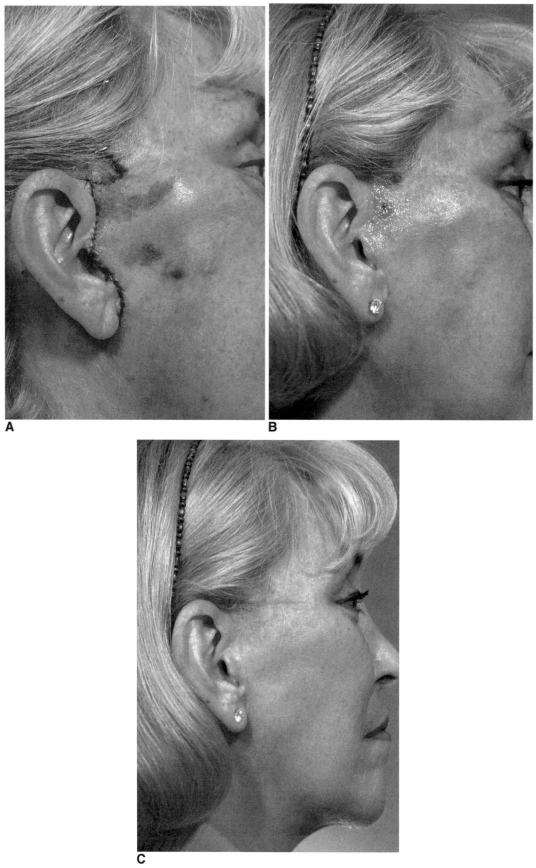

Figure 30-29. Partial-thickness necrosis of skin after rhytidectomy. Conservative treatment led to complete healing without hypertrophic scars or hypopigmentation. **A,** Two days postoperative. **B,** Three weeks postoperative. **C,** Six weeks postoperative. To view this image in color, please go to *www.ototext.com* or the Electronic Image Collection CD, bound into your copy of Cummings Otolaryngology—Head and Neck Surgery, 4th edition.

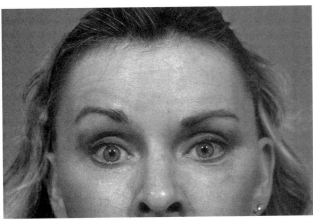

Figure 30-30. Paralysis of left temporal branch of facial nerve after endoscopic forehead lift and mid-facelifting. To view this image in color, please go to *www.ototext.com* or the Electronic Image Collection CD, bound into your copy of Cummings Otolaryngology—Head and Neck Surgery, 4th edition.

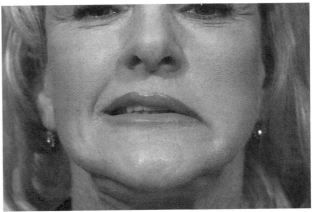

Figure 30-32. Paralysis of buccal branch of facial nerve after rhytidectomy. To view this image in color, please go to *www.ototext.com* or the Electronic Image Collection CD, bound into your copy of Cummings Otolaryngology—Head and Neck Surgery, 4th edition.

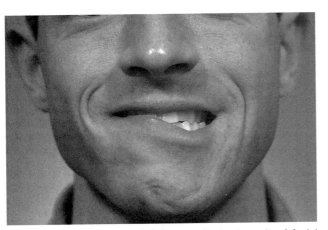

Figure 30-31. Paralysis of right mandibular branch of facial nerve. To view this image in color, please go to *www.ototext.com* or the Electronic Image Collection CD, bound into your copy of Cummings Otolaryngology—Head and Neck Surgery, 4th edition.

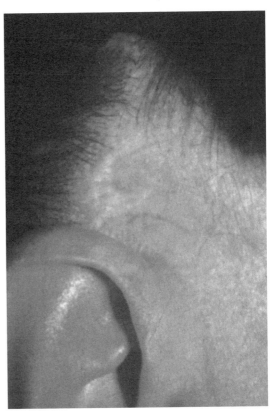

Figure 30-33. Unnatural appearance of temporal hair tuft from excessive elevation after rhytidectomy. To view this image in color, please go to *www.ototext.com* or the Electronic Image Collection CD, bound into your copy of Cummings Otolaryngology—Head and Neck Surgery, 4th edition.

Injury can occur either to the parenchyma or the ductal system and may result in a parotid pseudocyst or fistula formation.[23] Salivary collections beneath the facelift flap may delay the healing process by preventing the facial skin from adhering to the underlying tissue. This may prevent sealing of the injured glandular parenchyma and may eventually lead to the development of a pseudocyst. When dissecting beneath the SMAS over the parotid gland, it is important to recognize that parotid tissue has a gray or pink color and should not be confused with the more yellow fat that may be in the vicinity. If parotid gland parenchyma is inadvertently injured, it should be cauterized in an attempt to seal any ductules that have been violated.[34] After SMAS dissection is completed, a secure closure of the SMAS over the area of parotid injury is performed. Should a pseudocyst develop, serial percutaneous aspirations can be performed. Large pseudocysts greater than 3 cm and persistent salivary fistulas should be treated with closed suction drainage.

Pigmentary Changes

Darker complexioned individuals may have postinflammatory hyperpigmentation of scars or of the skin flap. This may persist for many months but eventually fades. Sun exposure during the first few months postoperatively may accentuate this problem. Hypopigmentation of skin adjacent to facelift incisions may occur if there is excessive skin tension on the wound closure. Skin necrosis and electrocautery of the dermis may also cause hypopigmentation. The severest postoperative pigmentary skin changes are observed in areas that have suffered partial or full-thickness skin necrosis. Facial skin telangiectasias are frequently increased in the skin undermined during dissection of the facelift flap. Patients prone to this problem should be advised of the possibility of accentuating telangiectasias.

Contour Deformities

Nodules and skin puckering can result from organization of localized hematomas not aspirated postoperatively. Most of these deformities will resolve with time, but resolution is hastened by use of warm compresses, massage, and subcutaneous injections of triamcinolone. A more diffuse but permanent depression or irregularity may result from suction-assisted liposculpturing. If severe, contour irregularities may require autogenous fat grafting. A major contour deformity can occur in the submentum if excessive subcutaneous fat or subplatysmal fat is removed. This is particularly accentuated if the platysmal muscles are not sutured together in the midline. In such instances, a hollow depression occurs above the hyoid in the midline of the upper neck and is referred as a cobra deformity.

Depression

Short-term situational depression occurs in approximately half of women undergoing rhytidectomy.[11] This develops within the first month postoperatively and is related to the distorted unnatural appearance of the face from edema and bruising. Patients should be given emotional support by reassuring them that depression is common after surgery and that they will improve as facial architecture returns to normal. Occasionally, a short course of antidepressant medication may be indicated.

REFERENCES

1. Baker DC: Lateral SMASectomy, *Plast Reconstr Surg* 100:509, 1997.
2. Baker DC, Conley J: Avoiding facial nerve injuries in rhytidectomy, *Plast Reconstr Surg* 64:781, 1979.
3. Baker SR: Triplane rhytidectomy: combining the best of all worlds, *Arch Otolaryngol Head Neck Surg* 123:1167, 1997.
4. Baker SR: Multiplane rhytidectomy, *Oper Tech Otolaryngol Head Neck Surg* 10:184, 1999.
5. Barton FE Jr.: The SMAS and the nasolabial fold, *Plast Reconstr Surg* 89:1054, 1992.
6. Barton FE Jr: Rhytidectomy and the nasolabial fold, *Plast Reconstr Surg* 90:601, 1992.
7. Cardoso de Castro C, Aboudib JH Jr.: Extensive cervical and lower face lipectomy: it's importance and anatomical basis, *Ann Plast Surg* 4:370, 1980.
8. Coleman SR: Facial recontouring with lipostructure, *Clin Plast Surg* 24:347, 1997.
9. Ellenbogen R, Karlin JV: Visual criteria for success in restoring the youthful neck, *Plast Reconstr Surg* 66:826, 1980.
10. Forrest CR and others: The bio-mechanical effects of deep tissue support as related to brow and facelift procedures, *Plast Reconstr Surg* 88:427, 1991.
11. Goin MK and others: A prospective psychological study of 50 female face-lift patients, *Plast Reconstr Surg* 65:436, 1980.
12. Gosain AK and others: Surgical anatomy of the SMAS: A reinvestigation, *Plast Reconstr Surg* 92:1254, 1993.
13. Gunter JP, Hackney FL: A simplified transblepharoplasty subperiosteal cheek lift, *Plast Reconstr Surg* 103:2029, 1999.
14. Hamra ST: The deep-plane rhytidectomy, *Plast Reconstr Surg* 86:53, 1990.
15. Hamra ST: Composite rhytidectomy, *Plast Reconstr Surg* 90:1, 1992.
16. Hamra ST: A study of the long-term effect of malar fat repositioning in facelift surgery: Short-term success but long-term failure, *Plast Reconstr Surg* 110:940, 2002.
17. Har-Shai Y and others: Mechanical properties and microstructure of the superficial musculoaponeurotic system, *Plast Reconstr Surg* 98:59, 1996.
18. Hester TR and others: Transorbital lower-lid and midface rejuvenation, *Oper Tech Plast Reconstr Surg* 5:163, 1998.
19. Hester TR and others: Evolution of technique of the direct transblepharoplasty approach for the correction of lower lid and midfacial aging: Maximizing results and minimizing complications in a 5-year experience, *Plast Reconstr Surg* 105:393, 2000.
20. Keller GS and others: Elevation of the malar fat pad with a percutaneous technique, *Arch Facial Plast Surg* 4:20, 2002.
21. Matarasso A and others: National plastic surgery survey: facelift techniques and complications, *Plast Reconstr Surg* 106:1185, 2000.
22. McKinney P: The management of platysma bands, *Plast Reconstr Surg* 98:999, 1996.
23. McKinney P and others: Management of parotid leakage following rhytidectomy, *Plast Reconstr Surg* 98:795, 1996.
24. Mitz V, Peyronie M: The superficial musculo-aponeurotic system (SMAS) in the parotid and cheek area, *Plast Reconstr Surg* 58:80, 1976.
25. Oliver DW and others: A prospective randomized, double-blind trial of the use of fibrin sealant for face lifts, *Plast Reconstr Surg* 108:2101, 2001.
26. Owsley JQ: Lifting the malar fat pad for correction of prominent nasolabial folds, *Plast Reconstr Surg* 91:4634, 1993
27. Paul MD: The periosteal hinge flap in the superisteal cheek-lift, *Oper Tech Plast Reconstr Surg* 5:145, 1998.
28. Psillakis JM, Rumley TO, Camargos A: Subperiosteal approach as an improved concept for correction of the aging face, *Plast Reconstr Surg* 82:383, 1988.
29. Ramirez OM, Maillard GF, Musolas A: The extended subperiosteal facelift: a definitive soft-tissue remodeling for facial rejuvenation, *Plast Reconstr Surg* 88:227, 1991.
30. Rogers, Blair O: History of the development of aesthetic surgery. In Regnault P, Daniel RK, editors: *Aesthetic plastic surgery*, Boston/Toronto, 1984, Little, Brown and Company.

31. Sasaki GH, Cohen AT: Meloplication of the malar fat pads by percutaneous cable-suture technique for midface rejuvenation: outcome study (392 cases, 6 years experience), *Plast Reconstr Surg* 110:635, 2002.

32. Seckel BR: *Facial danger zones: avoiding nerve injury in facial plastic surgery*, St. Louis, 1994, Quality Medical Pub Inc.

33. Skoog TG: *Plastic surgery: the aging face.* In Skoog TG, editor: *Plastic surgery: new methods and refinements*, Philadelphia, 1974, W.B. Saunders.

34. Stuzin JM, Baker JT, Baker TM: Discussion: iatrogenic parotid sialocele following rhytidectomy: diagnosis and treatment, *Plast Reconstr Surg* 108:1785, 2001.

35. Tessier F: *Facelifting and frontal rhytidectomy*. In Ely TF, editor: Transactions of the Seventh International Congress of Plastic and Reconstructive Surgery, Rio de Janeiro, 1980, Sociedade Brasileira de Cirurgia Plastica, p 33.

36. Yousif NJ and others: The nasolabial fold: an anatomic and histologic reappraisal, *Plast Reconstr Surg* 93:60, 1994.

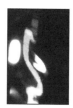

CHAPTER THIRTY ONE

MANAGEMENT OF THE AGING BROW AND FOREHEAD

Paul S. Nassif
J. Regan Thomas

PROPORTIONS OF THE AESTHETIC BROW AND FOREHEAD

The forehead, from the eyebrows to the hairline, makes up the upper third of the face. The aesthetically favored forehead produces a gentle convexity on profile; other forehead shapes include sloping, flat, and protruding. The eyebrows generally follow a smooth, gently curving arc that extends from the lateral eyebrow around the nasion and down the lateral nasal sidewall (see Figure 31-1, A). In women, the eyebrow should lie slightly above the supraorbital rim and follow a gently curving arc (see Figure 31-2). The eyebrow begins at a line drawn from the alar-facial groove through the medial canthus and ends at a line drawn from the alar-facial groove through the lateral canthus.[14] In females, the highest point of the eyebrow arc is at a line drawn tangential to the lateral limbus. The medial and lateral ends of the eyebrow should lie in a horizontal line. The medial end should have a club-like configuration that gradually tapers laterally. In men, the brow usually lies at the level of the supraorbital rim (see Figure 31-1, B).

THE AGING BROW AND FOREHEAD

Although different regions of the face age at variable rates and are influenced primarily by genetic factors, the upper third of the face ages in its own unique fashion (Figure 31-3).[12] As skin elasticity declines, the forehead, temple, and glabellar skin descend. The brow, especially in its temporal aspect, descends to or below the supraorbital rim, with the effects of gravity causing temporal hooding. If brow ptosis is severe, a visual deficit may develop in the superior and temporal quadrant. The supratarsal crease disappears under overhanging ptotic upper eyelid skin. Crow's feet (rhytids at the lateral canthus) appear secondary to gravity and repeated contraction of the orbicularis oculi muscle. Deep forehead creases appear as a result of the repetitive actions of the primary brow elevator,

the frontalis muscle, in its efforts to elevate the heavy, ptotic brow. Vertical, oblique, and horizontal rhytids appear in the glabella and nasion from contractions of the brow depressors: the corrugator, procerus, and depressor supercilii muscles.

PATIENT SELECTION
Psychological Considerations

As is true for any facial plastic surgery procedure, careful patient selection is paramount. Realistic expectations and proper motivations of the patient are extremely important for the achievement of a successful outcome, a satisfied patient, and a pleased facial plastic surgeon. If the surgeon, despite a visually pleasing surgical result, does not perform proper patient screening, patient dissatisfaction may be encountered. Educating patients about the different surgical procedures and goals requires excellent physician-patient communication and guidance. Computer imaging of the proposed brow elevation may enhance the communication of your surgical goals, because few patients are aware that brow ptosis is responsible for their orbital changes; often patients think and are told that droopy eyelid skin in the presence of a ptotic brow is the etiology of their "saddened" look. If upper blepharoplasty is performed in this situation, the eyebrow-lid margin is potentially narrowed, thereby obliterating adequate delineation of the supratarsal anatomy by sacrificing excessive upper eyelid skin.[2] After the education process, candidates for aging brow surgery must give informed consent following a discussion of possible adverse outcomes, complications, and risks of the selected surgical procedure.

Anatomic Considerations

Analysis of the upper third of the face, from the eyebrows to the hairline, should begin with the assessment of interpersonal factors that may significantly affect the patient's interpretation of successful surgical

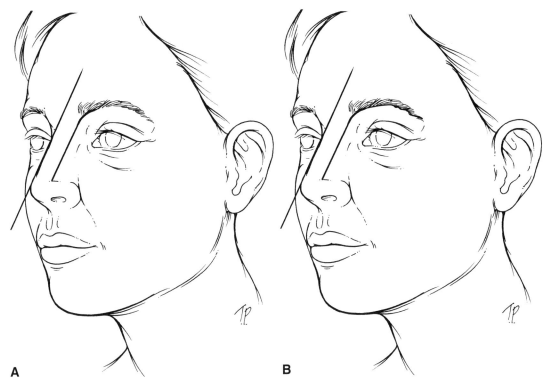

A   **B**

Figure 31-1. A, Smooth, gently curving line extending from eyebrow to nose. **B,** Sharp angle between eyebrow and nose. (Adapted from: Nassif PS, Kokoska MS: Aesthetic facial analysis, *Facial Plast Surg Clin North Am* 7:1, 1999, p 7. Used with permission from W.B. Saunders.)

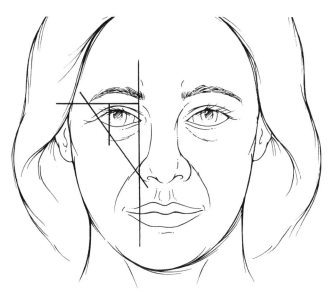

Figure 31-2. The ideal eyebrow. (Adapted from: Becker FF, Johnson CM Jr.: *Surgical treatment of the upper third of the aging face.* In Cummings CW and others, editors: *Otolaryngology—head and neck surgery, ed 3,* St Louis, 1998, Mosby, p 661. Used with permission from Mosby.)

intervention and, as such, must be carefully examined. Age, gender, race, body habitus, and personality are the main interpersonal components that must

receive consideration when assessing the eyebrow complex.[8]

When determining which brow lifting procedure should be employed, specific anatomic criteria should be evaluated when examining the patient. The patient should be examined in a sitting position and in facial repose. Manually elevating the brow will reveal the favorable effect of brow elevation. Individuals with ptotic eyebrows often involuntarily attempt to elevate the brow with frontalis muscle contraction. To eliminate "pseudoelevation" of the brow, have the patient close his or her eyes and then slowly open them after allowing the frontalis muscle to relax; the true position of the eyebrow can than be evaluated in repose by the surgeon. Additionally, the eyebrow position can be examined with the eyes closed. Listed below are anatomic and physiologic factors that need to be evaluated when considering a patient for aging forehead rejuvenative surgery:

- location of frontal and temporal hairline
- quality of hair: alopecia, thinning, or abundant hair
- forehead height relative to facial proportions
- severity of forehead, temporal, and lateral canthal (crow's feet) rhytids

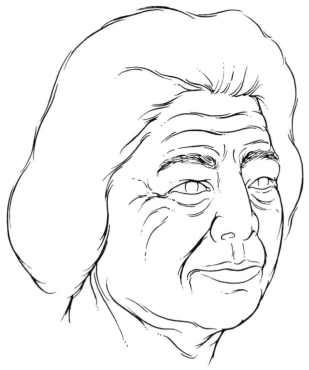

Figure 31-3. Characteristics of the aging brow, temple, eyelids, and face. Although environmental influences may worsen or hasten aging changes, each person's genetic disposition plays the predominant role in the aging process. (Adapted from: Tardy ME, Alex J, Hendrick D: *Rejuvenation of the aging brow and forehead.* In Putterman AM, Warren LA, editors: *Cosmetic oculoplastic surgery: eyelid, forehead, and facial techniques, ed 3,* Philadelphia, 1999, W.B. Saunders, p 269. Used with permission.)

- eyebrow aesthetics: shape, symmetry, quality, texture, position, and mobility
- presence of prominent supraorbital ridge or hollow orbit
- degree of dermatochalasis: excess skin, tone, lateral canthal hooding, and presence of medial fat pad
- previous eyelid or eyebrow surgery and scars
- presence of lagophthalmos (inability to close the upper eyelid completely)
- scalp mobility
- lateral canthus position
- skin elasticity and texture
- history of ocular disease or dry eyes.

SURGICAL GOALS

The goals associated with rejuvenation surgery of the brow and upper third of the face include the following[17]:

- elevation of ptotic eyebrows
- reduction of lateral hooding and redundant upper eyelid skin

- elevation of lateral canthus, if needed
- reduction of glabellar and corrugator rhytids
- reduction of transverse forehead rhytids
- reduction of lateral canthal "crow's feet" rhytids
- correction of eyebrow asymmetry.

In general, the selected brow elevation procedure should be performed before upper blepharoplasty so that the facial plastic surgeon can judge the precise amount of upper eyelid skin to be removed. This helps prevent the excessive elevation of the brow-lid complex with the potential for causing lagophthalmos. In some cases, the need for upper blepharoplasty maybe eliminated after brow lifting procedures.

Overall, selection of the specific brow procedure will be determined by integrating the psychological and anatomic considerations together with the proposed surgical goals.

SURGICAL TECHNIQUES

Traditional methods of forehead and brow rejuvenation, such as coronal, pretrichal, and direct brow lifts, have provided facial plastic surgeons with effective brow elevation for many years. In the past decade, the endoscopic forehead and brow lift has rapidly become accepted as part of the surgical armamentarium and is frequently the technique of choice.[5,15,18] The indications and contraindications for each forehead and brow lifting procedure are described in Table 31-1.[17]

Coronal Forehead Lift

For total forehead and brow elevation with excellent longevity, the coronal lift should be considered. The coronal incision is posterior to the frontal and temporal hairline, generally follows the shape of the hairline, and extends from the superior helical of one ear to the other; the subgaleal plane is used for the dissection. Redundant and excess skin and galea are excised, and the wound is closed in layers. Typically, 4-0 absorbable sutures are used in the galeal layer, and the skin is closed with skin staples. All aspects of the aging forehead and brow, including rhytids and ptosis, are effectively treated with this approach.

Pretrichal Forehead Lift

In patients with an elongated forehead and a high hairline, the pretrichal forehead lift may be used. The pretrichal incision, which is created in an irregularized pattern, is located at the junction of the cephalic aspect of the forehead and hairline or is placed just within the hairline to further camouflage the scar. A beveled incision is used to allow for hair-follicle growth through the scar, thus adding additional camouflage. The temporal component of the incision is

TABLE 31-1

INDICATIONS AND CONTRAINDICATIONS FOR INDIVIDUAL FOREHEAD AND BROW-LIFTING PROCEDURES

Procedure	Indications and Advantages	Contraindications and Disadvantages
Coronal forehead lift	• Treats all aspects of the aging forehead and brow	• Limited use in males • Elevates the hairline • Vertically lengthens the upper third of the face • Elongated scar • Possible prolonged hypesthesia of the scalp • Less fine-tuning of the brow position
Pretrichal forehead lift	• High hairline • No vertical forehead lengthening • Preserves the hairline • Treats all aspects of the aging forehead and brow	• Possible visible (exposed) scar • Possible prolonged hypesthesia of the scalp
Midforehead lift	• Prominent horizontal forehead creases • Preserves the hairline • Improved fine-tuning of the brow position • Corrects brow asymmetry	• Possible visible (exposed) scar • Avoid in areas of oily, thick skin
Midforehead brow lift	• Prominent horizontal forehead creases • Improved fine-tuning of the brow position • Corrects brow asymmetry	• Possible visible (exposed) scar • Treats brow only • Avoid in areas of oily, thick skin
Direct brow lift	• Accurate brow elevation • Preserves forehead and scalp sensation • Patients with abundant or thick brow hair preferred • Immediate scar camouflage (with hair) • Corrects brow asymmetry	• Possible visible (exposed) scar • Treats brow only
Temporal lift	• Ideal and immediate scar camouflage (with hair) • Improves lateral hooding	• Not useful for midforehead glabellar creases • No effect on medial aspect of the brow
Browpexy	• Performed through the upper blepharoplasty incision • Indicated for mild brow ptosis	• Possible prolonged eyelid edema • Possible brow asymmetry • Possible unsatisfactory results
Endoscopic brow lift	• Less invasive with small incisions • Excellent scar camouflage • High hairline • No vertical forehead lengthening • Preserves the hairline • Treats most aspects of the aging forehead and brow	• Less fine-tuning of the brow position • Possible depressions in the soft tissue of the scalp as a result of screw fixation

Adapted from: *Forehead-lift.* In Tardy ME, Thomas JR, Brown R, editors: *Facial aesthetic surgery, ed 1,* St Louis, 1995, Mosby, p 163.

connected to the pretrichal incision and is posterior to the temporal hairline, similar to a coronal lift. Excess skin and galea are resected from the anterior flap. Closure is beveled to accommodate the hair-follicle growth through the scar. The galeal and dermal layers are closed with 4-0 absorbable suture, and the skin is closed with 6-0 minimally reactive suture, which is removed in one week.

The advantage of the pretrichal incision is that the forehead is not elevated and the frontal hairline is pre-served. The pretrichal forehead lift treats all aspects of the aging forehead and brow.

Midforehead Lift

The midforehead lift is rarely performed. The typical patient must have prominent forehead creases, because the incision and ultimate scar are placed in an elongated, central transverse rhytid that crosses the midline. The subcutaneous plane is used for the dissection.

Midforehead Brow Lift

The midforehead brow lift is similar to the midforehead lift except that the forehead incisions are bilateral and do not cross the midline or interconnect. Forehead and glabellar rhytids are not treated with this brow-lifting procedure. The procedure may be unilateral, as in cases of hemifacial paralysis with brow ptosis on one side.

Direct Brow Lift

In certain situations, the direct brow lift may be used. The incision follows the eyebrow and is placed within and parallel to the uppermost hair follicles of the brow. Even in the best of meticulous closures, the fine scar may be visible. This procedure may also be useful for the facial paralysis patient.

Browpexy

Following the standard blepharoplasty excision of the skin and orbicularis muscle, the dissection is extended superiorly toward the brow in the submuscular postorbicularis plane.[1] Dissection should extend approximately 1 to 1.5 cm above the superior orbital rim (Figure 31-4, A). One to three 4-0 permanent sutures are passed transcutaneously from the lower edge of the brow hairs into the previously dissected subbrow space approximately 1 cm apart (Figure 31-4, B). This transcutaneous introduction of the sutures allows the surgeon to mark the position of the brow hairs while working underneath the dissected flap.

Each suture is then passed through periosteum approximately 1 to 1.5 cm above the supraorbital rim (Figure 31-4, C). At this stage of the procedure, the height and curvature of the brow can be adjusted according to the patient's gender. Placing the more central suture slightly higher allows the characteristic arch of the female brow to be restored or preserved.

The sutures are then passed again into the subbrow muscular tissue at the level of the original transcutaneously passed marking suture (Figure 31-4, D). It is important to engage into firm muscular-subcutaneous tissue with each suture and avoid suturing into superficial subbrow tissue to avoid dimpling of the skin.

The original transcutaneous suture ends are then pulled through the skin under the flap. The surgeon ties the suture in a loop over a 4-0 silk knot, releasing the suture if adjustment is necessary (Figure 31-4, E). Care is taken to avoid overtightening the suture once adequate placement is achieved, which may immobilize the brow. The upper lid blepharoplasty incision may then be closed.

Endoscopic Brow Lift

Endoscopic brow-lifting techniques have been progressively refined through experience and improvements in equipment.[5,15,18] In general, the temporal dissection and temporal fixation have been standardized; however, different options for forehead dissection are available. Subperiosteal dissection with release (elevation, incision, and spread) of periosteum or subgaleal dissection and release of brow depressor musculature to the supraorbital rim are both effective techniques used in endoscopic brow lifts.[9] Methods of bony fixation remain a controversial topic, because there are numerous methods. Some of these methods include absorbable and nonabsorbable screws,[5] bone tunnels with sutures, fixation to soft tissue using absorbable attachment devices such as Endotine (Coapt Systems, Inc; Palo Alto, Ca), and fibrin glue.[3,7] The primary author of this chapter advocates deep temporal fixation only without any bone fixation.[10]

The technique that achieves excellent brow elevation is the release of the periosteum from one inferolateral orbit to the other and the release of the brow depressor musculature (corrugator, procerus, depressor supercilii, and supraorbital orbicularis oculi) (Figure 31-5).[4,9,11] After the brow lift, all depressor vector forces should be eliminated to promote the maintenance of the newly elevated brow position, because periosteal reattachment to bone takes approximately 6 to 12 weeks.[16]

Temporal Lift

For patients with adequate medial brow position and ptotic lateral brow and lateral canthal hooding, an endoscopic temporal (temple) lift may be performed. A temporal lift is performed with the same principles and technique as the endoscopic brow lift (surgical technique described below) except that the medial border of the periosteal and brow depressor musculature release is the supraorbital neurovascular complex. The supraorbital orbicularis oculi muscle is the only brow depressor treated. The medial brow and glabellar region is not dissected, thereby resulting in elevation of the lateral two thirds of the brow-lateral canthal complex.

Treatment of the Depressor Muscles with Botulinum Toxin

Botulinum toxin may be used synergistically with the surgical brow depressor musculature release in an effort to weaken the inferior vector forces and promote the maintenance of the newly elevated brow. Botulinum toxin is used to block the depressor function of the corrugator, procerus, depressor supercilii, and lateral supraorbital orbicularis oculi muscles.[19] Two weeks before surgery, patients are injected with botulinum toxin. The corrugator, procerus, and depressor supercilii muscles (medial brow depressors) are typically injected with a total of 18 units of botulinum toxin, and the lateral supraorbital orbicularis oculi muscles (lateral brow depressor) are injected with about 4 units of botulinum toxin on each side (Figure 31-6). No botulinum toxin is injected into the frontalis muscle, because it acts as the only brow elevator. If an upper blepharoplasty is to be performed with the brow lift, botulinum toxin should be injected approximately 1 week following the procedure because upper eyelid levator ptosis may occur and subse-

quently interfere with the amount of upper eyelid skin to be removed.

ENDOSCOPIC BROW LIFT SURGICAL TECHNIQUE

Following photographic documentation of the patient's forehead and brows, the patient is brought into the operating suite. In most situations, an anesthesiologist administers general anesthesia with a laryngeal mask

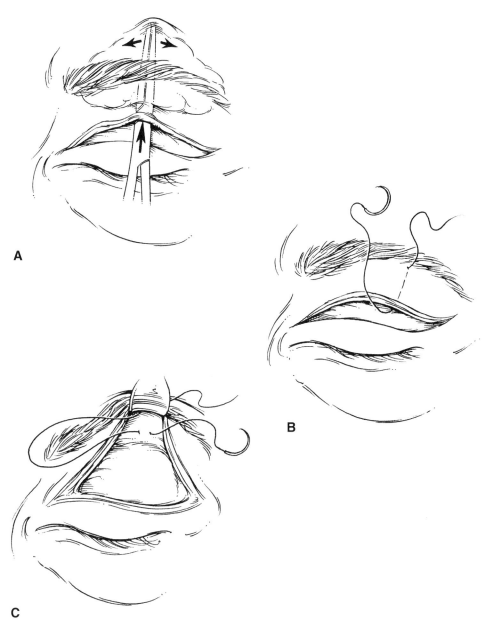

Figure 31-4. A, Frontal illustration of browpexy. A skin-muscle eyelid crease approach is used to expose the subbrow fat pad. The plane of dissection is in the submuscular postorbicularis fascia. **B,** A 4-0 polypropylene suture is passed transcutaneously from the lower edge of the brow hairs into the previously dissected subbrow space. **C,** The suture is sewn through the subbrow tissue and the periosteum above the orbital rim.

Continued

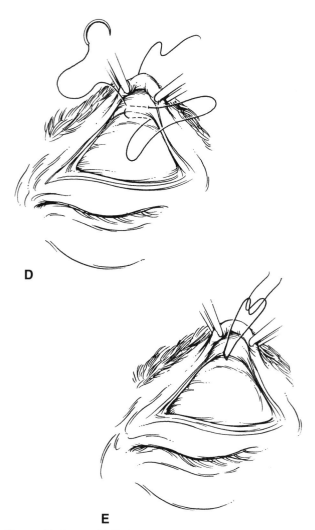

D

E

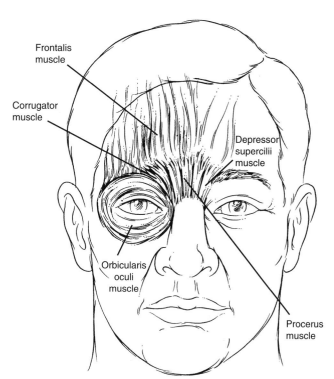

Figure 31-5. Frontal illustration of brow muscles. (Adapted from: Keller GS, Hutcherson R: *Endoscopy-assisted small-incision forehead and brow lift.* In Putterman AM, Warren LA, editors: *Cosmetic oculoplastic surgery: eyelid, forehead, and facial techniques, ed 3,* Philadelphia, 1999, W.B. Saunders, p 315. Used with permission.)

Figure 31-4, cont'd D, The suture is then passed again into the subbrow muscular tissue at the level of the original transcutaneously passed marking suture; the transcutaneous suture is removed. **E,** The suture is tied in a loop over a 4-0 silk knot, allowing for release of the suture if adjustment is necessary. Care is taken to avoid overtightening the suture after adequate placement is achieved, which may immobilize the brow. (Adapted from: Bowman CB, Tanenbaum M, McCord CD: *Internal brow lift: browplasty and browpexy.* In Putterman AM, Warren LA, editors: *Cosmetic oculoplastic surgery: eyelid, forehead, and facial techniques, ed 3,* Philadelphia, 1999, W.B. Saunders, p 117, 119–120. Used with permission.)

Incisions

The incisions are then marked: one midline and two temporal (two paramedian incisions are made if bone fixation is to be performed). The anteroposterior midline incision is approximately 2 cm posterior to the hairline and is 1 cm in length, which is just large enough to allow for the introduction of periosteal elevators into the subperiosteal space. The temporal incisions are 3 cm in length and are approximately

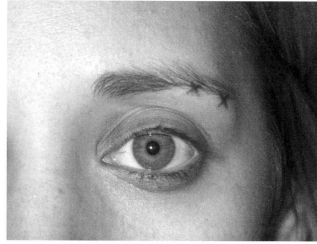

Figure 31-6. Supraorbital orbicularis oculi Botox injection sites (X). Two injections for a total of 4 units. (Adapted from: Zimbler MS, Nassif PS: Adjunctive applications for botulinum toxin in facial aesthetic surgery, *Facial Plast Surg Clin North Am,* in press. Used with permission.)

2 cm posterior to the hairline. The key to obtaining a natural-looking brow is to create a temporal incision that is parallel to the tail of the brow, with its medial extent at the temporal conjoint fascia (Figure 31-7). The temporal incision orientation will help elevate the lateral half of the brow in a superolateral vector.

Local Anesthesia

The local anesthesia consists of 15 cc of 1% lidocaine with 1:100,000 epinephrine injected into the corrugator, procerus, and depressor supercilii muscles, the proposed incision sites and for supraorbital and supratrochlear nerve blocks. The rest of the central forehead, the parietal scalp, and the temporal region are infiltrated with approximately 50 cc of a solution consisting of 500 cc of normal saline mixed with 0.5 cc of 1:1000 epinephrine, 5 cc of sodium bicarbonate, and 25 cc of 2% lidocaine without epinephrine. The high volume of the above solution acts as a vascular tourniquet to be used primarily in the temporal region. The patient is prepared and draped in the usual sterile fashion, and approximately 15 minutes are allowed for anesthesia and hemostasis to take place.

Dissection Over the Frontal and Parietal Bones

The midline vertical incision is made and extended through the periosteum. Without the use of the endoscope, a periosteal elevator is used to create a subperiosteal pocket posteriorly over the parietal forehead and anteriorly over the central forehead to approximately 1 cm above the brow, with care taken not to injure the supraorbital and supratrochlear neurovascular bundles.

Temporal Dissection and Release of the Periosteum and Lateral Supraorbital Orbicularis Oculi Muscle

The temporal incisions are made and extended to the deep temporal fascia (Figure 31-8). A blunt elevator dissects over the deep temporal fascia inferiorly until a branch of the zygomaticotemporal vein, called the *sentinel vein,* is encountered (Figure 31-9). This is the inferior limit of the dissection without the use of the endoscope. Facelift scissors are used to connect the temporal incision to the central forehead incision by severing the temporal conjoint fascia (fusion of the galea and the temporoparietal fascia). The conjoint

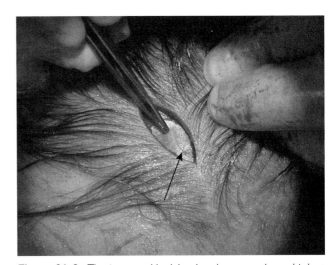

Figure 31-8. The temporal incision has been made and taken down to the deep temporal fascia *(arrow).*

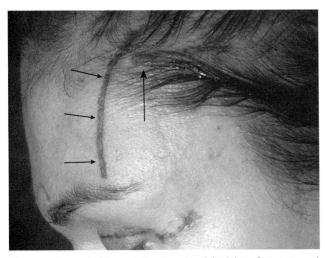

Figure 31-7. Marking of the temporal incision *(large arrow)* parallel to the tail of the brow with its medial extent at the temporal conjoint fascia *(small arrows).*

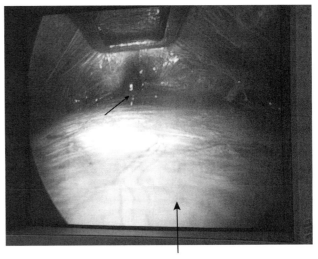

Figure 31-9. Endoscopic photograph of dissection over the deep temporalis fascia *(large arrow),* exposing the sentinel vein *(small arrow).*

fascia is released with a periosteal elevator in an inferior direction to the level of the supraorbital rim. Near the supraorbital rim, a thickening of periosteum called the *conjoint tendon* is incised sharply or bluntly. Adequate release of the conjoint tendon at the lateral supraorbital rim is an essential factor of the periosteal release.

The endoscope is placed into the temporal dissection along with the elevator visualizing the sentinel vein. This vein is a reliable marker for the frontal branch of the facial nerve, which lies superficial to the dissection on the undersurface of the temporoparietal fascia.[6,13] If possible, the sentinel vein is preserved, and the dissection is performed medial and inferior to the vein. If the vein is cauterized, the bipolar forceps are placed at the base of the sentinel vein to help prevent a thermal neuropraxic injury to the frontal branch of the facial nerve. Lateral and slightly inferior to the sentinel vein, the zygomaticotemporal sensory nerve is encountered and is usually considered the lateral border of the dissection.

Continuing dissection in a medial diagonal direction toward the malar eminence over the superficial temporal fat pad, the periosteum is penetrated just inferomedial to the lateral canthus over the frontal process of the zygoma and malar eminence. To prevent elevation of the lateral canthus, an assistant places his or her finger in the interior aspect of the lateral rim at the lateral canthus (Figure 31-10). If the surgical plan calls for lateral canthal angle elevation, the lateral canthus is released. The periosteal release (elevation, incision, and spreading) begins inferior to the lateral canthus onto the medial malar eminence and extends medially to the supraorbital neurovascular complex, with care taken to not injure the nerve.

After the periosteal release, the lateral supraorbital orbicularis oculi muscle is meticulously released from the inferomedial orbit to the supraorbital nerve, thus exposing the yellow brow fat. This same procedure is performed on the contralateral temporal region.

Release of the Brow Depressor Muscles

For the temporal lift, this portion of the procedure is eliminated. The endoscope remains placed through the temporal incision, and the periosteal elevator is placed through the central incision. The dissection is carried out to the central supraorbital region and radix of the nose, thus releasing the periosteum, with care taken to avoid injury to the supraorbital and supratrochlear nerves. Thorough corrugator, procerus, and depressor supercilii myotomies are performed. To ensure that complete myotomies have been performed, each nerve of the supratrochlear and supraorbital neurovascular complexes (Figure 31-11) should be easily visualized without obstruction from overlying muscle fibers. Finally, harvested deep temporalis fascia placed at the myotomy site of the corrugator muscles may prevent the reanastomosis of muscle fibers.

Brow Elevation and Fixation

In males and in patients with a moderate amount of bleeding, a drain is placed for approximately 24 hours. *If a complete release of all periosteum and brow depressor musculature is performed, the entire brow complex will elevate to an unnaturally high position without any tension* (Figures 31-12, *A* through *C*, and 31-13). Brow fixation is achieved by securing the superficial temporal fascia medially to the deep temporal fascia

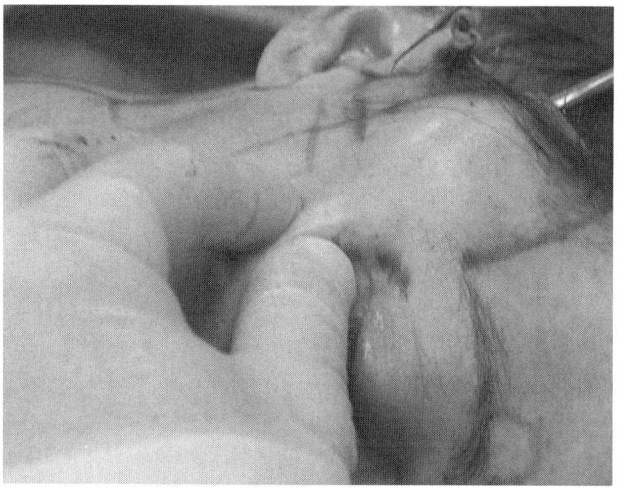

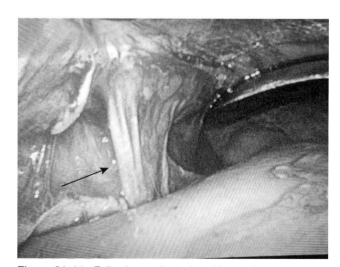

Figure 31-10. To prevent elevation of the lateral canthus, the surgeon or the assistant places a finger in the interior aspect of the lateral rim at the lateral canthus.

Figure 31-11. Following periosteal and brow depressor muscle release, the supraorbital neurovascular complex *(arrow)* is visualized without obstruction from overlying muscle fibers.

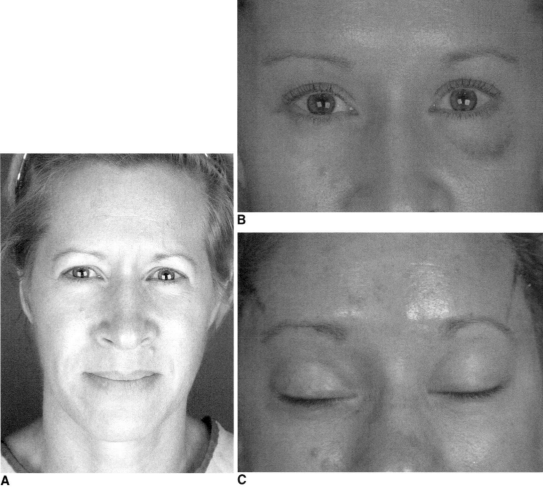

Figure 31-12. **A,** Patient before and **B,** 1 week after endoscopic brow lift with deep temporal fixation only. **C,** Intraoperative photograph of the patient's elevated brow complex to an unnaturally high position after a complete release of all periosteum and brow depressor musculature before fixation.

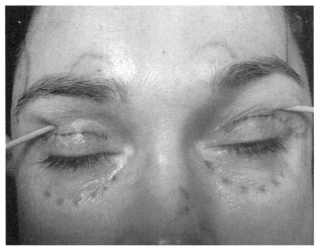

Figure 31-13. Intraoperative photograph of a patient's elevated left brow complex after a unilateral complete release of all periosteum and brow depressor musculature before fixation. Q-tips are positioned at the inferior border of the supraorbital rim.

in a superolateral vector with 2 2-0 Polydioxanone (PDS) (Ethicon, Somerville, NJ) horizontal mattress sutures while the brow is lifted laterally and overcorrected. The overcorrected brow will gradually drop to its final position after 3 weeks. The incisions are closed with surgical staples.

POSTOPERATIVE CARE PRINCIPLES

Incisions are dressed with antibiotic ointment without a head dressing. Patients may experience headaches and minimal pain initially. Shampooing with gentle cleaning of the hair occurs at 48 hours, when the hair may be blow-dried on a cool setting. For 4 days, patients are instructed to maintain a semi-upright position when sleeping or resting. The staples are removed at 7 days, and full activities may resume after 3 weeks.

RESULTS (BEFORE AND AFTER PHOTOGRAPHS) COMPLICATIONS

Few complications result from brow lifting. It has been our experience that fewer complications occur with the endoscopic brow lift as compared with the coronal lift. Hematoma, seroma, hypesthesia, tingling, pruritus,

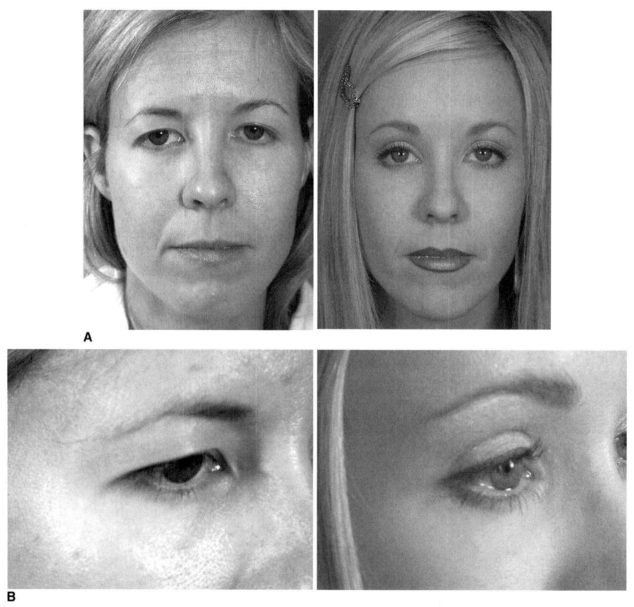

Figure 31-14. A, Frontal of before **(1)** and after **(2)**. **B,** Right oblique, before and after. A 32-year-old-woman with severe brow ptosis and blepharochalasis. Before *(left)* and 1 year postoperatively *(right)* following deep temporal fixation only endoscopic brow lift and bilateral upper blepharoplasty. The oblique view documents significant improvement in the temporal hooding, lateral canthal, and eyelid regions.

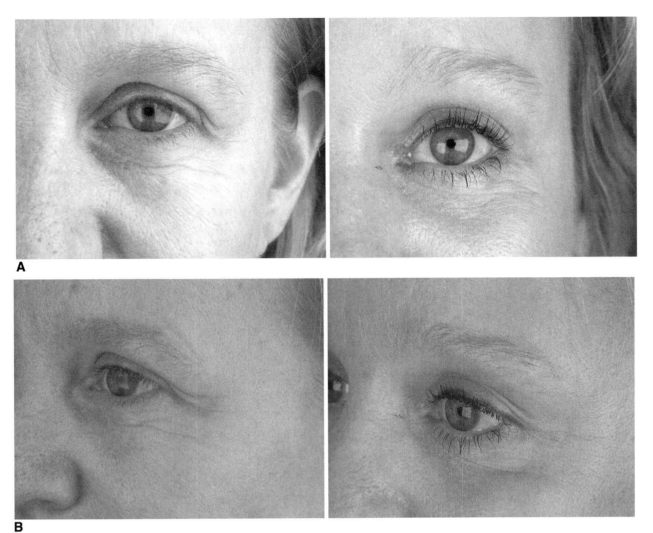

Figure 31-15. A, Frontal of before **(1)** and after **(2)**. **B,** Left oblique, before and after. A middle-aged patient with brow ptosis and fat herniation of the lower eyelids. Before *(left)* and 20 months postoperatively *(right)* following deep temporal fixation only endoscopic brow lift and bilateral lower fat repositioning blepharoplasty. Notice that the orbital region is rejuvenated, with the natural shape of the eyebrow kept intact.

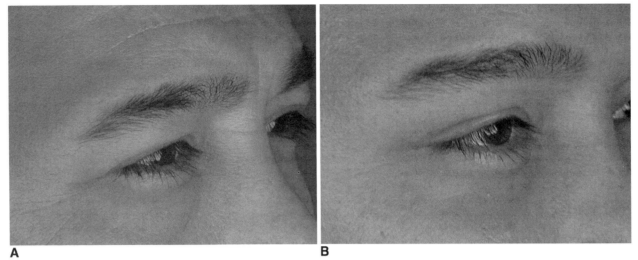

A

B

Figure 31-16. A, Right oblique before and B, after. A 43-year-old male who had an upper blepharoplasty 4 years previously was complaining of a "tired look." The brow, especially in the temporal region, descends below the supraorbital rim, causing temporal hooding, and the supratarsal crease is covered by overhanging ptotic upper eyelid skin. After a deep temporal fixation only endoscopic brow lift, the patient's brow ptosis is moderately improved.

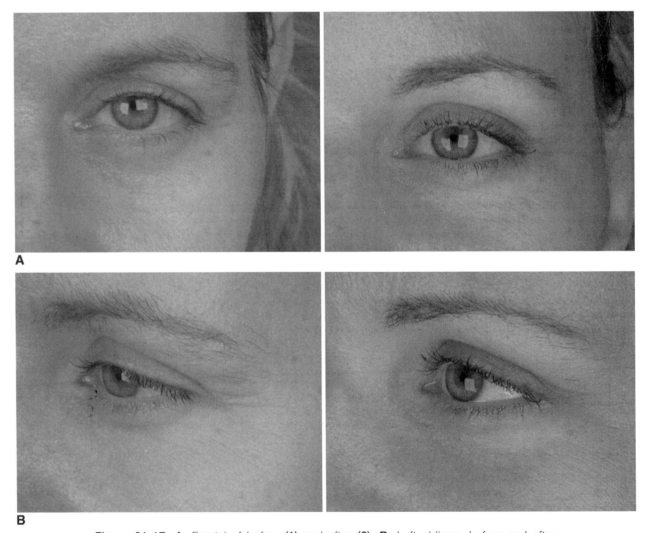

A

B

Figure 31-17. A, Frontal of before (1) and after (2). B, Left oblique, before and after. A 41-year-old patient with brow ptosis and fat herniation of the lower eyelids. After deep temporal fixation only endoscopic brow lift and bilateral lower transconjunctival blepharoplasty, notice the significant medial brow elevation.

"band-like" forehead sensation, temporary frontal branch of the facial nerve paresis, temporary or permanent alopecia, infection, stitch abscess, brow asymmetry, relapse of brow ptosis, paramedian incision depressions with screw fixation, and hypertrophic scars have been reported.[10,17]

REFERENCES

1. Bowman CB, Tanenbaum M, McCord CD: *Internal brow lift: browplasty and browpexy.* In Putterman AM, Warren LA, editors: *Cosmetic oculoplastic surgery: eyelid, forehead, and facial techniques, ed 3,* Philadelphia, 1999, W.B. Saunders, p 113–120.

2. Castanares S: Forehead wrinkles, glabellar frown and ptosis of the eyebrows, *Plast Reconstr Surg* 34:406, 1964.

3. Cousin JN, Ellis DA: *Fibrin glue as the sole fixator in endoscopic forehead lift.* Presented at the Canadian Society of Otolaryngology—Head & Neck Surgery annual meeting, Toronto, Ontario, May 30, 2000.

4. De La Fuente A, Santamaria AB: Facial rejuvenation: a combined conventional and endoscopic assisted lift, *Aesthetic Plast Surg* 20:471, 1996.

5. Isse NG: Endoscopic facial rejuvenation: endoforehead, the functional lift: case reports, *Aesthetic Plast Surg* 18:21, 1994.

6. Larrabee WF, Makielski KH, Cupp C: Facelift anatomy, *Facial Plast Surg Clin North Am* 1:135, 1993.

7. Marchac D, Ascherman J, Arnaud E: Fibrin glue fixation in forehead endoscopy: evaluation of our experience with 206 cases, *Plast Reconstr Surg* 100:704, 1997.

8. Nassif PS, Kokoska MS: Aesthetic facial analysis, *Facial Plast Surg Clin North Am* 7:1, 1999.

9. Nassif PS and others: Comparison of subperiosteal vs subgaleal elevation techniques used in forehead lifts, *Arch Otolaryngol Head Neck Surg* 124:1209, 1998.

10. Nassif PS, Massry GG: *Endoscopic brow lift: is bone fixation necessary?* Presented at the Seventeenth Annual Symposium on the Latest Advances in Cosmetic Surgery of the Face, Newport Beach, California, August 8, 2003.

11. Oslin B, Core GB, Vasconez LO: The biplanar endoscopically assisted forehead lift, *Clin Plast Surg* 22:633, 1995.

12. Pitanguy I: Indications and treatment of frontal and glabellar wrinkles in an analysis of 3,404 consecutive cases of rhytidectomy, *Plast Reconstr Surg* 67:157, 1981.

13. Pitanguy I, Ramos AS: The frontal branch of the facial nerve: the importance of its variations in face lifting, *Plast Reconstr Surg* 38:352, 1966.

14. Rafaty FM, Brennan HG: Current concepts of browpexy, *Arch Otolaryngol* 109:152, 1983.

15. Ramirez OM: Endoscopic subperiosteal browlift and facelift, *Clin Plast Surg* 22:639, 1995.

16. Sclafani AP and others: Strength and histological characteristics of periosteal fixation to bone after elevation, *Arch Facial Plast Surg* 5:63, 2003.

17. Tardy ME, Thomas JR, Brown R, editors: *Facial aesthetic surgery, ed 1,* St. Louis, Mosby, 1995.

18. Vasconez LO and others: Endoscopic techniques in coronal brow lifting, *Plast Reconstr Surg* 94:788, 1994.

19. Zimbler MS, Nassif PS: Adjunctive applications for botulinum toxin in facial aesthetic surgery, *Facial Plast Surg Clin North Am,* 11(4):477–482, 2003.

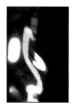

CHAPTER THIRTY TWO

MANAGEMENT OF THE AGING PERIORBITAL AREA

Oren Friedman
Tom D. Wang
Ted A. Cook

INTRODUCTION

The eyes are often said to be the doorway to a person's soul. When considering facial plastic surgery, this statement holds true. The eyes play a central role in human communication. They are capable of expressing emotions such as anger, sadness, happiness, surprise, disappointment, hatred, and love. However, it is not the globe of the eye itself or the color of the pupil that is responsible for expressing these emotions; rather, it is the dynamics of the periorbital region that allow us to convey our feelings through our eyes—alterations in the shape of the palpebral fissure, the positioning of the brows, the furrowing in the glabella, and the redundancy and fullness in the lids.

The aging process affects the skin and underlying tissues by both intrinsic and extrinsic factors. Intrinsic aging refers to the effects of time on the skin. Over the course of one's lifetime, the epidermis and subcutaneous fat layers become thinner, and there is effacement of the dermal-epidermal junction. There are fewer Langerhans' cells and melanocytes, and the morphology of the keratinocytes changes. There is a progressive loss of organization of the elastic fibers and collagen (elastosis) and a weakening of underlying muscles. Extrinsic factors such as gravity, smoking, and sun exposure may result in keratinocytic dysplasia and accumulation of solar elastosis. Taken together, the intrinsic and extrinsic aging processes create pigmentary changes, rhytids, and texture irregularities of the skin (Figure 32-1).[12,13]

On a macroscopic level, aging results in brow ptosis, lateral brow hooding, crow's feet, fine and deep rhytids, and loss of elasticity. Although the effects of aging are normal, ubiquitous, and acceptable to many individuals, others find such changes to be an area of concern. In the periorbital region, the effects of aging may cause an individual to unintentionally convey external expressions of boredom, fatigue, and sadness, despite the fact that these are not the emotions that he or she feels internally (Figure 32-2). Due to the

importance of the eyes in the conveyance of emotions, aging of the upper third of the face is almost always more visible and of greater impact than is aging in the lower face and neck. To fully address the periorbital region surgically, it is essential to first understand its anatomy and aesthetic ideals.[27]

ANATOMY
Orbital Anatomy

The orbits are pyramidal bony structures composed of seven different bones: the frontal, maxillary, sphenoid, zygomatic, ethmoid, palatine, and lacrimal. Each orbit is 30 cm^2 in volume and lies 25 mm from the other. The entrance of the orbit is 40 mm in height and 35 mm in width, and the widest part of the orbit lies 1 cm posterior to the anterior orbital margin. The orbital periosteum, called the periorbita, is firmly adherent to the bone, especially at the suture lines between the seven constituent bones of the orbit. The lacrimal gland fossa, which is located in the anterior-superior-lateral aspect of the orbit, houses the lacrimal gland. The supraorbital nerve and artery are transmitted through a true foramen in 25% of cases and through a notch in most cases. The frontal sinus lies superior to the orbits, and the ethmoid sinuses lie medial to the orbits.

The lateral orbital wall is formed by the greater wing of the sphenoid and zygoma, and it is 47 mm long. The lateral orbital tubercle (Whitnall's tubercle) is 10 mm below the zygomaticofrontal suture and 4 mm behind the anterior lateral orbital rim. The lateral canthal tendon (Whitnall's ligament) and Lockwood's ligament attach here. The medial orbital walls are 45 mm long. The medial wall is composed of the frontal process of the maxilla, the lacrimal bone, the lamina papyracea (ethmoid bone), and the lesser wing of the sphenoid bone. The anterior lacrimal crest forms the attachment for the medial canthal tendon. The lacrimal fossa and sac lie between the anterior and posterior lacrimal crests. The anterior and posterior

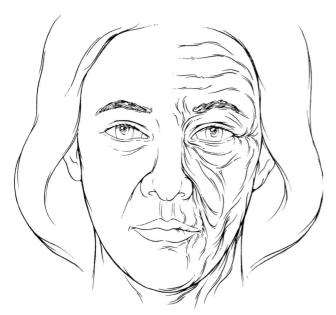

Figure 32-1. The aging face.

ethmoid foramina transmit the anterior and posterior ethmoid arteries and demarcate the level of the cribriform plate and floor of the cranial fossa. The average distance from the anterior lacrimal crest to the anterior ethmoid foramen is 24 mm; to the posterior ethmoid foramen is 36 mm; and to the optic foramen is 42 mm.[4]

The orbital floor is formed by the zygomatic bone, the orbital plate of the maxilla, and the orbital process of the palatine bone. The orbital floor ends at the inferior orbital fissure posteriorly (which transmits the sphenopalatine ganglion) and the maxillary division of the trigeminal nerve. The infraorbital neurovascular bundle travels through the infraorbital groove, canal, and foramen. The infraorbital foramen lies 8 mm inferior to the inferior orbital rim.[4]

The optic foramen, which is within the lesser wing of the sphenoid, transmits the optic nerve, the ophthalmic artery, and the sympathetic fibers to the orbit. The superior orbital fissure is bounded by the greater and lesser wings of the sphenoid. The annulus of Zinn is a fibrous ring that surrounds the optic foramen and the superior orbital fissure. The superior orbital fissure transmits cranial nerves IV; ophthalmic and mandibular divisions of V; VI (the nasociliary nerve); the superior and inferior ophthalmic veins; the lacrimal nerve; and the frontal nerve.[4]

Eyebrow Anatomy
Sensory Innervation

Sensation of the brow and anterior scalp region is provided by the ophthalmic division of the trigeminal nerve. The ophthalmic division divides into the lacrimal nerve, which provides sensation to the skin and conjunctiva of the upper eyelid, and the frontal nerve, which further divides into the supraorbital and supratrochlear nerves. The supratrochlear nerve innervates the conjunctiva, upper eyelids, and inferomedial aspect of the forehead, whereas the supraorbital nerve innervates the upper lid skin, forehead, and anterior scalp. The supratrochlear nerve lies 1.7 cm from the midline, and the supraorbital nerve lies 1 cm lateral to the supratrochlear nerve (Figure 32-3).[16]

Motor Innervation

The temporal (or frontal) division of the facial nerve supplies the muscles of the forehead and the orbicularis oculi muscle. This division of the facial nerve courses from the parotid gland (anterior to the superficial temporal artery) toward its final destination, where it pierces the undersurface of the frontalis muscle 1.5 cm above the lateral canthus. The frontal branch of the facial nerve lies deep to the superficial musculoaponeurotic system fascia (SMAS) and its continuation in the temporal region, the temporoparietal fascia (Figure 32-4). The course of the nerve may be approximated by a line drawn from a point 0.5 cm anterior to the tragus to a point 1.5 cm lateral to the lateral brow. The danger zone for the temporal branch of the facial nerve has been further described by others in the accompanying image (Figure 32-5). The nerve enters the orbicularis oculi muscle and frontalis muscle along the deep surface of the muscles. As the nerve crosses over the zygomatic arch, it lies between the periosteum of the zygoma and the SMAS. Dissection in the region of the zygomatic arch requires caution to avoid injury to the nerve and should be carried out either subcutaneously or subperiosteally.[4,16]

Fascial Layers of the Forehead and Temporal Region

The scalp consists of 5 layers: the skin, the subcutaneous tissue, the galea aponeurosis, loose areolar tissue, and the periosteum. The galea is a tendinous, inelastic sheet of tissue that connects the frontalis muscle of the forehead with the occipitalis muscle. The frontalis muscle originates from the galea and inserts into the forehead skin. At the superior orbital rim, the galea becomes tightly adherent to the periosteum. Laterally, the galea continues as the temporoparietal fascia, which lies in the immediate subcutaneous plane in the temporal region. The temporoparietal fascia is continuous with the SMAS layer of the face and the platysmal layer of the neck (Figure 32-6). Deep to the temporoparietal fascia lies the deep temporal fascia, which envelopes the temporalis muscle. The temporal fascia is contiguous with the calvarial periosteum at the temporal line of the skull, which is the

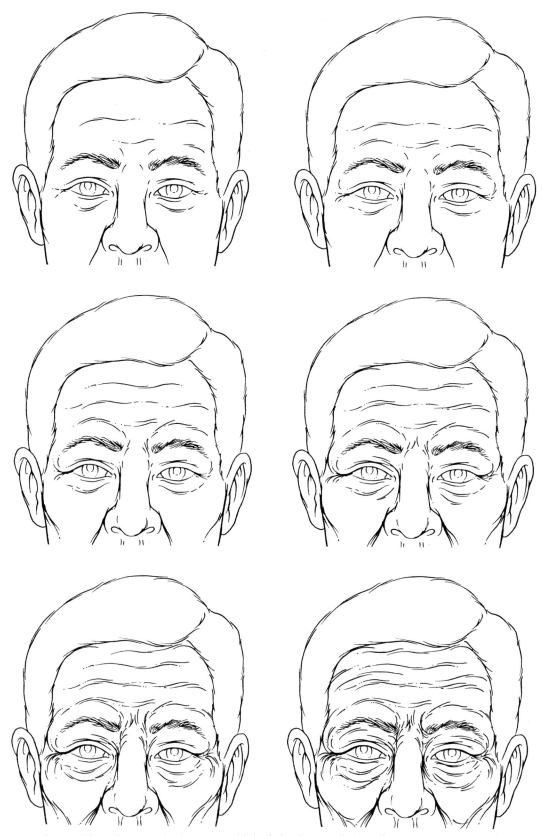

Figure 32-2. Changes in the upper third of the face and the effects of aging on facial expression.

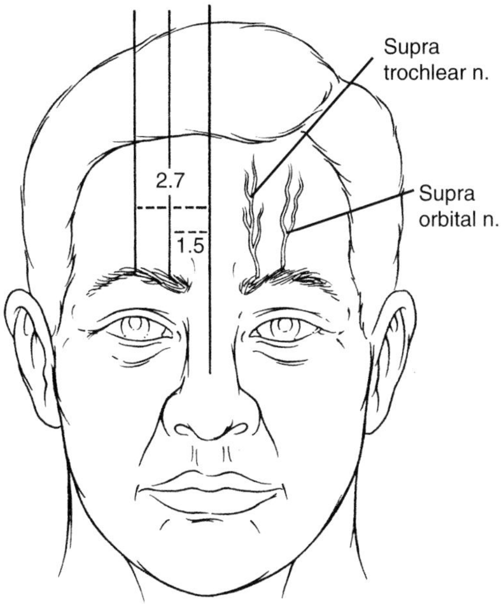

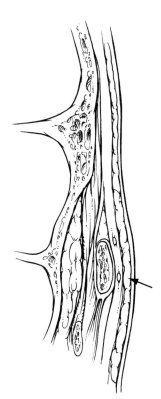

Figure 32-3. Sensory nerves of the forehead.

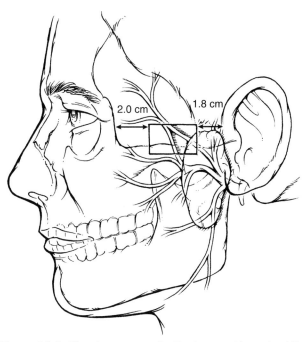

Figure 32-5. The danger zone for the temporal branch of the facial nerve, defined as the region overlying the zygomatic arch between 1.8-cm anterior to the helical root and 2-cm posterior to the anterior end of the arch. (From Weinberger MS, Becker DG, Toriumi DM: *Rhytidectomy.* In Cummings CW and others, editors: *Otolaryngology—head and neck surgery,* ed 3, St Louis, 1998, Mosby, p 650, Figure 33-2.)

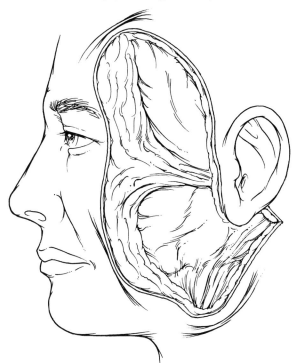

Figure 32-4. Temporal branch of the facial nerve deep (*arrow*) to the SMAS and TP fascia. (From Weinberger MS, Becker DG, Toriumi DM: *Rhytidectomy.* In Cummings CW and others, editors: *Otolaryngology—head and neck surgery,* ed 3, St Louis, 1998, Mosby, p 650, Figure 33-3.)

Figure 32-6. The superficial musculoaponeurotic system and the temporoparietal fascia is one continuous layer. (From Weinberger MS, Becker DG, Toriumi DM: *Rhytidectomy.* In Cummings CW and others, editors: *Otolaryngology—head and neck surgery,* ed 3, St Louis, 1998, Mosby, p 649, Figure 33-1.)

conjoint tendon. The temporal fat pad, which is just superior to the zygomatic arch, is ensheathed by the temporal fascia inferior to the level of the supraorbital ridge. At that point, the temporal fascia splits to become the intermediate temporal fascia and the deep temporal fascia, with the fat pad between them. The intermediate fascia layer attaches to the superior aspect of the zygoma laterally, whereas the deep layer attaches medially.[4,16]

Musculature

There are four muscles in the eyebrow: frontalis, procerus, corrugator supercilii, and orbicularis oculi (Figure 32-7). The frontalis is a paired subcutaneous muscle that inserts into the skin of the eyebrow; it is the continuation of the galea aponeurotica from the coronal suture downward, and it inserts in the dermis at the level of the supraorbital ridge. Laterally, the frontalis terminates at the conjoined tendon. The frontalis muscle has no bony insertions, and its only action is brow elevation. Horizontal forehead rhytids correspond with the long-term effects of frontalis activation. Inferonasally, the frontalis muscle extends to form the procerus muscle. The procerus originates on the caudal aspect of the nasal bones and cephalic margins of the upper lateral cartilages, and it inserts onto the medial belly of the frontalis muscle and the dermis between the eyebrows. The action of the procerus muscle produces inferior brow displacement and is responsible for horizontal glabellar wrinkles (Figure 32-8).

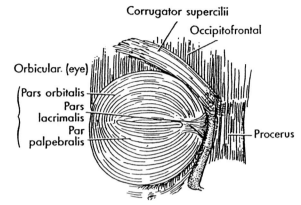

Figure 32-8. Corrugator supercilii contraction causes vertical glabellar rhytids, and procerus contraction causes horizontal glabellar rhytids. (From Graney DO, Baker SR: *Anatomy.* In Cummings CW and others, editors: *Otolaryngology—head and neck surgery,* ed 3, St Louis, 1998, Mosby, p 404, Figure 21-2.)

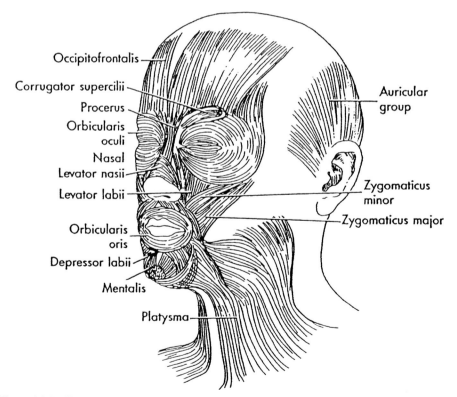

Figure 32-7. Eyebrow muscles include the frontalis procerus, corrugator supercilii, and orbicularis oculi. (From Graney DO, Baker SR: *Anatomy.* In Cummings CW and others, editors: *Otolaryngology—head and neck surgery,* ed 3, St Louis, 1998, Mosby, p 404, Figure 21-1.)

The corrugator muscle originates from the nasal process of the frontal bone near the superomedial orbital rim and inserts into the dermis at the middle third of the eyebrow after blending with the frontalis and orbicularis muscles. Its action produces inferior and medial forehead and brow movement and results in vertical glabellar wrinkles.[4,16]

Blood Supply

The internal and external carotid artery systems supply the blood to the forehead. The internal carotid artery, via the ophthalmic artery, branches to form the frontal, supraorbital, and supratrochlear arteries. The external carotid artery system supplies the largest area of the scalp via the superficial temporal artery; thus there is a rich anastomotic complex of vessels that provides adequate nutrients to the forehead, thereby allowing for safety during aesthetic surgery of the forehead and scalp.

Eyelid Anatomy

The eyelids are the protective covering of the eyes. They consist of an anterior and posterior lamella. At the level of the tarsal plates, the upper and lower eyelids consist of the same basic components; the anterior lamella consists of skin and the orbicularis oculi muscle, and the posterior lamella consists of the tarsus and conjunctiva. The two lamellae are separated by finely interdigitating eyelid retractors. The anterior and posterior lamellae have separate blood supplies, which is important to recognize when approaching eyelid reconstruction (Figure 32-9).[4]

Surface Anatomy of the Eyelids

The normal horizontal palpebral fissure is 28 to 30 mm, whereas the normal vertical palpebral fissure is 9 to 10 mm. The intercanthal distance (the distance between the medial canthi of the two eyes) is approximately 25 to 30 mm. The upper eyelid margin

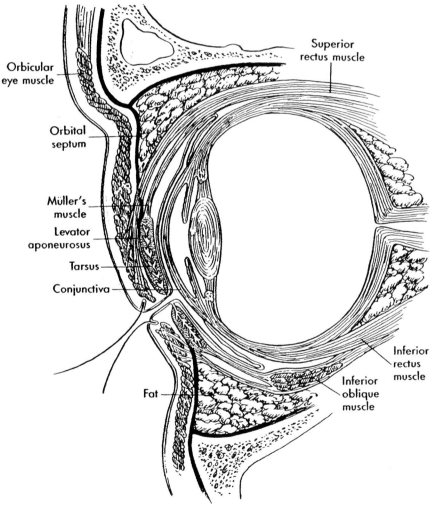

Figure 32-9. The cross section of the orbit and eyelid. (From: Colton JJ, Beekhuis GJ: *Blepharoplasty.* In Cummings CW and others, editors: *Otolaryngology—head and neck surgery,* ed 3, St Louis, 1998, Mosby, p 680, Figure 35-6.)

normally rests at a point midway between the superior corneal limbus and the pupil, and the lower eyelid margin typically abuts the inferior corneal limbus. The apex of the upper eyelid is located midway between the medial papillary margin and the medial corneal limbus. The nadir of the lower eyelid is at the lateral corneal limbus.[19]

The upper lid crease is the line that is formed by the insertion of the levator aponeurosis and orbital septum into the orbicularis oculi muscle and skin. In women, the lid crease is 10 to 12 mm above the lid margin, whereas in men it is 7 to 8 mm above the lid margin. The lateral canthal angle is more acute and 2 mm higher than the rounded and lower medial canthal angle (Figure 32-10).[4,19]

A number of anatomic differences exist between the Asian and occidental eyelids. In the Asian eyelid, the orbital septum and levator aponeurosis attach to the skin further inferiorly, anterior to the tarsus. As a result, orbital fat prolapses anteriorly, thereby preventing the formation of a prominent upper eyelid crease and creating a fullness of the upper eyelid.[4,16]

The Anterior Lamella

The skin of the eyelids is the thinnest skin of the body with almost no reticular dermis, and it is highly vascular. These factors allow the eyelid skin to heal rapidly and with minimal scar. As it approaches the orbital rim and the hair-bearing areas of the periorbital region, the skin of the eyelids thickens rapidly. The changes in skin thickness are important to consider when planning incisions during periorbital surgery (see Figure 32-9).[4,16,19]

The orbicularis oculi muscle is a subcutaneous muscle that serves as the sphincter of the eyelid. It is innervated by the temporal and zygomatic branches of the facial nerve. In addition to its function in eye closure, the orbicularis oculi muscle is essential for the proper functioning of the lacrimal pump apparatus, which propels tears into the puncta, canaliculi, and lacrimal sac. Failure of the pump mechanism, which can be a result of facial nerve paralysis, may result in epiphora.[4,16,19]

The orbicularis oculi muscle is divided into three segments: pretarsal, preseptal, and orbital (Figure 32-11). All of these segments act to close the eye, but each segment plays a unique role. Blinking is an involuntary action that depends on the contraction of the pretarsal orbicularis; winking is a voluntary action that is dependent on the same thing. The preseptal fibers contribute to both the involuntary and voluntary functions of the eyelids.[4,16,19]

The origin of the pretarsal orbicularis arises from two heads: one that inserts into the posterior lacrimal crest and the other that inserts into the anterior lacrimal crest and the anterior limb of the medial canthal tendon. The preseptal orbicularis also has two heads at its origin: the deep portion attaches to the lacrimal sac, and the superficial segment attaches to the anterior limb of the medial canthal tendon. The orbital orbicularis originates at the anterior limb of the medial canthal ligament and interdigitates with the frontalis, corrugator, and procerus muscles. Laterally, the three orbicularis segments fuse to form the inferior and superior crura of the lateral canthal tendon, which insert into Whitnall's tubercle. The lateral attachments of the lateral canthal tendon to

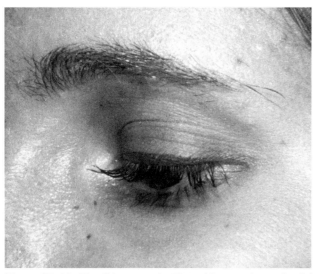

Figure 32-10. The lid crease is 10 to 12 mm above the lid margin in females and 7 to 8 mm above the lid margin in males. (From Colton JJ, Beekhuis GJ: *Blepharoplasty.* In Cummings CW and others, editors: *Otolaryngology—head and neck surgery,* ed 3, St Louis, 1998, Mosby, p 678, Figure 35-3.)

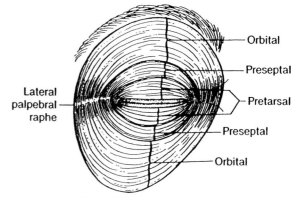

Figure 32-11. The sphincter mechanism of the eyelids depends on the three divisions of the orbicularis oculi muscle. (From Colton JJ, Beekhuis GJ: *Blepharoplasty.* In Cummings CW and others, editors: *Otolaryngology—head and neck surgery,* ed 3, St Louis, 1998, Mosby, p 679, Figure 35-5.)

Whitnall's tubercle are responsible for eyelid and globe apposition.[4,16,19]

The Orbital Septum

The orbital septum, which lies just deep to the orbicularis oculi muscle, forms the anterior border of the orbit and confines the orbital fat (see Figure 32-9). It is a fibrous sheath that is formed at the orbital rims as the arcus marginalis, and it is an extension of the orbital periosteum. In Caucasian upper lids, the septum fuses with the levator aponeurosis approximately 3 mm above the superior tarsal border. In Asian upper lids, the septum fuses with the levator aponeurosis further inferiorly, below the superior tarsal border; this allows orbital fat to lie anterior to the tarsal plate, thereby preventing the attachment of the levator to the skin and preventing the formation of an upper eyelid crease. In the lower lids, the septum fuses with the underlying orbital retractor (capsulopalpebral fascia) 5 mm below the inferior tarsal border. The orbital septum acts as a barrier to the spread of infection and neoplasms between the preseptal space and the orbital space.[4]

The Orbital Fat Pads

All of the eyelid fat pads lie deep to the orbital septum. The upper eyelid contains two fat pads medially and centrally and the lacrimal gland laterally (Figure 32-12). The lacrimal gland should be avoided during eyelid surgery to prevent postoperative dryness; it can be identified by its pink rather than yellow color and its firm rather than soft texture.[4,19]

The lower eyelid contains three fat pads: medial, central, and lateral. The medial and central fat pads are separated by the inferior oblique muscle, which should be identified during lower eyelid surgery to help prevent its disruption. Disruption of this muscle may result in postoperative diplopia (see Figure 32-12).[4,19]

Upper Eyelid Retractors

Deep to the fat pads are the eyelid retractors. In the upper lid, the levator palpebrae superioris (the levator muscle) is the major retractor, and it originates from the lesser wing of the sphenoid bone at the orbital apex (see Figure 32-9). The levator is innervated by the oculomotor nerve (cranial nerve III). The horizontal posterior segment of the levator consists of muscle fibers that extend anteriorly along the orbital roof for 36 mm until it reaches Whitnall's ligament. At Whitnall's ligaments, the levator changes its course by approximately 90 degrees and becomes an aponeurosis, which travels vertically for a length of 14 to 20 mm until its insertion into the upper third of the tarsal plate. Some fibers of the levator aponeurosis fuse with the orbital septum approximately 2 to 5 mm

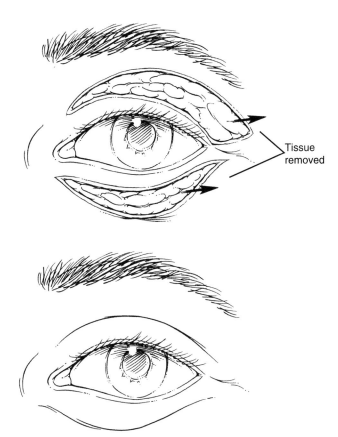

Figure 32-12. Fat pads of the upper and lower eyelids.

above the superior tarsal border and then together insert into the skin to create the upper eyelid crease. In addition to its inferior attachments to the septum, tarsal plate, and skin, the levator aponeurosis attaches medially to the medial canthal tendon and laterally to the lateral canthal tendon.[4]

Mueller's muscle (the superior tarsal muscle) arises from the undersurface of the levator aponeurosis just below Whitnall's ligament and courses inferiorly 10 to 12 mm to attach to the superior tarsal plate (see Figure 32-9). Mueller's muscle is innervated by sympathetic nerve fibers, and its action produces 2 to 3 mm of eyelid retraction. This muscle is adherent to the levator aponeurosis anteriorly, and it is loosely adherent to the conjunctiva on its posterior surface.[4]

Lower Eyelid Retractors

The capsulopalpebral fascia and inferior tarsal muscle are the lower eyelid retractors. The capsulopalpebral fascia originates from the fascia of the inferior rectus muscle and inserts on the inferior tarsal border. This fascia does not move independently but rather mimics the movement of the inferior rectus muscle from which it originates. The inferior tarsal muscle arises from the undersurface of the capsulopalpebral fascia, and the two are tightly adherent to each other and to the lower lid conjunctiva. The inferior tarsal muscle is sympathetically innervated.[4,19]

The Tarsus

The tarsal plates are dense fibrous connective tissues that form the skeleton of the eyelids (see Figure 32-9). Each plate is 25 to 30 mm in horizontal dimension. The upper eyelid tarsal plate is 10 to 12 mm in vertical height, whereas the lower eyelid tarsal plate is 3 to 5 mm in vertical height.[4]

The Conjunctiva

The conjunctiva is the innermost surface of the eyelid, which is in contact with the globe (see Figure 32-9). It is composed of nonkeratinized stratified squamous epithelium with goblet cells that produce the mucus layer of the tear film. The bulbar conjunctiva is that portion of the conjunctiva that lines the globe, whereas the palpebral conjunctiva lines the eyelid. These two segments meet at the conjunctival fornix at the base of the upper and lower eyelids. Dispersed throughout the conjunctiva are numerous additional glands that produce the aqueous layer of the tear film. The lacrimal gland secretes additional lacrimation in response to stimuli such as ocular irritant and emotional triggers.[4]

Midface Anatomy

With aging, the malar prominences descend inferomedially to deepen the nasolabial crease and expose the inferior and lateral orbital rims to a greater degree. In addition to the underlying bony malar eminence, the malar prominence is formed by a variety of soft-tissue components. The orbicularis oculi muscle extends beyond the eyelids to lie over the malar eminence. In youth, the orbicularis maintains a sling around the orbital rim but, with the loss of orbicularis tone associated with aging, descent of the malar soft-tissue complex prevails (Figure 32-13). Both the superficial and deep surfaces of the malar orbicularis oculi muscle are associated with a fat pad. Superficial to the orbicularis is the subcutaneous malar fat pad. Deep to the orbicularis lies the suborbicularis oculi fat (SOOF) layer. The SOOF layer is in close contact with the periosteum of the inferior orbital rim as well as with the insertions of the zygomaticus muscles. The zygomaticus major and minor muscles are innervated by the zygomatic and buccal branches of the facial nerve and enter the muscle on its deep surface.[24]

AESTHETIC CONSIDERATIONS AND IDEALS IN THE PERIORBITAL AREA

In an attempt to rejuvenate the periorbital area in the most natural and aesthetically pleasing way, consideration must be given to all of the elements that consti-

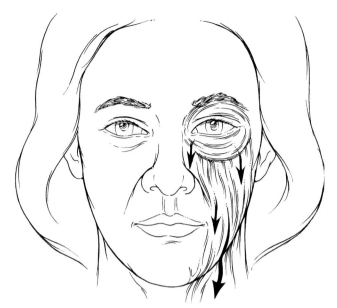

Figure 32-13. Descent of the midface with aging.

tute this region. If the ravages of aging have caused upper face and midface changes, the surgeon must recognize that correcting the ocular problems alone will not give the patient a harmonious cosmetic result. Rather, the contributions of both the upper face and the midface to the aging periorbital area must be considered. Brow position, glabellar rhytids, dermatochalasia, pseudoherniation of fat, lateral crow's feet, inferior malar displacement, ptotic lacrimal gland, and eyelid laxity should all be taken into account when addressing the periorbital complex.[14,15]

Brow Position

Management of brow malposition necessitates an understanding of the ideal brow position. Evaluation of the patient should include an examination in front of a mirror in both animation and repose. The patient's eyes should be closed for 10 to 20 seconds to allow for full relaxation of the forehead musculature. Upon eye opening, the true position of the brow will be noted, with minimal contribution to the brow position from the forehead muscles. The ideal brow anatomy in the male differs from that of the female. The classical brow position in women describes the medial brow as having its medial origin at the level of a vertical line drawn to the nasal alar-facial junction. The lateral extent of the brow should reach a point on a line drawn from the nasal alar-facial junction through the lateral canthus of the eye. The medial and lateral ends should lie on the same horizontal plane (Figure 32-14). The medial end should have a club head appearance, and the lateral end should gradually taper to a point. The brow should arch superiorly, well above the supraorbital rim, with the highest point classically described as lying at the

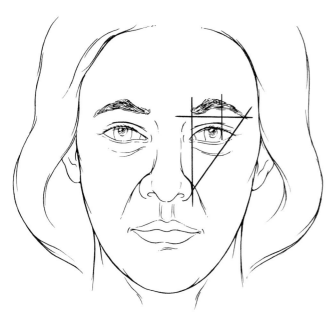

Figure 32-14. Ideal brow position. The classic description places the peak of the brow at the lateral limbus, whereas more recent ideals of beauty place the peak at the lateral canthus.

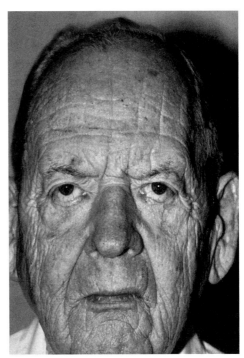

Figure 32-15. Elongation of the upper third of the face, with associated wrinkles at rest and ptotic brows.

lateral limbus and more recently described as lying at the lateral canthus. In men, there should be less of an arch to the brow position and more of a horizontal contour along the supraorbital ridge. The distance between the midpupillary line and the inferior brow border should be approximately 2.5 cm. The distance from the superior border of the brow to the anterior hairline should be 5 cm.[10,16]

The upper third of the face elongates with aging as a result of the hairline moving upward and the brow drifting downward (Figure 32-15). In addition to brow ptosis, the aging brow may reveal dynamic wrinkles or even wrinkles at rest. These furrows in the glabella and forehead are caused by the repeated pull on the skin by the facial mimetic muscles. The distance between the two eyebrows should be the same as the distance between the alar-facial junctions on the two sides of the nose.

Brow ptosis not only gives the face a tired, crowded, angry, and unattractive appearance, but it may also accentuate upper eyelid skin redundancy. As the brow descends below the supraorbital rim, it pushes additional skin over the upper eyelid, thereby worsening the cosmetic appearance of the eyelids and aggravating the functional deficits in the peripheral visual fields. Upper eyelid blepharoplasty alone will not correct the patient's problem and may even worsen the degree of brow ptosis by fixing the brow in an inferior position. Therefore, attention to the repositioning of the brow is essential and should be achieved before the blepharoplasty is performed.[20]

Eyelid Aesthetics

Several reproducible themes have been noted in the analysis of beautiful eyes and eyelids. The palpebral fissure should be almond shaped and symmetric between the two sides. The highest point of the upper eyelid is at the medial limbus, and the lowest point of the lower eyelid is at the lateral limbus. Sharp canthal angles should exist, especially at the lateral canthus. The lateral canthus should lie 2 to 4 mm superior to the medial canthus. The horizontal dimension of the palpebral fissure is 25 to 30 mm, whereas its vertical dimension is approximately 10 mm. Vertical palpebral asymmetry may indicate the presence of true ptosis of the eyelid, which would necessitate ptosis repair at the time of surgical intervention. The upper eyelid orbicularis muscle should be smooth and flat, and the upper eyelid crease should be crisp. The upper lid crease should lie between 8 and 12 mm from the lid margin in the Caucasian patient. A more inferior position of the upper lid crease gives a heavy and tired appearance to the eye. Excessive lid folds (tissue prolapsing over the upper eyelid crease) should be minimal to avoid the aged and tired look (Figure 32-16). The upper lid margin should cover 1 to 2 mm of the superior limbus, and the lower lid margin should lie at the inferior limbus or 1 mm below the inferior limbus. Note should be made of excessive skin, muscle, and orbital fat. A pinch test helps determine the degree of excess lid skin that is present. The snap test helps

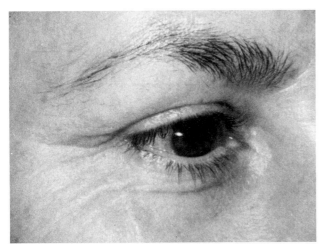

Figure 32-16. Prolapsing tissue over the upper eyelid crease resulting in a tired and aged look may be the result of skin, soft tissue, hypertrophied orbicularis muscle, and fat herniation. (From: Colton JJ, Beekhuis GJ: *Blepharoplasty.* In Cummings CW and others, editors: *Otolaryngology head and neck surgery, ed 3,* St Louis, 1998, Mosby, p 678, Figure 35-4.)

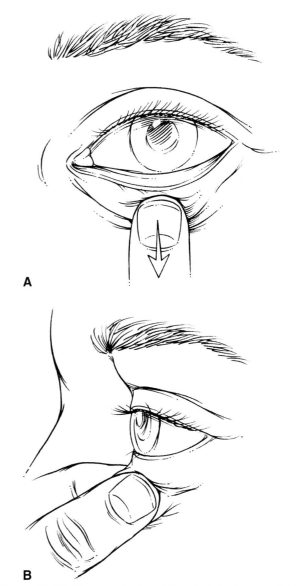

Figure 32-17. The snap test and the pinch test are useful for the determination of the degree of lid laxity and excess skin.

determine the degree of lower lid laxity and is useful in preoperative planning (Figure 32-17). Additionally, a ptotic lacrimal gland must be recognized for potential correction at surgery. Excessive lateral skin hooding may require skin excision beyond the lateral orbital rim, and prolonged wound healing would be expected in this area of greater skin thickness, which is a point that must be relayed to the patient before surgical intervention.[22,23]

The lower eyelid should closely appose the globe without any drooping of the lid away from the globe (ectropion) or in toward the globe (entropion). Excessive lower eyelid laxity should be recognized with the snap test and, when it is present, a lid shortening/tightening procedure should be performed in conjunction with blepharoplasty. Exophthalmos and enophthalmos should be recognized, because neither is favorable, and each may represent an underlying disorder. Visual acuity should be evaluated, and so should the presence of Bell's phenomenon. The absence of Bell's phenomenon places the patient at increased risk for the development of postoperative corneal abrasions if temporary or permanent lagophthalmos exists after surgery. If the patient exhibits signs of a dry eye, the Schirmer test should be performed, and caution should be used when making a decision about surgical intervention.[22,26]

Midface Aesthetic Ideals

The presence of a prominent cheek bone and malar eminence conveys a youthful appearance. As time advances, the tone of the orbicularis oculi muscle is

weakened, and the sling that helped maintain the soft-tissue fullness in the malar eminence can no longer support the underlying structures. The inferior and lateral orbital rims should be padded with malar fat and SOOF. Descent of the subcutaneous malar fat pads and the suborbicularis oculi fat results in a flattened malar eminence and prominent orbital rims that are not aesthetically pleasing (see Figure 32-13). In cases of ptotic midfacial structures and exposure of the orbital rim, the juxtaposition of prolapsed orbital fat and the fallen SOOF results in a double contour. Restoring the fallen SOOF to its more youthful position with a midface lift eliminates the double contour.[24]

PREOPERATIVE PLANNING

As is the case for all patients who present for cosmetic surgery, stable mental health and healthy motivations for the surgery should be determined. It is essential to establish in the patient realistic expectations for the surgical procedure. A complete history and physical examination is essential to elicit any signs or symptoms of visual field defects, dry eye symptoms, seasonal allergic symptoms, or thyroid dysfunction. Past medical and surgical histories must expose any prior issues relating to the periorbital region or to systemic disease that may preclude the use of general and local anesthetics. A history of connective tissue disorders, collagen vascular disorders, Graves' disease, or prior facial nerve paralysis should be determined. The medication history should not only include traditional allopathic preparations but also herbal and homeopathic preparations. Information about the use of eyeglasses, contact lenses, and eye medications and a family history of glaucoma should be elicited.

Before planning surgery, informed consent must be given to the patient in completely understandable terms and in a thorough manner. All of the risks of surgery should be explained fully. The patient should be cautioned about medications that may cause an increased risk of bruising and bleeding. The expected postoperative course and ultimate results should be described to the patient to prevent any misconceptions or disappointments.

Preoperative and postoperative photography should be obtained. The patient's head should be in the Frankfurt horizontal plane, and the hair should be pulled back to show the entire forehead and hairline. Standard views for the periorbital area include the following: anteroposterior full face portrait with the patient in repose and while smiling; anteroposterior full face portrait with the patient raising the eyebrows to accentuate the forehead rhytids and to demonstrate normal facial nerve function; anteroposterior full face portrait with the patient squinting to accentuate vertical and horizontal glabellar rhytids; and bilateral lateral profile full-face portraits. In addition, close-up photographs of the forehead, eyes, and glabellar region are useful to fully show the fine and deep forehead and glabellar rhytids.

SURGICAL TECHNIQUES-BROWLIFT

After the appropriate candidate has been selected, the surgeon has a number of options to consider regarding surgical technique. The type of anesthetic, incision locations, dissection planes, management of forehead muscles, and need for skin excision should all be addressed. Regardless of the technique employed, it is essential that the browlift be performed before the blepharoplasty, because upward repositioning of the brow reduces the amount of upper eyelid skin excess, thereby resulting in a decrease in the amount of skin to be excised with the blepharoplasty. Failure to adhere to this principle may result in the development of postoperative lagophthalmos.

Anesthesia and Skin Markings

All of the procedures described in this chapter may be performed under either local or general anesthesia, depending on patient and physician preferences. Regional block anesthesia combined with diffuse infiltrative anesthesia provides adequate anesthetic to perform the surgery. Skin markings should be completed prior to injection of the local anesthetic to avoid the distortion of landmarks and surgical misjudgment. The skin markings are best performed with the patient in the upright position to allow the soft tissues to drape in their natural positions under the influences of gravitational forces. Incision locations are determined on the basis of the type of browlift planned. It is generally believed that, the farther away an incision is placed from the brow, the less effective the pull that can be generated on the brow (Figure 32-18). After the browlift is complete, skin markings and incisions are made for the blepharoplasty.[16]

Planes of Dissection

Subcutaneous dissection allows for sparing of the sensory nerve branches, which are otherwise transected with the deeper dissection planes. Sensation posterior

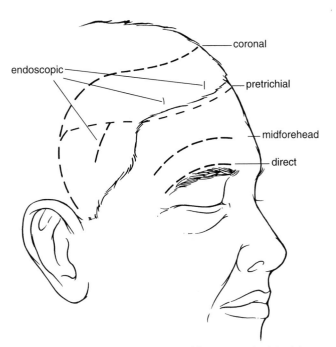

Figure 32-18. Illustration of the different surgical incisions used for brow elevation.

to the incision line will be maintained immediately postoperatively, whereas sensation below the incision line will return after a variable period of temporary paresthesia. The subcutaneous plane provides a most effective method of abolishing forehead rhytids and moderate to severe brow ptosis. Many believe that the subcutaneous plane provides the greatest degree of accuracy and control over brow position, thus enabling a great degree of postoperative brow symmetry. Additionally, dissection in the subcutaneous plane protects the facial nerve branches from injury. The primary disadvantage of the subcutaneous dissection plane rests in the higher incidence of skin slough and hair loss due to vascular compromise. The major vascular supply lies within the subcutaneous fat and the superficial fascia of the frontalis muscle; therefore, the subcutaneous plane is most useful in browlifting techniques that involve incisions anterior to the hairline, where hair loss is not an issue.[10,16]

Subgaleal dissection browlift techniques are simple and fast and provide for a nearly bloodless plane. A thick and well-vascularized flap is elevated, which leads to a low incidence of hair loss and skin slough. However, because a thicker flap is elevated, the degree of freedom for skin unfurling to treat rhytids or to elevate brow ptosis is not as great as with subcutaneous dissection techniques. The primary disadvantage of dissection in this plane lies in the fact that, although sensation is maintained anterior to the incision line, complete sensory denervation occurs posterior to the incision. The subgaleal plane is useful for patients with mild to moderate brow ptosis.[10,16]

Subperiosteal dissection, much like the subgaleal dissection plane, is a technically fast and simple approach with potential for limited brow elevation and rhytid correction. The inelastic periosteum limits the amount of elevation that is possible. In cases of mild to moderate brow ptosis, the subperiosteal plane is a very effective approach.[10,16]

Direct Browlift

The direct browlift is the simplest and longest-standing approach to the ptotic brow. It entails the excision of an ellipse of skin from just above the eyebrow. An incision site is marked, with the lower limb of the ellipse at the upper brow margin. The upper limb of the incision is determined by the estimated amount of desired brow elevation. The high point of the elevated brow should rest between the lateral limbus and the lateral canthus, and the ellipse should taper in both the medial and lateral extensions. The greatest amount of skin should be excised at the desired high point of the newly created brow (Figure 32-19). Skin and subcutaneous tissue are excised, and the orbicularis muscle is left intact (Figure 32-20). Permanent or

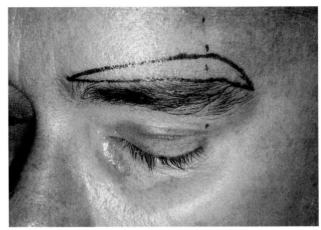

Figure 32-19. Skin markings for a direct browlift. Note that the planned peak of the new brow position will be at a point that corresponds with the lateral canthus. To view this image in color, please go to *www.ototext.com* or the Electronic Image Collection CD, bound into your copy of Cummings Otolaryngology—Head and Neck Surgery, 4th edition.

slowly absorbing sutures suspend the orbicularis muscle to the frontalis fascia or periosteum. This layer of closure should approximate the wound well, with buried dermal sutures used to help reduce the tension. Finally, skin closure is achieved in a tension-free method.[3,10,16,21]

Direct browlift allows for a fast, accurate, and long-lasting brow elevation with low morbidity. The risk of injury to the supraorbital, supratrochlear, and frontal nerves is minimal, and the risk of hematoma is low as a result of the minimal amount of undermining required. This technique should be used in patients

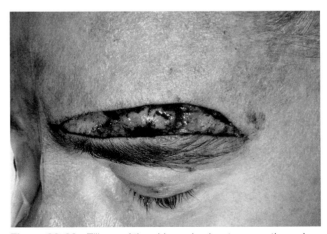

Figure 32-20. Ellipse of the skin and subcutaneous tissue has been excised, leaving the orbicularis oculi muscle intact. To view this image in color, please go to *www.ototext.com* or the Electronic Image Collection CD, bound into your copy of Cummings Otolaryngology—Head and Neck Surgery, 4th edition.

who are not prone to the development of hypertrophic scars; it is most useful in cases of lateral brow hooding.[3,10,16,21]

A number of shortcomings are associated with the direct browlift. It does not address forehead rhytids, and, as such, it should not be recommended for patients with extensive and deep forehead furrows. In addition, the procedure does not reposition the medial-most aspects of the brow. The most obvious disadvantage of this technique is the visible scar that remains, the severity of which depends on the soft-tissue techniques used and on the individual's healing properties. Scar revision and dermabrasion may be necessary to create an acceptable scar.[3,10,16,21]

Midforehead Browlift

The midforehead browlift has evolved over the years to the point where it is now recognized as a desirable procedure for the male patient with a receding hairline and deep horizontal forehead rhytids. With the patient in an upright position and the brow at rest, two separate horizontal skin creases at different vertical heights on either side of the forehead are chosen for incision marking (Figure 32-21). The area of greatest width of fusiform excision correlates with the point of greatest desired brow elevation, along the lateral aspects of the brows. The length of the fusiform excision extends from the medial-most to the lateral-most parts of the brows overlying each of the eyebrows. Connecting the two fusiform excisions across the midline of the forehead makes the entire incisional scar more visible. To further hide the inci-

sion, two horizontal rhytids located at two different vertical levels of the forehead are chosen on either side (see Figure 32-21). The skin is then excised along with subcutaneous tissue, thereby leaving the frontalis muscle uninterrupted. Sharp dissection with the scalpel is then used to undermine in the subcutaneous plane from the inferior border of the incision to the point where the horizontal fibers of the orbicularis oculi muscles are identified (Figure 32-22). To provide a long-lasting effect, we do not depend on the skin excision and skin suturing alone. Rather, deep horizontal mattress 4-0 PDS sutures from the orbicularis oculi muscle to the periosteum at the superior border of the fusiform excision provide permanent repositioning of the brow. Two separate sutures are placed: one at the midpupillary line and the other at the peak of the desired brow elevation. Two-layer skin closure is then achieved including 5-0 PDS subcuticular and 6-0 fast-absorbing gut sutures (Figure 32-23).[3,10]

There are a number of advantages to the midforehead browlift. It is a fast, relatively easy procedure with little morbidity. By placing the incision in a natural skin crease, the incisions are very well hidden, even in a patient with a receding hairline. Only a moderate amount of undermining is required, which results in a low risk to the frontal and other nerves, and there is a lower risk of hematoma as compared with longer flap techniques. In addition, there is no distortion of the hairline and no vascular compromise to the hair follicles. Sensation superior to the incision is maintained intact, and the sensation inferior to the incision returns after a variable amount of time.

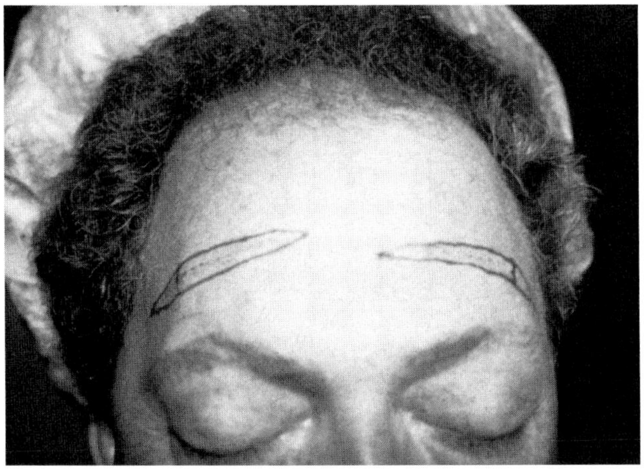

Figure 32-21. Skin markings for a midforehead browlift. Note the differences in the vertical position of the ellipse on either side of the forehead; this optimizes scar camouflage. To view this image in color, please go to *www.ototext.com* or the Electronic Image Collection CD, bound into your copy of Cummings Otolaryngology—Head and Neck Surgery, 4th edition.

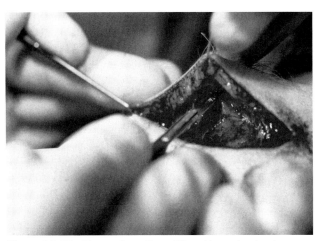

Figure 32-22. Sharp dissection of the skin and subcutaneous tissue off of the frontalis muscle down to the orbicularis fibers at the level of the eyebrow. To view this image in color, please go to *www.ototext.com* or the Electronic Image Collection CD, bound into your copy of Cummings Otolaryngology—Head and Neck Surgery, 4th edition.

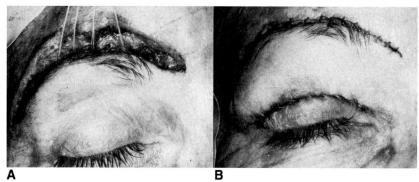

Figure 32-23. A, Fixation of the new brow position is achieved with three simple interrupted sutures securing the orbicularis oculi muscle at the level of the brow, with the periosteum at the region of the excised ellipse. **B,** Skin closure is then achieved in two layers to reduce the tension on the wound and promote scar-free wound healing. (From Becker FF, Johnson CM, Mandel LM: *Surgical management of the upper third of the face.* In Cummings CW and others, editors: *Otolaryngology—head and neck surgery,* ed 3, St Louis, 1998, Mosby, p 663, Figure 34-4.)

Precise control over brow position is easily achieved, which allows for the correction of preoperative brow asymmetries.

The primary disadvantages relate to the postoperative scar. This procedure should be avoided in patients with smooth, non-wrinkled forehead skin or in those patients with a history of hypertrophic scarring.

High Forehead Browlift

During the 1980s and 1990s, the coronal browlift became the gold standard against which to compare all other forms of browlift procedures. The coronal approach avoids the visible scars of the direct and mid-forehead browlifts and reduces the amount of forehead creases with the associated forehead lift. Glabellar rhytids due to corrugator and procerus contraction may be easily addressed with this technique.[18,28]

The patient's hair is parted 5 cm posterior to the hairline in the coronal incision approach or at the hairline in the trichophytic approach (Figure 32-24). After the patient has been prepared, draped, and injected with local anesthetic and vasoconstrictors, the incision is made. A number of different philosophies exist with regard to the method of incising the skin. Beveling the incision from anterior to posterior parallels the hair follicles and may help to prevent the cutting and resultant loss of the follicles. Alternatively, beveling from posterior to anterior allows the new hair growth to extend through the incision line, which may help hide the incision. Either way, the incision should go to the depth of the subgaleal level so that elevation of the flap may proceed in the subgaleal-supraperiosteal level, where injury to the frontal branch of the facial nerve is avoided (Figure 32-25). The extent of elevation proceeds to the root of the nose and beyond the

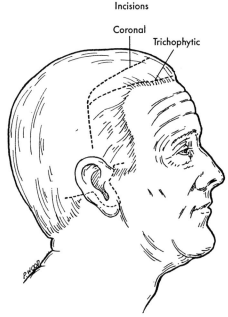

Figure 32-24. The coronal incision is made 5-cm posterior to the anterior hairline. The trichophytic incision is made to follow the natural contour of the anterior hairline. (From Becker FF, Johnson CM, Mandel LM: *Surgical management of the upper third of the face.* In Cummings CW and others, editors: *Otolaryngology—head and neck surgery,* ed 3, St Louis, 1998, Mosby, p 668, Figure 34-12.)

supraorbital rims. The supraorbital neurovascular bundles are identified and preserved. After undermining is complete, horizontal galeatomies are performed in the region that is medial to either midpupillary line. The corrugator and procerus may be transected as needed to help control the glabellar frown lines.

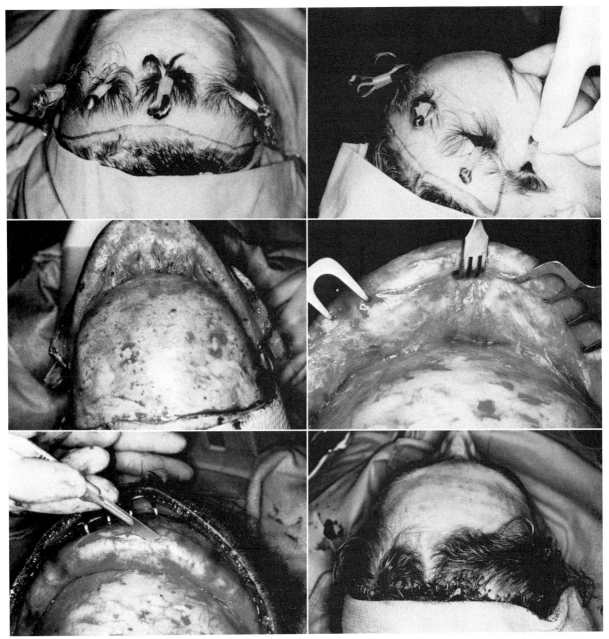

Figure 32-25. High forehead browlift. (From Becker FF, Johnson CM, Mandel LM: *Surgical management of the upper third of the face.* In Cummings CW and others, editors: *Otolaryngology—head and neck surgery,* ed 3, St Louis, 1998, Mosby, p 669, Figure 34-13.)

Upward pull on the flap helps to demarcate the amount of skin excision required. After skin excision, the flap is secured to its original position with slow-absorbing or permanent sutures in multiple layers of closure. The galeal layer is reapproximated, and the skin may be closed with a single layer of staples or subcuticular 5-0 PDS and cuticular 6-0 fast-absorbing gut sutures. A drain may be needed, and compressive dressings are recommended.

There are a number of disadvantages to this procedure, including length of operation and greater complexity. The length of flap undermining is extensive and results in an elevated risk of hematoma formation and supraorbital nerve injury. Because the incision is a greater distance from the brows, the surgeon has less control over the final position of the brow, and less-aggressive brow elevation may be achieved. The coronal incision causes an elevated frontal hairline, and there is a greater risk of hair loss along the incision line as a result of devascularization and direct follicle injury.[18] The pretrichial incision does not raise the hairline, but it may cause alopecia in the periincisional area and may result in a visible scar (Figure 32-26).[6] Loss of sensation is present superior to the incision, and patients must be cautioned of this fact so that they may avoid hairdryer injury to the scalp.[3,10]

Endoscopic Browlift

Until recently, the coronal approach to the forehead and brow was the gold standard. In recent years, with the development of endoscopic techniques, the endoscopic browlift has become increasingly popular. The long and potentially visible incisions of the coronal and trichophytic browlift, the high rate of alopecia, the widening of the scar, and the potential for pruritus and numbness promoted the demand for endoscopic techniques by the patient. The following is a standard technique; however, a number of subtle differences may exist among different surgeons.[17,25]

Before administering sedation in the holding area, the patient is assessed in the sitting position. Brow positioning and the degree of desired brow elevation are determined. Skin marking may be performed in the holding area or in the operating room. Incision markings are 1 to 1.5 cm in length and 1.5-cm posterior to the anterior hairline. They are located in the midline and in the paramedian areas that correspond to the sites of desired vectors of pull (Figure 32-27). Generally the paramedian incision should be placed at the desired peak of the lateral brow. Incisions are carried down through all layers of the scalp to the skull with a No. 15 scalpel blade. Temporal incisions are made 1-cm posterior to the temporal hairline, in the region that is anterior to the superficial temporal vessels (Figure 32-28). These incisions are carried down to the level of the superficial layer of the deep temporal fascia. Elevation of the temporal region is achieved directly on the superficial layer of the deep temporal fascia (deep to the temporoparietal fascia) to avoid injury to the frontal branch of the facial nerve. Identification of the sentinel vein is then achieved, with bipolar cautery performed at the deepest level possible to avoid frontal nerve injury (Figure 32-29). The temporal line at the medial-most extent of the temporalis fascia is separated from the periosteum in the forehead region by entering a subperiosteal plane at the conjoint tendon. The skull is exposed at the central and paramedian incisions—thereby allowing for the subperiosteal elevation of the forehead to a point just beyond the supraorbital rim—under endoscopic visualization with a 30-degree endoscope to avoid injury to the supraorbital neurovascular bundle. If necessary, the corrugator and procerus may be addressed at this time, with transection. After the supraorbital neurovascular pedicle is identified and preserved, periosteal relaxation incisions are made

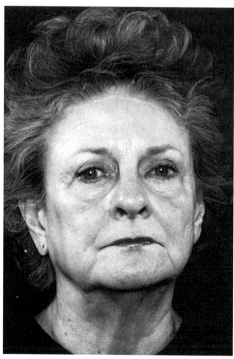

Figure 32-26. Visible pretrichial incision scar for which the patient was referred to our care. To view this image in color, please go to *www.ototext.com* or the Electronic Image Collection CD, bound into your copy of Cummings Otolaryngology—Head and Neck Surgery, 4th edition.

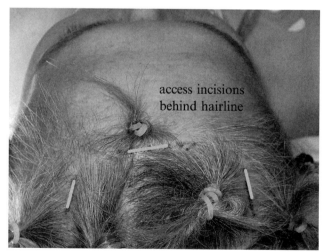

Figure 32-27. Paramedian access incisions for the endoscopic browlift technique. To view this image in color, please go to *www.ototext.com* or the Electronic Image Collection CD, bound into your copy of Cummings Otolaryngology—Head and Neck Surgery, 4th edition.

below the level of the brow with the cautery to allow for superior traction on the brows (Figure 32-30); this is achieved along the entire width of the brow on either side of the forehead. After adequate relaxing

incisions are made in the periosteum, brow elevation is secured by the fixation of the galea to the skull through the paramedian incisions. Lateral traction is supplied by the fixation of the temporoparietal fascia to the deep temporal fascia through the temporal incision line. Our preferred method for fixation of the forehead and brow to the skull involves using the drill to create a bone bridge to which we secure a permanent suture (2-0 Ethibond; Ethicon [Johnson & Johnson Health Care Systems]; Piscataway, NJ) and then tie it to a sizable bite of galea aponeurosis (Figure 32-31). All incisions are closed in a single layer of 5-0 Rapide (Ethicon) suture.[24]

The advantages of endoscopic forehead and browlifts are multiple. The incision lines are well hidden and may even be used in bald patients, because they heal inconspicuously. There is minimal alopecia and hairline alteration, there is less numbness in the forehead and scalp, and recovery time is less than with the open approach. Glabellar furrows are easily addressed through the endoscopic route.[17,24,25]

The disadvantages of this procedure lie primarily in the learning curve required for facility with endoscopic techniques. In addition, specialized, expensive instrumentation is required for this procedure. Because the endoscopic browlift procedure has only been used in the recent past, data regarding the best method for fixation is still pending. Alternatives include sutures, screws, and specialized absorbable fixation techniques. In addition, the longevity of the

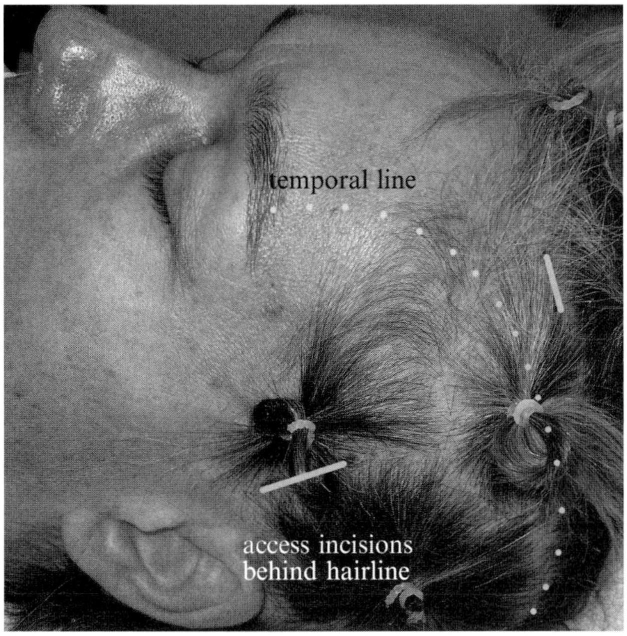

Figure 32-28. Temporal access incisions for the endoscopic browlift technique. To view this image in color, please go to *www.ototext.com* or the Electronic Image Collection CD, bound into your copy of Cummings Otolaryngology—Head and Neck Surgery, 4th edition.

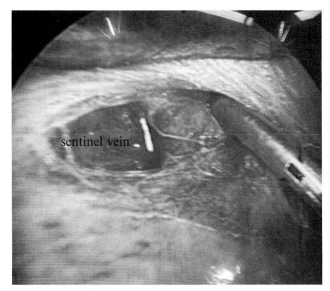

Figure 32-29. The sentinel vein is identified and cauterized to prevent bleeding that will obscure the operating field. To view this image in color, please go to *www.ototext.com* or the Electronic Image Collection CD, bound into your copy of Cummings Otolaryngology—Head and Neck Surgery, 4th edition.

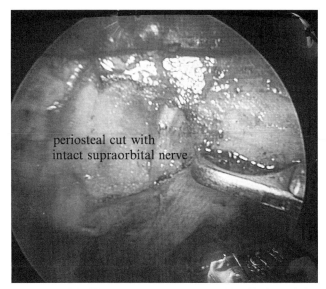

Figure 32-30. The supraorbital nerve is identified, and the periosteum along the inferior brow line is sectioned. To view this image in color, please go to *www.ototext.com* or the Electronic Image Collection CD, bound into your copy of Cummings Otolaryngology—Head and Neck Surgery, 4th edition.

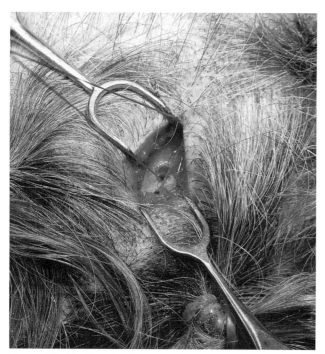

Figure 32-31. Bone bridge and suture are used to secure the brows and forehead in their elevated positions. To view this image in color, please go to *www.ototext.com* or the Electronic Image Collection CD, bound into your copy of Cummings Otolaryngology—Head and Neck Surgery, 4th edition.

browlift has not yet been definitively established. In ways that are similar to the open coronal and pretrichial browlifts, the increased distance from the brow makes for greater difficulty in the adequate elevation of the brows.[17,24,25]

MIDFACE LIFT

Midface suspension may be performed by the extension of endoscopic forehead lifting procedures or through a subciliary approach to lower eyelid blepharoplasty. If lower eyelid fat removal is indicated, it may be performed in the routine fashion if the subciliary approach is utilized, but it should be performed through a transconjunctival approach if the endoscopic technique is used for the midface lift. Regardless of which approach is used, skin of the lower eyelid must be addressed either with a pinch technique or with resurfacing techniques, because lifting the midface will result in bunching and redundancy of the lower eyelid skin.[7,24]

Endoscopic Midface Lift

The lateral temporal incision used for the endoscopic browlift approach is used for endoscopic access to the midface. The skin incision is carried down to the superficial layer of deep temporal fascia, thereby leaving the temporoparietal fascia attached to the skin

and subcutaneous tissue. A lighted converse retractor, a lighted Aufricht retractor, or endoscopic instruments may be used to elevate in this plane anteriorly toward the conjoined tendon and inferiorly along the temporal line to the superior orbital rim (Figure 32-32). Multiple vessels will be seen during the course of this dissection, and they act as indicators of the proximity to the frontal branch of the facial nerve. These vessels are cauterized with bipolar cautery at the deepest plane possible so as to remain at a distance from the frontal branch. The conjoined tendon is then divided with blunt and sharp dissection, thereby allowing for access to the subperiosteal plane and subsequent identification of the zygomaticofrontal suture line. Dissection continues in the subperiosteal plane from the zygomaticofrontal suture inferiorly along the lateral orbital rim and inferior orbital rim and then to the malar eminence and the face of the maxilla. Care is taken to preserve the infraorbital nerve by placing a finger over the foramen or by directly visualizing it with the endoscope. Dissection continues to the pyriform aperture and nasal bones to allow the greatest degree of mobility to the midface structures. A heavy absorbable suture is used to secure the periosteum of the midface to the superficial layer of the deep temporal fascia; the skin is then closed. We do not routinely place drains in facelifts, browlifts, or midface lifts.[7,24]

Subciliary Approach

The subciliary approach to the midface lift is a simple extension of the subciliary blepharoplasty technique that will be described in the next few sections.

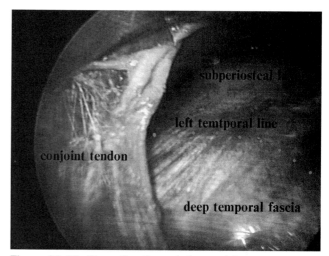

Figure 32-32. Dissection through the conjoint tendon allows access to the orbital rim and midface in the endoscopic approach. To view this image in color, please go to *www.ototext.com* or the Electronic Image Collection CD, bound into your copy of Cummings Otolaryngology—Head and Neck Surgery, 4th edition.

After access has been obtained, the arcus marginalis is released at the inferior orbital rim. Subperiosteal dissection of the midface structures is then achieved beyond the infraorbital foramen to the pyriform aperture and nasal bones. After adequate elevation has been achieved, suture fixation of the midface periosteum to the orbital periosteum allows for midface suspension. The remainder of the procedure is the routine subciliary blepharoplasty, which is described below.

Complications of Midface Lift

The recovery following a midface lift is somewhat prolonged as compared with browlift or forehead lift alone. The patient will feel presentable after 2 to 3 weeks, but the edema will persist for 6 to 8 weeks. If dissection along the temporalis muscle is extensive, masticatory pain may occur after the procedure. Periorbital edema and ecchymosis also remain for 6 weeks. Temporary ectropion may occur as a result of periorbital edema, which generally resolves in 6 weeks.[24]

BLEPHAROPLASTY
Upper Eyelid

Successful blepharoplasty requires that the surgeon understand the aesthetic relationships between the eyelids, eyebrows, forehead, orbit, and midface. These aesthetic ideals have been discussed earlier in this chapter and may be reviewed. After the individual patient's medical health, psychological motivations, and expectations about the surgery are understood to be reasonable, the surgery may proceed. Typically blepharoplasty is performed as outpatient surgery under either local or general anesthesia.[23]

If performed in conjunction with a browlift, the blepharoplasty incision markings are placed after the browlift is complete and all incisions have been closed. Marking the eyelids is the single most important step of a blepharoplasty, and, as such, great care must be taken to ensure precision (Figure 32-33). The initial lid marking is made at the natural skin crease or 1 mm above the natural crease. Making the incision 1 mm above the natural crease allows for wound contracture to bring the ultimate lid scar into the proper position at the natural crease. Generally the lid crease is at the same level bilaterally, but, if not, the incisions may be designed to create lid symmetry with the use of a caliper. The medial end of the incision is carried to the punctum of the medial canthus but not beyond the punctum. Incisions medial to the punctum and beyond the nasal orbital depression cause irreversible webbing. The lateral extent of the incision curves upward slightly, within a natural crease in the sulcus, between the orbital rim and the

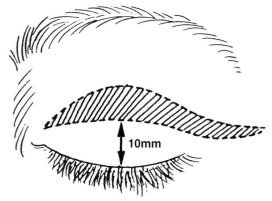

Figure 32-33. Upper eyelid skin is marked. (From Colton JJ, Beekhuis GJ: *Blepharoplasty.* In Cummings CW and others, editors: *Otolaryngology—head and neck surgery,* ed 3, St Louis, 1998, Mosby, p 686, Figure 35-19.)

eyelid. The lateral extent is determined by the degree and location of lateral hooding and may even extend beyond the lateral orbital rim. The patient must be told preoperatively that the skin incision lateral to the lateral orbital rim will take longer to heal, because the skin thickens beyond the lateral orbital rim. To determine the amount of redundant skin to excise, the pinch test is performed (Figure 32-34). One blade of a forceps grasps the skin at the previously marked lid crease, and the other blade grasps the skin at a point superiorly, which just smooths out the skin of the eyelid until slight eversion of the lid occurs. This technique helps to prevent postoperative lagophthalmos. Both the medial and lateral ends of the upper lid fusiform excision should form 30-degree angles.[9,23]

After the markings are complete, local infiltrative anesthesia is injected into the immediate subcutaneous plane. After adequate time is given for the

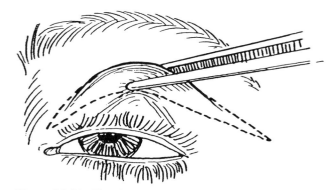

Figure 32-34. The pinch test helps in the determination of the amount of lid skin to be excised. (From Colton JJ, Beekhuis GJ: *Blepharoplasty.* In Cummings CW and others, editors: *Otolaryngology—head and neck surgery,* ed 3, St Louis, 1998, Mosby, p 687, Figure 35-20.)

anesthetic to take effect, the skin incisions are made with a fresh blade of the surgeon's choice, and the skin is taken as a single layer or as a two-layer skin-orbicularis unit (Figure 32-35). After this, a determination is made regarding the amount of orbicularis oculi muscle to excise. Resection of a strip of orbicularis along the inferior length of the skin excision helps to recreate a distinct upper eyelid skin crease. A variable amount of orbicularis oculi muscle should be resected, depending on the degree of muscle hypertrophy. Resection of orbicularis exposes the orbital septum and allows for the visualization of the orbital fat through the septum. Two different techniques may be used to address the pseudoherniation of fat. Bovie cautery of the orbital septum contracts the septum and reduces the degree of fat pseudoherniation (as has been described for lower lid blepharoplasty).[11] Alternatively, opening the orbital septum and removing fat from the medial and central compartments may be achieved (Figure 32-36). Clamping the fat that will be removed and then cauterizing the

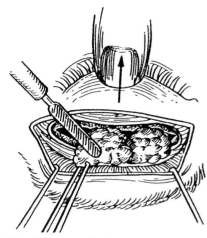

Figure 32-36. After the orbital septum is opened, orbital fat may be excised with the cautery and gentle digital pressure on the globe. (From Colton JJ, Beekhuis GJ: *Blepharoplasty.* In Cummings CW and others, editors: *Otolaryngology—head and neck surgery,* ed 3, St Louis, 1998, Mosby, p 687, Figure 35-22.)

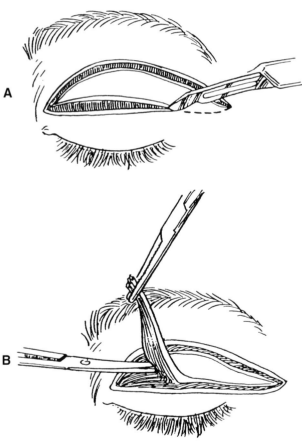

Figure 32-35. A, The skin incision is made. **B,** The skin is excised. (From Colton JJ, Beekhuis GJ: *Blepharoplasty.* In Cummings CW and others, editors: *Otolaryngology—head and neck surgery,* ed 3, St Louis, 1998, Mosby, p 687, Figure 35-21, *A* and *B*.)

fat in the clamp helps to prevent postoperative hematomas. Do not place anterior traction on the clamp to prevent avulsion, bleeding, and excessive resection. Only fat that protrudes into the wound with gentle globe pressure should be clamped and excised to avoid the overaggressive removal of orbital fat and a hollowed postoperative look. However, care should be taken to help avoid the common error of upper eyelid blepharoplasty of failing to remove enough of the medial orbital fat. Laterally the lacrimal gland may come into view and should be recognized to avoid its injury. The lacrimal gland is more pink, vascular, and firm than fat. After excellent hemostasis is achieved, wound closure proceeds with a single-layer closure of the skin with a 6-0 fast-absorbing gut suture.[9,23]

Lower Eyelid Blepharoplasty
Transconjunctival

The transconjunctival blepharoplasty has become increasingly popular during the past few years due to the hidden incision, the maintenance of the orbicularis support structure for the lower eyelid, and a reduced rate of postoperative ectropion. Proper patient selection is required for the successful use of this technique in blepharoplasty; patients with pseudoherniation of fat and little need for skin excision are good candidates. In addition, patients who heal with hypertrophic scars and patients who will not accept an external incision are good candidates. The presence of a mild to moderate amount of excess skin in the lower eyelid does not preclude the transconjunctival approach, because a pinch excision of skin and lid resurfacing techniques may be used to address the lower lid skin changes.[26]

After local anesthetic is injected and adequate time is allowed for the vasoconstriction to take effect, the lower eyelid conjunctival surface is exposed. Either a preseptal or postseptal approach may be used, depending on the surgeon's preference (Figure 32-37). A 4-0 silk suture is placed through the eyelid margin for traction. The traction suture, together with a Desmarres retractor, helps to evert the lower eyelid. The preseptal approach involves a transconjunctival incision made at the inferior margin of the tarsal plate. A plane is developed just superficial to the conjunctiva in an avascular plane, down to the level of the orbital rim, without exposing the orbital rim. A 4-0 silk suture is then passed through the conjunctival edge to provide traction and corneal protection. The orbital septum is now in clear view and may be entered with the Bovie cautery. Alternatively, the postseptal approach may be used; this entails a single incision placed 4 mm below the inferior tarsal margin and directly through the conjunctiva and lower eyelid retractors to expose orbital fat from the posterior aspect. The orbital septum is maintained completely intact with the use of this technique. Traction sutures of 4-0 silk or nylon are placed on either side of the transconjunctival incision to allow for blunt and sharp

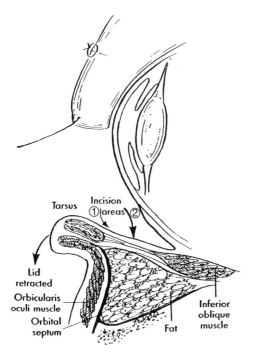

Figure 32-37. Preseptal (1) and postseptal (2) transconjunctival approaches to blepharoplasty. (From Colton JJ, Beekhuis GJ: *Blepharoplasty.* In Cummings CW and others, editors: *Otolaryngology—head and neck surgery,* ed 3, St Louis, 1998, Mosby, p 693, Figure 35-39.)

dissection to the orbital fat. Identification of the inferior oblique muscle, which separates the medial from the middle fat pads, should be performed in both the preseptal and postseptal methods to avoid injury to this structure. The fat is excised as described for the upper eyelid blepharoplasty, using a clamp and Bovie cautery. The lower eyelid fat pads communicate directly with the deeper orbital fat, so excessive traction on the fat should be avoided to help prevent orbital hemorrhage. The incisions may be left open to heal spontaneously, or loosely applied fast-absorbing sutures may be used. If redundant skin is present, it may be excised with the scalpel, and the incision can be closed with 6-0 fast-absorbing gut sutures (Figure 32-38).[9,26]

Subciliary Approach

The subciliary approach is most useful for those patients with large amounts of excess skin. A subciliary incision is made 2 mm below the lash line, extending from 1-mm lateral to the inferior punctum to 10-mm lateral to the lateral canthus. The incision extends through the skin and orbicularis muscle along the entire length of the incision (Figure 32-39). A skin-muscle flap is elevated to the orbital rim, thereby exposing the orbital septum in its entirety. The skin-muscle flap is extended over the rim so that the muscle is separated from the arcus marginalis to allow for proper skin redraping (Figure 32-40). The orbital septum is then approached either with Bovie cauterization of the intact orbital septum or by excising the orbital fat that is bulging. After hemostasis is achieved in the fat compartment, a variable amount of skin and muscle is excised, as needed (Figure 32-41). Closure of the incisions is accomplished in two layers. Laterally, the orbicularis fibers are reattached with a 5-0 PDS suture to help prevent tension on the lateral-most aspect of the incisions; this allows the skin edges of the incision to approximate one another closely. Finally, the skin layer is closed with 6-0 fast-absorbing gut suture.[9,26]

Lid-Shortening Procedure

If preoperative evaluation determines that the lower eyelid is excessively lax by the snap test, a lid-shortening procedure is indicated to prevent postoperative ectropion. We prefer to perform a lateral tarsal strip procedure with reattachment of the tarsus to the superior and inner aspect of the lateral orbital rim. This step is performed before closure of the lower eyelid blepharoplasty incision.

Complications

Orbital hemorrhage is a complication that is most commonly seen after lower eyelid blepharoplasty. The

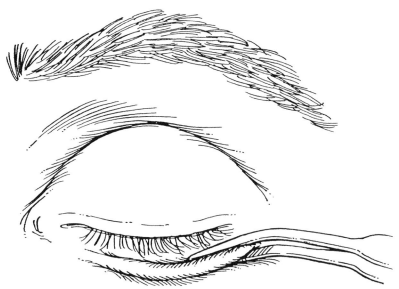

Figure 32-38. Resection of skin is achieved as needed after the completion of fat removal. (From Colton JJ, Beekhuis GJ: *Blepharoplasty.* In Cummings CW and others, editors: *Otolaryngology—head and neck surgery,* ed 3, St Louis, 1998, Mosby, p 694, Figure 35-43.)

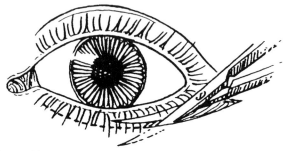

Figure 32-39. The lower eyelid incision may be made with scissors or a knife. Care is taken to avoid cutting the eyelashes. (From Colton JJ, Beekhuis GJ: *Blepharoplasty.* In Cummings CW and others, editors: *Otolaryngology—head and neck surgery,* ed 3, St Louis, 1998, Mosby, p 688, Figure 35-25.)

presence of orbital hemorrhage is first noted by the patient in the forms of increasing edema, ecchymosis, and severe pain. If vision remains intact, the patient simply has swelling and slight pain and the bleeding has stopped; ophthalmology consultation for funduscopic examination and close observation should be employed. Occasionally steroids may be used in combination with mannitol to help reduce the swelling; however, there are no prospective studies that demonstrate an advantage of this protocol. If there are signs of optic neuropathy (including severe pain and vision loss), immediate lateral canthotomy with cantholysis, mannitol, and intravenous steroids is instituted. If no resolution ensues, orbital decompression is

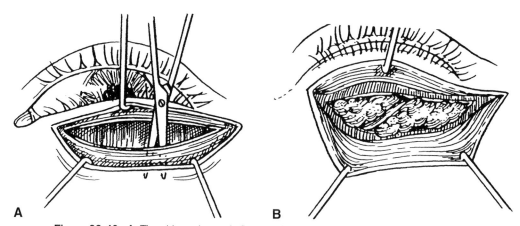

A   **B**

Figure 32-40. A, The skin and muscle flap are dissected bluntly and sharply. **B,** Access is gained to the septum and fat compartments for subsequent fat removal or cauterization of the septum. (From Colton JJ, Beekhuis GJ: *Blepharoplasty.* In Cummings CW and others, editors: *Otolaryngology—head and neck surgery,* ed 3, St Louis, 1998, Mosby, p 689, Figure 35-26.)

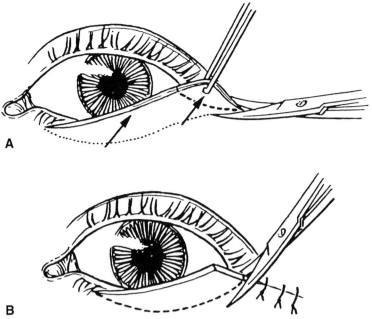

Figure 32-41. A, The flap is repositioned. **B,** Excess skin and muscle are excised. Care is taken to excise slightly more muscle than skin to ensure that there is no bunching of tissue at the incision line. (From Colton JJ, Beekhuis GJ: *Blepharoplasty.* In Cummings CW and others, editors: *Otolaryngology—head and neck surgery,* ed 3, St Louis, 1998, Mosby, p 689, Figure 35-28, *A* and *B*.)

advised. Failure to address this complication within 90 minutes of its onset may result in permanent blindness.[1,8]

Lagophthalmos, which is the failure of complete eye closure, is a common finding after upper lid blepharoplasty. It is frequently seen in the immediate postoperative period as a result of orbicularis paresis and possibly levator spasm. Over the next few postoperative weeks, periorbital edema may cause persistence of the lagophthalmos. Such patients should be managed with eye care precautions to prevent corneal exposure complications, including lubrication with ointment at night and artificial tears throughout the day. Additionally, a humidification chamber and taping the eyelids closed may be useful. If lagophthalmos persists beyond 6 to 8 postoperative weeks, an excess of upper eyelid skin may have been removed at the time of surgery. This would require surgical intervention for correction, including the use of a skin graft to replace the missing skin.[1,8]

Eyelid malposition is one of the most common complications after blepharoplasty and may range in severity from scleral show to frank lower eyelid eversion. Ectropion and lower eyelid retraction may result from two primary causes, both of which are quite common and easy to prevent. Overaggressive skin resection may lead to ectropion, because contraction of the shortened lower eyelid anterior lamella may progress to ectropion with wound healing. The second cause of ectropion is a failure to recognize and address excessive lower lid laxity in an effective manner. At the time of blepharoplasty, a lid-shortening procedure should be done in cases of excessive lower lid laxity. Failure to perform a lid-tightening procedure will result in wound contracture, thereby causing lower lid ectropion. Ectropion can usually be corrected by addressing the cause of the problem with either a tarsal strip for excessive laxity or with lysis of cicatricial adhesions that are causing the persistence of the ectropion.[1,8,9,26]

Entropion results from excessive shortening of the posterior lamella of the eyelid and the effects of long-term scar contracture. It is corrected by lysis of cicatricial adhesions and the placement of a hard palate mucosal graft to help prevent recurrent cicatrix and entropion.

Epiphora, in the absence of preoperative dry eye syndrome, is typically the result of a dysfunctional lacrimal collecting system. Causes of a dysfunctional lacrimal apparatus include punctual eversion as a result of wound contracture or edema; impairment of the lacrimal pump system as a result of atony, edema, or injury to the orbicularis oculi muscle; or outflow obstruction as a result of a lacerated canaliculus at the time of incision. If laceration has occurred, placement of a silastic stent is recommended. Persistent eversion of the lid may be corrected with cauterization or excision of the conjunctival surface below the canaliculus to cause inversion of the lid, punctum, and canaliculus.[1,8,9,26]

Excess skin that remains after blepharoplasty (i.e., failure to remove adequate skin at the time of blepharoplasty) is an easy complication to correct. After the swelling has completely subsided (4–6 weeks postoperatively), additional skin may be excised in the office, under local anesthesia.

Asymmetry during the early postoperative period may be the result of asymmetric soft tissue edema. If after the swelling has completely resolved the asymmetry persists, using the caliper and excising the appropriate amount of skin and fat will help to reestablish symmetry to the lids.[1,8,9,26]

Skin discoloration that persists after the incisions are well healed may be treated with topical Retin-A, hydroquinones, chemical peels, laser resurfacing, or dermabrasion. Milia may occur along incision lines and may be treated by unroofing with a scalpel or an 18-guage needle. Skin incisions that extend medial to the punctum of the lids not only increase the risk of lacrimal apparatus injury but also increase the risk of web formation in the epicanthal region; webs may be corrected with Z-plasty.

ADJUNCTIVE PROCEDURES
Skin Resurfacing

Facial resurfacing procedures may be used safely in conjunction with surgery of the periorbital area. They produce their effects by ablating skin to variable depths, thereby allowing for collagen regeneration and skin tightening. Different agents and techniques produce varying degrees of penetration and results. Although resurfacing cannot replace surgery for the treatment of deep hyperfunctioning rhytids, laser, chemical peels, and dermabrasion may be used to treat fine wrinkling, acne scarring, telangiectasias, and photodamaged skin. Care should be exercised when resurfacing skin that has been undermined in the immediate subcutaneous plane for fear of devascularizing the tissue and causing resultant flap necrosis. The resurfacing should be feathered into the hairline and eyebrows to avoid evident lines of demarcation. Birth control pills should be stopped 2 months before facial resurfacing to prevent pigment changes. Isotretinoin should not have been used during the year preceding skin resurfacing to avoid the increased risks of hypertrophic scarring associated with its use. An antiviral agent is prescribed by many physicians for use during the periprocedure period as prophylaxis against herpetic reactivation. Preoperative tretinoin is felt by many to accelerate wound healing.[2]

Milia, which are 1- to 2-mm pustules that originate from the skin adnexa, frequently occur after resurfacing procedures. They often resolve without treatment, but, if they persist, they may be unroofed with a scalpel or an 18-guage needle. Failure to treat the milia may result in permanent scar formation. Pigmentary changes are expected after resurfacing procedures; however, they should resolve by four to six weeks. If the erythema associated with the resurfacing procedure seems to be excessive, topical steroids may be applied to reduce the erythema. Prolonged discoloration occurs most commonly in patients with Fitzpatrick IV, V, and VI skin types and may be the result of sun exposure during the period that follows resurfacing. Persistent hyperpigmentation may require bleaching with hydroquinone or retinoic acid, whereas hypopigmentation may require serial excision and punch-graft replacement of the discolored skin. There is no data at present to suggest that pretreatment with any topical agent will help prevent pigment changes after resurfacing.[2]

Injectable Filler

Although the ideal implantable or injectable material has not yet been developed, collagen, silicone, fat, and polytetrafluoroethylene have been used extensively as filler material for facial rhytids. Injectable fillers provide a relatively easy and noninvasive approach to rhytids in facial locations that are difficult to access. Augmenting the soft tissues in these areas may eliminate the shadowing caused by the rhytids, thereby making the rhytid less visible. Forehead rhytids are less amenable to these techniques, whereas glabellar rhytids are well treated by these techniques. Each of the different injectable and implantable materials has its own safety and use profile, and a discussion of each is beyond the scope of this chapter.

Botox

Botulinum exotoxin A (Botox), which is produced by the bacteria *Clostridium botulinum,* is useful for the reduction of facial wrinkles that are associated with facial muscle contractions. Botox is safe, easy to administer, and reversible with time, thus making it a very attractive cosmetic adjunct for the treatment of the periorbital region. It reversibly blocks the release of acetylcholine from the presynaptic neuromuscular junction, thereby temporarily paralyzing the effected muscle. The affects of Botox are observed two to three days after injection, with maximal weakness occurring one to two weeks after its injection. The effects last for 3 to 6 months. Botox is useful for the treatment of glabellar frown lines, crow's feet, horizontal forehead rhytids, smile lines, horizontal neck lines, and unilateral facial paralysis to reduce the asymmetry between the normal and paralyzed side; it may also be used as a browlift procedure. Injection into the orbicularis oculi muscle inferior to the lateral brow allows for unopposed frontalis muscle action, which produces brow elevation. Similarly, frontalis injection along the medial aspect of the brow allows for unopposed orbicularis muscle activity, thereby producing a slight ptosis of the medial brow and a relative elevation of the lateral brow. Complications from Botox use include ptosis and lagophthalmos with inadvertent injection into deeper muscles. Additionally, erythema and bruising may occur.[5]

REFERENCES

1. Adams BJS, Feurstein SS: Complications of blepharoplasty, *Ear Nose Throat J* 65:11, 1986.

2. Alster TS, Lupton JR: Treatment of complications of laser skin resurfacing, *Arch Facial Plast Surg* 2:279, 2000.

3. Becker FF, Johnson CM, Mandel LM: *Surgical management of the upper third of the face.* In Cummings CW and others, editors: *Otolaryngology—head and neck surgery,* ed 3, St Louis, 1998, Mosby, p 660.

4. Bergin DJ: *Anatomy of the eyelids, lacrimal system, and orbit.* In McCord CD, Tanenbaum M, Nunery WR, editors: *Oculoplastic surgery,* New York, 1995, Raven Press, p 51.

5. Binder WJ, Blitzer A, Brin MF: Treatment of hyperfunctional lines of the face with botulinum toxin A, *Dermatol Surg* 24:1198, 1998.

6. Brennan HG: Pretrichial coronal lift, *Facial Plast Surg* 3:13, 1985.

7. Byrd HS: The extended browlift, *Clin Plast Surg* 24:233, 1997.

8. Castanares S: Complications in blepharoplasty, *Clin Plast Surg* 5:149, 1978.

9. Colton JJ, Beekhuis GJ: *Blepharoplasty.* In Cummings CW and others, editors: *Otolaryngology—head and neck surgery,* ed 3, St Louis, 1998, Mosby, p 676.

10. Cook TA and others: The versatile midforehead browlift. *Arch Otolaryngol Head Neck Surg* 115:163, 1989.

11. Cook TA, Dereberry J, Harrah ER: Reconsideration of fat pad management in lower lid blepharoplasty surgery. *Arch Otolaryngol* 110:521, 1984.

12. Ellis CN: *Management of aging skin.* In Cummings CW and others, editors: *Otolaryngology—head and neck surgery, ed 3,* St Louis, 1998, Mosby, p 629.

13. Gilchrest BA: Skin and photoaging: an overview, *J Am Acad Dermatol* 21:610, 1989.

14. Hamra ST: Composite rhytidectomy, *Plast Reconstr Surg* 90:1, 1992.

15. Hamra ST: The deep plane rhytidectomy, *Plast Reconstr Surg* 86:53, 1990.

16. Howard BK, Leach J: *Aesthetic surgery of the upper third of the face. A self instructional package.* Washington, D.C. American Academy of Otolaryngology Head and Neck Surgery Foundation, Inc.

17. Isse NG: Endoscopic facial rejuvenation: case reports, *Aesthetic Plast Surg* 18:21, 1994.

18. Kerth JD, Toriumi DM: Management of the aging forehead, Arch Otolaryngol Head Neck Surg 116:1137, 1990.

19. Kikkawa DO, Lemke BN: *Orbit and eyelid anatomy.* In Dortzbach RK, editor: *Ophthalmic plastic surgery: prevention and management of complications,* New York, 1994, Raven Press, p 1.

20. Koch RJ, Troell RJ, Goode RL: Contemporary management of the aging brow and forehead, *Laryngoscope* 107:710, 1997.

21. Lewis JR: Methods of direct eyebrow lift, *Ann Plast Surg* 10:115, 1983.

22. Moses JL, Tanenbaum M: *Blepharoplasty: cosmetic and functional.* In McCord CD, Tanenbaum M, Nunery WR, editors: *Oculoplastic surgery,* New York, 1995, Raven Press, p 285.

23. Pastorek NJ: *Upper lid blepharoplasty.* In Papel ID and others, editors: *Facial plastic and reconstructive surgery,* ed 2, New York, 2002, Thieme Medical Publishers, p 185.

24. Quatela VC, Graham D, Sabini P: *Rejuvenation of the brow and midface.* In Papel ID and others, editors: *Facial plastic and reconstructive surgery,* ed 2, New York, 2002, Thieme Medical Publishers, p 171.

25. Ramirez OM: Why I prefer the endoscopic forehead lift, *Plast Reconstr Surgery* 100:1033, 1997.

26. Rankin BS, Arden RL, Crumley RL: *Lower eyelid blepharoplasty.* In Papel ID and others, editors: *Facial plastic and reconstructive surgery,* ed 2, New York, 2002, Thieme Medical Publishers, p 196.

27. Sherris DA, Otley CC, Bartley GB: Comprehensive treatment of the aging face—cutaneous and structural rejuvenation, *Mayo Clin Proc* 73:139, 1998.

28. Wejtanowoski MH: Bicoronal forehead lift, *Aesthetic Plast Surg* 18:33, 1994.

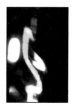

CHAPTER THIRTY THREE

SUCTION-ASSISTED LIPOCONTOURING

Edward H. Farrior
Stephen S. Park

INTRODUCTION

Having long been a part of cosmetic surgery, lipocontouring has continued to progress with the ever-changing technology of cosmetic surgery. Initially, lipocontouring was accomplished with the direct excision of fat through an open surgical approach; it now includes suction lipectomy, small cannula lipectomy, and, most recently, liposhaving and ultrasonic assisted liposuction. The goal of these procedures is to change the contour of the face or neck through the removal of localized fat deposits.

Suction lipectomy is an effective means of recontouring the face that has been popularized and refined over the past 30 years.[3,4,6,7,11] As with all cosmetic surgery, understanding the anatomy, physiology, and changes that result from the aging process is imperative. On the basis of these changes, a logical approach to the integration of suction-assisted lipocontouring into the practice of facial plastic and reconstructive surgery is possible (Figure 33-1).

The distribution of body fat is a consequence of genetics and is influenced by hormones, diet, exercise, medications, and patient age. It has become apparent through tissue culture studies that, after a critical mass within an adipocyte has been reached, hyperplasia can occur.[14] Although the mechanism of adipocyte hyperplasia has not yet been determined, the consensus remains that any significant change in fat deposition occurs through the enlargement rather than the addition of cells.[9] Diet-resistant localized fat deposits, which are ideal for lipocontouring, may represent localized adipocyte hyperplasia. Liposuction reduces the number of adipocytes regardless of their size and therefore should yield a lasting result, unless excessive weight gain occurs. The liposuctioned regions of hypertrophy should respond to weight gain in a fashion that is similar to adipocytes in other regions of the body and, therefore, should be resistant to significant contour changes that are out of proportion with overall weight fluctuation.

Liposuction involves the application of negative pressure through a hollow cannula with a 3- to 6-mm lumen in the subcutaneous plane. Fat is then avulsed as atraumatically as possible. Because of the loose intercellular connections, fat cells are more easily aspirated than tissues with greater structural integrity (e.g., muscle, vessels, nerves). Because the standard suction cannula has no cutting surface, structures with more integrity are protected. Liposhaving has recently been advocated as an alternative to liposuction. In this technique, a soft-tissue shaver is used with minimal suction to gently shave adipocytes.[4] The safety of this technique is of concern, and further investigation is under way. With liposuction and liposhaving, preserving important structures and maintaining bridges of uninterrupted tissue between the deep and superficial layers in an effort to maintain a healthier skin flap are the principles to be followed. Ultrasonic liposuction adds the mechanical agitation of the canula to assist in the dissection and release of adiposits and is usually done in conjunction with tumescent infiltration.[5] Recently the use of ultrasonography has been used both internally and externally to assist with liposuction. The ultrasonic energy is transferred into mechanical vibrations that cause the microcavities in the adipocytes to implode, thereby resulting in the liquefaction of the fat.[8] Multiple studies have shown potential complications with the use of subcutaneous ultrasonic energy resulting from heat generated at the cutaneous incision site and the more distal subdermal sites.[5,8,13] To date there are no controlled studies that demonstrate any added benefit from ultrasonic-assisted liposuction in the face and neck as compared with the standard technique.

PATIENT SELECTION

One of the greatest challenges with facial plastic surgery is the art of proper patient selection, and lipocontouring is no exception. Patient selection begins with an informal interview to get a sense of the patient's

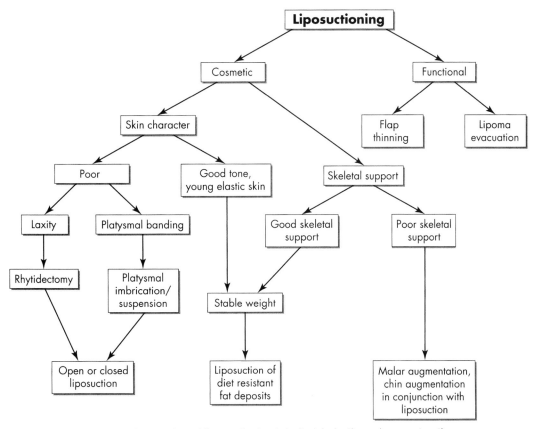

Figure 33-1. The integration of liposuctioning into facial plastic and reconstructive surgery.

motivation, expectation, and cooperation. The patient's motivation for pursuing a cosmetic procedure should be investigated. Some patients expect a change in external appearance to have a significant impact on their personal or professional lives (e.g., to get a promotion at work, to dissuade a spouse's infidelity); these patients are bound to be disappointed. A patient's expectations should be precise and realistic. Lipocontouring allows for the removal of a particular area of subcutaneous fullness; although it will not have a direct impact on other areas, the change in contour may create the illusion of affecting surrounding areas and thereby influence the overall balance of the face. For example, a submental lipectomy may appear to enhance chin projection (Figure 33-2), shorten the vertical height of the face, and create a wider and more cherubic-appearing face. Likewise, facial and jaw lipocontouring may create a more angular facial contour (Figure 33-3) but will not increase malar projection and could create a wasted appearance. The patient's expectations should be communicated preoperatively. Computer imaging can aid in communication, but it can also be misleading if not used prudently. Cooperation is imperative during the postoperative phase. A patient who cannot avoid the sun or continue with a pressure dressing postop-

eratively is a poor candidate for lipocontouring and should be dissuaded from pursuing surgery.

The ideal patient is not particularly overweight and has a localized fullness that is the result of an isolated pocket of subcutaneous adipose tissue refractory to weight loss. A patient who reports a familial pattern or who has had a double chin since childhood is a good candidate. The submental, melolabial, submandibular, and buccal areas lend themselves well to lipocontouring. Younger patients tend to have greater skin elasticity, which contracts better on the new subcutaneous contour; these candidates are ideal for isolated lipocontouring. Conversely, the loss of skin elasticity and turgor in older patients will necessitate a skin-tightening procedure (see Figure 36-1). Obese patients have excess adipose tissue in multiple layers and do not respond well to lipocontouring. Moreover, this procedure is not intended to replace general weight control.

Common Pitfalls

Patient evaluation may yield common pitfalls that lead to untoward effects: (1) Significant ptosis of facial skin may appear accentuated after lipocontouring, thereby creating a more aged appearance; these problems are best addressed with a formal facelift.[8]

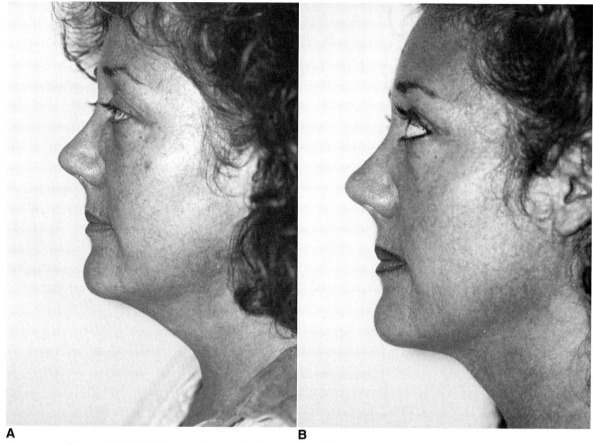

Figure 33-2. A, Preoperative and **B,** postoperative photographs show the illusion of enhanced chin projection after submental and submandibular liposuction, as well as the enhancement of the mandibular margin with improvement of the cervicomental angle.

(2) Lipocontouring depends on the skin's ability to contract and adhere to the new subcutaneous bed, and several factors may interfere with this intrinsic property of the skin (e.g., age, radiation, scarring, actinic injury, smoking). (3) Skeletal insufficiency may reduce structural definition and give the illusion of excess fullness of a certain area (e.g., the retrusive chin and low hyoid bone causing the blunted cervicomental angle); ancillary chin implantation or genioplasty may significantly improve the aesthetic contour (Figure 33-4). (4) Muscular problems (e.g., platysmal lift, platysmal plication, imbrication) may be present. (5) Ptotic submandibular glands and hypertrophy of parotid glands can mimic areas of excess adipose collection and should be appreciated and not traumatized.

INSTRUMENTATION

The instrumentation for lipocontouring the face and neck remains uncomplicated: a vacuum generator with the capability of reaching 1 atmosphere of negative pressure, a disposable canister to function as a

trap for the aspirated fat, sterile tubing, and relatively few liposuction cannulas. The cannulas are available from multiple manufacturers. Some surgeons prefer the round over the spatulated tip, and some prefer the cannulas in which the distal 1.5 to 2 cm is slightly angulated. Angulation of the distal portion allows the positioning of the aspiration port (on the deep surface away from the skin) to be determined on palpation. Cannulas that are 3 to 6 mm are most useful for liposuction. For liposuction, a soft-tissue shaver is used (Figure 33-5), such as the endoscopic soft-tissue shaver or the cartilage shaver used in joint surgery. Cannula size varies from 2.9 to 4.8 mm for liposhaving.

TECHNIQUE
Patient Preparation

Preoperatively, the patient is given routine instructions, such as to take nothing by mouth after midnight, to avoid any medications that alter platelet function, and to avoid the consumption of alcohol. Patients are instructed to wash their face and hair

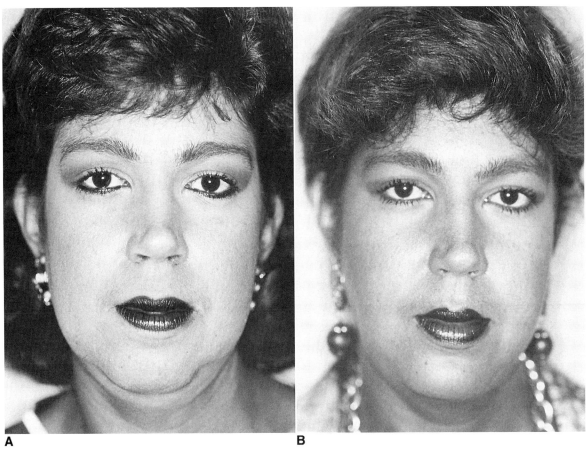

A   **B**

Figure 33-3. A, Preoperative and **B,** postoperative photographs show elimination of the double chin and augmentation of the facial skeleton status after jowl, submental, and submandibular liposuction.

with an antiseptic soap and to remove all makeup and hair-care products. Prescriptions for antibiotics and pain medicine are given to the patient preoperatively to fill before the surgical procedure. When the patient arrives for surgery, an intravenous line is started and preoperative antibiotics are administered. The patient is marked in the upright position, with the areas to be suctioned circumscribed and the zones of feathering indicated (Figure 33-6). Anatomic landmarks (e.g., the angle of the mandible, the anterior border of the sternocleidomastoid muscle, the hyoid bone and thyroid notch) may also be marked (see Figure 33-6). After marking has been completed, the patient is taken to the operative suite, where sedation and infiltration are carried out before preparing and draping the patient. This approach allows additional time for vasoconstriction to occur before surgery.

Anesthesia

Cosmetic procedures (by themselves or in conjunction with other such procedures) are performed under intravenous sedation and infiltration anesthesia. Sedation is administered by an anesthetist with close

monitoring of the patient, allowing for the virtually painless infiltration and nerve block. Submental and submandibular sculpturing are done with a block of the cervical plexus and mental nerve and with direct infiltration. Facial and melolabial contouring is accomplished with mental and infraorbital nerve block with infiltration. Block and infiltration are achieved using 0.5% lidocaine with 1:200,000 epinephrine. Long-acting agents are unnecessary for these patients.

Adequate sedation is paramount but generally needs to be heavy only during nerve block and infiltration of the local anesthetic. Midazolam, fentanyl, and propofol are short-acting agents and combine sedation with analgesia and amnesia. When necessary, these procedures are performed under general anesthesia. In this case, infiltration without nerve block is sufficient to obtain vasoconstriction and improve hemostasis.

Surgery

The location of incisions depends on the site to be contoured, and marking and infiltration are done accordingly. Incisions are limited to 5 to 10 mm and

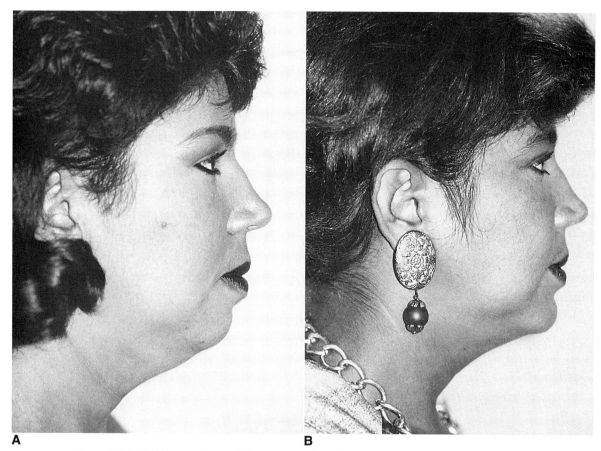

A   **B**

Figure 33-4. A, Preoperative and **B,** postoperative photographs show chin augmentation in conjunction with cervical liposuction.

are made within relaxed skin tension lines. The submental region will usually be done first, then the jaw and posterior cervical areas, followed by the region of the melolabial fold, as indicated. Flaps are then elevated, starting with a small cannula and graduating to the cannula size to be used for the lipectomy. A 5-mm cannula is usually used in the submandibular, submental, and jowl areas, and a 3-mm cannula is used for the melolabial fold.

A nonaspirative cannula is used to make multiple interconnecting tunnels throughout the region to be aspirated. During the nonaspirative phase of flap elevation, it is important to follow the same technique that would be followed when aspirating. The aspiration port should be kept on the deep surface. The skin incision is stabilized with countertraction using a skin hook, and the correct plane is identified with scissors (Figure 33-7). Graduating cannula sizes are used to develop the tunneling after the cannula is in the correct plane (Figure 33-8). The free hand is used to palpate the cannula tip and determine the depth of dissection (Figure 33-9). Dissection is carried out in a

spoke-like fashion from the incision; multiple distal pseudopods from each spoke are used to ensure that lateral aspiration with feathering is executed thoroughly (Figure 33-10). Additionally, nonaspiration tunneling is performed beyond the margins of the area to be aspirated to allow for complete redraping. The surgeon should concentrate on distal aspiration, because each repetitive motion (Figure 33-11) of the cannula will cross over the proximal adipose tissue in the region adjacent to the original insertion, possibly resulting in a hollowed appearance at that point. Hollowing and inconsistent flap elevation can also be avoided by palpating the cannula tip and preserving some fat on the undersurface of the flap.

After complete nonaspiration elevation has been accomplished, the suction is applied at an atmosphere of negative pressure, and multiple passes are re-executed. The assessment of evacuated fat may require the release of the vacuum so that any fat in the cannula and tube may be drawn into the canister; this approach may be necessary when the volume removed is small. Aspiration from the postauricular

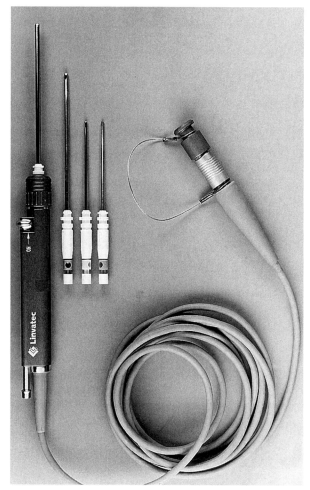

Figure 33-5. Soft-tissue shavers and cannulas of various sizes.

incision includes the jowl, posterior cervical, and submandibular regions (Figure 33-12). Crosshatching occurs with the submandibular portions aspirated from the submental incision. In aspiration of the jowl, it is imperative to release suction when withdrawing the cannula over the posterior facial soft tissue and masseter because this area may not require aspiration, and a groove may be created in the posterior face. The margins can be tapered with a smaller cannula or with fewer passes. Liposuction of the melolabial fold or, more appropriately, of the superior border of the fold is performed with a small cannula through an incision in the nasal vestibule (Figure 33-13).

Submental lipectomy should extend inferiorly to the level of the thyroid cartilage, posteriorly to the anterior border of the sternocleidomastoid muscle (with feathering over the muscle), and superiorly to the margin of the mandible. Lipectomy directed from the postauricular incision can extend anteriorly to

the submandibular area to the anterior border of the platysmas muscle and superiorly to the margin of the mandible. In the jowl, the specific deposit is aspirated, and feathering should be extended to the oral commissure and inferiorly to the margin of the mandible.

With liposhaving (Figure 33-14), flap elevation is done in a similar fashion. The cannula is inserted with the blade inactive. After the blade is activated, extreme care should be taken at the incision to avoid damage to the skin margins. The cannula is passed in a more delicate fashion and at a slower rate than it is with liposuction, because shaving—rather than avulsion—is occurring. Minimal amounts of suction are applied, and the cannula must remain in motion when the blade is active, because it will shave progressively deeper, thereby jeopardizing other structures.

Lipocontouring can augment other cosmetic procedures. In conjunction with cervicofacial rhytidectomy, the cannula can be used to elevate the flap while sculpting the fatty tissue. The authors prefer to perform open liposuction for sculpturing after flap elevation; this approach frequently requires the extension of liposuction tunnels beyond the limits of skin-flap elevation. Open liposuction with cervicofacial rhytidectomy allows the surgeon to completely crosshatch each area, thereby reducing the risk of banding. Additionally, uniform flap thickness can be ensured at the time of sharp elevation, thereby reducing the risk of dimpling of the skin. By combining lipocontouring with mentoplasty, the surgeon need only extend the submental incision to about 3 cm to allow for the placement of the implant. All wounds are closed in a layered fashion.

Dressing

Postoperatively, all patients require a pressure dressing circumferentially around the head and neck. Antibiotic ointment is first applied to the incision and then covered with a nonadhesive dressing. Fluffs are then placed over the region that has been aspirated, and a rolled cotton gauze is used to hold these fluffs in place. Coban R (3M; St Paul, Mn) dressing is applied using light but continuous pressure (Figure 33-15). The dressing is left undisturbed for two to three days and then removed. After this, an elastic dressing is used at night and when indoors, changed by the patient as needed (Figure 33-16). Antibiotics are used in all elective surgeries; drains are not routinely used. Liposuction is usually not painful, but the circumferential dressing can be uncomfortable and produce anxiety for some patients. For this reason, mild analgesics are helpful. Elevation of the head and the continuous use of ice packs minimize swelling.

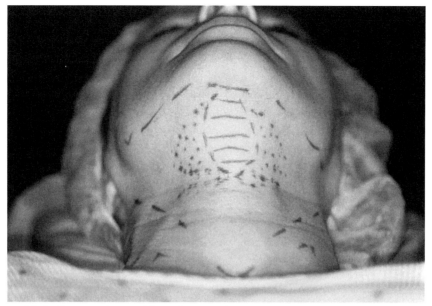

Figure 33-6. Preoperative marking of anatomic structures, including the margin of the mandible, the sternocleidomastoid muscle, and the hyoid bone, with stippling of lateral feathered regions and a vertical line through prominent submental fat pad.

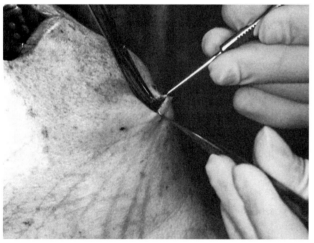

Figure 33-7. Identification of the plane of dissection using Metzenbaum scissors.

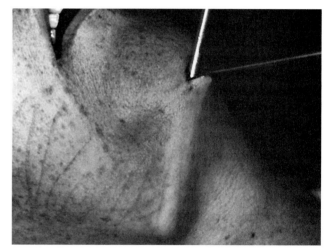

Figure 33-8. Use of the suction cannula to develop subcutaneous tunnels while stabilizing the skin with a skin hook.

Recovery Phase

Diligent patient education about the recovery phase can be very comforting for all involved. Some degree of bruising and facial edema is to be expected and may last for a week; the elevated skin may be numb for 3 to 9 weeks. As the facial skin scars and adheres to the new underlying contour, patients often note some firmness and tightness that diminishes over the subsequent months. Pain is usually minimal and sufficiently relieved with acetaminophen. When larger volumes of fat are removed, shallow dimpling and wrinkling from excess skin can occur as the skin adheres; diligent massage and patience will lead to a smoother final contour. Exercise is to be avoided for three weeks after surgery and should be resumed gradually, beginning with aerobic activities and progressing to more strenuous exercise.

COMPLICATIONS

Complications from lipocontouring are uncommon but may be dramatic. The most frequent complication is hematoma or seroma, which is evacuated by

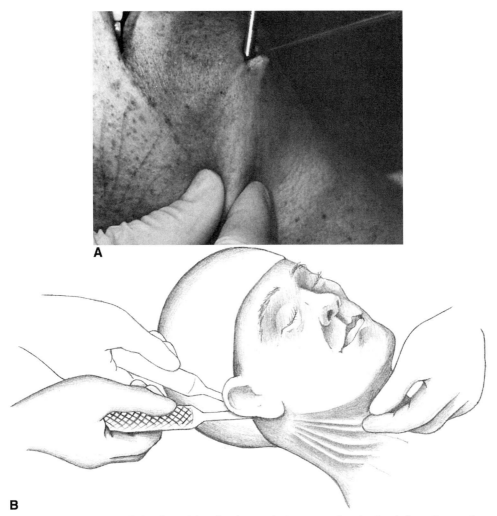

A

B

Figure 33-9. **A** and **B,** Palpation of the distal cannula to ensure the depth of dissection and the location of the distal cannula lumen.

needle aspiration, and then a pressure dressing is reapplied. If a hematoma accumulates acutely, there should be a low threshold for drainage and exploration in the operating room. Infections or cellulitis usually arise from a preexisting hematoma and should be managed aggressively to reduce the risk of skin-flap necrosis or scarring. Pigment changes can follow an undiagnosed hematoma and result from a breakdown in hemoglobin products. Contour irregularities and asymmetries may manifest after all swelling has subsided and are more likely to occur as residual fullness on the right neck area because most surgeons are right-handed, which makes the left side of the neck more accessible to them than the right side. If significant, this complication is best repaired with minor touch-up procedures using the handheld syringe technique, but not before six months have passed since the original operation to allow the full skin flap to soften as much as possible. For subtle areas, small quantities of corticosteroids

can be injected to induce fat atrophy. This approach should be used conservatively, because its effects continue for many months and are not reversible. Minor depressions can be remedied with autologous fat injection, but the longevity of the procedure is unknown. Motor or sensorineural injuries are rare but more serious, and they usually appear as transient neuropraxias. Cardiovascular instability is associated with total body liposuction and results from massive fluid shifts; this complication does not occur from lipectomy in the head and neck areas. Pulmonary fat embolism can theoretically occur during any surgical procedure but has not been reported after liposuction alone.

SUMMARY

Lipocontouring is a necessary adjunct to a facial plastic and reconstructive practice. Multiple tools are available and should be judged individually. Patient selection and education are paramount to achieving

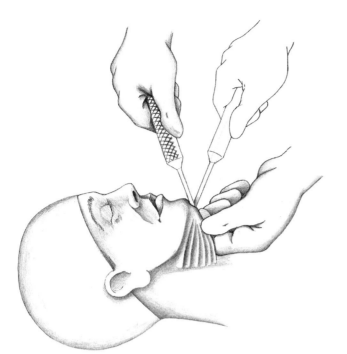

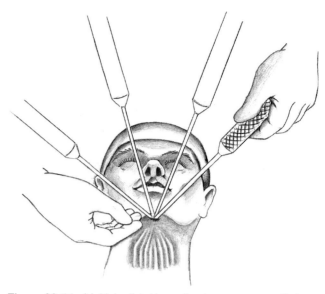

Figure 33-11. Multiple distal tunneling to ensure smooth transition in all regions and to avoid overreduction of the immediate submental adiposity.

Figure 33-10. Distal feathering to ensure smooth transition to nonaspirated sites.

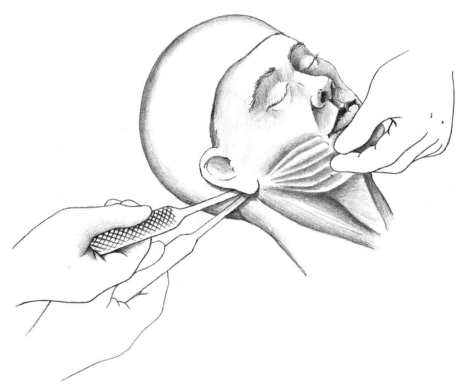

Figure 33-12. Suction lipectomy of the jowl, posterior cervical, and submandibular regions, which can be approached through the postauricular incision.

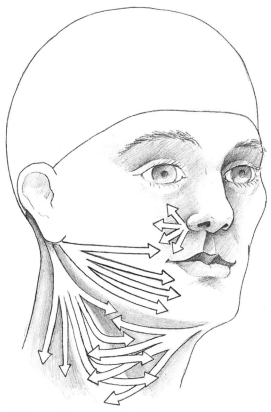

Figure 33-13. Sites that can be approached through the submental, postauricular, and vestibular incisions.

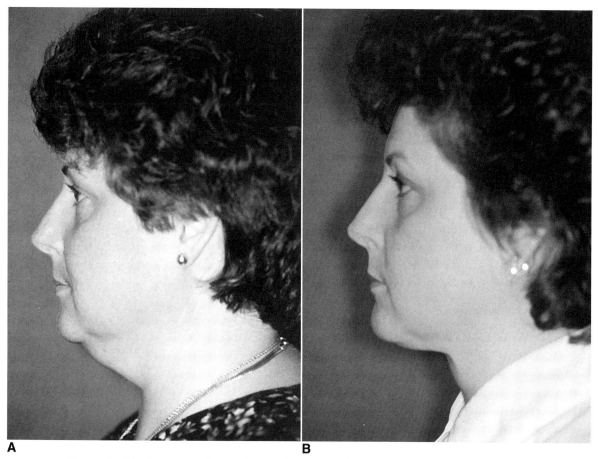

A   B

Figure 33-14. A, Preoperative and **B,** postoperative photographs show a patient who has undergone submental liposhaving with the illusion of enhanced chin projection caused by augmentation of the cervicomental angle.

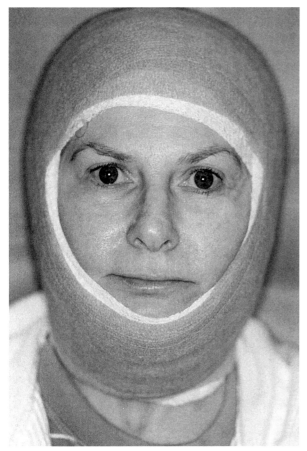

Figure 33-15. Immediate postsurgical dressing.

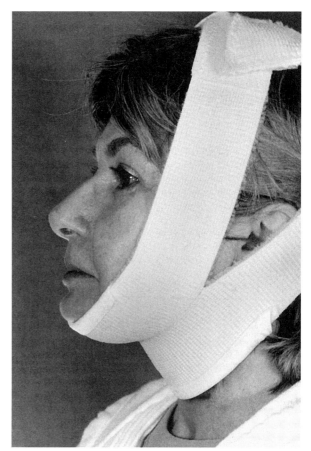

Figure 33-16. A light dressing can be applied by the patient after the immediate postsurgical dressing is removed.

satisfaction. The judicious use of liposuction in conjunction with other cosmetic procedures will enhance the results and the satisfaction of both the patient and the surgeon.

REFERENCES

1. Becker D, Park SS, Gross CW: Results from current investigation, 1995, University of Virginia.
2. Cueva R, Thomas JR, Davidson M: Liposuction to debulk the pectoralis major myocutaneous flap, *J Otolaryngol* 9:106, 1988.
3. Fournier PF: Why the syringe and not the suction machine? *J Dermatol Surg Oncol* 14:1062, 1988.
4. Gross CW and others: The soft-tissue shaving procedure for removal of adipose tissue: a new, less traumatic approach than liposuction, *Arch Otolaryngol Head Neck Surg* 121:1117, 1995.
5. Igra H, Satur NM. Tumescent liposuction versus internal ultrasonic-assisted tumescent liposuction: a side to side comparison, *Dermatol Surg* 23:1213, 1997.
6. Illouz YG: Body contouring by lipolysis: a 5 year experience with over 3000 cases, *Plast Reconstr Surg* 72:591, 1983.
7. Kesselring UK, Meyer R: A suction curette for removal of excessive local deposits of subcutaneous fat, *Plast Reconstr Surg* 63:305, 1978.
8. Kloehn RA. Commentary on ultrasound-assisted lipoplasty: task force July 1966 report to membership [letter], *Plast Reconstr Surg* 99:1198, 1997.
9. Kridel RWH, Pacella BL: *Complications of liposuction.* In Eisele D, editor: *Complications of head and neck surgery,* St Louis, 1992, Mosby–Year Book, p 791.
10. Markman B: Anatomy and physiology of adipose tissue, *Clin Plast Surg* 16:235, 1989.
11. Mladick RA: Lipoplasty: an ideal adjunctive procedure for the face lift, *Clin Plast Surg* 16:333, 1989.
12. Schrudde J: Lipexeresis as a means of eliminating local adiposity, *Aesthetic Plast Surg* 4:215, 1980.
13. Setliff RC: The hummer, *Otolaryngol Clin North Am* 29:93, 1996.
14. Van R: *The adipocyte precursor cell.* In Cryer A, Van R, editors: *New perspectives in adipose tissue,* London, 1985, Butterworths.

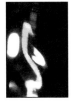

CHAPTER THIRTY FOUR

MENTOPLASTY AND FACIAL IMPLANTS

Jonathan M. Sykes
Travis T. Tollefson
John L. Frodel, Jr.

MENTOPLASTY

The chin prominence is not present in any four-legged mammal.[12] During evolution, with the adoption of an upright posture and with verticalization of the face; the chin became an important facial feature. The events contributing to the evolutionary development of the chin in humans are open to speculation; however, the importance of the chin in the overall appearance of the face cannot be overstated.

In general, when patients inquire about improving their facial appearance, they rarely ask about surgical correction of the chin. More commonly, requests focus on seemingly more obvious problems, such as reduction of a large nose or correction of sagging skin of the neck and jowls. However, recognition, evaluation, and treatment of chin abnormalities often has a great impact on facial appearance. It is clear that all attractive faces have an underlying balance and structural symmetry to their facial skeletons.[19] Proper balance of the facial skeleton requires harmony and proportion of all bones of the face in all three planes of space. The chin should therefore be evaluated as it relates to important adjacent structures, such as the lips, teeth, and nose.[35] Appropriate treatment of aesthetic deformities of the chin will contribute to facial harmony and will often improve the appearance of the mouth, the lips, and the nose. It is for these reasons that every face should be carefully studied to determine why the chin appears unattractive. This will enable the surgeon to correct the deformity and improve facial proportion.

Surgical correction of aesthetic deformities of the chin can be performed by either chin augmentation with an implant or by osteotomy and advancement (or reduction) of the bony mentum. Augmentation using alloplastic implants can camouflage a horizontal (anterior-posterior [AP]) bony deficiency.[38] However, this technique is not effective in correcting vertical (superior-inferior) or transverse deformities of the lower face and chin. Horizontal bony osteotomy of the chin (osseous genioplasty) is a simple and versatile procedure. This technique allows horizontal advancement or reduction of the chin, vertical lengthening or shortening of the chin, and correction of transverse deformities of the chin. The procedure chosen to correct the specific aesthetic problem is based on the type and extent of the deformity[35] (Table 34-1). If carefully evaluated and planned, aesthetic correction of chin deformities can provide significant improvement in the overall balance and proportion of the face.

Patient Evaluation

To precisely correct any chin deformity, careful preoperative analysis of the deformity is essential.[34,35] Specifically, the chin should be evaluated as it relates to other skeletal and soft tissue structures, including the lips, teeth, nose, and soft tissues of the neck. A detailed history of past trauma, orthodontic treatment, or prior oral surgery is essential. This is important because many patients with dental malocclusion and underlying facial skeletal abnormalities are treated with orthodontics. This method of dental compensation may correct the malocclusion, but it fails to improve the underlying skeletal deformity. It is therefore important to discuss prior therapy, including orthodontics, with the patient.

Physical examination should include inspection and palpation of the chin, lips, nose, and teeth. The entire face should be observed at rest and during animation to evaluate the mentalis soft tissue mound and its support. With aging, patients may develop ptosis of the soft tissue pad of the chin. In patients with open bite deformities and lip incompetence, hyperactivity of the mentalis muscles ("mentalis strain") can occur (Figure 34-1). For this reason, the dental occlusion

TABLE 34-1

MENTOPLASTY PROCEDURES

Horizontal (Anterior-posterior)	Vertical	Transverse	Procedure
D	N or sl D	N	Chin implant or genioplasty
D	E	N	Genioplasty (advancement with possible ostectomy if significant vertical excess)
D	D	N	Bony advancement (with downgrafting for chin lengthening)
N	N	Asymmetric	Bony osteotomy (with resection of downgrafting)
E	N	N	Bony osteotomy (with setback)
E	E	N	Bony osteotomy (with ostectomy)

D, Deficient; E, excessive; N, normal; sl, slight.
Modified from Sykes J, Frodel J: *Op Tech Otolaryngol* 6:319, 1995.

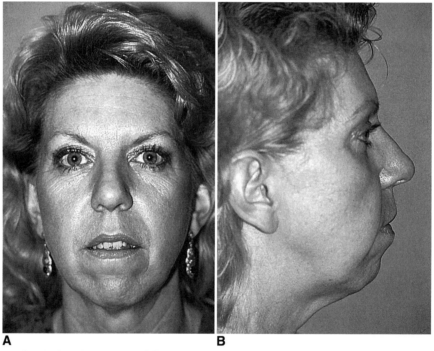

A   **B**

Figure 34-1. Anterior-posterior **(A)** and lateral **(B)** photograph of a patient with posterior vertical maxillary access and an open bite deformity. Note the mentalis strain caused by the patient trying to close her lips at rest.

should be carefully examined to determine whether orthodontics or orthognathic surgery is needed.

The evaluation of all patients for possible chin surgery should include consistent and reproducible clinical photographs in three views: AP (frontal), lateral (profile), and oblique. These photographs allow analysis of the contour and projection of the chin as it relates to the lips, nose, labiomental groove, and soft tissues of the neck. If the physical evaluation and clinical photographs show a minor deformity requiring augmentation with an alloplast, radiographs of the chin are usually not necessary. However, if the deformity is more complex, (e.g., vertical chin excess with horizontal deficiency or transverse bony asymmetry), radiographic analysis is essential.

Radiographic evaluation of the chin routinely includes a panoramic radiograph (Panorex) and cephalometric radiographs in the AP and lateral views. The panoramic radiograph shows the cortical outline of the mandible and the vertical mandibular height (Figure 34-2). The Panorex also delineates the position of the tooth roots and of the inferior alveolar canals and mental foramina. It is important to know the exact position of the mental foramen and canal preoperatively so intraoperative damage to the mental nerve can be prevented. The inferior alveolar nerve, a branch of the third division of the fifth (trigeminal) cranial nerve, travels through the mandibular canal and exits the mental foramen as mental nerve. The mental nerve supplies sensation to the skin and mucous membranes of the lower lip and chin. The mandibular canal is often located 2 to 3 mm below the level of the mental foramen.[12] Bony osteotomies should therefore be performed at least 5 mm below the mental foramen to avoid injury to the neurovascular bundle.

If bony genioplasty is considered, AP and lateral cephalometric radiographs should be performed (Figure 34-3). AP views allow detection and evaluation of transverse skeletal asymmetries of the chin. Transverse asymmetries are common in patients with Goldenhar's syndrome or hemifacial microsomia, but they are also commonly seen in nonsyndromic patients considering aesthetic surgery. When transverse bony or soft tissue asymmetries are overlooked preoperatively in a patient with microgenia, augmentation with an alloplastic chin implant can accentuate the deformity.[35]

Lateral cephalometric radiographs allow detailed analysis of both the soft tissues and the facial skeleton. The cephalogram should be obtained at a standard distance with the head positioned so that the Frankfort horizontal line is parallel to the floor.[27] From this standardized lateral radiograph, a series of soft tissue and skeletal points can be identified. This allows various analyses of the chin as described by Ricketts,[28] Steiner,[33] Burstone,[5] Gonzalez-Ulloa and Stevens,[10] and others. Ricketts' analysis (Figure 34-4) uses a tangent connecting the soft tissue pogonion

(most projecting point) of the chin with the most projecting point of the nasal tip.[28] In this system, the upper lip should lie about 4 mm behind the line, whereas the lower lip is ideally located 2 mm behind the line. While the Ricketts analysis correctly evaluates the

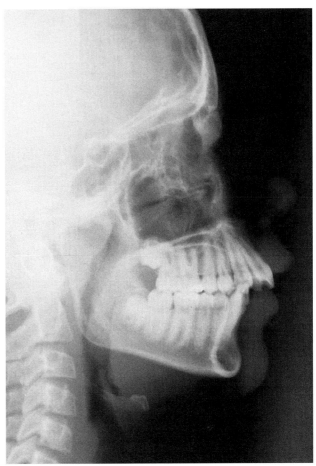

Figure 34-3. Lateral cephalometric radiograph showing the bony and soft tissue outline of a patient with a class II malocclusion and mild open bite deformity.

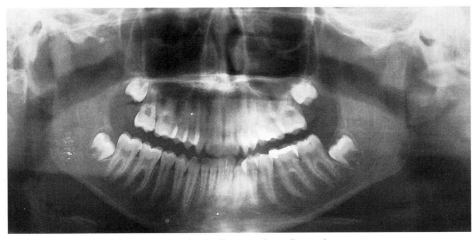

Figure 34-2. Panoramic radiograph.

lower face in profile, it places great importance on the projection of the nasal tip. The Steiner analysis uses the columellar inflection point(s) to identify the correct position for the chin point.[33] This method places importance on the lip position. The Holdaway "H" angle (Figure 34-5) relates the position of the soft tissue pogonion with important skeletal points on the mid and lower face. No single analysis is ideal, but each method attempts to determine the "ideal" positions for the soft tissues and skeleton of the chin because these structures relate to the remainder of the face.

An accurate chin analysis using the lateral cephalogram involves dropping a vertical line from the Frankfort horizontal (porion-infraorbitale) through the soft tissue subnasale.[16] With ideal horizontal chin projection, the soft tissue pogonion should lie approximately 4 mm behind this line (Figure 34-6). The most frequently used evaluation of the chin drops a perpendicular line from the vermillion border of the lower lip and compares the AP position of this line with the soft tissue pogonion (the anterior-most projecting chin point) (Figure 34-7). A general guideline for aesthetic chin position in this method is for the pogonion in a male patient to be positioned at the level of this vertical line and for the pogonion in a female patient to be just posterior to the line. If the position of the soft tissue pogonion is anterior to the proposed line, horizontal macrogenia is diagnosed, whereas microgenia is present if the chin is positioned posterior to the ideal line. Although this method is effective for AP deformities (microgenia or macrogenia), it does not account for vertical or transverse discrepancies. Because many surgeons primarily use this evaluation method, vertical or transverse chin problems are often overlooked.

Analysis of vertical facial heights is also essential in determining the appropriate heights of the lower facial third and the chin. Various methods for evaluating vertical facial heights have been used. The simplest technique involves division of the face into three equal thirds: the upper third, from the frontal hairline to the glabella; the middle third, from the glabella to the soft tissue subnasale; and the lower third, from the subnasale to the menton (the lowest point of the chin) (Figure 34-8). Because frontal hairline can vary significantly, an alternate method described by Powell and Humphreys[24] more accurately analyzes the vertical heights of the lower two thirds of the face. This method describes the middle third as the distance from the nasion to the subnasale and the lower third as the distance from the subnasale to the menton (Figure 34-9). The middle third distance in this analysis ideally represents 43% of the total height of the lower two thirds of the face, that is,

$$\frac{\text{Nasion} - \text{Subnasale}}{\text{Nasion} - \text{menton}} = 0.43$$

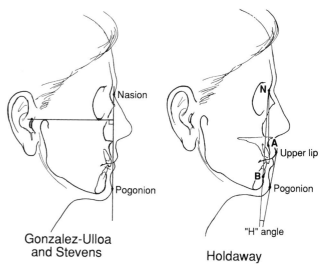

Figure 34-5. The Gonzalez-Ulloa and Stevens and the Holdaway analyses of the chin and lower third of the face.

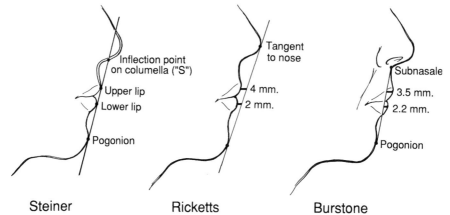

Figure 34-4. Steiner, Ricketts, and Burstone analysis of the ideal relationship of the chin as it relates to the lips and other lower facial structures.

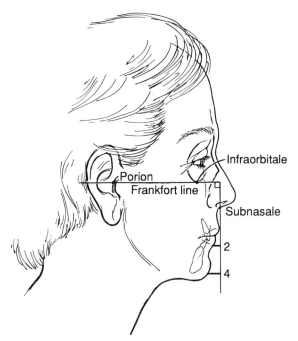

Figure 34-6. Horizontal relationships of the chin and upper and lower lips as they relate to the nasal perpendicular line.

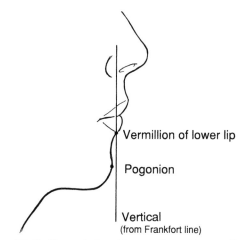

Figure 34-7. The relationship of the chin position to a perpendicular passing through the vermillion border of the lower lip.

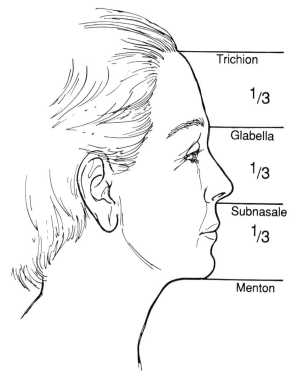

Figure 34-8. Vertical heights (thirds) of the face.

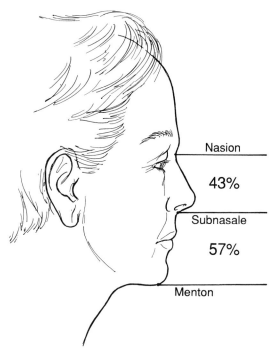

Figure 34-9. Vertical relationship of the face without accounting for the upper facial third.

whereas the lower third distance should approximate 57% of the total vertical height.

Other analyses of the vertical dimensions of the face have been described. One method includes inspection of the face in repose, when the maxillary incisor teeth should show 0 to 3 mm (Figure 34-10). If more than 3 mm of the maxillary incisors are visible at rest, excessive facial length (usually in the midface) is sometimes present. Additional analysis of the lower face includes subdividing the lower third of the face. Two methods exist for subdivision of lower facial heights. The first includes a vertical third from sub-nasale to upper lip stomion and two thirds from upper lip stomion to the menton (Figure 34-11). The second method divides the lower third into two equal parts, from the subnasale to the vermillion border of the

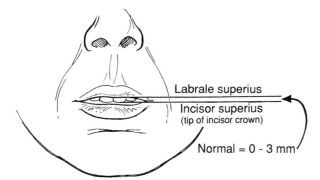

Figure 34-10. Schematic diagram of incisor show of the maxillary teeth. A normal relationship would be 0 to 3 mm of central incisor visible.

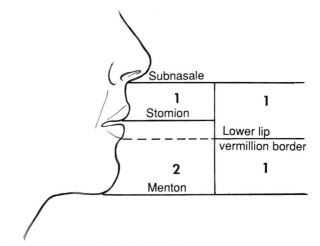

Figure 34-11. Vertical relationships of the lower third of the face.

lower lip and from the lower lip vermillion border to the menton. All of these analyses relate the height of the chin and lower face to the total facial height. In complex chin deformities, a vertical discrepancy as well as a horizontal deficiency or excess may often be present.

Another parameter that should be assessed is symmetry in the sagittal plane. Transverse asymmetries of the chin exist in many patients with cogenital anomalies (Goldenhar's syndrome, hemifacial microsomia) or in patients who have had significant skeletal facial trauma. However, many patients with only aesthetic concerns have minor but definite transverse asymmetries of the chin. In patients with asymmetry of the facial midline, chin augmentation with an implant may correct the horizontal deficiency but accentuate the skeletal asymmetry. AP cephalometric radiographs allow a comparison of the bony midline of the chin with the dental midlines of the maxilla and the mandible. If the skeletal and soft tissue midline of the chin are not aligned with the dental midlines and with the upper facial skeletal midline (e.g., nasion), an asymmetric bony genioplasty or chin implant can be performed.

Each of the systems of analysis relates the soft tissue pogonion with other facial structures. No single method provides comprehensive evaluation of the chin, but each allows a reference for assessing the bony and soft tissues of the chin and lower face. Using a variety of methods, appropriate evaluation of chin deformities can be achieved.

Chin Deformities

Deformities of the chin and lower face may be related to either bony abnormalities or to soft tissue malposition. The chin should be analyzed in all three planes of space: horizontal (AP), vertical (superior-inferior), and transverse. The horizontal and vertical dimensions can each be deficient, normal, or excessive. Simple deformities such as mild horizontal chin defi-

ciency (microgenia) are easily corrected using either an implant or bony advancement. More complex deformities, such as in a patient with horizontal deficiency and vertical excess, usually require horizontal osteotomy for adequate correction.[25]

Soft tissue deformities of the chin and submental region also exist. Ptosis of the soft tissues of the chin often accompanies other signs of facial aging. This condition, commonly called *witch's chin* or *senile chin deformity*, is caused by a weakening of the muscular attachments of the mentalis and depressor labii inferioris muscles. In this deformity, the soft tissue pad of the chin falls below the mandibular line, and a deep horizontal crease develops in the submental region. Descent of the soft tissue chin pad is accentuated with smiling (Figure 34-12, *A* through *C*). This deformity can be inadvertently created or worsened surgically if the mentalis muscles are not reapproximated while inserting a chin implant (Figure 34-12, *D*).

Procedure Selection

The selection of the best procedure to correct a given deformity of the chin should be based on the type and extent of the deformity (see Table 34-1). Augmentation of the chin with an alloplastic implant is a simple and effective method of correcting a horizontal chin deficiency. This technique is limited by the availability of various sizes and shapes of alloplastic implants. An infinite number of shapes and sizes of implants may be required. However, most implants are manufactured in only three or four sizes and one or two shapes. Additionally, chin augmentation with implants is less effective in patients with significant vertical discrepancies (vertical excess or deficiency). Placement of an implant in such a patient may exacerbate the vertical excess and make the chin appear longer. For these reasons, implant augmentation is an effective method

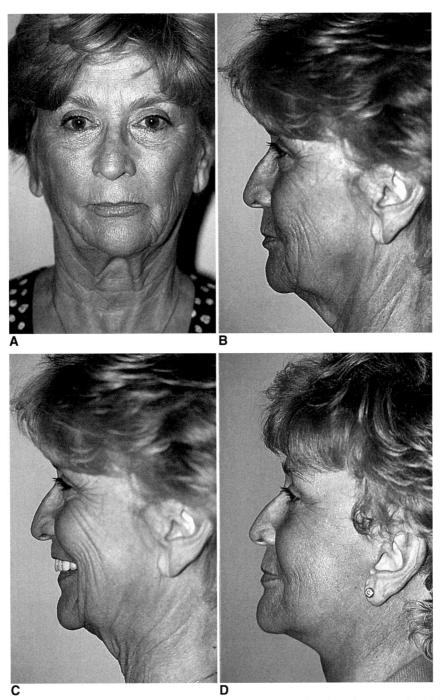

Figure 34-12. A, B, and **C,** Anterior-posterior lateral and smiling lateral preoperative views of a patient with senile ptosis of the chin. Note the deepened submental crease when smiling. **D,** Postoperative lateral view after deep plane facelift and soft tissue correction of the ptotic mentalis pad.

of camouflage for minor chin deformities, but may not be satisfactory for complex deformities.

Osteotomy of the bony mentum (osseous genioplasty) is a versatile and reliable procedure for correcting a variety of skeletal chin deformities. First described by Hofer in 1942,[15] this technique involves horizontal osteotomy and downfracture of the chin, with repositioning and fixation of the distal segment. Osseous genioplasty allows advancement or retrusion in the AP direction, as well as lengthening or shortening in the vertical direction.[6,32,39] Additionally, the genioplasty procedure provides an approach for correction of transverse asymmetries of the chin. Although customized chin implants can be made to correct chin asymmetries, preformed implants are usually symmetrical.

Correction of soft tissue ptosis has been described by Peterson[22] and other authors. The technique involves the removal of an ellipse of submental skin, creation of a flap of chin soft tissue, and advancement and plication of the soft tissue flap inferiorly. This technique tightens the soft tissue pad and obliterates the horizontal submental crease. However, the soft tissue pogonion is effectively moved posteriorly, and some form of simultaneous augmentation (implant or bony advancement) is usually required.

Surgical Technique
Chin Implant

To ensure precise midline placement of the chin implant, the midline of the chin, lower lip, and neck (thyroid cartilage) are marked externally before the infiltration of local anesthesia. A mental nerve block is then performed using xylocaine 1% with epinephrine 1:100,000. Additional infiltration of anesthesia into the submental region, the gingivolabial sulcus, and the central portion of the lower lip and chin is performed to ensure adequate anesthesia and vasoconstriction.

Either an intraoral or external (submental) incision and approach can be used to place a chin implant. If an extraoral approach is used, an incision (approximately 2 to 3 cm) is made in the submental crease and carried through the dermis and subcutaneous fat (Figure 34-13). The mentalis muscles are then divided to enter a dissection plane just superficial to the periosteum of the anterior face of the mandible. The chin implant can be placed in either the subperiosteal or the supraperiosteal plane. The advantage of placing an implant beneath the periosteum is improved fixation of the implant. However, subperiosteal placement has been shown to result in some erosion of the anterior mandible. For these reasons, most surgeons advocate dissection in the supraperiosteal plane centrally, with subperiosteal placement laterally (Figure 34-14). This will theoretically minimize mandibular erosion, while maximally fixing the implant.

Many sizes, shapes, and types of implants have been used for chin augmentation. In general, the two shapes of implants are the central "button" implant and the extended "anatomic" implant. Longer tapered implants have the advantages of being able to be placed in the subperiosteal plane laterally, and they allow for lateral mandibular augmentation (Figure 34-15). Most importantly, extended implants have the advantage of not being as apparent if 1 to 2 mm of displacement occurs. Smaller, central implants are more obvious if slight postoperative displacement of the implant occurs.

During the lateral subperiosteal dissection, the mental nerves should be identified and preserved. The implant should be placed along the inferior border of the mandible. If the implant extends laterally beyond the mental foramina, it should be positioned below the exit of the mental nerve (Figure 34-15). After placement of the implant, the mentalis muscles should be reapproximated and the soft tissue resuspended meticulously. If the mentalis muscle is not carefully realigned, postoperative ptosis of the soft tissues of the chin may occur. Closure of the mentalis muscle is performed with a No. 4-0 braided absorbable suture. The subcutaneous tissues and dermis are reapproximated with a No. 5-0 chromic suture, followed by skin closure with an interrupted No. 6-0 monofilament nonabsorbable suture. A secure chin strap dressing is

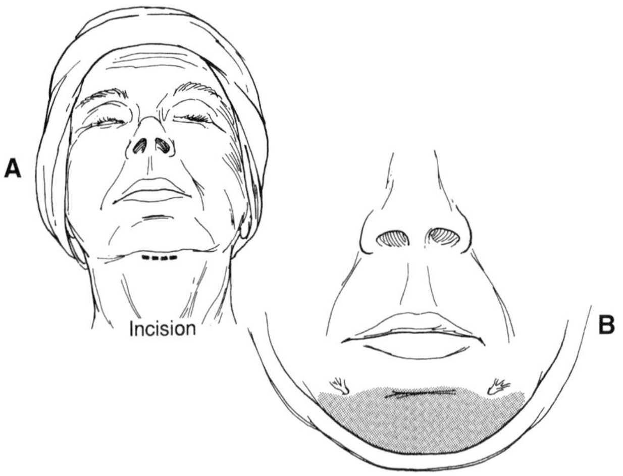

Figure 34-13. A, Horizontal submental incision in the crease for placement of a chin implant. B, Schematic diagram indicating the extent of dissection (stippled area) for placement of a chin implant.

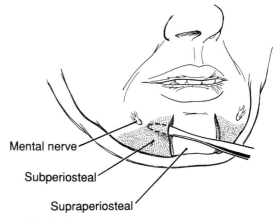

Figure 34-14. Dissection planes for placement of a chin implant with the central dissection being supraperiosteal and the lateral pockets in the subperiosteal plane.

Mental nerve
Subperiosteal
Supraperiosteal

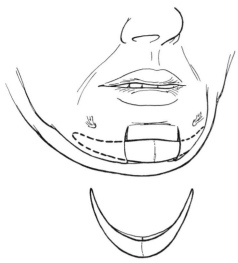

Figure 34-15. Lateral subperiosteal placement of an extended alloplastic chin implant.

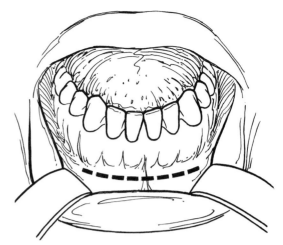

Figure 34-16. Schematic diagram of a horizontal gingivolabial incision for bony genioplasty.

placed for 3 days to ensure immobility of the implant. Perioperative antibiotics are used for 48 hours.

If an intraoral approach is used, the gingivolabial incision can be either horizontal or vertical. In either case, dissection through the mentalis muscles again occurs with placement of the implant in a supraperiosteal plane centrally and a subperiosteal pocket laterally. Closure is accomplished in two layers with the muscle closure achieving soft tissue resuspension. A chin strap dressing is used for 3 days to secure the position of the implant.

Osseous Genioplasty

Horizontal bony osteotomy of the chin (osseous genioplasty) is a versatile procedure that can be performed under general anesthesia or intravenous sedation with metalis nerve block. If general anesthesia is used, nasotracheal intubation is preferred; however, if rhinoplasty is to be performed with the genioplasty, orotracheal intubation should be used.

A gingivolabial incision is made from one canine tooth to the other (Figures 34-16 and 34-17). The incision is made on the labial side of the gingivolabial sulcus to allow an adequate mucoperiosteal soft tissue cuff for wound closure. Dissection is then carried through the soft tissues and mandibular periosteum. Subperiosteal dissection is performed laterally with identification and preservation of both mental nerves (Figures 34-18 and 34-19). A small inferior segment of soft tissue is preserved over the central segment (bony mentum) of the mandible to provide vascular supply to the distal segment after osteotomy.[1]

After the lateral subperiosteal dissection is completed, the proposed osteotomy is carefully measured and marked (Figures 34-20 and 34-21). The bony

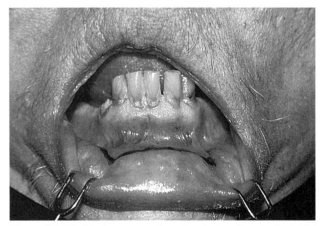

Figure 34-17. Marking on cadaver illustrating the gingivolabial incision not in the crease to facilitate later closure.

midline is vertically inscribed with a side-cutting burr (Figure 34-22) to allow the proximal and distal segments to be precisely aligned after osteotomy and repositioning. The osteotomy site is then measured and marked with calipers to ensure a symmetrical osteotomy. The horizontal osteotomy should be placed below the level of the tooth roots to prevent dental injury.

During the preoperative assessment, a decision is made on the 3D movement of the chin that is required. This treatment plan will affect the orientation of the osteotomy as well as the actual movement after the osteotomy. If only AP advancement is needed, the osteotomy is made with a horizontal orientation. If vertical movement (shortening) is needed in addition, the osteotomy is made in a more oblique orientation. An oblique osteotomy allows some vertical shortening because the distal segment is advanced.

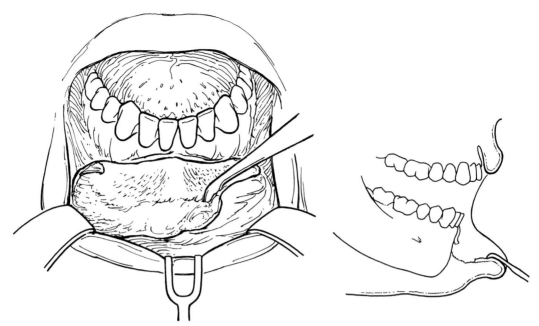

Figure 34-18. Schematic illustration of the subperiosteal plane of dissection for genioplasty. Note the mental nerves are isolated, identified, and preserved and an inferior cuff of central soft tissue is maintained on the distal segment of the chin to increase vascularity.

If the chin length is excessive and significant shortening is planned, two oblique osteotomies are made and the intervening bone is removed.

After the osteotomy is marked, the bone cut is created with a reciprocating saw blade in a lateral-to-medial direction (Figure 34-23). The lateral extent of the osteotomy should be made at least 5 mm below the mental foramen to avoid injuring the mental nerve. Gentle digital pressure is used to down-fracture the bony segment. A small amount of soft tissue must usually be separated from the posterior aspect of the distal segment to facilitate movement.

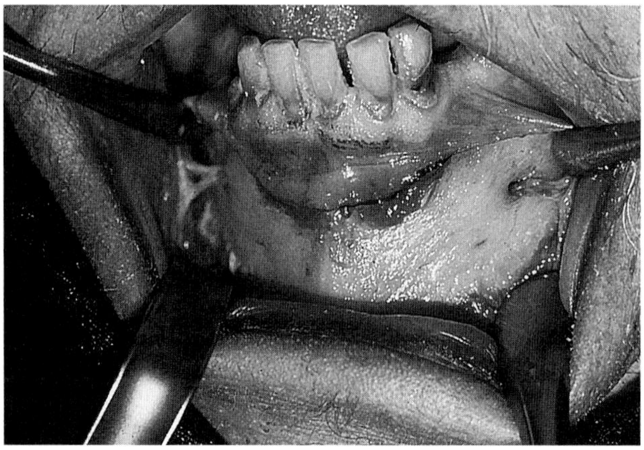

Repositioning of the distal segment is performed according to the preoperative treatment plan. If vertical lengthening is required, grafts are placed using autogenous bone or allogenic bone (Figure 34-24). If vertical shortening is planned, a second parallel osteotomy is made above the first, or the intervening bone is burred away (Figure 34-25). After the segment

Figure 34-19. The cadaver dissection of the subperiosteal plane of dissection for genioplasty.

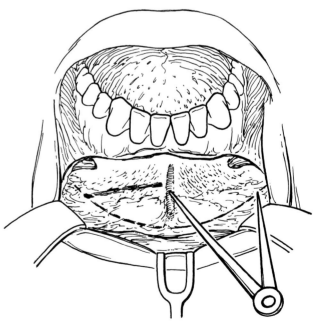

Figure 34-20. Schematic illustration indicating measurement of the osteotomy site from the middle line to ensure symmetry.

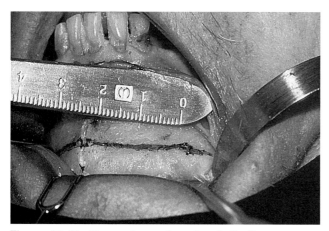

Figure 34-21. The cadaver dissection indicating measurement of the osteotomy site from the middle line to ensure symmetry.

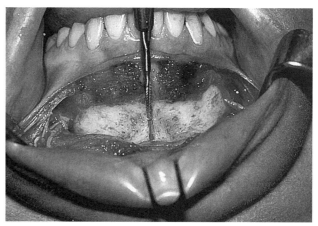

Figure 34-22. Inscription of the bony midline with a sidecutting burr to facilitate later accurate approximation after osteotomy.

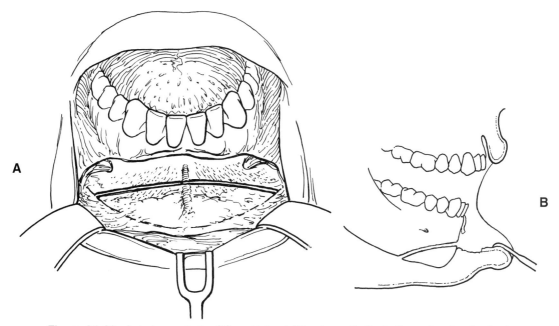

Figure 34-23. Anterior-posterior **(A)** and lateral **(B)** schematic illustrations showing the horizontal mandibular osteotomy of the mentum well below the mental foramena.

is repositioned, it is fixed in position using adaptation plates, positional screws, or interosseous wires (Figures 34-26 and 34-27). Adaptation plates can be preshaped and provide excellent fixation. The soft tissues of the chin and lips are then replaced, and the new contour is assessed.

The wound is closed in two layers with care taken to resuspend the soft tissues of the chin. Interrupted No. 3-0 catgut is used for the mentalis muscle, and a running locking stitch of No. 3-0 chromic catgut is used for the mucosa. A pressure chinstrap dressing is applied for 5 days, and the patient should eat a soft diet for 2 weeks.

Clinical Examples
Case 1

A 22-year-old woman presented for rhinoplasty. She had had orthodontic treatment to correct a class II malocclusion. She desired chin augmentation but refused bony genioplasty. At the time of rhinoplasty, chin augmentation was accomplished using an extended anatomic implant (Figure 34-28).

Case 2

A 42-year-old woman with a nasal deformity and significant microgenia underwent advancement genioplasty and open rhinoplasty (Figure 34-29).

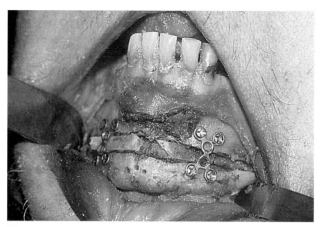

Figure 34-24. Vertical lengthening of the chin by inserting bone grafts into the down grafted osteotomy site.

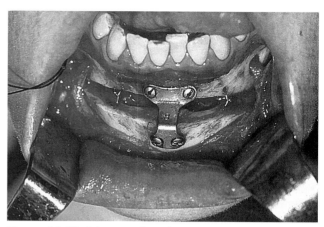

Figure 34-27. Intraoperative photograph of the preformed rigid genioplasty plate. Note that two small wires are used in this patient to insure stability of the bony movement.

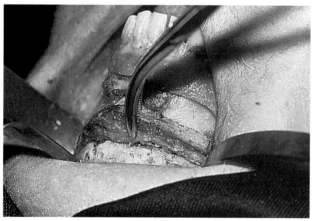

Figure 34-25. Bony ostectomy for shortening of the chin with removal of a segment of bone from the ostectomy site.

Case 3

A 25-year-old woman with class III malocclusion, bilateral crossbite, chin asymmetry, and temporomandibular dysfunction underwent Le Fort I maxil-

lary osteotomy with advancement, bilateral sagittal split ramus osteotomy of the mandible with setback and rotation, and asymmetric advancement genioplasty (Figure 34-30).

Complications

Complications after mentoplasty are uncommon. Chin implants can become malpositioned and occasionally are bothersome to patients with a thin overlying soft tissue pad. Infections are infrequent with either the intraoral or the submental approach. There have been reports of anterior mandible resorption with subperiosteal implant placement, occasionally causing secondary chin deformities.[17]

Complications after genioplasty include mental nerve injury and malunion or nounion of the bony segments. Nerve damage is extremely uncommon with careful dissection. Malunion of the bone segments can occur, but the excellent vascularity and the

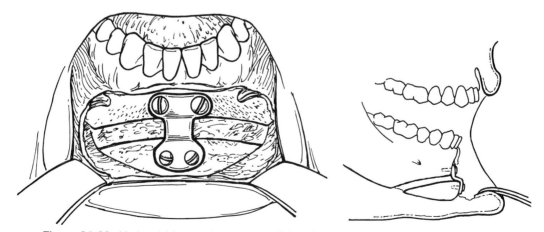

Figure 34-26. Horizontal bony advancement of the chin with fixation with a prebent genioplasty plate. If bony contact is good, a single plate can be used.

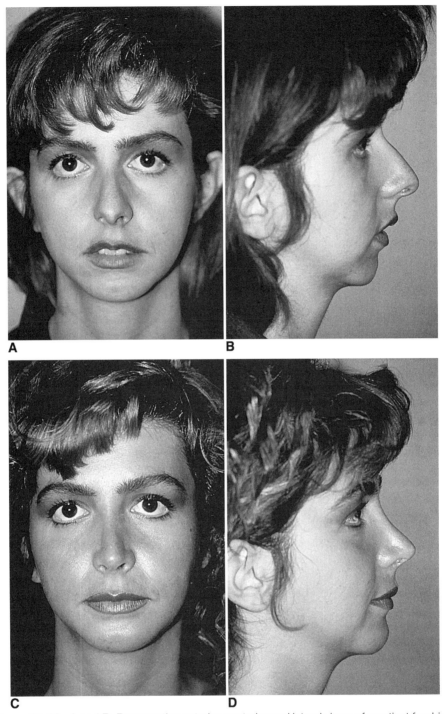

Figure 34-28. **A** and **B,** Preoperative anterior-posterior and lateral views of a patient for rhinoplasty and chin augmentation. **C** and **D,** Six-month postoperative photograph of a patient after open rhinoplasty and chin augmentation with alloplastic implant.

lack of direction force on the osteotomy site make this an infrequent problem.

Summary

Aesthetic surgery of the chin is extremely rewarding when performed in a carefully selected patient. Chin augmentation with alloplasts is a simple and effective means to correct mild to moderate horizontal microgenia. Horizontal osteotomy of the bony mentum (osseous genioplasty) is a more flexible and versatile procedure that can correct chin deformities in all three planes of space. When properly planned and

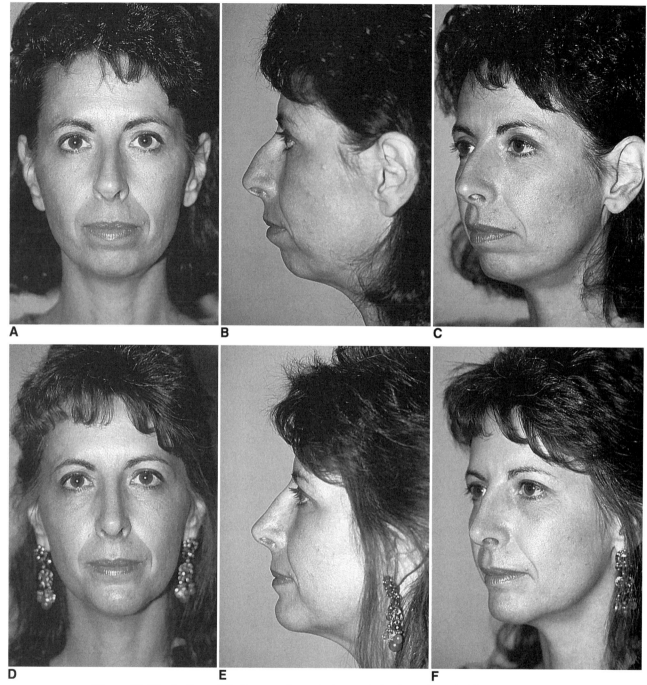

Figure 34-29. A, B, and **C,** Preoperative anterior-posterior, lateral, and oblique views of a patient for rhinoplasty and sliding advancement genioplasty. **D, E,** and **F,** Six-month postoperative views of the patient after open rhinoplasty and advancement genioplasty.

executed, either procedure provides an important adjunct for the facial plastic surgeon.

FACIAL IMPLANTS

Balanced proportion of facial features is a key component of beauty. Careful analysis of separate facial structures (i.e., nose, midface, and chin [jawline]) is important; however, a facial plastic surgeon must consider facial proportions and overall balance of all individual facial features to achieve optimal outcomes.[35]

Augmentation of deficient facial features can reduce the perceived size of prominent features and improve overall appearance. For example, a patient with a prominent nasal dorsum and a small chin (microgenia) can be treated with either a nasal hump reduction or a chin augmentation; however, performing both procedures will result in a more balanced aesthetic result.[11] Furthermore, a patient with a prominent nasal dorsum, flattened cheeks, and recessive chin will require less nasal reduction with concomitant chin and malar augmentation.

Implant Materials

Facial augmentation has been described for many facial aesthetic subunits including mandible (angle, jowl, chin), lips, nose, malar and submalar. Autologous grafts such as calvarial bone, cartilage (e.g., costal, auricular, septal), and fat are used for augmentation. This section will focus on augmentation of the face with alloplasts.

When alloplasts were initially described, they were composed of various metals. Today, most alloplasts are synthetic. Many different types of alloplasts have been developed to optimize success for specific regions of the face. One characteristic of a facial implant is the interaction between the alloplast and the surrounding tissue. Biocompatibility can be defined as "a state of affairs when a biomaterial exists within a physiologic environment without either the material adversely and significantly affecting the body, or the environment of the body adversely and significantly affecting the material."[37] This homeostatic relationship will ideally ensure that the patient's inflammatory reaction will not unfavorably affect the implant's substrate, position, contour, or stability. An ideal implant would be nonimmunogenic, durable, capable of being

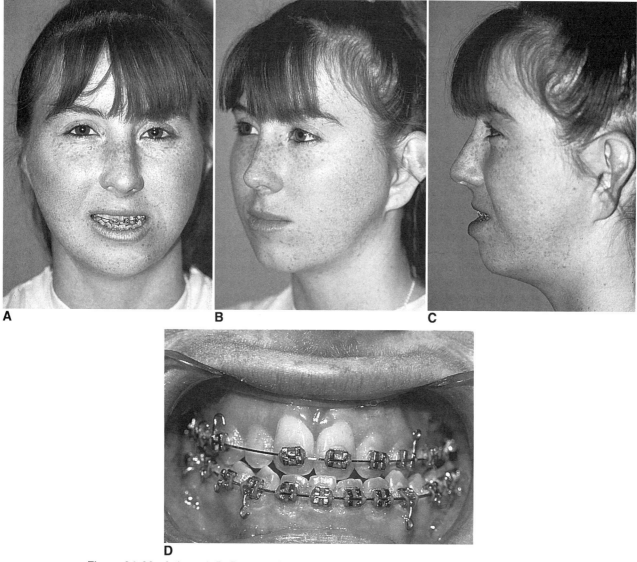

Figure 34-30. **A** through **D,** Preoperative anterior-posterior (AP), oblique, lateral, and occlusal views of a patient with significant congenital asymmetry, class III malocclusion, bilateral crossbite, and microgenia.

Continued

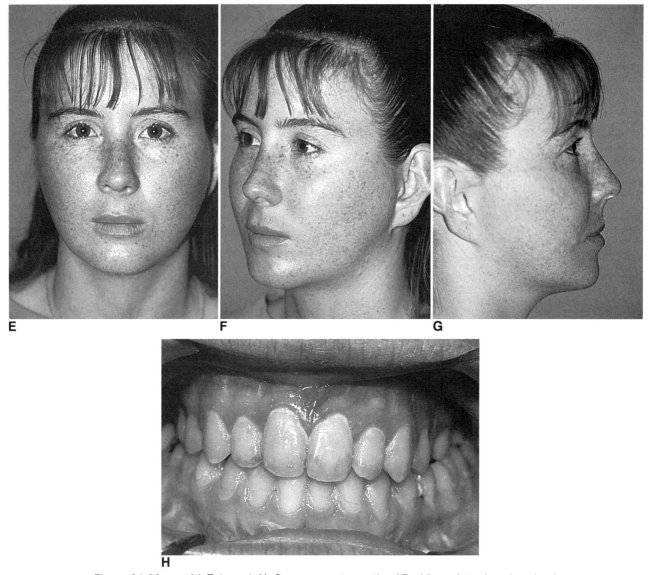

Figure 34-30, cont'd E through H, One-year postoperative AP, oblique, lateral, and occlusal views of the patient after Le Fort I maxillary osteotomy with advancement bilateral sagittal split, ramus osteotomy of the mandible with setback and rotation, and advancement genioplasty with rotation of the chin point.

sculpted, and resistant to infection (Table 34-2). Usually, it is desirable to maintain original implant size and shape (i.e., minimize implant resorption). However, two implant types exist in which resorption is expected. Absorbable craniofacial hardware is designed to completely resorb and bone cements are made that will integrate into new bone formation.

Silastic

A variety of implant materials are available. Solid implants include non–carbon-based polymers composed of silicone (polydimethylsiloxane). Silicone's viscosity increases with increased polymerization allowing liquid silicone to be vulcanized into a silicone rubber called Silastic (Dow Corning, Midland, Mi). Silastic is often used for mentoplasty and lateral mandibular augmentation. Silastic implants develop a fibrous capsule. Supraperiosteal placement is suggested to prevent underlying mandibular resorption and to minimize implant mobility (see Figure 34-14).

Fibrillated Expanded Polytetraflouroethylene

Fibrillated expanded polytetraflouroethylene (ePTFE, Gore-Tex, WL Gore, Flagstaff, Az) is a carbon-based polymer widely used in vascular surgery. Neel[21] suggested its use in facial augmentation in 1983. Tissue ingrowth, capsule formation, and resorption are

TABLE 34-2

FACIAL IMPLANT CHARACTERISTICS

Material	Polydimethyl-siloxane	Fibrillated ePTFE	High-density Polyethylene	Hydroxyapatite/ Carbonated Apatite
Trade name	Silastic (silicone rubber)	Gore-Tex	MEDPOR	Bone Source/Norion CRS
Tissue interface	Fibrous capsule	Limited tissue ingrowth	Fibrovascular ingrowth	Osseointegration
Advantages	Can be carved and removed	Sheets or tubular (lips)	Versatile, resistant to infection	Paste consistency can be molded
Disadvantages	Bone resorption, exposure	Palpable	Difficult to remove	Exposure or infection
Complications	Malposition, extrusion, infection	Malposition, extrusion, infection	Malposition, extrusion	Exposure, infection (i.e., frontal sinus)
Common sites for use	Chin, malar, nasal	Lips, nose	Malar, orbit, chin, nasal	Craniofacial, forehead

Trade names include Silastic (Dow Corning, Midland, Mi), Gore-Tex (ePTFE, Gore Tex, WL Gore, Flagstaff, Az), MEDPOR (Porex Surgical, Newnan, Ga), Norian CRS (Synthes-Stratec, Paoli, Pa), and BoneSource (Stryker Leibinger, Flint, Mi).

limited. Nasal dorsal augmentation can be performed using 1- to 2-mm ePTFE sheets.[8] A hollow, tubular ePTFE allows tissue ingrowth for soft tissue augmentation (SoftForm, Tissue Technologies, San Francisco, Ca). The author's preference for a softer, less palpable implant is a dual porosity lip implant (Advanta, Atrium Medical, Hudson, NH) with a highly porous core and medium porosity outer surface. The advantages of ePTFE as a facial implant include its preformed contour, stability, and relative ease of removal. However, extrusion and infection are seen.[29]

Porous Polyethylene

Porous polyethylene, a carbon-based polymer, was introduced in an ultra high-density form for weight-bearing joint reconstruction. The high-density form has pores of >100 microns that permit direct fibrovascular ingrowth and stabilization. MEDPOR (Porex Surgical, Newnan, Ga) is available in a variety of preformed sizes and shapes and can be customized for malar, submalar, orbital floor, ocular, auricular, mandibular,[41] or even large zygomaticomaxillary defects (Figure 34-31). In comparison to encapsulated silastic implants, polyethylene implants can be more difficult to remove due to tissue ingrowth.

Calcium Hydroxyapatite

Calcium hydroxyapatite bone cement is available for craniofacial augmentation and can become incorporated into bone.[7] Original ceramic varieties of hydroxyapatite were brittle and difficult to contour. Newer nonceramic bone cements can be mixed at the time of surgery into a paste-like consistency that can be molded and contoured into the craniofacial defect.

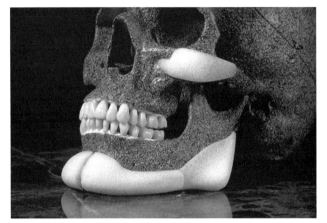

Figure 34-31. Porous polyethylene implants are shown. From left to right, a two-piece anatomic chin implant enhances chin projection while contouring onto mandibular body to prevent a chin "button" appearance as was seen with older implants. Mandibular angle implants help create an angulated jawline. A custom malar implant is also shown. (Medpor, Porex Surgical, Newnan, Ga. Used with permission.)

Two forms are commercially available. Hydroxyapatite (BoneSource, Stryker Leibinger, Flint, Mi) has tetracalcium phosphate and dicalcium phosphate dihydrate. Carbonated apatite (Norian CRS, Synthes-Stratec, Paoli, Pa) uses monocalcium phosphate, tricalcium phosphate, and calcium carbonate.[18]

Malar Augmentation

High cheekbones are often recognized as aesthetically pleasing in modern westernized culture. The malar eminence is often highlighted by makeup artists. Patients can present with a specific request for malar augmentation. On the other hand, a patient presenting for aging face consultation may not have considered the possibility of malar augmentation. Recognition of the patient's deficient and excessive attributes is paramount to achieving a balanced, aesthetically pleasing result for both the patient and surgeon. Enhancement of the malar prominence performed at the time of rhytidectomy was originally suggested in 1971.[14,31] Malar augmentation has also been suggested for congenital defects, posttraumatic bony deficiencies, and cheek soft tissue ptosis.[3,11,20] Submalar wasting (lipodystrophy) can also be improved with submalar implants.[30]

Midface Analysis

Several methods of malar aesthetic analysis have been suggested. Hinderer[13] recommended that the ideal malar eminence on a frontal view should rest posterior and superior to the intersection of a line drawn from the lateral canthus to the lateral commissure and a line extending from the tragus to the inferior alar-facial groove (Figure 34-32). Powell and colleagues[23] studied CT reconstructions and created a method to

define an ideal malar prominence. On frontal view, a curved line (see Figure 34-32, line A) is created from tragus to tragus at a vertical position located at the midpoint of the nasion and nasal tip. A second line (see Figure 34-32, line B) is drafted from the lateral canthus to inferior ala. The final line is created starting at the lateral commissure extending parallel to line B until it reaches the curved line A. The malar eminence would ideally be located at this intersection (Figure 34-33). Prendergast and Schoenrock[26] suggested that the most prominent part of the malar complex should rest below the lateral canthus on an oblique photograph. A line is drawn from the lateral canthus to lateral commissure and divided into thirds. The ideal malar prominence would occur at the upper third mark.

Another useful classification system introduced by Terino and colleagues[2] suggests five "architectural and functional zones" of the malar space. By defining these zones, precise implant types can help create balanced midface contours. Zone one makes up the majority of the malar bone and extends laterally from the infraorbital nerve to the first third of the zygoma. Augmentation in this region creates a sharp malar

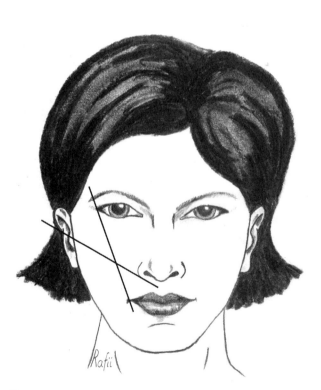

Figure 34-32. Hinderer recommended the ideal malar eminence on a frontal view should rest posterior and superior to the intersection of a line drawn from the lateral canthus to the lateral commissure and a line extending from the tragus to the inferior alar-facial groove.

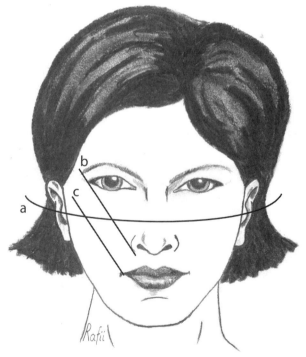

Figure 34-33. Powell and colleagues analysis technique. On frontal view, a curved line (A) is created from tragus to tragus at a vertical position located at the midpoint of the nasion and nasal tip. A second line (B) is drafted from the lateral canthus to inferior nasal ala. The final line (C) is creating starting at the lateral oral commissure extending parallel to line B until it reaches the curved line A. The malar eminence would ideally be located at this intersection.

projection. The middle third of the zygomatic arch (zone two) increases cheek width with augmentation. The malar bone medial to the infraorbital foramen (zone three) is less commonly augmented. The inherent thin skin in this region must be considered. Zone four (posterior third of zygoma) essentially designates an unsafe area due the close proximity of the frontal branch of the facial nerve to the zygomatic periosteum. Submalar (zone five) implants are used to treat a hollow cheek appearance from mid-face soft tissue ptosis in association with adequate malar projection. A wide variety of malar implants are available for specific malar contouring (Figure 34-34).[4]

Surgical Technique for Malar Contouring

Current trends in surgery have shifted from direct transcutaneous approaches to minimal incision and even endoscopic techniques.[7] Malar implant placement can be performed with a subciliary (blepharoplasty), rhytidectomy, coronal, or even transconjunctival approach. Intraoral placement negates the need for external skin incisions, minimizes risk to the facial nerves, allows direct visualization of the infraorbital neurovascular bundle, provides excellent access for direct positioning of the implant, and is the most com-

mon approach. Securing the implant with temporary sutures, cutaneous buttons, or craniofacial screws[8,40] has been suggested to minimize implant motion and subsequent inflammation, malposition, or exposure.

Intraoral Approach to Malar Implant Placement

Local, intravenous, or general anesthesia may be chosen. One percent lidocaine (Xylocaine) with 1/100,000 epinephrine should be infiltrated approximately 1 cm superior to the upper gingivobuccal sulcus. After appropriate vasoconstriction and sterile preparation, a mucosal incision is made with fine-tip cautery, with careful attention paid to avoid the parotid duct orifice at the level of the upper second molar. Standard malar subperiosteal dissection is performed to create a precise pocket with identification of the infraorbital nerve when appropriate for the implant positioning. Some implants have a preformed notch to fit around the foramen, and thus dissection must closely match the subperiosteal dissection. Porous polyethylene (Porex Surgical, Newnan, Ga) implants should not be placed on towels or gauze to prevent lint collecting on the implant. The implant should be handled with clean instruments. Antibiotic irrigation is used, and the implant is placed into

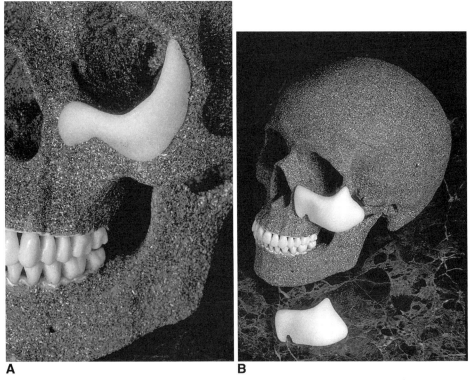

Figure 34-34. A, A variety of porous polyethylene malar implant sizes and shapes are available. A malar implant extending onto the lateral and inferior orbital rim is shown (zone one). **B,** A malar implant can be carved to custom fit the zones of augmentation needed. (Medpor, Porex Surgical, Newnan, Ga. Used with permission.)

the dissection pocket. One or two craniofacial screws are placed through the implant into the zygomaticomaxillary complex to secure the implant. The mucosal incision is closed with a running absorbable suture, and the patient is treated with oral antibiotics and chlorhexidine oral rinse for 5 to 7 days.

Complications

Inadequate preoperative analysis can lead to improper implant selection and can result in an undesirable aesthetic appearance. Malpositioned implants can occur from improper placement but may also occur due to scar contraction. Porous implants can be difficult to reposition due to tissue ingrowth. Soft tissue inflammation overlying the implant can occur but usually responds to oral antibiotics. Salvage of an exposed, intraoral implant is more likely with porous polyethylene implants and can be achieved by altering the implant size to allow meticulous mucosal closure. Infraorbital nerve hypesthesia can occur but is often transient.

Summary

Although a variety of implant materials are available, each implant characteristic should be considered. The evolution of facial implant materials provides more alternatives for each facial implantation site. These new technologies emphasize the importance of a facial plastic surgeon's knowledge of the characteristics, advantages, and disadvantages of each implant.

REFERENCES

1. Bell WH, Gallagher DM: The versatility of genioplasty using a broad pedicle, *J Oral Maxillofac Surg* 41:763, 1983.
2. Binder WJ, Schoenrock LD, Terino EO: Augmentation of the malar-submalar/ midface, *Facial Plast Surg Clin North Am* 2:265, 1994.
3. Binder WJ: Submalar augmentation a procedure to enhance rhytidectomy, *Ann Plast Surg* 24:200, 1990.
4. Binder WJ: A comprehensive approach for aesthetic contouring of the midface in rhytidectomy, *Facial Plast Surg Clin North Am* 1:231, 1993.
5. Burstone CJ: Lip posture and its significance in treatment planning, *Am J Orthod* 53:262, 1967.
6. Converse JM, Wood-Smith D: Horizontal osteotomy of the mandible, *Plast Reconstr Surg* 34:464, 1964.
7. Friedman CD, Constantino PD: Alloplastic materials for facial skeletal augmentation, *Facial Plast Surg Clin North Am* 10:325, 2002.
8. Godin MS, Waldman SR, Johnson CM: The use of expanded polytetrafluoroethylene (Gore-Tex) in rhinoplasty, *Arch Otolaryngol Head Neck Surg* 121:1131, 1995.
9. Goldman ND and others: Malar augmentation with self-drilling single screw fixation, *Arch Facial Plast Surg* 2:222, 2000.
10. Gonzalez-Ulloa M, Stevens E: Role of chin correction in profileplasty, *Plast Reconstr Surg* 41:477, 1968.
11. Gonzalez-Ulloa M: Building out the malar prominences as an addition to rhytidectomy, *Plast Reconstr Surg* 53:293, 1974.
12. Guyuron B: *Genioplasty*, Boston, 1993, Little, Brown.
13. Hinderer UT: Malar implant for improvement of the facial appearance, *Plast Reconstr Surg* 56:157, 1975.
14. Hinderer UT: Profileplasty, *Int Macro J Aesthetic Plast Surg* 1:12, 1971.
15. Hofer O: Operation der prognathie und mikrogenie, *Deutsche Zahnarztl Mund Kief* 9:121, 1942.
16. Lehman JA: Soft-tissue manifestations of aesthetic defects of the jaws: diagnosis and treatment, *Clin Plast Surg* 14:767, 1987.
17. Li K, Cheny M: The use of sliding genioplasty for treatment of failed chin implants, *Laryngoscope* 106:363, 1996.
18. Mathur KK, Tatum SA, Kellman RM: Carbonated apatite and hydroxyapatite in craniofacial reconstruction, *Arch Facial Plast Surg* 5:379, 2003.
19. McCarthy JG, Ruff G: The chin, *Clin Plast Surg* 15:125, 1988.
20. Metzinger SE and others: Malar augmentation: a 5 year retrospective review of the silastic midfacial malar implant, *Arch Otolaryngol Head Neck Surg* 125:980, 1999.
21. Neel HB: Implants of Gore-Tex, *Arch Otolaryngol Head Neck Surg* 109:427, 1983.
22. Peterson RA: Correction of the senile chin deformity in face lift, *Clin Plast Surg* 19:433, 1992.
23. Powell N, Riley RS, Laub DR: A new approach to evaluation and surgery of the malar complex, *Ann Plast Surg* 20:206, 1988.
24. Powell N, Humphreys B: *Proportions of the aesthetic face.* New York, Thieme-Stratton, 1984.
25. Precious DS, Delaire J: Correction of anterior mandibular vertical excess: the functional genioplasty, *Oral Med* 59:229, 1985.
26. Prendergast M, Shoenrock LD: Malar augmentation, *Arch Otolaryngol Head Neck Surg* 115:964, 1989.
27. Rakosi T: *An atlas and manual of cephalometry radiography.* Philadelphia, Lea & Febiger, 1982.
28. Ricketts RM: Esthetics, environment and the law of lip relation, *Am J Orthod* 54:272, 1968.
29. Rubin JP, Yaremchuk MJ: Complications and toxicities of implantable biomaterials used in facial reconstructive and aesthetic surgery: a comprehensive review of the literature, *Plast Reconstr Surg* 100:1336, 1997.
30. Schoenrock LD: *Malarplasty.* In Krause CJ, Mangat DS, Pastorek N, editors: *Aesthetic facial surgery,* New York, 1991, JB Lippincott.
31. Spadafora A De los Rios E, Toledo Rios R: Poulos planos (platizigion): endoprotesis dopolietileno insertadads pos via sub periostica de arco cigomatico, *Prensa Med Argent* 58:1946, 1971.
32. Spear SL, Kassan M: Genioplasty, *Clin Plast Surg* 16:695, 1989.
33. Steiner CC: Cephalometrics in clinical practice, *Angle Orthod* 29:8, 1959.
34. Sykes J, Donald PJ: Orthognathic surgery. In Papel I, Nachlas NE, editors: *Facial plastic and reconstructive surgery.* St. Louis, 1992, Mosby.
35. Sykes J, Frodel JL: Genioplasty, *Op Tech Otolaryngol* 6:319, 1995.
36. Terino EO: Three-dimensional facial contouring : alloplastic augmentation of the lateral mandible, *Facial Plast Surg Clin North Am* 10:249, 2002.

37. Williams DF: Implantable prostheses, *Phys Med Biol* 4:611, 1980.

38. Wolfe A: *The genioplasty: an essential tool in the correction of chin deformities.* In Ousterhout DK, editor: *Aesthetic contouring of the craniofacial skeleton,* Boston, 1991, Little, Brown.

39. Wolfe SA: *The chin.* In Wolfe SA, Berkowitz S, editors: *Plastic surgery of facial skeleton,* Boston, 1989, Little, Brown.

40. Yaremchuk MJ: Facial skeletal reconstruction using porous polyethylene implants, *Plast Reconstr Surg* 111:1818, 2003.

41. Yaremchuk MJ: Improving aesthetic outcomes after alloplastic chin augmentation, *Plast Reconstr Surg* 112:1422, 2003.

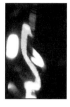

CHAPTER THIRTY FIVE

REHABILITATION OF FACIAL PARALYSIS

Roger L. Crumley
William B. Armstrong
Patrick J. Byrne

INTRODUCTION

Unilateral facial paralysis is usually a devastating emotional ordeal. The ability to restore symmetry and motion to patients afflicted with facial paralysis is one of the most rewarding skills of the well-trained reconstructive surgeon. This chapter discusses rehabilitation of facial nerve injuries. Many of the diagnostic considerations and surgical techniques described are applicable to otogenic paralyses (intratemporal), as well as injuries and diseases that affect the parotid and facial portions of the facial nerve.

The facial nerve, once damaged, rarely attains full recovery of function. The slightest injury to one branch, even if the nerve is not divided, may produce permanent weakness or another dysfunction, such as spasm or synkinesis. Any patient sustaining facial nerve injury or contemplating parotidectomy, as well as any preoperative patient with the slightest chance of sustaining surgical facial nerve injury, should be told that his or her face might never regain normal movements. It is worthwhile for the surgeon to take an extra moment to confirm that the patient understands this concept. It sometimes necessary to show patients videotapes, photographs, or movies of other patients before the true meaning of facial paralysis is conveyed to the patient.

Many patients listen to the physician's words yet are unable to fully understand the visual impact of facial paralysis or synkinesis. Therefore, it is unwise and unfair to describe hypoglossal-facial anastomosis or muscle transposition in such a way that the patient may believe that the facial nerve and movements will be restored. A realistic approach yields the rewards of patient compliance, understanding, satisfaction, and acceptance of reality. A recent review of all state and federal civil trials alleging malpractice and facial nerve paralysis demonstrates the importance of careful explanation and documentation, as well as the impor-

tance of good patient rapport and bedside manner in preventing lawsuits.[60]

CAUSES OF FACIAL PARALYSIS

The pathogenesis and eventual course of facial paralysis vary depending on the causative injury or disease. This chapter focuses on clinical situations requiring surgical reanimation.

PATIENT ASSESSMENT

Complete patient assessment is critical to attain optimal rehabilitation of facial paralysis. It is critical to properly understand the nature of the injury and the resulting defect, to know the viability of the proximal and distal facial nerve segments, to properly assess the viability of potential donor nerves and facial musculature, and to thoroughly assess both the patient's health status and personal desires for rehabilitation.

An outline of assessment of facial nerve paralysis follows:

I. **History**
   A. Type of injury
   B. Time since injury
   C. Age, overall health, and life expectancy
   D. Radiation therapy (past or planned)
   E. Nutritional factors
   F. Prior operative report
II. **Physical examination**
   A. Prior incisions and scars
   B. Integrity of trigeminal, vagal, and hypoglossal nerves
   C. Facial motion (is entire face paralyzed?)
   D. Status of eye (lagophthalmos, ectropion?)
   E. Facial tone, structure (habitus, etc.)
III. **Electromyography** (perform on all patients who have had paralysis for more than 1 year), computed tomography (CT) scan, temporal bone

(if there is any question about the cause of paralysis)

IV. **CT scan of temporal bone and magnetic resonance scan of parotid gland** (if there is any question about the cause of paralysis)

Assessment of the Deformity

Thorough history and physical examination are imperative to properly select appropriate rehabilitation options for facial paralysis. The type of injury, time since injury, age and health of the patient, coexisting medical problems, and life expectancy are key facts to ascertain. In addition, prior surgical therapy, rehabilitative procedures, and radiation therapy are ascertained. Swallowing and speech function are assessed in anticipation of possible use of the hypoglossal nerve. Whenever possible, the operative report(s) is(are) reviewed.

Physical examination includes complete head and neck examination with attention to cranial nerve function and the presence of functional masseter and temporalis muscles. The degree of facial nerve function is globally recorded using the House-Brackmann Facial Grading System (Table 35-1).[48] A number of facial nerve grading scales have been developed, but the House-Brackmann scale was adopted by the Facial Nerve Disorders Committee of The American Academy of Otolaryngology—Head and Neck Surgery in 1985 because of its reproducibility and ease of use.[48] This global scale is useful for evaluation of overall function, but it is insufficient for precise assessment of defects affecting one or more branches of the facial nerve, and it does not allow precise measurement of effectiveness of treatments isolated to one region of the face. Therefore, it is important to also assess deformity of the upper, middle, and lower thirds of the face independently. This allows more precise characterization of defects, aids the decision-making process for rehabilitation, and allows more precise assessment of treatment results. Facial tone is also noted, as is the presence of any reinnervation. Thorough assessment of the eye is also performed. Visual acuity, corneal integrity, eyelid closure, tearing, Bell's phenomenon, lagophthalmos, lower lid laxity, position of the lacrimal puncta, and eyebrow position are noted. Nasal examination focuses on the position of the ala and nasal septum and the presence or absence of nasal obstruction. Oral competence, height, and position of the lower lip are carefully noted. In long-term (>1 year) paralysis, electromyography

TABLE 35-1

THE HOUSE-BRACKMANN GRADING SYSTEM[48]

Grade	Description	Characteristics
I.	Normal	Normal facial function in all areas
II.	Slight	Appearance: slight weakness noticeable on close inspection; may have very slight synkinesis At rest: normal symmetry and tone Forehead motion: moderate to good function Eyelid closure: complete with minimal effort Mouth motion: slight asymmetry
III.	Moderate	Appearance: obvious but not disfiguring weakness between the two sides; noticeable but not severe synkinesis, contracture, and/or hemifacial spasm At rest: normal symmetry and tone Forehead motion: slight to moderate movement Eyelid closure: complete with effort Mouth motion: slightly weak with maximal effort
IV.	Moderately severe Dysfunction	Appearance: obvious weakness and/or disfiguring asymmetry At rest: normal symmetry and tone Forehead motion: none Eyelid closure: incomplete Mouth motion: asymmetric with maximal effort
V.	Severe	Appearance: only barely perceptible motion At rest: asymmetric Forehead motion: none Eyelid closure: incomplete Mouth motion: slight movement
VI.	Total	No facial function

(EMG) of the facial muscles is performed before performing reinnervation procedures. Occasionally, muscle biopsy provides additional information about the presence of viable muscle for innervation. If nerve fibrosis is suspected, nerve biopsy is occasionally indicated.

The patient's smile pattern is assessed. The smile is created by the muscles of the lips, and smile patterns can be classified into one of three types.[82] The "Mona Lisa" smile is the most common smile pattern (67%). It is dominated by action of the zygomaticus major muscle. The corners of the mouth move laterally and superiorly, with subtle elevation of the upper lip. The canine smile (31%) is dominated by levator labii superiorus action, appearing as vertical elevation of the upper lip, followed by lateral elevation of the corner of the mouth. The least common smile is the full denture smile (2%) or "toothy smile," produced by simultaneous contraction of the elevators and depressors of the lips and angles of the mouth. Knowledge of facial muscle anatomy and the smile pattern exhibited by the patient are important when considering rehabilitation techniques other than nerve grafting to recreate a balanced facial appearance at rest and the simulation of a symmetric smile.

Considerations in Facial Nerve Rehabilitation

A number of factors come into play in designing a management plan for a patient with facial paralysis. In clinical situations requiring facial reanimation, the technique used often depends on the availability of a viable proximal facial nerve.

Tumor ablation with facial nerve sacrifice (as in radical parotidectomy for parotid malignancy) dictates immediate facial nerve restitution, usually by cable grafting. When the nerve's continuity and viability are in question, however, as may be seen during and following cerebellopontine angle surgery, it is wise to wait 9 to 12 months before an extratemporal facial nerve operative procedure is undertaken. Hence, no modality is universally appropriate for all afflictions of facial nerve function. Static procedures are generally used when no viable reinnervation options exist, but can also be integrated with dynamic procedures to provide immediate restoration of facial symmetry.

Generally, however, the order of preference is as follows:

1. Spontaneous facial nerve regeneration (observation)
2. Facial nerve neurorrhaphy
3. Facial nerve cable graft
4. Nerve transposition
5. Muscle transposition
6. Microneurovascular transfer
7. Static procedures

A wide array of facial reanimation operations are available to the surgeon. Many of these procedures provide dramatic corrective results when appropriately applied, but their use may be injudicious in other patients. Factors influencing the timing and performance of facial reanimation procedures follow:

- Etiology, location, and severity of injury
- Time elapsed since injury
- Presence of partial regeneration
- Proximal and distal nerve integrity
- Viability of facial muscles (no denervation atrophy)
- Donor site morbidity
- Status of donor nerves
- Age of patient
- Health status of patient
- Radiation injury
- Patient desires and goals

Etiology of Paralysis and Location of Injury

Management of facial paralysis is highly dependent on the etiology of the paralysis. Bell's palsy is generally observed because partial or complete return of function occurs. Acute penetrating traumatic lesions are explored and repaired acutely, ideally before loss of electrical stimulability of the distal nerve fibers. The management of blunt temporal bone trauma is dependent on the presence or absence of complete facial paralysis immediately after injury. Surgical trauma from tumor resection in the parotid and mastoid segments of the nerve is treated by immediate nerve grafting. To the contrary, facial nerve paralysis from neurotologic procedures is observed if nerve integrity remains, but may often require nerve transposition procedures due to lack of availability of intact proximal facial nerve.

Time Since Transection

A chronic, longstanding paralysis with complete muscle degeneration creates several problems with regard to eventual reinnervation surgery. The facial muscles may undergo *denervation atrophy*. Severe atrophy renders the muscles incapable of reinnervation and contraction. Such severe atrophy may occur after 18 months of complete denervation, although in some clinical situations muscles have been known to persist inexplicably for many years without incurring such atrophy.[43] EMG is the most helpful method for assessing facial muscle atrophy and is therefore a preoperative prerequisite for all reanimation candidates if the paralysis is of more than 12 months' duration. The presence of nascent, polyphasic, or normal voluntary action potentials seen in a patient with facial paralysis indicates reinnervation. If more than 12 months have passed since the facial nerve injury, the situation can be assumed stable and an operative procedure may be warranted. However, in the first 12 months, these potentials may mean that reinnervation is occurring and that facial movements may return in the next few months. Reanimation surgery should therefore be postponed. Fibrillation or denervation potentials mean that the EMG electrode is positioned in denervated muscle. This is an optimal situation for cable nerve grafting, or, when no viable proximal facial nerve is available, for hypoglossal-facial anastomosis.

One of the most significant EMG findings is electrical silence. The absence of all electrical EMG potentials usually means that the muscles of facial expression have undergone denervation atrophy. The surgical implication is that nerve grafting or transfer is futile and thus contraindicated. If the facial muscles are absent or atrophied, muscle transfers are indicated.

Another effect of time includes endoneural scarring in the distal nerve segment. It is not known whether endoneural scarring acts as an impediment to nerve regeneration, but when associated with muscular atrophy, it probably further precludes nerve grafting or transfer.

Presence of Partial Regeneration

Partial regeneration is often overlooked, but it is extremely important in understanding which operation to perform. If the facial nerve has undergone enough regeneration to permit a few axons to reach the facial muscles, this partial innervation may be sufficient to preserve the muscles for many years, even though they may be totally paralyzed. This situation will optimize results from hypoglossal-facial anastomosis, which is generally preferable to muscle transfer.

Status of the Proximal and Distal Facial Nerve

As a rule, the most desired neural source for rejuvenation of the paralyzed face is the ipsilateral facial nerve. Anastomosis or grafting to the ipsilateral nerve has no donor consequence (other than the minor hypesthesia or anesthesia from the harvesting of a nerve graft) and allows at least some degree of voluntary and involuntary control of facial movement. Exceptions to this general rule are those situations in which the patient needs prompt relief from corneal exposure or drooling, and a tissue transfer/sling technique may be preferred because its effects are immediate.

For these reasons, the integrity of the proximal facial nerve is most important. As with other motor nerves, no reliable electrical tests exist to confirm the viability of the proximal nerve when it is discontinuous with its distal portion. Factors that affect proximal nerve viability, thereby enabling the clinician to make a qualified

assessment,[31] include (1) nature of nerve injury, clean transection, crush, and so forth; (2) location of injury (proximal vs distal); (3) age (younger nerves tend to regenerate more quickly and fully); (4) nutritional status (directly affects nerve regeneration); and (5) history of radiation (may impede neural regeneration).

The facial nerve distal to the injury site serves as a conduit for neural regeneration to the facial muscles following neurorrhaphy, grafting, or hypoglossal-facial anastomosis. Consequently, the anatomic integrity and continuity of the distal nerve to the facial muscles is critical. When the surgeon is dealing with acute injuries (<72 hours old), the electrical stimulator may be used to identify the distal nerve and the muscular innervation of distal branches. After this "golden period," however, the surgeon must rely on visual identification of the divisions and branches of the distal nerve because the ability to be stimulated electrically is generally lost after approximately 72 hours. For this reason, transected nerve branches in trauma or tumor cases should be tagged for identification by placing a small colored suture around or adjacent to each nerve branch. Any anatomic or surgical landmarks should be precisely dictated in the operative note. If no suture markers are available, and the golden period has elapsed, careful surgical searching (preferably with loupes or an operating microscope) may reveal each of the divisions or branches of the facial nerve. A topographic map is essential in guiding the dissection. A review by Bernstein and Nelson[10] describes the variability with which these branches are placed. The following landmarks are helpful (Figure 35-1).

1. The pes anserinus can be found 1.5 cm deep to a point 1 cm anterior and 2 cm inferior to the tragal cartilage.
2. The superior division courses from the pes anserinus to the lateral corner of the eyebrow, convex posterosuperiorly (see Figure 35-1). Bernstein and Nelson[10] stressed that these temporal branches may be multiple and as far posterior as the superficial temporal vessels.
3. The buccal branch courses superiorly then anteromedially, passing 1 cm inferior to the inferior border of the zygomatic arch (see Figure 35-1).
4. The marginal mandibular branch passes from the pes anserinus directly over the angle of the mandible and then under the inferior border of the mandible for approximately 3 cm. It then crosses above the mandible at the level of the facial vessels. Several anatomic variations may exist, requiring ingenuity in nerve grafting. When

the facial nerve trunk and pes anserinus are intact, a cable graft (or hypoglossal nerve) should be sutured to that portion of the main nerve trunk. However, certain injuries and surgical procedures may sacrifice important individual portions of the nerve, requiring selective routing of reinnervation to specific divisions. The order of priority for reinnervation of facial nerve branches is as follows: (1) buccal and zygomatic branches (equal), (2) marginal mandibular, (3) frontal, and (4) cervical (the latter may be disregarded or excluded).

As an example of selective routing, when a parotid tumor operation results in excision of the pes anserinus and the proximal facial branches, a branched nerve graft may be placed to reinnervate the zygomatic and the buccal branches, excluding the less important branches.

When nerve grafts are sutured to the entire facial nerve trunk, the relatively unimportant cervical

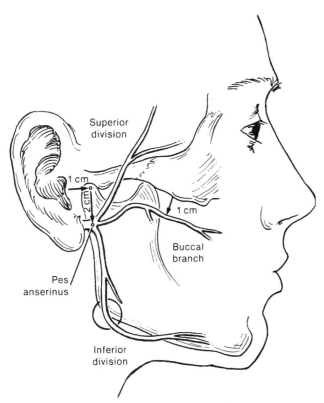

Figure 35-1. Topographic map of distal facial nerve anatomy, useful as a guide in finding nonstimulatable nerve branches for grafting. Pes anserinus is 2 cm inferior to a point 1 cm anterior to tragus. Marginal mandibular branch courses from the pes anserinus to the angle of the mandible: buccal branch parallels the zygomatic arch 1 cm below its inferior border. Superior division arcs from pes anserinus toward lateral end of the eyebrow, under line that is convex superiorly. (From House JW, Brackmann DE: *Otolaryngol Head Neck Surg* 93:146, 1985.)

branch appears to be the most easily innervated and may steal reinnervation axons needed for more important facial muscles. Fisch[34] advises clipping this branch to route innervation to the more important portions of the face. Minimal data exists, however, to confirm the efficacy of this technique.

If no nerve branches are found, and EMG shows that denervated facial muscles are present, the nerve graft may be sutured directly to the muscles that the surgeon wants to reinnervate. This technique is known as *muscular neurotization*. In these instances, the most important muscles are those of the mid-face (zygomaticus major and minor, levator labii superioris) and orbicularis oculi muscles. Reinnervation will not be as complete as in routine nerve grafting because the regenerating axons must form new connections to the old motor endplates, or they must create their own.[1]

Viability of Facial Muscles

Several variables affect the facial muscles and the results of nerve grafting and transfer procedures. Variables that can limit the results of the most precisely performed operation are scar tissue, congenital absence, denervation atrophy, and subclinical innervation.

EMG is an indispensable tool in determining whether denervation atrophy or subclinical innervation exists. EMG is the single most important test in determining the type of operative procedure to be performed. It is important that the surgeon knows and works well with the electromyographer so that facial muscles are correctly mapped, and nerve grafting or transfer is carried out in appropriate situations. If communication is poor between the surgeon and the electromyographer, the data from EMG may result in the wrong operative procedure being performed. For example, the electromyographer might fail to report denervation atrophy of the facial muscles (a contraindication to hypoglossal-facial anastomosis), and the surgeon might inappropriately perform it as a XII-VII anastomosis procedure.

Four types of information are generally available from EMG. *Normal voluntary action potentials* indicate that functioning motor axons have connections with and are stimulating motor units of facial muscle. *Polyphasic potentials* are seen during reinnervation and may precede visible evidence of reinnervation. *Denervation* or *fibrillation potentials* indicate that otherwise normal denervated muscle exists. *Electrical silence*, with no potentials seen, indicates atrophy or congenital absence of muscle, provided that the electromyographer has positioned the electrode correctly.[92]

Preexisting innervation prevents reinnervation by another neural source. Frequently, facial paralysis is associated with complete denervation of all facial muscles. However, in certain instances (e.g., otologic procedures, "failed" nerve grafts, acoustic neuroma surgery) a small number of axons may regenerate to the facial muscles and innervate motor endplates. If this axon population fails to reach a "critical mass," the innervation may not be sufficient to invoke facial movement. However, most or all of the motor endplates may be occupied by this subclinical innervation. In these cases, it is inappropriate to attempt reinnervation by neurotization procedures (e.g., introduction of nerve, innervated muscle, or neuromuscular pedicles into the paralyzed muscle) because innervated motor endplates reject new innervation. Usually this is not a problem because, in the performance of cable grafts or nerve substitution procedures, the distal facial nerve containing the subclinical innervation will be transected in preparation for the suture anastomosis of the graft or transposed hypoglossal nerve.

Donor Consequences

Many surgical procedures designed for facial reanimation borrow neural elements or signals from other systems (i.e., the hypoglossal and trigeminal systems). The consequences of sacrificing the donor nerve (known as *donor deficit*) are most important in planning for the overall needs of the patient. Certainly, the surgeon must assess the donor nerve preoperatively in all cases. The hypoglossal nerve must be tested for strength and vitality before it is transected and anastomosed to the distal facial nerve. Similarly, the trigeminal nerve must be intact and functional when its muscles, either masseter or temporalis, are considered for transposition into the facial muscle system.

The donor effects of facial reanimation surgery may be quite detrimental to the patient's welfare. For example, a patient with prior hypoglossal nerve injury on the opposite side could become an "oral cripple" if the remaining hypoglossal nerve is transected for use in a XII-VII anastomosis.

The ideal reanimation procedure is one with the following characteristics: (1) no donor deficit; (2) immediate restitution of facial movement; (3) appropriate involuntary emotional response; (4) normal voluntary motion; and (5) facial symmetry.

No currently available operative procedure satisfies all parameters. In fact, even a bacteriologically sterile and precise surgical transection and immediate microsurgical repair of the facial nerve will not allow a normal result. Therefore, the surgeon must clearly understand all operations available as well as his or her potential results and sequelae.

Status of Donor Nerves

The hypoglossal nerve is the most frequently used nerve source for transfer. Several reflex and physiologic similarities between the hypoglossal and facial nerves have been described by Stennert.[94] However, the integrity of the hypoglossal nerve must be determined before it is transferred for reinnervation. Irradiation of the brain stem, lesions of the skull base and hypoglossal canal, and surgical procedures of the upper neck may affect the integrity and function of this nerve. Preoperatively, the surgeon should ask the patient to protrude the tongue and wiggle it back and forth. The surgeon should then push against the ipsilateral half of the tongue to determine whether its musculature is vital.

The trigeminal nerve has been used for facial reanimation in many ways. The methods currently used most often involve the masseter or temporalis muscle transfer. Obviously, if either of these procedures is contemplated, the motor portions of the trigeminal nerves must be intact. Palpation of the muscle during jaw clenching will easily confirm whether the muscle is functional.

The cross-face nerve graft procedure (facio-facial anastomosis) was initially thought to be the most appropriate and ingenious facial reanimation procedure.[87,93] The procedure is unique in that it borrows appropriate neural input from the contralateral normal side and routes it to the paralyzed side. Obviously, for the purposes of this discussion, a strong donor (contralateral) facial nerve would be required if cross-face reinnervation were to be attempted.

Age

The proximal neuron's ability to regenerate declines with time because of denervation and with advancing age of the patient. This is probably because of the diminishing regenerative vitality of the perikaryon (cell body), although peripheral scarring may play a role. The clinical implication is that facial reanimation surgery should always be performed as soon as possible, provided that the operative procedure does not interfere with or injure existing innervation or ongoing reinnervation.[31]

Health Status

Patients with diabetes are notoriously poor at regenerating injured nerves, possibly because of cellular biochemical processes that result in a lack of neuronal vitality in the regenerative effort. Microangiopathy is an additional factor that may affect the grafted segment. These factors would not preclude a nerve graft procedure in a diabetic patient, but when combined with radiation, advancing age, and other factors, they might cause the surgeon to consider muscle transfer or a suspensory operation rather than a neural anastomosis. Nerve grafting might be followed by delayed reinnervation and poorer results in diabetic patients.

Prior Radiotherapy

Radiotherapy, a necessary component of treatment of certain salivary gland malignancies, appears to have a deleterious effect on reinnervation through facial nerve grafts. McGuirt and McCabe[65] demonstrated satisfactory muscle reinnervation from grafting despite irradiation in animals. Their group has subsequently documented return of facial function in nine patients receiving post-grafting radiotherapy. McGuirt and McCabe[65] and Conley and Miehlke[26] have published reports indicating that facial nerve grafts function well even though irradiated, and that nerves are among the most radio-resistant tissues of the human body. Pillsbury and Fisch[81] found that radiotherapy reduced the average outcome from 75% to 25% of nerve function recovery in a review of 42 grafted patients. Irradiation probably affects the neovascularization of the nerve graft by decreasing vascularity of the tissue bed, and probably injures the proximal and distal segments of the nerve as well. The most sensitive portion of the nerve to radiation—the pontine nucleus—is usually spared high doses because most salivary gland tumors do not require irradiation of the brain stem.

Patient Desires and Expectations

The patient's needs should be paramount in surgical planning for facial paralysis. Naturally, if the patient demands that normal function be restored, no operation will prove satisfactory because normal function is generally irretrievable.

Any single protocol is ill advised for the management of facial paralysis because patients' needs vary. The high school student with a parotid malignancy deserves the best long-term reanimation result possible; the ipsilateral nerve should be used in such cases. A nerve graft or substitution in an elderly person with a malignancy would be ill advised because the immediate result gained from a fascia or muscle sling would be preferable. Cosmetic results are not as important for this latter patient, so the most expeditious procedure to restore function should be selected. All of the factors determining the outcome of rehabilitation should be considered before any facial reanimation procedure is undertaken. Many of these procedures depend on the status of the existing muscles and nerves; other procedures depend on the patient's ability to achieve animation after the procedures and factors such as age, radiation exposure, and any preexisting disease, such as diabetes.

Congenital Paralysis

Of 95 cases of neonatal paralysis, Smith and others[92] found 74 to be secondary to intrauterine injury or birth trauma, whereas 21 were thought to be congenital. These infants should be studied with nerve excitability and EMG tests early in life to ascertain the status of nerves and muscles. Most patients with cases of injury-related neonatal paralysis recover rapidly, whereas instances associated with other congenital anomalies (such as Möbius' syndrome) are permanent. Nerve exploration or transfer is generally futile in the latter cases.

EARLY CARE OF FACIAL NERVE INJURY

Early management of facial nerve injury focuses on status of hearing and the status of the eye. Failure to recognize and treat eyelid dysfunction will result in devastating ocular complications that are entirely preventable. Ocular symptoms in facial palsy arise from several mechanisms. The ability to prevent, diagnose, and treat paralytic eyelid sequelae before major complications occur is essential in treating any patient with facial paralysis. In most patients, the outcome of the paralyzed eyelid is directly related to patient education and compliance. It is therefore the physician's responsibility to work closely with the patient to ensure understanding of the goals of eye care as well as the potential for serious ocular complications.

Eye Protection: Evaluation and Treatment of Eyelid Paralysis

Paralysis of the orbicularis oculi results in exposure and drying of the cornea. Patients at increased risk for exposure keratitis may be identified by recalling the acronym "BAD," which stands for (1) absence of Bell's phenomenon, (2) corneal Anesthesia, and (3) history of Dry eye. An inability to protect the cornea occurs because of incomplete eye closure, preventing effective distribution of the tear film across the surface of the eye, and ectropion occurs because the atonic lower lid and lacrimal punctum fail to appose the globe and bulbar conjunctiva. This causes faulty eyelid closure and improper distribution of tears across the cornea.

Epiphora may result from failure of tears to enter the lacrimal punctum, caused by pooling of tears due to ectropion and the loss of the orbicularis oculi tear-pumping mechanism. The response to abnormal corneal sensation may be reflex tear hypersecretion, which further increases the epiphora.

Any facial paralysis patient with a poor Bell's phenomenon is at risk for developing exposure keratitis. Eye pain may herald the onset of keratitis. However, in patients with diminished corneal sensation, exposure keratitis may asymptomatically progress to corneal ulceration. Thus, all patients with diminished orbicularis oculi function should have ophthalmologic consultation.

Initial efforts in eye care should be directed toward moisturizing the dry eye and preventing exposure. In terms of patient education, it is important to convey the risks of failure to protect the eye in hopes of improved compliance. If the eyelid paralysis is temporary or partial, these local measures may be all that are necessary to adequately protect the eye. Artificial tears are commonly the first method used to keep the eye moist. Ointments also may be used, but they are less practical in the daytime because they tend to blur vision.

Lacriserts, contact lenses, and occlusive bubbles are commonly used, although patient compliance may be problematic[38] (Figure 35-2). The eyelids are frequently patched or taped, but if incorrectly used, these methods may result in corneal injuries. Tape should

not be placed vertically across the eyelashes, but applied horizontally above the eyelashes on the upper eyelid, or supporting the lateral canthal portions of the lower eyelid.[102] When an eye patch is used, care must be taken that the eye cannot open because this allows contact between the patch and the cornea.

Procedures to Treat the Paralyzed Lower Lid (Ectropion)
Tarsorrhaphy

The temporary lateral tarsorrhaphy is an expeditious and effective method for protecting the eye in patients with mild lagophthalmos and mild corneal exposure. A horizontal mattress suture of 7-0 silk or nylon is placed laterally to approximate the gray line (mucocutaneous junction) of the upper and lower lids. Tarsorrhaphy sutures will remain effective longer if they are placed through bolsters made of rubber (Robinson) catheters.

For longer-lasting protection, the lid adhesion tarsorrhaphy is preferred. The lid margin (gray line) of each lid is denuded 4 to 6 mm from the lateral canthus, and a similar suture technique is used to approximate the denuded mucocutaneous junctions of upper and lower lids (Figure 35-3). Like the temporary lateral tarsorrhaphy, this procedure can be reversed if function returns. Cosmetic concerns as well as greatly improved alternative techniques to treat the upper and lower lids have led to a marked decrease in the use of tarsorrhaphies.

Wedge Resection and Canthoplasty

Wedge resection and canthoplasty are highly effective methods in the repair of paralytic ectropion. Wedge resection of all layers of the lower lid is a simple and expeditious procedure, but it can result in notching of the eyelid margin. A more effective option for lower lid laxity is the lateral canthoplasty, which is more reliable and less noticeable. Several techniques have been described for lid shortening and resuspension. They share the goal of eliminating laxity of the lateral canthal tendon by shortening and/or resuspending the tendon posteriorly behind and above Whitnall's tubercle. The modified Bick procedure consists of lateral canthotomy and inferior cantholysis, followed by conservative resection of the lateral canthal tendon and fixation to the medial aspect of the lateral orbital wall above and posterior to Whitnall's tubercle. The Tarsal strip procedure described by Anderson[2] modifies the previously described technique by denuding the conjunctiva over the lateral tendon and separating the posterior lamella and the tendon from the anterior lamella. The isolated tarsal strip is then suspended to the lateral orbital rim. Correct suture placement is difficult to attain. A solution to this problem has been

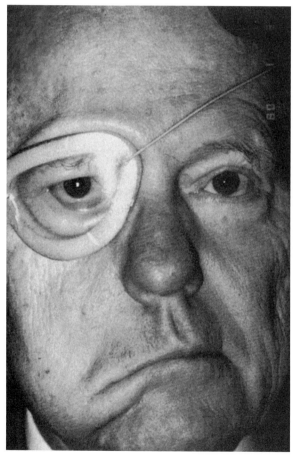

Figure 35-2. Occlusive bubble worn by a patient following acoustic neuroma surgery. The appliance has a foam rubber skin contact surface that is firmly attached to a thin Plexiglas lens. The authors have found that patient compliance is relatively high with this type of device. (Courtesy of Moisture Chamber, Pro-optics, Palatine, IL.)

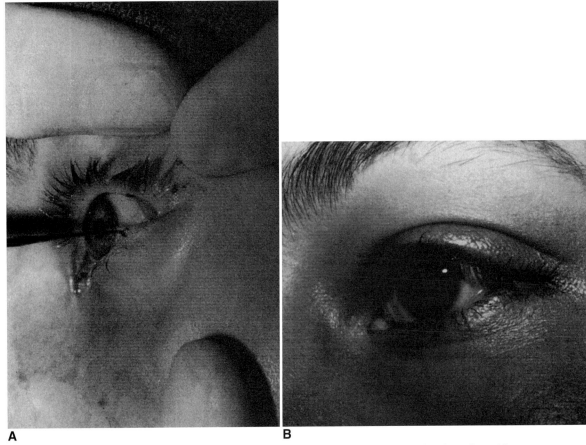

Figure 35-3. A, Tiny single skin hook being used to evert the lower lid for denuding of "gray line" (mucocutaneous junction). Note that a gray line of upper lid has been denuded. **B,** Healed tarsorrhaphy at 4 months. Increased eye closure may be achieved by extending the denudation and sutures medially.

described by Moe and Linder.[70] The lateral canthal tendon is secured to the orbital rim through two drill holes into the orbit through the lateral orbital rim. In cases of severe ectropion, the lower lid punctum may be everted and displaced laterally following lateral canthoplasty. In these instances, a medial canthoplasty is used to restore the physiologic relationship of the punctum to the globe.[49,52]

Procedures to Treat the Paralyzed Upper Lid (Lagophthalmos)
Weights, Springs, and Slings

Eyelid closure in patients exhibiting lagophthalmos can be obtained in several ways. Gold weight insertion is extremely effective and very popular because of its reliability, minimal cosmetic deformity, and relative ease of insertion. The implant weight used is determined preoperatively by taping a weight to the upper eyelid and assessing eyelid closure. The smallest weight that allows comfortable eyelid closure and does not cause fatigue of the levator muscle is selected.

Under local anesthesia, an incision is made extending equally between the medial third and middle third of the supratarsal crease, and the skin is elevated to the superior border of the tarsus. A pocket is formed immediately superficial to the tarsus to accommodate the dimensions of the weight. The weight is placed so that its inferior border is parallel to and just above the eyelash line. It is important to create a pocket directly on the tarsal plate, taking care to preserve a thin cuff of tissue at the lid margin to prevent inferior extrusion of the implant. The implant position is checked and is carefully secured with clear nylon sutures superior and inferior to the tarsal plate, the orbicularis-levator complex is reapproximated, and the skin is closed.[38]

Gold weights have some disadvantages. There is a very low incidence of extrusion associated with their use when inserted properly. In addition, weights depend on gravity and therefore do not effectively protect the cornea when the patient is supine, so a nighttime ointment is often required. If the weight is placed too far superior, it can result in paradoxical opening of the eye in the supine position. Finally, the gold weight can occasionally be noticed by the casual observer as a bump in the eyelid.

Palpebral springs and silastic slings as described by Morel-Fatio[72] and Arion,[4] respectively, have also been used for lagophthalmos. The palpebral spring technique has undergone several modifications since it was originally described, yet it remains the procedure of choice for some surgeons treating severe lagophthalmos. Silastic slings are used less frequently and are complicated by lateral ectropion.[57] Both procedures share the disadvantage of extrusion, and they are more difficult to place than eyelid weights.

FACIAL NERVE GRAFTING

Cable or interposition nerve grafts are frequently the desired approach to facial muscle reinnervation. The most common setting for this procedure is likely in combination with radical parotidectomy and facial nerve sacrifice. The clinical uses of interposition grafts are as follows: (1) radical parotidectomy with nerve sacrifice; (2) temporal bone resection; (3) traumatic avulsions; (4) cerebellopontine angle tumor resection; and (5) any other situation in which viable proximal nerve can be sutured and distal elements of facial nerve can be identified. Very short nerve gaps can be successfully treated by facial nerve rerouting. However, this is generally not possible after tumor resection. Tension-free repair is a critical element to successful nerve anastomosis. When tension-free apposition cannot be attained using existing nerve ends, cable grafts are used.

Facial nerve grafting for acute causes such as parotid malignancy requires the surgeon to customarily identify the distal facial nerve trunk divisions or branches for the distal anastomosis. Nerve restitution should be performed at this time unless extenuating circumstances (e.g., anesthetic complications, intraoperative emergencies) rule out immediate grafting.[7] If grafting is not undertaken at the time of nerve sacrifice, it should be completed within 72 hours thereafter so that the facial nerve stimulator may be used to identify the distal branches. When grafting is not done, the distal branch becomes nonstimulatable, thus much more difficult to locate and identify.

Surgical Planning

In planning the surgical procedure, the surgeon frequently finds the proximal site in the intraparotid portion proximal to the pes anserinus. This may present technical difficulties because there may not be a sufficient proximal stump for technical ease in suturing. In other instances, the nerve may be transected at the stylomastoid foramen. If transected at the stylomastoid foramen, a mastoidectomy should be performed and the facial nerve located in its midmastoid portion. Distal to this portion, the nerve's sheath merges with periosteum of the stylomastoid foramen and temporal bone, making this portion difficult to dissect free for suture. This difficult region exists roughly from 1 cm above to 1 cm below the stylomastoid foramen. Use of the mastoid portion of the facial nerve may require use of the longer sural or medial antebrachial cutaneous nerve rather than the greater auricular nerve as a cable graft.

Distally, several situations may be encountered that require some ingenuity in effecting reanimation. When the distal anastomotic site is at or proximal to the pes anserinus, a simple nerve-to-nerve suture will suffice. More frequently, however, after resection for parotid malignancy, several branches or divisions may present for anastomosis. In these cases, priority must be given to the zygomatic and buccal branches, sometimes to the exclusion of other less important facial nerve branches, because of the branching pattern of the nerve graft. Frequently, a two-branch graft can be prepared from the greater auricular or the sural nerve. This situation favors suturing of one branch of the nerve graft to the buccal branch and the other graft branch to the zygomatic branch or superior division. This technique will direct innervation to the important orbicularis oculi muscle and the muscles of the buccal-smile complex (Figure 35-4).

In the rare instance when time has elapsed and distal nerve branches cannot be found, it is acceptable to route the necessarily longer nerve grafts directly to the important muscles cited, usually the orbicularis oculi and the zygomaticus major. Attachment of the graft into a denuded portion of muscle will allow neurotization to occur.

Choosing a Donor Nerve

Several donor nerves are available for facial nerve grafting. Three of the most common nerves used are the greater auricular nerve, the sural nerve, and the medial antebrachial cutaneous nerve. Because each has distinctive advantages and limitations, the reconstructive surgeon should be familiar with each of these donor nerves to allow greater flexibility in graft reconstructions.

When harvesting the greater auricular nerve, tumor considerations mandate that the ipsilateral nerve not be used. Consequently, the opposite neck should be prepped and draped for harvesting the contralateral nerve in parotid malignancy cases. The nerve is easily identified, arising from the posterior surface of the sternocleidomastoid muscle at Erb's point and traveling

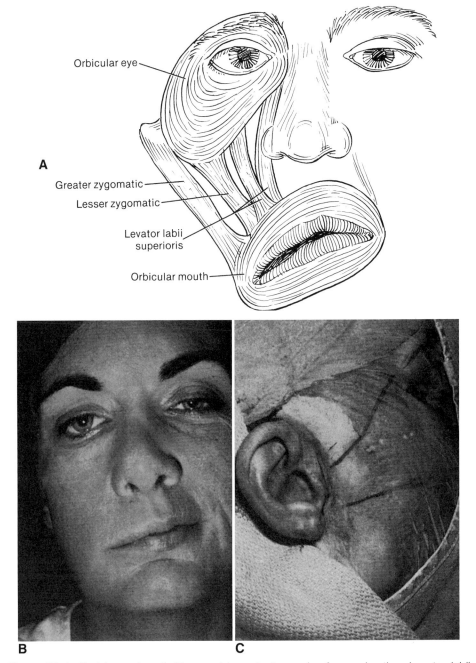

Figure 35-4. Facial muscles. **A,** The most important muscles for reanimation. Levator labii superioris, along with lesser zygomatic muscle, is probably the most significant muscle for elevation of upper lip. Greater zygomatic muscle is also critical as the strongest elevator of oral commissura. **B,** Example of a delayed nerve graft. A patient with parotid malignancy removed without immediate reconstruction (because of intraoperative anesthesia considerations). Patient was referred for nerve grafting after 9 months elapsed. Note elongation of buccal-smile complex of muscles (greater and lesser zygomatic, levator labii superioris) and paralysis of orbicular eye muscle. **C,** Preoperative surface markings for nerve branches. Nerve stimulator cannot be used to locate distal branches after 9-month time lapse. Markings are for superior division and buccal branch, based on landmarks described in Figure 35-1 and prior operative report.

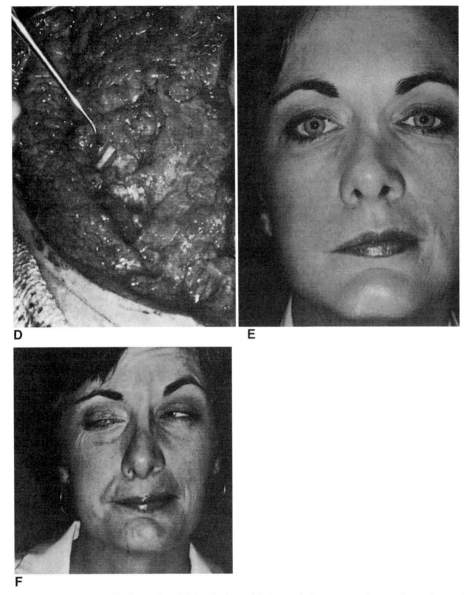

Figure 35-4, cont'd D, Superior division is found; it is ready for transection and anastomosis to sural graft (from midmastoid nerve segment). **E,** One year after operation. This is the typical result of a nerve graft when *delayed*. Orbicular eye and buccal branch muscles are improved but not normally or completely reinnervated. **F,** Voluntary motion in both zygomatic and buccal branches, with synkinesia. This result is also typical of most nerve grafts in that the temporal branch (to occipitofrontal muscle) shows no reinnervation. Note hairstyle designed to camouflage occipitofrontal muscle paralysis.

obliquely along the sternocleidomastoid muscle toward the ear. The surgical landmarks are well defined: a line drawn from the mastoid tip to the angle of the mandible is then bisected by a perpendicular line that crosses the sternocleidomastoid muscle from inferoposterior to anterosuperior, passing toward the parotid gland. A small horizontal incision in an upper neck skin crease is made along the path of the nerve. The nerve is identified in the subcutaneous tissues and followed superiorly

to the parotid gland dissecting each of the three branches, and inferiorly to the posterior border of the sternocleidomastoid muscle. Up to 10 cm of nerve can be harvested. The greater auricular nerve has several advantages: its size and fascicular pattern are similar to the facial nerve, it is easily harvested in familiar anatomy, and it has a favorable distal branching pattern for facial nerve grafting. The main limitation of this graft is the maximum of 10 cm available for grafting.

The sural nerve is also commonly used for facial nerve grafting. In contrast to the greater auricular nerve, the sural nerve is the longest donor nerve available, with up to 70 cm of graft available when all branches are dissected into the popliteal fossa. The donor site is located distant from the surgical resection, allowing a second team to simultaneously harvest nerve tissue. Donor site morbidity is low. However, caution should be exercised when working with diabetics or patients with peripheral vascular disease because ischemic pressure necrosis could result in the area of sensory deficit along the lateral aspect of the foot. The sural nerve is of larger diameter than the greater auricular nerve or the facial nerve, and it has more prominent connective tissue than the greater auricular nerve or medial antebrachial cutaneous nerve.

The sural nerve is formed by the junction of the medial sural cutaneous nerve and the peroneal communicating branch of the lateral sural cutaneous nerve between the two heads of the gastrocnemius muscle. The nerve lies immediately deep to and behind the lesser saphenous vein. Multiple nerve branches arise near the lateral malleolus. A pneumatic tourniquet should be applied to the thigh and a transverse incision made immediately behind the lateral malleolus. "Stair-step" horizontal incisions along the course of the nerve provide nerve exposure during the harvesting procedure. It is important to avoid stretching the nerve while harvesting. The nerve should be harvested immediately before grafting and placed in lactated Ringer's solution after débriding away any small pieces of fat or other soft tissue that might interfere with graft revascularization.

The medial antebrachial cutaneous nerve has been described in the orthopedic literature for peripheral nerve repairs and is used in situ with forearm microvascular flaps for sensory innervation in head and neck cancer reconstruction. This nerve has several properties that warrant consideration for use in facial nerve reconstruction.[19] The medial antebrachial cutaneous nerve arises from the medial cord of the brachial plexus, contains fibers from C-8 and T-1, and supplies sensation to the medial aspect of the forearm. This nerve has a consistent anatomy traveling in the bicipital groove immediately adjacent to the basilic vein. Nerve diameter and branching pattern are similar to the facial nerve, and there is minimal donor site morbidity with nerve harvest.

The entire arm is prepped and placed in a stockinette. The use of a tourniquet aids dissection. A linear incision is made in the bicipital furrow of the medial aspect of the arm. The nerve is located in the subcutaneous tissue immediately adjacent to the basilic vein. The median nerve lies deep to the basilic vein, and is readily identified and preserved. The medial antebrachial cutaneous nerve divides into anterior and posterior branches in the distal third of the arm. These can be dissected into the forearm to obtain adequate length. More than 20 cm of nerve can be harvested without difficulty. See Cheney[19] for further anatomic details.

Surgical Technique

For the surgical technique of neurorrhaphy, interrupted sutures of 9-0 or 10-0 monofilament nylon are preferred. A 75- or 100-micron needle is appropriate. A straight and a curved pair of jeweler's forceps as well as a Castroviejo needle holder are satisfactory instruments for performing the anastomosis. Both ends of the nerve graft and the proximal and distal stumps should be transected cleanly with a fresh sterile razor blade.[65] Some oozing of axoplasm will usually be seen at the proximal stump after preparation, but this generally can be ignored. For nerve trunk anastomosis, four simple epineural sutures will usually coapt the nerve ends accurately. However, obvious discrepancies in size or other epineural gaps should be closed with additional sutures. The needle should pass through epineurium only to avoid injury to the fascicular neural contents. The nerve graft should lie in the healthiest possible bed of supporting tissue, with approximately 8 to 10 mm of extra length for each anastomosis. Thus, the graft should lie in a somewhat "lazy S" configuration (see Figure 35-4), which appears to minimize tension during healing. Hemovac and other suction drainage systems should be placed away from any portions of the nerve graft. When adequate nerve stumps exist, securing them with a special microneural nerve clamp is helpful. This facilitates the anastomosis in a manner similar to a microvascular anastomosis.

When one division is excised or injured and other portions of the nerve remain intact, it may be desirable to graft from a fascicle within the pes anserinus to a distal branch. It is possible to dissect the nerves and divisions proximally into the pes anserinus and perform fascicular dissection at this point. Curved jeweler's forceps used for dissecting in the plane and in a direction parallel to the nerve fascicles will allow this dissection (Figure 35-5). The distal buccal branch often has several small filaments, so it may be necessary to select the larger of these for distal anastomosis.

Approximation of the nerve ends using an acrylic glue has been described (Histacryl or cyano-butyl-acrylate).[67] Subsequent investigators have shown that neural anastomosis with this tissue adhesive yields results similar to nerve suture. The technique is most helpful in tight temporal bone anatomic surgical situations rather than in distal facial anastomosis.[91]

Following temporal bone resection, the nerve may be routed from the tympanic or the labyrinthine portions directly to the face through a bony window near the posterior root of the zygomatic arch. This will shorten the necessary length of the nerve graft. However, when using this technique it is important to ensure the nerve graft's protection from trauma at the temporomandibular joint if the joint is preserved. Conley and Baker[23,24] have reported excellent results using similar techniques.

Millesi[69] introduced interfascicular nerve repair, reasoning that the exact microsurgical approximation of nerve fascicles or fascicle groups might minimize synkinesis or mass movement. It is well known that this type of repair is preferred in nerve injuries in the extremities; however, such repairs have not been universally accepted for use in the facial nerve. Several

reasons exist for this limited acceptance. The tympanic, and in many cases, the mastoid portions of the nerve have only one or two fascicles, and the intraneural topography is questionable. There are few, if any, sensory fibers in the facial nerve in its extratemporal portion, so performing sensory-to-sensory fascicular repair is not of value.

The authors, as well as May and Miehlke (in independent reports), have reported that discrete, spatially oriented fascicles are present in the nerve near the stylomastoid foramen.[28,61,66] Other authors, notably Sir Sidney Sunderland[95] and Tomander and others,[98] have reported conflicting data demonstrating that various portions of the face are represented in a random fashion in the proximal nerve. Presently, it is probably best to perform fascicular repair when the injury obviously lends itself to the technique (e.g.,

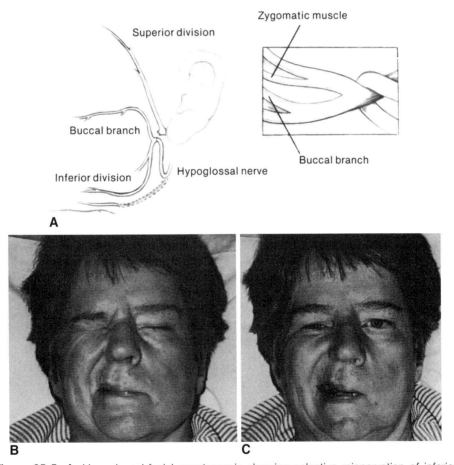

Figure 35-5. A, Hypoglossal-facial anastomosis showing selective reinnervation of inferior division, leaving superior division innervation intact. *Inset* shows fascicular dissection before anastomosis (see **D** and **E**). **B** and **C,** Preoperative view of patient with long-standing segmental paralysis of inferior division of facial nerve. Zygomatic branch to orbicular eye muscle shows preservation of innervation.

Continued

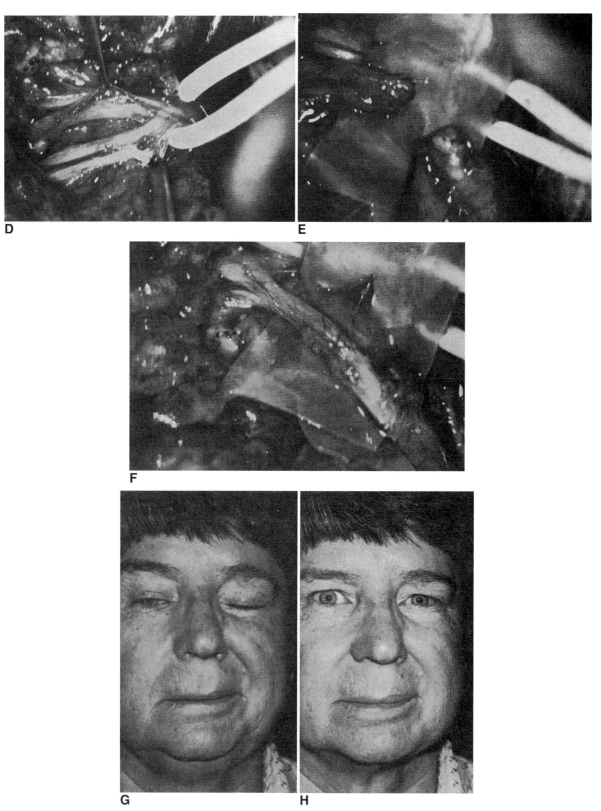

Figure 35-5, cont'd D, Perineural dissection of pes anserinus reveals fascicles destined for zygomatic and buccal branches (see **A**). **E,** Buccal branch and inferior division transected. Neurosurgical loop protects intact superior division under background piece of polymeric silicone (Silastic). Hypoglossal nerve *(lower right)* is ready for anastomosis. **F,** Completed anastomosis of hypoglossal nerve to buccal branch and inferior division of facial nerve. Superior division intact in continuity with proximal facial nerve. **G,** Strong reinnervation to entire face, 1 year after operation. Patient uses hypoglossal innervation to buccal branch muscles to enhance eye closure. **H,** Upward movement of oral commissura mediated by hypoglossal nerve, without associated or synkinetic eye closure.

clean lacerations through the pes anserinus and branch nerve grafts that require fascicular dissection in the pes). Basic research has yet to reveal the exact neural topography of the more proximal portions of the nerve.

Cross-Face Nerve Grafting

The creative and physiologic method of cross-face nerve grafting provides the possibility for facial nerve control of previously paralyzed facial muscles. It is the only procedure that has the theoretic ability of specific divisional control of facial muscle groups (e.g., the buccal branch controlling the buccal branch distribution, the zygomatic branch innervating the orbicularis oculi). Originally described by Scaramella[87] and Smith[93] in independent reports in 1971, the technique has not proved to be as advantageous as first thought. Anderl[2] subsequently described his own results as good in 9 of 23 patients, whereas Samii[86] reported that only 1 of 10 patients had good movement as a result of this technique. A more recent update by Ferreira[32] indicates that those patients operated on within the first 6 months of the paralysis did better than those operated on at a later date; however, some of these patients may have undergone partial spontaneous reinnervation because they appeared to have had lesions without total palsy, and the traditional waiting period of 1 year was not allowed to elapse.

Surgical Technique

The operative technique of cross-face grafting consists of transection of several fascicles, usually of the buccal branch, on the nonparalyzed side through a nasolabial fold incision. One to three sural nerve grafts are approximated to these normal contralateral branches. The nerve grafts are then passed through subcutaneous tunnels, usually in the upper lip. Cross-face grafts for the eye region are often passed above the eyebrow.

The anastomosis with the paralyzed facial nerve branches is done by most surgeons at a second stage, 6 to 12 months after the first. As described by most authors, the first stage is performed in the first 6 months of paralysis. This is not advisable unless the paralysis is of known permanence; for example, if spontaneous ipsilateral facial nerve regeneration may induce reanimation, then the surgeon should wait. Tinel's sign may often be elicited on the paralyzed side after several months because of sensory fibers accompanying the motor fibers through the cross-face graft. At this time, the cross-face graft is explored and sutured to the appropriate branches on the paralyzed side. This is approached through a parotidectomy/rhytidectomy approach and is usually performed within the parotid portion of the paralyzed side.

The cross-face technique suffers from a lack of sufficient axon population and neural excitatory vitality. It is of marginal value when used alone, but when combined with microvascular transfer of muscle (see below), it can provide suitable innervation. Conley[21,24] has discussed the shortcomings and unproven status of cross-face grafting. Cross-face grafting currently is only used in conjunction with free muscle transfers. Reinnervation of paralyzed facial muscles has not proven sufficient to justify use of this procedure without muscle transfer.

NERVE TRANSPOSITION

Reinnervation by connecting an intact proximal facial nerve to the distal ipsilateral facial nerve is generally the preferred method for facial paralysis rehabilitation. Only when a proximal facial nerve stump is not viable or available should attention be turned to other strategies, for example, muscle or nerve transfer.

Hypoglossal Nerve Transfer

Of the various nerves available for anastomosis with the facial nerve, the hypoglossal nerve is preferred because an anatomic and functional relationship exists between the facial and hypoglossal nerves. They both arise from a similar collection of neurons in the brain stem, and they also share similar reflex responses following trigeminal nerve stimulation.[94] In addition, the hypoglossal nerve is in close anatomic proximity and is readily available during other operations on the facial nerve. Hypoglossal nerve transection results in less donor disability than sacrifice of the spinal accessory, phrenic, or other regional nerves that have been used for facial reanimation. The most common criticism of hypoglossal nerve transfer is that it results in a lack of voluntary emotional control. Although this is true, it is also usually true of ipsilateral facial nerve anastomosis as well, in that mass movements and spasms preclude any voluntary control of eye closure, smiling, or other emotional movements.

May and others[64] attempted to decrease morbidity from tongue atrophy by performing partial transection of the hypoglossal nerve with use of a jump graft from the partially transected nerve to the distal facial nerve. Decreased effectiveness of partial transection with jump graft has been observed by some authors.[5] When the facial nerve is available for mobilization, proximal dissection into the mastoid and transection at the second genu of the facial nerve with mobilization can be performed to directly insert the facial nerve into the partially transected hypoglossal nerve.[5]

Recently, "pure" end-to-side anastomosis of the facial nerve or a jump graft into the donor hypoglossal nerve has been rediscovered[9] and reported in a small series of patients.[53] The authors report anastomosis of facial nerve either mobilized from the mastoid or bridged by interposition graft into the intact hypoglossal nerve, without removal of epineurium or perineurium. Two patients underwent direct end-to-side anastomosis of facial nerve into the hypoglossal nerve. Both regained tone and volitional motion after 8 months. Two other patients undergoing a similar procedure with an interposition graft developed facial tone but poor function. This technique relies on the presumed axon sprouting across intact epineurium of the hypoglossal nerve. There is evidence to indicate lateral axonal growth after end-to-side nerve anastomosis occurs. Rat studies demonstrate axonal penetration of endoneurium, perineurium, and epineurium.[75,76,105] Whether this technique will be applicable in humans who have decreased nerve regenerative capacity and much thicker perineurium and epineurium compared with the rat remains to be seen. It may be more effective to remove an epineural window and perform the anastomosis without disruption of nerve fibers, yet still induce enough axonal regrowth to provide tone and function. Further animal and human studies will be necessary to determine the utility and role of end-to-side neurorrhaphy for facial rehabilitation.

Surgical Technique

A parotidectomy incision with an extension made inferiorly toward the hyoid bone is usually used in hypoglossal nerve transfer. The procedure also may be performed with somewhat more difficulty through a modified facelift incision. The parotid gland is dissected forward from the sternocleidomastoid muscle, and the facial nerve is identified in its trunk–pes anserinus region. The posterior belly of the digastric muscle is then identified and the hypoglossal nerve is dissected free immediately medial to the tendon of the latter muscle. The ansa hypoglossi should be identified and dissected free so that, if desired, it may be sutured to the distal hypoglossal stump for reinnervation of the tongue musculature. The hypoglossal nerve should be transected as far distally as possible to provide extra length for the anastomosis. It is advisable then to dissect the nerve and pass it superiorly, deep to the posterior belly of the digastric muscle, to facilitate anastomosis. After the nerve ends are prepared carefully under high power using a blade breaker knife, four to eight epineural sutures of 10-0 monofilament nylon complete the anastomosis.

The procedure for the hypoglossal-facial nerve jump graft is similar to pure hypoglossal-facial nerve transfer. A greater auricular nerve graft is harvested for use as a jump graft. The facial nerve is transected on the main trunk. The hypoglossal nerve is incised in a beveled fashion to expose about 30% of the nerve fibers. The jump graft is secured to the proximal edge of the hypoglossal nerve and to the distal end of the transected facial nerve. If the facial nerve is mobilized proximally from the mastoid, it can be directly anastomosed to the partially transected hypoglossal nerve, avoiding placement of a jump graft.

Results

In the largest series to date involving 137 patients, approximately 95% regained satisfactory tone in repose and regained some mass facial movement.[6] Among these patients, 15% demonstrated hypertonia and excessive movement in the middle third of the face; however, none of these patients requested that the transferred nerve be reoperated. This excessive movement was found to decrease gradually over 10 to 20 years. However, Dressler and Schonle[30] and Borodic and others[16] have had success treating facial hyperkinesia with selective injection of botulinum toxin. Seventy-eight percent of the patients had moderate to severe tongue atrophy, whereas 22% showed minimal atrophy; this wide variability in response of the tongue to hypoglossal nerve transection has been confirmed by other series[68] (Figure 35-6). Lingual Z-plasty has been shown to minimize difficulties with tongue movement when the entire hypoglossal nerve is transected.[83] Use of the interpositional jump graft with partial hypoglossal nerve preservation preserved tongue function in the majority of patients and provided satisfactory function. In 20 patients followed up, every patient developed facial tone and symmetry, and 13 of 20 had "excellent" restoration of facial movement, with only three patients developing 12th nerve deficits.[64]

When desirable, the hypoglossal nerve can be used to reanimate only one portion of the paralyzed face. Stennert[94] used the hypoglossal nerve to reanimate the lower face while existing elements of the ipsilateral facial nerve were routed to the upper division for eye and forehead rejuvenation. Sachs and Conley[85] described a combination of the hypoglossal nerve with masseter transfer in a similar combined technique. The authors have used hypoglossal nerve transfer for reanimation of the upper or lower division selectively by performing fascicular dissection in the pes anserinus to identify the specific fascicles that required reinnervation (see Figure 35-5).

Other Nerve Transfers

The spinal accessory nerve was used before the hypoglossal nerve in nerve transposition techniques. Drobnik performed the first XI-VII anastomosis in 1879.[94] The phrenic nerve has been similarly used, but this technique causes paralysis of the diaphragm and induces undesirable involuntary inspiratory

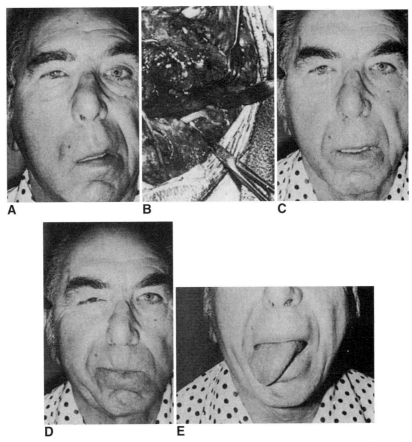

Figure 35-6. A, Patient with facial paralysis after acoustic neuroma excision. Lateral tarsor-rhaphy in place. **B,** Exposure of hypoglossal nerve. Note exit of ansa cervicalis branch to lower right of photograph. This may be transected and sutured to the distal hypoglossal, although preservation of tongue innervation is usually weak when this is performed. **C,** Repose. Note elevated commissura and reconstitution of nasolabial fold. **D,** Movement, instigated by pushing tongue tip against lingual aspect of mandible in canine region. This maneuver usually results in strongest facial movement following 12th nerve–7th nerve anastomosis. **E,** Typical lingual deviation following procedure.

movements in the facial muscles.[44] The technique is now obsolete. The neuromuscular pedicle technique described by Tucker transfers a branch of the ansa hypoglossi nerve and a small muscle block directly to paralyzed facial muscles. According to Tucker,[99] this procedure is only valuable for the perioral muscles, depressor anguli oris, and the zygomaticus muscles. The procedure is described as transferring innervated motor endplates to the denervated facial muscles without the usual delay period seen with free nerve grafts and nerve transfers. The technique allows limited reanimated strength because of the small number of axons present in the donor nerve. In addition, sound electrophysiologic confirmation that the technique produces reinnervation is somewhat lacking, despite a report by Anonsen and others on this topic.[3] Until physiologic data are presented and confirma-

tion by other surgeons is made, the procedure has potential but remains unproven. Recently, Goode has described use of a neuromuscular pedicle from the masseteric branch of V_3 to reinnervate the upper lip elevators (Richard Goode, 2002 personal communication).

MUSCLE TRANSFERS
Masseter Transfer

Although masseter and temporalis muscle transfer techniques are effective, they should generally be used only if ipsilateral cable nerve grafting is not possible. For most patients with viable facial muscles, a nerve transfer such as hypoglossal facial anastomosis is also preferable to muscle transposition. However, when the proximal facial nerve and the hypoglossal nerve are unavailable, or when facial muscles are surgically absent or atrophied, new contractile muscle must be delivered into the face. A large group of patients who fit into this category are those whose complete paralysis has lasted 2 years or more. These patients are usually characterized by severe denervation atrophy as noted through EMG. In these situations, muscle transfer is the preferred technique of reanimation.

Since the masseter was first used for facial reanimation in 1908, many modifications have been described.[58] Many authors, notably Conley, prefer the masseter muscle for rehabilitation of the lower and mid-face.[22]

The masseter transfer procedure is generally performed for rehabilitation of the sagging paralyzed oral commissure and the buccal-smile complex of muscles. The masseter's upper origin from the zygomatic arch allows a predominantly posterior pull on the lower mid-face. Transfer of the muscle can be accomplished externally through a rhytidectomy/parotidectomy incision, or intraorally using a mucosal incision in the gingivobuccal sulcus lateral to the ascending ramus of the mandible (Figure 35-7). The masseter's blood supply is medial and deep, and its nerve supply passes through the sigmoid notch between the condylar and coronoid processes of the mandible to reach the upper deep surface of the muscle. The nerve supply then ramifies and courses distally and inferiorly, terminating near the periosteal attachments on the lateral aspect of the mandibular angle and body. In general, the external approach is preferred, insofar as the intraoral approach is associated with somewhat limited access, poorer muscle mobilization, and less vascular control. The troublesome facial artery branches may be difficult to secure when using this limited exposure, thus the external approach is preferred.

A generous parotidectomy incision is made and extended inferiorly below the mastoid tip. The parotid gland and masseteric fascia are exposed. The posterior border of the muscle is freed from the mandible's ascending ramus, and the inferior attachments at the lower border of the mandible are also detached using electrocautery. The nerve supply courses along the deep surface approximately midway between the anterior and the posterior borders of the muscle (see Fig. 35-7). It is advisable to transfer the entire anterior-posterior diameter of the muscle and preserve the deep fascial layer when dissecting the muscle free from the mandible. Mobilization of the periosteal attachments along the inferior border will provide secure tissue for anchoring sutures and will provide greater length of the transposed muscle.

Continued dissection is then carried forward to the nasolabial fold in the subcutaneous plane using large Metzenbaum or rhytidectomy scissors. The external

incisions are made at or just medial to the nasolabial fold, the lateral oral commissure, and at the vermilion cutaneous junction of the lower lip. Each of these incisions is connected to the cheek tunnel, allowing transfer of slips of the masseter muscle. The muscle may be divided into three slips for attachment at these three sites, or the entire periosteal end of the muscle may be used to suture the remnants of the orbicularis oris muscle from the lateral upper lip to the commissure and below. These muscle slips are sutured to the dermis and the orbicularis oris muscle using 4-0 clear nylon sutures. May[62] reported that suturing to the mucocutaneous line deep to the orbicularis muscle promotes a more healthy nasolabial fold and more positive results overall, compared with suturing to the dermis. The best results depend on the following:

1. Gross overcorrection: no matter how this procedure is performed, gravity and natural laxity of the tissues will allow for sagging of the oral commissure, so that the intraoperative result should be a contorted hyperelevation of the oral commissure.
2. Preservation of masseteric nerve supply.
3. Placement of many sutures in the transposed muscle: the surgical assistant should hold the oral commissure at the exaggerated overcorrected level during attachment of the muscle.
4. After skin closure (the commissure should continue to be held upward), the skin of the perioral and cheek region should be painted with benzoin or Mastisol, and a tape dressing (which maintains overcorrection) should be left in place for 7 days to retain overcorrection. Perioperative antibiotics are recommended. The patient should not be given anything orally; nasogastric feedings should be administered for the first 5 days to minimize masseter movement.

Results from the masseteric procedure are quite gratifying and usually yield a high degree of facial symmetry. However, the masseter's arc of rotation will not allow for rehabilitation around the orbit. For this reason, the temporalis transfer can be combined with masseter transfer, or the orbital region can be treated separately with such procedures as canthoplasty and gold weights.

Temporalis Transfer

Although Gillies[41] is usually given credit for introducing the temporalis procedure, Rubin[83,84] deserves much credit for refining the goals of the procedure and the operative technique in the United States. Like the masseter transfer, the temporalis transfer

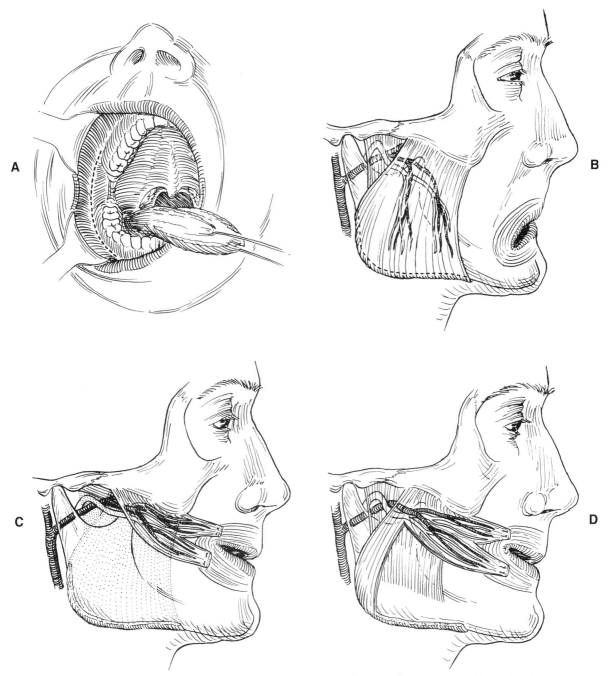

Figure 35-7. Masseter transfer procedure. **A,** Intraoral approach to masseter. Procedure is more difficult when performed in this manner; external approach is preferred. **B,** Correct incisions in muscle and periosteum. Periosteum must be incorporated in the lower portion of the muscle flap to leave the tissue secure for suturing to the lip region. **C** and **D,** Entire muscle, rather than only anterior elements, is transposed, so that the masseteric nerve supply is transferred intact with muscle belly.

Continued

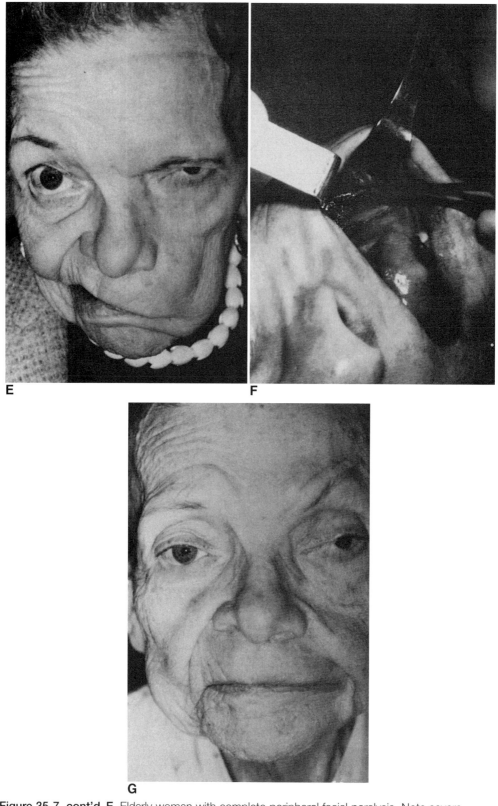

Figure 35-7, cont'd E, Elderly woman with complete peripheral facial paralysis. Note severe brow ptosis, medial tarsorrhaphy, and severe redundancy of cheek, paranasal, and lateral lip tissues on the left. **F,** Intraoperative photograph showing intraoral masseter transfer. Large Kelly clamp is used to grasp the inferior portion of the masseter, which will be passed through the cheek tissues to a nasolabial fold incision (see **A** through **D**). **G,** Photograph taken after brow-lifting procedure (tarsorrhaphy has been left for eye safety). Masseter transfer has successfully raised the corner of the mouth and the nasolabial fold. The patient declined further excision of the nasolabial fold for improved cosmesis.

procedure requires an intact ipsilateral trigeminal nerve. The nerve supply to the temporalis lies along the deep surface of the muscle. The upper origin of the temporalis muscle is fan-shaped and arises from the periosteum of the entire temporal fossa. The muscle belly converges on a short tendinous portion deep to the zygomatic arch and inserts on the coronoid process and a portion of the ascending ramus of the mandible. The muscle is best exposed through an incision that passes above the ear, slightly posteriorly, and then in an anteromedial arc. This will expose the entire upper portion of the muscle (Figure 35-8). A convenient aponeurotic dissection plane exists lateral to the temporalis fascia.

In Rubin's technique, the muscle is dissected free from the periosteum and attached to fascial strips, which are turned down inferiorly to reach the oral commissure and eyelid area. If these fascial strips are omitted, the transposed muscle's length is insufficient to reach the lateral oral commissure.

More recently, Rubin[84] refined his temporalis transfer technique by including a slip of masseter muscle that is sutured to the oral commissure and lower lip. The resulting masseteric pull improves results by providing more posterior and lateral vectors to the oral commissure.

We prefer to use the technique described by Baker and Conley,[6] who describe retaining the integrity of the upper muscle and its overlying fascia. The latter is dissected free, then turned inferiorly for suturing to the oral commissure.

A tunnel at least 1- to 1.5-inches wide must be made over the zygomatic arch to allow the muscle to turn inferiorly and eliminate an unsightly bulge. The attachment of the strip should be just medial to the nasolabial fold so that the natural crease is reproduced by the muscle pull. As with the masseteric procedure, a marked overcorrection is necessary on the operating table. A soft silicone block may be used to fill the depression in the donor defect. Alternatively, the temporoparietal fascia flap may be used to fill the temporal hollow.

Several modifications of the temporalis transfer have been reported in attempts to avoid folding of the temporalis muscle over the zygomatic arch. Labbé and Huault[56] describes partial inferior mobilization of the temporalis muscle from the skull by elevation of the posterior and superior attachments of the muscle. The coronoid attachments of the muscle are detached, and the muscle is inferiorly mobilized towards the upper lip. The coronoid insertion of the inferiorly displaced muscle is secured to the perioral musculature. In a variation on this theme, Croxson and others[27] describe mobilization of the coronoid

attachment of the temporalis muscle through a nasolabial fold approach. Fascial strips are attached to the coronoid insertion of the temporalis muscle and attached to the soft tissues around the oral commissure to produce balanced elevation of the corner of the mouth.

Although the gold weight–canthoplasty technique is often preferred, the temporalis muscle can be used for orbital rehabilitation. The anterior third of the temporalis muscle is turned laterally into the eyelids (see Figure 35-8). Subcutaneous tunnel dissection between the paralyzed orbicularis oculi and the eyelid skin allows passage of the fascial strips medially through both eyelids to the medial canthus, where they are sutured. As with any reconstructive procedure, adjustments and suture revisions should be checked carefully on the operating table to ensure proper eyelid contour.

With both masseter and temporalis transfer, facial muscle activation originates from the trigeminal nerve. Patients need to learn through videotape, biofeedback, or similar methods the proper way to contract the muscles by chewing or biting. Some younger patients may actually learn how to incorporate these movements into their own facial expressions (e.g., smiles, grimaces). However, patients should be told preoperatively that muscle transfer procedures will not allow any emotional or involuntary reanimation. In the best hands, these techniques provide symmetry and tone in repose, with some learned and induced movements on attempted chewing.

Microneurovascular Muscle Transfer

Microneurovascular muscle transfer was popularized in the 1970s and has been combined with cross-face nerve grafting to restore some facial movement.[46] Because facial movements are highly complex and interrelated, enthusiasm for free muscle transfer was stimulated by the potential to use muscles that might provide isolated or independent segmental contractions, such as for superior elevation of the oral commissure. In patients with absence of facial musculature (such as those with congenital paralysis as in Möbius syndrome), microneurovascular muscle transfer seems to have strong potential. A number of muscles have been used for microneurovascular transfers. The most popular muscles include the gracilis, latissimus dorsi, and inferior rectus abdominis muscle flaps.[90] Along with viable muscle, nerve supply must be brought into the transplanted muscle. Ideally, the proximal stump of the facial nerve is used, but this is often not possible, and the contralateral facial nerve is used. Traditionally, reinnervation has been accomplished in two stages, with a preliminary cross-face nerve graft

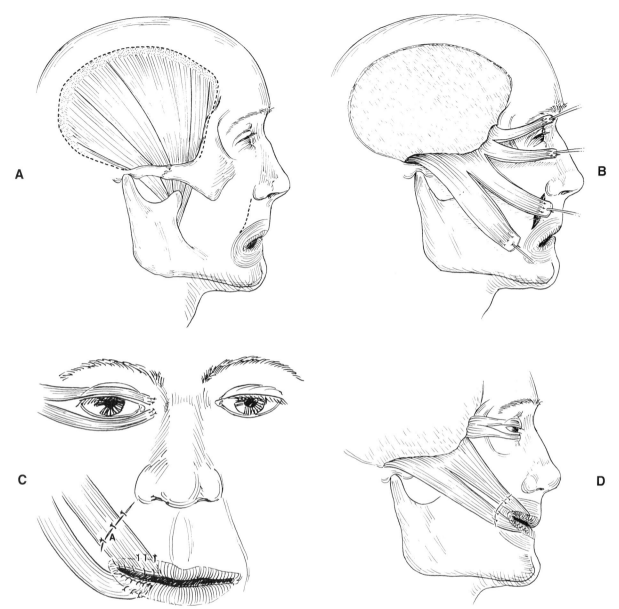

Figure 35-8. Temporalis muscle transposition. **A,** *Dotted line* illustrates incision in pericranium peripheral to edge of muscle. This results in strong periosteum to hold sutures in transposed position. Nerve supply on deep side of muscle is not shown. **B,** Temporalis muscle divided into four slips. Note pericranium at the end of the slips sutured to the muscle to reinforce the suture site. Temporal fascia superficial to the muscle can be used in the same way. **C,** Transposed slips sutured to perioral muscles. Creativity and compulsivity must be used during this portion of procedure. Overcorrection is mandatory. Sutures *(A)* must be placed in subdermis inferior to incision or in submucosal portion of wound deep to orbicularis oris muscle.[36] **D,** Completed procedure. Wide tunnel over the zygomatic arch precludes an unsightly bulge of muscle, which would otherwise be produced. Superior pull of temporalis muscle is somewhat preferred to the posterolateral pull of masseter muscle (see Figure 35-7).

performed about 1 year before muscle transfer. Neural ingrowth within the grafted nerve is monitored by recording progression of Tinel's sign along the path of the graft. When reinnervation of the graft has occurred, microvascular muscle transfer is then performed. More recently, one-stage procedures using long neurovascular pedicles connected directly to the contralateral facial nerve have become popular.[45,50,51,55] A recent comparison study found favorable a outcome with the one-stage reconstruction compared with the more traditional two-stage reconstruction.[55] Muscle preservation using implantable intramuscular stimulators is under investigation and may allow preservation of facial muscles while reinnervation occurs.[74] This technique shows promise in management of peripheral nerve injuries, and exploratory studies on the facial nerve have been initiated.[74] When facial nerve input is not available, alternative nerves can be used for input, including the masseteric branch of V_3, ansa hypoglossi, or the hypoglossal nerve.[90,100]

Significant advances in microvascular techniques and one-stage microneurovascular facial rehabilitation have greatly improved the functional outcome for appropriately selected patients. These techniques are complex, requiring expertise in both microvascular techniques and facial reconstruction. In the face of very effective alternative techniques, careful patient selection limits the number of patients who are candidates for these procedures. In general, patients with absent distal facial nerve fibers or intact facial musculature who are motivated to attain dynamic function are potential candidates for these procedures. If the patient is a candidate for temporalis or masseter transfer, careful assessment of patient goals must be made preoperatively.

STATIC PROCEDURES

Although reinnervation techniques and dynamic slings (muscular transfers) generally provide the best functional outcomes, a number of static procedures are indicated for selected patients. Use of static techniques is indicated in debilitated persons with poor prognosis for survival and in those for whom nerve or muscle is not available for dynamic procedures. Static procedures are also useful as adjunctive procedures to provide immediate benefit in conjunction with dynamic techniques. The primary benefit of static procedures is immediate restoration of symmetry in the mid-face. Success depends on mastering several techniques and selective application using sound clinical judgment. Static suspension relies on elevation and positioning the soft tissues of the oral commissure and/or nasal ala, most commonly by attaching graft materials, which are elevated and secured to the

temporal-zygomatic region. There are several major benefits arising from the use of static slings. First, facial symmetry at rest can be achieved immediately. Second, complaints associated with ptosis of the oral commissure (e.g., drooling, disarticulation with air escape, difficulty with mastication) are improved. Finally, nasal obstruction caused by alar soft tissue collapse can be dramatically improved by re-suspension and fixation of the nasal alar complex.

Several materials have been used for static suspension. The most common have been fascia lata[17] and expanded polytetraflouroethylene (PTFE or Gore-Tex).[77] More recently, acellular human dermis (AHD, or Alloderm) has been used with success.[36] Gore-Tex and Alloderm have the advantage of avoiding donor site morbidity, but use of foreign materials carries a small risk of infection, which is of greater concern in persons undergoing radiation therapy.

Autologous materials such as fascia lata require a significant overcorrection due to stretching of the implant material. This introduces undesirable predictability to the procedure. Delayed sagging as well as increased surgical time and donor site morbidity associated with autologous grafts have stimulated the search for alternative materials. Gore-Tex grafts have been used with considerable success.[11,80] Less overcorrection is necessary, and there is no need for a harvest procedure. Although Gore-Tex grafts are very well tolerated in the body, there has been concern about the incidence of infection and extrusion. Recent results for facial slings report a postoperative infection rate of 9%.[54,73] These observations, along with the further technologic developments have stimulated the use of Alloderm for static facial slings. Fisher and Frodel[36] reported good to excellent results in 9 of 10 patients who underwent static slings with Alloderm with no infections. They also report that no overcorrection is necessary, but this has not been our experience.

Static Facial Sling: Technique

The implant can be placed through a preauricular or temporal incision. In patients with a well-developed contralateral nasolabial fold, a nasolabial incision can be used instead. Additional incisions are made at the vermilion border of the upper and lower lips, adjacent to the commissure. A subcutaneous dissection plane is created to connect the temporal region to the oral commissure. In selected patients with nasal alar collapse and nasal obstruction from soft tissue ptosis, the dissection is extended to include the mid-face immediately adjacent to the nasal ala. A single strip of implant material is adequate for the procedure. This is cut to appropriate size and can be split near the end to include slips for attachment to the upper and lower lips. Permanent sutures are placed to secure the implant to the orbicularis oris muscle and deep dermis. Resorbable sutures are placed in the deep dermis to fixate the material just medial to the proposed nasolabial fold. Similar fixation is performed for a strip to the ala if desired. The sling is then suspended and fixated with permanent suture to the superficial layer of the deep temporal fascia or the periosteum of the zygomatic arch. The sling can also be secured to the malar eminence securing the graft to a miniplate or by fixation using a miniature bone anchor screw.[63] If fascia lata or AHD are used, overcorrection of the smile is achieved before fixation. Additional procedures such as a facelift may be performed simultaneously. The wound is typically closed over a suction drain. Alternatively, fibrin sealant sprayed in the wound bed as a fine mist, with our without a drain, has been a helpful adjunct to seal the flaps.[33]

ADJUNCTIVE PROCEDURES

A number of adjunctive procedures are available to fine-tune the results in persons undergoing facial rehabilitative procedures. Optimizing the care of patients with facial paralysis requires having a full range of techniques in the surgical armamentarium. Although reinnervation techniques and measures to protect the eye take precedence, there are a number of options that allow "fine-tuning" of results for the patient with facial paralysis. They can be broadly subdivided into procedures to rehabilitate the upper, middle, and lower thirds of the face. Finally, synkinesis can be a major concern, and treatment options for synkinesis are outlined.

Upper Third of the Face

Paralysis of the upper third of the face produces significant functional and cosmetic deformities. Brow ptosis may cause superior visual field deficits as well significant facial asymmetry. This asymmetry may be further accentuated after procedures to address the lower face. Browlift techniques to manage paralytic ptosis are the same as for a cosmetic browlift, the only significant technical difference being exercise of restraint to avoid further compromising eyelid closure. Direct, mid-forehead, endoscopic, or indirect browlifts are all effective. When not overdone, a browlift in conjunction with lid loading, lower eyelid tightening, or both generally produces satisfactory cosmetic and functional results. Brow ptosis associated with normal aging may be accentuated unnaturally by a unilateral lift, and in older patients, improved results are seen when bilateral browlifts are performed.[20] Younger patients do not have the same degree of unilateral brow ptosis and generally do not require bilateral elevation. Rubin[85] has described the addition of a slip of

contralateral frontalis muscle to provide some motion and correction the medial brow. Since much of the aesthetic deformity is secondary to asymmetry, manipulations on the normal side of the face including selective myectomies and botulinum toxin injections can help camouflage the paralysis. Recently, endoscopic frontal branch neurectomy combined with corrugator myectomy and browlift has been described.[71] However, as will be discussed in the section on synkinesis, caution should be exercised when considering a permanent nerve ablative procedure.

Many patients with facial paralysis, particularly older individuals, will express interest in additional adjunctive procedures in the periocular region. In certain patients with excessive redundant eyelid skin, conservative blepharoplasty can not only provide additional cosmetic benefit, but it can also further decrease superior visual field defects caused by brow ptosis and excessive folds of upper eyelid skin. Extreme caution is necessary when performing blepharoplasty in conjunction with browlift procedures. The risk of further impairing eye closure mandates a conservative approach. Maneuvers to help assess the amount of skin to be safely removed include manually holding the paralyzed brow in the normal position with observation for impairment of eyelid closure. Similarly, it is also helpful to pinch together the excessive eyelid skin to be resected while holding the brow superiorly and observing its effect on eye closure.

Middle Third of the Face

The middle third of the face is most commonly rehabilitated using reinnervation techniques, dynamic slings, or static slings. A number of additional procedures are available to fine-tune the results obtained with these procedures, and selection of the appropriate procedure(s) is determined by both the defect and the desires of the patient.

Nasal obstruction following facial paralysis can occur because of collapse of the alar sidewall from adjacent soft tissue ptosis and loss of intrinsic dilator naris tone. As described, a properly designed static sling may alleviate this problem. Alar batten grafting may also provide relief.

Mid-face soft tissue laxity and sagging characteristic of the aging mid-face is abnormally pronounced in the paralyzed face. In older patients with significant skin laxity, performing a facelift enhances the results of other treatments for mid-face deformity. Facelifts can be performed concurrently with other procedures, whether dynamic or static, and some patients will benefit from and prefer a bilateral facelift (Figure 35-9). As with aging patients, in a patient with facial paralysis the palpebral-malar and nasojugal sulci become ptotic, producing a hollowed out appearance

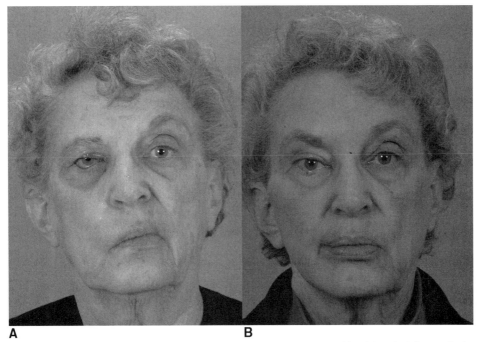

Figure 35-9. Static rehabilitation techniques in a patient with right facial paralysis. Preoperative **(A)** and postoperative **(B)** views. Patient underwent direct browlift, lateral transorbital canthopexy, alloderm facial sling, and gold weight placement.

to these areas. The lower eyelid fat may bulge, and the suborbicularis oculi fat (SOOF) descends, producing a "double convexity" sign on lateral view. In the youthful patient, the suborbicularis oculi fat typically lies at the inferior orbital rim between the orbicularis oculi muscle and the periosteum. The mid-face lift, also called the *SOOF lift*, repositions the SOOF and associated soft tissue superior to its preexisting position. The SOOF lift has become a popular technique in facial rejuvenation surgery, and has also shown utility in the treatment of facial paralysis, because of the support provided to the lower eyelid because these tissues are in continuity with the SOOF.[47,78] The SOOF lift can be performed through a transconjunctival incision, with a lateral canthotomy and inferior cantholysis. The periosteum is incised near the orbital rim and is elevated down to the inferior maxilla, where it is released. Care is taken to avoid injury to the infraorbital nerve. The periosteum and overlying soft tissue are then elevated and fixated superiorly to the deep temporal fascia.

Lower Third of the Face

The functional deficits with paralysis of the lower face are dominated by manifestations of oral incompetence. Drooling, air escape with speech, and difficulty with mastication may be present. The asymmetry also produces a significant aesthetic deformity. This is due to the lack of a smile (loss of zygomaticus function) as

well as the lack of depressor anguli oris (marginal mandibular nerve) function. These defects can be worsened by performance of static procedures on the middle third of the face, which can produce a troublesome gap in the region of the commissure from elevation of the upper lip.

Reinnervation, free tissue transfer, dynamic slings, and to some degree even static slings assist in repositioning the oral commissure to recreate a more symmetric smile. The asymmetry of depressor function; the so-called "marginal mandibular lip," is more troublesome and difficult to improve. The most commonly used procedures are wedge resection and transposition of the anterior belly of the digastric muscle. The wedge resection with or without supplemental cheiloplasty technique to improve symmetry and oral competence has been described by Glenn and Goode.[42] A 2- to 2.5-cm full-thickness excision is performed, with the lateral portion of the resection 7 to 10 mm from the commissure (Figure 35-10).

The most common dynamic technique for depressor dysfunction is the digastric transposition, first described by Conley.[25] The digastric tendon is identified via a submandibular approach. It is released from the hyoid bone, transected, transposed superiorly, and attached to the orbicularis oris via a separate vermilion border incision. Care is taken to preserve the mylohyoid nerve innervating the anterior belly of the digastric muscle. The anterior belly of the digastric

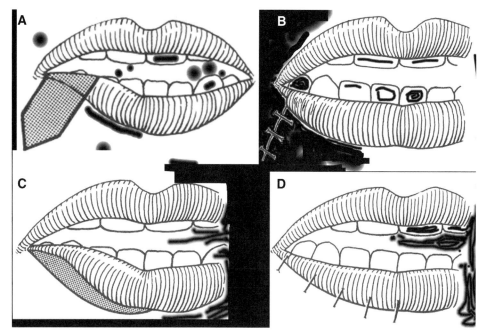

Figure 35-10. Lip wedge excision and cheiloplasty. **A,** Outline of incisions for lip wedge excision. Excision tightens the lower lip, and removes part of the denervated muscle. **B,** Appearance after lip resection. Note the intentional asymmetry of vermilion border during closure to evert the lower lip. **C,** Outline of incisions for cheiloplasty. **D,** Appearance of cheiloplasty after resection. Note lowering and outward rotation of the lower lip. (Adapted from Glenn MG and Goode RL. *Otolaryngol Head Neck Surg* 97:464-465, 1987.)

muscle might not be available after extirpative cancer surgery, however.[96] The transfer of pedicled platysma has been described with some success.[97] A technique more recently described by Yavuzer and Jackson[103] uses the contralateral functional lower lip orbicularis muscle to provide symmetry and function. A wedge is removed from the paralyzed lower lip and the orbicularis is advanced to the modiolus to provide a functional orbicularis all the way across the lower lip up to the angle of the mouth.

Synkinesis

Patients with incomplete recovery from facial paralysis are typically troubled by both weakness and hyperkinesis (synkinesis). Synkinesis develops in many patients after facial paralysis of any cause. These uncoordinated mass movements may begin within weeks after paralysis as regeneration occurs. Although the classic description of synkinesis places the etiology in aberrant axonal regeneration, it is now known that the sites of pathology are multiple. Synaptic stripping also occurs in the facial nucleus of the brain stem, and ephaptic (non-synaptic) transmission among axons contributes to synkinesis. Future efforts to prevent or treat synkinesis will require addressing each of these areas. Synkinesis ranges in severity from a mild, barely noticeable tick to painful and debilitating mass facial movements.

Careful assessment of each region of the face is performed. It is incumbent upon the physician to carefully evaluate the individual to identify the most troublesome symptoms and determine which symptoms result from decreased function and which from synkinesis. One must therefore individualize the treatment plan to address the patient's needs.

Traditionally, neurolysis has been a mainstay in the management of synkinesis, but it has been largely abandoned as safer and more conservative yet effective techniques have evolved. These include chemodenervation with botulinum A toxin injections and selective myectomies to target affected muscles.

Botulinum A Toxin

Botulinum A toxin is the most potent poison known to man, yet it has been used effectively for over two decades to treat a variety of hyperfunctional disorders including torticollis,[15] blepharospasm,[89] spasmodic dysphonia,[37] strabismus,[88] hyperhidrosis,[59] hyperdynamic skin creases,[14] palatal myoclonus,[101] hemifacial spasm,[104] and facial synkinesis.[13] Botulinum toxin causes paralysis by blocking the presynaptic release of acetylcholine at the neuromuscular junction. This typically results in paralysis of the treated muscle for approximately 3 months. Botulinum toxin A is produced in vials containing 100 U of lyophilized toxin. This preparation is stable up to 4 years in a −5°C freezer. After reconstitution it degrades rapidly, and the manufacturer recommends use within 4 hours. Systemic weakness can occur with doses greater than 200 U. The lethal dose is approximately 40 U/kg.[12]

Botulinum toxin has dramatically improved the management of patients with facial movement disorders. It is now a first-line treatment for facial synkinesis. In most persons, surgical treatment is not necessary or desired. Synkinesis after facial nerve injury can occur in any region of the face, and botulinum toxin can be used to denervate specific muscle groups. The location of the injections is targeted to the muscles causing synkinesis. Typically, 3 to 5 U are injected per site.

Initial treatments use conservative doses, which can be subsequently titrated upwards. No anesthesia is generally necessary, but many patients prefer pretreatment of the area with ice or a topical anesthetic. Patients are asked to remain upright and avoid strenuous exercise for 4 to 6 hours after the injections. Drug effects are first seen several days after the injection, with a maximal effect observed at 5 to 7 days. Additional toxin can be injected after this time if the initial effect is insufficient.

Adverse effects can occur, related to the diffusion of toxin into surrounding muscles. An example is the development of ptosis after periocular injection. This is uncommon, occurring in perhaps 5% of cases. It can be treated with apraclonidine 0.5% drops administered to the affected eye three to four times a day until the ptosis resolves.[18] Apraclonidine causes contraction of Müllers muscle to elevate the upper eyelid. Other complications from botulinum toxin treatment of the face include diplopia, further impairment of eyelid closure, lower eyelid ectropion, brow ptosis, and drooling.

In some patients, the effectiveness of botulinum toxin decreases over time. This could be the result of resprouting of motor endplates or the development of neutralizing antibodies. This may not be overcome with increased doses of the toxin.[29] Patients who do not benefit from botulinum toxin treatments, develop resistance, or desire a more permanent solution may be candidates for selective myectomy.

Selective Myectomy

The development of botulinum toxin has significantly expanded the options available to the surgeon caring for a patient with synkinesis. It may be considered the first-line treatment, and for many it may the only treatment necessary. However, there are patients who will prefer something more permanent or for whom the results of botulinum toxin injection are unsatisfactory. These patients may be candidates for selective myectomy.

Neurolysis was for many years the procedure of choice for these patients. Although Fisch[35] reported excellent results, others did not have the same success.[79] Paralytic ectropion, lagophthalmos, lip paresis, oral incompetence, blunted facial expression, and other complications from neurolysis have been reported.[8,40] Myectomy has been offered as a safer, more specific procedure for permanent resolution of synkinesis after facial paralysis.[79] Myectomy results in a more predictable result because the removed muscle does not re-grow, a phenomenon that can be seen with neurolysis. In patients desiring no further treatment with botulinum toxin, or for whom botulinum toxin was ineffective, a myectomy may be performed. In this procedure a brow incision is performed, extending to the periosteum, while the supraorbital and supratrochlear neurovascular bundles are preserved. The orbicularis oculi muscle, the corrugator supercilii, and procerus muscles are excised. Brow ptosis is addressed at the same time by excising skin and full-thickness soft tissues from the superior flap of the brow incision. A more limited myectomy can be offered to selected patients who have a good response to botulinum toxin, have limited brow ptosis, and are willing to continue receiving botulinum toxin injections. The limited myectomy does not resect the corrugator or procerus muscles and does not address brow ptosis.[79] A lid crease incision provides exposure to the orbicularis oculi, which is dissected free from the surrounding tissue. The preseptal and orbital portions of the muscle are excised, including the lateral raphe. Repair of the levator aponeurosis is performed to prevent eyelid ptosis. Selective myectomies can also be performed on other synkinetic facial muscles. Chin dimpling can be addressed by excision of the mentalis, an exaggerated nasolabial fold, by excision of the zygomaticus, and inferior displacement of the lower lip by depressor anguli oris excision.

SUMMARY

A variety of techniques are available for facial nerve rehabilitation after paralysis. The surgeon should know the advantages and disadvantages of the various techniques to apply them properly in each clinical situation. Thorough knowledge of neuromuscular pathophysiology is also important in the understanding of how time affects the available rehabilitative procedures. When properly informed of the limitations of these operative procedures, most patients can be rehabilitated and many of their symptoms can be alleviated.

REFERENCES

1. Aitken JT: Growth of nerve implants in voluntary muscle, *J Anat* 84:38, 1950.
2. Anderl H: Cross-face nerve transplant, *Clin Plas Surg* 6:433, 1973.
3. Anderson RL, Gordy DD: The tarsal strip procedure, *Arch Ophthalmol* 97:2192, 1979.
4. Anonsen CK and others: Reinnervation of skeletal muscle with a neuromuscular pedicle, *Otolaryngol Head Neck Surg* 93:48, 1985.
5. Arion HG: Dynamic closure of the lids in paralysis of the orbicularis muscle, *Int Surg* 57:48, 1972.
6. Atlas MD, Lowinger DS: A new technique for hypoglossal-facial nerve repair, *Laryngoscope* 107:984, 1997.
7. Baker DC, Conley J: Regional muscle transposition for rehabilitation of the paralyzed face, *Clin Plast Surg* 6:317, 1979.
8. Barrs DM: Facial nerve trauma: optimal timing for repair, *Laryngoscope* 101:835, 1991.
9. Bates AK and others: Surgical management of essential blepharospasm, *Br J Ophthalmol* 75:487, 1991.
10. Battal MN, Hata Y: A review on the history of end-to-side neurorrhaphy, *Plast Reconstr Surg* 99:2110, 1997.
11. Bernstein L, Nelson RH: Surgical anatomy of the extraparotid distribution of the facial nerve, *Arch Otolaryngol* 110:177, 1984.
12. Biel MA: GORE-TEX graft midfacial suspension and upper eyelid gold-weight implantation in rehabilitation of the paralyzed face, *Laryngoscope* 105:876, 1995.
13. Biglan AW and others: *Botulinum A toxin*. In May M, Schaitkin BM, editors: *The facial nerve*. New York, Thieme, 2001, p 441.
14. Biglan AW, May M, Bowers RA: Management of facial spasm with Clostridium botulinum toxin, type A (Oculinum), *Arch Otolaryngol Head Neck Surg* 114:1407, 1988.
15. Blitzer A and others: Botulinum toxin for the treatment of hyperfunctional lines of the face, *Arch Otolaryngol Head Neck Surg* 119:1018, 1993.
16. Borodic GE, Mills L, Joseph M: Botulinum A toxin for the treatment of adult-onset spasmodic torticollis, *Plast Reconstr Surg* 87:285, 1991.
17. Borodic GE and others: Botulinum A toxin for treatment of aberrant facial nerve regeneration, *Plast Reconstr Surg* 91:1042, 1993.
18. Brown JB: Support of the paralyzed face by fascia, *JAMA* 135:18, 1947.
19. Carucci JA, Zweibel SM: Botulinum A exotoxin for rejuvenation of the upper third of the face, *Facial Plast Surg* 17:11, 2001.
20. Cheney ML: *Medial antebrachial cutaneous nerve graft*. In Urken ML, editor: *Atlas of regional and free flaps for head and neck reconstruction*. New York, 1995, Raven Press.
21. Clark JM, Shockley W: *Management of reanimation of the paralyzed face*. In Papel I and others, editors: *Facial plastic and reconstructive surgery*. New York, Thieme, 2001, p 660.
22. Conley J: *Facial rehabilitation: new potentials*. In Baker CD, editor: *Clinical plastic surgery*. Philadelphia, 1979, WB Saunders.
23. Conley J, Baker DC: The surgical treatment of extratemporal facial paralysis: an overview, *Head Neck Surg* 1:12, 1978.
24. Conley J, Baker DC: Hypoglossal-facial nerve anastomosis for reinnervation of the paralyzed face, *Plast Reconstr Surg* 63:63, 1979.
25. Conley J, Baker DC: Myths and misconceptions in the rehabilitation of facial paralysis, *Plast Reconstr Surg* 71:538, 1983.
26. Conley J, Baker DC, Selfe RW: Paralysis of the mandibular branch of the facial nerve, *Plast Reconstr Surg* 70:569, 1982.
27. Conley J, Miehlke A: *Factors influencing results in extratemporal facial nerve repair*. In Fisch U, editor: *Facial nerve surgery*. Birmingham, Ala, 1977, Aesculapius Publishing.
28. Croxson GR, Quinn MJ, Coulson SE: Temporalis muscle transfer for facial paralysis: a further refinement, *Facial Plast Surg* 16:351, 2000.
29. Crumley RL: Spatial anatomy of facial nerve fibers: a preliminary report, *Laryngoscope* 90:274, 1980.
30. Dressler D and others: Antibody-induced botulinum toxin therapy failure: can it be overcome by increased botulinum toxin doses? *Eur Neurol* 47:118, 2002.
31. Dressler D, Schonle PW: Botulinum toxin to suppress hyperkinesias after hypoglossal-facial nerve anastomosis, *Eur Arch Otorhinolaryngol* 247:391, 1990.
32. Ducker TB, Kempe LG, Hayes GJ: The metabolic background for peripheral nerve surgery, *J Neurosurg* 30:270, 1969.
33. Ferreira MC: Cross-facial nerve grafting, *Clin Plast Surg* 11:211, 1984.
34. Fezza JP and others: The use of aerosolized fibrin glue in face-lift surgery, *Plast Reconstr Surg* 110:658, 2002.
35. Fisch U: *Facial nerve surgery*. Birmingham, Ala, 1977, Aesculapius Publishing.
36. Fisch U: *Extracranial surgery for facial hyperkinesis*. In May M, editor: *The facial nerve*. New York, 1986, Thieme, p 535.
37. Fisher E, Frodel JL: Facial suspension with acellular human dermal allograft, *Arch Facial Plast Surg* 1:195, 1999.
38. Ford CN, Bless DM, Lowery JD: Indirect laryngoscopic approach for injection of botulinum toxin in spasmodic dysphonia, *Otolaryngol Head Neck Surg* 103:752, 1990.
39. Freeman MS and others: Surgical therapy of the eyelids in patients with facial paralysis, *Laryngoscope* 100:1086, 1990.
40. Frueh BR and others: The effects of differential section of the VIITH nerve on patients with intractable blepharospasm, *Trans Am Acad Ophthalmol Otolaryngol* 81:OP595, 1976.
41. Gillies H: Facial paralysis, *Proc R Soc Med* 27:1372, 1934.
42. Glenn MG, Goode RL: Surgical treatment of the "marginal mandibular lip" deformity, *Otolaryngol Head Neck Surg* 97:462, 1987.
43. Gutman E, Young J: The reinnervation of muscle after various periods of atrophy, *J Anat* 78:15, 1944.
44. Hardy R, Perret G, Myers RD: Phrenicofacial anastomosis for facial paralysis, *J Neurosurg* 14:400, 1957.
45. Harii K and others: One-stage transfer of the latissimus dorsi muscle for reanimation of a paralyzed face: a new alternative, *Plast Reconstr Surg* 102:941, 1998.
46. Harii K, Ohmori K, Torii S: Free gracilis muscle transplantation, with microneurovascular anastomoses for the treatment of facial paralysis: a preliminary report, *Plast Reconstr Surg* 57:133, 1976.
47. Horlock N, Sanders R, Harrison DH: The SOOF lift: its role in correcting midfacial and lower facial asymmetry in patients with partial facial palsy, *Plast Reconstr Surg* 109:839, 2002.
48. House JW, Brackmann DE: Facial nerve grading system, *Otolaryngol Head Neck Surg* 93:146, 1985.
49. Jelks GW, Smith B, Bosniak S: The evaluation and management of the eye in facial palsy, *Clin Plast Surg* 6:397, 1979.

50. Jiang H and others: One-stage microneurovascular free abductor hallucis muscle transplantation for reanimation of facial paralysis, *Plast Reconstr Surg* 96:78, 1995.
51. Jones BM: Cross-face reanimation of the paralysed face, with single stage microneurovascular gracilis transfer without nerve graft, *Br J Plast Surg* 48:519, 1995.
52. Kazanjian VH, Converse JM: *Facial palsy*. In Converse JM, editor: *Surgical treatment of facial injuries*. Baltimore, Md, 1974, Williams & Wilkins.
53. Koh KS and others: Hypoglossal-facial crossover in facial-nerve palsy: pure end-to-side anastomosis technique, *Br J Plast Surg* 55:25, 2002.
54. Konior RJ: Facial paralysis reconstruction with Gore-Tex Soft-Tissue Patch, *Arch Otolaryngol Head Neck Surg* 118:1188, 1992.
55. Kumar PA, Hassan KM: Cross-face nerve graft with free-muscle transfer for reanimation of the paralyzed face: a comparative study of the single-stage and two-stage procedures, *Plast Reconstr Surg* 109:451, 2002.
56. Labbé D, Huault M: Lengthening temporalis myoplasty and lip reanimation, *Plast Reconstr Surg* 105:1289, 2000.
57. Levine R: *Eyelid reanimation surgery*. In May M, editor: *The facial nerve*. New York, 1986, Thieme.
58. Lexer E, Eden R: Uber die Chirurgische Behandlung der Peripheren Facialislahmung, *Beitr Klin* 73:116, 1911.
59. Lowe NJ and others: Efficacy and safety of botulinum toxin type a in the treatment of palmar hyperhidrosis: a double-blind, randomized, placebo-controlled study, *Dermatol Surg* 28:822, 2002.
60. Lydiatt DD: Medical malpractice and facial nerve paralysis, *Arch Otolaryngol Head Neck Surg* 129:50, 2003.
61. May M: Anatomy of the facial nerve (spatial orientation of fibers in the temporal bone), *Laryngoscope* 83:1311, 1973.
62. May M: Muscle transposition for facial reanimation. Indications and results, *Arch Otolaryngol* 110:184, 1984.
63. May M: *Regional reanimation: nose and mouth*. In May M, Schaitkin BM, editors: *The facial nerve*. New York, 2001, Thieme, p 775.
64. May M, Sobol SM, Mester SJ: Hypoglossal-facial nerve interpositional-jump graft for facial reanimation without tongue atrophy, *Otolaryngol Head Neck Surg* 104:818, 1991.
65. McCabe BF: Facial nerve grafting, *Plast Reconstr Surg* 45:70-75, 1970.
66. Miehlke A: A topography of the course of fibers in the fascialis stem, *Arch Klin Exp Ohren Nasen Kehlkopfkunde (Berlin)*:171, 1958.
67. Miehlke A: Probleme Beider Naht der Feinstenperipheren Neruen im Bereich der Otolaryngologie, *Melsunger Med Mitteilungen* 42:71, 1968.
68. Miehlke A, Stennert E, Chilla R: New aspects in facial nerve surgery, *Clin Plast Surg* 6:451-486, 1979.
69. Millesi H: *Facial nerve suture*. In Fisch U, editor: *Facial nerve surgery*. Birmingham, Ala, Aesculapius Publishing, 1977.
70. Moe KS, Linder T: The lateral transorbital canthopexy for correction and prevention of ectropion: report of a procedure, grading system, and outcome study. *Arch Facial Plast Surg* 2:9, 2000.
71. Moody FP and others: Endoscopic frontal branch neurectomy, corrugator myectomy, and brow lift for forehead asymmetry after facial nerve palsy, *Plast Reconstr Surg* 108:218, 2001.
72. Morel-Fatio D, Lalardrie JP: Palliative surgical treatment of facial paralysis: the palpebral spring, *Plast Reconstr Surg* 33:446, 1964.
73. Moser G, Oberascher G: Reanimation of the paralyzed face with new gold weight implants and Goretex soft-tissue patches, *Eur Arch Otorhinolaryngol* 254 (Suppl 1):S76, 1997.
74. Nicolaidis SC, Williams HB: Muscle preservation using an implantable electrical system after nerve injury and repair, *Microsurgery* 21:241, 2001.
75. Noah EM and others: A new animal model to investigate axonal sprouting after end-to-side neurorrhaphy, *J Reconstr Microsurg* 13:317, 1997.
76. Noah EM and others: End-to-side neurorrhaphy: a histologic and morphometric study of axonal sprouting into an end-to-side nerve graft, *J Reconstr Microsurg* 13:99, 1997.
77. Okamura H, Yanagihara N: Multiple facial suspensions in protracted facial palsy, *Auris Nasus Larynx* 14:105, 1987.
78. Olver JM: Raising the suborbicularis oculi fat (SOOF): its role in chronic facial palsy, *Br J Ophthalmol* 84:1401, 2000.
79. Patel BCK, Anderson RL, May M: *Selective myectomy*. In May M, Schaitkin BM, editors: *The facial nerve*. New York, Thieme, 2001, p 467.
80. Petroff MA, Goode RL, Levet Y: Gore-Tex implants: applications in facial paralysis rehabilitation and soft-tissue augmentation, *Laryngoscope* 102:1185, 1992.
81. Pillsbury HC, Fisch U: Extratemporal facial nerve grafting and radiotherapy, *Arch Otolaryngol* 105:441, 1979.
82. Rubin LR: The anatomy of a smile: its importance in the treatment of facial paralysis, *Plast Reconstr Surg* 53:384, 1974.
83. Rubin LR: *Reanimation of the paralyzed face: new approaches*. St. Louis, 1977, Mosby.
84. Rubin LR: *Reanimation of total unilateral facial paralysis by the contiguous facial muscle technique*. In Rubin LR, editor: *The paralyzed face*. St. Louis, 1991, Mosby.
85. Rubin LR, Lee GW, Simpson RI: Reanimation of the long-standing partial facial paralysis, *Plast Reconstr Surg* 77:41, 1986.
86. Sachs ME, Conley J: Dual simultaneous systems for facial reanimation, *Arch Otolaryngol* 109:137, 1983.
87. Samii M: *Nerves of the head and neck: management of peripheral nerve problems*. In Omer G and Spinner M, editors: *Management of peripheral nerve problems*. Philadelphia, 1970, WB Saunders.
88. Scaramella LL: L'anastomosi tradue nervi facciali, *Arch Otologia* 82:208, 1971.
89. Scott AB: Botulinum toxin injection into extraocular muscles as an alternative to strabismus surgery, *Ophthalmology* 87:1044, 1980.
90. Scott AB, Kennedy RA, Stubbs HA: Botulinum A toxin injection as a treatment for blepharospasm, *Arch Ophthalmol* 103:347, 1985.
91. Shindo M: Facial reanimation with microneurovascular free flaps, *Facial Plast Surg* 16:357, 2000.
92. Siedentop KH, Loewy A: Facial nerve repair with tissue adhesive, *Arch Otolaryngol* 105:423, 1979.
93. Smith JD, Crumley RL, Harker LA: Facial paralysis in the newborn, *Otolaryngol Head Neck Surg* 89:1021, 1981.
94. Smith JW: *A new technique of facial reanimation*. Transactions of fifth international congress of plastic and reconstructive surgery, Chatswood, MSW, Australia, Butterworths, 1971.
95. Stennert EI: Hypoglossal facial anastomosis: its significance for modern facial surgery: II. Combined approach in extratemporal facial nerve reconstruction, *Clin Plast Surg* 6:471, 1979.
96. Sunderland S: *Mass movements after facial nerve injury*. In Fisch U, editor: *Facial surgery*. Birmingham, Ala, Aesculapius Publishing, 1977.

97. Tan ST: Anterior belly of digastric muscle transfer: a useful technique in head and neck surgery, *Head Neck* 24:947, 2002.

98. Terzis JK, Kalantarian B: Microsurgical strategies in 74 patients for restoration of dynamic depressor muscle mechanism: a neglected target in facial reanimation, *Plast Reconstr Surg* 105:1917, 2000.

99. Tomander L, Aldshogius H, Grant G: *Motor fiber organization of the facial nerve in the rat*. In House W, editor: *Disorders of the facial nerve*. New York, Raven Press, 1980.

100. Tucker HM: The management of facial paralysis due to extracranial injuries, *Laryngoscope* 88:348, 1978.

101. Ueda K, Harii K, Yamada A: Free neurovascular muscle transplantation for the treatment of facial paralysis using the hypoglossal nerve as a recipient motor source, *Plast Reconstr Surg* 94:808, 1994.

102. Varney SM and others: Palatal myoclonus: treatment with Clostridium botulinum toxin injection, *Otolaryngol Head Neck Surg* 114:317, 1996.

103. Wesley RE, Jackson CG: *Facial palsy*. In Hornblass A, editor: *Oculoplastic, orbital and reconstructive surgery, vol I, Eyelids*. Baltimore, Md, Williams & Wilkins, 1988.

104. Yavuzer R, Jackson IT: Partial lip resection with orbicularis oris transposition for lower lip correction in unilateral facial paralysis, *Plast Reconstr Surg* 108:1874, 2001.

105. Yoshimura DM and others: Treatment of hemifacial spasm with botulinum toxin, *Muscle Nerve* 15:1045, 1992.

106. Zhao JZ, Chen ZW, Chen TY: Nerve regeneration after terminolateral neurorrhaphy: experimental study in rats, *J Reconstr Microsurg* 13:31, 1997.

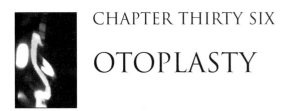

CHAPTER THIRTY SIX

OTOPLASTY

Peter A. Adamson
Suzanne K. Doud Galli

INTRODUCTION

Although protruding ears are considered a sign of good fortune by some Asians, in most other cultures, they are associated with feelings of anxiety, social discomfort, and even abnormal behavior.[1] They are frequently a source of teasing or social ridicule, especially for young children.

Fortunately, today there are techniques that allow for correction of this deformity with minimal pain and disruption of lifestyle. Achieving success as an otoplasty surgeon requires an appreciation of facial aesthetics, intimate knowledge of ear anatomy, a firm understanding of the rationale for the surgical technique employed, and meticulous attention to technical detail (Figure 36-1).

HISTORY

Otoplasty has a long history. The Indian method of auricular reconstruction was described as early as the 7th century, in the writings of Sushruta.[26] Sushruta's writings were some of the earliest on the topic of Ayurveda (Indian medicine), and many of modern plastic surgery's roots stem directly from these ancient Indian teachings. In 1597, Tagliacozzi[43] published "De Curtorum Chirugia," which described techniques of auricular and other reconstruction and became known as the Italian method. However, in the early 1800s, the Prussian surgeon Johann Friedrich Dieffenbach described the first technique for treating prominent ears. His techniques were published in the treatise "Die Operative Chirugie," an extraordinary two-volume work that encompassed all types of reconstructive and general surgical methods.[14] He specified setting back the pinna by suturing the auricular cartilage to the mastoid periosteum once the postauricular skin had been excised.

A few years later, Ely described his treatment of protruding ears with an anterior approach involving a fusiform excision of skin and cartilage.[15] Monks redefined this approach and treated children with a skin-only excision in the cephaloauricular sulcus and adults with an excision of skin with cartilage.[34]

In the early 1900s, Morestin[35] devised a method of excising the conchal cartilage at the medial wall to break the "spring" of the cartilage; this served to medialize the antihelix and decrease the projection of the concha. In 1910, Luckett[30] reported on his method of reestablishing the antihelix with an excision of cartilage and plication of the edges. In 1937, Davis and Kitlowski[12] reported on their technique, which combined cartilage excision, incision, and shaving; these, in addition to postauricular skin removal and sutures through the cartilage, were used to create a new antihelix. Becker[7] sought to avoid unnatural cartilaginous ridging with incisions through the cartilage and reported on his technique in 1949. In 1955, Converse[11] created a new antihelix with two parallel incisions along with suturing; he used a wire brush to round off the edges. In 1958, Gibson and Davis[22] reported that making relaxing incisions in the cartilage resulted in a bending on the opposite side. Farrior,[18] in 1959, recorded his excision of cartilage wedges to break the cartilage spring before stabilizing the antihelix with a suture. In 1963, Stenstrom[42] reported his findings that scoring the cartilage anteriorly facilitated the posterior plication; this method was particularly applicable to strong, stiff cartilage. In 1967, Kaye[29] reported on his technique, which involved anterior scoring and posterior plication with removal of a vertical ellipse of the conchal cartilage (Figure 36-2).

Surgery for the treatment of protruding ears has since evolved. More modern techniques center on less invasive therapies and recognize the underlying anatomical defects. This is evident, in particular, with the Mustarde method of reestablishing the antihelical relief and the Furnas conchal setback method.

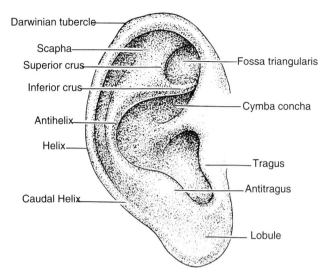

Darwinian tubercle

Scapha

Superior crus

Inferior crus

Antihelix

Helix

Caudal Helix

Fossa triangularis

Cymba concha

Tragus

Antitragus

Lobule

Figure 36-1. Anatomic landmarks of the normal ear. (Adapted from Adamson PA, Tropper GJ, McGraw BL: *Otoplasty.* In Krause CJ, Mangat DS, Pastorek N, editors: *Aesthetic facial surgery.* Philadelphia, 1991, J.B. Lippincott, Figure 40-1, p 709.)

Mustarde[36] published his method in 1963 and described using suture plication at three points without incision of the cartilage. Furnas'[21] technique was published in 1968 and introduced correction of conchal excess by suturing the concha to the mastoid (Figure 36-3).

INCIDENCE

The incidence of microtia is 1 in 20,000; however, protruding ears are much more prevalent and may be the most common congenital deformity of the head and neck.[5] In the Caucasian population, the incidence

is 5%,[5] with the unfurled helix being the most common abnormality.[21] The hypertrophic protruding conchal bowl is the second most common deformity and is often present with the deformity of the antihelix.[49]

ETIOLOGY

Genetic predisposition plays a role in this development; this is clearly seen in families with auricular deformities in both the parents and the children. In one study, 59% of otoplasty patients had a positive family history,[39] and it has been shown that the inheritance is autosomal dominant with variable penetrance.[38]

ANATOMY AND EMBRYOLOGY

The pinna is an appendage that is composed of fibroelastic cartilage covered in very thin skin. On the anterior aspect, the skin attaches to the perichondrium, whereas posteriorly there is a thin layer of areolar connective tissue underlying the skin. The auricular cartilage is an extension of the cartilage of the external auditory canal; it is invested in perichondrium and secured to the head by several ligaments and muscles. An anterior ligament stabilizes the tragus and helical root at the zygomatic process, and a posterior ligament stabilizes the concha to the mastoid. The "bowl" of the ear consists of three component concavities: the cavum concha inferiorly and the cymba concha and fossa triangularis superiorly. The pinna is defined by the series of folds and prominences on its anterior surface, with the major landmarks being the lobule, the helix and the antihelix, the tragus and the antitragus, the triangular fossa, the scapha, and the helical crus. Sensory innervation is through cranial nerves V (the auriculotemporal

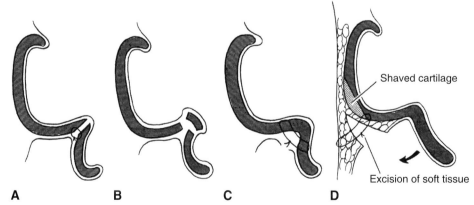

Shaved cartilage

Excision of soft tissue

A   B   C   D

Figure 36-2. Historical techniques in otoplasty. **A,** Cartilage incision to recreate antihelical fold. **B,** Parallel cartilage incisions. **C,** Mustarde suture technique. **D,** Conchal cartilage shaving with excision of postauricular soft tissues. (Adapted from Adamson PA, Tropper GJ, McGraw BL: *Otoplasty.* In Krause CJ, Mangat DS, Pastorek N, editors: *Aesthetic facial surgery.* Philadelphia, 1991, J.B. Lippincott, Figure 40-5, p 721.)

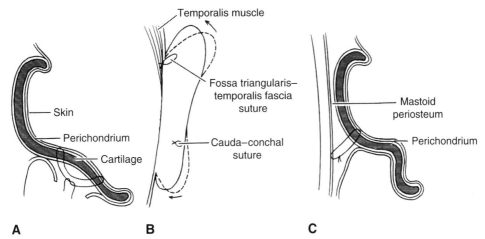

Figure 36-3. Suture techniques in otoplasty. **A,** Scapha-conchal sutures. **B,** Effects of fossa triangularis-temporalis fascia and cauda-conchal sutures. **C,** Concha-mastoid sutures. (Adapted from Adamson PA, Tropper GJ, McGraw BL: *Otoplasty.* In Krause CJ, Mangat DS, Pastorek N, editors: *Aesthetic facial surgery.* Philadelphia, 1991, J.B. Lippincott, Figure 40-10, p 721.)

nerve), VII (the facial nerve) and X (Arnold's nerve), and also C2 and C3 (the cervical plexus). The main blood supply comes from the external carotid artery via the posterior auricular and the superficial temporal arteries, with additional contributions from the occipital artery. The lobule, which lies caudal to the cartilaginous structure, is made up of soft fibrofatty tissue and typically can protrude slightly. A cartilaginous protuberance at the helix is called "Darwin's tubercle" and is the vestigial remnant that corresponds with the tip of an animal's ear.[45]

The otic placode is the first hint of a future ear and is present during the third week of intrauterine growth. The auricle emanates from the mesoderm of the first and second branchial arches; its growth occurs through the development of the six hillocks of His at week six.[27] The following six structures evolve from these hillocks: (1) the tragus; (2) the helical crus; (3) the helix; (4) the antihelix; (5) the antitragus; and (6) the lobule. By week 12, the hillocks have fused. When these fuse inappropriately, a preauricular sinus tract can result.

Cartilage formation begins at week seven. The concha derives from the ectoderm of the first branchial groove. The upper portion forms the cymba concha, the middle portion forms the cavum concha, and the lowest portion forms the intertragal incisura. Malformation of the conchal bowl contributes to excessive protrusion of the pinna from the head. Additionally, the helical margin may develop separately from a skinfold caudal to hillocks four and five,[40] which then develops rapidly during weeks eight through 12. Finally, the helix furls during the sixth month. The antihelix furls

during weeks 12 through 16; it is the failure of it to do so that results in a protruding scapha.

Normally the pinna is positioned about 15 to 20 mm from the helical rim to the scalp. From the frontal view, the rim is posterior to the antihelix laterally by about 2 to 5 mm. The auriculocephalic angle is 30 degrees in the cosmetic ideal, with the normal range being between 25 and 35 degrees. Ears that exceed 40 to 45 degrees are typically considered abnormal.[31]

In patients with protruding ears, the most common underlying anatomic abnormalities are either an insufficiency in the furl at the antihelix or a misshapen conchal bowl with a high conchal wall. There is often a combination of the two abnormalities, and there can be inappropriate folding of the elastic cartilage at the helix and antihelix to varying degrees. Otoplastic techniques are employed to reestablish the normal anatomic landmarks and/or to adjust the angulation of the pinna in relation to the head at the conchal cartilage. From an embryologic point of view, understanding that there are distinct anatomic bases for the protruding ear leads to choosing the appropriate technique or combination of techniques necessary for repair.

By the time a person is three years old, 85% of auricular growth is complete,[2,3] and the cartilaginous growth is almost complete by age five.[33] The average vertical dimension is 5 cm in infants, whereas in adults it is 6 cm.[31] Because of these growth characteristics, surgical intervention can be accomplished at the age of five or six without hindering additional growth; this is also the time that other children start to note such abnormalities in others, and, in the social milieu of school, teasing may begin.

CARTILAGE-CUTTING VS CARTILAGE-SPARING TECHNIQUES

The ultimate goal of otoplasty is to achieve a permanent aesthetic result by reintroducing normal anatomy and normal anatomic position into the deformed auricle. Cartilage-cutting techniques derive from the observation that the cartilage will bend away from the cut side. Physical modification of the cartilage includes techniques that involve cutting the cartilage in either partial- or full-thickness processes, either on the anterior or posterior side. Cartilage can be excised partially to adjust the framework, or it can be sculpted by scoring or abrading the surface. These types of techniques are often appropriate for cartilage that is stiff and thick; however, there is a risk of developing irregularities at the surface or sharp edges, especially over the long term. Additionally, excisions can result in a diminished pinna, and any of these techniques may cause scarring.

The cartilage-sparing techniques involve suturing to maintain the position and contour of the newly shaped pinna. The final result can be readjusted easily, and there is minimal cartilage damage or scarring. Bilateral symmetry can be established by adjusting the sutures after comparing the two sides. Mustarde[36] advised the use of permanent sutures to resculpt the antihelical relief. Multiple horizontal mattress sutures of permanent suturing material were organized posteriorly along the antihelical fold. Furnas[21] also used horizontal mattress sutures, but he used them to anchor the conchal bowl to the mastoid periosteum to relieve mastoid cupping. Since the descriptions of these techniques, many modifications and combinations have been tried and established (Figure 36-4).

GRADUATED-APPROACH OTOPLASTY

With a graduated approach, auricular deformities are addressed in a stepwise and logical process that entails carefully assessing the deformity and correcting each of its aspects precisely.[2,3]

Local anesthesia is infiltrated before excising a fusiform section of skin from the postauricular sulcus. The precise amount is determined by manipulating the ear to the desired position and identifying the redundant skin. The excision is eccentric and positioned over the posterior aspect of the pinna so that the resultant scar lies in the sulcus. A superiorly placed releasing incision facilitates suture placement. In continuity with the skin excision, variable amounts of soft tissue can be removed from the postauricular sulcus to treat conchal protrusion in addition to the three Furnas-type horizontal mattress sutures of the

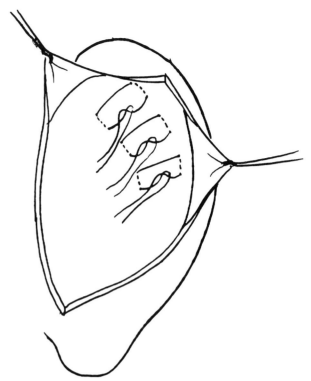

Figure 36-4. Scapha-concha sutures. One to three Mustarde sutures are positioned as required. (Adapted from Adamson PA, Tropper GJ, McGraw BL: *Otoplasty.* In Krause CJ, Mangat DS, Pastorek N, editors: *Aesthetic facial surgery,* Philadelphia, 1991, J.B. Lippincott, Figure 40-13, p 723.)

mastoid periosteum. These sutures are placed at the fossa triangularis, the cavum concha, and the cymba concha to address the superior conchal bowl, the inferior conchal bowl, and the mid bowl, respectively. Additional shave excisions at the ponticulus, triangular, and conchal eminences are reserved for very deep conchal bowls.

The conchal-mastoid sutures are placed without excessive overcorrection in the middle third of the ear to prevent the telephone ear deformity. Additionally, by pulling superiorly and posteriorly on the bowl, stenosis of the external auditory canal is avoided.

After the conchal bowl has been repositioned, the antihelix is treated with two to four Mustarde-type horizontal mattress sutures. These sutures are placed after simulating the desired furl manually, and then they are tied in order. The sutures require a 4- to 6-mm bite through the cartilage and anterior perichondrium. Rasping or scoring may be required for particularly stiff cartilage.

When these therapies are complete, the skin is closed with dissolvable sutures. These are placed in an interrupted and inverted fashion to allow egress of blood. Bolsters of cotton soaked in mineral oil and hydrogen peroxide are molded against the ear, and a mastoid-type dressing is secured. Scaphal reduction, helical refinement, and lobe reduction are carried out as required (Figure 36-5).

OTHER OTOPLASTY TECHNIQUES

Caouette-Laberge[10] reported on a scoring technique that was in use in Quebec, Canada, for more than 30 years. The auricle was approached posteriorly. Then, through a transcartilage incision at the cauda helicis, the antihelical cartilage was exposed, cut, and scored; this served to eliminate the intrinsic memory of the cartilage. With dissolvable sutures, the antihelix was then recreated. Nordzell[37] reported on his scoring technique, which was in use in Sweden for more than 30 years. With an anterior approach, the cartilage was accessed and incised. Abrasion of the cartilage allowed the antihelix to be recreated easily as it folded backward naturally; then absorbable sutures were used to anchor the medial edge of the incised cartilage over the lateral edge. Spira[41] reported on his 30-year experience in otoplasty in Houston, Texas. He depended on a revised Mustarde technique. His four-step technique included anterior otobrasion, posterior suture placement at the antihelix and at the concha and, finally, anterior suture placement at the root of the helix, with a hatch suture to prevent telephone ear. Bauer and colleagues[6] also reported on a combined otoplastic technique to address conchal hypertrophy. The conchal deformity was addressed first through an anterior excision of skin and cartilage. A greater width of cartilage was excised to facilitate skin closure; then the deformity was addressed from the posterior aspect with a "squid-shaped" section of skin removed and sutures used to affect the conchal setback.

Erol[17] described an approach through an anteriorly based skin flap through which the conchal cartilage was incised and freed. After excising the necessary amount, the cartilage was scored. Suturing of the cartilage was arranged posteriorly. He reported that this approach was suited to all modern methods of otoplasty and contributed greatly to the protection of the shape of the cartilage and the avoidance of scarring (e.g., posterior keloids). Horlock and colleagues[28] described the addition of a posterior fascial flap to protect the sutures from extruding; this flap can be applied to both Furnas- and Mustarde-type sutures.

Fritsch[20] described a technique of incisionless otoplasty in which the correction of the auricular protuberance was effected with precise placement of percutaneous retention sutures. In this method, incisions were avoided as suture material was placed subcutaneously to reshape the cartilage; the knots were buried. de la Torre[13] and colleagues described the use of temporary Kaye sutures to make precise adjustments to the antihelix. Three silk sutures were placed percutaneously from the posterior aspect of the auricle; these were left untied until all three were in place, and then secured to recreate the antihelical fold. They served as a guide for permanent nylon suture placement and were especially useful for bilateral correction and assurance of symmetry. After the permanent sutures were placed, the temporary silk sutures were removed.

Epstein and colleagues[16] reported on the use of electrocautery to weaken and sculpt the cartilage. From the posterior approach, an ellipse of skin was excised. Electrocautery was then used to create a partial-thickness Y-shaped trough. Horizontal mattress sutures were placed next, through the cartilage, to recreate the antihelical fold. Azuara[4] described his method of otoplasty with multiple transfixion incisions. The initial incision was from the posterior aspect of the auricle, preserving as much of the underlying connective tissue and perichondrium as possible. The dissection was subperichondrial anteriorly after an initial transfixion incision had been made. Transfixion incisions were then made in a multidirectional but precise manner; they were to be in the newly formed antihelix. These incisions served as relaxing incisions that allowed the cartilage to be rolled into a new antihelix. Permanent suture was used to secure the new antihelix.

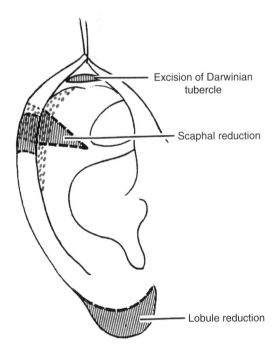

Figure 36-5. Otoplasty refinement. Wedge resection *(stripes)*, fusiform scaphal excision with block helix resection *(dotted)*, lobe reduction, and helical trimming may be performed as necessary. (Adapted from Adamson PA, Tropper GJ, McGraw BL: *Otoplasty.* In Krause CJ, Mangat DS, Pastorek N, editors: *Aesthetic facial surgery.* Philadelphia, 1991, J.B. Lippincott, Figure 40-14, p 724.)

Octyl-2-cyanoacrylate is a tissue adhesive that has been used for neonatal otoplasty.[25] The antihelical fold can be recreated as the ear is secured to the mastoid with a drop of this glue; the skin and adhesive slough in a week or two. This simple procedure may relieve the child from further surgical intervention. Finally, endoscopy has been proposed as a method to avoid certain incisions and potential unnecessary scarring during otoplasty. In a report by Graham and Gault,[24] an incision was made in the temporal scalp with an anterior stab incision at the hairline. An optical pocket was formed, and, through the second incision, the cartilage was abraded. Sutures were placed posteriorly through small stab incisions and under endoscopic vision. Sutures maintained the new antihelix and were secured to the mastoid fascia.

COMPLICATIONS

Complications can be classified as early or late. The main early complications are hematoma, pain, infection, perichondritis, and cartilage necrosis. Late complications include problems with sutures, keloids and hypertrophic scars, hypoesthesia, cold susceptibility, and, of course, unsatisfactory results.

Early hematoma is a significant complication that, if left untreated, may progress to infection and cartilage necrosis, or even to the cauliflower ear deformity. Causes of hematoma formation are improper tissue dissection, inadequate hemostasis, and inadequate pressure dressings. The incidence is about 3%, with potentially higher rates seen with cartilage-cutting techniques.[23,32] If a hematoma develops, pain is often the presenting symptom. The collection should be drained immediately under sterile conditions, and any active bleeding should be controlled with electrocautery. The incision should be closed either over a drain or with interrupted sutures to allow egress of any additional blood. The ear should be dressed again with a conforming dressing, and the patient should receive a broad-spectrum antibiotic.

Pain is often equated with hematoma presentation or infection; other causes are dressing problems such as a bent ear, or even pressure necrosis. For the most part, pain should be minimal after otoplasty. If pain is progressive, dressing removal is mandated.

The risk of infection is reduced with sterile technique, intraoperative antibiotics, antibiotic wound irrigation before closure, and antibiotic ointment applied to the suture line. If an infection develops, treatment is by evacuation of any collection and antibiotic use. The typical pathogens are *Staphylococcus aureus, Escherichia coli,* and *Pseudomonas aeruginosa;* these are seen as either acute or chronic infections (e.g., an infected suture, granuloma).[23,32]

Perichondritis may follow any infection or hematoma. It requires treatment under sterile conditions with the débridement of necrotic tissue and the administration of intravenous antibiotics. Cartilage necrosis may result also from infection or hematoma. Additionally, improper surgical technique, cautery use, or even dressing placement may cause cartilage necrosis.

Late suture complications can occur with many types of suturing material. Chromic catgut can cause a localized skin reaction and inflammation. Certain sutures (e.g., braided as compared to monofilament) are more reactive and have the potential to initiate a foreign-body granuloma; if this happens, the granuloma and suture material should be removed. Removal can be postponed for several months postoperatively and thus diminish the potential for a negative impact on the cosmetic result. Another suture complication is loss of correction with the suture techniques. In these techniques, overcorrection is recommended to account for the expected loss of correction, which can be up to 40%.[2] This type of complication is minimized by placing an appropriate number of sutures and employing cartilage-weakening modalities for stiffer cartilage.

Hypertrophic scarring or keloid formation may develop, especially after a postauricular incision.[9] Patients at risk are younger patients and those with more pigmented skin, particularly blacks with a history of keloid formation. Preventive modalities include avoiding overaggressive skin resection and ensuring an absolutely tension-free closure.

Injury to the greater auricular nerve may lead to hypoesthesia after otoplasty. Although a nuisance, it is of minimal significance clinically; sensory function often returns within weeks to months postoperatively. Disruption of the auricular blood supply may lead to recurrent frostbite and a higher susceptibility to cold temperatures after otoplasty.[8]

Perhaps the most complicated complication is patient dissatisfaction. Preoperative discussion requires dialogue to establish realistic expectations. Patients need to be advised that improvement—not perfection—is the goal. Small asymmetries (i.e., up to 2 or 3 mm when comparing one side with the other) are accepted to be within the norm of the human condition. It is our experience that overcorrection is better tolerated as compared with undercorrection; the patient will require reassurance postoperatively if the expectation is not met. If the deformity can be corrected surgically, then revision can be undertaken when appropriate. Continued reassurance may be needed when correction is not possible.

Several postoperative scenarios have been observed in otoplasty patients. One of the most common is loss of correction. This problem may imply a technical deficiency, because it is more often seen in the suture technique and usually during the first three months postoperatively.[19] It may imply that the sutures were not placed properly or that not enough sutures were placed. Alternatively, failure may occur if the cartilage is too stiff or insufficient conchal setback was obtained. In approximately half of the cases in which there has been a loss of correction, there is a history of associated trauma to the ear.[2]

The telephone ear deformity occurs when there has been overaggressive conchal setback or postauricular skin excision in the central portion of the ear. Other conchal deformities include buckling of the concha or impingement on the external canal. Conchal hypertrophy may limit conchal setback if not addressed surgically either by excision or suture methods. In addition, there is a risk of overcorrection resulting in a "stuck down" look if the conchal bowl is overresected and the antihelix excessively furled.

In the case of the overcorrected antihelix, the ear may appear "stuck down" if excess conchal wall height has not been addressed. Additionally, the helix may appear hidden as the antihelix is more laterally positioned. A vertical post deformity in the scapha may result with overcorrection as well; this refers to an unnatural vertical fold in the scapha and buckling of the helix if sutures are placed incorrectly. Finally, undercorrection and asymmetry are potential complications that may cause dissatisfaction; both may obligate surgical revision.

SUMMARY

Protruding ears are a common congenital condition that cause significant emotional discomfort for many individuals. Numerous techniques—from very simple to very complex—have been described over the years to correct this deformity. Cartilage-cutting incisions may result in less frequent loss of correction but increased cartilage irregularities in the long term. Cartilage-sparing suture techniques primarily leave the cartilage intact, thereby reducing the incidence of these irregularities. Our experience of using the soft-tissue conchal bowl setback and horizontal mattress antihelical fold suture technique in a graduated approach has proved very successful (Figures 36-6 and 36-7). Cartilage scoring is reserved for thicker cartilage that may be more refractory to suture-only techniques. Complications are not common and are usually minor. Creating a natural ear brings harmony to the face and requires an appreciation of the finer

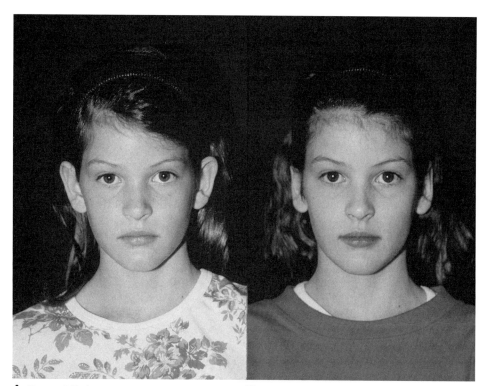

A, Pre-op A-P view   **B,** Post-op A-P view

Figure 36-6. A, This 10-year-old girl had a minimal soft tissue bowl excision for conchal setback and minimal modified Mustarde sutures to recreate the antihelical fold to set back the superior pole.

Continued

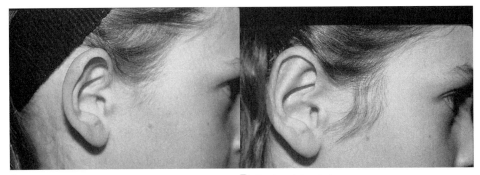

A, Pre-op lateral view   **B,** Post-op lateral view

Figure 36-6, cont'd B, Results one year later.

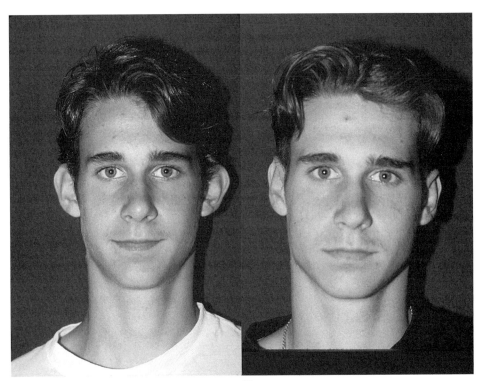

A, Pre-op A-P view   **B,** Post-op A-P view

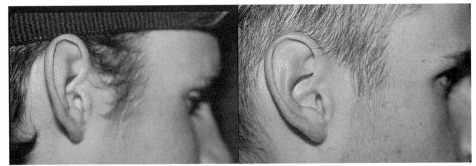

A, Pre-op lateral view   **B,** Post-op lateral view

Figure 36-7. A, This 15-year-old young man had a moderate soft tissue bowl excision for conchal setback and minimal modified Mustarde sutures to recreate his antihelical fold and superior pole protrusion. **B,** Results two years later.

aspects of ear anatomy and attention to surgical detail; the surgeon who is so committed is rewarded with a high degree of patient satisfaction.

REFERENCES

1. Adamson JE, Horton CE, Crawford HH: The growth pattern of the external ear, *Plast Reconstr Surg* 36:466, 1965.
2. Adamson PA, McGraw BL, Tropper GJ: Critical review of clinical results, *Laryngoscope* 101:883, 1991.
3. Adamson PA, Tropper GJ, McGraw BL: *Otoplasty.* In Krause CJ, Pastorek N, Mangat DS, editors: *Aesthetic facial surgery.* Philadelphia, 1991, Lippincott, p 707–734.
4. Azuara E: Aesthetic otoplasty with remodeling of the antihelix for the correction of the prominent ear: criteria and personal technique, *Arch Facial Plast Surg* 2:57, 2000.
5. Bardach J: *Surgery for congenital and acquired malformation of the auricle.* In Cummings C, editor: *Otolaryngology—head and neck surgery,* St Louis, 1986, Mosby, p 2861.
6. Bauer BS, Song DH, Aitken ME: Combined otoplasty technique: chondrocutaneous conchal resection as the cornerstone to correction of the prominent ear, *Plast Reconstr Surg* 110:1033, 2002.
7. Becker OJ: Surgical correction of the abnormally protruding ears, *Arch Otolaryngol* 50:541, 1949.
8. Bruck HG: Correction of prominent ears, *Arch Otolaryngol* 98:10, 1973.
9. Calder JC, Naasan A: Morbidity in otoplasty: a review of 562 consecutive cases, *Br J Plast Surg* 47:170, 1994.
10. Caouette-Laberge L and others: Otoplasty: anterior scoring technique and results in 500 cases, *Plast Reconstr Surg* 105:504, 2000.
11. Converse JM and others: A technique for surgical correction of lop ear, *Plast Reconstr Surg* 15:411, 1955.
12. Davis JS, Kilwoski WA: Abnormal prominence of the ears: a method of readjustment surgery, *Surgery* 2:835, 1937.
13. de la Torre J and others: A simplified technique of otoplasty: the temporary Kaye suture, *Ann Plast Surg* 41:94, 1998.
14. Dieffenbach JF: *Die operative chirugie,* Leipzig, Germany, F.A. Brockhaus, 1845.
15. Ely ET: An operation for prominence of the auricles, *Arch Ophthalmol Otolaryngol* 10:97, 1881.
16. Epstein JS, Kabaker SS, Swerdloff J: The "electric" otoplasty, *Arch Facial Plast Surg* 1:204, 1999.
17. Erol OO: New modification in otoplasty: anterior approach, *Plast Reconstr Surg* 107:193, 2001.
18. Farrior RT: A method of otoplasty, *Arch Otolaryngol* 69:400, 1959.
19. Feuerstein SS: Revision techniques in otoplasty: evaluation and management, *Otolaryngol Clin North Am* 7:133, 1974.
20. Fritsch MH: Incisionless otoplasty, *Laryngoscope* 105(5 Pt 3 Suppl 70):1, 1995.
21. Furnas DW: Correction of prominent ears by conchamastoid sutures, *Plast Reconstr Surg* 42:189, 1968.
22. Gibson T, Davis WD: The distortion of autogenous cartilage grafts, its cause and prevention, *Br J Plast Surg* 10:257, 1958.
23. Goode RL, Profitt SD: Complications of otoplasty, *Arch Otolaryngol* 91:352, 1970.
24. Graham KE, Gault DT: Endoscopic assisted otoplasty: a preliminary report, *Br J Plast Surg* 50:47, 1997.
25. Hallock GG: Expanded applications for octyl-2-cyanoacrylate as a tissue adhesive, *Ann Plast Surg* 46:185, 2001.
26. Hauben DJ: Sushruta Samhita (Sushruta'a Collection) (800-600 B.C.?). Pioneers of plastic surgery, *Acta Chir Plast* 26:65, 1984.
27. His W: *Die formentwicklung des ausseren ohren.* In *Anatomie menschlicher embryonen,* part III. Leipzig, Germany, 1985, F.C.W. Vogel.
28. Horlock N, Misra A, Gault DT: The postauricular fascial flap as an adjunct to Mustarde and Furnas type otoplasty, *Plast Reconstr Surg* 108:1487, 2001.
29. Kaye BL: A simplified method for correcting the prominent ear, *Plast Reconstr Surg* 52:184, 1967.
30. Luckett WH: A new operation for prominent ears based on the anatomy of the deformity, *Surg Gynecol Obstet* 10:635, 1910.
31. Mallen RW: Otoplasty, *Can J Otolaryngol* 3:74, 1974.
32. Maniglia AJ, Maniglia JV: Otoplasty: an eclectic technique, *Laryngoscope* 87:1359, 1977.
33. Maniglia AJ, Maniglia JV: Congenital lop ear deformity, *Otolaryngol Clin North Am* 14:83, 1981.
34. Monks GH: Operations for correcting the deformity due to prominent ears, *Boston Med Surg* 124:84, 1891.
35. Morestin H: De la reposition et du plissement cosmetiqies du pavillon de l'oreille, *Revue Orthop* 4:289, 1903.
36. Mustarde JC: The correction of prominent ears using simple mattress sutures, *Br J Plast Surg* 16:170, 1963.
37. Nordzell B: Open otoplasty, *Plast Reconstr Surg* 106:1466, 2000.
38. Potter EL: A hereditary ear malformation transmitted through 5 generations, *J Hered* 28:255, 1937.
39. Rhys Evans PH, Bull TR: Correction of prominent ears using the buried suture technique: a ten year survey (unpublished). Cited in Rhys Evans PH. Prominent ears and their surgical correction, *J Laryngol Otolaryngol* 95:881, 1981.
40. Schwalbe G: *Die ohrmuschel. Handbuch der anatomie des menschen,* vol 5. Jena, Germany, G. Fischer, 1987.
41. Spira M: Otoplasty: what I do now—a 30-year perspective, *Plast Reconstr Surg* 104:834, 1999.
42. Stenstrom SJ: A natural technique for correction of congenital ear deformities, *Br J Plast Surg* 99:562, 1963.
43. Tagliacozzi G: de Curtorum chirurgia per Institionem Libri Duo, Venice, 1597.
44. Tanzer RC: *Congenital deformities. Deformities of the auricle.* In Converse JM, editor: *Reconstructive plastic surgery.* Philadelphia, 1977, W.B. Saunders, p 1671.
45. Webster RC, Smith RC: *Otoplasty for prominent ears.* In Goldwin RM, editor: *Long-term results in plastic and reconstructive surgery.* Boston, Little Brown and Company, 1980, p 146–186.

Index

Note: Page numbers set in italic indicate figures; those followed by *t* indicate tables, those followed by *b* indicate boxes.

Peripheral T-cell neoplasms
clinical diagnosis of, 940–941
treatment of, 941
Peripheral vestibular disorders,
3209–3238
basic principles of, 3209–3210
clinical relevance of, 3210
Peripheral vestibular system, dizziness and,
3160
Peritonsillar infections, tonsillitis and,
4143–4144, *4144*
Peroxynitrite, ototoxicity and, 2936
Persistent generalized lymphadenopathy
(PGL), 319
Pertechnetate thallous chloride imaging, for
hyperparathyroidism, 2741–2742
PET. *See* Positron emission tomography
Petrositis, chronic otitis media and, *3004,*
3004–3006, *3005, 3006t*
anatomy of, *3004,* 3004–3005, *3005*
diagnosis of, 3005–3006, *3006t*
history of, 3004
management of, 3006
tests for, 3005–3006, *3007*
Petrous apex, transsphenoidal/transclival
approaches to, *3864,* 3870–3871, *3872*
Petrous apex lesions, *3725,* 3725–3726,
3819–3820
asymmetric petrous apex pneumatization
and, 3819, *3821*
cholesterol granulomas and, 3819, 3819t,
3820
giant cell tumors and, 3820
mucocele/mucus retention cysts and,
3819–3820, *3821*
petrous carotid artery aneurysms and, 3820,
3822
Petrous apicitis
symptoms of, 3006t
temporal bone infections and, extracranial
complications of, *3024,* 3024–3027,
3025, 3026
Petrous bone
inferior surface of, osseous anatomy of,
2802, 2803, 2804, *2809, 2810, 2812*
medial surface of, osseous anatomy of, *2802,
2803,* 2804, *2808, 2809, 2810, 2811*
osseous anatomy of, *2802,* 2803, *2803, 2808,
2809,* 2810, *2811, 2812*
superior surface of, osseous anatomy of,
2802, 2803–2804, *2810, 2813*
Petrous carotid artery aneurysms, petrous apex
lesions and, 3820, *3822*
Peyer's patches, immune system and, 282
Pfeiffer's syndrome, craniofacial abnormalities
and, 4035
Phagocytes, innate immune system and,
294–295
Pharmacokinetics, ototoxicity and,
2933–2934
Pharmacologic toxicity
SNHL and, 3540–3541
SSNHL and, 3553
Pharmacology, of free tissue transfer, 204
Pharyngeal abscess, *1805,* 1805–1806
Pharyngeal flap, VPD and, 4094–4095
Pharyngeal function
articulation and, 1973
in breathing, 1968–1970, *1969, 1970*
expiratory force and, 1971
in phonation, 1970–1971, *1970b, 1971*
pitch control and, 1972
resonance and, 1972
in speech, 1970–1973, *1970b, 1971*
vocal fold positioning and, 1972
vocal fold shape and, 1972
vocal folds vibratory capacity and, 1972

Pharyngeal imaging, 1785–1821
barium swallow and, 1788
CT and, 1789–1790
fluoroscopy in, 1785–1786
MRI and, 1790–1791
oral contrast agents and, 1788–1789
pharyngoesophagram and, *1786–1787,*
1786–1788, *1788–1789, 1789, 1790*
radiography in, 1785, *1786*
techniques of, 1785–1791
ultrasound and, 1791, *1792*
Pharyngeal neurology
acoustic analysis and, 2061
aerodynamic assessment and, 2061
cineradiography and, 2063
edrophonium and, 2063
electromyography and, 2062–2063
photoglottography/electroglottography and,
2062
sensory assessment and, 2063–2064
Pharyngeal pouches, 1798, *1799, 1800, 1880*
Pharyngeal pressure generation, in swallowing,
1439–1440
Pharyngeal reconstruction, in total
laryngectomy, 2389–2391, *2390*
Pharyngeal stage, of swallowing, 1438–1440
Pharyngeal surgery
for childhood obstructive sleep apnea, 4176
swallowing disorders from, 1444
Pharyngeal tonsils. *See* Adenoids
Pharyngitis
adenovirus and, 1695
in adults, 1685–1698
arcanobacterium haemolyticum and, 1688
bacterial infection of, 1685–1692
chlamydia pneumoniae and, 1689–1690
coronavirus and, 1692–1693
corynebacterium diphtheriae and,
1691–1692
definition of, 1685
EBV and, 4140
Epstein-Barr virus and, 1695–1696, *1696*
etiologies of, 1685, 1686t
francisella tularensis and, 1690–1691
fungal infection and, 1697–1698
GABHS and, 1685–1687, 1686t
herpes simplex virus and, 1697, *1697*
HIV and, 1694–1695
influenza virus and, 1693–1694
mycobacterium tuberculosis and, 1690
mycoplasma pneumoniae and, 1690
neisseria gonorrhoeae and, 1688–1689,
1689
non-group A-β hemolytic streptococcus
infections and, 1688–1692
parainfluenza virus and, 1692–1693
pediatric, 4135–4161
management algorithm for, *4136–4137*
viral, *4139,* 4139–4140
rhinovirus and, 1692–1693
treponema pallidum and, 1689
viral infections and, 1692–1698
yersinia enterocolitica and, 1692
Pharyngocele, left lateral, *1879*
Pharyngocutaneous fistula, total laryngectomy
and, 2392–2393
Pharyngoesophageal foreign bodies, 1812,
1812, 1813
Pharyngoesophageal mass lesions, 1812–1819,
1813, 1814, 1815, 1816, 1817, 1818, 1819
benign neoplasms and, 1817, *1818*
esophageal carcinomas and, 1815, *1815,
1816*
hypopharyngeal carcinomas and, *1814,*
1814–1815, *1815*
lymphadenopathy and, 1815–1817, *1817*
malignant neoplasms and, 1813

Pharyngoesophageal mass lesions *(Continued)*
nasopharyngeal carcinomas and, *1813,*
1813–1814
nonneoplastic mucosal masses and,
1817–1819, *1818, 1819*
oropharyngeal carcinomas and, 1814, *1814*
Pharyngoesophageal stenosis/stricture, total
laryngectomy and, 2393
Pharyngoesophageal web, esophageal
narrowing and, 1806, *1807*
Pharyngoesophagram, *1786–1787,* 1786–1788,
1788–1789, 1789, 1790
Pharyngoplasty, VPD and, 4095–4096
Pharyngoscopy, 1825–1834
complications of, 1829–1830
contraindications for, 1827–1828, 1827t
flexible, 1828, *1828, 1829*
history of, 1825
indications for, 1826, 1826t
rigid, 1829, *1829*
Pharynx
abnormal deglutition of, 1795–1796
brainstem lesions and, 2056
cerebellar lesions and, 2056
diffuse central nervous system lesion and,
2057
extrapyramidal system defects and, 2056
lesion site identification in, 2056–2057,
2056b
lymphatic drainage of, 3946
motility disorders of, 1795
neurologic evaluation of, 2054–2064
neuropathological symptoms of, 2054, 2055b
normal function of, 2055
peripheral nerve injuries and, 2056–2057
radiographic anatomy of, *1789,* 1791,
1792–1793, 1794
Phenol toxicity, chemical peel agents and, 701
Phenytoin, 456t
Pheochromocytoma, case study of, 269–270
Phobic postural vertigo, psychophysiological
dizziness and, 3284
Phonation, pharyngeal function and,
1970–1971, *1970b, 1971*
Phonation threshold pressure, voice analysis
and, 2022
Phospholipase C system, salivary glands and,
1300–1301
Photoaging groups, Glogau classification of,
696t
Photodynamic therapy, flexible fiberoptic
bronchoscopy and, 2471t, 2472–2473
Photoglottography/electroglottography
laryngeal neurology and, 2062
pharyngeal neurology and, 2062
Photography/imaging, rhinoplasty and, 1035,
1038
Photon
absorption of, 214–215, *215*
stimulated emission of, 214–215, *215*
Phrenic nerve, neck neural complications of,
2655
Physical dysmorphology, voice analysis and,
2015
Physical examination
of adenopathy, 6–7
of auricles, 8
of ears, 8–11
of external auditory canal, 8–9
of face, 5, 5t
general appearance and, 4–5, 4b
hearing assessment and, 9–11, 10t
of hypopharynx, 12
of larynx, 12, 12–13
of lymph node regions, 7–8, 8
of nasopharynx, 14
of neck, 5–8, 6, 7, 8

Round window membrane (RWM), 2944–2949, *2945, 2946*
  adhesions of, 2947
  anatomy of, 2944–2945, *2945*
  delivery methods to, *2947,* 2947–2949, *2948*
  kinetics of, *2946,* 2946–2947
  permeability of, 2945–2946, *2946*
  physiology of, 2945, *2946*
RPC. *See* Recurrent parotitis of childhood
RS. *See* Rhinosinusitis
RSI. *See* Reflux Symptom Index
RSTL. *See* Relaxed skin tension lines
RSV. *See* Respiratory syncytial virus
RWM. *See* Round window membrane

S

Saccade testing, of vestibular function, 3178, *3179*
Saccades, disorders of, 3166–3167
Saccadic eye movements, dizziness and, *3166,* 3166–3167
Saccular cysts, *2176, 2177,* 2177–2179, *2178*
  classification of, 2178
  clinical information of, 2178
  management of, *2178,* 2179
  physical examination of, *2177,* 2178
  workup of, 2178–2179
Saccular disorders, 2175–2184
Saddle nose deformity
  augmentation for, 1097–1099, *1098–1099, 1100*
  dynamic adjustable rotational tip graft and, 1099, *1102*
  indications of, 1099, *1101*
  special rhinoplasty techniques for, 1097–1099, *1098, 1099, 1100, 1101,* 1102
Saethre-Chotzen syndrome, craniofacial abnormalities and, 4035
Safety considerations, with surgical lasers, 226–230
Sagittal lingual marginal mandibulectomy, *1595*
Sagittal synostosis, craniofacial abnormalities for, 4039, *4040, 4041*
Salicylates
  ototoxicity and, 2938
  SNHL and, 3541
Saliva
  antibacterial activity of, 1306
  buffering/clearance role of, 1305–1306
  composition of, 1302–1305, 1302*t*
  flow rate of, 1301–1302, 1302*t*
  functions of, 1305–1307
  inorganic components of, 1302–1303
  lubrication/protection role of, 1305
  macromolecules in, 1303–1305, 1303*t,* 1304*t*
  organic components of, 1303–1305, 1303*t,* 1304*t*
  relative viscosities of, 1295, 1295*t*
  taste and, 1430–1431
  taste/digestive role of, 1306–1307
  tooth integrity and, 1306
Salivary duct carcinoma, of salivary glands, 1393
Salivary duct injury
  penetrating, 1342–1343
  repair of, *1342,* 1342–1343, *1343, 1344*
Salivary flow, facial nerve function tests and, 3329–3330
Salivary gland calculi, location of, 1307, 1308*t*
Salivary gland carcinomas, 135–136
  cervical lymph node carcinoma and, 2606–2607
  radiation for, 108–109, 109*t*

Salivary gland disease, 1307–1310, 4116–4133
  actinomycosis and, 4125
  acute inflammatory disease and, 4119–4126, *4120*
  acute suppurative sialadenitis, 4119–4121, *4120,* 4121*t*
  aging and, 1308–1309, *1310*
  bacterial, 4119–4121, *4120*
  biopsy of, 4118–4119
  cat-scratch disease and, 4125
  chronic inflammatory disease and, 4122–4123
  chronic sialectasis and, 4122–4123
  cystic fibrosis and, 1310
  cysts and, 4123
  differential diagnosis of, 4117*b*
  granulomatous and, 4123
  history of, 4117–4118
  laboratory studies on, 4117–4118
  mucoceles and, 4123
  mycobacterial disease and, *4124,* 4124–4125
  necrotizing sialometaplasia and, 4125–4126
  physical examination of, 4117
  radiology for, 4118
  sarcoidosis and, 4125
  sialadenosis as, 1307
  sialolithiasis as, 1307–1308, 1308*t,* 4123
  Sjögren's syndrome as, 1308, *1309*
  toxoplasmosis and, 4125
  tularemia and, 4125
Salivary gland injury
  blunt trauma and, 1345–1346
  by radiation, 1346
  radiologic evaluation of, 1342
Salivary gland malignancies, 1378–1401
  clinical presentation of, 1378–1379
  complications/morbidity of, 1400–1401
  deformity and, 1401
  diagnosis of, 1378–1382
  epidemiology of, 1378, 1379*b*
  facial nerve paralysis and, 1400
  fine needle aspiration of, 1381–1382
  Frey's syndrome and, 1401, 1401*b*
  frozen section biopsy of, 1382
  greater auricular nerve defect and, 1400
  hematoma and, 1401
  histologic subtypes of, 1383–1394, 1383*b,* 1383*t*
  imaging of, *1379,* 1379–1381, *1380, 1381*
  metastatic cancer and, 1393–1394, 1394*t*
  metastatic disease and, 1400
  pediatric
    histopathology/molecular biology of, 4201, *4201, 4202*
    management of, 4200–4201
    presentation/evaluation of, 4200, 4202*t*
  pediatric neck masses and, 4221
  staging of, 1382–1383, 1382*b*
  surveillance of, 1400
  trismus and, 1401
Salivary gland neoplasms, 4126–4131, 4126*t*
  acinic cell carcinomas and, 1384–1386, 1388*b,* 4128
  adenocarcinomas and, 1390–1391, 1391*b,* 1392*t,* 4128
  adenoid cystic carcinoma and, 1211, 1384–1386, *1385,* 1385*t, 1386, 1387, 1388,* 4128–4129
  allelic loss and, 1350
  arteriovenous malformations and, 1365
  basal cell adenoma and, 1362
  canalicular adenoma and, 1362
  clinical features of, 1351–1352, *1352, 1353*
  color Doppler sonography of, 1359
  CT/MRI of, 1354–1359, *1355, 1356, 1357, 1358*
  distribution of, 1351, 1351*t*

Salivary gland neoplasms (*Continued*)
  environmental factors of, 1349–1350
  etiology of, 1349
  FNAB of, 1352–1354
  genetic factors in, 1350
  hemangiomas and, 1364–1365, 4126–4127, *4127*
  histogenesis of, 1348–1349, *1349*
  imaging of, 1354–1359, *1355, 1356, 1357, 1358*
  incidence of, 1350–1351, *1351,* 1351*t*
  inverted ductal papilloma and, 1364
  lymphangiomas and, 4127–4128, *4128*
  lymphatic malformations and, 1365
  management principles for, 1365–1375
  monosomy/polysomy and, 1350
  mucoepidermoid carcinoma and, 4128
  myoepithelioma and, 1363–1364
  oncocytic papillary cystadenoma and, 1363
  oncocytoma and, 1363
  parapharyngeal excision of, 1371–1375, *1372–1373, 1373–1374*
  parotidectomy for, 1365–1371, *1366, 1367, 1368*
  pathology of, 1359–1365, *1360, 1361*
  patient evaluation for, 1351–1359, *1352, 1353, 1355, 1356, 1357, 1358*
  pleomorphic adenoma and, 1359–1362, *1360, 1361,* 4128–4129
  positron emission tomography of, 1359
  radiation exposure and, 1349
  sialadenoma papilliferum and, 1364
  sites of, 1351, *1351*
  structural rearrangement and, 1350
  submandibular gland excision of, *1369–1370,* 1371
  surgical techniques for, 1365–1375, *1366, 1368, 1369, 1370, 1372, 1373, 1374*
  tobacco use and, 1350
  ultrasonography of, 1359
  vascular malformations and, 1364–1365, 4128
  vasoformative neoplasms and, 4126–4128
  viruses and, 1349
  Warthin's tumor and, 1362–1363
Salivary gland trauma, patient workup for, 1341–1342
Salivary glands
  acinic cell carcinomas and, 1384–1386, 1388*b*
  acute suppurative sialadenitis of, 1323–1325
  adenocarcinoma of, 1390–1391, 1391*b,* 1392*t*
  adenylate cyclase system and, 1300
  agenesis of, 4130–4131
  allergic reaction of, 4132
  anatomy of, 1339, 1341
  autoimmune diseases of, 4131–4133
  bacterial infections of, 1323–1330
  benign lymphoepithelial disease, 4131
  benign neoplasms of, 1348–1375
  blunt trauma to, 4131
  branchial cleft cysts of, 4130
  branchial pouch cysts of, 4130
  cell surface receptors and, 1298–1300, *1299,* 1299*t*
  chemotherapy for, 1399–1400
  chronic sialorrhea of, 4132
  congenital cysts of, 4130–4131
  congenital ductal cysts of, 4130
  CT of, 39–41
  cystic fibrosis and, 4132
  dermoid cysts of, 4130
  drugs and, 4132
  ductal secretion mechanisms of, 1298
  G-proteins and, 1300
  granulomatous infections of, 1332–1333, *1333*